FUNDAMENTALS OF CUTANEOUS SURGERY

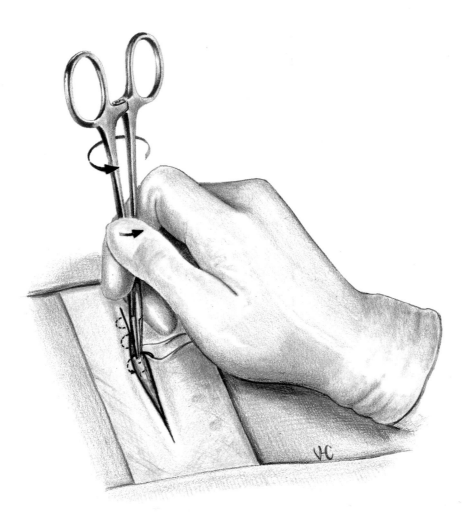

To place running intradermal suture, needle holder is held like pencil and rotated with thumb on second and third fingers.

FUNDAMENTALS
OF
CUTANEOUS SURGERY

RICHARD G. BENNETT, M.D.

Adjunct Associate Professor of Medicine (Dermatology)
University of California, Los Angeles
School of Medicine;
Consultant in Medicine (Dermatology)
University of Southern California
School of Medicine
Los Angeles, California

With 826 illustrations and 2 color plates
Drawings by Virginia Cantarella

THE C. V. MOSBY COMPANY
St. Louis • Washington, D.C. • Toronto • 1988

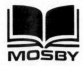

A TRADITION OF PUBLISHING EXCELLENCE

Editor: Eugenia A. Klein
Assistant Editor: Anne Gunter
Editorial Assistant: Ginny Wharton
Project Editor: Patricia Tannian
Production Editors: Stephen Dierkes, Celeste Clingan
Designer: Susan E. Lane

Printed in the United States of America

The C.V. Mosby Company
11830 Westline Industrial Drive, St. Louis, Missouri 63146

Library of Congress Cataloging-in-Publication Data

Bennett, Richard G.
  Fundamentals of cutaneous surgery.

  Includes bibliographies and index.
  1. Skin—Surgery.   I. Title.   [DNLM: 1. Skin—
Surgery.   WR 650 B472f]
RD520.B46 1987   617′.477   87-7941
ISBN 0-8016-0606-3

AC/MV/MV 9 8 7 6 5 4 3 2   02/C/210

To my best teachers of cutaneous surgery,
the dermatology residents:

at Emory 1978-1984
at UCLA 1984-present
at USC 1985-present

PREFACE

Surgery on the cutaneous surfaces is specialized, yet at the same time it requires a knowledge of general surgical principles. My experience during the last decade of teaching within academic dermatology has been that such principles are poorly understood and inadequately taught. The purpose of this book is to provide the reader with an in-depth understanding of those principles as they pertain to cutaneous surgery.

In 1982 the Board of Directors of the American Society for Dermatologic Surgery held a retreat to chart the future of teaching and research within the field of cutaneous surgery. From this meeting, at which I was present, a core surgical curriculum—which is currently an integral part of every major academic dermatologic residency program in the United States—was developed. This book was written with that core curriculum in mind.

The reader may ask why I have not included chapters on skin flaps and grafts, dermabrasion, or nail surgery. These topics and others are planned for a subsequent volume, which will discuss them in detail similar to that found in this volume. I believe that the fundamentals of cutaneous surgery must be understood and mastered before one undertakes complex procedures.

In my exploration of the fundamental principles of cutaneous surgery, I unexpectedly uncovered many significant concepts—some good, some bad—buried in the literature. These chance revelations are analogous to a phenomenon in art known as *pentimento* (from the Italian word for repentance). It was once common practice for impoverished artists to paint over earlier artwork on the same canvas (often an outline or change of mind). Many of these overlying paintings became masterpieces, but with time some of them began to chip and fade, and the underlying painting became apparent. The emergence of these hidden paintings is known as pentimento. On examination of the surgical principles that pertain to cutaneous surgery, an analogous pentimento effect occurs. As one examines some of the outstanding recent literature within surgery, the older works, somewhat obscured by more modern data, begin to shine forth and take on new meaning and importance. Many of the "truths" and "dogmas" that I hear continuously espoused and accepted as fact at meetings and in clinical settings need

to be carefully reevaluated. Only by scratching away at the canvas is it possible to uncover reasons for overlying principles; all too often we find nothing to support dogma. This book represents such a discovery process.

An additional benefit from careful review of the older literature is that one can appreciate that the principles and practice of cutaneous surgery did not evolve from only one specialty group. Cutaneous surgery is practiced by many different specialists, such as dermatologists, plastic surgeons, head and neck surgeons, ophthalmologists, general surgeons, and general practitioners. Each specialty has made its own contributions to surgery on the skin, and all have borrowed from each other to better their own surgical results.

Dermatologists in particular have acquired extensive background knowledge in both the biology and pathology of the skin, which has enabled them to develop surgical techniques quite apart from (as well as in conjunction with) other specialists. These developments have led to the emergence of a relatively new subspecialty within the specialty of dermatology called "dermatologic surgery." Such an evolution is a natural outcome of problems peculiar to the specialty and parallels to some extent similar evolution that occurred in ophthalmology, which is also both a medical and a surgical specialty.

Despite the foregoing, some physicians question the importance, or even the existence, of dermatologic surgery within the field of dermatology. Such skepticism can certainly be ascribed to resistance to change, but there is also an element reminiscent of the enduring differences that have existed for centuries between medically oriented physicians and those doing surgery. Negativism toward surgery reached its zenith in the middle ages and has persisted ever since. As the English poet Shelley eloquently stated, "History is a cyclic poem written by time upon the memories of man."

Writing this book required extensive research into many areas of basic science in addition to clinical investigation. My main effort has been to present this material so as to show its clinical relevance. I hope that this presentation will provide an impetus for future research within cutaneous surgery.

Richard G. Bennett, M.D.

ACKNOWLEDGEMENTS

Quite obviously this book represents the efforts of many people who believed in me and the goal I set forth to accomplish. Virginia Cantarella, the illustrator, is a true professional with whom it was delightful to work. Her illustrations are outstanding, and she took the extra effort to make sure we were both happy with each one. Several of the chapters were reviewed by the dermatology residents at UCLA and others who made many helpful suggestions. In particular, I wish to thank the following reviewers: Willard Marmelzat, M.D. (Chapter 1); Jouni Uitto, Ph.D., M.D., and Christine Kenney, Ph.D., M.D. (Chapter 2); Stuart Kaplan, M.D. (Chapter 5); Ronald Moy, M.D. (Chapter 6); Howard Sofen, M.D. (Chapter 7); Richard L. Kronenthal, Ph.D., of Ethicon, Inc. (Chapter 8); Lia van Rijswijk, RNET, and Richard Bradley, F.A.I.C., of ConvaTec (Chapter 9); Lisa Oki, M.D. (Chapters 10 to 15); Roger Odell, E.E., of Valleylab (Chapter 16); Mitchel Goldman, M.D. (Chapter 18); and Michael Borok, M.D. (Chapters 19 to 28).

The managing editors at Mosby, Eugenia Klein and Carol Trumbold, demonstrated extreme patience in allowing me as much time as I took to complete this first volume; Carol in particular pushed me to produce the best book I could write. Additional editing was done in Los Angeles by Judy Hohl. All the surgical photographs are of my work; I took a few in training as a chemosurgery fellow under the tutelage of Dr. Perry Robins in New York. Perry encouraged me to develop my surgical knowledge and skills. Anne Gunter is to be commended for coordinating the multitude of illustrations in this text. My nurses—Cindy Baggett, R.N., Nora Tabila, R.N., Linda Short, R.N., and Mary Beth Harbin, R.N.—all worked under extreme pressure; they knew my mind was always "on the book," but all were understanding and helped me through my clinical responsibilities. Most of the book was processed by three secretaries, Ginger Nerbonne in Atlanta, Ginny Wharton in St. Louis, and Rona Krasner in Los Angeles. Rona did the bulk of the typing and retyping and much library research. My good friends, Dr. Michael Albom of New York, Dr. Ricardo Mora of New Orleans, and Dr. Vincent Peng of Atlanta, gave me encouragement every step of the way. The faculty at UCLA were also particularly supportive, allowing me the latitude and time to write. In particular, I would like to thank Dr. Ronald Reisner, Chairman of the Division of Dermatology at UCLA, and Dr. Richard Strick, who along with myself is codirector of the dermatologic surgery program at UCLA.

Finally, I wish to thank my wife Laurie, who has been most patient during this project.

R.G.B.

CONTENTS

APPENDICES

FUNDAMENTALS OF CUTANEOUS SURGERY

BACKGROUND AND BASIC SCIENCE

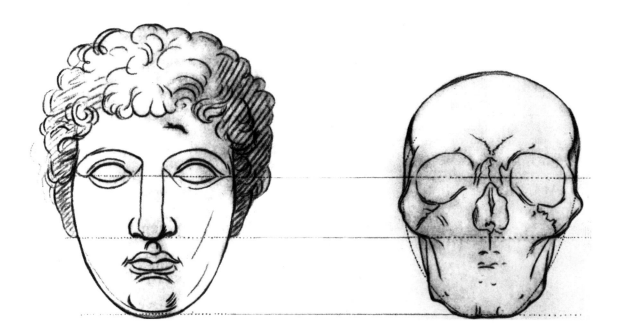

Illustration by Charles Bell demonstrating the correlation of clinical appearance with underlying anatomic structures. (From Bell, C.: Essays on the anatomy of the expression in painting, London, 1806, Longman, Hurst, Rees, and Orme.)

CHAPTER

1

Cutaneous Surgery: History and Development

Cutaneous surgery is surgery designed to correct or repair problems localized to the skin or mucous membranes. Its goal is to produce the best cosmetic and functional results. Because skin is so visible, the final appearance of scars is a major concern for both patient and physician.

Each tissue of the human body possesses unique characteristics that influence the tissue's response to different therapeutic methods. Such variations include, for instance, the anatomy, degree of vascularity, and reaction to foreign material such as sutures. Surgical principles, materials, and instruments have evolved to deal with each tissue.

The skin is unique because it is the covering of the human body; it is therefore relatively impermeable, helping to maintain the homeostasis of the body it invests. Also unique to the skin are its anatomic connections with underlying structures such as muscle, nerves, and blood vessels. One cannot consider the skin to exist in isolation. The underlying fibrous attachments to muscles and other structures must be appreciated to produce the best surgical results.

The cutaneous surface is readily accessible to observation and thus over the course of centuries has been the most closely and perhaps most accurately studied organ. Certain concepts have therefore developed and form the basis of cutaneous surgery—the understanding of which is essential to the performance of the highest quality work.

Cutaneous surgery is rapidly expanding because of the increasing desire of patients to improve or at least maintain their outward appearance. Moreover, economic factors have brought pressure on those performing surgery to do so less expensively. This has resulted in a greater emphasis on skin surgery within teaching programs, both in dermatology and in other specialties. Surgical research involving the skin is being done by many different disciplines, each making unique contributions.

Physicians who practice excellent cutaneous surgery have more than mere technique; they have aesthetic judg-

ment. Aesthetic judgment can be defined as the ability to visualize the end result.[15] Physicians who acquire the skills of different treatment modalities for any one cutaneous problem have a more highly developed aesthetic judgment than do physicians who are confined within the narrow framework of their specialties.

Equally important to aesthetic judgment is an understanding of cutaneous biology. Appreciation of skin physiology, anatomy, and pathology is necessary to achieve consistently good results. The nature of cutaneous lesions must also be known, since this knowledge provides the basis of treatment, whether surgical or otherwise.

I must emphasize at the outset that surgical principles and procedures of the cutaneous surface developed because of the contributions of many different physicians and scientists, from many specialties and disciplines. Major contributions have been made by dermatologists, ophthalmologists, oral surgeons, otolaryngologists, plastic surgeons, and even internists. The best patient management results from an exchange of ideas and experience rather than the jealous guarding of information. The team approach to patient care has always existed to some degree; with it, medical care has shown the most progress.

This chapter traces some of the major developments in surgery that have contributed to current concepts of cutaneous surgery (Table 1-1). Exploration and understanding of the problems that confronted our forebears can enhance our appreciation for current knowledge, which is often taken for granted. In addition, such examination puts into perspective the status of cutaneous surgery, within dermatologic surgery and medicine in general. The novelist and physician Oliver Wendell Holmes, Jr., once stated, ''When I want to understand what is happening today or try to decide what will happen tomorrow, I look back.'' Thus I offer the following brief account. Many other chapters in the text also include historical data.

TABLE 1-1

Major developments in surgery that contributed to cutaneous surgery

Date	Development	Source	Country
1800 BC	Sutures, dressings	Edwin Smith Surgical Papyrus	Egypt
700 BC	Skin flaps, cautery, instruments	Sushruta *Samhita*	India
400 BC	Instruments, tables, cauterization	Hippocrates (480-377 BC)	Greece
AD 50	Local skin flaps, ligation of vessels	Celsus (25 BC–AD 50)	Rome
AD 200	Placements of incisions	Galen (130-200)	Rome
	Excisional surgery, layered wound closure		
1547	Wound healing studied; "dry sutures"	Paré (1510-1590)	France
1597	Distant and local skin flaps	Tagliacozzi (1546-1599)	Italy
1804	Experimental skin grafts	Baronio (1759-1811)	Italy
1814	Forehead flap nasal reconstruction	Carpue (1746-1848)	England
1823	First skin graft	Bünger (1782-1842)	Germany
1840	Advancement flap	Warren (1778-1856)	United States
1842	General anesthesia	Long (1815-1878)	United States
1867	Antisepsis	Lister (1827-1912)	England
1869	Pinch graft	Reverdin (1842-1930)	France
1872	Split-thickness skin graft	Ollier (1825-1900)	France
1874	Split-thickness skin graft	Thiersch (1822-95)	Germany
1876	Full-thickness skin graft	Wolfe (1823-1904)	England
1884	Local anesthesia	Koller (1857-1944)	Germany
1890	Complete hemostasis	Halsted (1852-1922)	United States
	Gentle manipulation and close approximation of tissue		
	Surgical gloves and asepsis		
1893	Pedical flap	Dunham (1862-1951)	United States

HISTORICAL DEVELOPMENT
Ancient history

The Egyptian practice of medicine and surgery is best revealed in the Ebers Papyrus and the Edwin Smith Papyrus, probably written around 1800 BC or earlier.[9] These documents are the earliest medical textbooks and reveal the sophistication apparent at that time in treating afflictions medically or surgically. Herodotus, the famous Greek traveler and essayist, tells us that the Egyptians had specialists in certain areas of medicine, such as ophthalmology and gastroenterology.[27]

The Edwin Smith Papyrus is important because it is the first known reference to suturing wounds. One case report in this papyrus describes a gaping wound above the eyebrow, penetrating to the bone.[9] It was recommended that the wound be sutured and a dressing applied. If the sutures became loose, the wound should be treated with grease and honey and held together by two strips of linen. The linen strips were similar to modern skin tape closures. Gum was probably applied to make them stick.[40] Honey has been demonstrated to have antibacterial properties and ointments have been shown to promote wound healing.[24] A mummified example of what probably represents Egyptian suturing techniques is shown in Fig. 1-1.

Egyptians were greatly concerned about their cosmetic appearance. Some of the earliest facial abrasives described in the Egyptian papyri are not unlike modern formulations.[7]

Ancient Indian medicine was also quite sophisticated, as recorded in Sanskrit about 700 BC in the Sushruta *Samhita*.[6] This document, written by the Indian Hindu physician Sushruta, gives a precise description of cheek and forehead flaps for nasal reconstruction.[52] Apparently nasal repair was a frequent operation in ancient India, since nasal amputation was a common punishment for infidelity and criminal acts.[78] Nasal repairs were performed by specialists belonging to a caste of potters, the Koomas, who transmitted their skills from one generation to the next.[56] Such operations succeeded despite the lack of adequate anesthesia, asepsis, antibiotics, and instruments.

The *Samhita* also describes the first antiseptic measures taken at the time of surgery, such as the fumigation of operating rooms, and the first use of anesthetics (alcoholic drinks) before and during operations. The use of ant pinchers to close wounds is mentioned. Sushruta records a detailed list of 125 surgical instruments (some of which are shown in Fig. 1-2) and wisely states at the end that the physician's hand is the most important instrument of all.[52]

Early Greek medical thought is reflected in the writings

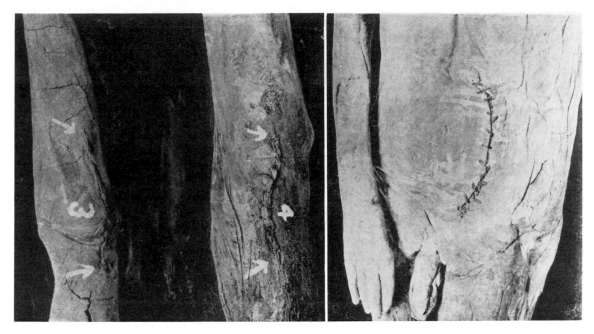

Fig. 1-1. Egyptian mummy with sutures, perhaps early examples of Egyptian suturing techniques (From Breasted, J.H.: The Edwin Smith surgical papyrus, vol. 1, Chicago, 1930, University of Chicago Press.)

of Hippocrates (480 to 377 BC). Although best known for his scientific approach to the study of disease, Hippocrates reported in great detail on operations and included remarks on instruments, lighting, and assistants.[40] He mentioned the use of wine for irrigating open wounds and described wound healing by primary and secondary intention.[70]

Medicine and surgery at the time of Hippocrates were intertwined and complementary. Greek physicians did not look down on surgery but rather viewed it as a necessary form of treatment in some circumstances. This is illustrated in a quotation of Hippocrates: "What drugs fail to cure, that the knife cures; what the knife cures not, that the fire cures; but what the fire fails to cure, this method must be called incurable."[40] The fire mentioned by Hippocrates as a third method of treatment refers to cautery. This form of therapy was later developed by Arabic physicians[56] and has survived in that part of the world even to this day as a method of treatment for various illnesses.[44]

Rome became the next great learning center in medicine. The famous Roman physician Celsus (25BC to AD 50) suggested the use of ligatures and local skin flaps.[59] These skin flaps were either H-advancement flaps or island pedicle flaps and were fashioned to repair defects on the ears, nose, or lips.[43] Celsus described the use of relaxation incisions if the flap was too tight (Fig. 1-3). He is also credited with having devised an operation for surgically restoring foreskin to Jews in Rome who sought acceptance by the Romans.[31]

Another famous Roman physician, Galen (AD 130 to 200), was an important surgeon. For more than 1500 years his writings were considered to be authoritative in many countries.[40] Galen was the physician assigned to the gladiators of Pergamon in Asia Minor. While there he developed concepts of wound repair that have survived to the present day. He advocated primary approximation of tendons, the trimming of ragged edges of wounds, the closing of wounds in layers, and the proper placement of incisions.[65]

Dark and middle ages

With the fall of Rome, the Western world entered a period of history in which learning was scarce and civilization advanced slowly. Little advancement occurred in medicine because religion was looked on as the substitute for medicine. The teachings of medical authorities were preserved in monasteries by the monks, who provided much of the medical and hospital care, based on the principles of Christian charity; however, with time the Church began to limit this work. In 1163 at the Council of Tours, Pope Gregory III forbade surgical practice by monks and issued the famous proclamation, "Ecclesia abhorret a sanguine [The Church hates blood]."[82]

The church's removal of surgery from medieval medical science was a great misdeed with serious consequences: the medical schools of the time could not teach surgery and even forbade their graduates to practice it. This led to the establishment of a separate guild of individuals, who eventually were called barber-surgeons. Many of the barber-surgeons were itinerants, which added to the disrepute of surgery. The surgical profession was divided into the surgeons with formal medical school education ("gentlemen of the long coat") and the barber-surgeons ("gentlemen of the

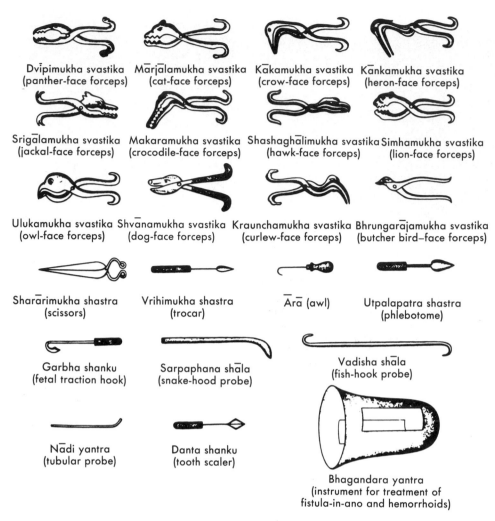

Fig. 1-2. Instruments described in detail in the *Samhita*. (From Prakash, U.B.: Surg. Gynecol. Obstet. **146**:263, 1978.)

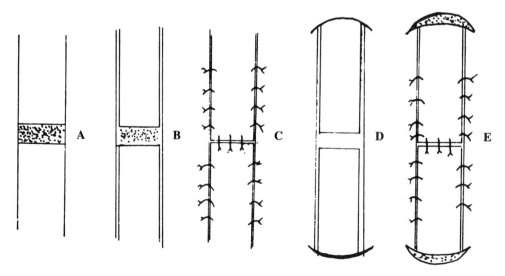

Fig. 1-3. Advancement flaps described by Celsus. **A,** H-advancement flap incisions. **B,** Skin and underlying tissue raised. **C,** Flaps advanced and sutured together. **D,** Semilunar incisions made to relieve tension. **E,** Relaxed flaps drawn together. (From Spencer, E.G.: Celsus: de medicina, with an English translation, Cambridge, Mass., 1938, Harvard University Press. Reprinted by permission.)

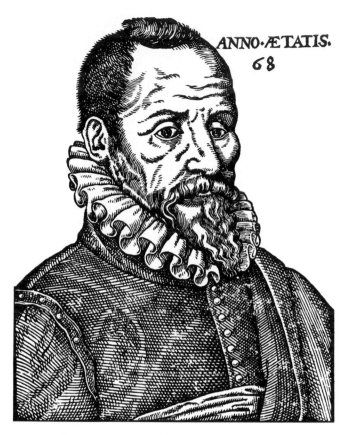

ANNO·ÆTATIS.
68

Fig. 1-4. Ambroise Paré at age 68; woodcut. (From Lyons, A.S., and Petrucelli, R.J.: Medicine: an illustrated history, New York, 1978, Harry N. Abrams, Inc., Publisher. Courtesy New York Academy of Medicine.)

short coat''). The former acted in the capacity of advisors to the latter; that is, physicians themselves did not do the surgery. The tradition of the senior physician wearing the longer coat and the younger less educated physician wearing the shorter coat has survived to this day in medical institutions.[82]

Three surgeons of note during this bleak period of history were Guglielmo Salicet (1210 to 1277) of the medical school in Bologna, Henri de Mondeville (1260 to 1320) of the medical school of Montpellier, and Guy de Chauliac (1300 to 1368), who studied at several schools in France and Italy. Salicet preferred the knife to the cautery, and de Mondeville advocated simple cleanliness in treating wounds and the avoidance of pus. It was de Mondeville who suggested that the surgeon consider cosmetic results when planning excision; he advised his students to make incisions horizontally on the forehead and to remove sutures from the face in 4 to 5 days.[33] Guy de Chauliac was the most erudite authority on surgery during the fourteenth century. He took surgery out of the hands of traveling quacks and gave it legitimacy. Unfortunately, he embraced the doctrine of suppurative wound healing. This concept originated with Galen, who wrote that "no wound can heal unless an evil

smelling laudable pus appears.'' This idea survived for centuries after de Chauliac because surgeons knew that pus-forming wounds (presumably caused by *Staphylococcus aureus*) would drain, whereas those developing great erythema (presumably caused by *Streptococcus*) would extend and possibly kill the patient.

Renaissance

The Renaissance, or rebirth of civilization, gained momentum in the fourteenth century and continued into the fifteenth and sixteenth centuries. Cultural enlightenment in both the humanities and science spread throughout Europe. Galileo, Copernicus, Michelangelo, and Shakespeare flourished and dared to confront the established order. Martin Luther initiated the Reformation in 1517. In medicine, however, change was resisted. Physicians continued to embrace Hippocratic and Galenic dicta while discouraging independent observation, the questioning of dogma, or experimentation.

An exception to medicine's resistance to change was Ambroise Paré (1510 to 1590), who can be considered a true Renaissance physician (Fig. 1-4). He distinguished himself by contending that a system of observation was preferable to blind adherence to an ancient dogma. In 1537 Paré was not permitted to enter medical school, so he joined the army. In 1547 he published *The Method of Treatment for Wounds Caused by Firearms,* which detailed his experiences as a medic in battle. This work is considered to be one of the first on experimental wound healing. The standard method of treating gunshot wounds had been to apply boiling oil. One day while treating casualties Paré ran out of oil. Therefore he cleaned the remaining wounds and dressed them with lard. It was with some trepidation that he retired to bed that evening. The next day to his surprise the soldiers who had been treated with boiling oil were feverish and in pain, whereas those treated with lard were resting comfortably.[40] When complimented later by another physician on a good job helping a patient's wound to heal, Paré answered, "Je le pansey, Dieu le guarit. [I dressed it, God healed it.]''[20] A French Hugenot, Paré was the only Protestant spared by royal mandate at the St. Bartholomew's Day Massacre in 1572.

Paré was not only a keen observer but an innovator as well. He described "dry sutures," which are similar in principle to modern-day butterfly sutures (Fig. 1-5), as well as several types of nasal prostheses. Sensitive to cosmetic results after surgery, Paré advised, "If they require suturing, it should be dry suturing so that the scars will not remain ugly, as there are many who fear such happening, particularly the belles demoiselles.''[31]

Among Paré's other surgical insights was his advice to use ligatures instead of cautery for hemostasis and to guide wounds together with sutures even if the edges could not be absolutely apposed. He advocated use of a turpentine mixture on wounds[71]; this topical preparation—composed of

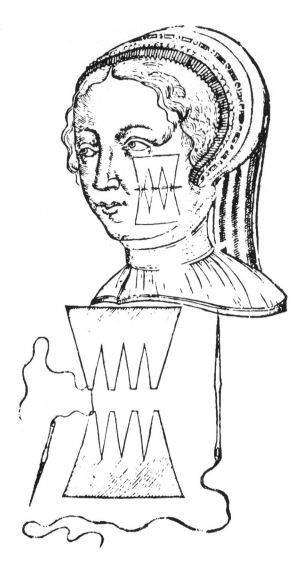

Fig. 1-5. Dry suture technique of Ambroise Paré. (From Lyons, A.S., and Petrucelli, R.J.: Medicine: an illustrated history, New York, 1978, Harry N. Abrams, Inc., Publisher. Courtesy New York Academy of Medicine.)

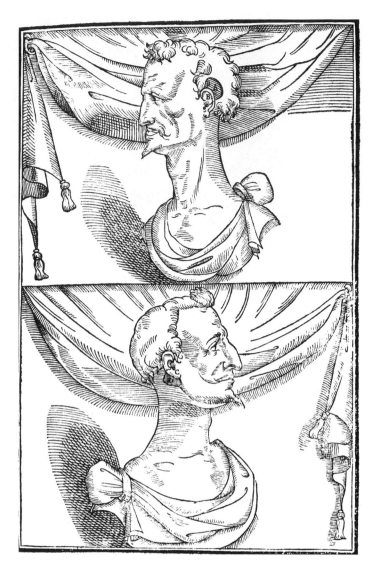

Fig. 1-6. Tagliacozzi's donor areas for local flaps for ear repair. (From Tagliacozzi, G.: De curtorum chirurgia per insitionem, Venice, 1597, Gaspare Dindoni. Courtesy Washington University School of Medicine, Rare Book Collection.)

turpentine, oil of lilies, and fat from newborn puppies—has since been shown to be bacteriostatic for *Escherichia coli* and *Staphylococcus aureus*.[3]

Through his work and publications, Paré brought a renaissance to surgery. He was one of the first great surgeons to emphasize the humane treatment of patients as an integral part of his profession. He was a simple, kindly man whose goal was to cure his patients with as little suffering as possible. He made no distinction between rich and poor. Needless to say, he was at odds with the medical establishment, the Faculté de Médecine.

A few years after the death of Paré a physician in Bologna named Gaspare Tagliacozzi published a monumental work entitled *De Curtorum Chirurgia per Insitionem*.[63] Basically this is a description of a method, now known as

the Tagliacozzi method, of rebuilding nasal tips and ears. The donor skin is taken from the inner aspect of the arm. Delay in lifting the flap and delay in cutting the flap are described in detail and beautifully illustrated in woodcuts. Tagliacozzi's observations regarding tissue transfer are unique and of value to all physicians performing skin flaps.

Among the woodcuts in Tagliacozzi's work is one showing donor areas for local flaps for ear reconstruction (Fig. 1-6). Although this local method of repair did not work well for the superior part of the ear, apparently the lower ear was successfully repaired in this manner.

Tagliacozzi's perspective on reconstruction was best summarized when he said, "We restore, repair and make whole those parts of the body which nature has given but fortune has taken away [to] buoy up the spirit and help

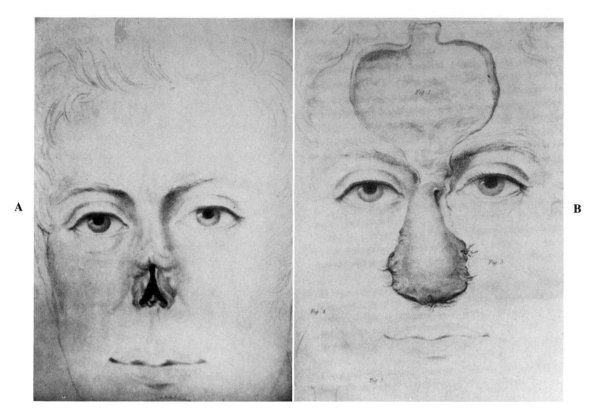

Fig. 1-7. Forehead flap performed by Carpue in 1814. **A,** Preoperative engraving. **B,** Postoperative engraving. (From Carpue, J.C.: An account of two successful operations for restoring a lost nose from the integuments of the forehead, London, 1816, Longman.)

the mind of the afflicted.'' Unfortunately, the church's teaching was that such surgery was tampering with God's will; because of his work, Tagliacozzi's remains were exhumed and moved to unconsecrated ground.

Seventeenth and eighteenth centuries

In the seventeenth and eighteenth centuries corrective surgery was ridiculed by most physicians and by laymen, such as Voltaire. Strife and rivalry between physicians, surgeons, and barbers continued in full force.[20]

Nineteenth century

During the nineteenth century a rebirth of skin flap surgery took place, set in motion by a chance event that occurred in 1794. A letter appeared in the October issue of *The Gentleman's Magazine,* published in London.[21] The letter detailed an operation that was witnessed in India during the Third Mysire War. The enemy captured a bullock driver named Cowasjee and cut off his nose, which was reconstructed by an Indian physician. An English physician named Carpue was inspired by the letter and sought out the physician who had witnessed the surgery. This led him to perform the same operation in England in 1814.[12]

The operation that Carpue performed was a forehead flap procedure,[12] an operation still used to reconstruct the nose

(Fig. 1-7). Amazingly this operation took Carpue only 15 minutes to perform, with no anesthesia.[5] That Carpue performed the operation in two stages shows his understanding of flap physiology—the blood supply must not be interrupted until the flap has ''taken.''[19]

As the nineteenth century progressed, so did the performance of skin flap surgery. In 1840 Warren described the ''Tagliacotian operation'' for nasal reconstruction, as well as the use of advancement or rotation cheek flaps for nasal reconstruction.[72] Shortly afterward, in 1842, Pancoast also discussed both rotation and advancement flaps.[50] Because of the lack of anesthesia, only patients who were quite disfigured and highly motivated were considered candidates for such operations.

In 1893 Dunham[16] described a pedicle flap based on the temporal artery for reconstruction of the nose and cheek after resection for a recurrent basal cell carcinoma. Dunham emphasized that survival of the flap was based on maintenance of the blood supply. A few years later, in 1898, Monks[46] reconstructed a lower eyelid, following the principles set forth by Dunham. Monks's patient also had a basal cell carcinoma of the lower eyelid (Fig. 1-8).

The development of skin grafts followed that of skin flaps. One must remember that early in the nineteenth century there was no anesthesia or antisepsis. Performing a skin

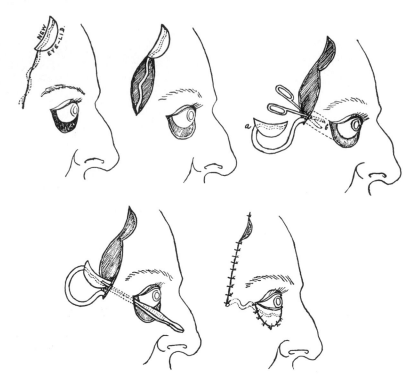

Fig. 1-8. Reconstruction of lower eyelid by vascular pedicle flap following excision of skin cancer in 1898. (From Monks, G.H.: The restoration of the lower eyelid by a new method, Boston Med. Surg. J. **139**:385, 1898.)

graft meant creating a second wound for the patient. Because every wound was susceptible to infection, physicians preferred not to take the chance. Those who did were only partially successful.

In 1804 Baronio described the successful results of experimental skin grafting in sheep[4] (Fig. 1-9). Bünger[10] in 1823 reported the first successful skin graft in modern medical literature, from the buttock to the nose. The technique used was similar to the ancient Indian method in which the buttock was beaten to increase the blood supply before the graft was harvested.[55]

Reverdin, a Swiss intern at the Hospital Necker in Paris, described the first pinch grafts to a granulating wound in 1869. He explained that they led to more rapid healing.[53] Interestingly, Reverdin's method was criticized by his contemporaries because the donor site wounds could possibly become infected (''ouvert une porte a l'erysipele [open the door for erysipelas]'').

Ollier de Lyon is credited with the first split-thickness graft, in 1872.[48] His contribution to the field of skin grafting included the discovery that immobilization of the skin graft increased the likelihood of success—''pour assurer le succes des graffes, il faut immobilizer la region operee.'' [to ensure success of grafts, it is necessary to immobilize the surgical area.].''

The first full-thickness skin graft was described by J.R. Wolfe in 1875.[77] A skin graft from the forearm to the lower eyelid was performed to repair an ectropion. Wolfe con-

tended that the previous unsuccessful grafts had been caused by failure to remove the subcutaneous fat. He explored the relationship of graft thickness to likelihood of take in his patient by varying the thickness of the graft in three separate areas. Where the graft was thickest, Wolfe observed signs of the greatest difficulty in taking compared to the other areas.

In 1886 Karl Thiersch described a split-thickness graft and was initially given credit for the procedure.[64] However, when Ollier's earlier work was discovered, these grafts came to be known as Ollier-Thiersch grafts.

Two other developments in the nineteenth century that greatly influenced surgery were the discoveries of anesthesia and antisepsis.[79] In 1842 Dr. Crawford Long of Danielsville, Georgia, removed a small cutaneous cyst from the back of a patient's neck with ether as an anesthetic.[13] The first public demonstration of general anesthesia did not occur until 1846 when Dr. John C. Warren at the Massachusetts General Hospital removed a small cutaneous tumor just below the jaw on the left side of the patient's neck. Afterward Warren commented, ''Gentlemen, this is no humbug.'' This operation is the subject of a famous painting. Both hypnosis and acupuncture were also used in the nineteenth century. Cloquet in 1826 experimented with acupuncture and in 1829 used hypnosis to perform a mastectomy.[14]

Local anesthesia was not introduced until later in the nineteenth century. Freud was the first to suggest that co-

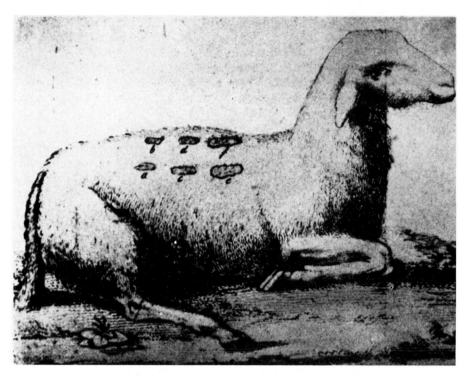

Fig. 1-9. Full-thickness skin autotransplants on a sheep performed by Baronio in 1804. (From Baronio, G.: Delgi innesti animali, Milano, 1804, Stamperia e Fonderia del Genio.)

caine be tried as a local anesthetic, and in 1884 Karl Koller reported its success in ophthalmology.[34] Physicians in other specialties, including dermatology and general surgery, soon began to use local anesthesia for excisions.[29] It was not used sooner for intracutaneous injection because the syringe was not widely available until the 1890s. Probably one of the reasons that many operations are currently performed on patients under a general anesthetic is that general anesthesia was developed first, and the early local anesthetics were less safe than they have become. It is also interesting to note that local anesthetics for dental procedures were pioneered by a general surgeon, William Halsted, whereas dentists initiated the use of general anesthetics.

The introduction of antisepsis met with intense resistance by surgeons. In the early 1840s Ignas Semmelweis, a Hungarian physician, was appointed assistant obstetrician at the Allgemeines Krankenhaus, a Viennese maternity hospital. He observed a lower incidence of patients dying from childbed fever if he washed his hands before attending to them. Semmelweis instituted the use of a chlorinated lime solution for handwashing by all house officers and other physicians at his institution. Unfortunately, this produced antagonism on the part of the faculty, despite the fact that the death rate was markedly reduced. Semmelweis's chief, Professor Klein, denounced the "hand-washing theory," and although Semmelweis was permitted to maintain his position as professor, he was prohibited from treating patients. Disillusioned, he left the hospital for seclusion in private practice.

Between 1857 and 1863 Louis Pasteur developed the theory that germs cause milk to spoil. Since Pasteur was a scientist and not a physician, however, he did not immediately relate his work to wound infection.

In 1860 Joseph Lister, a surgeon at the Glasgow Royal Infirmary, became interested in the widespread problem of wound infection in hospitals. It was not uncommon to clean the wounds of all the patients on a ward with a single piece of gauze.[67] By chance, a professor of chemistry at Glasgow pointed out to Lister Pasteur's current research work. Lister grasped the parallel between the fermentation process described by Pasteur and wound putrefaction. He reasoned that if germs cause wound infection, he needed to find a chemical to destroy the germs. He tried carbolic acid because of its success in treating sewage at a nearby town. Initially he packed wounds with lint soaked in carbolic acid and covered them with tinfoil, which caused a dramatic decrease in the number of cases of gangrene and erysipelas on his ward. This was the beginning of the listerian principle of antisepsis, defined as preventing suppuration by preventing the growth of bacteria and first reported in 1867.[39] In 1883 the majority of speakers at the American Surgical Association opposed the theory of antisepsis,[74] in part because they believed that cleanliness rather than antisepsis was the proper method to arrest putrefaction.[66]

In 1882 the Prussian scientist Robert Koch isolated the tubercle bacillus, the cause of tuberculosis, and suggested that different microorganisms could cause infection independently and with different characteristics. This led to the development of Koch's postulates, a system for determining that a given microorganism has caused a given disease that is still considered valid.

Among the first bacteria to be demonstrated on the body (in 1875 by Eberth) were those on the skin, sweat glands, and hair follicles. Eberth's findings led to the practice of scrubbing the hands with soap and water to prevent the transmission of infection. Thus a transformation occurred in attitudes toward aseptic techniques, which included not only hand washing but sterilization of instruments. Koch developed the first steam sterilizer in 1881, and in 1886 Kummel showed, as had Semmelweis 40 years previously, that hand washing prevents infection. In 1895 Schimmel-busch published a book that outlined aseptic techniques and popularized the sterilizer.[57]

During the nineteenth century medical specialization first began to appear formally and become widespread. Dermatology evolved from the English, German, and French schools. At first dermatology in the United States (mainly in New York City) was associated with urology, as can be seen in the *Journal of Dermatology and Genitourinary Diseases,* first published in 1882. However, with time dermatologists became less surgically oriented and took up the challenge of syphilology, a major public health problem at the turn of the century. In Europe dermatology has retained its connection with urology, and to this day European dermatologists perform a number of urologic procedures.

That the early dermatologists were concerned by cosmetic surgery is evidenced by the origins of the cutaneous punch. Edward L. Keyes, a professor of dermatology and urology, developed this instrument to punch out areas on the face of a patient who had been tattooed with gunpowder; he reported this method in 1887.[30] Unknown to Keyes, a similar instrument, called the discotome, was described for the same purpose in 1878 by Dr. B.A. Watson.[73]

The dermal curette was developed as a simple instrument to treat both superficial and deep cutaneous problems. Henry G. Piffard in 1870 and Edward Wigglesworth in 1876 popularized this instrument and the technique for its use.[51] Wigglesworth used it for literally everything: eczema, psoriasis, and even syphilitic condylomata (rubber gloves were not yet available). Occasionally patients were curetted under general anesthesia.[76]

It is fascinating to leaf through Louis A. Duhring's classic textbook, *Cutaneous Medicine,* published in 1905.[17] Much space is devoted to dermatologic surgery. For instance, the use of cocaine for local anesthesia is discussed at length and compared with the anesthesia produced by plain water (which Duhring terms "anesthesia dolorosa" and says is very painful). Both pinch grafting and Thiersch (split-thickness) grafting are well described, and Duhring apparently thought they belonged within the scope of dermatology. The lines of skin excision are discussed in detail.

Twentieth century

The dominant force in the development of surgery in the twentieth century was William Halsted. Halsted was an indifferent student at Yale, more attracted by athletics than books. As a student at Columbia Medical School, however, he became interested in anatomy and did quite well. In the 1880s, while still in New York, he began an investigation of the local anesthetic properties of cocaine. This led to an addiction that Halsted battled for the remainder of his life and for which he was hospitalized at least twice.

In 1890 Halsted's friend William H. Welsh invited him to Johns Hopkins Medical School to head a new department of surgery. Halsted was an individualistic thinker and did not readily accept dogma. He established a long surgical residency program that became the model for surgical residency programs in the United States.

Halsted's contribution to cutaneous surgery was his insistence on a slow, methodical technique. Until Halsted a surgeon was judged by how fast he could operate. Halsted, however, was tediously slow in his work and would not be rushed. He realized that absolute hemostasis, careful handling of tissue, conservation of tissue, careful suturing technique, and meticulous closure of wounds in layers all had great benefits for the patient.[28] Dr. Charles Mayo facetiously commented that Halsted was the only surgeon he knew who was still suturing the bottom of a wound when the top had already healed.

Halsted was responsible for the introduction of rubber gloves into the operating room. Interestingly the use of gloves had a dermatologic origin.[80] In 1894 a nurse in Halsted's operating room developed a dermatitis of the hands from exposure to mercuric chloride, which was used as an antiseptic solution to disinfect instruments. No dermatologic compound Halsted could devise seemed to help, but then he had the idea of using rubber gloves to protect the nurse's hands. He had plaster casts made of her hands and sent to the Goodyear Rubber Company in New York. With the use of these specially made rubber gloves, her dermatitis cleared up. It soon became apparent that rubber gloves served a useful purpose in making surgical operations more sterile. After rubber gloves were used in the operating room, they could be either boiled or placed in carbolic acid as a means of disinfection. Halsted later married this nurse; one might say that infatuation produced the first rubber gloves in the operating room.

The routine use of rubber gloves in surgery took place over several years. Halsted himself wore them only occasionally and did not realize the importance of invariably wearing them during surgery.[26] It was Bloodgood, one of Halsted's first residents, who reported in 1899 the results of routine use of rubber gloves by both surgeon and assistant in surgery.[8] Ironically, rubber gloves, which were developed to protect the care-giver from caustic solutions and later came into general use to protect the patient from infection, again have recently been emphasized as a means of protec-

**MAJOR DEVELOPMENTS IN
DERMATOLOGIC SURGERY**

Dermabrasion (Kromayer, 1905)
Chemical peels (MacKee and Karp, 1952; Ayres, 1960)
Hair transplantation (Orentreich, 1959)
Laser surgery (Goldman, 1964)
Cryosurgery (Zacarian, 1966)
Microscopically controlled surgery
    Fixed-tissue technique (Mohs, 1941)
    Fresh-tissue technique (Tromovitch, 1976)

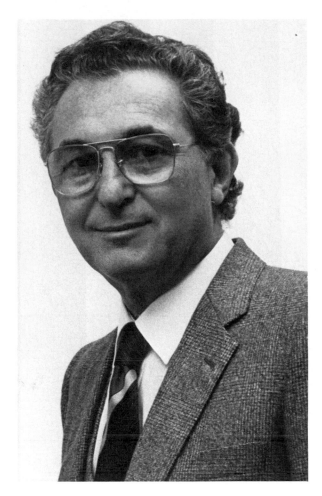

Fig. 1-10. Norman Orentreich, M.D., circa 1983. (Courtesy Norman Orentreich, New York.)

tion for surgeons, this time against hepatitis[58] and AIDS.[47]

Dermatologists continued their interest in developing methods for the elegant removal of cutaneous lesions or scars (see box on p. 13). An electrosurgical apparatus was pioneered by MacKee[41] and liquid nitrogen by White-house.[75] Dermabrasion was essentially a dermatologic procedure first employed by Kromayer in Germany in 1905.[35] He used motor-driven rotary steel burs to remove pitted acne scars or tattoos by cutaneous abrasion. In 1930 Kromayer[36] described his techniques in a book entitled *Cosmetic Treatment of Skin Complaints*. Kromayer's techniques received mixed interest and acceptance among dermatologists in the United States. A few proponents, such as Eller,[18] Kurtin,[38] Burks,[11] and Ayres,[2] did promote his work and advanced both the equipment and methods used.

Dermatologists who are well trained in the basic sciences of cutaneous medicine and pathology are likely to solve cutaneous problems from a rational scientific approach. An excellent example of such an approach can be found in the field of hair transplantation. Norman Orentreich (Fig. 1-10) in the 1950s investigated cutaneous punch autotransplants for various dermatologic conditions.[49] He realized that transplanting hair from hair-bearing areas of the scalp to areas of hair loss caused by male pattern alopecia resulted in permanent growth of hair in the donor skin. Orentreich developed techniques and equipment for transplanting large numbers of hair-bearing "plugs," resulting in hair growth in previously balding individuals. Other dermatologists[62,69] have since extended Orentreich's initial discoveries by developing both scalp-reduction and scalp-flap techniques. Dr. S. Ohmari, formerly a dermatologist and now a plastic surgeon in Japan, reported the first completely successful free flaps in 1973.[25] He has since used free flaps to create natural-appearing anterior hairlines for patients with male pattern alopecia.

The field of skin cancer has always been of interest to dermatologists, who have generated a number of techniques for the treatment of neoplasms. These forms of therapy include curettage and electrodesiccation, cryosurgery,[81] 5-fluorouracil,[32] radiotherapy, and excisional therapy. Dermatologists were among the first to employ the technique of skin cancer excision known as Mohs chemosurgery, after its originator, Dr. Frederic Mohs (Fig. 1-11).

In the late 1930s Mohs was doing research on mammary sarcoma in rats. This led him to develop a technique for the fixation of tissue in vivo before removal and microscopic examination. Although dermatologists became interested in this technique early, it was not widely used because of the time required to perform the surgery and then carry out microscopic examination. In 1974 Tromovitch and Stegman published a paper demonstrating that for many tumors the fixation of tissue was unnecessary to provide the high rate of cure Mohs had reported.[68] Elimination of this step was a tremendous advance because it shortened the procedure and made the technique widely available. This technique is currently available in most major medicl centers largely as a result of persistent efforts of a handful of dedicated dermatologists.

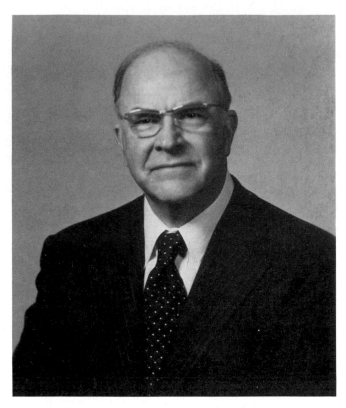

Fig. 1-11. Frederic Mohs, M.D., circa 1983. (Courtesy Frederic Mohs, Madison, Wisc.)

In 1978 Robins summarized the feelings of many dermatologists toward Mohs[54]:

> By his meticulous, painstaking and skillful efforts, Dr. Mohs has maintained cure rates for cutaneous cancers that exceed those achieved by practitioners of other methods. . . . Patients were referred to Dr. Mohs' office in Madison, Wisconsin from all over the world. Dr. Mohs' motto ''can do'' brought him the most extensive, the most difficult and seemingly hopeless cases. Dr. Mohs frequently salvaged patients who had been judged by others to be inoperable.

The advance of fresh-tissue Mohs surgery brought the benefit that reconstruction could be performed immediately after surgery. Although this may not always be the wisest course of action, dermatologists have been quite thoughtful in their approach to the problem.[60] Modifications of standard surgical repairs are currently made by dermatologists for cutaneous defects of unusual size and location as an outgrowth of this approach.

Two further advances in cutaneous surgery in which dermatologists have played a major role are chemical peeling of the skin for wrinkles or blemishes and laser surgery. Initial pathologic and early cosmetic results with superficial chemical peels were reported by George M. MacKee in 1954[42] and Samuel Ayres in 1960.[1] Dr. Leon Goldman in Cincinnati pioneered the use of lasers on the skin for treatment of port-wine stains.[23] Lasers are increasingly useful as new applications are found in all fields of surgery.[22]

SCOPE OF DERMATOLOGIC SURGERY

As one can see from the foregoing brief history of cutaneous surgery, a modern dermatologist may be qualified by virtue of training to perform all of the surgery used in cutaneous surfaces, including not only simple excisions and biopsies but more extensive cosmetic surgery. Since dermatologists have been instrumental in the development of many techniques currently used by other specialists, such as plastic surgeons, there is justification in the sharing of techniques and knowledge from these other fields. No one knew this better than Dr. John Converse, who said, ''It is the intradisciplinary interchange that makes for surgical progress and provides for the optimal care of the patient.''[15]

Modern dermatology departments offer training specifically devoted to dermatologic surgery. This training encompasses the basic science of tumor biology and wound healing, as well as active participation in various surgical techniques on the skin. The free exchange of ideas with other surgical departments having common interests, such as otolaryngology or plastic surgery, is encouraged and demonstrated by collaborative care of patients.

Dermatologists are therapeutically eclectic. Not only are they well grounded in dermatopathology, but they are versatile in choosing procedures. They are neither plastic surgeons nor cosmetic surgeons, but rather specialists in surgery of the cutaneous surfaces. The term *plastic* comes from the Greek word $\pi\lambda\acute{\alpha}\sigma\sigma\omega$, meaning to mold or to shape. Although this applies to ''molding'' a nose or breast, it does not apply to hair transplantation. The term ''cosmetic'' comes from the Greek $\kappa o\sigma\mu\acute{e}\omega$, meaning to adorn or beautify. Actually the origin of the term in Greek itself meant to set in order, since cosmos ($\kappa\acute{o}\sigma\mu\acute{o}\varsigma$) means order. ''Cosmetic'' is preferable to ''plastic,'' but because of its other Greek meaning (to adorn) it is less than perfect. I propose the word *corrective* as the most suitable term, and *corrective cutaneous surgery* as most applicable to the work performed by dermatologic surgeons as well as plastic or cosmetic surgeons. This term is equally applicable to hair transplantation, scar surgery, dermabrasion, flaps, and grafts. The current status of cosmetic surgery in dermatology has been summarized by Stegman.[61]

FUTURE OF DERMATOLOGIC SURGERY

The relationship of dermatology with other specialties in surgery will be strengthened as more patients are jointly managed to provide better patient care. The concept of the team approach to the management of extensive cutaneous malignancies is becoming well established in major medical centers. Dermatologists are an important part of this team. Krull said, ''Rather than squandering our efforts in the self-serving arguments over territorial practice privileges, all physicians performing some skin surgery should direct and unite their efforts into improving the quality of patient care and the reduction of its cost.''[37] Interdiscipliary interchange leads to surgical progress and choices in patient care.

Dermatologic surgery is a rapidly growing field, with increasing interest being shown within residency training programs, as well as by dermatologists in practice. This textbook lays a firm foundation for knowledge in this area. Knowledge is, however, no substitute for experience; only with experience can a good sense of judgment be gained. However, everyone needs a starting point—and I hope this book will be that starting point in the field of dermatologic surgery.

REFERENCES

1. Ayres, S., III: Dermal changes following application of chemical cauterants to aging skin (superficial chemosurgery), Arch. Dermatol. **82:**578, 1960.
2. Ayres, S., III, Wilson, J., and Luikart, R., II: Dermal changes following abrasion, Arch. Dermatol. **79:**553, 1959.
3. Bagwell, C.E.: Ambroise Paré and the renaissance of surgery, Surg. Gynecol. Obstet. **152:**350, 1981.
4. Baronio, G.: Degli innesti animali, Milano, 1804, Stamperia e Fonderia del Genio.
5. Bennett, J.P.: Aspects of the history of plastic surgery since the 16th century, J. R. Soc. Med. **76:**152, 1983.
6. Bhishagratna, K.C.: An English translation of the Sushruta Samhita, based on original Sanskrit text, Calcutta, 1916, Bose.
7. Blau, S., and Rein, C.R.: Dermabrasion of the acne pit, Arch. Dermatol. Syph. **70:**754, 1954.
8. Bloodgood, J.C.: Operations on 459 cases of hernia in the Johns Hopkins Hospital from June 1889 to January 1899, Johns Hopkins Hosp. Rep. **7:**223, 1898-99.
9. Breasted, J.H.: The Edwin Smith surgical papyrus, vol. 1, Chicago, 1930, University of Chicago Press.
10. Bünger, C.: Gelungener Versuch einer Nasenbildung, J. Chir. Augenk. **4:**569, 1823.
11. Burks, J.W.: Abrasive removal of scars, South. Med. J. **48:**452, 1955.
12. Carpue, J.C.: An account of two successful operations for restoring a lost nose from the integuments of the forehead in the cases of two officers of his majesty's army, in which are included historical and physiologic remarks on the nasal operation, including descriptions of the Indian and Italian methods, London, 1816, Longman Hurst, Kees, Orme, and Brown.
13. Cartwright, F.: The development of modern surgery, London, 1967, Arthur Baker Ltd.
14. Chertok, L.: Surgery using hypnosis in 1829 (letter), Am. J. Psychiatr. **131:**721, 1974.
15. Converse, J.M.: Introduction to plastic surgery. In Reconstructive plastic surgery, Philadelphia, 1977, W.B. Saunders Co.
16. Dunham, T.: A method for obtaining a skin flap from the scalp and a permanent buried vascular pedicle for covering defects of the face, Ann. Surg. **17:**677, 1893.
17. Duhring, L.A.: Cutaneous medicine, Philadelphia, 1905, J.B. Lippincott Co.
18. Eller, J.J.: Developments in rotary abrasive techniques for removing acne scars and other cosmetic defects, N. Engl. J. Med. **253:**11, 1955.
19. Freshwater, M.F., et al.: Joseph Constantine Carpue—first military plastic surgeon, Milit. Med. **142:**603, 1977.
20. Garrison, F.H.: An introduction to the history of medicine, Philadelphia, 1929, W.B. Saunders Co.
21. Gentleman's Magazine: A communication to the editor, Mr. Urban, signed B.L.; engraved illustration between pp. 882 and 883. **64**(pt. 2):891, 1794.
22. Goldman, L., and Rockwell, R.J.: Lasers in Medicine, New York, 1971, Gordon & Breach.
23. Goldman, L., and Richfield, D.F.: The effects of repeated exposure to laser beam, Acta Derm. Venereol. [Stockh.] **44:**264, 1964.
24. Goldwyn, R.M.: Is there plastic surgery in the Edwin Smith Papyrus? Plast. Reconstr. Surg. **70:**263, 1982.
25. Harii, K., and Ohmori, S.: Use of gastroepiploic vessels as recipient in donor vessels in the free transfer of composite flaps by microvascular anastomoses, Plast. Reconstr. Surg. **52:**541, 1973.
26. Harvey, A.M.: Early contributions to the surgery of cancer: William S. Halsted, Hugh H. Young, and John G. Clark, Johns Hopkins Med. J. **135:**399, 1974.
27. Herodotus: The Persian wars, New York, 1942, Random House. (Translated by George Rawlinson.)
28. Holman, E.: William Steward Halsted, Johns Hopkins Med. J. **135:**418, 1974.
29. Horowitz: Local cocaine anaesthesia (correspondence), J. Cutan. Genito-Urinary Dis. **5:**231, 1887.
30. Keyes, E.L.: The cutaneous punch, J. Cutan. Genito-Urinary Dis. **5:**98, 1887.
31. Khoo, C.T.: Cosmetic surgery: where does it begin? Br. J. Plast. Surg. **35:**277, 1982.
32. Klein, E., et al.: Tumors of the skin. Part 12. Topical 5-fluorouracil for epidermal neoplasms, J. Surg. Oncol. **3:**331, 1971.
33. Klein, M.D.: The practice of surgery in the fourteenth century, Am. J. Surg. **131:**587, 1976.
34. Koller, K.: Ueber die Verwendungen des Cocaine zur Anasthesirung am Auge, Wien Med. Wochenschr. **34:**1276, 1884.
35. Kromayer, E.: Rotationsinstrumente: ein neues technisches Verfahren in der dermatologischen Kleinchirurgie, Derm. Z. **12:**26, 1905.
36. Kromayer, E.: Cosmetic treatment of skin complaints, New York, 1930, Oxford University Press.
37. Krull, E.A.: Reflections on skin surgery, J. Dermatol. Surg. **2:**400, 1976.
38. Kurtin, A.: Corrective surgical planing of skin, Arch. Dermatol. Syph. **68:**389, 1953.
39. Lister, J.: On the antiseptic principle in the practice of surgery, Lancet **2:**353, 1867.
40. Lyons, A.S., and Petrucelli, R.J.: Medicine: an illustrated history, New York, 1978, Harry N. Abrams, Inc., Publishers.
41. MacKee, G.M.: Fulguration: the local application of a current of high frequency by means of a pointed metallic electrode—its use in dermatology, J. Cutan. Dis. **27:**245, 1909.
42. MacKee, G.M., and Karp, F.L.: The treatment of post-acne scars with phenol, Br. J. Dermatol. **64:**456, 1952.
43. Marmelzat, W.L.: Medicine in history—Celsus (AD 25), plastic surgeon: on the repair of defects of the ears, lips, and

nose, J. Dermatol. Surg. Oncol. **8**(12):1012, 1982.

44. Mohammad, A., et al.: Skin cauterization marks on patients in Saudi Arabia (letter to the editor), Lancet **1:**714, 1983.

45. Mohs, F.E., and Guyer, M.F.: Pre-excisional fixation of tissues in treatment of cancer, Cancer Res. **1:**49, 1941.

46. Monks, G.H.: The restoration of the lower eyelid by a new method, Boston Med. Surg. J. **139:**385, 1898.

47. Morbidity and Mortality Weekly Report: Acquired immune deficiency syndrome (AIDS): precaution for health care workers and allied professionals, M.M.W.R. **32:**450, 1983.

48. Ollier de Lyon: Greffes cutanées ou autoplastiques, Bull. Acad. Med. **1:**243, 1872.

49. Orentreich, N.: Autografts in alopecias and other selected dermatologic conditions, Ann. N.Y. Acad. Sci. **83:**463, 1959.

50. Pancoast, J.: Plastic operations, Am. J. Med. Sci. **4:**337, 1842.

51. Piffard, H.G.: Histological contribution, Am. J. Syph. Dermatol. **1:**217, 1870.

52. Prakash, U.B.: Shushruta of ancient India, Surg. Gynecol. Obstet. **146:**263, 1978.

53. Reverdin, J.L.: Bulletin de la Impériale Société de chirurgia de Paris, **10:**511, 1869.

54. Robins, P.: A tribute to Dr. Frederic E. Mohs, J. Dermatol. Surg. Oncol. **4:**37, 1978.

55. Rogers, B.O.: Historical development of free skin grafting, Surg. Clin. N. Am. **39:**289, 1959.

56. Rogers, B.O.: The historical evolution of plastic and reconstructive surgery. In Wood-Smith, D., and Porowski, P.C., editors: Nursing care of the plastic surgery patient, St. Louis, 1967, The C.V. Mosby Co.

57. Schimmelbusch, C.: A guide to the antiseptic treatment of wounds, New York, 1895, Putnam.

58. Smith, J.G., Jr., and Chalker, D.K.: A glove upon that hand (editorial) South. Med. J. **75:**129, 1982.

59. Spencer, E.G.: Celsus: de medicina, with an English translation, vol. 3, Cambridge, Mass., 1938, Harvard University Press.

60. Stegman, S.J.: Fifteen ways to close surgical wounds, J. Dermatol. Surg. **1:**25, 1975.

61. Stegman, S.J.: Cosmetic dermatologic surgery, Arch. Dermatol. **118:**1013, 1982.

62. Stough, D.B., III: Punch scalp autografts for bald spots, Plast. Reconstr. Surg. **42:**450, 1968.

63. Tagliacozzi, G.: De Curtorum chirurgia per Insitionem, Venice, 1597, Gaspare Dindoni.

64. Thiersch, C.: Über die feineren anatomischen Veränderungen bei Aufheilung von Haut auf Granulationen, Arch. Klin. Chir. **17:**318, 1874.

65. Toledo-Pereyra, L.H.: Galen's contribution to surgery, J. Hist. Med. **28:**357, 1973.

66. Toledo-Pereyra, L.H., et al.: Anticontagionism in the opposition to Lister, Curr. Surg. **36:**78, 1979.

67. Treves, F.: The elephant man and other reminiscences, New York, 1923, Henry Holt and Co.

68. Tromovitch, T.A. and Stegman, S.J.: Microscopically controlled excision of skin tumors, Arch. Dermatol. **110:**231, 1974.

69. Unger, W.P.: Hair transplantation, New York, 1979, Marcel Dekker.

70. Wangensteen, O.H.: Some early Greek heroes of medicine: the training of surgeons and some post-Hunterians schools of surgery, J. Hist. Med. Allied Sci. **34:**211, 1979.

71. Wangensteen, O.H., Wangensteen, S.D., and Klinger, C.F.: Wound management of Ambroise Paré and Dommique Larrey, great French military surgeons of the 16th and 19th centuries, Bull. Hist. Med. **46:**207, 1972.

72. Warren, J.M.: Taliacotian operation, Boston Med. Surg. J. **22:**261, 1840.

73. Watson, B.A.: Gunpowder disfigurements, St. Louis Med. Surg. J. **35:**145, 1878.

74. Wheeler, E.S.: The development of antiseptic surgery, Am. J. Surg. **127:**573, 1974.

75. Whitehouse, H.H.: Liquid air in dermatology: its indications and limitations, J.A.M.A. **49:**371, 1907.

76. Wigglesworth, E., Jr.: The curette in dermal therapeutics, Boston Med. Surg. J. **94:**143, 1876.

77. Wolfe, J.R.: A new method for performing plastic operations, Br. Med. J. **2:**360, 1875.

78. Wood-Smith, D.: History of plastic and reconstructive surgery, J. Dermatol. Surg. **1:**45, 1975.

79. Wyman, M.: Medicine and surgery in 1881, N. Engl. J. Med. **305:**1059, 1981.

80. Young, A.: Scalpel: men who made surgery, New York, 1956, Random House.

81. Zacarian, S.A., and Adham, M.I.: Cryotherapy of cutaneous malignancy, Cryobiology **2:**212, 1966.

82. Zielonka, J.S.: The barber-surgeons, J. Hist. Med. **29:**330, 1974.

2

Cutaneous Structure, Function, and Repair

Cutaneous surgery, like other forms of surgery, is a mixture of science and art. It is the science of fission and fusion and the art of wound creation and repair. The well-educated surgeon interested in cutaneous surgery must have a broad background of fundamental knowledge not only in cutaneous biology, but also in repair mechanisms of the skin. However, such knowledge by itself does not tell one how to repair damaged tissue, just as an understanding of thermodynamics does not make it possible for one to repair a broken automobile engine. Understanding the scientific basis of wound repair helps one to appreciate the victories and defeats we all see surgically.

Wound repair represents the main point of convergence of all the disciplines of surgery; it may therefore be viewed as the foundation of surgery. How to maximize the human body's capacity to heal disrupted tissue with the optimal restoration of form and function is the concern of all who perform surgery, regardless of the tissue on which one works.

Wound repair is one of the fundamental processes of life. The mysteries of wounds and the mechanisms of repair are slowly being unraveled, but it appears that the more one gains knowledge about them, the more questions seems to arise. Understanding of the cellular and biochemical mechanisms involved in wound healing is far from complete. Indeed, many individuals have spent their lifetimes exploring wound healing, and many careers, both academic and nonacademic, have been based on exploration of this subject. Knowledge of the practical aspects of wound repair requires a continuous process of observation and learning throughout one's medical career, moving from the patient to the literature or laboratory and back to the patient.

Philosophically wound healing can be considered an extension of morphogenesis because it is more than merely the formation of new tissue and cells; it is an awakening of cellular states that existed at an earlier time ontogenetically.

Cellular mitosis, formation of intercellular substances, and cellular migration are found both embryologically when tissue is first formed and in the reformation of tissue, which allows wound healing to proceed.

Howes, Sooy, and Harvey[215] in 1929 described a surgical wound as the simplest form of an acute disease. They justified this concept on the basis that a wound is self-limiting, occurring as a result of mechanical damage, and that normally the reparative processes are not subject to further injury to interfere with healing. Thus this "disease" has a definite beginning and usually a predictable ending.

Although much of our knowledge of surgical management of wounds is based largely on empiric observations, there exists a substantial amount of scientific data that helps to support mere clinical impressions. This chapter explores much of this information as it relates to surgery of the cutaneous surfaces. Indeed, much of the knowledge of wound healing in general surgery is based on knowledge of the healing of cutaneous surfaces, since these are readily accessible to investigation.

Most of the scientific data widely quoted regarding wound repair have been exclusively the result of animal experimentation. Although one may gain valuable information and helpful indications from animal experimentation, its applicability to human patients must be made with reservation. It is not possible to extrapolate completely information based on animal experimentation to clinical situations. There are many differences between research animals and humans regarding the location, anatomy, and function of the skin, its response to injury, and its subsequent repair process. Therefore one must be cautious in the interpretation of such data, particularly if they do not fit the clinical situation with patients.

The topic of wound repair is immense and the amount of literature on it is staggering. I have therefore attempted to choose only a small portion of the total topic to discuss and have selected many important references that are relevant to an understanding of this problem with special reference to the skin, based largely on my own clinical experience. For those who wish to explore wound healing in greater depth, there are several excellent books that are more comprehensive.[107,219,234,365]

HISTORY AND BACKGROUND

Physicians have concerned themselves with wounds on the skin since the earliest medical writings of antiquity. Although many of the wounds described are the result of battle injuries, physicians' accounts of management evoke images of modern problems. The Edwin Smith Papyrus, an Egyptian document written perhaps over 3400 years ago, describes wounds from combat and testifies to the pharmacologic usefulness of ointments such as honey for wounds.[49] Recently there has been a resurgence of interest in sugars and honey to stimulate wound healing; somewhat surprisingly such substances have been shown to have inherent antibacterial qualities.[265]

The earliest Greek physicians were recognized for their ability to administer to battle wounds, applying ointments and dressings. Early on, a physician was viewed in ritualistic terms, particularly with respect to wounds. Homer[206] describes a physician as a man who "is worth many men for he can cut out arrows and sprinkle mild remedies." The concept of the physician having magical healing powers for wounds has survived to this day.

One of the basic threads winding through history from the Greeks to modern medicine is conflict over the way in which wounds are best managed. On one side are those who believe that wounds should be left to heal by themselves without interference. Here we find such physicians as Hippocrates (460 to 370 BC), Ambroise Paré (1510 to 1590), John Hunter (1729 to 1793), Alexis Carrel (1873 to 1944), and Frederic Mohs (1910-   ). On the other side are physicians who feel it is best to intervene in a wound healing naturally. One of the first in this group was Galen (AD 131 to 201), whose writings were interpreted to mean that open wounds should be made to suppurate, producing "laudable pus." Originally this was done with cautery, boiling oil, or other caustics. More recently the interfering method has been to cover all wounds with skin grafts or flaps.

In this context it is interesting (and humbling) to review a quotation of John Hunter[228]:

> Many wounds ought to be allowed to scab in which this process is now prevented; and this arises, I believe, from the conceit of surgeons who think themselves possessed of powers superior to nature and therefore have introduced the practice of making sores of all wounds.

John Hunter was perhaps the first thoughtful researcher in wound healing. He began his medical career working as an

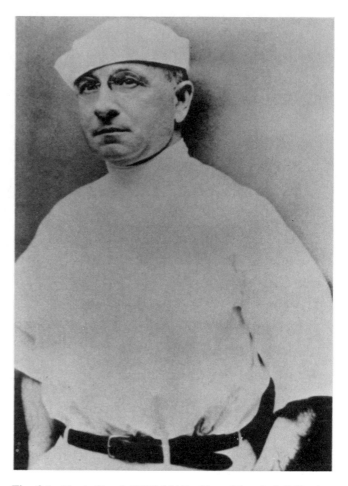

Fig. 2-1. Alexis Carrel (1873-1944). (From Historical Collection of the College of Physicians, Philadelphia.)

anatomist in London. He decided to leave the dissection laboratory and joined the British army. He was fortunate to be involved in the cure of many battle injuries, particularly those from the 1761 British invasion of the then French island, Belle-Île, off the southern coast of Brittany. Hunter was inspired to document his experiences in the management of many cases of injury in a medical classic, *A Treatise of Blood, Inflammation, and Gun-Shot Wounds,* published in 1794.[227] This book documents the advisability of conservative wound management and, in addition, records a number of animal experiments.

Another thread that becomes apparent in the history of wound healing is that the advances and research were the direct result of war. Paré, Hunter, and Carrel made their brilliant observations on natural wound healing during war. Carrel[64] (Fig. 2-1) made his observations during World War I and calculated, along with LeComte du Noüy, the rate of healing of wounds allowed to heal by granulation and epithelialization.[284] Born in France, Carrel immigrated to the United States in 1906 to accept a research position at the

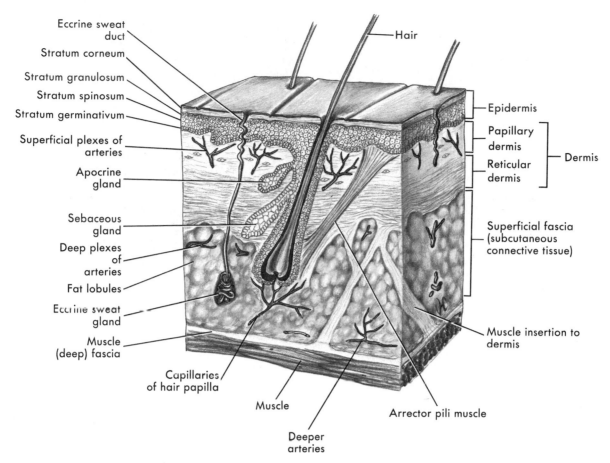

Eccrine sweat duct
Stratum corneum
Stratum granulosum
Stratum spinosum
Stratum germinativum
Superficial plexes of arteries
Apocrine gland
Sebaceous gland
Deep plexes of arteries
Fat lobules
Eccrine sweat gland
Muscle (deep) fascia
Capillaries of hair papilla
Muscle
Deeper arteries
Arrector pili muscle
Muscle insertion to dermis
Superficial fascia (subcutaneous connective tissue)
Dermis
Reticular dermis
Papillary dermis
Epidermis
Hair

Fig. 2-2. Structure of skin on face and its relationship to underlying musculature. Note fibrous insertions of muscles to dermis through subcutaneous layer. These insertions are abundant on head and neck. Note that stratum corneum is outer layer; stratum granulosum is 1 cell thick; stratum spinosum is 2 cells thick in drawing; and stratum germinativum is bottom epidermal cell layer.

Rockefeller Institute in New York City. His initial interest was in wound healing, and he single-handedly was responsible for the institution of its scientific study, thus making him the father of modern wound healing research. His classic paper "The Treatment of Wounds" appeared in 1910.[62]

Carrel was instrumental in the development of cell culture techniques, which enabled later researchers to study the process of epithelial and fibroblastic growth in vitro. Carrell received the Nobel prize in 1912, the first American to be so honored. His work is reviewed later in this chapter.

Many other researchers in the twentieth century have been instrumental in various aspects of wound healing research, and their contributions are also reviewed in detail later in this chapter. Of importance are Howes,[211-217] who investigated techniques for the measurement of tensile strength; Arey,[16] for his remarkable insights into the mechanisms of wound healing; and Dunphy,[105] for progress on measuring the collagen content of wounds.

ANATOMY OF THE SKIN

The skin is the covering of a person, and it has several functions. It protects that person from and permits communication with the environment. The skin contains and maintains an internal environment that prevents life-threatening desiccation. It functions as the thermoregulatory blanket of the body and is capable of allergic and immunologic responses. It serves to convey both beauty and ugliness: its perfect conformity to the underlying contours of the body early in life heightens the sense of aesthetic beauty; its slackening with age results in a draping effect between points of tension. Such unique changes in the skin with time are particularly human. Its adornment with makeup and jewelry is a means of sexual attraction. Scars on the skin are readily apparent and therefore undesirable, usually more from a cosmetic than from a functional standpoint.

Although the skin may be the heaviest organ, it is not the largest in surface area, since it is only slightly plicated and measures only about 2 square yards.[329] In comparison,

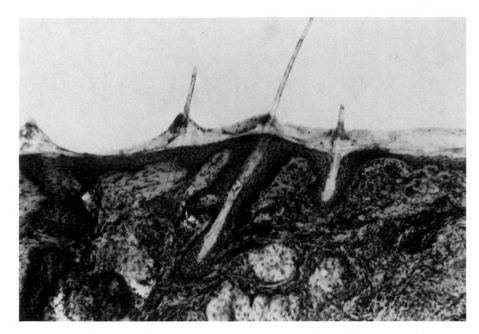

Fig. 2-3. Frozen section of skin from scalp. Note stratum corneum, which is exaggerated in its appearance and appears to be draped from the hairs. (×100.)

the lungs on expiration measure 5 square yards. Skin is by no means an inert tissue, but rather a complex structure that is undergoing continuous metabolic activity.

The general structure of the skin is shown in Fig. 2-2. Basically, it can be divided into three layers, the epidermis, the dermis, and the subcutaneous connective tissue (superficial fascia).

The epidermis forms an outer veneer and is divided into four zones. A basal cell layer (the stratum germinativum) is comprised of a single layer on the bottom of the epidermis. It is composed of basal cells, which undergo mitosis to produce the next zone above, the prickle cell layer. Intermixed in the basal cells are melanocytes (pigment-forming cells). A second type of specialized cell in the basal cell layer is Merkel's cells, which are associated with neural terminations. The basal cell layer is attached below to the basement membrane, which separates the epidermis above from the dermis below. The zone of cells immediately above the basal cell layer is the prickle cell layer (the stratum spinosum). It is usually three or four cells thick and given this name because of the intercellular bridges (prickles) seen in this layer on light microscopy. These bridges help to maintain the integrity of the epidermis. Intermixed with the prickle cells are Langerhans' cells, thought to be important mediators of immune response. On top of the prickle cell layer is a thin zone, one or two cells thick, the granular cell layer (the stratum granulosum). Here keratin, the main product of the epidermis, is first seen as keratohyalin granules. Finally, a keratin cell layer (the stratum corneum), the fourth layer of the epidermis, is formed. This layer varies

greatly in thickness and is composed of a number of layers of precisely stacked units. It is very thick in the palms and soles but very thin in the eyelids. On frozen sections it may become more apparent (Fig. 2-3).

Piercing the skin are hair follicles and eccrine sweat ducts, which vary in density on the surface of the skin. Of particular importance are the density and size of the sebaceous-follicular apparatus on some areas of the body such as the central face. Here in some individuals the follicular orifices are rather large and the sebaceous glands rather prominent histologically. Such individuals are said to have "porous" skin, which must be viewed as a separate aesthetic cosmetic territory. When attempting to match skin with skin grafts or flaps, such cutaneous characteristics must be taken into account.

The hair is variable in extent and density and shows differences of distribution, which are genetically determined. Women, for instance, usually maintain a good frontal hairline until late in life, whereas almost all men have some recession of the hairline beginning in their midtwenties. Some men develop baldness of the scalp, the type and extent of which are genetically controlled.

The dermis is composed mainly of collagenous tissue and may be divided into two zones. The upper portion of the dermis is known as papillary dermis. It is made up of a loose arrangement of thin collagen fibers with some fibrocytes (more in this portion of the dermis than in the reticular dermis below) and lies directly underneath the epidermis. Beneath the papillary dermis lies the reticular dermis, composed of rather thick collagenous bundles and very sparse fibrocytes. In addition to collagen fibers, elastic and reticular fibers are also present in both the papillary and reticular dermis. These fibers are embedded in an amorphous acellular ground substance. Traversing the dermis are blood vessels, lymphatics, and nerves important for nourishment and sensitivity of the skin. Also present are eccrine sweat ducts, as well as hair follicles with their attached sebaceous and apocrine glands. The apocrine duct empties into the hair follicle superior to the sebaceous gland. Although not fully shown in Fig. 2-2, the apocrine gland is situated in the subcutaneous tissue at about the level of the eccrine sweat gland. The apocrine glands are found only in certain areas, such as the axillae, groin, and nipples. The smooth muscles (arrectores pilorum) attached to the hair follicles are also found in the dermis.

The two-tier arrangement of the dermis helps to explain the rates of wound healing in various tissues of the body. As Ordman and Gillman[355] have elegantly shown, a wound going through the whole dermis is vascularized from the fatty subcutaneous tissue below and the papillary dermis above. The reticular dermis makes only a minimal initial contribution to a healing wound because it is relatively avascular and acellular. Therefore wherever the reticular dermis is thin (for instance on the eyelids), wound healing is very fast and sutures may be removed in 3 days; however, on the back, where the reticular dermis is thick, wound healing proceeds much more slowly because the granulation tissue must bridge the broad gap of the reticular dermis. Here sutures need to be left longer, from 7 to 10 days. This concept is discussed in greater detail later.

Beneath the dermis is the superficial fascia, also known as the subcutaneous connective tissue layer. It is comprised of both fat and fibrous tissue in varying degrees. When the fibrous tissue is minimal and the fat comprises most of this layer, it appears as a grossly fatty layer. This is the situation over the trunk and extremities. However, on the face and scalp the fibrous tissue is much more abundant, and this layer becomes somewhat fibrous. On the scalp this layer is largely fibrous.

One should also notice in Fig. 2-2 that there are discrete fibrous connections between the deep fascial layer covering the muscles below and the overlying dermis. These connections are well developed on the face and represent insertions of the underlying muscles. Their presence therefore makes it more difficult to undermine tissue in this location. On the trunk and extremities such connections are almost absent; as a consequence, it is relatively easy to undermine in these sites.

The thickness of the epidermis and dermis are important determinants of the tensile strength of wounds, the amount of scar tissue produced, and the rapidity with which wounds heal. Their thickness is not uniform but varies not only with the anatomic location on the body (Fig. 2-4) but also with age and sex. The epidermis is thin at birth, becomes thicker in childhood and puberty, and then becomes thin in the fifth

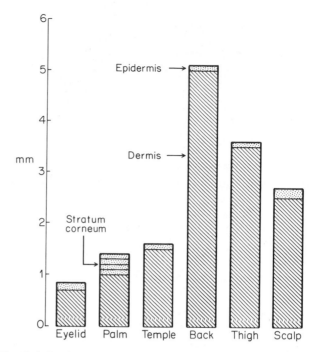

Fig. 2-4. Regional variations in thickness of epidermis and dermis. (Modified from Odland, G.F.: In Fitzpatrick, T.B., et al., editors: Dermatology in general medicine, New York, 1971, McGraw-Hill Book Co.)

or sixth decade of life. One also sees flattening of the dermal papillae with age.[438]

The thickness of the epidermis is relatively stable over most of the body and measures 75 to 150 μm (0.075 to 0.15 mm), except on the palms and soles, which may be 400 to 600 μm (0.4 to 0.6 mm) thick.[350] The glabrous skin's epidermis tends to be thick compared with that of hairy skin.[329] Moreover, the undersurface of the nonhairy epidermis tends to be more complex with many undulations. Such complexity helps to hold the thicker attached epidermis in place and to provide nutrients.

The dermis, unlike the epidermis, varies greatly in thickness from one region of the body to another. It measures from less than 1 mm on the eyelid to over 4 mm on the back[350] and is responsible for the main strength of the skin. It is thickest on the extensor dorsal surfaces, and thinner ventrally. The back has the thickest dermis and the eyelid the thinnest. The dermis is thicker in men than in women; like the epidermis, it is thin at birth, but it gradually increases in thickness to a maximum in the fourth or fifth decade, after which it decreases in thickness.

The skin is a mobile tissue capable of extension when pulled and resisting compressive forces when pushed inward. Extensibility of the skin is the basis for staged excision of skin lesions and scalp reductions for baldness. Some primitive peoples stretch the skin of the lips or ears gradually for cultural beautification. Its great capacity for stretching is commonly seen over the abdomen of pregnant women.

However, there are limits to such stretching: with extreme extension the dermis tears and stretch marks appear. In pregnancy with stretching of the abdomen these stretch marks, known as striae gravidarum, appear first as red streaks but with time fade to become white and then are more properly referred to as lineae albicantes. Stretch marks also appear in skin that has been stretched by weight gain or expansion of muscles (seen in weight lifters). Striae may also be found in patients with Cushing's disease or those on chronic steroid therapy (Fig. 2-5).

The extensibility and strength of the skin depend largely on the collagen fibers. These properties are the result of intrinsic mechanical behavior and the pattern in which collagen fibers are woven.[149] These fibers are oriented parallel to the surface of the skin. The directional variations in skin extensibility are not uniform but vary from one area of the body to another and even within the same area. This is shown by puncturing the skin with a skin punch or an awl. Langer[274] in 1861 punctured the skin of cadavers with an awl and found that in general the round holes were converted into elliptic ones. The forces of the collagen were thus found to be greatest in one direction, along the long axes of the ellipses.

Other factors also help to determine skin extensibility, for instance, the age, the genetic makeup of the individual, and underlying attachments to muscles or fascia. With aging the skin loses its elasticity.

When the skin is stretched, the loose collagen fibers at first take up the slack and rearrange themselves parallel to the direction of pull[51,148] (Fig. 2-6). In scar collagen, fibers are generally found oriented parallel to the direction of the scar.[336] With increased stretch beyond a certain limit, slippage and rupture between collagen bundles occur. Such rupture is irreversible and clinically is seen as striae (stretchmarks), which usually are oriented *perpendicular* to the maximal skin tension lines (Fig. 2-5).

The elastic fibers in skin are found in the dermis and form only a small portion of the skin. Their origin is unclear, but they probably arise from fibroblasts. Elastic fibers are thought to provide the force that restores the deformed collagen network to its normal morphology.

The collagen of the dermis is set within the ground substance comprised by proteoglycans, which are composed of carbohydrate and protein. The ground substance helps to maintain the resiliency of the compressed skin by redistributing the forces of pressure. A fairly well-localized pressure force that ordinarily might cause damage is converted to a diffuse, harmless pressure.

When a person sleeps on a hard surface that indents the skin, a visible depression may be left temporarily. This may be easily massaged out. Such depressions are partially related to ground substance redistribution in the skin.

If pressure on the skin exists for a continuous time, necrosis may occur. Decubitus ulcers are the result of such

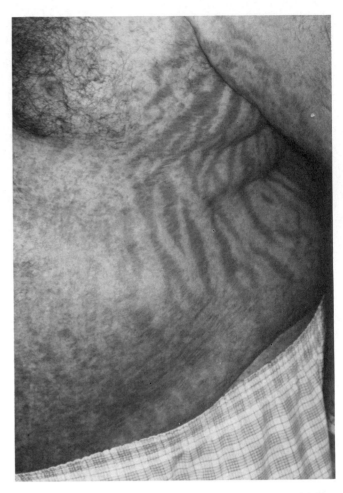

Fig. 2-5. Striae may be found in patients on chronic steroid therapy, as shown, or in patients with Cushing's disease. Note that striae are oriented perpendicular to maximal skin tension lines.

pressures. In such cases the forces of distribution of pressure are limited by bony prominences.

The structure of the skin is thus complex in both form and function. Its intimate relationship with the underlying muscles, particularly on the face, makes it more than just an organ of investiture. Furthermore, definitions as to the true cutaneous boundaries in depth are arbitrary because of the ''subcutaneous'' connections between the dermis and underlying muscle. Such realizations are essential in understanding and evaluating both the mechanisms of wound healing and the results of cutaneous surgery.

CHARACTERIZATION OF WOUNDS

Before beginning a discussion of the mechanics of wound healing, it is necessary to define the types of wounds. This is of great relevance because research into wound healing should compare comparable types of wounds; extrapolation of data from one wound type to another should be made with caution.

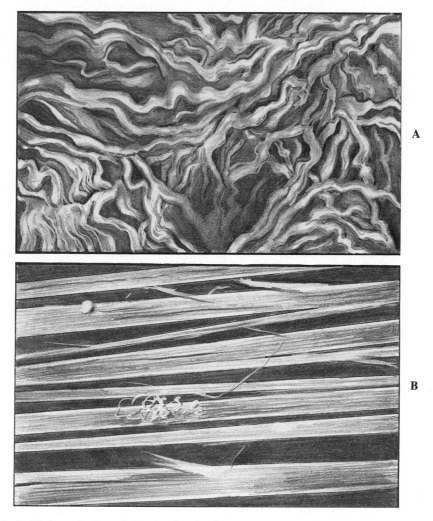

Fig. 2-6. A, Horizontal view of dermis, showing loose arrangement of collagen fibers. **B,** Same collagen fibers orienting themselves parallel to line of stretch force. (Modified from Brown, J.A.: Br. J. Dermatol. **89:**383, 1973.)

A wound is defined simply as the disruption of the cellular and anatomic continuity of tissue. Wounds may be characterized by the anatomic site, the method of creation, the degree of contamination, the depth and lateral extent of tissue loss, and the method of closure or wound repair. All these factors are interrelated and influence wound repair.

Anatomic site

The anatomic site of a wound is important because wounds in some areas heal faster and with fewer problems than in other locations. For instance, wounds of the head and neck readily heal with less chance of wound infection than wounds on the extremities. Wounds across joints are more subject to scar contracture than elsewhere.

Method of creation

Wounds may also be described by the method of their creation, for instance by burn, surgery, gunshot, and so forth. The method of injury has certain important implications. Burn wounds may destroy more tissue than is initially apparent, producing areas of tissue infarcts. Traumatic wounds are potentially contaminated. Suture needles also create their own type of wound, which allows epidermization of suture tracts with time.[356]

Degree of contamination

As is stressed in Chapter 4, wounds can be classified as clean, clean-contaminated, contaminated, and dirty, depending on the degree of contamination—potential or known—that has occurred. The greater the level of bacterial contamination in a wound, the greater the likelihood of significant wound infection, which impairs wound healing.

Depth and lateral extent

Wounds should also be characterized by their true depth and lateral extent. The depth may be full thickness of the

TABLE 2-1

Types of wound repair

	Synonyms	Depth	Wound edges approximated	Closure	Example	Wound type*
Primary (first) intention	Primary union; primary closure ("secondarily closed" if dehisces)	Superficial or deep dermis or below	Yes	Immediate suturing or other closure (graft, flap)	Excision wound sutured closed; skin graft; skin flap	IIA and IIB
Secondary (second) intention						
Superficial		Epidermis and superficial dermis	No	Epithelialization	Dermabrasion; donor site of split-thickness skin graft	I
Deep		Entire dermis or below	No	Granulation, contraction, and epidermization	Third-degree burn; defect from Mohs surgery (fresh or fixed technique)	IIA and IIB
Tertiary (third) intention	Delayed primary closure; delayed suture ("secondarily closed" is a misnomer)	Deep dermis or below	Yes	Delayed suturing or other delayed closure (graft, flap)	Contaminated wounds	IIA and IIB

*See Table 2-2.

dermis to the superficial fascia, or into muscle or even bone. The breadth (lateral extent) of a wound should be expressed as its two longest diameters measured perpendicular to each other (for example, 2 cm × 4 cm). It should be noted that largest diameters may not be perpendicular to each other; the measureres must find the two largest diameters that *are* perpendicular. Such measurements are artificially high because the skin normally retracts when cut. The significance of the depth and lateral extent in classifying wounds is discussed in greater detail in the following sections.

Types of wound repair (Table 2-1)

Wound repair restores the continuity of tissues. A wound that is closed by apposition of fresh skin surfaces on the day of its creation is said to heal by *primary intention.* Intention does not mean purpose but rather the process of closing a wound, coming from the Latin *intendere,* meaning to stretch out. Such wounds may be deep into the deep dermis or below and may be wide; they are closed with either simple suturing or more complex skin flaps or grafts. Sometimes primary intention wounds may be just superficial, and the skin edges stick together by themselves with no great tissue loss or can be brought together with skin tape.[16] Such wounds are not allowed to granulate. An example of a wound healing by primary intention is a simple excision of a nevus with immediate linear closure by means of sutures.

Other names for primary intention wound healing are primary closure and primary union.

Wounds that are not surgically closed but allowed to heal naturally by epithelialization or epidermization with or without granulation and contraction are said to heal by *secondary intention.*[16] One must be specific regarding the depth of the wound. A wound involving only the epidermis and papillary portion of the dermis is superficial. Such a wound epithelializes both from the wound edges and from the follicular and eccrine sweat ducts, which are still left in the wound bed. Granulation and contraction do not occur in superficial wounds or are very minimal. Such wounds include those produced by dermabrasion or thin split-thickness skin graft donor sites.

A wound involving the whole dermis or deeper heals by a process of granulation, contraction, and subsequent epidermization if not closed surgically. Such a wound includes a third-degree burn or surgical defects resulting from Mohs surgery (fresh or fixed-tissue technique). Because such wounds are different from superficial wounds, which heal only by epithelialization, data from animal or human studies cannot be extrapolated from one wound type to another.

Wounds that are surgically closed after the day of their creation are said to heal by *tertiary intention.*[125] Sometimes it is desirable to allow a wound to granulate before closure.

TABLE 2-2

Classification of wounds

			Usual method of repair	Events in healing by secondary intention		
				Epidermization	Granulation	Contraction
Type I	Superficial		Secondary intention	+	−	−
Type IIA	Deep		Primary intention (suturing)	+	+	−
Type IIB	Deep and wide		Primary (suturing, graft, or flap) or secondary intention	+	+	+

This is particularly true of potentially contaminated wounds, which may be closed 4 to 6 days after their creation, assuming that minimal bacterial growth has occurred.[304] This gives the surgeon the opportunity to observe the wound for signs of infection and to weigh the risk of repair versus functional impairment. Another example of third intention wound healing is closure of a surgical defect with a skin graft after granulation has taken place, to create a good vascular bed for the transplanted skin. Synonyms for this type of wound healing include delayed primary closure and delayed suture.

Occasionally a wound that is primarily sutured and thus allowed to heal by primary intention will dehisce or need to be opened to evacuate blood and stop bleeding. At that point the wound may be allowed to heal by secondary intention or may be resutured. If resutured, the wound is said to be secondarily closed. This is really a variant of primary intention healing, since granulation tissue is not allowed to occur and the reclosure occurs within a short time after dehiscence. Occasionally the term "secondarily closed" is misused in the literature to mean delayed primary closure (tertiary intention) wound healing.[241] Therefore when evaluating studies, one should pay particular attention to what the authors mean by their own terms for types of wounds.

CLASSIFICATION OF CUTANEOUS WOUNDS

Cutaneous wounds may be conveniently classified into one of three main groups (Table 2-2), depending on their depth and lateral extent. Type I wounds have only a superficial loss of tissue involving the epidermis and superficial (papillary) dermis. The deeper portions of the pilosebaceous

apparatus and sweat ducts are not destroyed. Although superficial wounds may be thin, usually they are wide. Examples of such wounds include those produced by abrasions, chemical peels, or the harvesting of superficial split-thickness skin grafts. Type I wounds heal mainly by epithelialization alone.

Type II wounds are deep into the dermis, usually involving its full thickness, and into the subcutaneous tissues. In addition, type II wounds may also be of great width. Those without tissue loss should be designated IIA wounds. An example of such a wound is a traumatic laceration. Where substantial tissue loss occurs, a type IIB wound is produced—for example with a fusiform excision.

The importance in distinguishing these three types of wounds is that the major forces which by themselves unite these wounds—that is, to reform the tissue integrity by secondary intention—are different for each (Table 2-2). Type I wounds heal mainly by epithelialization, with negligible granulation and no contraction. *Epithelialization* is a process whereby the epidermis resurfaces a wound from the wound edges at the sides *and* adnexal structures from below, and thus results in a new epithelium (Fig. 2-12). Type IIA wounds heal by epidermization and minimal granulation. In contradistinction to epithelialization, *epidermization* is the process whereby the epidermis resurfaces a wound without the reformation of glandular and follicular structures. Since the wound edges here are almost completely apposed from the time of wound creation, contraction is unnecessary and negligible. Type IIB wounds, on the other hand, depend on the forces of contraction to bring the wound edges together. This occurs through granulation tissue, which acts like a contractile organ. Epidermization occurs as a later phenomenon, which bridges the gap that cannot close by contraction alone.

Although the distinctions between types I, IIA and IIB wounds are arbitrary and artificial, it is useful to classify wounds into one of these three categories when evaluating data on wound healing. Whatever variables may facilitate wound healing for a type I wound may not necessarily enhance wound healing for a type II wound.

HEALING BY PRIMARY INTENTION

The healing of cutaneous wounds involves repair of the epidermis, the dermis, and the subcutaneous tissue, depending on the depth of the surgical defect. This section considers the sequence of events that occurs in an ordinary wound involving both the epidermis and dermis and in which the skin edges are relatively close together or are apposed by sutures. Healing of other types of wounds is considered in separate sections.

Ordman and Gillman[355] properly emphasize that wound healing should be considered in four dimensions: length, depth, width, and time. Vertical incisions closed primarily are not "invisible scars" but are most properly represented as a vertically placed block of new tissue extending down to the subcutaneous fat. This block of tissue has a certain length, width, and height (depth). In addition, modifications in these dimensions occur over time, and therefore the time when a wound is analyzed or photographed should be specified and taken into account.

Wound healing follows an orderly, regular, and predictable sequence of events, which are characterized by both inflammation and regeneration of tissue. The inflammatory events that characterize wound healing are the same inflammatory processes that occur in any inflammation.[69,358] In general, substances that induce inflammation accelerate wound healing, whereas substances that decrease inflammation, such as cortisone, depress healing. If the inflammatory process is too prolonged, the repair process is also lengthened.[305] Less collagen is produced during periods of inflammation.[353] The regeneration of tissue is thus intimately involved with the inflammatory process by which it is stimulated, modulated, and terminated.

The older beliefs that wounds are "localized in space and restricted in time"[1] are giving way to newer concepts. It is known, for instance, that surgical scars are constantly undergoing collagen degradation and synthesis over the lifetime of an individual and therefore are not restricted in time. In addition, a surgical scar cannot be considered in isolation from the individual or species of animal. Different individuals or animal species show variations from the norm, which must be taken into account.

Phases of wound repair

Since the early twentieth century, the cellular and extracellular events in a healing wound have been arbitrarily

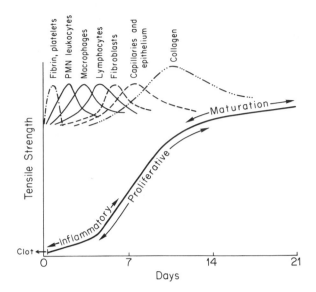

Fig. 2-7. Relationship between cellular and extracellular events in wound healing and grain in tensile strength of wounds. Note overlap between inflammatory, proliferative, and maturation phases of early wound healing. (Modified from Schilling, J.A.: Surg. Clin. N. Am. 56(4):859, 1976.)

divided into three or four stages.[103,104,215,355] Although this is conceptually convenient, there is considerable overlap between these different stages of repair (Fig. 2-7). It should also be stressed that the known sequence of events in wound healing is based on studies mainly in rats[29,89,104,305] and guinea pigs.[104,355]

Inflammatory phase. Immediately after a wound is created and blood vessels are cut, the first reaction is vascular. Initially there is vasoconstriction followed by vasodilation. The dilation of venules allows escape of serum, plasma, proteins, and blood cells. Polymorphonuclear leukocytes (PMNLs), red blood cells, and blood migrate to fill the wound (Fig. 2-8). A coagulum of fibrin is formed, which initially helps to hold the wound together. This is spoken of as the agglutination of a wound. The polymorphonuclear leukocytes preferentially increase in the wound for 1 or 2 days and then decrease in number. Concomitant with the decrease in PMNLs, lymphocytes and monocytes become the dominant cells, increasing in number from the second day to peak on the third or fourth day. The monocytes are transformed into macrophages engaged in phagocytosis. As we shall see, the macrophages are the dominant cells in early wound healing, directing the next phase (proliferative phase) and helping to terminate the inflammatory phase. The main inflammatory phase normally lasts up to 5 days.

During the inflammatory phase fibroblasts first appear at 24 to 48 hours; it has been shown that collagen synthesis and the laying down of proteoglycans are beginning. Some new blood vessel formation also occurs. As shown in Fig.

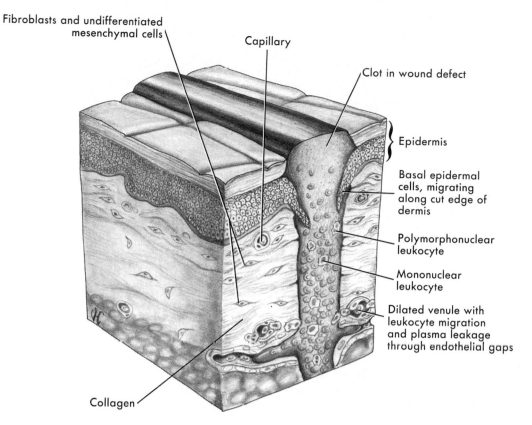

Fibroblasts and undifferentiated mesenchymal cells

Capillary

Clot in wound defect

Epidermis

Basal epidermal cells, migrating along cut edge of dermis

Polymorphonuclear leukocyte

Mononuclear leukocyte

Dilated venule with leukocyte migration and plasma leakage through endothelial gaps

Collagen

Fig. 2-8. Inflammatory phase of wound repair. (Modified from Bryant, W.M.: Clin. Symp. [Ciba] **29**(3):1, 1977).

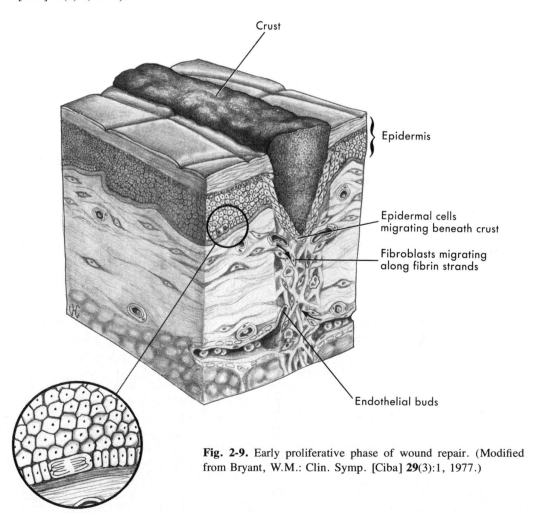

Crust

Epidermis

Epidermal cells migrating beneath crust

Fibroblasts migrating along fibrin strands

Endothelial buds

Mitosis

Fig. 2-9. Early proliferative phase of wound repair. (Modified from Bryant, W.M.: Clin. Symp. [Ciba] **29**(3):1, 1977.)

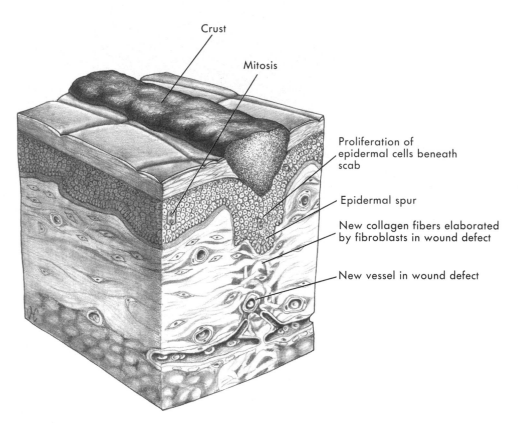

Fig. 2-10. Late proliferative phase of wound repair. (Modified from Bryant, W.M., Clin. Symp. [Ciba] **29**(3):1, 1977.)

2-7 there is overlap between this phase and the proliferative phase.

During the inflammatory phase the epidermis begins to thicken and migrate into the wound, eventually crossing the surgical defect. This migration takes place in the midst of the clot that has formed in the surgical defect and is directed in a downward fashion into the wound. In a well-sutured wound epithelial migration may be complete in as soon as 24 hours.[355]

Proliferative phase. In the early proliferative phase, there is intense proliferation of fibroblasts and capillaries (Fig. 2-9). The fibroblasts at first migrate along fibrin strands, most of which have oriented vertically in the wound. Capillary endothelial budding occurs particularly in the subcutaneous tissue and papillary dermis. The epithelium from each side continues to grow and eventually unites in the upper dermis. Note that in Fig. 2-9 mitoses occur not within the epidermal tongues moving under the scab but peripheral to the wound. Also the epidermis begins to thicken in the wound, a process that continues into the next phase.

Later in the proliferative phase collagen is laid down by the fibroblasts, increasing the tensile strength of wounds. Note that in Fig. 2-9 the direction of fibroblastic migration and vascular proliferation into the wound is from the papillary dermis above and from the subcutaneous tissue below.

Thus at first the collagen laid down is *vertical,* but as the wound tension increases, the collagen becomes more *horizontal*[355] (Fig. 2-10). Mucopolysaccharides are also synthesized and secreted by fibroblasts. The wound is filled with granulation tissue and new collagen, which has poor tensile strength because the fibers lack orientation and extensive linkage. Therefore this phase represents a quantitative phase of collagen production. The duration of this phase is variable, lasting from 4 days to 2 weeks after wound creation.

During the time after the scab is shed (usually 1 to 2 weeks), the surface of the wound appears as a depressed furrow. This gradually becomes level at about 3 weeks.

Early maturation phase (Fig. 2-11). During the early maturation phase, which lasts from 2 weeks to 3 months, the collagen is remodeled along the lines of tension. There is also a gradual gain in tensile strength of wounds as more cross-linking occurs and covalent bonds are formed between collagen fibrils. The number of cells in the wound decreases.

Late maturation phase. All scars go through changes that continue for the lifetime of the individual. The vascular network of the scar decreases over 6 months to a year, and the redness of the scar gradually fades. With time the scar becomes white. Collagen is also continually synthesized

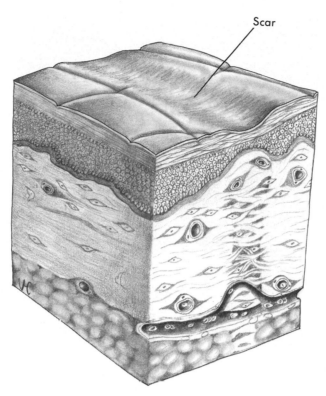

Scar

Fig. 2-11. Early maturation phase of wound repair. (Modified from Bryant, W.M.: Clin. Symp. **29**(3):1, 1977.)

and broken down. If the scar is at first hypertrophic, it may flatten out on its own as breakdown becomes greater than synthesis of collagen. Other, less appreciated facts about this late maturation phase are the late appearance of elastic fibers (at about 2 months) and the ingrowth of nerve fibers. Regardless of all the remodeling that occurs, the collagen of a wound always appears abnormal and never looks exactly like unwounded tissue.

HEALING BY SECONDARY INTENTION

Wound healing by secondary intention implies that a wound is allowed to heal without further surgical intervention. Usually such wounds may be classified as either broad superficial (type I) wounds or deep (type IIB) wounds (Table 2-2). Superficial wounds extend no deeper than papillary dermis. Deep wounds extend well into the reticular dermis and usually into the subcutaneous tissue. Deep wounds may also penetrate into muscle, bone, tendon, or cartilage.

As mentioned previously, the reason for dividing the wounds that heal by secondary intention into superficial and deep is that the mechanism of healing is not the same for each. A superficial wound heals by a resurfacing of epidermis from both the wound margins and adnexal structures. A deep wound through to the subcutaneous tissue is

resurfaced by epidermis only from the wound margins.

The new skin over superficial type I wounds closely resembles normal epidermis both histologically and functionally. Therefore this process of resurfacing is true epithelialization, in that a normal functional epithelium is reproduced. Healing by epidermization from the adnexal structures is unique to this form of wound healing. There is little or no granulation and no contraction.

A deep wound, on the other hand, is resurfaced by epidermis from the skin margins only. The final epidermis is quite different from normal cutaneous epithelium. There is a lack of rete pegs and adnexal structures. Therefore the process of resurfacing in this case is properly called epidermization. In addition, granulation and wound contraction play a prominent role in the healing of deep wounds by secondary intention.

Superficial wounds

Superficial wounds that are broad heal by true epithelialization. Examples of such wounds include those resulting from dermabrasion or the harvest of a thin split-thickness skin graft. Initially exudate and blood clots cover the wound surface. There is minimal organization of the clotted blood into granulation tissue. Epidermis from the wound edges, but also from the undestroyed adnexal structures, covers the

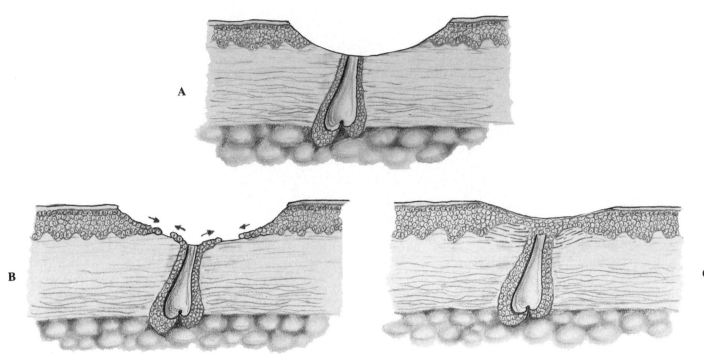

Fig. 2-12. Epithelialization of superficial wound (type I) allowed to heal by secondary intention. Note that new epidermis is derived from both epidermis at wound margin and adnexal structures. Hair follicle is shown. **A,** Superficial wound; **B,** epidermal migration from hair follicle and adjacent epidermis; **C,** healed wound.

wound surface—usually in 6 to 10 days (Fig. 2-12).

A scab may or may not be allowed to form. There is some evidence to suggest that not allowing a scab to form results in quicker resurfacing of this type of wound.[194,495] This is partially caused by the fact that the epidermis in regrowing does not need to grow as deeply into the dermis (Fig. 2-24). This results in less loss of dermis, so theoretically there is less likelihood of scarring (visibly abnormal skin).

In superficial wounds that heal by true epithelialization, some minimal granulation tissue forms. Thus there is capillary ingrowth as well as fibroblastic proliferation leading to new connective tissue accumulation.[152] This explains the persistent erythema sometimes seen with dermabrasion.

The new epidermis that results from secondary intention healing of superficial wounds is not completely normal. There are fewer rete pegs, but because of the presence of adnexal structures this epidermis is functionally close to normal cutaneous epithelium. In time it may appear histologically somewhat hyperplastic, forming the ''pseudo-rete'' pegs.[153] This is caused by the invasion of the hyperplastic epidermis into the granulation tissue itself.

The superficial dermis of such superficial wounds is also not completely normal. Nor does it return to normal even after many years.[152] There is a different pattern of organization of the collagen fibers, as well as blood supply. Occasionally on biopsy one may see the presence of epithelial fragments in the dermis, caused not by implantation but by invasion from the overlying epidermis.[152] The degree of dermal changes in superficial wounds depends on the depth of the wound.

Deep wounds

Deep wounds that are allowed to heal by secondary intention do so by the processes of granulation, contraction, and epidermization (Fig. 2-13). Usually such wounds result from extensive tissue loss. Although any wound may be closed and made to heal by primary intention, there are circumstances where this is unnecessary and undesirable. If the ultimate cosmetic result will be superior and one does not wish to change tissue planes, healing by secondary intension should be considered.[30] For instance, a wound resulting from a multiple recurrent skin tumor in the posterior auricular sulcus can be allowed to heal by secondary intention. The cosmetic as well as functional result is excellent, and the patient can forego any further surgery. This is of particular value in the elderly because it precludes possible hospitalization.[86] Allowing such wounds to heal by secondary intention has recently been popularized by Mohs.[328] However, some experience is necessary to be able to predict which sites will heal with good functional and cosmetic results.[505]

On creation of a deep, broad tissue defect, the wound cavity is lined with wound exudate and blood clot. The

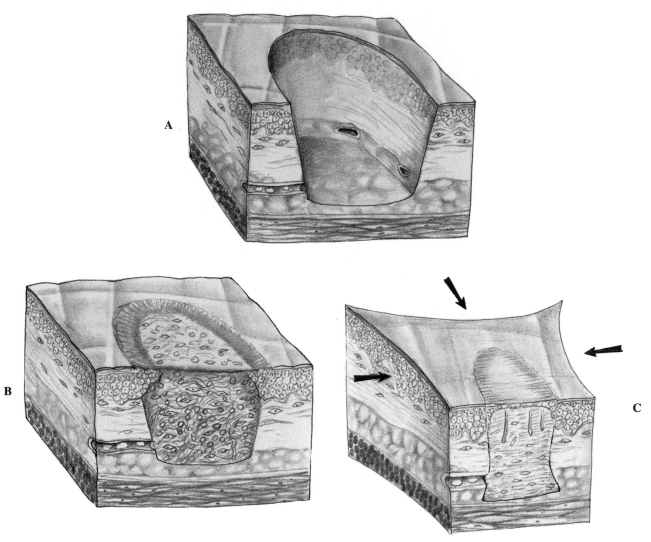

Fig. 2-13. Secondary wound healing of deep and broad wound (type IIB). **A,** Wound after creation. **B,** Wound cavity filled with granulation tissue. Epidermis is beginning to migrate from periphery. **C,** Wound closed by contraction and epidermization. Note contracture of surrounding tissue.

latter results in a fibrin layer, which forms the initial network on which the granulation is built. During the first week the wound continues to ooze because it is left open, increasing the vascular permeability. The wound exudate is rich in a variety of blood proteins, other substances, and cells concerned with the initial inflammatory reaction common to all wounds.

The fibrinous coagulum that forms on an open wound helps to wall off the new wound surfaces from the external environment. Part of its function is to surround bacteria physically and to keep them from penetrating the underlying vasculature.

Within a few days to weeks granulation tissue forms in the wound. "Granulation" comes from the Latin *granum,* meaning grain. Small hillocks of red, proliferating vascular buds appear, which coalesce into a sheet of proliferating vascular tissue. Intermixed in this granulation tissue are fibroblasts, as well as more specialized fibroblasts called myofibroblasts. Myofibroblasts are contractile and probably are responsible for the contraction that occurs with granulation tissue.

The process of contraction of granulation tissue begins when sufficient granulation tissue has formed. Usually this occurs at about 1 to 2 weeks after the wound was formed, depending on the depth and lateral extent of the wound. The contraction process occurs at a logarithmic rate, progressing rapidly at first, but more slowly as the wound edges come closer together.[62,379] Larger wounds have been found to heal at a faster rate by contraction than smaller wounds.

Wounds that are allowed to form granulation tissue are a good barrier to infection.[179] In addition, such wounds are a barrier that prevents systemic antibiotics from reaching the microbes that may be present.[113,396] Therefore granulating wounds are a good, relatively clean base for skin grafts.

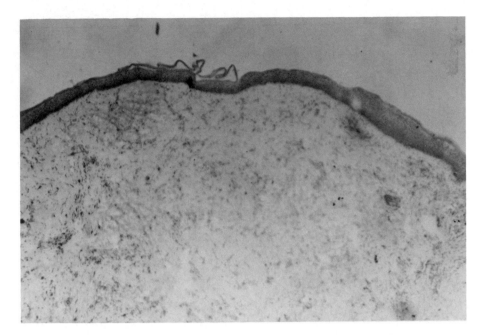

Fig. 2-14. Epidermis over scar tissue. Note lack of rete pegs and absence of adnexal structures. (×100.)

Migration of the epidermis across the wound surface begins within a few days after contraction has begun and when the granulation tissue is almost flush with the surrounding skin (Fig. 2-13, *B*). At that point epidermization proceeds concomitantly with wound contraction. Usually in 4 to 6 weeks the wound has resurfaced with epithelium.

Two objections are raised by some physicians concerning the scars that result from healing by secondary intention. The first is that the newly formed epidermis tends to break down; the second is that the contraction process distorts and functionally impairs surrounding structures. For example, Cohen and McCoy[77] state that ''if epithelial cells cover the granulating surface without dermal approximation, the wound will predictably break down.'' This is not true in the experience of those who have had a chance to observe many wounds that are allowed to heal by secondary intention. However, because the epidermis is not anchored to the underlying dermis by rete pegs or adnexal structures (Fig. 2-14), it is *at first* more susceptible to trauma, such as a shearing force, and may be loosened. Sometimes a blister may form as the new epidermis is lifted up by blood or exudate from trauma. However, in my experience this delicateness of the epidermis lasts only for the first month or two after initial wound healing. Once the underlying vascular response recedes and the bonds between the new epidermis above and the dermis below are strengthened, the epidermis is rather stable.

The second objection to allowing wounds to heal by secondary intention—the distortion of surrounding structures—may or may not occur, depending on the size and location of the surgical defect. As mentioned previously, it takes some experience to predict the likelihood of such distortion. Areas that heal with the least distortion and the smallest scars, yielding the best cosmetic results, are those able to contract the most. These areas include the neck, the nasolabial fold, the inner canthus, and the preauricular and postauricular areas. Fig. 2-15 shows a surgical wound on the neck that was allowed to heal by secondary intention. The scar, which is thin and linear, is hardly visible and aligns itself along the maximal tension lines in the skin. This scar is narrow because the wound healed almost entirely by contraction with little epidermization. This should be compared with Fig. 2-16. Here the contraction occurred only to a point, and much of the wound was resurfaced by epidermis from the wound edges. Thus this almost circular wound healed into a broad elliptic scar, with its long axis directed along the lines of maximal tension.

Occasionally wounds allowed to heal by secondary intention may result in distortion of surrounding structures. Such distortion is known as *contracture,* the end result of *contraction.* An ectropion (an example of contracture) caused by scar contraction is shown in Fig. 2-17. Such contracture would have been prevented by closure of the surgical defect by means of a skin graft or skin flap.

Once contraction has occurred maximally, there is frequently relaxation of the scar. Such relaxation is known as retraction. Some of this relaxation is caused by the countertension of the surrounding skin and muscle groups. With relaxation the scar tissue widens and, if hypertrophic, often flattens out. Retraction is discussed later (Fig. 2-27, *E*).

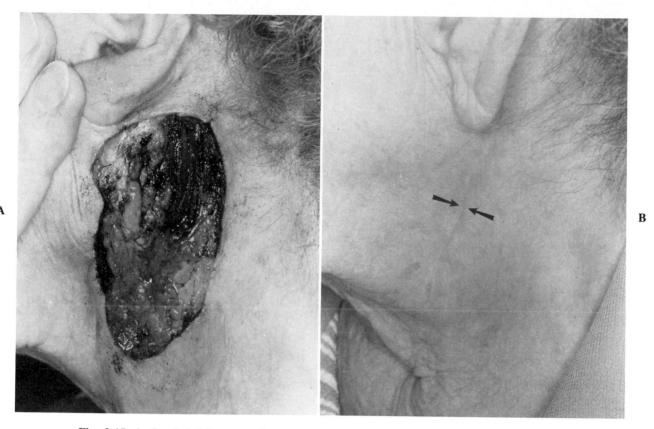

Fig. 2-15. A, Surgical defect on neck resulting from extirpation of extensive recurrent basal cell carcinoma. Note exposed muscle fibers, fat, and portion of parotid gland. **B,** Healed surgical defect 6 weeks later. Note thin linear scar *(arrow)* following lines of maximal tension and perpendicular to lines of minimal tension. There is so little tension perpendicular to this wound that contraction closed practically whole defect with minimal contribution from epidermization.

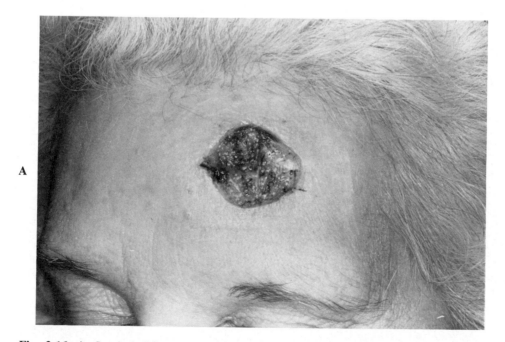

Fig. 2-16. A, Surgical defect (practically round) on left forehead resulting from extirpation of recurrent basal cell carcinoma. This wound extends to depth of whole dermis.   *Continued.*

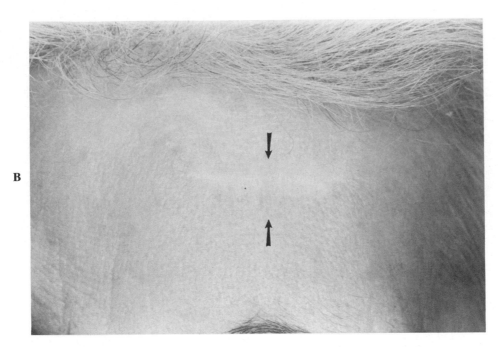

Fig. 2-16, cont'd. B, Healed surgical scar *(between arrows).* Wound healing took 6 weeks and resulted in elliptic scar that is broad but oriented along lines of maximal tension in area. Concept that circular wounds heal more slowly than other-shaped wounds is not true when wound contraction makes significant contribution to closure.

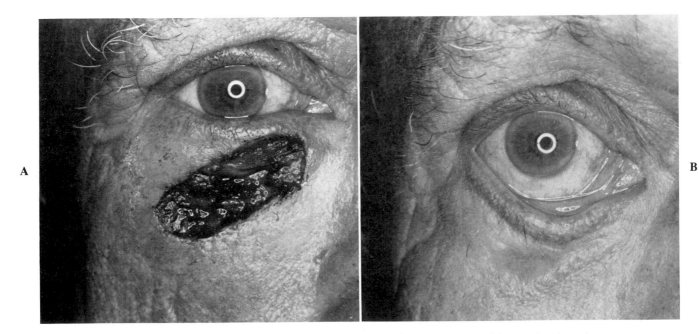

Fig. 2-17. Contracture of lower eyelid, an ectropion caused by contraction with secondary intention wound healing. **A,** Immediate postoperative surgical defect. **B,** Ectropion.

Wounds that penetrate muscle require special comment. Here myocytes proliferate in response to injury, usually within a week, and new muscle fibers are present within 2 weeks.[89] Muscle tends to granulate rapidly.

Cartilage and bone may be exposed on the head and will granulate. However, cartilage exposed on both sides necroses (for instance on both sides of the helix of the ear). Bone usually granulates by itself and does not necrose if exposed on the face or scalp, partially because of the rich vascular supply in this area. If bone does not show signs of granulation by itself after a suitable time (3 to 4 months), removing a superficial layer of cortical bone will uncover blood vessels, which may be then allowed to proliferate and form granulations. One exception to bone's ability to granulate is bone that has been previously irradiated, for instance, to treat an overlying malignancy. In this circumstance bone is so avascular that granulations may not occur even with removal of cortical bone.

A major difference between wounds that heal by primary intention and those that are allowed to heal by secondary intention is the degree and amount of granulation tissue formed. In both types of wounds it should be stressed that granulation tissue bridges the gap between the skin edges. However, in wounds allowed to heal by secondary intention, this granulation tissue helps to close the surgical defect by contraction. Wounds allowed to heal by primary intention do not need granulation tissue to contract to close the surgical defect and thus are more quickly healed.

HEALING BY TERTIARY INTENTION

Occasionally it is desirable to allow wounds to granulate before closure by wound edge approximation or a skin graft. The granulation tissue that forms helps to fill in the surgical wound defect so that a contour defect is absent when a graft is placed. The sequence of healing here is the same as that for secondary intention healing, except wound contraction usually either does not occur or occurs to a lesser degree. Wounds closed by approximation of the wound edges in 4 to 6 days have some granulation tissue, which is absent if wound edges are approximated on the day of surgery. If a full-thickness skin graft is placed on a granulating surface, the granulation tissue may partially resorb but will not contract. If a thin split-thickness skin graft is placed on granulation tissue, the granulation tissue may contract, particularly if contraction has already begun (usually after 1 week).

CLOSER INSPECTION OF SOME EVENTS IN WOUND HEALING
Hemorrhage, thrombosis, platelet aggregation

Bleeding from skin wounds is usually stopped in 3 minutes by platelet plugs in the free ends of vessels. This aggregation of platelets occurs because of exposure of platelets to fibrillar collagen in the vessel walls.[421] There is some evidence that a local increase in norepinephrine with tissue injury causes changes in endothelial cells, which enhance platelet adherence to the vascular surface.[46] After the bleeding stops, the platelets separate and fibrin appears between the platelets, soon taking over the function of hemostasis.[486]

Platelets are known to transport many substances as they pass through blood vessels. They contain over 60 enzymes and clotting factors.[268] Circumstantial evidence suggests that platelets are a source of a growth-promoting substance for both fibroblasts[239,268,408] and capillaries.[268] This substance has been called platelet-derived growth factor (PDGF). In addition, platelets probably secrete substances that are chemotactic for polymorphonuclear leukocytes (PMNLs) and activate factor XII (Hageman factor), which in turn activates the intrinsic coagulation pathway, kinin system, and complement system.

Blood coagulation in the wound results in the formation of fibrin strands, which serve as a scaffold for fibroblast migration and help to bridge a wound, holding it together during the earliest inflammatory phase of wound repair. If fibrin is absent from a wound, granulation tissue forms but is delayed. Moreover, if fibrin is added to experimental wounds in rats, one sees a faster appearance of granulation tissue. Therefore fibrin has been found to be helpful in wound healing but not necessary.[187,188]

Vasodilation

The initial vascular contraction that occurs with wounding is soon followed by vascular dilation. This vasodilation can be caused by several possible factors. Both histamine and kinins are known vasodilators, as are prostaglandins of the E series. Histamine may be released either from tissue mast cells or from platelets. It appears to act on the small venules, causing separation of the endothelial cells.[365] However, its period of action is short, only about 30 minutes. Serotonin is also a vasodilator released from the same cells as histamine and having about the same duration of action.

Kinins are peptides that induce vasodilation and capillary permeability; like histamine they are short-lived. Kinins (particularly bradykinin) is released from the α_2 globulin fraction of plasma by kallikrein, which is in turn activated by Hageman factor (XII).[38] Hageman factor may be activated directly by injury or via platelets.

Prostaglandins are also produced at sites of injury. Prostaglandin E_1 and E_2 (PGE$_1$ and PGE$_2$) have strong vasodilation properties. In addition, PGE, increases the cyclic AMP (cAMP), which in turn helps to mediate the effects of histamine. PGE, may also have chemotactic and growth-stimulatory effects (through cAMP).

Chemotaxis

With vasodilation there occurs a diapedesis of white blood cells into the wound. This is not merely caused by cells being swept into the wound by the force of blood flow; it involves substances that induce cells to migrate preferentially into the wound. Such substances are known as chemotactic agents, and in a wound there are several possible sources of such mediators. Complement—in particular, the C3a and C5a fractions—is particularly chemotactic. C3a and C5a may be produced by the action of various tissue proteases on C3 and C5.[201] In guinea pigs that are depleted of complement by cobra venom factor, an approximately 50% reduction in PMNLs occurs at 24 hours after production of a wound. However, despite this decrease in PMNLs, wound debridement and subsequent fibrogenesis proceed as on controls. Therefore complement is helpful but not necessary.[478]

Other known chemotactic factors include prostaglandin E, bacterial factors, kinins, and fibronectins.

Function of polymorphonuclear leukocytes

As pointed out previously, PMNLs are the initial cells in quantity in a wound. These cells are important but not essential, at least not in noninfected wounds. In rats[448] or guinea pigs[431] made neutropenic by antineutrophil serum, wounds healed normally, as judged by rate of debridement, extent of repair, or tensile strength measurements. Therefore a neutrophil response in early wounds is not a necessary antecedent to the infiltration of monocytes. However, should infection be present, the infiltration of PMNLs may be more important.

PMNLs function as phagocytes, ingesting debris and microorganisms. After ingestion, PMNLs must kill their prey by superoxide and hydrogen peroxide production, a process requiring oxygen.[201,203] It is interesting to note that in the studies already quoted (in which PMNLs were eliminated from wounds)[431,448] heavy bacterial colonization did not exist. One wonders what the results would have been if such colonization had been present. For patients receiving steroids or with diabetes, leukemia, or neutropenia there is a decreased neutrophil response.[201] Patients with chronic granulomatous disease cannot increase their oxidative metabolism in leukocytes to kill ingested microbes. This may help to explain the increased numbers of infected wounds in such patients.

PMNLs also contain substances important for wound repair, such as collagenase, proteolytic enzymes, and prostaglandins. It has been suggested that injured tissue (including collagen) is phagocytized by PMNLs and that amino acids useful in repair are subsequently processed and put back into the wound. Most of the granulocytes become lysed in time and release their cytoplasmic contents into the extracellular space. Therefore PMNLs do not function purely as phagocytes but may make other important contributions to the healing wound. Fromer and Klintworth[138] found that PMNLs or the supernatant fluid from PMNLs induced vascularization in rat corneas. Thus PMNLs may also promote wound blood vessel growth.

Wound transudate

The fluid in a wound is not inert but contains many biologically active substances. For instance, human serum contains growth-promoting substances, perhaps caused by platelet release, that stimulate the growth of fibroblasts and maintain capillary stability.[268] Separate factors that stimulate collagen synthesis but not fibroblast proliferation have also been detected.[351]

Wound fluid has also been shown to have antibacterial activity. Hohn et al.[204] demonstrated that human wound fluid contains two proteins, one being heat stable and having specific antibacterial activity against *Staphylococcus aureus*. This activity was found to be greater than that in normal serum and different from that in other bacterial substances in normal serum, such as complement, properdin, or immunoglobulins. This challenges the concept that wound fluid is an ideal culture medium.

The action of vasodilators on venules results in leakage into the wound of many larger macromolecules than would otherwise have extravascular access. Albumin transports amino acids and binds zinc and fatty acids (a source of energy). Protease inhibitors, which include α_1 antitrypsin and α_2 macroglobulin, accumulate at the site of inflammation and prevent further damage to tissue. Haptoglobin removes free hemoglobins released by hemolysis and reduces the iron available in the wound, thus decreasing the likelihood of significant infection. Fibrinogen is converted to fibrin, which provides the initial strength in a wound. Fibrin-stabilizing factor (factor XIII) converts the soluble, noncovalently linked fibrin to an insoluble, covalently bonded form, which helps to stabilize the wound.[382] A cold-soluble globulin fraction of the plasma, fibronectin, is also found in the wound fluid and is thought to act as a glue to the wound scaffold, aiding in cell attachment and movement during wound repair.[477]

Macrophage

The macrophage is emerging as the pivotal cell in wound healing (Fig. 2-18). Its antiinflammatory activity of phagocytosis helps to quell the inflammatory events while stimulating fibroblastic growth, collagen synthesis, and vascular proliferation. Tissue injury by itself is not a stimulus for repair but stimulates macrophages, which appear to direct repair. Hunt[226] feels that wound repair is excessive when macrophages are stimulated beyond normal. Pathologic stimulants, such as antigen-antibody complexes and endotoxin, result in prolonged macrophage activation.

The origin of wound macrophages is mainly from the transformed monocytes, which are of hematogenous origin. Blood monocytes, after entering the wound environment, are transformed into both histiocytes and macrophages.[55,441] The immigration of monocytes into a wound does not appear to depend on PMNLs, because in animals depleted of PMNLs, wound monocytes and macrophages appear at normal levels at the appropriate time.[287] Probably

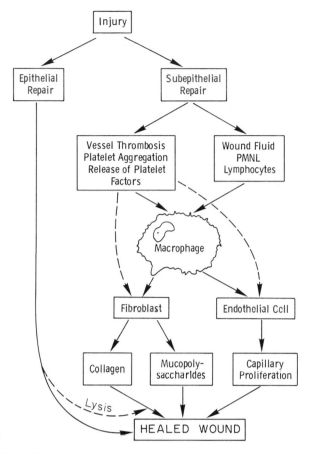

Fig. 2-18. Central role of macrophage during wound repair, linking early inflammatory activity to later reparative events.

fibrin or fibrin degradation products are chemotactic for macrophages.[262]

Another source of wound macrophages may be the tissue adjacent to a wound. Although this tissue is usually thought to be a minor source, tissue macrophages exist in such areas at all times and may undergo mitosis, thus contributing to the wound pool of macrophages.

Besides phagocytosis and modulating information with lymphocytes in the area, there is increasing evidence that macrophages are important factors in both the fibroblastic and angiogenic responses.[72] If animals are depleted of macrophages by antimacrophage serum, wound fibrin has been found to increase (indicating a depressed phagocytic activity), and wound fibroblasts are sparse compared to normal. Both the onset and proliferation of fibroblasts are delayed.[287] It is thought the macrophages stimulate the fibroblasts by means of a substance found in the plasma and transformed by macrophages. The macrophages do not produce this stimulatory substance by themselves.[286,288]

Macrophages also have been found to stimulate the growth of blood vessels.[72,378] If macrophages from a 3-week-old wound are injected into a 2-day-old wound in rabbits, vascularization occurs at an earlier time.[464] The

angiogenesis factors elaborated by macrophages appear to be particularly sensitive to oxygen concentrations. When macrophages are cultured at low oxygen concentrations, as might be found in a wound, angiogenesis is stimulated, but when they are cultured at higher oxygen concentrations, as found in arterial blood, angiogenesis stimulation is absent.[262] Fibrin or fibrin degradation products may also stimulate macrophages to produce an angiogenesis factor.[263]

Epidermal coverage

The epidermis covers a simple incision wound long before the tensile strength of a wound reaches a maximum and collagen production is complete. Using pig skin, Ordman and Gillman[355] found that the epidermis grows across the sutured wound within 24 hours. The stimulus for epidermal migration is thought to be lack of contact inhibition.[484] This term means that once similar cells are disrupted and are no longer positioned beside each other, the loss of contact stimulates migration. After this migration occurs and the cells once again make contact, migration is inhibited. Some investigators believe that migration occurs by detachment of the epidermis as a whole and the movement of a whole sheet of cells.[484] Others feel that migration occurs by cells sliding over each other.[272] These theories are discussed in detail later (see p. 48).

Scab

Histologically the scab or crust on a wound contains clotted blood, elastic tissue, collagen fibers, and dead epithelium.[355] The presence of part of the dermis is thought to be caused by the epidermis tunneling its way through the upper dermis by way of collagenolytic enzymes. Once formed, a scab separates with the stratum corneum of the new epidermis, a process that takes about a week.

Fibronectin

A glycoprotein—fibronectin—is emerging as an important substance in wound healing. Fibronectin is found in plasma as a cold-insoluble globulin and has a high molecular weight (440,000). This sticky substance is the only plasma component binding to the gelatin Sepharose.[477] Fibronectin is a connecting material thought to be a prerequisite for wound repair and responsible for the initial strength of wounds.

Fibronectin is found both free within plasma (plasma fibronectin) and on the surface of cells (cell membrane–bound fibronectin); these are the same substance. On the surface of cells, fibronectin helps dividing cells remain attached. It can cause the agglutination of erythrocytes and may function in platelet-collagen adhesion in thrombus formation.[368] Fibroblasts are also helped to adhere to collagen partially by fibronectin.[261,368] This assists fibroblasts during migration and wound contraction. Therefore cell membrane–bound fibronectin serves a number of purposes during wound repair: assisting in cell-to-cell aggregation, cell-substrate adhesion, cell motility, and the binding to macromolecules such as fibrin or heparin. Fibroblasts in culture have been shown to attach to collagen types I through IV, but only if serum (with glycoprotein) is present.[261] The fibronectin binds to the collagen first; then in the presence of Ca^{++} and Mg^{++} the fibroblasts adhere to the fibronectin-collagen complex. The sialic acid portions of gangliosides may block this attachment of fibroblasts by attaching to fibronectin.[260] Fibronectin has been shown in vitro to be chemotactic for fibroblasts.[381] An increase in fibronectin is also found in proliferating capillary endothelial cells in granulating wounds and may function there in a manner similar to that with fibroblasts.[74]

In wound studies on humans, fibronectin appeared as early as 1 hour after injury. It peaked at 24 to 48 hours and then gradually declined.[477] Thus the rapid appearance, the large amount present on the second day, and the gradual reduction are consistent with the supposition that fibronectin functions as a biologic guide for the cellular activity in wound repair.

Capillary migration

The growth of capillaries in a wound provides nutrients for both the dermis and epidermis. Myers and Wolf[339] found that the earliest complete vascular crossing occurs in a wound at 3 days, and thereafter these crossings increase, becoming greatest at 7 days. Although collagen deposition was initiated by 3 days, complete bridging across the wound did not occur until 5 days. Therefore complete vascular crossing of a wound precedes complete collagen crossing.

Most new capillaries do not migrate horizontally across a deep dermal incisional wound but rather upwards from its base and down from its surfaces[151,355] (Fig. 2-9). This is caused by the large proliferation of vessels in the superficial papillary dermis and subcutaneous tissue, compared with that in the rather acellular and avascular reticular dermis. However, in the subcutaneous tissue or superficial papillary dermis, blood vessels may grow straight across.

In a microscopic study of granulation tissue, Branemark[48] made some interesting observations on the development of capillary growth. He observed extraluminal red blood cells (RBCs) moving through fibrous tissue from capillaries to venules in a pulsating manner. This ''open circulation'' appeared to precede and served as a pathway for the sprouting of capillaries across the wound. More recently fibronectin has been found to increase in blood vessel walls before endothelial cell proliferation.[74] Such fibronectin may provide a provisional substrate for capillary growth.

SYNTHESIS AND STRUCTURE OF CONNECTIVE TISSUE

The production of connective tissue occurs in all wounds, although the new tissue produced differs in some respects from normal connective tissue. Connective tissue in scars is more fibrous and lacks the amount of elastic tissue in normal dermis. Because scars are formed in response to tissue tension, orientation of their collagen fibrils may be different from that found normally in a given area.

Connective tissue consists of collagen and fibrocytes, which are embedded in a ground substance. Reticulin fibers and elastic fibers are also present. Blood vessels and nerves form a network in connective tissue, and a few fixed histiocytes and mast cells are also present.

Fibroblast

The fibroblast is the major cell involved in the production of connective tissue. It has been described as the architect[473] of connective tissue and the ubiquitous ally of the surgeon for the production of scars.[102] The fibroblast is responsible for the synthesis and secretion of collagen and mucopolysaccharides.[446] In addition it produces reticulin fibers and probably elastic fibers.

The fibroblast plays a number of distinct roles in wound repair and differentiates into cellular types that appear different ultramicroscopically for each of these roles. The fibroblasts that are concerned mainly with the metabolic function of laying down collagen and mucopolysacchrides have an extensive endoplasmic reticulum with many ribosomes (Fig. 2-19). The fibroblasts that are concerned with contraction and drawing the wound edges together have well-developed microfilaments on the cytoplasm. Such fibroblasts are known as myofibroblasts and are discussed later. Fibroblasts also migrate into the wound as they lay down collagen and serve to direct the collagenous structure of the wound. For this movement fibroblasts use microfibrils.

The origin of the fibroblasts in wounds is thought to be fibrocytes in the adjacent tissue, particularly in the perivascular connective tissue, the adventitia of hair follicles, and the subdermal tissue and adjacent to wounds.[307,402] Grillo[163] irradiated wounds in guinea pigs and found the reduction of fibroblasts at 5 days to be similar regardless of whether the irradiation was given 20 minutes or 28 hours after wounding. Therefore most wound fibroblasts do not arrive immediately by the vascular route. Similar conclusions have been based on studies of parabiotic rats.[401]

The stimulus to fibroblastic reproduction appears to be from several sources, including platelet-derived growth factors (PDGF),[239,262] macrophage-dependent factors,[286,288] prostaglandins, and insulin.

The movement of fibroblasts is thought to take place along fibrin strands in the wound (Fig. 2-9). Weiss has termed this process *contact guidance*,[483] meaning that a cell orients itself along a given oriented substrate and moves along a line determined by the substrate. The forces of a wound tend to orient the fibrin fibers, and the fibers in turn orient the cells, such as fibroblasts.[484]

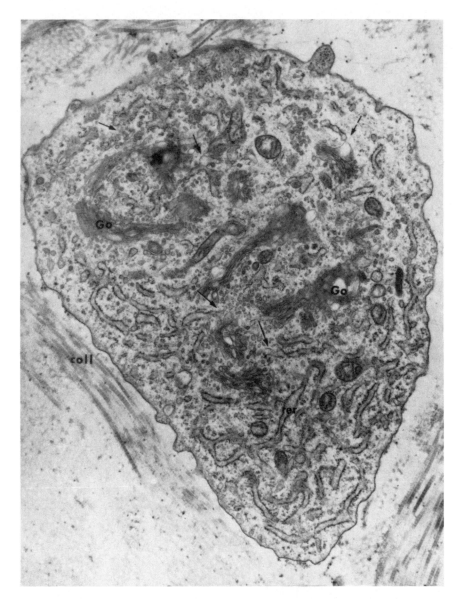

Fig. 2-19. Ultrastructural appearance of wound fibroblast, sectioned so that nucleus is not shown. Note extensive Golgi *(Go)* apparatus and prominent rough endoplasmic reticulum *(rer)*. In several areas *rer* appears to pinch off smooth vesicles to Golgi complex *(arrows)*. Outside cell are numerous collagen fibrils *(coll)* that demonstrate the characteristic 640 Å banded periodicity. ($\times$ 18,000.) (From Ross, R. Biol. Rev. **43:**51, 1968.)

Importance of collagen

Collagen is the major macromolecule of most connective tissue and all scars. It is the major fibrous protein in the human body and constitutes about one quarter of the total body protein.[316] In the skin it accounts for about 70% of the dry weight. Its omnipresence makes it an important constituent in wound repair.

Connective tissue is necessarily strong because it functions to bind and support structures in the body. This strength is mainly caused by collagen, which is a very strong substance. To break a collagen fiber 1 mm in diameter requires a weight of 10 to 40 kg.[160] The ground substance is a complex mixture of glycoproteins and other miscellaneous substances, which helps to bind collagen and give further strength to connective tissue.

Structure of collagen

Collagen is a fibrous protein. It is unique in that it contains almost all the hydroxyproline in the human body. The hydroxyproline content of collagen is about 15%, and analysis of a wound for hydroxyproline content serves as an index of the collagen content.

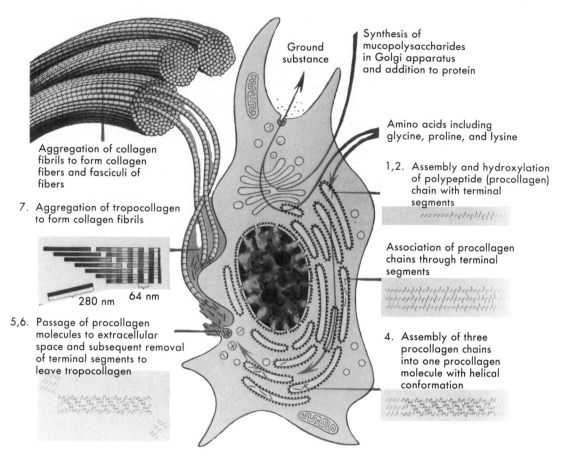

Aggregation of collagen fibrils to form collagen fibers and fasciculi of fibers

7. Aggregation of tropocollagen to form collagen fibrils

280 nm   64 nm

5,6. Passage of procollagen molecules to extracellular space and subsequent removal of terminal segments to leave tropocollagen

Ground substance

Synthesis of mucopolysaccharides in Golgi apparatus and addition to protein

Amino acids including glycine, proline, and lysine

1,2. Assembly and hydroxylation of polypeptide (procollagen) chain with terminal segments

Association of procollagen chains through terminal segments

4. Assembly of three procollagen chains into one procollagen molecule with helical conformation

Fig. 2-20. Major steps in synthesis of collagen. Step 3, glycosylation, is not depicted. (Modified from Williams, P.L., and Warwick, R.: Gray's anatomy, ed. 36, Philadelphia, 1980. W.B. Saunders Co.)

TABLE 2-3

Types of collagen

Type	Molecular form	Tissue distribution
I	$[\alpha1(I)]_2$, $\alpha2$	Skin, tendon, bone, dentin
II	$[\alpha1(II)]_3$	Hyaline cartilage
III	$[\alpha1(III)]_3$	Skin wounds, arteries, fetal skin, granulation tissue
IV	$[\alpha1(IV)]_3$	Basement membrane
V	αA, αB	Basement membrane and interstitial tissues
VI	$\alpha1(VI)$, $\alpha2(VI)$, $\alpha3(VI)$	Interstitial tissues
VII	Unknown	Anchoring fibrils
VIII	$[\alpha1(VIII)]_3$	Some endothelial cells
IX	$\alpha1(IX)$, $\alpha2(IX)$, $\alpha3(IX)$	Cartilage
X	$[\alpha1(X)]_3$	Calcifying endochondrial cartilage

The basic component of collagen is the monomeric tropocollagen molecule, which measures approximately 300 nm long and 1.5 nm wide, with a molecular weight of 300,000[362,383] (Fig. 2-20). It consists of three polypeptide (alpha) chains twisted around each other into a right-handed superhelix. Each alpha chain consists of about 1000 amino acids with every third amino acid being glycine. The remaining amino acids include proline and hydroxyproline, which help to give the molecule structural stability, and other amino acids with side groups which help to form crosslinks that determine how the collagen molecules become associated with one another.

The tropocollagen molecules become associated in a staggered arrangement, polymerizing to form banded collagen fibrils with a periodicity of about 640 Å[170] (Fig. 2-19). The smallest structures seen on electron microscopy are microfibrils, the smallest seen on light microscopy are fibrils, and the smallest seen with the unassisted eye are fibers.[160]

Collagen may be heated with either an acid or an alkali. This solubilizes some of the collagen into solution, which cool to gelatin. Collagen that is so well cross-linked that it is difficult to solubilize is known as insoluble collagen. In early wounds most of the collagen is soluble because cross-linkage has not occurred, but with time a greater proportion becomes insoluble as cross-links develop. This correlates somewhat with size. New collagen fibrils are 8.1 to 13.7 μm wide, whereas more mature normal and relatively insoluble collagen is 27.2 μm in width.[89]

Types of collagen

There are 10 distinct types of collagen, which differ in the composition of the alpha chain amino acid sequences.[319] These are listed in Table 2-3. The major significance of these different types of collagen is that they are found in different tissues. Furthermore, different types of collagen form unique structures, which include fibers (collagens I, II, III), sheets (IV), or short, insertional fibrils (VII). Type I collagen is the main collagen in skin. It is found in bone and tendon as well. Type II collagen is found in cartilage, particularly hyaline cartilage. Healing wounds and fetal skin contain significant amounts of type III collagen.[123] It is thought that the fine reticulin fibers are composed of type III collagen and that this collagen may be important in establishing the initial wound structure by providing a latticework for events in wound repair. Type III collagen is structurally more stable than type I collagen but is readily degraded by collagenases.[29] It may rapidly disappear from wounds within a few days after it is deposited.[67,76] Therefore from a teleologic point of view this stronger collagen serves a useful purpose when needed during embryonic development and in early wound healing; it is then readily disposable.

In normal skin, type I and type III collagen exist together, usually in a ratio of about 3.5:1. In embryonal skin the amount of type III collagen is increased, resulting in a ratio of 1:1.[20,122] Wounds also have an increased percentage of type III collagen.[21] Although normal scars usually lose the increased type III collagen, hypertrophic scars continue to contain a larger percentage of type III collagen in a ratio of about 2:1; this increase in type III collagen persists for many months or years.[20] Ten-year-old hypertrophic scars in humans have been reported to have increased type III collagen.[29]

Type IV collagen is found in basement membranes. Type IV collagen has three identical alpha chains and has been identified in the lens and Descemet's membrane.[247] Type V collagen is composed of two different alpha chains. It is known to be synthesized by epidermal cells and is found in the basement membrane zone of human skin.[450] Type V collagen is also known to be a component of capillary basement membrane.[191] Therefore this collagen type is important and may play a role in epidermal cell migration, as well as angiogenesis. Type V collagen has also been detected in hypertrophic scar tissue.[119]

Types VI to X collagen have been only recently de-

scribed. Type VII collagen is longer than the other collagens and visually resembles the anchoring fibrils linking the epithelial basement membrane to underlying dermis.

Synthesis of collagen

Collagen undergoes separate and well-defined steps in its synthesis, which requires a number of enzymes (Table 2-4 and Fig. 2-20). Many of these steps can be influenced by various agents or deficiencies, resulting in a number of clinical syndromes. It is important to understand the sequence of events in the production of collagen, since it is central to wound repair.

Step 1: Assembly of polypeptide chains. Messenger RNA (mRNA) in the nucleus transcribes the genetic code for the alpha chain. Each alpha chain has a separate mRNA. The mRNAs then go to the ribosomes in the cytoplasm, where with amino acids and transfer RNA (tRNA), transcription occurs to produce the alpha chains. Each alpha chain has an amino terminal end and a carboxyl terminal end. At the amino terminal end a "signal" sequence is produced, which helps in orientation of the alpha chains.

Step 2: Hydroxylation. The proline and lysine on the alpha chains (protocollagen) are hydroxylated to hydroxyproline and hydroxylysine. This step occurs before complete alpha chain assembly,[316] and the proline and lysine must be incorporated into the peptide sequence before hydroxylation.[245] Free hydroxyproline or hydroxylysine is not incorporated into the alpha chains. Hydroxylation also occurs before helical formation of the alpha chains. Helical formation prevents further hydroxylation from occurring.

There are two types of prolyl hydroxylase and one type of lysyl hydroxylase.[383] Prolyl hydroxylase (PH) requires ferrous iron, alpha-ketoglutarate, ascorbic acid (vitamin C), and atmospheric oxygen.[229,254,453] Normally this enzyme is in excess in fibroblasts synthesizing collagen, so the lack of cofactors may be rate limiting.[155] The lack of vitamin C as occurs in scurvy leads to collagen that is underhydroxylated. Such underhydroxylated collagen is nonhelical and cannot be used for the later assembly of collagen fibrils. The PH is increased in wounds, scars, keloids, and hypertrophic scars.[78,82] Therefore where collagen is being synthesized, PH is increased. Recent evidence suggests that there exist in wounds specific stimulating factors, "collagen-stimulating factors," that specifically stimulate prolyl hydroxylase.[351]

Pinnell et al.[375] described a syndrome characterized by collagen deficient in hydroxylysine. The patients had hyperextensible joints and skin, easy bruisability, and kyphoscoliosis from birth. It was surmised that these individuals were deficient in lysyl hydroxylase. This condition has since been designated Ehlers-Danlos syndrome type VI.

Step 3: Glycosylation. Sugar residues are next added to the alpha peptide chains. Either galactose (by galactosyltransferase) or glucose (by glucosyltransferase) are added to the hydroxylysine. These enzymes usually act on the helical

TABLE 2-4

Steps in synthesis of collagen

Step	Mechanism	Metabolic interference	Clinical relevance
1. Assembly of polypeptide chain with terminal segments (protocollagen)	Transcription (mRNA) Translation (tRNA)	Genetic defect	Marfan's syndrome, pseudoxanthoma elasticum, osteogenesis imperfecta, Ehlers-Danlos syndrome type IV
2. Hydroxylation of protocollagen	Prolyl hydroxylase	Lack of vitamin C	Scurvy
	Lysyl hydroxylase	Low O_2	Ehlers-Danlos syndrome type VI (hydroxylysine deficiency)
3. Addition of carbohydrate to protocollagen	Glycosylation (galactosyl transferase, glucosyl transferase)	—	—
4. Assembly of procollagen (triple helix)	—	—	—
5. Secretion of procollagen	Microtubules and microfilaments	Colchicine, vinblastin	—
6. Hydrolysis of extension peptides (cleavage) of procollagen to yield tropocollagen	Procollagen peptidase	Procollagen peptidase deficiency	Dermatosparaxis (cattle); Ehlers-Danlos syndrome type VII
7. Polymerization of tropocollagen	Lysyl oxidase R-COH (aldehyde) RCH=NR' (Schiff base) RCHoHCH$_2$CHO (Aldol)	BAPN; Cu deficiency; lysyl oxidase deficiency; d-penicillamine; homocysteine	Lathyrism; Menkes' kinky-hair syndrome; cutis laxa (X-linked); Ehlers-Danlos syndrome type V; fragile skin

configuration, and therefore glycosylation occurs before formation of the triple helix.

Step 4: Formation of triple helix. The alpha chains are released from the polyribosomes of the rough endoplasmic reticulum and form triple helical configurations. This is partially accomplished by disulfide bonds. Three alpha chains become intertwined and form a *procollagen* molecule. The procollagen molecule has a large carboxyl terminal end and an amino terminal. However, the carboxyl end is probably the last to be formed on the ribosomes and is mainly responsible, through its well-developed disulfide bonds, for holding the alpha chains together.[59]

Step 5: Secretion. The assembled procollagen passes to the Golgi apparatus and is then secreted into the extracellular space. This processing is facilitated by microtubules and microfilaments, which may be disrupted by colchicine, slowing down the excretion of procollagen.

Step 6: Cleavage. The procollagen molecule is bound together at both end by peptides (also called telopeptides). These are cleaved off in the extracellular space by procollagen peptidases. There exists a peptidase for the peptides at both the amino end and the carboxyl end (procollagen aminoprotease, procollagen carboxyprotease).[383] Once the terminal peptides are cleaved off, the collagen molecule is known as *tropocollagen.*

Diseases associated with a deficiency in procollagen peptidase have been described. In newborn calves this deficiency results in dermatosparaxis.[275] Here the skin is fragile and may be literally wiped off. In humans the deficiency results in Ehlers-Danlos syndrome type VII.[294]

Step 7: Polymerization. Assembly of cleaved procollagen (tropocollagen) into fibrils occurs next. Initially these polymerized fibrils are weak because they lack intermolecular cross-linking. Cross-linking by covalent bonds occurs but requires further chemical modification first. Lysyl oxidase, a copper-containing enzyme, catalyzes the oxidative deamination of the ϵ-amino groups of certain lysyl and hydroxylysyl residues of collagen-yielding aldehydes.[19] Once the aldehydes are formed, cross-links may occur by means of aldol condensation or Schiff bases.[43] This covalent intermolecular cross-linking occurs mainly during the first month of wound healing and accounts for the early gain in strength of collagen.[131] This intermolecular cross-linking also results in insolubility of collagen fibers and is vital for fibrillar tensile strength and stability.[457]

Since biblical times it has been known that ingestion of *Lathyrus odoratus,* the sweet pea, may lead to connective tissue problems. The sweet pea contains β-aminopropionitrile (BAPN), which acts as a competitive inhibitor of lysyl oxidase, and thus interferes with the oxidative deamination of lysine in newly formed collagen. This results in collagen with few cross-links, since the subsequent aldol and Schiff bases can no longer be formed. However, BAPN does not appear to affect earlier-formed fibrils,[458] and has no effect on wound contraction.[85]

Problems arising from sweet pea ingestion were first observed in cattle and occur in young animals fed BAPN; they include aortic rupture, abdominal herniations, knock-knees, dislocated lenses, and ultimately severe bony defects. Collectively this constellation of problems with connective tissue instability is known as lathyrism. Lathyritic animals in addition have wounds with reduced tensile strength.

Penicillamine is another substance known to interfere with cross-linking of collagen but by a separate mechanism. Penicillamine is a metabolic byproduct of penicillin but at the usual dosage of antibiotics does not accumulate to any significant extent.[146] However, penicillamine is used therapeutically for patients with Wilson's disease; these patients may have side effects such as increased skin fragility, as well as connective tissue problems such as elastosis perforans serpiginosa. This compound interferes with the cross-linking of collagen by chelating important cross-link sites produced by oxidative deamination of lysine. It may also preferentially act on the disulfide bonds of type III rather than type I collagen.[243] An additional mechanism of action for penicillamine is to chelate copper, which is required for lysyl oxidase. Wounds in guinea pigs and rats given penicillamine have a decreased breaking strength, although the hydroxyproline content is normal.[146,347] Moreover, the amount of soluble collagen increases because it is less cross-linked than insoluble collagen.[347] Therefore penicillamine results in a qualitative change in collagen.

Degradation of collagen

Collagen is not a static protein once it is deposited in the skin or scars but is continually broken down and replaced in both normal and pathologic conditions. Therefore the ''apparent'' metabolic inertness of collagen does not exist. Klein and Weiss[257] showed with ^{14}C-labeled proline that wounds in rats and guinea pigs were repaired with previously existing collagen. Therefore collagen in the body is reutilized.

The continued metabolic activity of collagen was further demonstrated in skin grafts. Using split-thickness and full-thickness skin grafts labeled with ^{14}C or ^{3}H, Klein and Rudolph[259] showed in rats a loss of up to 60% of the original graft collagen at 4 weeks and up to 88% by 20 weeks.

Collagen is degraded probably by collagenases, which may be found within the dermis, epidermis, or even bacteria or granulocytes. These collagenases are specific for collagen and exist because of the resistance of native collagen to general tissue proteases. Gross and Lapière[171] first demonstrated a diffusible collagenolytic factor in bullfrog tadpole tissue, which had been cultured on calf skin collagen (Fig. 2-21). These investigators reasoned that if a collagenase existed, it probably did so in the tadpole because of the rapid dissolution of such anatomic structures as the tail and fins during metamorphosis. Viable cell cultures were necessary to demonstrate collagenase, since cell extracts were initially unsuccessful. Gross and Lapière also observed collagenolysis in cultures of postpartum myometrium.

Collagenolytic activity on the human skin was first demonstrated in 1965,[139] and the enzyme activity was characterized by Eisen, Jeffrey, and Gross in 1968.[121] Collagenases from the epidermis have slightly different properties from those of the dermis.[165] Large amounts of collagenase are present in wound tissue, particularly the wound margins, and increased collagenolytic activity can be found in scars as old as 30 years.[394] Unwounded skin has weak collagenolytic activity, although some tissues—for instance scalp—seem to have more.[121] The upper or papillary dermis also has significantly more activity than the lower reticular dermis, at which location collagenase may be undetectable.[120]

There are thought to be three steps in the breakdown of collagen.[184] First, collagenase cleaves collagen at a specific site in the helical portion of the molecule. This is usually three quarters of the way down from the amino terminal, producing a 75% fragment with an amino terminal (TC^A_{75}) and a 25% fragment with a carboxyl terminal (TC^B_{25}).

The second step is natural denaturation or uncoiling of the cleavage products. This allows the third step, degradation by cellular proteases, to proceed. These latter enzymes are released into the extracellular space or may work on the denatured collagen subsequent to phagocytosis by cells.

Collagenolytic activity may be inhibited by certain globulins from the serum and from progesterone.[25] However, control of collagenase induction may reside within the epidermis. Ehrlich and Buttle[114] showed that hypertrophic scar epidermis controls the scar collagenase below. The epidermis as the control of collagenase induction is consistent with other findings that most of the collagenolytic activity takes place in the papillary dermis near the epidermis.[121]

Extracts of granulocytes also contain a collagenase.[280] This neutrophilic collagenase preferentially attacks type I rather than type III collagen[280] and probably acts within the cytoplasm rather than the extracellular space. Once the collagen is split by the intracellular collagenase, it is degraded further by intracellular proteases. The importance of this method of collagen breakdown is underscored by the presence of banded collagen observed with phagocytes in wounds particularly during the remodeling phase of wound repair.[320] Some of the degraded products of this collagen are undoubtedly released and used as substrates for further repair.

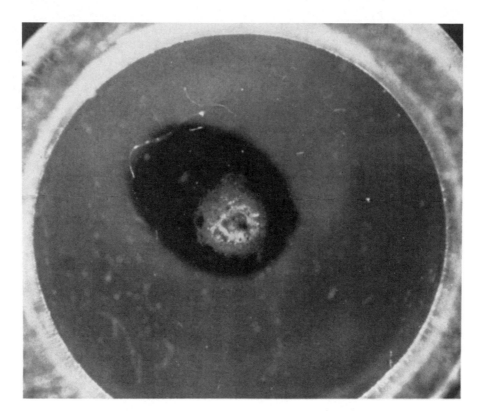

Fig. 2-21. Culture of tadpole fin skin on collagen gel. Note area of lysis *(clear area)* around explant. (From Gross, J., and Lapière, C.M.: Proc. Natl. Acad. Sci. **48:**1014, 1962.)

Reticulum fibers

Reticulum fibers are very fine fibers, which stain black with silver stains. These fibers are thought to be probably very thin collagen fibers. Some reticulum fibers are associated closely with the basement membrane and probably help to anchor the epidermis.

Elastic fibers

Elastic fibers are rather ill-defined, amorphous fibers that constitute only a small percentage of normal dermis (less than 2% dry weight). The origin of these fibers is unknown, but they are thought to be secreted by fibroblasts. Elastic fibers on electron microscopy are composed of two elements, an amorphous portion (elastin) and a microfibrillar portion. Elastin contains hydroxyproline and glycine but no cystine or hydroxylysine. Unique to elastin are the amino acids desmosine and isodesmosine, derived from lysine. Elastic fibers are not an important component of early wound repair but do appear much later in the healing process, after 2 months.[81,489]

Ground substance

The amorphous interfibrillar acellular material in collective tissue, whether normal or scarred, has been termed ground substance. As pointed out by Jackson[236] this is a mistranslation of the German word *Grundsubstanz,* which literally means fundamental substance.

Although its composition is complex and heterogeneous, ground substance behaves as a gel or sol. Therefore it does not leak, is impermeable to microbes, and gives some support to structures, such as vessels or nerves, that traverse it.

The ground substance is composed of colloid-rich phase and a water-rich phase.[156] The water-rich phase is composed of water, electrolytes, dissolved nutrients, metabolic products of cells, and gases traveling between the blood and tissue cells. Therefore the ground substance may be regarded as an extension of the vascular system.

The colloid-rich phase is composed of insoluble substances, mainly glycoproteins and proteoglycans. Glycoproteins and proteoglycans have similar structures, composed of a protein core attached to which are carbohydrate side chains. Thus the physical configuration is that of a bottle brush or pipe cleaner. The side chains of the glycoproteins are short, whereas the side chains of the proteoglycans are more complex. Glycoproteins and proteoglycans both help to cement the collagen together and are therefore important in the stabilization and maturation of connective tissue.

The terminology of connective tissue carbohydrate-pro-

TABLE 2-5

Glycosaminoglycans in the dermis

Name	Synonym	Hexuronic acid	Hexosamine	Repeating units	Molecular weight	Protein linked	Hyaluronidase susceptible	Location
Hyaluronic acid	—	Glucuronic acid	N-acetyl glucosamine	2500	500,000- 10 million	Little or none	Yes	Embryonic tissue, synovial fluid, vitreous humor, early healing (inflammatory states)
Chondroitin sulfate A	Chondroitin 4-sulfate	Glucuronic acid	N-acetyl- galactosamine	60	20,000- 40,000	Yes	Yes	Cartilage, skin bone, cornea, late healing (associated with collagen synthesis)
Chondroitin sulfate B	Dermatan sulfate	Iduronic acid	N-acetyl- galactosamine	60	20,000- 40,000	Yes	No	Skin, blood, vessels, scar, tendons
Chondroitin sulfate C	Chondroitin 6-sulfate	Glucuronic acid	N-acetyl- galactosamine	60	20,000 40,000	Yes	Yes	Skin, cartilage, late healing
Heparin	—	Glucuronic acid	Glucosamine	60	17,000- 20,000	No	—	Mast cells, cell surface components

tein complexes is confusing and requires further clarification. The side chains of proteoglycans are mucopolysaccharides, also called glycosaminoglycans (GAGs), which are secreted by fibroblasts. These substances are straight-chain molecules composed of repeating disaccharide units, described later. The side chains of the glycoproteins, on the other hand, are simpler oligosaccharide units. Although a protein chain is central to both glycoproteins and proteoglycans, it is more prominent in glycoproteins than in proteoglycans. Another term used is mucoprotein, which is simply a glycoprotein with a larger amount of hexosamine (less than 4%).

There are five different glycosaminoglycans in human skin: hyaluronic acid, chondroitin sulfate A, chondroitin sulfate B, chondroitin sulfate C, and heparin. These differ in basic structure, molecular weight, location, and susceptibility to hyaluronidase (Table 2-5). Although most GAGs are linked to protein, some are not, such as hyaluronic acid.

Glycosaminoglycans in ground substance are highly acidic because they contain many carboxylic acid groups. As these carboxylic acids dissociate, the connective tissue may be ionized, resulting in a fixed negative charge. In general, however, because dermis has abundant collagen and a small amount of acid mucopolysaccharides, there is a low net negative charge. GAGs therefore behave like polyanionic electrolytes. Probably the negative acid groups of the glycosaminoglycans are bound to the positive basic amino groups of collagen. The electrostatic binding of glycosaminoglycans to collagen is an important factor in connective tissue organization and structural stability.

Glycosaminoglycans and glycoproteins have been studied during wound healing. Glycoproteins appear first, but probably originate from the blood rather than being synthesized in the wound itself.[237,488] GAGs are readily formed during the first 1 to 2 weeks and decrease in amount thereafter.[31,267] Hyaluronic acid is the first to appear in significant quantities, followed by chondroitin sulfate A and B.[31,488] Hyaluronic acid may be associated with cellular proliferation and differentiation of fibroblasts. It decreases in amount during the first week concomitantly with an increase in hyaluronidase found in wounds.[35] In scorbutic[267] or cortisone-treated animals[462] the ground substance may be deficient.

Glycosaminoglycans are also increased in many scars. In hypertrophic scars, chondroitin sulfate A, B, and C and hyaluronic acid are all increased compared with that in normal skin.[97] Therefore the size of hypertrophic scars may in part be caused by the increased ground substance rather than by the collagen content alone.

EPIDERMAL RESURFACING OF WOUNDS

On the production of a cutaneous wound the surrounding epidermis migrates and proliferates within a short period of time to resurface the defect. This ability is undoubtedly of evolutionary significance, for without a rapid mechanism to repair the outer surface, survival would be difficult. The skin in particular is constantly subject to trauma and therefore continually needs such a mechanism for repair.

Epidermal resurfacing occurs through a process of cellular migration, proliferation, and differentiation. Although the term "epidermal regeneration" is sometimes used, a new normal epidermis is not formed by this process. The new epidermis lacks normal rete pegs and usually connections with adnexal structures such as eccrine sweat ducts or hair follicles (Fig. 2-14).

Migrating epidermis over a wound performs a number of functions besides merely restoring the integrity of skin.[40] It undermines, causing the dead superficial tissue that comprises a scab to slough away. The collagenous transformation of granulation tissue is facilitated, perhaps by the secretion of growth factors from the new epidermis. Exudation from the wound is reduced by the new epidermal cover, and the tissues below are sealed off from the environment, thereby reducing the risk of infection. Despite the fact that the new epidermis is feeble, it does provide some fortification against wound dehiscence.[404] Although some large wound defects may close almost solely by contraction, most do not in human beings. The epidermal resurfacing covers the portion of the wound that does not close by contraction.

Gross microscopy

On creation of a wound the epidermis surrounding the defect reacts quickly and in 12 to 24 hours begins thickening and migrating.[349] For a simple incisional type of wound, a "tongue" of stratified epidermal cells inverts and grows down into the incision a short distance (Fig. 2-8). If a scab is formed, the epidermis tunnels underneath. The epidermal cells from both sides meet in the upper reticular dermis in 1 to 5 days (Fig. 2-9). The epidermis is the first tissue in a wound to reconstitute itself and fill the wound gap. After the epidermis has bridged the surgical defect, it characteristically thickens,[349,440] and an epidermal "spur" is formed, invading into the subepidermal tissues close to the surface of the incision.[355] As the new epidermis differentiates back toward normal, keratin is formed, and the overlying attached scab is dislodged within 5 days of epidermal union. The epidermal spurs are remodeled during the second week and by 3 weeks the initial inverted epithelium is level.[355]

For wounds that are broad and superficial (type I) and allowed to heal by granulation, the epidermis grows not only from the surrounding epidermis but also from the pilosebaceous structures and eccrine sweat ducts.[153] For large deep surgical defects with extensive loss of tissue, it may take weeks, or even months, for full epidermization of the wound surface to occur because the wound cavity must first be filled with granulation tissue and a large amount of wound surface needs to be covered by new epidermis.

Migration

Almost immediately epidermis begins moving to resurface a wound before significant mitotic activity begins. This usually occurs in the first 24 hours.[349] It is important to realize the essential role played by epidermal migration alone in covering a wound, since mitosis alone cannot account for rapid coverage.

Stimulus for migration. The main stimulus for epidermal migration is unknown but is probably a combination of factors. When an injury occurs, cells are destroyed or damaged. The deficit of tissue and the altered tissue both trigger responses in local cells.[2] Epidermal cells have the capacity for migration and phagocytosis.[349] This latter function may be related to the damaged tissue and its elimination. Both migration and phagocytosis are morphogenetic functions of cells, and phagocytosis is a natural accompaniment to cellular movement. In other words, a cell moves to surround what it intends to engulf. Therefore since these are not everyday functions of normal epidermis, one may consider that a certain degree of dedifferentiation takes place before epidermal migration occurs.

Contact inhibition. The loss of contact inhibition provides a stimulus for cell movement. Like cells that are in contact with one another do not migrate, whereas when this contact is lost, cells begin to move. Simplistically stated, "An epithelium will not tolerate a free edge."[2] This phenomenon is seen in tissue culture with epidermal cells, fibroblasts, and capillaries, but not blood lymphocytes.

Contact inhibition is cell specific and requires a certain amount of cell differentiation. Therefore the dedifferentiation that occurs with migration of epidermis can proceed only to a limited degree. The onset of contact inhibition usually requires contact on all sides of the cell. Therefore in tissue culture this requires confluence of growth. In addition, the onset of contact inhibition is gradual. Both cell division and migration decrease but do not stop immediately on contact of cells.[65] This may explain the epidermal spur found in incision lines, as well as the hypertrophy of the epidermis where the advancing wound edges meet.

When a wound is created, the cells in the epidermis may be exposed to various substances in the serum that could promote cell migration. One such substance, epibolin, has been recently shown to enhance cell spreading and migration.[449] There may of course be many others.

Morphologic changes in migrating epidermal cells. Migrating epidermal cells appear morphologically distinct from nonmigrating epidermal cells. The cells elongate in the direction of movement, and both the nucleus and overall cell size increase.[16,303,440] This not only sustains increased metabolic activity but also helps cells to cover a larger area. Elongation of cells in the direction of cell growth is a phenomenon common to the epidermis.[374]

On electron microscopy the migrating epidermal cells are seen to have a "ruffled" cell membrane and cytoplasmic extensions in the direction of cell movement.[349] Filaments measuring 40 to 80 Å in diameter are seen just beneath the cell membrane[143,271,331] (Fig. 2-22). These filaments presumably are contractile in function. Staining of the cyto-

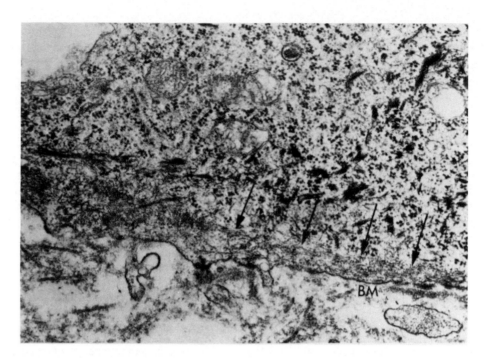

Fig. 2-22. Epidermal cell in portion of regenerating epidermis on 7-day-old human wound. Faint basement membrane material *(BM)* is seen underneath cytoplasm. Microfilamentous structures *(arrows)* are seen in lower portion of cell. (×32,000.) (From Montandon, D., and Gabbiani, G.: In Marchac, D., and Hueston, J.T., editors: Transactions of the Sixth International Congress of Plastic and Reconstructive Surgery, Paris, 1976, Masson.)

plasm of advancing epidermal cells has been demonstrated with AAA serum (containing antiactin antibodies).[142] Thus the pseudopodal extensions and contractile elements perhaps work in concert to mediate cell movement.

Substrate attachment. Epidermal cell migration requires attachment to an underlying substratum. If present, for instance in a blister, the basement membrane serves this purpose. However, the basement membrane is usually absent in surgical wounds, and therefore the epidermis must utilize other structures. Fibrin and fibronectin are currently thought to provide the provisional foundation to which epidermal cells may attach themselves and on which they move.[73,75,95] The importance of an underlying substratum is to provide direction and orientation for cell movement. Such a function has been termed contact guidance.[483]

Once migration is completed, a basement membrane appears underneath the epidermis. The origin of this basement membrane and of the provisional guiding substratum during cell movement appears to be the epidermal cells themselves. Epidermal cells have been shown to secrete fibronectin[75,352] and the components of normal epidermal basement membrane. The normal basement membrane is composed of four regions seen under electron microscopy: (1) the epidermal cell plasma membrane portion, (2) the lamina lucida, (3) the lamina densa, and (4) the sublamina densa.[500] The lamina lucida is composed of laminin, a very large glycoprotein thought to be useful in gluing the epidermal cell membrane onto the layer below (the lamina

densa).[130] Also present in the lamina lucida is bullous pemphigoid (BP) antigen, whose function is unknown.

The lamina densa is composed of type IV collagen.[501] This layer is thought to provide a cushion for the epidermis and to separate it from the tissue fluids below. In addition, epidermis has been shown to attach to type IV collagen preferentially.[261] An additional type of collagen synthesized by epidermal cells, type V, is also formed in the basement membrane, but its exact location is still unknown.[450] The lowest portion of the basement membrane, the sublamina densa, is composed of collagenous anchoring fibers between the lamina densa and the dermis below. These anchoring fibrils have been designated type VII collagen.[319]

All of the portions of the basement membrane except the sublamina densa have been shown to be produced by epidermal cells. These include laminin, type IV collagen, BP, and type V collagen.[73,450,500] Furthermore, epidermal cells, as already mentioned, secrete fibronectin, an important component of the provisional basement membrane.[75,352]

It is thought that initially migrating epidermal cells secrete fibronectin, to which they attach.[75] Although some of the fibronectin in the provisional substratum comes from the serum, much comes from the epidermal cell itself. This sticky substance allows the epidermal cell to move with some attachment below. The intracellular contractile (actin) microtubules of epidermal cells may be connected to the extracellular fibronectin by plasma membrane linkage. Once epidermization has been completed, type IV collagen and laminin appear.[73] These two substances are absent under migrating epidermal cells. Therefore the epidermis itself reconstitutes the major portion of the basement membrane.

The sublamina densa portion of the basement membrane is probably formed later. Because this zone is responsible for attaching the lamina densa to the dermis, new epidermis is at first more easily separated from underlying tissue. However, this zone eventually becomes more developed, resulting in an epidermis that is more resistant to detachment.

Hemidesmosomes are also produced by epidermal cells and assist them in attaching to the basement membrane.[271,349] Such attachments are perhaps helpful in cell movement, but they must also be broken for cell movement forward.

Mechanisms of epidermal movement. Early in the twentieth century, investigators believed that epidermal cells migrate by individual ameboid movement.[16,303] As more insight has been gained recently concerning cell attachments to substrates, newer mechanisms of movement have been proposed. Basically these fall into two categories: The new epidermis is either pushed forward or pulled forward (Fig. 2-23). Perhaps both of these mechanisms operate together.

One proposed mechanism of movement of the epidermis is by mass movement rather than by individual cell effort.[68] In this model the new epidermis is pushed forward (Fig. 2-23, *A*). Evidence for this is that cells appear to pile up at the points of contact of migrating epidermal edges. This helps to explain such phenomena as the hyperplastic skin edges of grafts and incision lines, as well as the epidermal spurs that are seen microscopically in incision lines.

The pulling of the epidermis forward by advancing basal cells is another proposed mechanism currently in vogue. Cells in the advancing basal cell layer migrate actively, whereas cells above and behind are passively pulled forward (Fig. 2-23, *B*). The epidermal cells in the vanguard attach to a substrate and pull forward the cells behind.[384] This attachment could be in the form of a hemidesmosome,[271] fibronectin,[75] or laminin with type IV collagen.[500] Here attachments to the substratum are made at the leading edge of the epidermis, while farther back such attachments are lost. This type of movement has been described as similar to that of a ratchet.

Important in the movement of cells, if they are pulled forward, are the contractile microfilaments near the plasma membrane of the epidermal cells (Fig. 2-22). These contract in the pseudopodal extensions, thereby advancing the cells forward.

An interesting variant of the pull mechanism of cell movement was described by Krawczyk[271] (Fig. 2-23, *C*), who proposed that epidermal cells glide or slide over each other to advance the tissue forward. An epidermal cell has pseudopodal attachments to a substrate. Because of cell attachments to other cells above and partially behind, the attached cells above are pulled forward as the pseudopodal attachments contract. These cells in turn form their own attachments and pull the next cell (above and slightly behind) forward. Thus the epidermis moves forward like a military tank tread.

Migration under a scab. The migration of epidermis occurs not only on a substrate but frequently beneath a scab (Fig. 2-24). Histologically a scab or crust is formed from collagenous tissue, elastic fibers, epithelial tissue, fibrin, and cellular components of the wound exudate.[9] The scab is formed partially by dehydration of the dermis and the leukocytes, which become trapped in this desiccating tissue. The epidermis then must negotiate a path between the dried-out collagen and the cellularly active connective tissue. This tunneling through collagen is perhaps accomplished by an enzyme, collagenase, which is known to be produced by epidermal cells and dissolves away collagen in its path.[165] With the production of keratin by the epidermis once epidermization has occurred, the scab is sloughed off.

The scab is often thought of as a physical barrier to epidermal migration, slowing down the growth of the migrating epidermis.[154,303,496] The leading edge of the epidermis is thicker and has a longer distance to migrate than if scab formation is prevented. When occlusion has been used to prevent scab formation, epidermization proceeds at a faster rate (Fig. 2-25).

Rate of epidermal cell migration. The rate of migration of epidermal cells varies with the type of wound and the distance that must be traversed. The terrain plays some role in influencing the rate as well. In 1936 Arey[16] noted that epidermal movement was faster in smooth and shallow wounds and slower in uneven wounds or wounds that had a firm, adherent scab. This was also confirmed by other extensive studies.[355,496] Epidermal resurfacing of superficial wounds through a scab takes approximately two[495] or three[291] times longer than if a scab is not present. Whether this increased time for resurfacing is caused by a longer pathway for the epidermis to migrate or by a slowing of the rate of movement has not been determined.

Investigators tend to imply that the rate of epidermization can be used as the unequivocal measure of wound healing; however, epidermization of wounds is only one component of wound repair. Although for superficial wounds it is probably the major biologic event, for full-thickness wounds other processes are equally if not more important.

Migration of melanocytes. Occasionally in scar epidermis one may see a pigmented streak from the skin edge to the center of the new epidermis. This is probably caused by the proliferation of epidermal melanocytes immediately adjacent to the wound and their migration into the regenerating epidermis.[197]

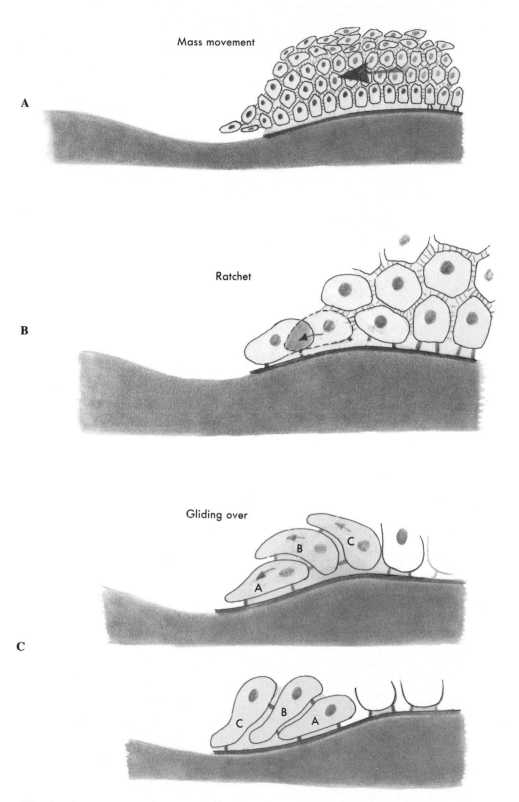

Fig. 2-23. Proposed mechanisms of epidermal cell migration over wound. **A,** Mass movement theory. **B,** Pulling (ratchet) theory. **C,** Gliding over.

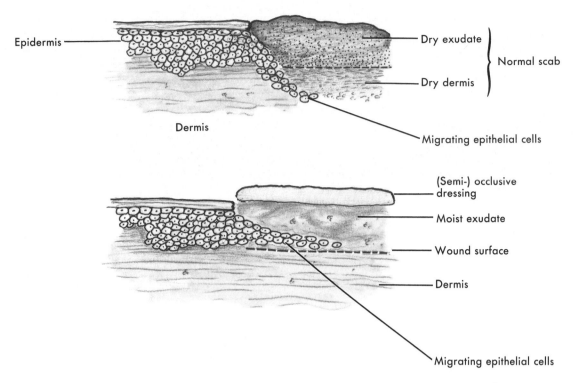

Epidermis ——

Dry exudate

Normal scab

Dry dermis

Dermis

Migrating epithelial cells

(Semi-) occlusive dressing

Moist exudate

Wound surface

Dermis

Migrating epithelial cells

Fig. 2-24. Deeper migration of epidermis underneath scab in unoccluded (dry) wound *(top)*, compared with wound that is occluded *(moist)* and thus keeps scab from forming *(bottom)*. (Data from Winter, G.D.: Nature **193:**293, 1962.)

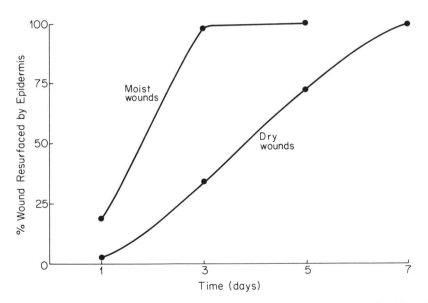

Fig. 2-25. Comparison between epidermization rates of superficial (type I) wounds with occlusion *(bottom)* and without occlusion *(top)*.

Proliferation

To cover a wound, the epidermis not only migrates but also has an increased mitotic rate. These two processes are intimately related.

Location of mitoses. The main location of mitoses in a wound initially is neither in nor close to the advancing epidermal tongue, but farther back and more proximal, extending into the "normal" epidermis[271,440] (Fig. 2-9). This locus of increased mitotic activity results in a microscopic hyperplasia of the skin to the sides of the wound. For a variable distance back from this hyperplastic epithelium, but within the epidermis, there is a decreasing mitotic cell rate among basal cells.[58] In a few days after the wounding, however, the mitotic rate increases in the advancing tongue of epidermis,[440] reaching a maximum just before complete epidermization and then sharply decreasing on closure.[16,440]

Time of mitotic activity. Increased epidermal mitotic activity does not occur for the first 24 to 48 hours after injury. Therefore initial movement of the epidermis, as already mentioned, occurs by migration and not proliferation. It has also been shown that when epidermal mitotic activity occurs, it does so in bursts rather than as a continuous period of high activity.[374,455]

Factors increasing mitotic activity. Injury to the epidermis alone will increase the mitotic rate.[57] If the skin is stripped with tape, removing the stratum corneum, and is then occluded, the mitotic rate is increased for 7 to 9 days. However, if the injured skin is allowed to dry out instead, the mitotic rate increases even more and persists longer, for 12 to 14 days. Therefore desiccation of epidermis plays a role in sustaining the increased mitotic rate.[403]

It has been suggested that within the unwounded epidermis there exists a mitotic inhibitor, which becomes absent when a wound occurs. Bullough and Laurence[57] observed that if the epidermis is stripped off one side of the ear of a mouse, mitotic activity is increased on the opposite side. They proposed that with the removed epidermis was also removed a potent epidermal mitotic inhibitor, which became known as a chalone.[56] This inhibitor was synthesized by the epidermis and inhibited activity only of the epidermis. Thus a chalone is a substance, usually a protein, which is synthesized by the same tissue on which it specifically acts to inhibit mitoses. Chalones act most strongly in the presence of epinephrine and glucocorticoids. This perhaps explains the delay of epidermal resurfacing of wounds by fluorinated steroids, which could act to enhance the chalone system at the surrounding edge of a wound, othewise the site of highest mitotic activity.

Specific epidermal growth factor (EGF) has also been recently described.[17] It is a single-chain polypeptide with a molecular weight of 5300 to 5500. EGF is found in human urine as well as the submaxillary glands of animals and presumably reaches the proliferating epidermis through the serum. Thus the usefulness of a dog's licking of its wounds or the old wives' tale of putting urine onto wounds might have a scientific basis. However, Greaves was unable to demonstrate a significant effect of ECF topically applied to epidermal wounds in man.[161]

Other mitotic stimulants have been found in the epidermis.[189] Their precise role in regulating epidermal growth is unknown. Some growth factors produced by the epidermis may also act on the collagenous tissue below to stimulate cellular activity.[442]

Factors depressing mitotic activity. Immediately after a wound is created, the mitotic rate may actually decrease. Arey[16] felt that this was caused by the shock of wounding, but it may also result from a decreased blood supply with nutrients essential for growth.

Movement and mitotic activity are slowed down when the epidermal edges meet from opposite sides of a wound. This contact between cell borders of like cells results in contact inhibition, stopping migration. As pointed out earlier, cell proliferation continues even after migration has ceased but at a reduced rate.[65]

Differentiation

On resurfacing a wound, the epidermis no longer plays a morphogenetic role but differentiates into nearly normal epidermis. As such it thickens at first but then thins out in 3 or 4 weeks. The new epidermis is somewhat friable at first, probably because the subdermal portion of the basement membrane is not totally developed until long after epidermization is complete.

FACTORS MODIFYING EPIDERMAL RESURFACING

Enhancement of epidermal coverage of wounds is the goal of wound care. In reality, however, it is probably wiser to concentrate on preventing factors that impede wound healing, since it is difficult to improve on nature.

Presence of a scab

A scab normally accompanies a wound and serves to protect the wound and underlying epidermis, once formed, from the external environment. One prevents its formation with occlusive dressings and frequent wound debridement, two artifacts of modern surgical care.

Desiccation of tissue causes a scab to form, which is composed not only of coagulated blood and fibrin but of dried-out collagen and any trapped debris.[9] Sitting in the center of a wound to be resurfaced, the scab represents an impediment to the migrating epidermis, which must navigate a course beneath it (Fig. 2-24). To do this, the epidermis must dissolve away collagen in its path, which it presumably does with collagenase.

A scab thus presents three potential problems for a healing wound. First, the epidermis must travel a longer distance, so it takes longer for a wound with a scab to resurface[195,495] (Fig. 2-25). Second, more dermis is sacrificed by the formation of a scab. This is usually not advantageous because it is difficult to predict the depth of tissue loss. Third, scabs occasionally provide a haven for bacterial proliferation.

Occlusion

Superficial wounds (type I) have been found to epithelialize faster if occluded than if exposed to air.[13,195,291,495] Gimbel et al.[154] observed in 1957 that blisters epithelialize 40% faster if the roof remains intact than if it is removed. Aspiration of the blister fluid slows the growth of the epidermis, but not as greatly as when the roof is removed.

The reasons why epidermization is faster under occlusion are unknown. Some authorities speculate that occlusion increases the humidity bathing the wound. This prevents the wound bed and superficial dermis from drying out and thus prevents scab formation.[154,497] As already mentioned, the scab acts as a barrier to advancing epidermis and forces the epidermis to migrate along a path that is longer to meet the epidermis on the opposite side of the wound (Fig. 2-24).

The effects of occlusion on enhancing epidermal coverage have been reported only in superficial (type I) wounds. Despite claims to the contrary,[496] full-thickness wounds may heal equally fast whether occluded or not.[264] With this wound type, though, the confounding variable of wound contraction occurs, so assessing the data is difficult. It should also be pointed out that the rate of epidermization cannot by itself be used as the determining sign of complete wound healing but only as a single component of the process.[41]

Oxygen concentration

As early as 1936 Arey[16] realized that an oxygen gradient may be an important factor in epidermal resurfacing. In cutaneous tissue cultures grown anaerobically, epidermal cell movement and cell division were shown by Medawar[323] to come to a standstill. Still, skin was able to survive for up to 1 week without oxygen. This is not surprising, since the basal cell portion of the epidermis must submit routinely to low oxygen tensions because of its relatively secluded position relative to the circulation.

In healing, energy production shifts from emphasis on the Krebs cycle and the Embden-Meyerhof pathway to the pentose phosphate shunt, which can act at low oxygen concentrations. Because of this change to anaerobic metabolic pathways, the consequences of decreased oxygen supply are minimized.

If full-thickness wounds are hyperoxygenated with 45% oxygen at atmospheric pressure, epidermization is accelerated by 15%.[359] The contraction rate, however, is not influenced by changes in oxygen tension.

The practical implications of all these studies may be that

dressings on wounds should be semi, not totally, occlusive. That is, free exchange of oxygen should be permitted to enhance epidermization. More details of the role of oxygen in wound healing are presented later.

Uneven skin edges

Ordman and Gillman[355] showed that wounds sutured with uneven wound edges resulted in prolonged epidermal resurfacing. Because one edge was higher than another, the epidermis had to travel a longer distance to reach its mate from the other side. In addition, loss of dermis in the higher side was greater since the epidermis from the lower side tended to tunnel deeper than that on the higher side and actually invaded the dermis on the higher side.

Drugs

Literally thousands of topical drugs have been proposed to enhance wound healing. Few, however, have been well studied. In an effort to dispel the confusion, Eaglstein and Mertz[108] developed an animal model in pigs and assessed the epidermal resurfacing of thin (type I) wounds. It should be pointed out that their data do not apply to open granulating wounds (type IIB wounds) or even wounds under pathologic conditions. These investigators confirmed that occlusion enhanced epidermal wound healing by as much as 40%. Moreover, both petrolatum and triamcinolone ointment (an antiinflammatory glucocorticoid) prolonged epidermal resurfacing.[108,110] Hydrocortisone had no effect on epidermization but did appear to decrease the wound collagen.[13,110] A base cream and lotion in this model system appeared to enhance reepithelialization, possibly because they are less occlusive than petrolatum. An anabolic steroid, nandrolone, had only a slight positive effect on epithelialization.

One interesting topical preparation investigated by the Eaglstein group[110] was Neomycin Ointment, which contains polymyxin sulfate, zinc bacitracin, and neomycin sulfate. Using their pig experimental model, they showed that the zinc bacitracin portion of Neomycin Ointment speeded up epithelialization. Perhaps the zinc portion of the bacitracin was responsible, for the preparations formulated with higher zinc levels seemed to work better.

I have for many years empirically used Polysporin Ointment for all wounds. This antibacterial preparation contains both polymyxin sulfate and zinc bacitracin and appears to promote wound healing with few complications. Therefore the studies by the Eaglstein group seem to support experimentally what I have seen clinically.

GRANULATION AND CONTRACTION

For many centuries physicians have known the process of wound healing by granulation, contraction, and epidermization. This process, also known as healing by secondary intention, may be allowed to occur when there is significant tissue loss (type IIB wounds; see Table 2-2) so the wound edges cannot be easily apposed. Unless such a defect is sutured or resurfaced with a skin graft or skin flap, it closes naturally, barring any pathologic obstacles such as infection or poor vascular supply. This closure occurs by two distinct events: contraction of the granulation tissue and epidermization. Both of these processes overlap in time.

After a large wound is created, it fills with granulation tissue, a process known as granulation (Fig. 2-13). This tissue becomes contractile and generates forces that bring the wound edges together. This process of the centripetal movement of tissue and skin edges is known as contraction. Contraction closes the wound at the expense of mobile skin surrounding the surgical defect. Concomitant with much of the contraction process is epidermization, which continues until the wound is completely closed. Usually in humans contraction does not completely bring the wound edges together. The remaining portion, which cannot be completely closed by contraction, is resurfaced by the migrating epidermis. Usually contraction by itself, however, is responsible for closing anywhere from 25% to 75% of the wound surface area.[62]

Wound healing by granulation, contraction, and epidermization is influenced by the tension of the surrounding tissue. The resultant scar formation is a function of the size, shape, depth, and location of the wound. Most wounds allowed to heal by this process do well over time and remain stable.

Secondary wound healing should not be regarded as a regeneration of normal tissue but rather as the generation of scar tissue. No true skin has formed anew; scar tissue restores *form* to the defect created by lost tissue, but *function* is always lessened. No scar performs like normal tissue. In addition, because contraction also pulls on surrounding tissues, contractures may result in impaired function of these tissues as well. How much this function is impaired of course depends on the factors already mentioned: the size, location, and depth of a wound. It should be pointed out that attempts to repair defects surgically rather than to allow granulation and contraction to take place always result in other scars, which in turn lead to their own set of difficulties with form and function. Sometimes this trade-off is in the patient's favor, sometimes it is an even trade, and sometimes there is a loss that results in more difficulties than if the wound had been allowed to heal naturally. Deciding when it is necessary to repair a wound and when it is acceptable to allow contraction and epidermization to occur is a matter of surgical experience.

It should be emphasized that many so-called definitive experimental studies done on healing by secondary intention have been done on laboratory animals, particularly rabbits, rats, and guinea pigs. These animals have a substantial layer of cutaneous striated muscle, the panniculus carnosus, which separates the skin above from the tissue below. This

allows plenty of give to the skin. Large wounds in such animals can heal almost entirely by contraction with little contribution by epidermization. Furthermore, contraction does not result in much distortion of adjacent structures.

In humans, the panniculus carnosus is absent, although Montagna and Parakkal[329] consider the platysma muscle of the neck the one vestigial muscle comparable to the panniculus carnosus of other animals. The skin of human beings is much more closely interconnected with the tissue below (Fig. 2-2), so contraction of wounds is more likely to lead to distortion of surrounding structures.

Sequence of events in granulation, contraction, and epidermization

The five distinct periods that occur during healing by secondary intention are granulation, contraction, epidermization, retraction, and remodeling. Although all these processes overlap to some degree, they are considered separately here.

This sequence of events in secondary wound healing can be seen graphically in Fig. 2-26 and photographically in Fig. 2-27. Carrel carefully plotted both decrease in wound size and size of the cicatrix (new epidermis) in patients with battle wounds suffered during World War I.[63,64] Fig. 2-26 represents the time sequence for secondary healing of a large (40 cm²) full-thickness shell wound on the back of a 21-year-old soldier.

Granulation. Immediately after the creation of a surgical defect, blood with fibrin enters the wound. This fibrin forms the scaffold upon which fibroblasts migrate and angiogenesis proceeds. The process of angiogenesis with fibroblastic growth proceeds to fill up the wound cavity (Fig. 2-27, *A*). The time it takes to do this is variable, depending on the wound size, depth, and location, but is usually about 1 week. Carrel[62] refers to this as the "quiescent period," since there is no change in wound size—but it is anything but quiescent with respect to the metabolic production of granulation tissue. Note that in Fig. 2-26 the time for building up granulation tissue lasted 4 days before contraction of the wound edges began.

Contraction. After sufficient granulation tissue is formed, the wound edges gradually begin to draw together (Fig. 2-27, *B*). This is caused by the contractile forces generated by the granulation tissue, which was poetically named by Billingham and Russell[41] "the ephemeral organ of contracture." This designation actually has much basis in fact, since the granulation tissue actually resorbs as it contracts. There does not appear to be a relationship between the amount of wound hydroxyproline or surface area of granulation tissue and the force of wound contraction.[168,193] Thus no difference is found in the hydroxyproline content per unit weight during contraction.[5] The actual force of wound contraction is best related to the thickness of the granulation tissue.

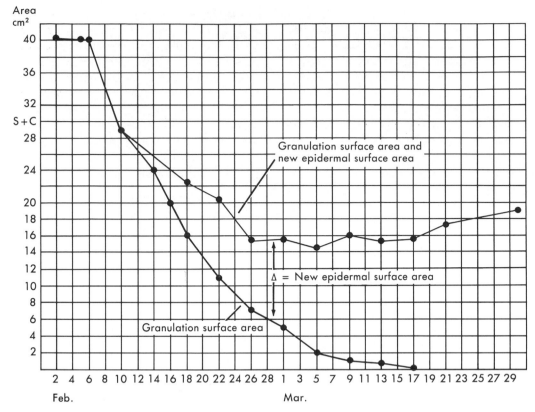

Fig. 2-26. Contraction and epidermization of 40 cm² wound in 21-year-old man. Lower curve represents granulation surface area, whereas upper curve is granulation surface area plus new epidermis. Difference between two curves is surface area of new epidermis. (From Carrel, A.: Reproduced from *The Journal of Experimental Medicine* **24:**429, 1916, by copyright permission of the Rockefeller University Press.)

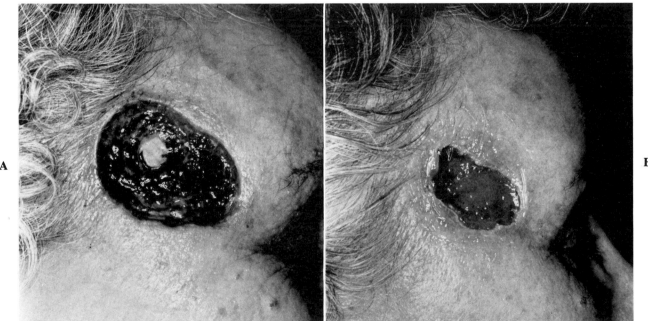

Fig. 2-27. A, Chemosurgical wound subsequent to extirpation of lentigo maligna melanoma of right temple. At time of slough of zinc chloride fixative, exuberant granulation bed is already formed. **B,** Within 10 days granulation tissue contraction has already occurred. Compare size of wound to that in **A.** Epidermization is just beginning at wound edge.

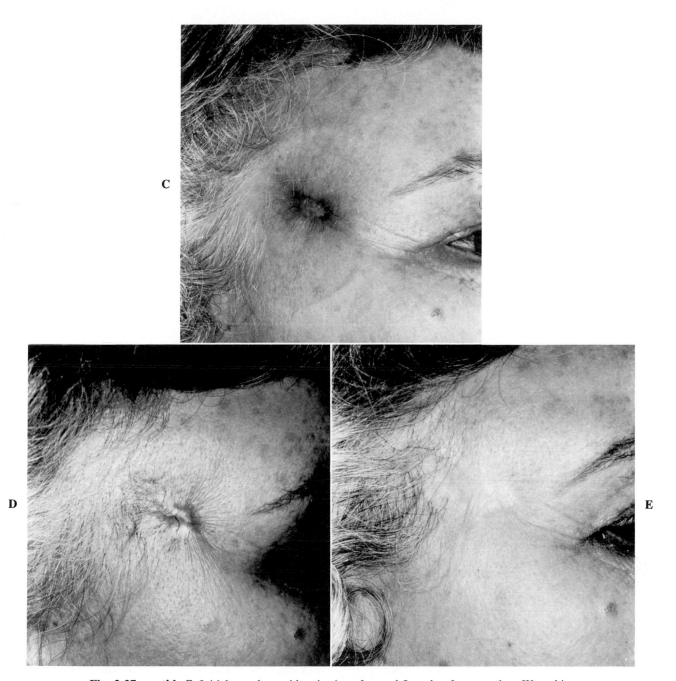

Fig. 2-27, cont'd. C, Initial complete epidermization of wound 5 weeks after operation. Wound is erythematous because of increased vasculature of underlying tissue. Note that there are many ingrowing, dilated vessels from wound edges visible through epidermis. **D,** Initial flat scar becomes hypertrophic as contraction process continues despite complete epidermization of wound (shown 3 months after surgery). Note increased prominence of tension lines surrounding wound. This process of continued contraction may persist for 1 to 3 months after epidermization. Patient experiences sensation of ''drawing,'' or tightening of wound. **E,** With time (6 months to 1 year after surgery), wound scar flattens out, caused by countertraction of surrounding muscles and skin. This relaxation of scar is called retraction. Scar becomes hypopigmented but blends in well with surrounding skin.

The time contraction takes to occur was worked out empirically by Carrel[62-64] and mathematically by LeComte du Noüy.[282-284] In general these investigators found that the rate of contraction and the percentage of a wound closed by contraction are a function of wound size. The larger the wound, the faster the rate of contraction and the quicker the wound diminishes in size. As the wound progressively becomes smaller, the rate of closure becomes less (decreased slope of bottom curve in Fig. 2-26). In addition, contraction was found to play a comparatively greater role in larger wounds and a lesser role in smaller wounds. For instance, a large, 6 cm wound is closed to a third or a fourth of its original size by contraction alone, whereas a wound measuring approximately 3 cm is closed to half its original size.[62]

Wound contraction should be viewed not only within the context of the initial wound size but also relative to the size of a planned excision before cutting the skin. On excision of a full-thickness piece of skin, the resultant wound normally expands. Catty[66] performed an interesting experiment on human volunteers; 1×1 cm squares were tattooed on their forearms. On full-thickness excision of the squares, the wound expanded by one third. Subsequent healing by contraction resulted in a wound that was 20% to 25% smaller, but this was still larger than the originally marked 1×1 cm square.

As a wound contracts, if the skin is quite mobile as in animals and in some areas in humans, it transforms into a pyramidal scar with outwardly slanted sides rather than a scar with vertical sides (Fig. 2-13, C and D). That is, the skin is pulled over the deeper scar tissue to some extent.[44] The less mobile the skin, the less this phenomenon occurs. With subsequent relaxation of the contracted skin, this effect is less exaggerated.

Epidermization. The covering of a wound healing secondarily with epidermis from the skin edges begins usually after a wound has begun to contract and proceeds concomitantly with this process (upper curve in Fig. 2-26). Carrel[62] found that the rate of epidermization was inversely proportional to the size of the wound. In other words it usually is tardy if the wound is large but occurs much earlier if the wound is smaller. Carrel calculated the rate of epidermization and found that if the distance between the wound edges was more than 1.5 cm, the epidermis grew slowly. However, if the wound edges were less than 1 cm apart, the epidermis grew quickly.

Since wounds in human beings usually cannot completely heal by contraction, epidermization completes the closure that contraction fails to close (Fig. 2-27, C). As pointed out previously, the new epidermis that forms is not normal. It is loosely attached at first to the underlying connective tissue but in time adheres more firmly.

Many investigators use the time for complete epidermal closure as the end point of wound healing. However, this is hardly the completion of the healing process. As we shall see, significant events still occur once the epidermis is reconstituted over a wound.

It has been stated that once complete, epidermization stops the process of contraction.[62] This is not totally true. Contraction may continue for a month or two after the new epidermis covers a wound. This may result in scar hypertrophy and the sensation of pulling or drawing that patients experience (Fig. 2-27, D). With time this additional contraction relaxes, giving way to the next phase, the relaxation phase.

Relaxation. As just mentioned, subsequent to contraction (which ends after epidermization), there is a relaxation of the scar (Fig. 2-27, E). Sometimes the scar becomes hypertrophic during the contraction phase but flattens out with relaxation (also called "retraction"). This is partially the result of the counterforces of the surrounding skin and muscle groups opposing the forces generated by the contractile tissue in the wound. A measurement of the new epidermis at the end of the contraction phase shows that it actually expands in this phase of relaxation. Billingham and Medawar[40] call this expansion of the skin "intussusceptive growth."

Relaxation of the epidermis and dermis may occur at different times. The relaxation of the epidermis begins soon after epidermization has been completed and continues for 3 to 6 months. The relaxation of the dermis, however, does not occur until after contraction has ceased, which may not happen for 2 to 3 months after the wound has healed. Usually by 6 months the wound is fully relaxed.

Remodeling. After the wound healing is complete, all scars go through a remodeling phase, which lasts up to 6 months in some wounds but 2 years in many wounds. This process is particularly apparent with scars resulting from second intention healing. Remodeling involves changes in the collagen arrangement, the vascular content, and the overlying epidermis. The collagen arrangement becomes more stable with time in any scar, resulting in increased tensile strength. This arrangement of collagen is caused by the most efficacious alignment of collagen and the formation of stable crosslinks. The vasculature decreases in time, having outlived its usefulness. This is seen as a whitening of the scar. The epidermis also changes in time, becoming more firmly anchored to the underlying dermis, which has in turn become more securely organized.

In Carrel's curves for secondary intention wound healing (Fig. 2-26) several of the stages just mentioned are seen graphically. The contraction process is reflected in the top curve; this is a measurement of the total surface area of the wound, which includes both granulation tissue and the new epidermis. The bottom curve represents the surface area of granulation tissue alone. Therefore the difference between the upper and lower curves represents the surface area of new epidermis. As can be seen, the new epidermis appears

1 week after the wound occurs. It gradually proceeds to take over the function of closing the wound as the process of contraction (top curve) slows down at about 4 weeks (on February 26). At that point the upper curve flattens out, and the difference between the two curves gradually increases. Thus closure of the wound during the last 2 weeks is caused almost solely by new epidermis (represented by the difference between the two curves).

At about 4 weeks the wound (granulation surface and new epidermis) is at its smallest—about 38% of its initial size—but is still not completely healed. It takes another 2 weeks to complete closure of the wound, mostly by epidermization at this point. This final phase of wound closure is the slowest phase of the healing process.

At first the slopes of the curves for contraction (top curve) and granulation surface area (bottom curve) are relatively steep, but as the wound becomes smaller, the curves flatten out with the decreased rate of healing. Thus the rate of secondary intention healing is not linear but rather progresses exponentially.[282] It has been estimated that granulation tissue has to contract by 2% every 3 days to account for the observed contraction rate in large human wounds.[436] The wound healing reflected in the graph was complete in about 6 weeks, which in my experience is the average for most wounds over 2 cm.

On total wound closure the scar (new epidermis) covering the wound still measures about 38% of the initial wound size. However, there occurs a period of relaxation (retraction), which is seen by the scar's actual increase in size (top curve). The scar at 8 weeks measures 47% of the initial wound size and has relaxed about 26% from its size at 6 weeks. The process of relaxation may proceed for months.

Fig. 2-27 also illustrates the phases of healing by secondary intention. Initially granulation tissue fills the surgical wound (Fig. 2-27, *A*). Within a week after granulation has begun, epidermization is just beginning (Fig. 2-27, *B*). On total closure of the wound 5 weeks later, the epidermis is thin and appears erythematous (Fig. 2-27, *C*). The underlying blood vessels are proliferative at this point and may be seen through the overlying epidermis. The new epidermis is thin and loosely attached to the underlying tissue and therefore easily damaged. Within the next few months the scar continues to contract, causing hypertrophic scar tissue despite epidermal coverage (Fig. 2-27, *D*). Within a year after the surgery the wound relaxes, flattens out, and becomes white, as the vascular hyperplasia recedes (Fig. 2-27, *E*).

Location of contractile force

Three main theories attempt to explain the contraction of wounds and the location of forces capable of bringing the dermal wound edges toward one another: the push theory, the pull theory, and the picture frame theory. The push theory proposes that the tissue outside the wound pushes the wound edges together. However, Cuthbertson showed that if the skin of rats is tattooed in a grid fashion and a wound created on the center square, the lines parallel to the wound separate as contraction takes place.[88] Therefore the site of action of the contracting force is in the wound itself. This makes the push theory unlikely.

The pull theory proposes that the granulation tissue in the wound itself pulls the wound edges together. This pull from the granulation tissue was termed "granulous retraction" by Carrel.[62] This theory is consistent with the work of Cuthbertson[88] just mentioned. Other studies also support this theory. Abercrombie, James, and Newcombe[5] splinted full-thickness wounds in rabbits. This prevents wound contraction. When the splints are removed at 10 days, the wounds immediately contract. If the central granulation tissue is removed, contraction is prevented. Furthermore, if the central granulation tissue is isolated by incisions, the isolated tissue still contracts, bulging above the surface of the wound. These experiments have been confirmed by others using slightly different techniques.[297,502]

The picture frame theory proposes that the main force of contraction in a wound resides in a narrow band of connective tissue beneath the wound edge, which adheres to the base of the epidermis. This band of tissue moves with the skin edge as contraction proceeds. This theory was popularized by Watts, Grillo, and Gross in 1958.[167,168,481] These investigators, using guinea pigs, excised the central granulation tissue in contracting open wounds and found, contrary to other studies, that doing this did not seem to interfer with either the rate or extent of wound contraction. However, excision of the wound edge caused immediate retraction of the resultant wound edge and delayed subsequent contraction. Separation of the wound edge from the underlying tissue also inhibited contraction. Thus they concluded that the contractile apparatus was situated in a narrow zone along the wound margin and not in either the central granulation tissue or the peripheral skin tissue. Subsequent studies by other investigators[193,372] supported the picture frame theory by showing that incisions perpendicular to the "picture frame" caused a decrease in wound tension and a decreased rate of wound contraction.

Source of contractile force. Within granulation tissue there are three elements that can conceivably produce contractile forces: collagen, fibroblasts, and vascular tissue with smooth muscle cells. The possibility of collagen shortening being the main contractile force was proposed by Arey[16] and Majno.[312] However, the weight of current evidence is against such a theory. First, the amount of collagen in a granulating wound does not correlate with contraction.[3,168] Second, drugs known to interfere with collagen synthesis, such as β-aminopropionitrile (BAPN), do not affect wound contraction.[85] Third, the decreased collagen formation in wounds of vitamin C–deficient animals does not interfere with wound contraction.[4] Therefore collagen does not appear to play a central role in wound contraction.

The fibroblast has emerged as the main contractile force in wounds; this realization is a natural outgrowth of the recognition of this cell's importance in wound healing.[186] Fibroblast growth and multiplication are intimately connected with the development of a healing wound as it gains tensile strength. These cells were shown to arise from the connective tissue adjacent to the wound.[163] They migrate into the wound from this peripheral location, probably using fibrin strands for guidance and fibronectin for adherence. Fibroblasts undergo changes seen in electron microscopy, which differentiate them from fibrocytes. These changes indicate an active metabolic process and include the marked development of an endoplasmic reticulum (Fig. 2-19). The fibroblasts become the central architects for wound healing, synthesizing and excreting not only collagen fibrils but mucopolysaccharides and probably elastin as well.[473]

Fibroblasts in wounds are also known to take on other morphologic features, which are more compatible with a role as a contractile element in wounds.[332] A well-formed fibrillar system is seen on electron microscopy. In addition, other changes in the nucleus and cell surface occur (Fig. 2-28). These changes include nuclear deformation and cell surface differentiation.[145] The surface changes are similar to hemidesmosomes or maculae adherentes—structures that probably help to transmit the mechanical pull of the surrounding tissue. Since the fibrillar system in these specialized fibroblasts resembles the fibrils in smooth muscle cells, these "modified fibroblasts" are named myofibroblasts.[140] In rats these anatomic modifications in the fibroblasts become apparent usually between 7 and 21 days after wound creation, at the same time that contraction occurs.[144]

As early as 1956 it was realized that granulation tissue by itself was capable of contraction when exposed to certain chemicals.[200] This idea was expanded in 1971 by Majno,[314] Gabbiani,[143-145] and their coworkers. They reported the contraction of granulation tissue by exposure to vasopressin, bradykinin, or angiotensin. This contraction could be reversed by papaverine (Fig. 2-29). Since fibroblasts are the most common extravascular cells in connective tissue, they are the most likely candidates for generation of the contractile force. These investigators proposed that fibroblasts could modulate toward a cell type that morphologically and functionally resembled smooth muscle cells.[314,410] Since it was known that fibroblasts in vitro develop an extensive fibrillar system, it was proposed that this system is responsible for contraction. The idea that some fibroblasts behave as smooth muscle cells was further supported by the demonstration that actively contracting granulation tissue could be inhibited from contracting by the topical application of the smooth muscle antagonist thiphenamil (Trocinate).[309]

To make sure that the blood vessels were not partially responsible for contraction, or solely responsible instead of

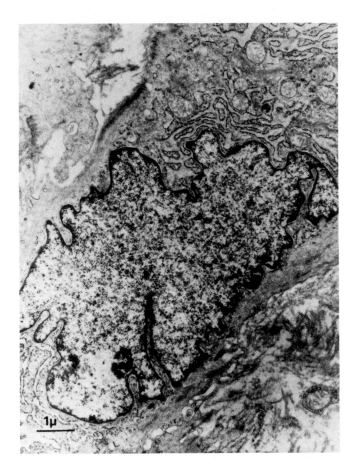

Fig. 2-28. Myofibroblast from granuloma pouch of rat. Note nuclear folds and indentations as well as bundles of densely packed filaments in cytoplasm (×13,000.) (From Gabbiani, G., and Montandon, P.: Int. Rev. Cytol. **48:**187, 1977.)

fibroblasts, Ryan et al.[409] investigated avascular connective tissue. They found that this tissue contracted pharmacologically in a manner similar to that of normal granulation tissue. Therefore, since this tissue contained no blood vessels but abundant fibroblasts, the fibroblast as the force responsible for contraction seemed logical.

The next bit of evidence linking the myofibroblast to contractile smooth muscle cells was immunologic.[144] Myofibroblasts were demonstrated to fluoresce with the use of serum containing anti–smooth muscle antibodies.[144] A more specific antiserum against actin filaments of smooth muscle cells, antiactin serum, has been tested on these modified fibroblasts as well and found also to result in positive fluorescence when the appropriate fluorescein-tagged antibodies were used.[443] Since the serum attaches to actin filaments in smooth muscle, the filaments in the myofibroblast are thought to be actin filaments as well. Thus the evidence for myofibroblasts being the contractile cells in granulation tissue is morphologic, pharmacologic, and immunologic. Myofibroblasts have also been

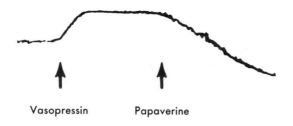

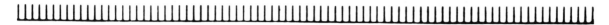

Fig. 2-29. Contraction of granulation tissue of 11-day-old skin wound with vasopressin. Subsequent relaxation induced with papaverine. (From Gabbiani, Reproduced from *The Journal of Experimental Medicine* **135:**719, 1972 by copyright permission of the Rockefeller University Press.)

noted in abundance in early hypertrophic scar tissue.[26]

The myofibroblast probably has a life cycle that correlates with the needs of the wound relative to contraction. The initial proliferation corresponds to the onset of wound contraction, whereas the decline in myofibroblast numbers signifies a lessening of tissue contractility. This life cycle may also be related to the natural cycle of cell differentiation and dedifferentiation.[472] In other words the myofibroblast ''turns into a pumpkin'' after a certain predetermined time, becoming a mundane fibroblast. In granulating wounds of rats, the myofibroblast population peaks at about 3 weeks and subsequently decreases over a 20-week period.[406] At its zenith the myofibroblast population comprises about 70% to 100% of the fibroblasts in a wound.[27,472] This persistence of myofibroblasts in wounds for 2 to 3 months after wound healing is compatible clinically with the continued scar contraction that occurs after epidermization and other remodeling changes, described earlier.

The cytoskeleton of the myofibroblast probably plays an important role in modulating the contractile forces in granulation tissue.[407] There are three systems of tubules and filaments to consider. The largest are the microtubules, which are 250 Å in diameter and are thought to help maintain the general shape of the cell. Treatment of cells with colchicine leads to loss of microtubules and cell shape.

The second system is comprised of filaments measuring about 100 Å in diameter. These filaments are seen on spreading cells in culture and are probably involved with intracellular transport.

A third type of intracellular system is the microfilaments, 60 Å in diameter. Microfilaments appear to be concerned with cell movement and are associated with membrane ruffling at the leading edge of cell movement. In myofibroblasts these microfilaments are actinlike protein.

Thus myofibroblasts have the machinery for either motility or contraction. Whether they are mobile is a matter for speculation, but the fact that they are responsible for wound contractile forces is fairly well accepted. The myofibroblast

is thought to anchor itself either to collagen or fibrin through small anchoring strands: myofibroblast-anchoring strands (MASs)[27] (Fig. 2-30). Myofibroblasts may also attach themselves directly to other myofibroblasts by way of intercellular attachments such as desmosomes or tight junctions.[141] The MASs appear to be either collagen or fibronectin. Because of the presence of MASs, Baur and Parks hypothesize that the myofibroblasts migrate along structures to which they are attached, and that the migration is responsible for wound contraction.[27] Moreover, these investigators feel that MASs become a focal point of collagen extrusion from myofibroblasts and intrusion into collagen fibrils.

Certain proteins in saliva may be important in facilitating wound contraction in animals. Epidermal growth factor (EGF) is one factor previously discussed in the section on epidermal resurfacing of wounds. Another protein recently isolated from saliva and shown to accelerate wound contraction in mice is nerve growth factor (NGF). NGF is a 116,000–molecular weight protein secreted in saliva; it has been purified from the submandibular gland of the mouse. Animals that have been sialoadenectomized have been shown to heal their wounds more slowly than normal animals. When NGF was applied to a group of animals that had been sialoadenectomized, wound contraction occurred at a normal rate.[293]

Factors influencing wound contraction

Granulating wounds do not heal at the same rate in each individual. Just as no two individuals are alike, neither are two wounds. Some of the modifying factors have already been discussed but are discussed here relative to secondary wound healing.

Age. Granulating wounds have been found to contract faster in young laboratory animals[41] and young soldiers[282,283,284] compared to their older counterparts. The data of LeComte du Noüy[284] are shown in Fig. 2-31. The reasons for this phenomenon are unclear but may be related

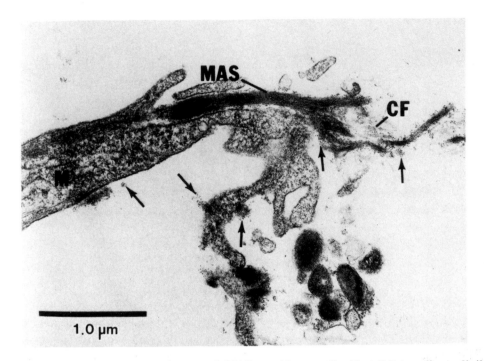

Fig. 2-30. Myofibroblast-anchoring strand *(MAS)* attaching myofibroblast *(M)* to collagen fibrils *(CF)* in a granulating wound. *Arrows,* ferritin-labeled antihuman fibronectin IgG. (×35,000.) (From Baur, P.S.: J. Trauma **23:**853, 1983.)

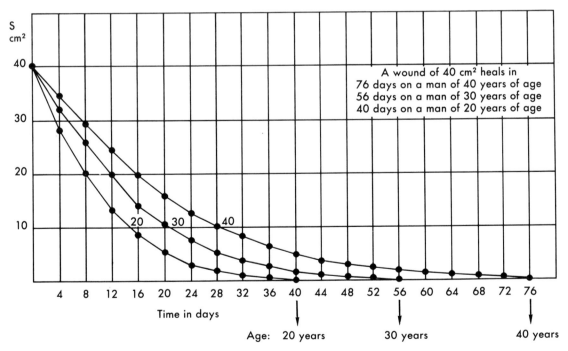

Fig. 2-31. Rate of healing of granulating wounds as function of age. *S,* Surface area. (From LeComte du Noüy, P.: Biological time, New York, 1937, Methuen & Co.)

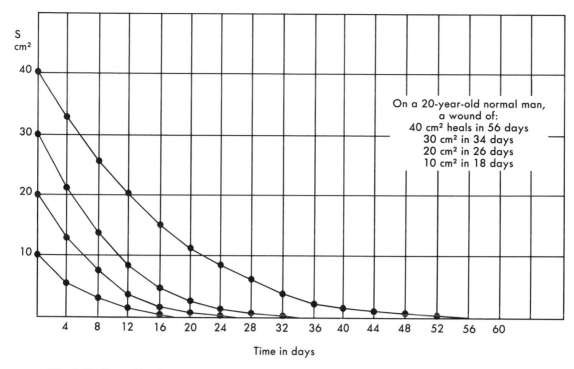

Fig. 2-32. Rate of healing of granulating wounds as function of initial wound size. *S*, Surface area. (From LeComte du Noüy, P.: Biological time, New York, 1937, Methuen & Co.)

to the decrease in fibroblast turnover with age.

Size of wounds. The larger the wound, the faster is the rate of contraction compared to that of smaller wounds.[64,440] The data on calculations of the healing rate for different size wounds that were allowed to heal by second intention in man are shown in Fig. 2-32. As one can see, the smaller wounds heal in less time, but the rate of healing is faster for larger wounds. In other words a wound one quarter the size of another heals in about one third the time instead of one quarter the time. Also illustrated in Fig. 2-32 is the fact that as the size of the wound decreases, the rate of healing slows.

Carrel points out in regard to the size of wounds that the law discovered by Spallanzani for the tails of salamanders holds equally well for human wounds.[62] Spallanzani found that if the tail of a salamander is cut off near its base, the new part grows faster than if its tail is cut off near the tip. The general law of regeneration is that the rate of regeneration is proportional to the work to be done. Therefore for human wounds, the larger the wound is, the faster is the regeneration rate.

Epidermization also appears to be related to the size of a wound, but in an inverse manner.[62] If the size of the wound is large, the epidermis grows slowly. If the wound is small (less than 1 cm), the epithelium quickly migrates. Thus small wounds epidermize quickly and contract little.

Because a larger wound contracts more readily than a smaller wound, the resultant scar formation for a larger wound is proportionately less than for a smaller wound.[62]

Depth. Wounds that are superficial, such as defects from dermabrasion, heal almost exclusively by epidermization. Granulation may be minimal in wounds from donor sites of split-thickness skin grafts, but contraction does not occur with such wounds. Wounds deep in the reticular dermis or below have elements of both granulation and contraction. However, if such wounds are primarily closed, the epidermal coverage is so rapid that the need for contraction is precluded. Nevertheless, some element of contraction may well exist for such wounds if the wound edges separate, and the phase of relaxation may occur if such wounds are under much tension. The latter is seen clinically as a spread scar.

Shape. Much has been written concerning the influence of a wound's shape on subsequent healing by granulation and contraction. Hippocrates noted that circular wounds healed more slowly than wounds of other shapes.[313] Paré[360,481] made the same clinical observation on the battlefield and stated, "A round ulcer does not heal, unless it is drawn into another shape." More modern researchers have produced data from animal studies to support the view that round ulcers heal more slowly.[41]

McGrath and Simon[321] investigated the effect of wound geometry on wound healing in rats. They found that square and circular wounds healed in the same time. In an attempt to reconcile their data with centuries of clinical observation, they suggest that a square, being larger in perimeter than a circle, actually contracts at a faster rate.

My own clinical experience is that the healing of round lesions does not necessarily take longer than wounds of other shapes. Round wounds on fixed surfaces—such as the ear cartilage, where contraction plays a small role in wound healing—do heal more slowly than other wounds, probably because the epidermis must make a greater contribution than normally required. Fig. 2-16 shows healing of a nearly round lesion on the forehead. The time of healing was 6 weeks, average for healing of lesions this size on the face. There were no problems.

Shape plays a role in the healing rate of wounds, but it is not a simple issue. Henshaw and Mayer proposed the concept of the "greatest inscribed circle."[190] If one considers two wounds of the same area but differing shape, for instance a square and a rectangle, the rectangle heals faster. This is because if one draws a circle inside each structure, the rectangle will have the smaller circle. These investigators found that the time for full healing was directly proportional to the radius of this circle, because the radius is the farthest distance that epidermis needs to grow before the wound area is completely covered. It is critical to define the size of the circle being studied. If the circle has the same area that a square has, it is larger than the greatest inscribed circle in the square. Thus its healing is slower.

Location. Wounds allowed to heal by secondary intention do so against the forces of the surrounding skin. Therefore the position of the lines of maximal and minimal skin tension relative to the wound determines the resultant scar.[454,480] In general a greater amount of contraction occurs perpendicular to the lines of maximal tension and parallel to the lines of minimal tension. This is illustrated in Figs. 2-15 and 2-16. Both of those wounds resulted from extirpation of recurrent basal cell carcinomas and were allowed to heal by granulation, contraction, and epidermization. Note that the wound on the forehead (Fig. 2-16, *A*) healed with an elliptic scar with its long axis oriented parallel to the crease lines (Fig. 2-16, *B*), the lines of maximal tension. The wound on the neck also healed parallel to the maximal tension lines (Fig. 2-15, *B*). Because of the greater laxity of skin in the neck, perhaps caused by the underlying platysma muscle, the resultant scar looks as though the wound has been primarily sutured. The wound on the forehead, however, healed with a wider scar because the skin is not nearly so mobile, and therefore epidermization plays a greater role here.

It should not be forgotten that the contraction of skin in one direction frequently results in expansion or at least relaxation in another direction.[454] This lateral expansion usually diffuses itself slowly and thus is not clinically evident. Consider, for instance, a round wound on the arm. If it is sutured primarily, it has dog ears on each end, seen as the expansion of skin perpendicular to the direction of closure. If such a wound is allowed to heal by itself, dog ears are not evident, despite the fact that there is expansion at the lateral ends of the long axis of the resultant scar.

Pathologic modifications. Slight infection or either chemical or mechanical irritation appears to shorten the lag period for contraction of open wounds.[63] However, once contraction has begun, significant bacterial proliferation slows or even impairs total epidermization.[64] The critical number for open wounds on the head and neck appears to be 40,000 colonies of *Staphylococcus aureus* per square centimeter. With more than this number of organisms, total wound epidermization is slowed or prevented.

Skin grafts. Full-thickness skin grafts stop contraction once it has begun, whereas split-thickness skin grafts do not.[41,96] Therefore if a split-thickness skin graft is to be placed on a wound, it should be done within a few days after the wound is created; otherwise contraction inevitably occurs.

The presence of the whole dermis in a graft is considered to be the critical factor acting to inhibit contraction.[96,258] Perhaps a full-thickness skin graft somehow prevents myofibroblasts from developing and thus prevents these cells from effecting contraction. Once a full-thickness graft is placed onto a granulating wound, the collagen content in the wound decreases as well as the collagenase activity. Therefore the decrease in collagen is probably caused by a decrease in collagen synthesis.[96]

Occlusion. Full-thickness wounds left uncovered have been observed to begin contraction sooner than if they are kept covered.[41,437] Zahir[502] feels that loss of moisture provides a powerful force for the movement of skin edges in a wound healing by secondary intention. If a wound in a guinea pig was kept moist when splinted, it contracted when the splint was removed and the wound allowed to dry out; however if a wound was allowed to dry out while splinted, it hardly contracted when the splints were removed. This initial greater decrease in wound size with dehydration does not mean the wound heals any sooner.

Other investigators claim that occlusion of full-thickness wounds leads to faster contraction and even less scarring.[297,496] Lindquist[297] found that in rats most rapid contraction and epidermization occurred with vaseline. Dry dressings or lanolin caused a significant decrease in the rates of both contraction and epidermization.

Perhaps the most instructive study was that of Knudsen and Snitker.[264] They compared punch biopsy sites in humans matched by location for healing time. One half the biopsy sites were allowed to scab—no dressing was used. The remainder of the biopsy sites were dressed with Telfa dressings. There was no difference between healing times of these two types of wound care. Similar findings have also been noted in comparable animal experiments[435]; scab formation in full-thickness wounds had little effect on the overall rate of wound contraction. Therefore for full-thickness wounds, occlusion may not necessarily hasten healing.

I prefer an occlusive dressing because in general the patients are more comfortable than if a scab is allowed to form on full-thickness wounds with significant tissue loss. In addition, bacteria are kept to a minimum; they are sometimes able to proliferate better underneath crusts. Furthermore, tissue loss due to dehydration is minimized.

BIOMECHANICS OF THE SKIN AND WOUND HEALING

Skin may be defined by its physical properties, such as its ability to stretch or to resist rupture. These physical properties change with scar tissue formation, usually for the worse. Scar tissue in general is stiff and relatively inelastic and thus frequently results in impaired function. The reparative process of wound healing, although essential to all living creatures, is still imperfect, particularly in humans. Complete restoration of normally functional tissue does not occur after wounding. This is probably related to the inability of scar tissue to reduplicate exactly the architecture of normal skin.

Biochemical properties of normal skin

If one pinches and picks up the skin, one gets a feeling for (and can thus estimate) the amount of skin tension and its ability to be stretched in a given area. This skin tension and extensibility show obvious anatomic and personal distinctions, varying with age and different states of disease, such as dehydration or obesity. The degree of skin extensibility and tension is important because it markedly affects the type and size of scar tissue that eventuates from a wound.

Skin is best characterized biomechanically as a viscoelastic structure. When stretched it demonstrates an elastic component and a nonelastic (viscous) component. These properties are caused mainly by the connective tissue (dermal) components, which demonstrate both viscous and elastic properties. Simplistically viewed the elastic property is related to the collagen and elastic fibers, whereas the viscous component is related to the ground substance. The viscoelastic forces are not evenly and equally distributed in all directions, thus explaining the variations in tension at different angles to any given point in the skin.

It is convenient to view skin behavior by using the Maxwell model[326] (Fig. 2-33). The elastic component is represented by the spring and the viscous component by the plunger. As the two ends of the model are pulled apart, the spring expands, and the plunger moves as well but more slowly. When released, the spring and plunger move in opposite directions.

The viscoelastic properties of the skin expressed with this model predict and explain certain time-dependent features seen clinically with skin stretching. For instance, the length of time the skin is stretched or a force is applied influences or changes the force required or the stretched length.[148] These properties are spoken of as stress relaxation and creep. *Stress relaxation* occurs when skin is sudden-

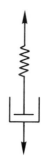

Fig. 2-33. Maxwell model, demonstrating cutaneous viscoelastic behavior.

ly stretched to a new position and held there indefinitely. The force required to keep it there decreases with time. *Creep* occurs when a given force is applied to skin and continues to be applied. The skin increases its extension with time.

In the model, as the ends are stretched suddenly *(arrows)* and held in the new position for an indefinite period of time, the spring is immediately stretched to the new position; but as the more slowly moving viscous component (the plunger) comes into action, it relaxes the tension generated between the spring and the stretching force. Thus less force is required to maintain the two ends in the new position because stress relaxation has occurred.

If a certain stretching force is applied to the model and maintained continuously at a certain level, the spring immediately stretches, but with time the plunger moves also and greater stretch occurs (creep). These two properties, stress relaxation and creep, help to explain the stretch of skin seen with staged excisions of lesions or the expanded abdominal skin of pregnant women.

Hooke's law, defined by Hooke in 1678, applies to materials that are elastic or partially elastic, such as skin—that is, materials that have the capacity to return to their normal shapes once a deforming force is removed. Algebraically, Hooke's law may be written as follows:

$$S = kE$$

S is the stress applied, E the extension, and k the proportionality constant (the coefficient of elasticity). This law states a proportional relationship between stretch *(E)* and force *(S)* when the force is not beyond the elastic limit, which would cause injury to the material. Unlike a spring, however, skin is more than just elastic. Since it has a viscous component, it does not obey Hooke's law in a linear relationship. Nevertheless, it is still helpful to use Hooke's law to measure certain physical characteristics of skin.

When discussing a tissue system such as skin, stress is defined as the force per unit of cross-sectional area.[242] The strain (extension) is the change in length $(L_1 - L_0)$ compared to the original length (L_0).[326] Therefore these may be

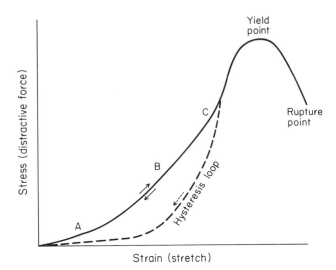

Fig. 2-34. Stress-strain curve for skin. Points *A*, *B*, and *C* are explained in text.

written as follows:

$$\text{Stress (S)} = \frac{\text{Force}}{\text{Cross-sectional area}} = \frac{F}{A}$$

$$\text{Strain (E)} = \frac{\text{Elongation}}{\text{Original length}} = \frac{L_1 - L_0}{L_0}$$

With Hooke's law, one arrives at the following:

$$\frac{F}{A} = k\frac{L_1 - L_0}{L_0}$$

Using Hooke's law and applying it to the study of a piece of skin, as a force is applied to a particular cross-sectional area to stretch the skin, a certain amount of elongation takes place. If the force is released, the skin returns to its original length. This can be seen graphically in Fig. 2-34. As the force is increased to a certain point (the yield point), the skin begins to break and collagen fibers rupture microscopically. If the skin is released at this point it does not return to its original length, as it did before. When the skin is stretched beyond the yield point, total visible tissue separation (rupture) occurs.

The force at the time of visible rupture (the rupture point) is used to measure skin or wound "strength." The force at the rupture point is less than the force at the yield point. Therefore use of the rupture point force gives an underestimate of the actual maximal strength (the force at the yield point) of a piece of tissue.[294]

Tensile strength is the ability of tissue of a given cross-sectional area to resist rupture when a force is applied. Usually the term is used loosely to mean the tensile strength at rupture in the tissue. Tensile strength is measured as the greatest longitudinal forces a material can bear without tearing apart. As just seen, tensile strength at rupture is slightly less than tensile strength at the yield point. In addition, it should be emphasized that the forces must be applied to a certain cross-sectional area of tissue. Tensile strength is thus measured in pounds/in² or kg/cm² or g/mm². In some earlier studies cross-sectional area of tissue was not taken into account, and authors were thus measuring breaking strength (defined later) rather than tensile strength and using the term *tensile strength* inappropriately.[132] Another common error was to assume that the rate of application of the force made no difference in the tensile strength. This is a false assumption, as we shall see.

Tissue can be described in terms not only of strength but also of *extensibility*. The longest length a material can be stretched without breaking is known as the elongation at break. This is related to how stretchable a tissue is and is expressed as the modulus (coefficient) of elasticity. For instance, compared with normal tissue, scars are less elastic. Therefore scar tissue is less extensible and has less elongation at break than normal tissue.

Breaking strength refers to the ability to resist rupture and is measured by the least force necessary to disrupt tissue or a wound of a given length. Taking cross-sectional area into account is not necessary. From a practical point of view, breaking strength is of more value to the clinician. Tensile strength is of value for a scientific analysis of biomechanical strength. Breaking strength is a function of the length of the incision, the skin thickness, and how the wound is put together; tensile strength is not.[348] Breaking strength varies in different areas of the body, but tensile strength tends to be the same, since variations in skin thickness are taken into account.

In human skin the collagen fibers are arranged somewhat randomly in a multidirectional manner; however, more fibers tend to be oriented in a longitudinal direction, which is parallel to Langer's lines or crease lines.[205] Thus the strength of the collagen network is parallel to the direction of Langer's lines or maximal skin tension lines. Skin tends to behave as a membrane that is under more tension in one direction than another. This explains Langer's findings of elliptically shaped defects when puncturing the skin of cadavers with a round awl. The round holes became converted into elliptic defects because the pull is greater parallel to the long axis of the ellipse.

Ragnell[386] excised circular portions of skin from the trunk and extremities and subjected them to forces in various directions perpendicular and parallel to Langer's lines. His results are shown in Fig. 2-35. Note that if a force is applied parallel to Langer's lines, less extension of the skin occurs, compared to a force perpendicular to Langer's lines. In general this investigator found that the forces of tension were a third greater along Langer's lines than perpendicular to these lines on the trunk. Therefore scars oriented along Langer's lines are under more tension along the long axis of the scar but under less tension perpendicular to the scar.

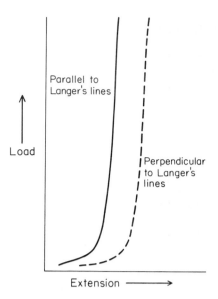

Fig. 2-35. Comparison of extensibility (tensibility) of human skin of trunk in relation to Langer's lines. (Modified from Ragnell, A.: Plast. Reconstr. Surg. **14:**317, 1954.)

Returning to our stress-strain curve (Fig. 2-34), one sees that there are different phases, which correspond histologically with the rearrangement of the collagen fibers as normal skin is stretched.[51,133,149] During the first phase *(A)* the curve is rather horizontal. There is relatively greater extension of tissue with a small load. The collagen fibers orient themselves to be almost parallel to the applied force, and the epidermis flattens. This occurs no matter which direction the skin has been stretched. In the second phase *(B)* the curve begins to move up. This is a transitional phase during which more fibers are oriented more parallel to the applied force, and fluid is displaced from the meshwork of fibers. The collagen fibers become compacted; this results in a decrease in volume of tissue and an increased stretch. Finally a third phase *(C)* is reached, at which the curve becomes very steep. A large increase in load is necessary for even a short increase in length. This last phase is thought to be caused by the elongation of the collagen fibers themselves. The epidermal cells are pulled progressively flatter. When the skin is released, elastic fibers in the skin as well as within blood vessels help to return the skin to its normal length and shape.

If a piece of skin is repeatedly stretched and relaxed (load cycled), two deviations from the typical stress-strain curve occur. First, a hysteresis loop develops—that is, the unloading curve becomes different from the loading curve (Fig. 2-34). Second, the first few curves during loading are not exactly the same until enough loading and unloading has occurred. This may be caused by the variations in collagen alignment during the early loading cycles.[150]

Normal skin may adapt to stretching in a number of

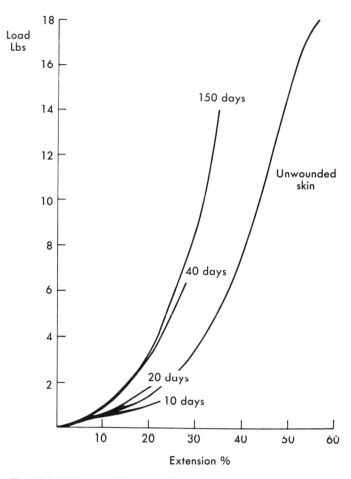

Fig. 2-36. Stress-strain curve for rat wounds of different ages compared to normal unwounded skin. (From Forrester, J.C., Zederfeldt, B.H., and Hunt, T.K.: J. Surg. Res. **9:**207, 1969.)

ways, depending on the force of the pull and on the laxity of the skin and surrounding tissue. If skin is stretched acutely and with enough force, it blanches. This occurs because blood vessels are narrowed by extension. If the stretch is maintained long enough, the prolonged vascular impairment may result in necrosis of the skin, as sometimes occurs with skin flaps. Excessive tension may also result in tears in the dermis as collagen bonds are ruptured and striae result. Skin may also adapt to stretching, since stress relaxation occurs over time. This hopefully is the case with staged excisions.

Scar tissue behaves differently from normal skin when stretched. Early in wound healing (after 10 days in rats), Forrester, Zederfeldt, and Hunt[133] found an increased extensibility of scar tissue compared with that of normal tissue with any given load (Fig. 2-36). They interpreted this to mean that there is no firm orientation of collagen fibers at that point. This is substantiated in scanning electron microscopy, with which collagen fibrils were seen at that point to be thinner and less discrete than those found in normal

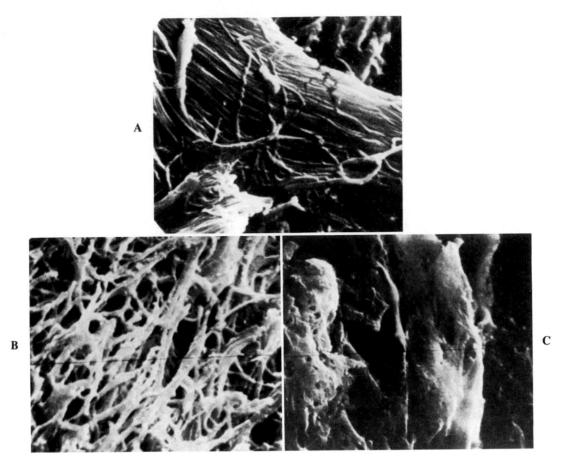

Fig. 2-37. Scanning electron microscopy of collagen in skin and wounds. **A,** Normal skin. Collagen fiber composed of many fibrils. (× 10,000.) **B,** Sutured wound at 10 days. Collagen fibrils predominate in haphazard array. (× 10,000.) **C,** Wound at 100 days. Collagen in irregular masses. (× 3000.) (From Forrester, J.C., et al.: Reproduced by permission from *Nature* **221**:373. Copyright © 1969. Macmillan Journals Limited.)

skin[134] (Fig. 2-37, *B*). They also lie quite haphazardly. At 20 days there is less extensibility than in normal skin. The normal architecture of collagen is not reestablished, but an orientation in the direction of pull appears. Collagen bundles in scars eventually form large irregular masses (Fig. 2-37, *C*). Therefore final scar tissue is less extensible than normal tissue and breaks sooner. Tensile strength measured in cutaneous scars is always less than normal skin in humans even after many years.

MEASURED STRENGTH OF WOUNDS AND SCARS

Soon after a wound is sutured, healing begins. One may measure the strength of the wound at various times during healing as well as after healing, when scar formation occurs. Usually strength is measured and expressed by tensile strength or breaking strength.

Tensile strength has already been discussed and defined as the force per unit of cross-sectional area that is neces-

sary to disrupt tissue. However, measurements of tensile strength are imprecise and subject to error.[326] Ideally a dumbbell-shaped piece of tissue of uniform length and width is clamped at both ends, and the skin is stretched at a given rate and temperature. However, some slippage of the clamped ends almost always occurs. The rate of stretch needs to be precisely defined, since different rates of stretch influence the tensile strength. In general the greater the rate of stretch, the higher the force necessary to lengthen tissue, mainly because of the viscous forces in skin. Temperature also affects tensile strength of tissue, since viscosity tends to increase with decreasing temperature.

Many measurements of wound or scar strength have been done in animals and only a few in humans. There is great variation in the wound strength between animals within one species, between species, in animals with multiple wounds, and between different tissues on the same animal.[45,99,214] Therefore wound strength measurements must be extrapolated from animals to humans with extreme caution.

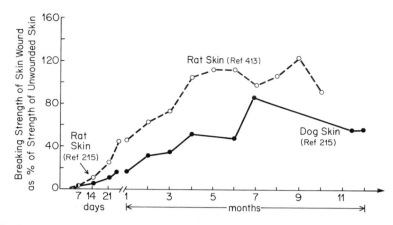

Fig. 2-38. Comparison of breaking strength gain in skin wounds of dogs and rats. (Data from Howes, E.L., Harvey, S.C., and Hewitt, C.: Arch. Surg. **38**:934, 1939; and Sandberg, N.: Acta Chir. Scand. **126**:294, 1963.)

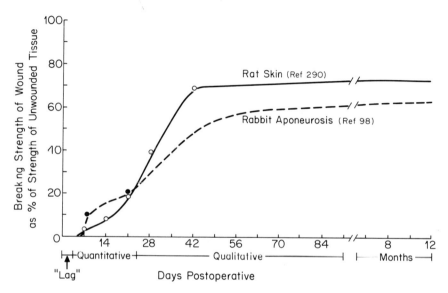

Fig. 2-39. Breaking strength gain in rat skin and rabbit aponeurosis as function of time. (Data from Levenson, S.M., et al.: Ann. Surg. **161**:293, 1965; and Douglas, D.M.: Br. J. Surg. **40**:79, 1952.)

Strength of wounds or scars is frequently expressed as a percentage of normal (unwounded) tissue strength or, less frequently, as a percentage of ultimate wound or scar strength. The former may be misleading because the unwounded tissue strength may vary from one region of the body to another and from one animal to another. In addition, the normal tissue strength of the skin may vary with the age of the animal.[290] Howes, Harvey, and Hewitt[214] found that in some animals (for instance, rats, rabbits, and guinea pigs) a wound regained or even exceeded the breaking strength of normal tissue, whereas in other animals (such as dogs), the normal breaking strength was never regained (Fig. 2-38). In general the repair of tissue to prewounding strength is inversely proportional to the strength of the wounded tissue or the hydroxyproline content of the

skin.[290] Where the strength of normal tissue is low initially, as in rats, a wound heals with a scar of normal strength. However, in humans the inherent tensile strength of normal tissue is so great that only a moderate return to prewound tensile strength is possible.

The breaking strength measurements for cutaneous wounds in rats and aponeurotic wounds in rabbits during the first 80 days are shown in Fig. 2-39. There are three phases. An early ("lag") phase is almost flat. This occurs during the first few days of wound healing, as collagen begins to be laid down and the wound has little if any appreciable strength. Sutures are necessary to maintain wound edge apposition. At 7 to 20 days there is a marked increase in breaking strength, greater in aponeurosis than in skin, and the curve deflects sharply up. Fibroblasts proliferate and lay

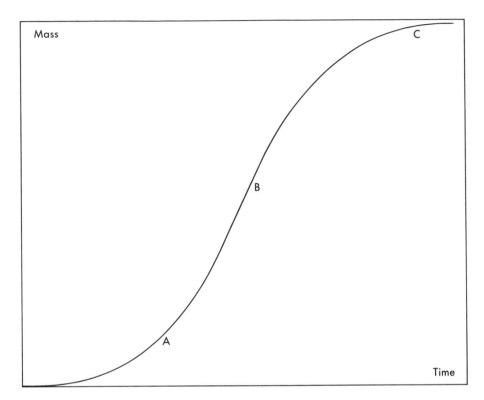

Fig. 2-40. General growth curve. *A,* Lag phase; *B,* growth phase; *C,* leveling-off phase (Modified from Harvey, S.C.: Arch. Surg. **18**:1227, 1929.)

down collagen, which begins to be organized.[104] This increase in wound strength continues until 40 to 50 days, at which time the curve again flattens out, as collagen is laid down at a lesser rate, and wound strength increases more slowly over time. This late increase in breaking strength is caused by better intermolecular links and stronger collagen bundles.

The early gain in wound strength as a function of time (shown particularly in rabbit aponeurosis 0 to 14 days after wounding in Fig. 2-39) resembles the general growth curve of many biologic processes, for instance, the curve for the multiplication of unicellular organisms such as bacteria[185] (Fig. 2-40). This curve is also seen with many monomolecular autocatalytic chemical reactions. There is a latent period or lag phase, during which the bacteria must synthesize enough proteins and accumulates energy for growth, followed by phases of sharp growth and then leveling-off.

The initial phase of apparent inactivity was called the "lag" phase by Harvey.[185] However, we currently know that there is much metabolic activity and proliferation of cells occurring during this phase. Fibroblast proliferation is found experimentally to peak 3 to 5 days after wounding,[307] although a much earlier increase in this cell population has been detected.

The production and organization of collagen in wounds occur in two separate but overlapping phases, which can be measured by and correlated with tensile strength changes.

The *quantitative* phase of collagen deposition correlates with the rapid rise in tensile strength. Here an increase in strength is correlated with an increase in the amount of collagen produced,[104] which may also be measured by the increase in hydroxyproline content.[99,308] This period lasts for 1 to 2 weeks but varies with the animal studied (Fig. 2-39). In this phase collagen fibers are poorly cross-linked between fibrils or fibers. Roughly 10% to 30% of the ultimate wound strength is attained at this point.[103,131] This period of delay in cross-linking may be the body's way of buying time so the organizational pattern of collagen fibers may be rearranged into a more functional pattern before being fixed irretrievably in the next phase.

The *qualitative* phase of collagen organization occurs from about 1 month after wounding until 3 to 4 months or indefinitely. In this phase the amount of collagen (measured by hydroxyproline content) does not increase appreciably, but the strength of wounds does[100,310] (Fig. 2-41). Therefore the amount of collagen does not correlate with the increase in breaking or tensile strength[236] Measurements of hydroxyproline during this phase do not show the marked increase found earlier during the quantitative phase, but the tensile or breaking strength rises nevertheless.[310] This disparity is attributed to the formation of stable intermolecular cross-links between collagen molecules and results in a more gradual increase in wound tensile strength.[103,412] Besides the formation of intermolecular cross-links, this slower, more gradual

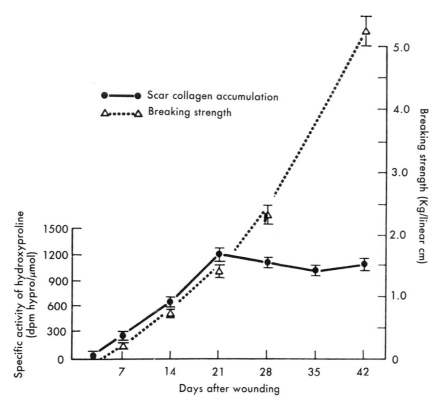

Fig. 2-41. Collagen accumulation in scars compared to breaking strength. (From Madden, J.W., and Peacock, E.E., Jr.: Ann. Surg. **174:**511, 1971.)

increase in tensile or breaking strength may be caused by collagenous interaction with ground substance material, such as proteoglycans.

Indirect evidence for the differences between these two phases is the reaction of collagen to formalin.[290] Formalin fixation of skin results normally in an increase in tensile or breaking strength. This occurs because formalin causes more cross-linking to occur between collagen bundles. This effect of formalin is much greater during the quantitative phase, when cross-linking is minimal, than during the qualitative phase.

Other evidence for the differences between the quantitative and qualitative phases of collagen is thermal rupture temperature. As the qualitative phase is reached, it is more difficult to rupture wounds.[366] This is probably a reflection of the increase in intermolecular cross-links that occurs.

The solubility of collagen itself is also different in these two phases. The quantitative phase is characterized by an increase in soluble collagen, which is newly deposited and nonbonded and therefore extractable in saline. Later in the qualitative phase the soluble collagen content of the wound decreases to that of normal tissue.[133,363]

RATE OF GAIN OF WOUND AND SCAR STRENGTH

The rate of gain of strength in wounds or scars is very slow. A freshly healed wound that is only a few months old

over a boxer's eye can be easily reopened with only a slight glancing blow. Even after many years the strength of human scars is far less than normal tissue[99]; the architectural configurations of collagen formed in response to tissue tension are never as good as the original arrangements.

Douglas et al. measured the breaking strength of excised scars of various ages in both men and women and found that after 2 years the strength of scars was only 20% of normal and even at 12 to 13 years was 40% to 80% normal[99] (Fig. 2-42). One 36-year-old scar was only 64% of normal. Therefore a skin wound is weaker than intact skin for a long period of time and probably never regain normal skin strength.

Other investigators have measured tensile or breaking strength of wounds as a function of age in animals, including guinea pigs,[45,100] dogs,[45,217] rats,[133,290,412] and rabbits.[99,124,294,340] As mentioned already, one should only cautiously extrapolate such data to humans, particularly in view of the work just mentioned.[99] In a similar manner, the percentage of gain in breaking or tensile strength varies widely among animals (Fig. 2-38). For instance, the early phase of wound healing, in which there is a rapid rise in breaking strength (the quantitative phase of collagen), occurs from 4 to 10 days in guinea pigs,[45] but from 10 to 60 days in rabbits.[99] Similar differences are also noted among other animals during both the early and late phases of wound healing (Fig. 2-38). Some often-quoted data[98] show that

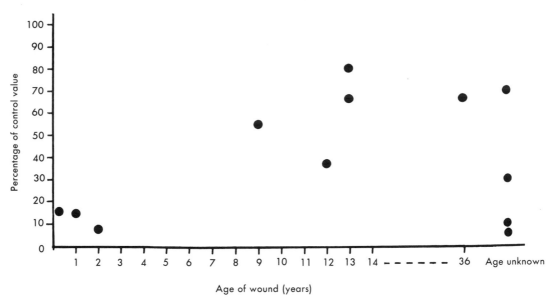

Fig. 2-42. Gain of breaking strength in human scars with time—measured postmortem and expressed as percentage of unscarred normal skin strength. Note that in first 2 years scars have less than 20% of normal (unwounded) tissue strength. Points on far right are from scars of unknown age. (From Douglas, D.M., Forrester, J.C., and Ogilvie, R.R.: Br. J. Surg. **56:**219, 1969.)

aponeurotic incisions in rabbits resulted in wounds in which breaking strength was about 20% of normal at 2 weeks, 60% to 80% of normal at 1 month, and 80% of normal strength in 1 year. Similar data were reported for healing wounds on rats.[290] Although rabbit aponeurosis and rat skin show similar gains in breaking strength compared to the normal control tissue, extrapolation of such data to man should be made cautiously. First, the available animal data show such wide variance that it is difficult to compare different studies from the same animal, let alone compare these studies with those on man. Some of the animals in Douglas' study had breaking strength measurements as low as 50% at 1 year, whereas other animals had values as high as 90%.[98] The curves in Fig. 2-39 represent only an average curve from the available data. Second, the rate of gain and ultimate gain of tensile or breaking strength appear to be related to how strong the tissue is initially. If unwounded tissue—for instance cutaneous tissue of the back—is very strong, the gain in wound strength is small on a percentage basis. If the tissue is relatively weak to begin with—for instance, rat skin—then the percentage gain is great. One can predict therefore that the percentage gain in man for wounds on the trunk is less than that in rabbit aponeurosis seen in Fig. 2-39, whereas wounds on human eyelids (where the skin is thin and weak have a greater percentage gain and more closely approximate the curves in Fig. 2-39.

FACTORS INFLUENCING WOUND AND SCAR STRENGTH
Age

Normal skin, as measured in cadavers, is more extensible in the young than the aged.[149] The breaking strength of wounds in older patients (older than 70 years) is less than in younger patients,[417] perhaps because older patients may produce less scar tissue that is stiff (and thus less extensible).[456]

Epidermis

The epidermis makes a contribution, albeit small, to the tensile strength of wounds. Initially the epidermis may well be one of the main forces holding a wound together, particularly in incisional wounds, where the epidermis may bridge the gap within the first 3 to 4 days.[357,404]

Dermis

The thickness of the dermis influences the tensile strength of skin. The skin of a boxer may become lacerated from a glancing blow around the eyes where the dermis is thin; however, the skin of the trunk has a thick dermis and is not easily ruptured. The tensile strength of scar tissue compared to normal tissue also varies with the thickness of the dermis, but inversely. The thicker the dermis, the less likelihood there is of scar tissue approximating the normal level of organization and strength.

Sutures

Sutures help to appose wound edges, thereby increasing the tensile strength and breaking strength of an incision. Sutures give a wound about 40% to 70% of the strength of unwounded tissue.[124,294] Contrary to popular belief,[212,340] if cutaneous sutures are left in place for 2 months, they increase the wound tensile strength about 30%.[294] That is, sutures do contribute to the strength of a wound even after initial wound healing has taken place in the first 2 to 3 weeks.

The type of cutaneous sutures influences the tensile strength. Sutures of catgut evoke an inflammatory response and produce wounds with less immediate tensile strength.[45] Paradoxically, tape-closed wounds have been found to have greater tensile strength than sutured wounds.[53] This has been ascribed to Wolff's law, which states that structure of tissue is altered to fit the functional demands.[136] Although this law was originally postulated in relation to the structure of bones, it is equally applicable to scar tissue. Tension in wounds results in the development of higher tensile strength and collagen fibers more suitably aligned to withstand the surrounding tissue tensions. Taped wounds are probably under more tension from the outset. The collagen fibers are thus under more force to become oriented along these lines of tension, creating stronger wounds.[135,136] Collagen fibers in taped incisions are found to be oriented almost parallel to the incision length. The collagen may be induced to organize and mature earlier and be more favorably aligned to withstand tension. However, taped wounds, though stronger, have been found to be less extensible,[132] perhaps because more scar tissue is produced.

Rate of strain

When coughing or straining, a patient may inadvertently cause a wound to dehisce. It is of some value, then, to understand the role of the rate of strain on tensile strength. The viscoelastic nature of skin results in a higher stress level for a given strain or stretch if the stretch is performed at a higher rate.[15] In other words, with a high rate of stretch, as with a cough, it takes more force to disrupt a wound than with a lower rate of stretch. However, rupture may still occur with less elongation because the viscous forces are larger with higher strain rates.[326]

Dehisced and resutured wounds

Wounds that are opened during the first week and resutured show a rapid gain in tensile strength, which actually exceeds the gain in strength of wounds that do not dehisce.[45] The older the wound is during the first week when disrupted, the greater is its tensile strength 3 days after resuturing.[61] This effect is thought to be caused by fibroblasts being mobilized and the production of collagen at the wound edges during the first few days after wounding. Pea-

cock[362] measured saline-extractable collagen from resutured wounds and found an earlier increase than that in primarily closed wounds. The rapid gain in tensile strength may be related also to organization and cross-linking of collagen molecules and not just the production of new collagen fibrils.

The chemically active zone of hydroxyproline production around wounds was most marked within 6 mm of the scalpel tract.[8] Therefore local excision of 5 to 10 mm of the wound margin abolishes the resuture effect. If the dehiscence and resuturing occur much later than 1 week, rapid increase in tensile strength is not seen, probably because of the demobilization of fibroblasts that has occurred by that time.

Delayed closure

A wound may be safely closed from 3 to 7 days after creation if no significant contamination exists. Such wounds do not show an increased incidence of dehiscence or infection.[426] Wounds closed by delayed closure rapidly gain tensile strength and within a few days have strength similar to control wounds that were created at the same time but sutured immediately. In one study wounds closed after 6 days did not gain tensile strength as rapidly but at about the same rate as if sutured primarily. Wounds closed after 6 days also tended to become infected.[425] Thus during the first 4 to 6 days the wound margins are prepared for closure, whether separated or apposed. Excision of these prepared edges abolishes the accelerated increase of tensile strength in the same way and for the same reasons as in wounds that are ruptured and resutured.

Occlusion

Rovee and Miller[404] showed that superficial wounds occluded with Saran Wrap had better breaking strength at 7 days than nonoccluded wounds had (Fig. 2-43). They suggest that this is caused by the earlier epidermal resurfacing and the thicker epidermis, which comes about earlier.

Ischemia

Wounds that are ischemic have a decreased tensile strength during the first few weeks, but then the tensile strength increases to a normal level at 1 month.[15]

Bacterial contamination

Contamination of wounds with nonpathogens, such as *Staphylococcus epidermidis,* makes little difference in the development of tensile strength.[45] However, pathogenic colonization of a significant degree prolongs the inflammatory phase of wound healing and perhaps results in additional scar tissue. If one measures infected wound tensile strength early, therefore, it is less than normal. If one checks the same wounds later, the tensile strength is greater than normal, with increased scar tissue.

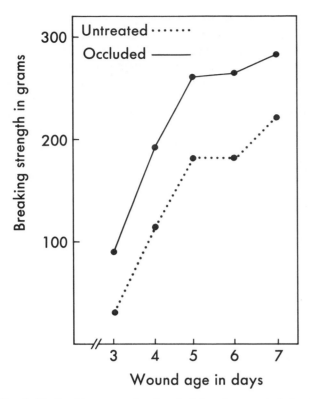

Fig. 2-43. Breaking strength of occluded and nonoccluded epidermal wounds as function of time. (From Rovee, D.T., and Miller, C.A.: Arch. Surg. **96:**43, 1968.)

SCARS

Every wound results in a scar, and any surgical procedure that begins with an incision must end with a scar. A scar remains for a lifetime; it grows older and matures with the individual. On the cutaneous surfaces, especially the face, scars are indelible signs of prior injury or surgery. The goal of the surgeon should be to minimize scar tissue as much as possible and to situate it as inconspicuously as possible. Very fine scars from well-performed surgical operations may be quite noticeable if unfavorably situated.

Superstitions and folklore of various cultures have attached meaning to certain scars. In Africa hypertrophic scars, or keloids, may be signs of beauty, whereas in the United States such growths are regarded as ugly. The Chinese regarded the bearer of smallpox scars as lucky; such scars showed that the individual had been fortunate enough to survive a commonly fatal disease. Scars from pinta used to bring a higher price for slaves because they reflected an immunity to it.[333]

When the full thickness of the dermis is injured, noticeable scar tissue results. Foerster and Jacques[129] made incisions at various levels in the skin of Berkshire pigs and showed that visible and microscopic scars were produced only when the full thickness of the dermis was incised. This implies that for scar formation more importance is attached to the skin layers penetrated than to the actual depth of penetration. Still, although this study is often quoted, actual depth of penetration does make a difference in the production of scar tissue. Curetting on the back (where the dermis is thick) can result in hypertrophic scars, even though one has injured only the top half of the dermis. Therefore the study by Foerster and Jacques cannot be completely extrapolated to man.

Scar tissue is biomechanically inferior to normal skin. Scar tissue has little elastin, so on deformation it does not reform its shape as easily. Although early scar tissue is more extensible than normal skin, after maturation it is less easily stretchable.[389] The strength of human scars determined by their tensile strength at rupture is always less than those of normal skin.[99]

Microscopically, collagen in scar tissue is oriented along the long axis of a scar, whether it is parallel to the crease lines or not.[205,336] In normal unscarred tissue, the collagen is arranged more haphazardly. This results in birefringence under polarized light seen with normal tissue but not with scar tissue[132,499] (Fig. 2-44). An additional reason for the lack of birefringence in scar tissue is the small caliber of the collagen fibers initially.[100]

Hypertrophic scars and keloids (Table 2-6)

Occasionally wounds do not result in flat scars but in raised scars. If the scar is elevated above the surface of the skin but confined within the boundaries of the wound, it is a hypertrophic scar. A keloid is a scar that extends not only above the surface of the skin but beyond the margins of the wound (Fig. 2-45).

Keloids are benign growths of connective tissue localized to the dermis.[34,269] The growth of connective tissue is thought to originate from the reticular dermis; histologically it is difficult to distinguish a keloid from a hypertrophic scar. Sometimes there are fingerlike extensions into the surrounding normal skin, which explains the origin of the name (from the Greek χηλη, meaning crab's claw). Early keloids are well vascularized, giving a red color, but eventually become white and avascular.

The etiology of keloids is unknown, although usually there is some history of preceding trauma or inflammation in the area. Keloids are more common in blacks and rare in those below 4 years of age or very old. In addition, true keloids do not form in the central face. Theories as to the pathogenesis of keloids have included histamine stimulation of fibroblasts,[467] immunologic mechanisms,[253] decreased vasculature,[253] increased melanocyte-stimulating hormone (MSH) activity,[269] foreign bodies,[315] or decreased collagen degradation.[132]

Histologically, collagen fibers in hypertrophic scars tend to orient the same way they do in normal scars: parallel to the long axis of the scars.[205,336] On scanning electron mi-

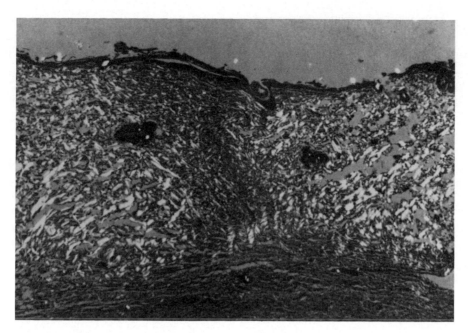

Fig. 2-44. A 100-day wound photographed under polarized light. Dermal wound collagen in center is not refractile compared to normal birefringence seen on each side. This lack of birifringence is thought to reflect the relatively organized structure of newly formed wound collagen. (From Dunphy, J.E., and Van Winkle, W., editors: Repair and regeneration, New York, 1969, McGraw-Hill Book Co. Reproduced with permission.)

TABLE 2-6

Comparison between normal scars, hypertrophic scars, and keloids*

	Appearance	Clinical progression	Behavior	Collagen amount	Collagen configuration	Collagen orientation	Collagen type	Glycos-amino-glycans	Hista-mine	Prolyl hydrox-ylase	Collage-nase
Normal scar	Flat	If slightly raised, flattens in few months	↓ Exten-sibility	N	Some fibrils small, hya-lin in 1-2 months	Parallel to long axis	↑ Type III	N or slight-ly ↑	N	↑	N
Hyper-tro-phic scar	Raised within scar borders	Progresses for few months, re-gresses in few years	↑ Exten-sibility	N	Fibrils large; hyalin late (months)	Parallel to long axis	↑ Type III	↑ (1.5-4 × N)	↑	↑↑	N
Keloid	Raised beyond scar borders	Progresses for many months, lasts many years or indefinitely	↑ Exten-sibility	N or ↑	Larger fibers; hyalin late (years)	Haphazard	↑ Type III	↑	↑	↑↑↑↑	↑

*N, Normal; ↑, elevated; ↓, decreased.

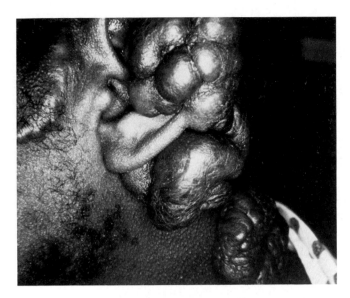

Fig. 2-45. Extensive keloid of ear of black man.

croscopy, hypertrophic scar collagen appears as a whorled pattern around a central mass or nodule; this was described by Larson et al.[276] to be like a hurricane viewed from high altitude. Collagen in keloids has little pattern.[205]

Mancini and Quaife[315] studied the progression of scars and keloids in patients, some of whom were known to have keloid-formation tendencies. They divided the evolution of scar tissue into fibrous and hyaline phases. During the fibrous phase the collagen fibers are relatively thin, and the scars and keloids appeared pink. As the vasculature regressed, the collagen became thicker and hyalinized, and the scars and keloids became white. For keloids the progression from the fibrous phase to the hyaline phase took much longer than it did for scars. Scars normally entered the hyaline phase in this study at about 35 days, whereas the keloids took months to years. It was also noted that keloids tended to be more vascularized earlier and more hyalinized later. Moreover, keloids tended to be pigmented.

Hypertrophic scars (compared to normal tissue) are characterized by an increased amount of glycosaminoglycans and water as well as type III collagen.[342] Therefore hypertrophic scars are partially produced by tissue swelling. The increase in glycosaminoglycans may result in firmer bonding of collagen fibers.

Hypertrophic scars and keloids are also known to contain higher levels of histamine than normal tissue and scar tissue. This may be related to the symptoms of pruritus experienced by many patients. Cultured fibroblasts from keloids were found to have some growth stimulated by histamine, and this effect could be suppressed with diphenhydramine.[467] It has previously been shown that histamine increases in skin wounds in rats and that the rates of healing can be increased by increasing the histamine-forming capacity of tissue.[244]

The itching or burning associated with keloids is most evident during the early fibroblastic phase, which may last months, and is consistent with the idea of histamine stimulation of fibroblasts.[315] I have noted an increased number of mast cells in scar tissue associated with previous therapy for skin cancers; such increased numbers of mast cells may be found in hypertrophic scars as well. An increase in mast cells is not seen in rat wounds, but the relevance of this to human wound healing is unknown.[371]

The surgical treatment of keloids and hypertrophic scars is described in later chapters. In addition to surgical treatment, the injection of steroids is widely used and accepted. The fluorinated antiinflammatory steroids, such as triamcinolone acetonide, have given good results.[251] Hydrocortisone is ineffective.[169] In 1966 an 88% regression of keloids with intralesional triamcinolone acetonide in doses ranging from 40 to 120 mg per injection was reported.[251] Injections were given at 3-week intervals. The investigators noted that the younger the patient and the younger the scar, the more response there was to steroids. This has also been shown by Bernstein.[34] Complications of injections included depigmentation of the skin (in blacks) and excessive atrophy of tissue. Telangiectasia may also be seen with intralesional injections but is more marked when the overlying epidermis has been damaged.[445] To prevent these problems, I inject 5 to 10 mg/ml of triamcinolone acetonide (Kenalog) directly into the scar tissue. For blacks the concentration should be reduced to 2.5 to 5 mg/ml, to prevent hypopigmentation. Injections are repeated at 3- to 4-week intervals until regression occurs. Interestingly, I have found that such injections into keloids or hypertrophic scars also decrease the pruritus and burning described by patients.

Recently Bhawan[37] reported that steroids injected into keloids caused the development of a mucinous acellular material, around which occurred a histiocytic granulomatous response. Whether this represents a tissue reaction to the drug or to the vehicle is unknown.

The most efficacious dose of steroid to be injected into a keloid has not been systematically studied. The higher doses (up to 120 mg) of Ketchum et al.[251] are interesting in this regard. Another interesting approach is the treatment of older keloids with oral steroids.[34] I have no personal experience with systemic therapy for this problem.

The action of steroid injections may be to solubilize the collagen. In a subsequent study, rat tails were injected with either hydrocortisone or triamcinolone.[250] An increase in the soluble fraction of collagen occurred at 2 to 3 weeks. Triamcinolone acetonide was also tested for collagenase activity but was found to have none. Another hypothesis concerning the action of steroids is that the steroid may act systematically to inhibit melanocyte-stimulating hormone (MSH), a substance that may play a role in the activation of keloids.[269]

Newer experimental approaches to treatment of keloids

include the use of β-aminopropionitrile (BAPN) in combination with colchicine after surgical extirpation.[364] Methotrexate has also been advocated.[354] Although these studies are encouraging, further trials are needed.

Hypertrophic scars may also be treated by both intralesional steroids and compression-type bandages if possible. The latter have been used for over 100 years and point up the response of scar tissue to the forces of tension and compression. Torring[468] describes the success of customized Jobst compression bandages, especially for burn scars.

For a more complete discussion of keloids and scars, see Chapter 23.

FACTORS AFFECTING WOUND HEALING AND SCAR FORMATION

Several factors affect wound healing, many of which have already been discussed. Fortunately, most wounds heal readily, so most of these factors need not be considered. The physician's goal in treating wounds is to minimize factors that are deleterious to rapid wound healing.

Physicians are constantly in search of substances or devices that speed up wound healing. Improvement of the normal repair process is rarely if ever obtained. Although it is intriguing to discuss factors, such as drugs, that may speed up normal wound healing, such interventions have not been shown to improve on the normal process to any significant degree.

I have divided the factors affecting wound healing into four sections: environmental factors, systemic factors, local factors, and systemic medications. Although there is some overlap in these four sections, such a categorization is useful for purposes of discussion. I have tried to indicate when areas in these sections are covered in depth elsewhere in the chapter.

Environmental factors

Temperature. Increased environmental temperature increases the wound's healing rate.[415] This is not surprising, since changes in the temperature will affect the metabolic rate. In one study rabbits were flown to Greenland, and the rate of wound healing on ear wounds was measured.[126] The rabbits in this cold environmental climate were found to have retardation of healing compared with rabbits kept at warmer temperatures. Similar findings were also found in alligators.[111]

Increasing the temperature locally over wounds by means of warm compresses, poultices, or heating pads increases the local blood flow and thus aids in wound healing. If the patient is receiving an antibiotic, heat also helps to concentrate the drug at the wound site.

Oxygen. Oxygen in the environment is known to affect the rate of healing of wounds. This topic is discussed later, in the section about local factors that affect wound healing.

Humidity. The increased local humidity under occlusive dressings leads to an increased rate of epidermization. Ambient environmental humidity's effect on wound healing, however, has not been well studied.

Systemic factors

Wounds should not be viewed in isolation but rather as part of the whole organism. The body's state of health greatly influences wound healing.

Age. Wounds heal more rapidly and with fewer problems in young patients than in the elderly. This is borne out by both clinical and experimental studies. In one study 10,668 patients were treated in a hand clinic.[281] The treatment time for hand infections and hand lacerations was extended as the patients' ages increased. Grove induced blisters in the outer forearm and inner arm and calculated time to healing.[172] He found that older individuals (65 to 75 years) uniformly lagged behind younger patients (18 to 25 years). Similar decreases in rates of wound healing by second intention with increasing age have been reported in human[282-284] and animal experiments.[41,158]

The scars produced by the wounds of older patients are not as strong as in the young. Old patients, particularly those older than 70 or 80 years, have a decreased tensile strength of wounds compared with that of younger age groups.[298,417]

Impaired wound healing in the elderly is probably the result of several factors. Vitamin and other nutritional deficiencies are common in this age group. Vascular occlusion also exists to some degree. Fibroblasts have become worn out.

Experimentally in vitro, fibroblasts synthesize less collagen with increasing age up to the age of 40.[470] Fibroblasts are also less proliferative and show a decreased life span in older patients. It has been found that fibroblasts in the papillary dermis are more proliferative than those in the reticular dermis. This may be explained by the fact that with increasing age the papillary dermis decreases in size and thus results in a decrease in the more actively proliferating fibroblasts.[183] The actual percentage of skin weight that consists of collagen also decreases with age.[504]

Among animals fibroplasia has been noted to occur earlier in younger animals, resulting in an increased rate of wound healing.[213] Although one study did not find such a difference,[405] the weight of evidence is in favor of faster wound healing in young animals. Collagen turnover in skin grafts also decreases with age.[259]

The types of scar formed in young and old animals are also markedly different. Younger rats produce more scar tissue than older rats do.[456] The breaking strength of the scar tissue is greater in younger animals, and the scars are more extensible. Thus there are both quantitative and qualitative differences in scar tissue produced by younger animals.

Genetics. Certain individuals tend to have a greater propensity for forming scars. Blacks are known to be more prone to the development of keloids. Patients with hyperextensible skin and joints usually develop spread scars.

Distant infection or inflammation. Sites of distant infection or inflammation have been associated with impaired wound healing. Bierens de Haan et al. made incisions in rats, which were sutured; they then injected the animals elsewhere with either *Pseudomonas* bacteria or turpentine.[39] These other sources of infection or inflammation impaired healing of the initial sutured wounds. The basis for this phenomenon is unknown. Some of the wounds were invaded by *Pseudomonas,* presumably from the bloodstream.

It used to be believed that if one had a wound in the process of healing and a second wound was made, the second wound would heal at a faster rate than usual.[416] The first wound was said to stimulate the healing of the second wound. This idea, however, has not been substantiated experimentally in animals.[419,423,503] In fact, wounding and stress seem to decrease the insoluble collagen elsewhere in animals.[209]

General nutritional status. Wound healing is an active process that requires energy and raw materials for reconstruction. The central factor in impaired wound healing is cellular privation, which may be caused by lack of nutrients, inaccessibility to nutrients, or inability to utilize nutrients. Malnutrition leads to defective fibroplasia and collagen as well as defective mucopolysaccharide synthesis.

The necessary requirements for normal wound repair include not only proteins, but fats and carbohydrates as well. Carbohydrates are particularly important as a source of energy. Important minerals include sodium, potassium, calcium chloride, phosphorus, and magnesium. Trace elements, such as iron, copper, zinc, and manganese, play a role as part of many enzyme systems (metalloenzymes). Important vitamins in wound repair include vitamins A, C, and E. These are discussed shortly.

Nutritional difficulties, although not common in outpatient surgical settings, can still affect even minor surgical procedures. Conversely, minor surgical procedures have been said to result in nutritional deficiencies that could theoretically interfere with wound repair. A study of patients in the hospital setting undergoing minor surgical procedures discovered patients with weight loss and decreases in hemoglobin, white blood cell count, vitamin C, folate, vitamin B_{12}, and albumin.[194] These changes were ascribed to the effects of surgery and remind us that surgical stress, even of a minor degree, can greatly affect the homeostatic balance. Patients should therefore be encouraged to eat well and have a well-balanced diet before and after surgery.

Prolonged starvation of experimental animals leads to impaired wound healing, but normally only when a significant weight loss has occurred (20% to 30% of body weight).[127,233] Wound collagen, tensile strength, and granulation tissue are all found to be decreased under such circumstances. Protocollagen proline hydroxylase, the enzyme

that hydroxylates peptide-bound proline, is decreased by starvation within a few days.[447] The effects of starvation are greater in young animals because they have greater demands for food for growth.[216] Chronic starvation has more negative influence on wound healing than acute starvation has.[432]

Protein deficiency. Protein is an essential ingredient of wound healing, since it supplies the building blocks for collagen. Therefore protein deficiency specifically has been a much-studied aspect of general nutrition deficiency in wound healing.

Experimental studies in animals that were given prolonged protein-free or protein-restricted diets have demonstrated impaired wound healing (Fig. 2-46). Collagen production and mucopolysaccharide deposition appeared to be decreased, leading to decreased granulation tissue,[127,397] delayed wound healing,[104,266,302,327] and wounds with less tensile strength.[60,367,370,494] The deleterious effects of protein depletion were particularly pronounced, with concomitant cortisone administration, which resulted in delayed wound healing.[127]

Specific correction of protein deficiency in animals has led to reversal of the effects of protein restriction in wound healing. Animals fed high-protein diets have wounds with increased tensile strength, compared with animals on low-protein diets.[494] Protein restriction extends the lag phase and prolongs the quantitative phase of collagen repair[104,186,266,302] (Fig. 2-46). This results in a delay of final healing.

An interesting phenomenon shown in some early animal experiments was the correction of impaired wound healing by feeding protein-depleted animals sulfur-containing amino acids such as methionine[302,370,469,493,494] or cystine.[492,493] Regenerating wound tissue has a high concentration of cystine and methionine compared with normal tissue, and these amino acids in particular are believed essential for the normal sequence of events in wound healing. Methionine is necessary in tissue culture for proliferation of fibroblasts and may play an important role in providing sulfate for the sulfated mucopolysaccharides in the ground substance. Protein sulfur thus appears to be more important than protein itself.[494]

Despite an abundance of data on the value of methionine in wound healing, more recent studies have not substantiated the earlier results.[60,232,233,397] Although to reverse wound healing problems in protein-depleted patients with a single amino acid is an attractive concept, the reversal process appears to be more complex.

Protein restriction in man has several effects besides interfering with wound repair. Cell-mediated immunity is impaired,[277] plasma cortisol may be increased, and the liver may undergo fatty metamorphosis.[434] All these changes can secondarily affect wound repair indirectly by leading to an increased risk of infection and a decreased supply of amino

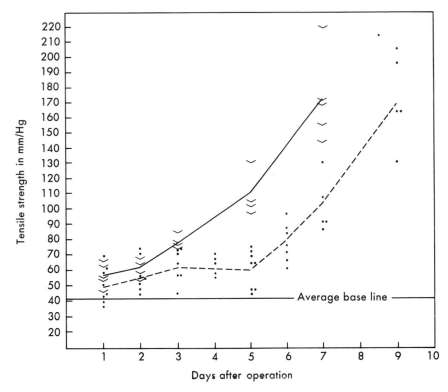

Fig. 2-46. Comparison of tensile strength of wounds of abdominal wall in protein-depleted and normal control rats. *Solid line,* Control diet. *Dashed line,* Low-protein diet. (From Kobak, M.W., et al.: Surg. Gynecol. Obstet. **85:**751, 1947.)

acids. In addition, as total body protein is reduced, so is the protein catabolism in general, further restricting amino acid availability.[373] With protein restriction, collagen is lost from the body; most of this loss (about 60%) is from the skin. It is estimated that the skin loses 16% of its collagen under such circumstances.[182]

Some physicians have suggested that the total serum protein and albumin be used as a rough guide to the protein state in the body. This was based on early studies showing impaired wound healing in dogs with hypoproteinemia.[466] Subsequent investigators failed to confirm a correlation between low serum protein and actual wound disruption or a decreased tensile strength.[266,270] Rhodes et al.[393] felt the effects of low serum albumin depended more on the decreased osmotic pressure and edema than on direct effects of protein nonavailability. More recently, however, Lindstedt and Sandblom[298] demonstrated decreased wound strength in patients with low serum albumin or protein. They found significantly weaker wounds in these patients compared with normal people.

One study discovered that the serum protein concentration may not be a true reflection of the tissue protein level.[301] The investigators proposed the concept of hypoproteinism—the decreased level of protein in tissue whether or not it is accompanied by a similar depletion in the serum. This helped to explain patients with low serum protein lev-

els but normal wound healing, as well as patients with normal serum protein levels with wounds that dehisced.

Probably a chronic lack of protein in the diet leads to less than optimal wound healing in patients. This long-term protein deficiency leads to hypoproteinism and less protein available for fibroblast utilization in tissue. Serum protein may be low, normal, or even high in a hypoproteinemic state, since it is influenced by the intake of proteins near the time of measurement. Low serum protein by itself means very little; and the state of nutrition behind the serum protein is of extreme importance. Patients with chronic low-protein diets should be given high-protein supplements if undergoing extensive cutaneous surgery. Consultation with a dietetic service should be obtained. Caloric intake should be recorded and supplementation, either oral or intravenous, should be given.

An interesting but as yet unsubstantiated approach to healing is to apply protein solutions topically to the wounds themselves. Kaufman et al. applied Revital, containing 19 amino acids, to second-degree burns in guinea pigs.[246] They found that this solution enhanced granulation tissue formation. Similar results were found in patients with a solution containing vitamin C and glucose in addition to amino acids.[430]

Zinc deficiency. Zinc is an important element and essential nutrient found roughly at the same concentration as iron in the blood and tissue. It is involved with the functioning of several enzyme systems, serving as either a cofactor or an essential component for metalloenzymes such as alkaline phosphatase, carbonic anhydrase, and some dehydrogenases. Zinc also is closely involved with protein synthesis, energy production, and cellular proliferation. It plays a role in the functioning of DNA polymerase and reverse transcriptase. Zinc deficiency may therefore result in a decrease in RNA and DNA synthesis, with a subsequent fall in protein synthesis, cell growth, and cell division. Zinc has also been shown to be involved in the mobilization of vitamin A from the liver, and thus in zinc deficiency the plasma vitamin A level may fall.[433] Zinc has been called "a potent catalyst of wound healing."[379]

Paradoxically zinc also has some effects that may be detrimental to wound healing. It stabilizes lysosomes, which are useful to macrophages for phagocytosis. High levels of zinc also inhibit lysyl oxidase in vitro.[70] Lysyl oxidase is a copper-dependent enzyme that helps to form the aldehyde groups necessary for establishing covalent crosslinks in collagen. Zinc probably competes with copper in the lysyl oxidase system if zinc levels are high enough. Ironically, zinc deficiency also interferes with lysyl oxidase synthesis, and thus weak collagen is formed.

The use of zinc to promote healing is not new. It was used in ancient Egypt in the form of calamine, which is a mixture of zinc oxide and ferric oxide. Calamine lotion has survived to this day. Application to injured tissue may result in systemic absorption or local beneficial effects on wound repair.

In animals with a zinc deficiency, surgical wounds heal with a delay in closure and a decrease in tensile strength after the first week.[387,420] If the animals are not zinc deficient, zinc supplementation has little effect on wound repair. However, it has been pointed out that since zinc-deficient animals become anorexic, such studies need to control for weight of the animals. Otherwise zinc deficiency could lead to malnutrition and thereby affect wound healing indirectly.

Zinc deficiencies occur in both humans and animals. In zinc-deficient cattle, sheep, and swine, ulcerating lesions develop on the legs. In humans, acrodermatitis enteropathica has been shown to be associated with zinc deficiency caused by poor intestinal absorption. Such patients develop eczematous lesions around the mouth, rectum, and fingers.

A 1967 report stated that oral zinc sulfate (220 mg three times a day) accelerated the healing of pilonidal sinuses that had been marsupialized in healthy young airmen.[379] The acceleration took place *not* during the stage of granulation but during epidermization. This acceleration was on the order of 43%. Barcia repeated that study and found that zinc did not increase the rate of wound healing.[23] Oral zinc supplementation has also been reported to be of value for ischemic leg ulcers, decreasing the healing time.[177]

Topical application of zinc to wounds has also been advocated and found to result in decreased wound healing time in rats.[437] However, Williams et al.[490] were unable to confirm these beneficial results unless a true zinc deficiency was present. Another interesting study showed that Neomycin Ointment accelerates wound epidermization,[147] Neomycin contains zinc bacitracin and other antibiotics. The zinc bacitracin appeared to be the factor promoting wound resurfacing; preparations with higher concentrations of zinc appeared to demonstrate a more enhanced effect.[110]

The confusion surrounding zinc supplementation in wound healing is thus the result of conflicting data as well as poorly designed studies. Zinc needs to be measured within both tissue and serum because serum levels do not necessarily reflect tissue levels. Zinc levels should be constantly monitored before, during, and after wound healing. Some other problems associated with studies of zinc and wound healing are discussed in detail by Haley.[178]

Based on the foregoing, zinc supplementation may possibly be valuable in promoting wound healing in patients known to be zinc deficient. Although such deficiency is undoubtedly rare, it should be kept in mind. One hopes that better-designed studies will someday shed more light on this confusing topic.

Vitamin deficiency

Vitamin A. Vitamin A is a known labilizer of lysosomes but under normal conditions has little effect on wound healing.[223] Given systemically to animals it does not affect the hydroxyproline content of wounds,[411] although it may help increase the number of cells and acid mucopolysaccharides in granulation tissue.[285] Tissue cultures of skin in vitro with vitamin A show decreased keratinization of the epidermis, but this is of little consequence for healing wounds. Topically applied vitamin A increases the number of cells in granulation tissue and possibly helps to promote the immune response.[411]

The importance of vitamin A in wound healing appears to be the antagonism it provides to lysosomal stabilizers. Glucocorticoids, aspirin, and vitamin E are all lysosome stabilizers that depress wound healing by interfering with the important functioning of lysosomes in macrophages as well as other cells. Such lysosomal stabilizers given to animals delay wound healing and decrease tensile strength of wounds. Systemic vitamin A given concomitantly with these stabilizers reverses their deleterious effects on wound repair. This has been shown for cortisone,[115,117,411,447] aspirin,[285] and vitamin E.[118] Beta-carotene has the same antagonistic effect as vitamin A toward cortisone.[172] Unfortunately, high levels of vitamin A are necessary to reverse the effects of glucocorticoids on wound healing, and the vitamin is effective only in the early stages, so its use clinically for this purpose is limited.[411] However, topical application of vitamin A has anecdotally been reported to accelerate wound healing when systemic steroids were given.[223]

Vitamin C. The deleterious effect of vitamin C deficiency on wounds has been known for over 200 years. Sailors in the eighteenth century were subject to scurvy, and the lives of many men were lost. In the British Royal Navy it was noted that limes could reverse this disease process. Because British sailors were thereafter prescribed limes while on long voyages, they became known as limeys.

An interesting phenomenon associated with scurvy is that old wounds break down. In his classic study Lind quotes Richard Walter's description of this situation during the voyage of Lord Anson around the world from 1740 through 1744[296]:

> The scars of wounds which had been for many years healed were forced open again by this virulent distemper [scurvy]. Of this there was a remarkable instance in one of the invalids on board the *Centurion,* who had been wounded above fifty years before at the battle of Boyne: for though he was cured soon after, and had continued well for a great number of years past, yet, on his being attacked by the scurvy, his wounds, in the progress of his disease, broke out afresh, and appeared as if they never had been healed. Nay, what is still more astonishing, the callus of a broken bone, which had been compleatly formed for a long time, was found to be hereby dissolved; and the fracture seemed as if it has never been consolidated.

Lind also describes hemorrhage underneath scars even when they did not totally break down.

Vitamin C (ascorbic acid) is one of the cofactors required for the proper functioning of proline hydroxylase and lysine hydroxylase, the enzymes that hydroxylate proline and lysine after incorporation into the collagen peptide.[453] The collagen formed in severe vitamin C deficiency is underhydroxylated and thus unable to form stable cross-links. Since collagen is constantly turning over in scars, vitamin C is also necessary for the proper formation and maintenance of collagen, even in old wounds.

One of the best studies on the effects of ascorbic acid deficiency on wound healing in humans was performed in 1940.[84] Crandon courageously served as the experimental subject, making himself deficient in vitamin C. At 3 months, although the plasma ascorbic acid level was undetectable, wound healing was normal; however, the white blood cell (buffy coat) ascorbic acid was still detectable. At 6 months wound healing did not occur. Instead only a clot formed inside an experimental wound cavity. At this point both plasma and white blood cell levels of ascorbic acid were undetectable. Vitamin C administration was then begun and wound healing proceeded normally.

This study points up several aspects of vitamin C deficiency. First, the white blood cell level of ascorbic acid is a better reflection of tissue levels than the plasma level is.[83] Second, ascorbic acid deficiency leads to fragility of blood vessels with hemorrhage into wounds. Third, ascorbic acid deficiency may be quickly reversed despite months of depri-

vation[105]; the building blocks for collagen are present but not utilized. Fourth, moderate vitamin C deficiency does not interfere with wound repair, but total deficiency does.[198]

Microscopically in animal wounds, vitamin C deficiency results in negligible collagen or capillary formation, but fibroblasts still proliferate.[24,400,498] Edema and hemorrhage are readily apparent.[337] Mucopolysaccharide formation in granulation tissue may also be impaired.[267] This results in a prolonged lag phase of wound healing, but the period of rapid gain in tensile strength is not delayed.[104] Thus vitamin C deficiency causes a problem with the formation of collagen; it plays less of a role once collagen is formed.[105] Wound contraction in scorbutic animals has been observed to proceed fully but is delayed.[4,164] This has already been cited as evidence against collagen and for fibroblast migration being mainly responsible for wound contraction. Once the wound is healed, ascorbic acid is necessary for the maintenance of scar tissue.

Clinically, vitamin C–deficient patients are eight times more likely to have dehiscence of their wounds.[83] If wounds are infected in scorbutic guinea pigs, the initial macrophage reaction is delayed, and the necrotic abscesses are not walled off as the collagen production is lowered.[325]

Ascorbic acid metabolism has been studied and found to be susceptible to a number of factors. After injury, ascorbic acid accumulates at the wound site along with fibrin clot and blood cells. The catabolism and excretion of ascorbic acid are decreased. If the experimental animal is depleted of vitamin C, the half-life of this substance is substantially increased as the requirements for vitamin C are increased.[7]

After surgery ascorbic acid levels decrease in the buffy coat layer of leukocytes, probably related to the leukocytosis associated with wound injury.[235] By the third postoperative day there is a 42% reduction in the circulating leukocyte ascorbic acid levels. Cortisone administration has also been reported to decrease the buffy coat ascorbic acid levels.[83] However, these transient depressions of the ascorbic acid levels are of unknown significance. Perhaps the patients who have very low ascorbic acid levels to begin with may have serious problems with wound repair after surgery. Moderate vitamin C deficiency, however, does not seem to interfere with wound repair.[198]

Some studies in the literature suggest that vitamin C supplementation helps wound healing. Taylor et al. reported good results with ascorbic acid given to patients with bed sores.[463] Although this was a double-blind study, buffy coat ascorbic acid levels were not recorded.

Vitamin E. Vitamin E is a biologic antioxidant that soaks up free radicals and thus protects cells from the harmful effects of such substances. It also functions, like cortisone, as a membrane stabilizer and thus helps to maintain the integrity of lysosomes. Given to rats, vitamin E results in wounds with decreased tensile strength compared to controls[118] because of a retardation of wound healing and collagen production. The effect can be overcome by the co-administration of vitamin A a membrane labilizer.

The topical application of vitamin E to wounds has been proposed on the basis that it may decrease scar formation, much like cortisone, but there is no evidence that this is of therapeutic benefit. In fact, patients may become allergic to any of several components used in topical vitamin E preparations.

Medical problems. Some medical problems are known to affect wound healing adversely. Patients with diabetes, for instance, are said to have a tendency toward prolonged wound healing. This tendency, however, is mainly in poorly controlled cases.[159] Patients with well-controlled diabetes have normal wound healing.

The effects of poorly controlled diabetes on wound healing are unknown but probably multifactorial, involving ischemia of both large and small vessels, as well as insulin deficiency in fibroblasts. Fibroblasts have been shown to have insulin receptors.[390] Epidermal cells may also be influenced by insulin, which helps to maintain these cells in cell culture.[47] There is also a decreased neutrophilic response in diabetic patients.[201]

An interesting approach to wound healing is the application of insulin. This was initially reported by Paul[361] in 1966 and was stated by Goodson and Hunt[159] to be possibly beneficial in diabetic wounds. Good results have been shown experimentally in mice, some of which were diabetic,[181] but in normal animals the effects may not be as pronounced.[398]

Uremia can also affect wound healing. Peacock found a decrease in the tensile strength of wounds in uremic rats.[362] There was a decrease in the amount of collagen in the wounds. A similar decrease in hydroxyproline, which reflects collagen content, has also been shown with topical urea applied to wounds.[482] The breaking strength of wounds in such animals was decreased up to the seventh day postoperatively, showing that the early phase of wound healing was negatively influenced. On the other hand, more recent studies have demonstrated that in uremic rats the hydroxyproline content of wounds was normal, but that cellular proliferation of fibroblasts decreased at the wound's edges.[80] Fibroblasts in culture with uremic plasma do not have a normal morphology.

Anemia was believed by some physicians in the past to influence wound repair adversely.[415] For purposes of discussion anemia is divided into that produced by acute blood loss and that caused by a chronic underlying pathology or by malnutrition. If animals are acutely bled, both blood volume and hemoglobin concentration fall. Although early investigators[36] showed that acute blood loss in dogs had no adverse effects on tensile strength of wounds, subsequent work by Zederfelt revealed that in rabbits tensile strength of wounds was impaired by acute blood loss.[503] However, tensile strength returned to normal when the blood volume (by use of a plasma expander) was restored, but not when the

hemoglobin concentration was increased. Therefore for acute blood loss situations it seems that blood volume rather than hemoglobin concentration is more important in influencing wound repair. Normovolemic anemia acutely produced does not appear to impair wound healing.[192] However, acute blood volume reduction results in reflex vasoconstriction and collapse of vessels, which lead to impaired capillary blood flow. This reduced blood flow is probably the main cause of delay in wound healing under such circumstances.[414]

Acute anemia caused by trauma may still possibly impair wound healing despite correction of blood volume.[503] This is because intravascular coagulation may occur and decrease the blood supply to the wound.

Chronic anemia appears to have a more profound adverse impact on wound repair. Chronic anemia in rats decreased tensile strength of wounds, even if blood volume was controlled.[22] Chronic anemia is more complicated than acute blood loss anemia. Chronic anemia is frequently associated with other factors, such as malnutrition, that also impair wound repair.

The mechanism of the negative influence of chronic anemia on wound repair is unknown. Oxygen diffusion into wounds is influenced more by its partial pressure than by the total amount of oxygen in the blood.[192] Therefore low hemoglobin by itself does not always play a significant role in limiting the oxygen supply to wounds.

Leukemia appears to be associated with delayed wound healing. This is commonly seen in lesions if such patients are infected with varicella-zoster virus. In this situation small vesicles become deep ulcerations, caused by the patient's inability to mount an effective inflammatory response initially. These ulcerations take a long time to heal.

Wounds left to heal by granulation subsequent to Mohs surgery have in my experience taken much longer to heal in patients with leukemia or polycythemia. The latter condition may result in decreased blood supply to the wound, caused by increased blood viscosity. Neutrophil response is also decreased in patients with leukemia, which could lead to increased wound infection problems.[201]

Cushing's syndrome is associated with hypersecretion of the adrenal cortex resulting in excessive production of glucocorticoids. Patients with this syndrome have thin, transparent skin, easy bruisability, and marked susceptibility to skin infections. Some of the first patients given adrenocorticotrophic hormone (ACTH) in the late 1940s were observed to have inhibition of wound healing.[87] Other studies measured breaking strength of wounds in patients with Cushing's disease and found it to be decreased[298] (Fig. 2-47). The problems with wound healing in such patients have been ascribed to the hypercortisolism, which accompanies either ACTH therapy or Cushing's disease. However, the problems of wound healing in patients on steroids is not nearly so simple or straightforward, as is described later.

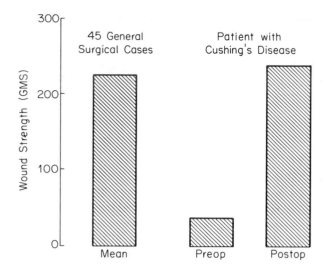

Fig. 2-47. Breaking strength wound measurements in patient before and after removal of tumor from adrenal cortex, compared with those of 45 surgical wounds in normal patients. (Modified from Sandblom, P.: Langenbeck Arch. Klin. Chir. **287:**469, 1957.)

Jaundice may be associated with impaired wound healing. Wounds in rats with obstructive jaundice have a decreased tensile strength.[28] Perhaps bilirubin or some other substance in bile has a depressant effect on fibroplasia or collagen synthesis.

Patients with coagulopathy are likely to bleed into their wounds, resulting in separation of wound edges, prolongation of wound healing, and less than desirable cosmetic results. A coagulopathy commonly seen is that associated with liver disease, usually alcoholic cirrhosis. Patients with this condition have a prolonged prothrombin time and partial thromboplastin time associated with a decrease in the vitamin K–dependent coagulation factors (VII, IX, X, prothrombin). Unfortunately, with liver disease the clotting abnormalities do not respond to vitamin K supplementation.

Patients with scleroderma sometimes have a decreased ability to heal wounds on the thickened skin. This is probably caused by the increased distance new blood vessels and fibroblasts must travel to bridge the gap and proliferate rather than any inability of fibroblasts themselves. Patients with scleroderma have been found to have normal levels of protocollagen proline hydroxylase (PPH).[447]

Cancer may also affect wound healing. A large tumor burden causes a decrease in wound breaking strength in animals.[42,50] Such decreases in wound strength may be exacerbated by cytotoxic agents, especially methotrexate or doxorubicin (Adriamycin).[90]

Malabsorption disease leads to wound healing problems indirectly by the nutritional deficiencies seen in such patients. Decreased absorption of fats, carbohydrates, and proteins, as well as vitamins and minerals, may occur with intestinal malabsorption.

Local factors

The immediate surrounding environment of a wound and how a wound is treated locally are important determinants of whether the process of wound repair proceeds normally. Many of the factors discussed here have already been discussed in greater detail in this chapter or are described elsewhere in the text.

Size. Wounds that heal by secondary intention do so at a rate determined by their size. Larger wounds heal at a faster rate than smaller wounds do. This was initially expressed mathematically by LeComte Du Noüy,[282-284] who formulated the following mathematical expression based on clinically observed rates of wound healing in men:

$$i = \frac{(S - S') \div S}{t + \sqrt{T}}$$

Here i is the index of cicatrization; S the initial area of the wound; S', the area of the wound t days later; t, the time interval between the initial size and the time of observation; T, the total time between wound formation and measurement. Du Noüy found it necessary to correct the time with the square root of time because the observed healing rate decreased with time. An assumption in some studies that granulating wounds heal at a constant rate is thus untrue.[178]

Depth. In general the more superficial the wound is, the less scar formation occurs. Experiments in animals suggest that the layers of the skin transected are of more importance in scar formation than the actual measured depth of an incision is.[120] This is not wholly applicable in humans. Paradoxically, some wounds with less measurable scar tissue are more unsightly than wounds with greater scar tissue. Consider, for instance, a lesion in the nose that is either curetted to the middermis or excised full thickness to subcutaneous tissue. Both wounds are allowed to heal by granulation and epidermization. The curetted wound results in a shallow but noticeable depression. The excised wound, on the other hand, heals in addition by contraction. This minimizes any depression, although it may result in more measurable scar tissue.

Shape. Excisional wounds closed as lines may be straight or curved. Since all scars contract, both straight and curved incisions shorten to some degree. If the shortening is pronounced, a trapdoor deformity may be produced in the curved incision. The shape of a wound should be viewed not two dimensionally but three dimensionally. The sides of incisions should be vertically straight rather than beveled toward the center of the wound. Such beveling tends to invert the skin edges as the skin is sutured. Beveled incisions also tend to form trapdoor deformities. This is explained later (Fig. 10-33, *D*).

Wounds allowed to heal by secondary intention are influenced by the shape. This is discussed in the section on granulation and contraction.

Location. Wounds in areas of little mobility with little tension and an excellent vascular supply heal with a minimum of problems. The scalp is such a location. Wounds in areas of high mobility with significant tension and a poor vascular supply frequently heal with problems. The lower extremity is such a site. Wounds in some locations, for instance over bony prominences, may undergo pressure from beneath if the patient is confined to bed.

Wounds directed along the lines of maximal tension result in less spreading of the scar than wounds perpendicular to them. The collagen in wounds directed along the lines of maximal tension is laid down parallel to the majority of the surrounding collagen, and thus such wounds result in the best ultrastructural reconstruction of the dermis.[205]

Vascular supply varies from one area of the body to another, being highest in the head and neck and lowest in the extremities. Areas of greater vascular supply are more rarely infected and heal faster.

Type of skin. The texture and thickness of the skin are not universally the same either from one region of the body to another or between individuals. Thick skin, such as on the back, takes longer to heal than the thin skin of the penis or eyelid does, because the thickness of the relatively avascular, acellular reticular dermis must be bridged from above and below by blood vessels and fibroblasts.

Oily, sebaceous skin heals with more visible scarring than does smooth telangiectatic skin. Sebaceous skin, with its patulous pores and arborizing glands, results in a thicker yet less tough skin. Such tissue is easily torn by sutures.

Skin may also be looser in some locations, such as the face, compared with others, such as the back. With age the tension of the skin also becomes less, particularly on the face, where it becomes draped across the cheeks and jaw. Scarred skin is less vascular and more difficult to heal.

Vascular supply. The better the vascular supply to a wound is, the less chance of infection exists and the faster the wound heals. The vascular supply may be decreased by scarring, for instance, from radiation. Extreme tension on wounds may also decrease the blood supply. Sympathectomies may increase the blood supply by decreasing vasoconstriction and thus speed up wound healing.[306,415]

Radiation. Skin that has been irradiated is a special type of injured tissue. Therapeutic radiation tends to produce tissue that in time is scarred and relatively avascular, although the remaining superficial blood vessels may dilate, producing telangiectasia. Such tissue heals slowly and is more susceptible to infection. These chronic effects (fibrosis and avascularity) from radiation begin 4 to 6 months after radiation and may progress with time.

The radiation effects on wound repair are proportional to the total dose and the time interval in which given.[334] Single doses of less than 300 rad cause little delay in wound healing, whereas doses above 1000 rad can cause significant morphologic and biochemical changes, resulting in early decreases

in tensile strength. Irradiation to wounds in rats slows the process of wound healing, but ultimately the wounds attain the same tensile strength that controls have.[278] Histologically radiation produces depression of the fibroblast proliferation and capillary formation, and results in disorganization of the normal repair structure.

The peak effect of radiation on wounds appears if it is given about 36 hours after wounding. However, when radiation is applied after the process of contraction has started, it has little effect. The main effect of irradiation appears to be on the fibroblasts, since the process of contraction is slowed as well.[166]

Oxygenation. Considerable investigation has been directed in recent years to the influence of oxygen on wound healing. For centuries the Indians living high in the mountains of South America have realized that wounds heal more quickly when they descend into the valleys, where the air is thicker. Some evidence exists that the rate of epidermization is slower at high altitudes than at sea level.[218]

The important role of oxygen in wound healing was surmised for many years as physicians realized that better-vascularized wounds healed faster and with less infection. Only recently has oxygen's role been worked out more exactly.

Inflammation and wound repair usually place high metabolic demands on the local microvasculature. Oxygen comes to the wound mainly from the blood and increases the rate of fibroblast reproduction, fibroblast production of collagen, and epithelial cell growth. Collagen production particularly depends on oxygen because proline and lysine hydroxylase, the enzymes responsible for hydroxylation of proline and lysine, require molecular oxygen for hydroxylation.[229,471] Without hydroxylation, intermolecular cross-linking does not occur. Therefore adequate oxygenation is important during the lag phase and early proliferative (quantitative collagen) phase. Primary intention wounds are not as susceptible to the changing oxygen environment as secondary intention wounds are, because the vascular connections are reestablished early in primary intention wounds, resulting in an early decreased need for additional oxygen.

Deep wounds routinely function under unfavorable oxygen concentrations, since the normal blood supply is disrupted. The center of the wound has the lowest O_2 tension, lower than the edges of the wound, which still have a lower O_2 tension than normal tissue. Thus an oxygen gradient exists in wounds. This hypoxic gradient disappears as new blood vessels grow completely across the wound.[391]

Epidermis does not usually function in high oxygen concentrations because it does not contain a blood supply. Therefore it relies largely on the glycolytic mechanism of metabolism and will switch from the Embden-Meyerhof pathway to the pentose phosphate pathway under conditions of low oxygenation.[240] Culturing skin under anaerobic conditions resulted in cessation of cell movement and cell division, but the skin was still capable of survival for up to 1 week.[323]

Hypoxia may be a stimulus for capillary growth in wounds. Macrophages secrete an angiogenesis factor only under hypoxic conditions.[263] Hypoxia also shifts the wound metabolism from the Krebs cycle toward anaerobic glycolysis (particularly the pentose phosphate shunt).[230] This shift in wound metabolism helps to minimize the consequences of a decreased oxygen supply. The increased activity of the pentose phosphate pathway can be seen by an increase in the glucose 6-phosphate dehydrogenase (G6PD) activity in healing wounds.[231] It is interesting to note that failure of skin flaps has been reported to occur with G6PD deficiency.[207]

With anaerobic glycolysis the wound edge becomes acidotic as lactic acid accumulates. This increased lactic acid level may be a signal for increased collagen synthesis in fibroblasts.[225] It has been shown that lactic acid may increase the activity of proline hydroxylase in cultured fibroblasts.[344] However, the shift away from the citric acid cycle yields less energy production per unit of glucose. This is overcome somewhat by the increased metabolic rate of wounded skin.[230]

Increasing the pO_2 in a wound shifts the metabolism from anaerobic glycolysis toward aerobic glycolysis with activation of the Krebs cycle. This gives the wound more energy to heal, since the energy yield per molecule of glucose is increased as lactic acid is broken down to CO_2 and H_2O.[475]

Oxygen is carried in blood by red blood cells and dissolved in plasma. This oxygen diffuses from the nearest functioning capillary down a concentration gradient to reach the least oxygenated areas of the wound. This rate of diffusion depends on the partial pressure of oxygen in the blood (rather than the concentration), which in turn helps to determine the steepness of the gradient. In addition, as oxygen is used by the wound, it drives the gradient downhill as well. Thus the oxygen tension in tissue is determined by the supply from the vascular system balanced against the wound's utilization of oxygen. This has led to speculation that the oxygen supply limits the wound-healing rate. Normally in wound dead space the O_2 tension is very low (less than 3 mm Hg), whereas in areas where fibroblasts are dividing, the O_2 tension is higher (more than 15 mm Hg). Collagen formation appears at tensions between 15 and 30 mm Hg.[429] The normal O_2 tension in mammalian subcutaneous tissue is 15 to 24 mm Hg.[71]

Although oxygen is required for the synthesis of collagen, the critical pO_2 requirement has not yet been determined.[222] Growth suppression of fibroblasts does not occur until oxygen concentrations are very low (less than 3%).[71] The optional or at least adequate O_2 tension for cell growth may actually be less than "air."[248,346]

If the oxygen concentration is increased in the air, sev-

eral changes take place in the healing wound in animals. Epithelialization,[359] collagen synthesis,[220] and wound closure rates are all increased. Some studies[343,452] have shown that tensile strength of wounds appears to be slightly increased; however, Kirk and Irwin[252] were unable to show such an increase in the tensile strength. Hyperoxia also appears to decrease bacterial proliferation in wounds.[203,224] This may be caused by enhanced killing of bacteria by the leukocyte oxidase system, which is oxygen dependent.[204] As one breathes pure O_2, the arterial pO_2 is raised; however, when the pO_2 rises above 140 mm Hg, arterial constriction occurs.[429] This limits the increased oxygen approach to wound healing.

In animals placed in hypoxic environments, collagen accumulation in wounds is decreased[256,306] and wound infection rates are increased.[224]

One method of increasing the oxygen available to tissue is to increase the pressure of oxygen in the air by means of a hyperbaric chamber. This is based on the concept that increasing the oxygen concentration alone in the ambient air does not increase the oxygen in tissue. Increasing oxygen under pressure does result in an increase in tissue oxygen tension.[174] Since the hemoglobin is saturated at normal atmospheric pressure, increasing the pressure in the air only increases the oxygen dissolved in plasma. This increase on a percentage basis is rather small. At 3 atmospheres, the arterial blood pO_2 is 2000 mm Hg but the oxygen in solution in plasma is only increased 6%.[249] Nevertheless, the tremendously high pO_2 in the arterial blood creates a force (pressure gradient) that favors diffusions of oxygen into an ischemic area.

Hyperbaric oxygen has been reported to be useful in increasing the oxygen tension of pedicle flaps as well as skin grafts and thus increasing the likelihood of their survival[428,479]; however, other studies have not been uniformly in accordance.[175,249] This is probably because hyperbaric oxygen by itself penetrates tissue poorly,[174] and skin flaps that are avascular are not perfused by the hyperoxygenated blood. Decreased healing time of open wounds have also been reported to occur with hyperbaric oxygen, even if the wound edges are devascularized[255,428] In addition, the tensile strength of wounds may actually be weakened by oxygen under pressure just as by air at half the atmospheric pressure.[306,343]

Various devices have been created to deliver oxygen to wounds directly with or without pressure. For instance, Fisher[128] reported good results on leg ulcers, using a system that delivered absolute oxygen at flow rates of 2 to 8 L/minute for 6 to 8 hours a day at 1.03 atmospheres of pressure. The early encouraging results have not stood the test of time; probably the results seen have more to do with the increased care given to the patients than with the type of care.

Type of injury. Some forms of injury are more destructive of tissue than others are. The basic types of injury include cold, heat, electrical, and mechanical. Cold injury is less injurious to fibroblasts than to epidermal cells.[427] Collagen is more susceptible to destruction by heat than by cold.[292] Burn wounds tend to produce nonviable tissue for some distance from the coagulated vessels; with physical injury there is little destruction beyond this point.[221]

A study compared the amount of tissue destruction and subsequent wound healing for the plasma scalpel, the electrosurgical apparatus, and the steel scalpel.[299] Wounds created with the steel scalpel showed the most rapid rate of epidermization and resulted in scars with the least spreading. In addition, the inflammatory response with the steel scalpel was confined to the immediate edges of the wound and there was no proximal tissue damage. The plasma scalpel and the electrosurgical apparatus both produced significant tissue damage and an inflammatory response beyond the wound edges. This resulted in slower epidermization and wider scars. It seems difficult to improve on the steel scalpel as an instrument for incising tissue.

Lasers have been recommended as a method to cut or destroy tissue because of the minimal and controllable destruction produced. In addition, lasers appear to have direct effects on fibroblasts. The Nd:YAG (neodymium–yttrium-aluminum-garnet) laser has been shown to suppress collagen production in both fibroblast cultures and normal skin. The helium-neon and gallium-arsenide lasers, on the other hand, were shown to stimulate collagen production.[6] Lasers, however, do not always miraculously cut without scarring; hypertrophic scars can certainly occur.[94]

Methods of handling tissue. The gentle handling of tissue probably is the single largest controllable factor contributing to excellent wound healing. Some surgeons get better results than others. This is well known but difficult to measure.

Factors known to be important in wound healing include the minimization of handling tissue with instruments or destroying tissue with the electrosurgical apparatus, meticulous hemostasis, good closure technique with proper apposition of wound edges, and knowledge of the type and number of sutures.[299] Sutures pulled too tightly enfeeble the circulation, as do excessive sutures used to obliterate dead space.[180,338] The least number and smallest caliber of sutures to appose tissue adequately should be used. Sutures that evoke a significant inflammatory response, such as catgut, tend to prolong wound healing and decrease the tensile strength of wounds.[211] Often sutures, such as those made of nylon, evoke little inflammatory response and result in a shorter period of initial wound healing and a stronger wound.[300] If convenient, sutures should be removed at the earliest possible time and skin tape applied. This results in less noticeable suture tracts or scars and less delay in wound healing without decreasing the tensile strength of wounds.[52,135,136,357]

Dehiscence. Wounds that dehisce may be safely closed if resutured in the first week. Such wounds have been shown to gain tensile strength rapidly, as though the wounds had not been disrupted.[61,100,432] This was shown in 1941[45] and investigated later in detail.[363,422,423] Collagen deposition as masured by hydroxyproline content was unaffected by disruption of wounds within 6 days followed by immediate resuturing.[311] Excision of the wound margin abolishes the rapid gain in tensile strength seen in such wounds and is therefore probably not advisable.[61]

Delayed closure. Wounds may be safely closed between 3 days and 6 or 7 days after the injury with rapid gain in tensile strength and no significant risk of infection, assuming that no gross contamination of the wound has occurred. Excision of the wound margin abolishes the rapid gain in tensile strength normally seen with delayed closure.[425,426]

Foreign bodies. Foreign bodies may prevent wound closure and lead to chronic drainage and hypergranulation tissue. Small pieces of silica can evoke granulomatous responses, which tend to persist unless the silica is removed. Some foreign bodies produce little inflammatory response and persist for years without problems. Such substances include carbon from pencil tips or in tattoos. Hair, nonabsorbable suture fragments, and even absorbable sutures behave like foreign bodies and can lead to persistent reactions until eliminated or removed.

Infection. Wound healing and wound infection are tightly interwoven: any factor that delays wound healing increases the risk of infection. Alternatively, infection delays wound healing. Although infection prolongs the inflammatory phase of wound healing, paradoxically it was noted early on that the resulting strength of infected wounds was greater than that of noninfected wounds.[176,241,415] This might be caused by an increase in scar tissue, however, so that such wounds are not as desirable cosmetically.

Infected wounds with a decreased production of collagen and local hypoxia also take longer to heal.[345] An increase in the healing time of open granulating wounds should alert the physician to the possibility of significant pathogen colonization.[317] Nonpathogens, such as *Staphylococcus albus,* appear to have little significant adverse influence on wound healing.[45]

The level of bacterial colonization has been shown to influence wound healing. More than 10^6 organisms of *Staphylococcus aureus* per square centimeter of wound surface for superficial wounds[291] or more than 10^5 organisms of *S. aureus* per gram of tissue for deep wounds adversely affect both the time and degree of wound healing.[395]

Remote infection also has been shown to impair wound healing. A decreased bursting strength of abdominal wounds was shown in rats when infection was induced elsewhere.[39] In all cases the same organisms were found in the wounds themselves. The investigators speculated that perhaps the negative influence of infection was caused by an increase in collagenase, an induced prolonged destructive phase of inflammation or hypersensitivity response against products of tissue breakdown. A similar effect of remote inflammation or infection has also been noted in secondary intention wounds.[63]

Occlusion. Wounds that are superficial and only into the top part of the dermis heal mainly by epithelialization. This epithelialization is more rapid if such wounds are occluded and a crust is prevented from forming.[108,154,195,495] Occlusion tends to increase the bacterial population under the dressing, but this does not usually interfere with wound healing.[324] However, if a significantly high number (10^5 or 10^6/cm^2) of pathogenic organisms proliferates, it could interfere with wound healing. Another benefit to occlusion of superficial wounds is that the epidermis has an increased tensile strength sooner.[404]

The influence of occlusion on full-thickness wound healing has been less well studied. Such wounds in rats healed faster with respect to both contraction and epidermization with Vaseline than with a dry dressing.[297] On the other hand, a study of the healing rate of punch biopsy wounds in humans compared similar sites with or without occlusion, and was unable to demonstrate a significant difference in healing time.[264] Scab formation has little effect on the overall rate of wound contraction of full-thickness wounds.[435]

Topical preparations. Numerous topical preparations are said to enhance wound healing. Such substances literally number in the thousands and include such items as gold foil, slime from the Arabian Gulf catfish,[10] and honey.[32] In evaluating such preparations one must consider the depth of the wound and whether any pathologic factors are influencing the healing of a wound. All too often clinical findings of the efficacy of some topical preparation are in reality simply the result of better nursing care and bed rest rather than a measurement of the substance's wound healing properties.

My usual topical preparation for routine use in uncomplicated acute wounds, both superficial and deep, is hydrogen peroxide and a topical antibiotic ointment, usually Polysporin Ointment. Empirically I have found this to lead to rapid wound healing with few problems for either superficial or full-thickness wounds. Since all wounds are kept occluded until wound healing is complete, this method is difficult to compare with experimental studies, which seem to separate occlusion from topical preparations.

Experimentally there is evidence against my own empiric expeirence. Eaglstein and Mertz[108] showed that petrolatum retarded epithelialization more than occlusive dressings did. It would have been interesting to see what effect occlusive dressings and petrolatum together had on wound healing, since that more clearly parallels actual clinical practice. In a later paper they showed that creams and lotions are more effective than petrolatum in speeding up superficial wound healing.[109]

Hydrogen peroxide has been shown to speed up the healing time of wounds in rats.[173] This is probably the result of the effervescent effect of the peroxide on cleaning the wound, although its oxidizing properties may be of benefit as well. However, in vitro hydrogen peroxide has been shown to decrease the ability of fibroblasts to proliferate.[199] Such effects must be minor in vivo, since I have found hydrogen peroxide to be quite useful. Some investigators recommend benzoyl peroxide to increase the rate of epidermization.[12] I have no experience in its use.

Recently there has been interest generated by the use of topical honey or other sugar compounds on wounds in imitation of the ancient Egyptians.[57] In mice, honey-treated wounds heal faster than in controls.[32] Good results were clinically reported with a sugar and povidone-iodine mixture in 605 patients.[265] The wound-healing properties of these sugar compounds are ascribed to their energy-producing properties, hygroscopic effects on draining wounds, and bacteriostatic properties. However, many of the patients would probably have healed with standard dressings; there was no comparable control group.[265]

Ulcers or other wounds that are not healing should be carefully cultured. An appropriate antibiotic or antiseptic solution and perhaps a systemic antibiotic should be used. Other topical preparations to consider that may influence nonhealing ulcers include topical insulin,[181,361] topical nutrient solutions,[430] topical minerals such as zinc, and wound-debriding agents such as Travase and Elase. These latter substances are discussed in Chapter 4.

Other interesting topical substances that affect wound healing are steroids and vitamins. They are discussed elsewhere.

Electrical current. Galvanic current has been known for a number of years to increase the rate of wound healing.[16] The human skin behaves as a battery; the voltage difference between the surface of the epidermis and the dermis is about -23 mV. The negative potential is in the outer stratum corneum with respect to the dermis. There is regional variation of such battery voltages; they are higher on the hands and feet.[137]

Alvarez et al.[14] have shown—using an anode in pigs' wounds—that a direct electrical current of 50 to 300 μA accelerated epidermal resurfacing of superficial partial-thickness wounds. Electrical stimulation has been used successfully in clinical situations such as ulcers. Its usefulness has been reported for an ulcer associated with the trigeminal trophic syndrome.[487]

The mechanism of electrical currents for stimulation of wound healing is unknown. Perhaps epidermal cells move under the influence of voltage gradients either by electrophoresis or by polarization of molecules in the cell membranes. Dry wounds apparently switch off the current that normally exists in a wound, and the lateral voltage gradient is eliminated.[238] This may help to explain why dry superficial wounds heal more slowly than moist wounds.

Ultrasound. The application of ultrasound to wounds is associated with acceleration of healing as well as increased tensile strength.[101,157] Ultrasound increases the temperature of tissue, increasing the blood supply. Pulsed ultrasound, on the other hand, has minimal thermal effects on tissue.

Pulsed ultrasound was used on skin graft donor sites and showed a significantly greater (59% versus 29%) number of patients, with more than 90% healing at 7 days.[157] Pulsed ultrasound has also been used successfully on ulcers on the legs.[106]

Ultrasound is thought to affect the cells of healing wounds in many different ways. Fibroblasts are stimulated toward protein synthesis.[106] Repolarization of depolarized damaged cells occurs, and the electrical field provides a directional polarity.[157]

Systemic medications

Anticoagulants. Although anticoagulants do not decrease the strength of wounds in animals,[415] patients receiving such medications are likely to bleed into their wounds. This leads to increased tension on wound edges and increased time for remodeling of the wound, since resorption of the blood clot will take time. Sometimes such bleeding underneath skin flaps gives rise to elevation of the skin, which resolves over several months.

Anabolic steroids. Anabolic steroids, such as testosterone, have improved the condition of patients with Cushing's disease. They are thought to be lysosomal labilizers, and they counteract the negative effects of cortisone on wound healing.[115,116]

Testosterone has been shown to have several effects on wound healing. Wound tensile strength is increased initially but falls to normal within a short period of time.[367] However, if animals are protein deficient, anabolic steroids noticeably increase the tensile strength.[367,476] Granulation is increased, as is the rate of wound contraction.[392,460] Topically applied nandrolone has been reported to increase the rate of epithelialization.[289]

In summary, testosterone by itself appears to have minor effects on wound healing. But under conditions of increased cortisone (endogenous or exogenous) or protein depletion, anabolic steroids may reverse the negative effects on wound healing.

Antiinflammatory drugs (nonsteroidal). The nonsteroidal antiinflammatory drugs retard wound repair, probably by a number of mechanisms. These medications are antiinflammatory by virtue of their ability to stabilize lysosomes and prevent the release from lysosomes of substances that participate in the inflammatory events of wound healing (see box). Phenylbutazone and indomethacin have been shown to increase the catabolism of collagen by inducing increased collagenolytic activity.[210] Both aspirin and phenylbutazone have been shown to decrease the tensile strength of wounds in rats.[285,474] Aspirin not only decreases the inflammatory

---

DRUGS AFFECTING LYSOSOMES

Lysosomal stabilizer (depresses wound healing)	Lysosomal labilizer (stimulates wound healing)
Glucocorticoids	Testosterone
Nonsteroidal antiinflammatory drugs (aspirin, indomethacin, phenylbutazone, colchicine)	Vitamin A
Vitamin E	
Zinc	

---

response in wounds, but decreases the acid mucopolysaccharide synthesis as well.[285]

Colchicine is an antimitotic, antiinflammatory drug with known effects on microtubular disruption of cells. Given to rats, it paradoxically has been shown to increase collagenase activity and collagen synthesis. However, the total collagen remains the same.[335] This ability to increase collagenase activity has led to its use in conditions of overproduction of collagen, such as keloids.[364] Colchicine also inhibits the release of histamine from mast cells. As discussed previously, histamine may stimulate fibroblasts. Such applications are intriguing, but it is too soon to say with certainty their ultimate applicability.

Antiinflammatory drugs (steroidal). Soon after cortisone was introduced into medical usage, it was clinically observed that patients with systemic lupus erythematosus or rheumatoid arthritis treated with this medication did not form granulation tissue easily in open wounds.[385] The action of this medication on these collagen diseases was thus thought to affect the local collagen-repair mechanisms. Anecdotal reports of poor wound healing, sepsis, and death have also been associated with cortisone use.[369] Further studies have shown that wounds in patients with Cushing's syndrome have decreased strength[417] (Fig. 2-47), and that patients having abdominal surgery and receiving steroids have a greater incidence of wound dehiscence than those not receiving steroids.[162] Administration of cortisone to humans results in loss of collagen from the skin.[210] The association of cortisone or steroid therapy and wound healing has been the object of extensive study.

Cortisone is a prototypic glucocortocoid hormone, which has an antiinsulin role in the body's metabolism. It is a naturally occurring glucocorticoid secreted by the adrenal gland and is converted to cortisol (hydrocortisone) before becoming biologically active. Thus it promotes gluconeogenesis in the liver, but at the expense of protein catabolism. Cortisone inhibits not only the synthesis of extrahepatic protein and nucleic acids, but long-chain fatty acids as well. Thus patients receiving cortisone or its related synthetic steroids develop protein-wasting. Moreover, cortisone inhibits utilization of glucose in peripheral tissues.

The systemic usage of cortisone is associated with several effects on wound repair. Cortisone decreases the number of monocytes and lymphocytes in the peripheral blood.[465] This leads to a decrease in the accumulation of these cells in wounds[411] and thus impedes the important inflammatory events in repair.

Cortisone has been shown mainly to decrease the elements of repair involving the mesenchymal tissues (the fibroblasts and blood vessels), although there is also some slowing of the rate of epidermal resurfacing.[11,217] Protocollagen proline hydroxylase (PPH), a useful indicator of collagen synthesis, is decreased, as is hydroxyproline in granulation tissue.[413,447] The development and amount of granulation tissue are markedly delayed.[217,369,385] This is thought to be caused not by delayed migration of fibroblasts but by suppressed synthesis within the fibroblasts, particularly of glycosaminoglycans and collagen.[112,279] Cortisone may also interfere with wound healing by interfering with histamine release. Histamine stimulation is known to be associated with an increased wound healing rate.[244]

Contraction of wounds is also inhibited by cortisone.[41,392] This phenomenon occurs in open wounds even if the cortisone administration is begun after contraction has started.[451]

Probably because of the decreased rate of fibroplasia, systemic cortisone results in wounds that are less strong, if measured early, than control wounds.[11,115,196,322,461] However, the changes seen in tensile strength depend on a number of variables and are usually marked only early on.[367] If cortisone was started 2 days after wounding in rats, there was no decrease in tensile strength, whereas if given before that time it decreased the tensile strength.[413] The effects of cortisone are thus thought to be limited to the first few days after wounding.[439]

The length of time cortisone is given before the surgery also affects the tensile strength.[377,423] Cortisone given in rabbits for at least 5 days before surgery had the greatest effect on wound strength.[196]

The fact that cortisone mainly inhibits the fibroplasia during the first few days of wound repair is dramatically illustrated by what happens if wounds are disrupted and then resutured. Normally such wounds rapidly gain tensile strength, so that at a week they are even stronger than primarily closed undisrupted wounds. However, if animals are given cortisone and their wounds are disrupted, this accelerated gain in tensile strength is abolished.[196,423]

The dosage of cortisone also influences to some degree its effect on wound repair.[92,115] The repair processes of humans are a well-designed response to trauma. Since such trauma may result in small increases in endogenous cortisone, it is not surprising that high and prolonged doses of cortisone are necessary to affect wound healing.

Protein depletion tends to potentiate the negative effects of cortisone on wound repair,[127] whereas testosterone or vitamin A may reverse the effects of cortisone.[115,116,411,447] Both vitamin A and β-carotene result in increased hydroxyproline in wounds when given with glucocorticoids.[117] Anecdotal but unproven reports have appeared, suggesting that topical vitamin A stimulates healing in patients receiving cortisone.[223]

Topical glucocorticoid steroids have been shown to decrease the rate of epidermization in superficial wounds. Whether this is caused by the catabolic effects of such steroids or their known local vasoconstrictive or antiinflammatory effects is unknown.[485] In one study triamcinolone ointment 0.1% decreased the rate of epidermal regeneration by 62%.[108] Hydrocortisone may have similar effects but not nearly as marked.[318] Some authors have not shown that hydrocortisone has any negative influence on epithelial repair.[13,289]

Topical steroids also affect collagen production in wounds. It is thought that the effects on collagen production occur independent of the epithelial effects.[289] Hydrocortisone, for instance, may decrease the wound collagen in some animal models without affecting the reepithelialization.[13] Fluorinated glucocorticoids are particularly effective in decreasing the collagen formation.[13,411] Tensile strength of such wounds is also decreased early.[93] However, some authors have suggested that since the ultimate strength of wounds treated with topical steroids is no different from that of controls, perhaps topical steroids could be used to advantage in inhibiting overproduction of scar tissue.[33]

Antineoplastic agents. The effect of antimetabolites and antimitotic agents on wound repair is not clear. In general this class of compounds does not profoundly impair wound healing, but there are some exceptions. As with other medications, the dose, route of administration, and time of treatment relative to the wound creation all influence wound healing.[341] Doxorubicin for instance, decreases wound breaking strength if given the day of wounding but has little effect if given 7 days earlier or 7 days later.[90]

Antineoplastic agents are given for systemic cancer. The patients who receive these medications may become cachectic and protein depleted. In addition, if the cancer is very widespread, it may also affect the body's ability to heal wounds. Wound tensile strength in rats was decreased in tumor-bearing animals given doxorubicin or methotrexate compared with normal animals treated with the same agents.[42] Apparently cancer potentiated the effect of these agents on impairment of wound healing. These effects occurred during the early phases of wound repair before the remodeling and cross-linking phases.

The antineoplastic agents are not uniform in their effects on wound repair. Vincristine and methotrexate, for instance, impair wound strength in mice early (at 3 days) but not if the wounds are tested at a later time (7 and 21 days). Actinomycin D, however, impairs wound strength both early and later.[79] In some studies systemic 5-fluorouracil impaired wound healing,[444] whereas in others it had no effect.[79] Azathioprine, which interferes with purine metabolism, does not seem to interfere with wound healing in rats.[18]

Dilantin. Dilantin has known effects on collagen tissue, and in a small percentage of patients who chronically take this drug gingival hypertrophy occurs. Nevertheless, the effect of dilantin on wound healing is negligible.

Hormones (miscellaneous). Several hormones may act individually, synergistically, or antagonistically to affect wound repair. Thyroid hormone appears to accelerate wound healing. In animals that have been hypophysectomized, granulation tissue is decreased in wounds.[459,460] If these animals are given thyroxin, granulation tissue is stimulated. Both ACTH and estradiol also inhibit granulation tissue.[460] Human growth hormone has no effect on wound healing.[388]

Penicillamine. As discussed earlier, penicillamine is a degradation product of penicillin. It is an effective chelator of metals such as copper, zinc, and mercury and facilitates their excretion in the urine. Penicillamine is used to treat Wilson's disease, cystinuria, and rheumatoid arthritis.

The medication *d*-penicillamine interferes with the biosynthesis of interchain cross-links in collagen.[243] Thus collagen in wounds may be poorly cross-linked in patients taking it. After prolonged administration, extravasation of red blood cells occurs in the skin caused by fragility of the dermis.

Vitamins. Vitamins A, C, and E can affect wound repair. They have already been discussed.

Zinc. Zinc affects wound repair if taken to remedy zinc depletion. This has already been discussed.

REFERENCES

1. Abercrombie, M.: Localized formation of new tissue in an adult mammal, Symp. Soc. Exp. Biol. **11:**235, 1957.
2. Abercrombie, M.: Behavior of cells toward one another, Adv. Biol. Skin **5:**95, 1964.
3. Abercrombie, M., Flint, M.H., and James, D.W.: Collagen formation and wound contraction during repair of small excised wounds in the skin of rats, J. Embryol. Exp. Morphol. **2:**264, 1954.
4. Abercrombie, M., Flint, M.H., and James, D.W.: Wound contraction in relation to collagen formation in scorbutic guinea pigs, J. Embryol. Exp. Morphol. **4:**167, 1956.
5. Abercrombie, M., James, D.W., and Newcombe, J.F.: Wound contraction in rabbit skin, studied by splinting the wound margins, J. Anat. **94:**170, 1960.
6. Abergel, R.P., et al.: Control of connective tissue metabolism by lasers: recent developments and future projects, J. Am. Acad. Dermatol. **11:**1142, 1984.
7. Abt, A.F., and Von Schuching, S.: Catabolism of L-ascorbic-1-C^{14} acid as a measure of its utilization in the intact and wounded guinea pig on scorbutic, maintenance and saturation diets, Ann. N.Y. Acad. Sci. **92:**148, 1961.
8. Adamsons, R.J., Musco, F., and Enquist, I.F.: The chemical dimensions of a healing incision, Surg. Gynecol. Obstet. **123:**515, 1966.
9. Ahmad, M.: Glucosamine and hydroxyproline content of granulation tissue on different days of wound healing in white albino rats, Ann. Biochem. Exp. Med. **21:**295, 1961.
10. Al-Hassan, J.M., Thomson, M., and Criddle, R.S.: Accelerated wound healing by a preparation from skin of the Arabian Gulf catfish (letter), Lancet **1:**1043, 1983.
11. Alrich, E.M., Carter, J.P., and Lehman, E.P.: The effect of ACTH and cortisone on wound healing, Ann. Surg. **133:**783, 1951.
12. Alvarez, O.M., et al.: Benzoyl peroxide and epidermal wound healing, Arch. Dermatol. **119:**222, 1983.
13. Alvarez, O.M., Mertz, P.M., Eaglstein, W.H.: The effect of occlusive dressings on collagen synthesis and reepithelialization in superficial wounds, J. Surg. Res. **35:**142, 1983.
14. Alvarez, O.M., et al.: The healing of superficial skin wounds is stimulated by external electrical current, J. Invest. Dermatol. **81:**144, 1983.
15. Apesos, J., Hamilton, R.W., and Korostoff, E.: Tensile strength in ischemic wounds in rats, Surg. Forum **19:**505, 1968.
16. Arey, L.: Wound healing, Physiol. Rev. **16:**327, 1936.
17. Arturson, G.: Epidermal growth factor in the healing of corneal wounds, epidermal wounds, and partial-thickness scalds, Scand. J. Plast. Reconstr. Surg. **18:**33, 1984.
18. Arumugam, S., Nimmannit, S., and Enquist, I.F.: The effect of immunosuppression on wound healing, Surg. Gynecol. Obstet. **133:**72, 1971.
19. Bailey, A.J., Robins, S.P., and Balian, G.: Biological significance of the intermolecular crosslinks of collagen, Nature **251:**105, 1974.
20. Bailey, A.J., et al.: Characterization of the collagen of human hypertrophic and normal scars. Biochim. Biophys. Acta **405:**412, 1975.
21. Bailey, A.J., et al.: Collagen polymorphism in experimental granulation tissue, Biochem. Biophys. Res. Commun. **66:**1160, 1975.
22. Bains, J.W., Crawford, D.T., and Ketcham, A.S.: Effect of chronic anaemia on wound tensile strength, Ann. Surg. **164:**243, 1966.
23. Barcia, P.J.: Lack of acceleration of healing with zinc sulfate, Ann. Surg. **172:**1048, 1970.
24. Barnes, M.J.: Function of ascorbic acid in collagen metabolism, Ann. N.Y. Acad. Sci. **258:**264, 1975.
25. Bauer, E.A., Eisen, A.Z., and Jeffrey, J.J.: Regulation of vertebrate collagenase activity in vitro and in vivo, J. Invest. Dermatol. **59:**50, 1972.
26. Baur, P.S., Larson, D.L., and Stacey, T.R.: The observation of myofibroblasts in hypertrophic scars, Surg. Gynecol. Obstet. **141:**22, 1975.
27. Baur, P.S., Jr., and Parks, D.H.: The myofibroblast-anchoring strand: the fibronectin connection in wound healing and the possible loci of collagen fibril assembly, J. Trauma **23:**853, 1983.
28. Bayer, I., and Ellis, H.: Jaundice and wound healing: an experimental study, Br. J. Surg. **63:**392, 1976.
29. Bazin, S., LeLous, M., and Delaunay, A.: Collagen in granulation tissues, Agents Actions **6:**272, 1976.

30. Bennett, R.G., and Robins, P.: Repair of tissue defects resulting from removal of cutaneous neoplasms, J. Dermatol. Surg. Oncol. **3**(5):512, 1977.
31. Bentley, J.P.: Rate of chondroitin sulfate formation in wound healing, Ann. Surg. **165**:186, 1967.
32. Bergman, A., et al.: Acceleration of wound healing by topical application of honey: an animal model, Am. J. Surg. **145**:374, 1983.
33. Berliner, D.L., et al.: Decreased scar formation with topical corticosteroid treatment, Surgery **61**:619, 1967.
34. Bernstein, H.: Treatment of keloids by steroids with biochemical tests for diagnosis and prognosis, Angiology **15**:253, 1964.
35. Bertolami, C.N., and Donoff, R.B.: Identification, characterization, and partial purification of mammalian skin wound hyaluronidase, J. Invest. Dermatol. **79**:417, 1982.
36. Besser, E.L., and Ehrenhaft, J.L.: The relationship of acute anaemia to wound healing, Surgery **14**:239, 1943.
37. Bhawan, J.: Steroid-induced "granulomas" in hypertrophic scars, Acta Derm. Venereol. [Stockh.] **63**:560, 1983.
38. Bhoola, K.D., Calle, J.D., and Schachter, M.: The effect of bradykinin, serum kallikrein, and other endogenous substances on capillary permeability in the guinea pig, J. Physiol. **152**:75, 1960.
39. Bierens de Haan, B., Ellis, H., and Wilks, M.: The role of infection on wound healing, Surg. Gynecol. Obstet. **138**:693, 1974.
40. Billingham, R.E., and Medawar, P.B.: Contracture and intussusceptive growth in healing of extensive wounds in mammalian skin, J. Anat. **89**:114, 1955.
41. Billingham, R.E., and Russell, P.S.: Studies in wound healing with special reference to the phenomenon of contracture of experimental wounds in rabbit skins, Ann. Surg. **144**:961, 1956.
42. Bland, K.I., et al.: Experimental and clinical observations of the effects of cytotoxic chemotherapeutic drugs on wound healing, Ann. Surg. **199**:782, 1984.
43. Bornstein, P., Kang, A.H., and Piez, K.A.: The nature and location of intramolecular cross-links in collagen, Proc. Nat. Acad. Sci. **55**:417, 1966.
44. Bothwell, J.W.: Collagen resorption in contracting guinea pig wounds, Nature **201**:825, 1964.
45. Botsford, T.W.: The tensile strength of sutured skin wounds during healing, Surg. Gynecol. Obstet. **72**:690, 1941.
46. Boucek, R.J.: Factors affecting wound healing, Otolaryngol. Clin. North Am. **17**:243, 1984.
47. Boyce, S.T., and Ham, R.G.: Calcium-regulated differentiation of normal human epidermal keratinocytes in chemically defined clonal culture and serum-free serial culture, J. Invest. Dermatol. **81**:33, 1983.
48. Branemark, P.I.: Capillary form and function: the microcirculation of granulation tissue, Bibl. Anat. **7**:9, 1965.
49. Breasted, J.H.: The Edwin Smith surgical papyrus, vol. 1, Chicago, 1930, University of Chicago Press.
50. Brennan, M.F.: Metabolic response to surgery in the cancer patient, Cancer **43**:2053, 1979.
51. Brown, I.A.: A scanning electron microscopic study of the effects of uniaxial tension on human skin, Br. J. Dermatol. **89**:383, 1973.
52. Brunius, U.: Wound healing impairment from sutures, Acta Chir. Scand. **395**:1, 1968.
53. Brunius, U., Zederfeldt, B., and Ahren, C.: Healing of skin incisions closed by nonsuture technique, Acta Chir. Scand. **133**:509, 1967.
54. Bryant, W.M.: Wound healing, Clin. Symp. (Ciba) **29**:1, 1977.
55. Büchner, T., et al.: Origin and formation of inflammatory cells in granulation tissue: autoradiographic investigation with thymidine-^{3}H on cotton pellet granuloma of the rat, Klin. Wochenschr. **48**:867, 1970.
56. Bullough, W.S.: The action of chalones, Agents Actions **2**:1, 1971.
57. Bullough, W.S., and Laurence, E.B.: The control of epidermal mitotic activity in the mouse, Proc. R. Soc. Lond. **151**:517, 1959.
58. Burrows, M.T.: Studies in wound healing, J. Med. Res. **44**:615, 1924.
59. Byers, P.H., et al.: Interchain disulfide bonds in procollagen are located in a large nontriple-helical COOH-terminal domain, Proc. Natl. Acad. Sci. **72**:3009, 1975.
60. Caldwell, F.T., et al.: Effect of single amino acid supplementation upon the gain of tensile strength of wounds in protein-depleted rats, Surg. Gynecol. Obstet. **119**:823, 1964.
61. Calnan, J., Fry, H.J.H., and Saad, N.: Wound healing and wound hormones: a study of tensile strength in rats, Br. J. Surg. **51**:448, 1964.
62. Carrel, A.: The treatments of wounds, J.A.M.A. **55**:2148, 1910.
63. Carrel, A.: Cicatrization of wounds. XII. Factors initiating regeneration, J. Expr. Med. **34**:425, 1921.
64. Carrel, A., and Hartmann, A.: Cicatrization of wounds. I. The relation between the size of the wound and the rate of its cicatrization, J. Exp. Med. **24**:429, 1916.
65. Castor, L.N.: Control of division by cell contact and serum concentration in cultures of 3T3 cells, Exp. Cell Res. **68**:17, 1971.
66. Catty, R.H.C.: Healing and contraction of experimental full-thickness wounds in the human, Br. J. Surg. **52**:542, 1965.
67. Celleno, L., et al.: Collagen deposition in skin wound healing (abstract), J. Invest. Dermatol. **80**:325, 1983.
68. Chiakulas, J.J.: The role of tissue specificity in the healing of epithelial wounds, J. Exp. Zool. **121**:383, 1952.
69. Chvapil, M.: Pharmacology of fibrosis: definitions, limits and perspectives, Life Sciences **16**:1345, 1975.
70. Chvapil, M., et al.: Pathophysiology of zinc, Int. Rev. Neurobiol. **1**:105, 1972.
71. Clark, M.E.: Growth and morphology of adult mouse fibroblasts under anaerobic conditions and at limiting oxygen tensions, Exp. Cell Res. **36**:548, 1964.
72. Clark, R.A., et al.: Role of macrophages in wound healing, Surg. Forum **27**:16, 1976.
73. Clark, R.A.F., et al.: Fibronectin and fibrin provide a provisional matrix for epidermal cell migration during wound reepithelialization, J. Invest. Dermatol. **79**:264, 1982.
74. Clark, R.A.F., et al.: Blood vessel fibronectin increases in conjunction with endothelial cell proliferation and capillary ingrowth during wound healing, J. Invest. Dermatol. **79**:269, 1982.

75. Clark, R.A., et al.: Fibronectin beneath re-epithelializing epidermis in vivo: sources and significance, J. Invest. Dermatol. **80:**265, 1983.

76. Clore, J.N., Cohen, I.K., and Diegelmann, R.F.: Quantitation of collagen types I and III during wound healing in rat skin, Proc. Soc. Exp. Biol. Med. **161:**337, 1979.

77. Cohen, I.K., and McCoy, B.J.: Wound healing. In Goldsmith, L.A., editor: Biochemistry and physiology of the skin, vol. 1, New York, 1983, Oxford University Press.

78. Cohen, I.K., Keiser, H.R., and Sjoerdsma, A.: Collagen synthesis in human keloid and hypertrophic scar, Surg. Forum **22:**488, 1971.

79. Cohen, S.C., et al.: Effects of antineoplastic agents on wound healing in mice, Surgery **78:**238, 1975.

80. Colin, J.F., Elliot, P., and Ellis, H.: The effect of uraemia upon wound healing: an experimental study, Br. J. Surg. **66:**793, 1979.

81. Converse, J.M., and Robb-Smith, A.H.T.: Healing of surface cutaneous wounds: its analogy with the healing of superficial burns, Ann. Surg. **120:**873, 1944.

82. Craig, R.D.P., Schofield, J.D., and Jackson, S.S.: Collagen biosynthesis in normal human skin, normal and hypertrophic scar, and keloid, Eur. J. Clin. Invest. **5:**69, 1975.

83. Crandon, J.H., et al.: Ascorbic acid economy in surgical patients, Ann. N.Y. Acad. Sci. **92:**246, 1961.

84. Crandon, J.H., Lund, C.C., and Dill, D.B.: Experimental human scurvy, N. Engl. J. Med. **223:**353, 1940.

85. Craven, J.L.: Wound contraction in lathyritic rats, Arch. Pathol. **89:**526, 1970.

86. Crawford, B.S., and Gipson, M.: The conservative management of pretibial lacerations on elderly patients, Br. J. Plast. Surg. **30:**174, 1977.

87. Creditor, M.C., et al.: Effect of ACTH on wound healing in adults, Proc. Soc. Exp. Biol. Med. **74:**245, 1950.

88. Cuthbertson, A.M.: Contraction of full-thickness skin wounds in the rat, Surg. Gynecol. Obstet. **108:**421, 1959.

89. Dann, L., Glucksmann, A., and Tansley, K.: The healing of untreated experimental wounds, Br. J. Exp. Pathol. **22:**1, 1941.

90. Devereux, D.F., et al.: The quantitative and qualitative impairment of wound healing by adriamycin, Cancer **43:**932, 1979.

91. Devito, R.V.: Healing of wounds, Surg. Clin. N. Am. **45:** 441, 1965.

92. DiPasquale, G., and Steinetz, B.G.: Relationship of food intake to the effect of cortisone acetate on skin wound healing, Proc. Soc. Biol. Med. **117:**118, 1964.

93. DiPasquale, G., Tripp, L.V., and Steinetz, B.G.: Effect of locally applied antiinflammatory substances on rat skin wounds, Proc. Soc. Exp. Biol. Med. **124:**404, 1967.

94. Dixon, J.A., et al.: Hypertrophic scarring in argon laser treatment of portwine stains, Plast. Reconstr. Surg. **73:**771, 1984.

95. Donaldson, D.J., and Mahan, J.T.: Fibrinogen and fibronectin as substrates for epidermal cell migration during wound closure, J. Cell Sci. **62:**117, 1983.

96. Donoff, R.B., and Grillo, H.C.: The effects of skin grafting on healing open wounds in rabbits, J. Surg. Res. **19:**163, 1975.

97. Donoff, R.B., Swann, D.A., and Schweidt, S.H.: Glycosaminoglycans of normal and hypertrophic human scar. Exp. Mol. Pathol. **40:**13, 1984.

98. Douglas, D.M.: The healing of aponeurotic incisions, Br. J. Surg. **40:**79, 1952.

99. Douglas, D.M., Forrester, J.C., and Ogilvie, R.R.: Physical characteristics of collagen in the later stages of wound healing, Br. J. Surg. **56:**219, 1969.

100. Douglas, D.M.: Acceleration of wound healing produced by preliminary wounding, Br. J. Surg. **46:**401, 1959.

101. Drastichova, V., Samohyl, J., and Slavetinska, A.: Strengthening of sutured skin wounds with ultrasound in experiments on animals, Acta Chir. Plast. [Praha] **15:**114, 1973.

102. Dunphy, J.E.: The fibroblast, a ubiquitous ally for the surgeon, N. Engl. J. Med. **268:**1367, 1963.

103. Dunphy, J.E., and Jackson, D.S.: Practical applications of experimental studies in the care of the primarily closed wounds, Am. J. Surg. **104:**273, 1962.

104. Dunphy, J.E., and Udupa, K.N.: Chemical and histochemical sequences in the normal healing of wounds, N. Engl. J. Med. **253:**847, 1955.

105. Dunphy, J.E., Udupa, K.N., and Edwards, L.C.: Wound healing: a new perspective with particular reference to ascorbic acid deficiency, Ann. Surg. **144:**304, 1956.

106. Dyson, M., and Suckling, J.: Stimulation of tissue repair by ultrasound: a survey of the mechanisms involved, Physiotherapy **64:**105, 1978.

107. Eaglstein, W.H., editor: Wound healing, Clin. Dermatol. **2:**1, 1984.

108. Eaglstein, W.H., and Mertz, P.M.: New method for assessing epidermal wound healing, J. Invest. Dermatol. **71:**382, 1978.

109. Eaglstein, W.H., and Mertz, P.M.: "Inert" vehicles do affect wound healing, J. Invest. Dermatol. **74:**90, 1980.

110. Eaglstein, W.H., Mertz, P., and Alvarez, O.M.: Effect of topically applied agents on healing wounds, Clin. Dermatol. **2:**112, 1984.

111. Ebeling, A.H.: Cicatrization of wounds. XIII. The temperature coefficient, J. Exp. Med. **35:**657, 1922.

112. Ebert, P.S., and Prockop, D.J.: Influence of cortisol on the synthesis of sulfated mucopolysaccharides and collagen in chick embryos, Biochim. Biophys. Acta **136:**45, 1967.

113. Edlich, R.F., Smith, Q.T., and Edgerton, M.T.: Resistance of the surgical wound to antimicrobial prophylaxis and its mechanism of development, Am. J. Surg. **126:**583, 1973.

114. Ehrlich, H.P., and Buttle, D.J.: Epidermis promotion of collagenase in hypertrophic scar organ culture, Exp. Mol. Pathol. **40:**223, 1984.

115. Ehrlich, H.P., and Hunt, T.K.: Effects of cortisone and vitamin A on wound healing, Ann. Surg. **167:**324, 1968.

116. Ehrlich, H.P., and Hunt, T.K.: The effect of cortisone and anabolic steroids on the tensile strength of healing wounds, Ann. Surg. **170:**203, 1969.

117. Ehrlich, H.P., and Tarver, H.: Effects of beta-carotene, vitamin A, and glucocorticoids on collagen synthesis in wounds, Proc. Soc. Exp. Biol. Med. **137:**936, 1971.

118. Ehrlich, H.P., Tarver, H., and Hunt, T.K.: Inhibitory effect of vitamin E on collagen synthesis and wound repair, Ann. Surg. **175:**235, 1972.

119. Ehrlich, H.P., and White, B.S.: The identification of αA and αB collagen chains in hypertrophic scars, Exp. Mol. Pathol. **34:**1, 1981.

120. Eisen, A.Z., Bauer, E.A., and Jeffrey, J.J.: Animal and human collagenases, J. Invest. Dermatol. **55:**359, 1970.

121. Eisen, A.Z., Jeffrey, J.J., and Gross, J.: Human skin collagenase: isolation and mechanism of attack on the collagen molecule, Biochim. Biophys. Acta **151:**637, 1968.

122. Epstein, E.H., Jr.: $[\alpha 1(\text{III})]_3$ Human skin collagen: release by pepsin digestion and preponderance in fetal life, J. Biol. Chem. **249:**3225, 1974.

123. Epstein, E.H., Jr., and Munderloh, N.H.: Isolation and characterization of CNBr peptides of human $[\alpha 1(\text{III}_3)]_3$ collagen and tissue distribution of $[\alpha 1(\text{I})]_2\alpha 2$ and $[\alpha 1(\text{III})]_3$ collagens, J. Biol. Chem. **250:**9304, 1975.

124. Fast, J., Nelson, C., and Dennis, C.: Rate of gain in strength in sutured abdominal wall wounds, Surg. Gynecol. Obstet. **84:**685, 1947.

125. Fernandez, A., and Finley, J.M.: Wound healing: helping a natural process, Postgrad. Med. **74:**311, 1983.

126. Filston, H.C., and Vennes, G.J., Jr.: Temperature as a factor in wound healing, Surg. Gynecol. Obstet. **126:**572, 1968.

127. Findlay, C.W., Jr., and Howes, E.L.: The combined effect of cortisone and partial protein depletion on wound healing, N. Engl. J. Med. **246:**597, 1952.

128. Fischer, B.H.: Topical hyperbaric oxygen treatment of pressure sores and skin ulcers, Lancet **2:**405, 1969.

129. Foerster, D.W., and Jaques, W.E.: Cutaneous scarring: a correlation between depth of penetration and scar formation, Plast. Reconstr. Surg. **30:**479, 1962.

130. Foidart, J.M., et al.: Distribution and immunoelectron microscopic localization of laminin, a non-collagenous basement membrane glycoprotein, Lab. Invest. **42:**336, 1980.

131. Forrest, L., and Jackson, D.S.: Intermolecular cross-linking of collagen in human and guinea pig scar tissue, Biochim. Biophys. Acta **229:**681, 1971.

132. Forrester, J.C.: Mechanical, biochemical and architectural features of surgical repair, Adv. Biol. Med. Phys. **14:**1, 1973.

133. Forrester, J.C., Zederfeldt, B.H., and Hunt, T.K.: A bioengineering approach to the healing wound, J. Surg. Res. **9:**207, 1969.

134. Forrester, J.C., et al.: Scanning electron microscopy of healing wounds, Nature **221:**373, 1969.

135. Forrester, J.C., et al.: Tape-closed and sutured wounds: comparison by tensiometry and scanning electron microscopy, Br. J. Surg. **57:**729, 1970.

136. Forrester, J.C., et al.: Wolff's law in relation to the healing skin wound, J. Trauma **10:**770, 1970.

137. Foulds, I.S., and Barker, A.T.: Human skin battery potentials and their possible role in wound healing, Br. J. Dermatol. **109:**515, 1983.

138. Fromer, C.H., and Klintworth, G.K.: An evaluation of the role of leukocytes in the pathogenesis of experimentally induced corneal vascularization, Am. J. Pathol. **82:**157, 1976.

139. Fullmer, H.M., et al.: Collagenolytic activity of the skin associated with neuromuscular diseases including amyotrophic lateral sclerosis, Lancet **1:**1007, 1966.

140. Gabbiani, G., Majno, G., and Ryan, G.B.: The fibroblast as a contractile cell: the myofibroblast. In Pikkarainen, J., and Kulonen, E., editors: Biology of fibroblast, New York, 1973, Academic Press.

141. Gabbiani, G., and Montandon, D.: Reparative processes in mammalian wound healing: the role of contractile phenomena. Int. Rev. Cytol. **48:**187, 1977.

142. Gabbiani, G., and Ryan, G.B.: Development of a contractile apparatus in epithelial cells during epidermal and liver regeneration, J. Submicr. Cytol. **6:**143, 1974.

143. Gabbiani, G., Ryan, G.B., and Majno, G.: Presence of modified fibroblasts in granulation tissue and their possible role in wound contraction, Experientia **27:**549, 1971.

144. Gabbiani, G., et al.: Granulation tissue as a contractile organ: a study of structure and function, J. Exp. Med. **135:**719, 1972.

145. Gabbiani, G., et al.: Human smooth muscle autoantibody: its identification as antiactin antibody and a study of its binding to "nonmuscular" cells, Am. J. Pathol. **72:**473, 1973.

146. Geever, E.F., et al.: Penicillamine and wound healing in young guinea pigs, J. Surg. Res. **7:**160, 1967.

147. Geronemus, R.G., Mertz, P.M., and Eaglstein, W.H.: Wound healing: the effects of topical antimicrobial agents, Arch. Dermatol. **115:**1311, 1979.

148. Gibson, T., and Kenedi, R.M.: Biomechanical properties of the skin, Surg. Clin. N. Am. **47:**279, 1967.

149. Gibson, T., Kenedi, R.M., and Craik, J.E.: The mobile micro-architecture of dermal collagen: a bioengineering study, Br. J. Surg. **52:**764, 1965.

150. Gibson, T., and Kenedi, R.M.: The structural components of the dermis and their mechanical characteristics. In Montagna, W., Bentley, J.P., and Dobson, R.L., editors: Advances in the biology of the skin, vol. 10, The dermis, New York, 1970, Appleton-Century-Crofts.

151. Gillman, T.: Some aspects of the healing and treatment of wounds, Triangle **4:**68, 1959.

152. Gillman, T., et al.: Reactions of healing wounds and granulation tissue in man to auto-Thiersch, autodermal, and homodermal grafts, Br. J. Plast. Surg. **6:**153, 1953.

153. Gillman, T., et al.: A reexamination of certain aspects of the histogenesis of healing cutaneous wounds, Br. J. Surg. **43:**141, 1955.

154. Gimbel, N.S., et al.: A study of epithelialization in blistered burns, A.M.A. Arch. Surg. **74:**800, 1957.

155. Goldberg, B., and Green, H.: Relation between collagen synthesis and collagen proline hydroxylase activity in mammalian cells, Nature **221:**267, 1969.

156. Goldin, E.G., and Joseph, N.R.: Responses of connective tissue ground substance in wound healing, Arch. Surg. **97:**753, 1968.

157. Goldin, J.H., et al.: The effects of Diapulse on the healing of wounds: a double-blind controlled trial in man, Br. J. Plast. Surg. **34:**267, 1981.

158. Goodson, W.H., III, and Hunt, T.K.: Wound healing and aging, J. Invest. Dermatol. **73:**88, 1979.

159. Goodson, W.H., III, and Hunt, T.K.: Wound healing and the diabetic patient, Surg. Gynecol. Obstet. **149:**600, 1979.

160. Grant, M.E., and Prockop, D.J.: The biosynthesis of collagen, N. Engl. J. Med. **286:**194, 242, and 291, 1972.

161. Greaves, M.W.: Lack of effect of topically applied epidermal growth factor (EGF) on epidermal growth in man in vivo, Clin. Exp. Dermatol. **5:**101, 1980.

162. Green, J.P.: Steroid therapy and wound healing in surgical patients, Br. J. Surg. **52**:523, 1965.

163. Grillo, H.C.: Origin of fibroblasts in wound healing: an autoradiographic study of inhibition of cellular proliferation by local x-irradiation, Ann. Surg. **157**:453, 1963.

164. Grillo, H.C., and Gross, J.: Studies in wound healing. III. Contraction in vitamin C deficiency, Proc. Soc. Exp. Biol. Med. **101**:268, 1959.

165. Grillo, H.C., and Gross, J.: Collagenolytic activity during mammalian wound repair, Dev. Biol. **15**:300, 1967.

166. Grillo, H.C., and Potsaid, M.S.: Studies in wound healing. IV. Retardation of contraction by local X-irradiation and observations relating to the origin of fibroblasts in repair, Ann. Surg. **154**:741, 1961.

167. Grillo, H.C., Watts, G.T., and Gross, J.: The marginal localization of the contraction mechanism in open wounds, Surg. Forum **8**:586, 1957.

168. Grillo, H.C., Watts, G.T., and Gross, J.: Studies in wound healing. I. Contraction and the wound contents, Ann. Surg. **148**:145, 1958.

169. Griswold, M.L., Jr.: Effects of adrenal cortical preparations on scar hypertrophy, Plast. Reconstr. Surg. **13**:454, 1954.

170. Gross, J., Highberger, J.H., and Schmitt, F.O.: Collagen structures considered as states of aggregation of a kinetic unit: the tropocollagen particle, Proc. Nat. Acad. Sci. U.S.A. **40**:679, 1954.

171. Gross, J., and Lapière, C.M.: Collagenolytic activity in amphibian tissues: a tissue culture assay, Proc. Nat. Acad. Sci. **48**:1014, 1962.

172. Grove, G.L.: Age-related differences in healing of superficial skin wounds in humans, Arch. Dermatol. Res. **272**:381, 1982.

173. Gruber, R.P., Vistnes, L., and Pardoe, R.: The effect of commonly used antiseptics on wound healing, Plast. Reconstr. Surg. **55**:472, 1975.

174. Gruber, R.P., et al.: Hyperbaric oxygen and pedicle flaps, skin grafts, and burns, Plast. Reconstr. Surg. **45**:24, 1970.

175. Gruber, R.P., et al.: Hyperbaric oxygenation of pedicle flaps without oxygen toxicity, Plast. Reconstr. Surg. **46**:477, 1970.

176. Gruber, D.K., et al.: Acceleration of wound healing by *Staphylococcus aureus,* Surg. Forum **32**:76, 1981.

177. Haeger, K., and Lanner, E.: Oral zinc sulphate and ischaemic leg ulcers, Vasa **3**:77, 1974.

178. Haley, J.V.: Zinc sulphate and wound healing, J. Surg. Res. **27**:168, 1979.

179. Halley, C.R.L., Chesney, A.M., and Dresel, I.: On the behavior of granulating wounds of the rabbit to various types of infection, Bull. Johns Hopkins Hosp. **41**:191, 1927.

180. Halsted, W.S.: The treatment of wounds with special reference to the value of blood clot in the management of dead space, Johns Hopkins Hosp. Reports **2**:255, 1891.

181. Hanam, S.R., Singleton, C.E., and Rudek, W.: The effect of topical insulin on infected cutaneous ulcerations in diabetic and nondiabetic mice, J. Foot Surg. **22**:298, 1983.

182. Harkness, M.L.R., Harkness, R.D., and James, D.W.: The effect of a protein-free diet on the collagen content of mice, J. Physiol. **144**:307, 1958.

183. Harper, R.A., and Grove, G.: Human skin fibroblasts derived from papillary and reticular dermis: differences in growth potential in vitro, Science **204**:526, 1979.

184. Harris, E.D., Jr., and Krane, S.M.: Collagenases, N. Engl. J. Med. **291**:557, 1974.

185. Harvey, S.C.: The velocity of the growth of fibroblasts in the healing wound, Arch. Surg. **18**:1227, 1929.

186. Harvey, S.C., and Howes, E.L.: Effect of high-protein diet on the velocity of growth of fibroblasts in the healing wound, Ann. Surg. **91**:641, 1930.

187. Hedelin, H., et al.: Influence of local fibrin deposition on granulation tissue formation, Eur. Surg. Res. **15**:312, 1983.

188. Hedelin, H., et al.: The influence of locally deposited fibrin on the biomechanical properties of developing granulation tissue in rats, Scand. J. Plast. Reconstr. Surg. **17**:179, 1983.

189. Hell, E.: A stimulant to DNA synthesis in guinea pig ear epidermis, Br. J. Dermatol. **83**:632, 1970.

190. Henshaw, P.S., and Meyer, H.L.: Measurement of epithelial growth in surgical wounds of the rabbit's ear, J. Nat. Cancer Inst. **4**:351, 1943.

191. Hering, T.M., Marchant, R.E., and Anderson, J.M.: Type V collagen during granulation tissue development, Exp. Mol. Pathol. **39**:219, 1983.

192. Heughan, C., Grislis, G., and Hunt, T.K.: The effect of anemia on wound healing, Ann. Surg. **179**:163, 1974.

193. Higton, D.I.R., and James, D.W.: The force of contraction of full-thickness wounds of rabbit skin, Br. J. Surg. **51**:462, 1964.

194. Hill, G.L., et al.: Malnutrition in surgical patients, Lancet **1**:689, 1977.

195. Hinman, C.D., and Maibach, H.: Effects of air exposure and occlusion on experimental human skin wounds, Nature **200**:377, 1963.

196. Hinshaw, D.B., Hughes, L.D., and Stafford, C.E.: Effects of cortisone on the healing of disrupted abdominal wounds, Am. J. Surg. **101**:189, 1961.

197. Hirobe, T.: Proliferation of epidermal melanocytes during the healing of skin wounds in newborn mice, J. Exp. Zool. **227**:423, 1983.

198. Hodges, R.E., et al.: Experimental scurvy in man, Am. J. Clin. Nutr. **22**:535, 1969.

199. Hoffmann, M.E., and Meneghini, R.: Action of hydrogen peroxide on human fibroblast in culture, Photochem. Photobiol. **30**:151, 1979.

200. Hoffmann-Berling, H.: Das Kontraktile Eiweiss Undifferenzierter Zellen, Biochim. Biophys. Acta **19**:453, 1956.

201. Hohn, D.C.: Leukocytic phagocytic function and dysfunction, Surg. Gynecol. Obstet. **144**:99, 1977.

202. Hohn, D.C., et al.: The effect of O_2 tension on microbicidal function of leukocytes in wounds and in vitro, Surg. Forum **27**:18, 1976.

203. Hohn, D.C., et al.: Antimicrobial systems of the surgical wound. I. A comparison of oxidative metabolism and microbicidal capacity of phagocytes from wounds and from peripheral blood, Am. J. Surg. **133**:597, 1977.

204. Hohn, D.C., et al.: Antimicrobial systems of the surgical wound. II. Detection of antimicrobial protein in cell-free wound fluid, Am. J. Surg. **133**:601, 1977.

205. Holmstrand, K., Longacre, J.J., and de Stefano, G.A.: The ultrastructure of collagen in skin, scars and keloids, Plast. Reconstr. Surg. **27**:597, 1961.

206. Homer: Illiadis, book 11 (Λ), London, 1957, Oxford University Press. (Translation by R.G. Bennett.)

207. Hoopes, J.E., Su C.-T., and Im, M.J.C.: Enzyme activities in hypertrophic scars and keloids, Plast. Reconstr. Surg. **47:**132, 1971.

208. Horwitz, A.L., Hance, A.J., and Crystal, R.G.: Granulocyte collagenase: selective digestion of type I relative to type III collagen, Proc. Natl. Acad. Sci. **74:**897, 1977.

209. Houck, J.C.: The effect of local necrosis upon the collagen content of uninjured dista skin, Surgery **51:**770, 1962.

210. Houck, J.C., and Sharma, V.K.: Induction of collagenolytic and proteolytic activities in rat and human fibroblasts by antiinflammatory drugs, Science **161:**1361, 1968.

211. Howes, E.L.: Effects of suture material on the tensile strength of wound repair, Ann. Surg. **98:**153, 1933.

212. Howes, E.L.: The immediate strength of the sutured wound, Surgery **7:**24, 1940.

213. Howes, E.L., and Harvey, S.C.: The age factor in the velocity of the growth of fibroblasts in the healing wound, J. Exp. Med. **55:**577, 1932.

214. Howes, E.L., Harvey, S.C., and Hewitt, C.: Rate of fibroplasia and differentiation in the healing of cutaneous wounds of different species of animals, Arch. Surg. **38:**934, 1939.

215. Howes, E.L., Sooy, J.W., and Harvey, S.C.: The healing of wounds as determined by their tensile strength, J.A.M.A. **92:**42, 1929.

216. Howes, E.L., et al.: Effect of complete and partial starvation on the rate of fibroplasia in the healing wound, Arch. Surg. **27:**846, 1933.

217. Howes, E.L., et al.: Retardation of wound healing by cortisone, Surgery **28:**177, 1950.

218. Hunt, T.K.: Recent advances in wound healing, Surg. Ann. **2:**1, 1970.

219. Hunt, T.K.: Wound healing and wound infection: theory and surgical practice, New York, 1980, Appleton-Century-Crofts.

220. Hunt, T.K., and Pai, M.P.: Effect of varying ambient oxygen tensions on wound metabolism and collagen synthesis, Surg. Gynecol. Obstet. **135:**561, 1972.

221. Hunt, T.K., Sheldon, G., and Fuchs, R.: Physiological mechanisms in repair of burns, Burns **1:**212, 1975.

222. Hunt, T.K., et al.: Respiratory gas tensions and pH in healing wounds, Am. J. Surg. **114:**302, 1967.

223. Hunt, T.K., et al.: Effect of vitamin A on reversing the inhibitory effect of cortisone on healing of open wounds in animals and man, Ann. Surg. **170:**633, 1969.

224. Hunt, T.K., et al.: The effect of differing ambient oxygen tensions on wound infection. Ann. Surg. **181:**35, 1975.

225. Hunt, T.K., et al.: Anaerobic metabolism and wound healing: an hypothesis for the initiation and cessation of collagen synthesis in wounds, Am. J. Surg. **135:**328, 1978.

226. Hunt, T.K., et al.: Studies on inflammation and wound healing: angiogenesis and collagen synthesis stimulated in vivo by resident and activated wound macrophages, Surgery **96:**48, 1984.

227. Hunter, J.: A treatise of blood, inflammation, and gun-shot wounds, London, 1794, Geo. Nicol.

228. Hunter, J.: Quoted in Strauss, M.B., editor: Familiar medical quotations, Boston, 1968, Little, Brown & Co.

229. Hutton, J.J., Jr., Tappel, A.L., and Udenfriend, S.: Cofactor and substrate requirements of collagen proline hydroxylase, Arch. Biochem. Biophys. **118:**231, 1967.

230. Im, M.J.C., and Hoopes, J.E.: Energy metabolism in healing skin wounds, J. Surg. Res. **10:**459, 1970.

231. Im, M.J.C., and Hoopes, J.E.: Enzyme activities in the repairing epithelium during wound healing, J. Surg. Res. **10:**173, 1970.

232. Irvin, T.T.: The effect of methionine on colonic wound healing in malnourished rats, Br. J. Surg. **63:**237, 1976.

233. Irvin, T.T.: Effects of malnutrition and hyperalimentation on wound healing, Surg. Gynecol. Obstet. **146:**33, 1978.

234. Irvin, T.T.: Wound healing: principles and practice, London, 1981, Chapman & Hall.

235. Irvin, T.T., Chattopadhyay, D.K., and Smythe, A.: Ascorbic acid requirements in postoperative patients, Surg. Gynecol. Obstet. **147:**49, 1978.

236. Jackson, D.S.: Some biochemical aspects of fibrogenesis and wound healing, N. Engl. J. Med. **259:**814, 1958.

237. Jackson, D.S., Flickinger, D.B., and Dunphy, J.E.: Biochemical studies of connective tissue repair, Ann. N.Y. Acad. Sci. **86:**943, 1960.

238. Jaffe, L.F., and Vanable, J.W., Jr.: Electric fields and wound healing, Clin. Dermatol. **2:**34, 1984.

239. Jalkansen, M., et al.: Wound fluids mediate granulation tissue growth phases, Cell Biol. Int. Rep. **7:**745, 1983.

240. Jarrett, A.: The pentose phosphate pathway in human and animal skin, Br. J. Dermatol. **84:**545, 1971.

241. Johnson, B.W., et al.: Primary and secondary healing in infected wounds: an experimental study, Arch. Surg. **117:**1189, 1982.

242. Ju, D.M.: The physical basis of scar contraction, Plast. Reconst. Surg. **7:**343, 1951.

243. Junker, P., and Lorenzen, I.: Reversibility of *d*-penicillamine–induced collagen alterations in rat skin and granulation tissue, Biochem. Pharmacol. **32:**1753, 1983.

244. Kahlson, G., et al.: Wound healing as dependent on rate of histamine formation, Lancet **2:**230, 1960.

245. Kao, K-Y.T., et al.: Connective tissue. VIII. Factors effecting collagen synthesis by sponge biopsy connective tissue, Proc. Soc. Exp. Biol. (N.Y.) **113:**762, 1963.

246. Kaufman, T., et al.: The effect of topical hyperalimentation on wound healing rate and granulation tissue formation of experimental deep second-degree burns in guinea pigs, Burns **10:**252, 1984.

247. Kefalides, N.A.: Isolation of a collagen from basement membrane containing three identical α chains, Biochem. Biophys. Res. Comm. **45:**226, 1971.

248. Kenny, G.E., and Fink, B.R.: The growth response of cells in culture to oxygen, Fed. Proc. **25:**297, 1966.

249. Kernahan, D.A., Zingg, W., and Kay, C.W.: The effect of hyperbaric oxygen on the survival of experimental skin flaps, Plast. Reconstr. Surg. **36:**19, 1965.

250. Ketchum, L.D., Robinson, D.W., and Masters, F.W.: Degradation of mature collagen: a laboratory study, Plast. Reconstr. Surg. **40:**89, 1967.

251. Ketchum, L.D., et al.: The treatment of hypertrophic scar, keloid and scar contracture by triamcinolone acetonide, Plast. Reconstr. Surg. **38:**209, 1966.

252. Kirk, D., and Irvin, T.T.: The role of oxygen therapy in the

healing of experimental skin wounds and colonic anasto-moses, Br. J. Surg. **64:**100, 1977.

253. Kischer, C.W., Shetlar, M.R., and Chvapil, M.: Hypertro-phic scars and keloids: a review and new concept concerning their origin, Scand. Electron. Microsc. Part **4:**1699, 1982.

254. Kivirikko, K.I., and Prockop, D.J.: Enzymatic hydroxyla-tion of proline and lysine in protocollagen, Proc. Natl. Acad. Sci. **57:**782, 1967.

255. Kivisaari, J., and Niinikoski, J.: Effects of hyperbaric oxy-genation and prolonged hypoxia on the healing of open wounds, Acta Chir. Scand. **141:**14, 1975.

256. Kivisaari, J., et al.: Energy metabolism of experimental wounds at various oxygen environments, Ann. Surg. **181:**823, 1975.

257. Klein, L., and Weiss, P.H.: Reutilization of mature collagen in vivo, Biochem. Biophys. Res. Commun. **21:**311, 1965.

258. Klein, L., and Rudolph, R.: ^{3}H-collagen turnover in skin grafts, Surg. Gynecol. Obstet. **135:**49, 1972.

259. Klein, L., and Rudolph, R.: Turnover of soluble and insol-uble ^{3}H collagens in skin grafts, Surg. Gynecol. Obstet. **139:**883, 1974.

260. Kleinman, H.K., Martin, G.R., and Fishman, P.H.: Gangli-oside inhibition of fibronectin-mediated cell adhesion to collagen, Proc. Natl. Acad. Sci. U.S.A. **76:**3367, 1979.

261. Kleinman, H.K., et al.: Connective tissue structure: cell binding to collagen, J. Invest. Dermatol. **71:**9, 1978.

262. Knighton, D.R., et al.: Role of platelets and fibrin in the healing sequence: an in vivo study of angiogenesis and col-lagen synthesis, Ann. Surg. **196:**379, 1982.

263. Knighton, D.R., et al.: Oxygen tension regulates the expres-sion of angiogenesis factor by macrophages, Science **221:**1283, 1983.

264. Knudsen, E.A., and Snitker, G.: Wound healing under plas-tic-coated pads, Acta Derm. Venereol. **49:**438, 1969.

265. Knutson, R.A., et al.: Use of sugar and povidone-iodine to enhance wound healing: five years experience, South. Med. J. **74:**1329, 1981.

266. Kobak, M.W., et al.: The relation of protein deficiency to experimental wound healing, Surg. Gynecol. Obstet. **85:**751, 1947.

267. Kodicek, E., and Loewi, G.: The uptake of (^{35}S) sulphate by mucopolysaccharides of granulation tissue, Proc. R. Soc. Lond. **144:**100, 1955.

268. Kohler, N., and Lipton, A.: Platelets as a source of fibro-blast growth-promoting activity, Exp. Cell Res. **87:**297, 1974.

269. Koonin, A.J.: The aetiology of keloids: a review of the litera-ture and a new hypothesis, S. Afr. Med. J. **38:**913, 1964.

270. Koster, H., and Kasman, L.P.: Relation of serum protein to well-healed and to disrupted wounds, Arch. Surg. **45:**776, 1942.

271. Krawczyk, W.S.: A pattern of epidermal cell migration dur-ing wound healing, J. Cell. Biol. **49:**247, 1971.

272. Krawczyk, W.S., and Wilgram, G.F.: Hemidesmosome and desmosome morphogenesis during epidermal wound heal-ing, J. Ultrastruct. Res. **45:**93, 1973.

273. Lampiaho, K., and Kulonen, E.: Metabolic phases during the development of granulation tissue, Biochem. J. **105:**333, 1967.

274. Langer, K.: Zur Anatomie und Physiologie der Haut: über die Spaltbarkeit der Cutis, S. B. Akad. Wiss. Wien **44:**19, 1861.

275. Lapière, C.M., Lenaers, A., and Kohn, L.D.: Procollagen peptidase: an enzyme excising the coordination peptides of procollagen, Proc. Natl. Acad. Sci. U.S.A. **68:**3054, 1971.

276. Larson, D.L., et al.: Mechanisms of hypertrophic scar and contracture formation in burns, Burns **1:**119, 1975.

277. Law, D.K., Dudrick, S.J., and Abdou, N.I.: Immunocom-petence of patients with protein-calorie malnutrition: the ef-fects of nutritional repletion, Ann. Int. Med. **79:**545, 1973.

278. Lawrence, W., Jr., Nickson, J.J., and Warshaw, L.M.: Roentgen rays and wound healing, Surgery **33:**376, 1953.

279. Layton, L.L.: Effect of cortisone upon chondroitin sulfate synthesized by animal tissues, Proc. Soc. Exp. Biol. Med. **76:**596, 1951.

280. Lazarus, G.S., et al.: Degradation of collagen by a human granulocyte collagenolytic system, J. Clin. Invest. **47:**2622, 1968.

281. Leaming, D.B., Walder, D.N., Braithwaite, F.: The treat-ment of hands: a survey of 10,668 patients treated in the hand clinic of the Royal Victoria Infirmary, New castle Upon Tyne, Br. J. Surg. **48:**247, 1960.

282. LeComte du Noüy, P.: Cicatrization of wounds. III. The relation between the age of the patient, the area of the wound, and the index of cicatrization, J. Exp. Med. **24:**461, 1916.

283. LeComte du Noüy, P.: A general equation for the law of cicatrization of surface wounds, J. Exp. Med. **29:**329, 1919.

284. LeComte du Noüy, P.: Biological time, New York, 1937, Methuen & Co.

285. Lee, K.H.: Studies on the mechanism of salicylates. III. Effect of vitamin A on the wound healing retardation action of aspirin, J. Pharmaceut. Sci. **57:**1238, 1968.

286. Leibovich, S.J.: Production of macrophage-dependent fibro-blast-stimulating activity (M-FSA) by murine macrophages, Exp. Cell. Res. **113:**47, 1978.

287. Leibovich, S.J., and Ross, R.: The role of macrophages in wound repair: a study with hydrocortisone and antimacro-phage serum, Am. J. Pathol. **78:**71, 1975.

288. Leibovich, S.J., and Ross, R.: A macrophage-dependent factor that stimulates the proliferation of fibroblasts in vitro, Am. J. Pathol. **84:**501, 1976.

289. Levendorf, K.D., et al.: Topical steroids alter dermal and epidermal healing [abstract], J. Invest. Dermatol. **80:**372, 1983.

290. Levenson, S.M., et al.: The healing of rat skin wounds, Ann. Surg. **161:**293, 1965.

291. Leyden, J.J.: Effect of bacteria on healing superficial wounds, Clin. Dermat. **2:**81, 1984.

292. Li, A.K.C., et al.: Differences in healing of skin wounds caused by burn and freeze injuries, Ann. Surg. **191:**244, 1980.

293. Li, A.K.C., et al.: Nerve growth factor: acceleration of the rate of wound healing in mice, Proc. Natl. Acad. Sci. U.S.A. **77**(7):4379, 1980.

294. Lichtenstein, I.L., et al.: The dynamics of wound healing, Surg. Gynecol. Obstet. **130:**685, 1970.

295. Lichtenstein, J.R., et al.: Defect in conversion of procolla-

gen to collagen in a form of Ehlers-Danlos syndrome, Science **182**:298, 1973.

296. Lind, J.: A treatise on the scurvy, ed. 3, London, 1772, S. Crowder.

297. Lindquist, G.: The healing of skin defects: an experimental study in the white rat, Acta Chir. Scand. **94**(107):1, 1946.

298. Lindstedt, E., and Sandblom, P.: Wound healing in man: tensile strength of healing wounds in some patient groups, Ann. Surg. **181**:842, 1975.

299. Link, W.J., Incropera, F.P., and Glover, J.L.: Plasma scalpel: comparison of tissue damage and wound healing with electrosurgical and steel scalpels, Arch. Surg. **111**:392, 1976.

300. Localio, S.A.: Wound healing: experimental and statistical study. IV. Results, Surg. Gynecol. Obstet. **77**:376, 1943.

301. Localio, S.A., Chassin, J.L., and Hinton, J.W.: Tissue protein depletion: a factor in wound disruption, Surg. Gynecol. Obstet. **86**:107, 1948.

302. Localio, S.A., Morgan, M.E., and Hinton, J.W.: The biological chemistry of wound healing: the effect of dl-methionine on the healing of wounds in protein-depleted animals, Surg. Gynecol. Obstet. **86**:582, 1948.

303. Loeb, L.A.: A comparative study of the mechanism of wound healing, J. Med. Res. **41**:247, 1920.

304. Lowry, K.F., and Curtis, G.M.: Delayed suture in the management of wounds: analysis of 721 traumatic wounds illustrating the influence of time interval in wound repair, Am. J. Surg. **80**:280, 1950.

305. Lundberg, C., et al.: Quantification of the inflammatory reaction and collagen accumulation in an experimental model of open wounds in the rat: a methodological study, Scand. J. Plast. Reconstr. Surg. **16**:123, 1982.

306. Lundgren, C.E.G., and Zederfeldt, B.: Influence of low oxygen pressure on wound healing, Acta Chir. Scand. **135**:555, 1969.

307. MacDonald, R.A.: Origin of fibroblasts in experimental healing wounds, Surgery **46**:376, 1959.

308. Madden, J.W.: Studies on the biology of collagen during wound healing. I. Rate of collagen synthesis and deposition in cutaneous wounds of the rat, Surgery **64**:288, 1968.

309. Madden, J.W., Morton, D., Jr., and Peacock, E.E., Jr.: Contraction of experimental wounds. I. Inhibiting wound contraction by using a topical smooth muscle antagonist, Surgery **76**:8, 1974.

310. Madden, J.W., and Peacock, E.E., Jr.: Studies on the biology of collagen during wound healing. III. Dynamic metabolism of scar collagen and remodeling of dermal wounds, Ann. Surg. **174**:511, 1971.

311. Madden, J.W., and Smith, H.C.: The rate of collagen synthesis and deposition in dehisced and resutured wounds, Surg. Gynecol. Obstet. **130**:487, 1970.

312. Majno, G.: Contraction of collagen fibers in vivo induced by inflammation, Lancet **2**:994, 1958.

313. Majno, G.: The healing hand: man and wound in the ancient world, Cambridge, Mass., 1977, Harvard University Press.

314. Majno, G., et al.: Contraction of granulation tissue in vitro: similarity to smooth muscle, Science **173**:548, 1971.

315. Mancini, R.E., and Quaife, J.V.: Histogenesis of experimentally produced keloids, J. Invest. Dermatol. **38**:143, 1962.

316. Manner, G., et al.: The polyribosomal synthesis of collagen, Biochim. Biophys. Acta **134**:411, 1967.

317. Marks, J., et al.: Prediction of healing time as an aid to the management of open granulating wounds, World J. Surg. **7**:641, 1983.

318. Marks, J.G., Jr., et al.: Inhibition of wound healing by topical steroids, J. Dermatol. Surg. Oncol. **9**:819, 1983.

319. Martin, G.R., et al.: The genetically distinct collagens, Trends Biochem. Sci. **10**:285, 1985.

320. McGaw, W.T., and Cate, A.R.: A role for collagen phagocytosis by fibroblasts in scar remodeling: an ultrastructural stereologic study, J. Invest. Dermatol. **81**:375, 1983.

321. McGrath, H.M., and Simon, R.H.: Wound geometry and the kinetics of wound contraction, Plast. Reconstr. Surg. **72**:66, 1983.

322. Meadows, E.C., and Prudden, J.F.: A study of the influence of adrenal steroids on the strength of healing wounds, Surgery **33**:841, 1953.

323. Medawar, P.B.: The behavior of mammalian skin epithelium under strictly anaerobic conditions, Q. J. Micros. Sci. **88**:27, 1947.

324. Mertz, P.M., and Eaglstein, W.H.: The effect of a semiocclusive dressing on the microbial population in superficial wounds, Arch. Surg. **119**:287, 1984.

325. Meyer, E., and Meyer, M.B.: The pathology of *Staphylococcus* abscess in vitamin C–deficient guinea pigs, Bull. Johns Hopkins Hosp. **74**:98, 1944.

326. Milch, R.A.: Tensile strength of surgical wounds, J. Surg. Res. **5**:377, 1965.

327. Modolin, M., et al.: The effects of protein malnutrition on wound contraction: an experimental study, Ann. Plast. Surg. **12**:428, 1984.

328. Mohs, F.: Chemosurgery: microscopically controlled surgery, Springfield, Ill., 1978, Charles C Thomas, Publishers.

329. Montagna, W., and Parakkal, P.F.: Structure and function of the skin, ed. 3, New York, 1974, Academic Press.

330. Montandon, D., and Gabbiani, G.: Contractile events during wound epithelialization. In Marchac, D., and Hueston, J.T., editors: Transactions of the Sixth International Congress of Plastic and Reconstructive Surgery, Paris, 1976, Masson.

331. Montandon, D., D'Andiran, G., and Gabbiani, G.: The mechanism of wound contraction and epithelialization: clinical and experimental studies, Clin. Plast. Surg. **4**:325, 1977.

332. Montandon, D., et al.: The contractile fibroblast, its relevance in plastic surgery, Plast. Reconstr. Surg. **52**:286, 1973.

333. Montgomery, D.W.: Cicatrix, Urol. Cutan. Rev. **43**:403, 1939.

334. Moore, M.J.: The effect of radiation on connective tissue, Otolaryngol. Clin. North Am. **17**:389, 1984.

335. Morton, D., Jr., et al.: Effect of colchicine on wound healing in rats, Surg. Forum **25**:47, 1974.

336. Motegi, K., Nakano, Y., and Namikawa, A.: Relation between cleavage lines and scar tissues, J. Maxillofac. Surg. **12**:21, 1984.

337. Myers, A.H., Postlethwait, R.W., and Smith, A.G.: Histologic grading of the experimental healing wound, Arch. Surg. **83**:771, 1961.

338. Myers, M.B., and Cherry, G.: Functional and angiographic vasculature in healing wounds, Am. Surg. **36:**750, 1970.

339. Myers, M.B., and Wolf, M.: Vascularization of the healing wound, Am. Surg. **40:**716, 1974.

340. Nelson, C.A., and Dennis, C.: Wound healing, Surg. Gynecol. Obstet. **93:**461, 1951.

341. Newcombe, J.F.: Effect of intra-arterial nitrogen mustard infusion on wound healing in rabbits: formation of granulation tissue and wound contraction, Ann. Surg. **163:**319, 1966.

342. Nicoletis, C., Bazin, S., and LeLous, M.: Clinical and biochemical features of normal, defective, and pathologic scars, Clin. Plast. Surg. **4:**347, 1977.

343. Niinikoski, J.: Effects of oxygen supply on wound healing and formation of experimental granulation tissue, Acta Physiol. Scand. **334:**1, 1969.

344. Niinikoski, J.: Cellular and nutritional interactions in healing wounds, Med. Biol. **58:**303, 1980.

345. Niinikoski, J., Grislis, G., and Hunt, T.K.: Respiratory gas tensions and collagen in infected wounds, Ann. Surg. **175:**588, 1972.

346. Niinikoski, J., Heughan, C., and Hunt, T.K.: Oxygen tensions in human wounds, J. Surg. Res. **12:**77, 1972.

347. Nimni, M.E., and Bavetta, L.A.: Collagen defect induced by penicillamine, Science **150:**905, 1965.

348. Nishihara, G., and Prudden, J.F.: A quantitative relationship of wound tensile strength to length, Surg. Gynecol. Obstet. **107:**305, 1958.

349. Odland, G., and Ross, R.: Human wound repair. I. Epidermal regeneration, J. Cell. Biol. **39:**135, 1968.

350. Odland, G.F., and Short, J.M.: Structure of the skin. In Fitzpatrick, T.B., et al., editors: Dermatology in general medicine, New York, 1971, McGraw-Hill Book Co.

351. O'Hare, R.P., et al.: Isolation of collagen-stimulating factors from healing wounds, J. Clin. Pathol. **36:**707, 1983.

352. O'Keefe, E.J., et al.: Production of soluble and cell associated fibronectin in cultured keratinocytes, J. Invest. Dermatol. **82:**150, 1984.

353. Olsen, C., and Forscher, B.K.: Soluble collagen in acute inflammation, Proc. Soc. Exp. Biol. **111:**126, 1962.

354. Onwuke, M.F.: Treating keloids by surgery and methotrexate [letter], Arch. Dermatol. **116:**158, 1980.

355. Ordman, L.J., and Gillman, T.: Studies in the healing of cutaneous wounds. I. The healing of excisions through the skin of pigs, Arch. Surg. **93:**857, 1966.

356. Ordman, L.J., and Gillman, T.: Studies in the healing of cutaneous wounds. II. The healing of epidermal, appendageal, and dermal injuries inflicted by suture needles and by the suture material on the skin of pigs, Arch. Surg. **93:**883, 1966.

357. Ordman, L.J., and Gillman, T.: Studies in the healing of cutaneous wounds. III. A critical comparison in the pig of the healing of surgical incisions closed with sutures or adhesive tape based on tensile strength and clinical and histological criteria, Arch. Surg. **93:**911, 1966.

358. Page, A.R., and Good, R.A.: A clinical and experimental study of the function of neutrophils in the inflammatory response, Am. J. Pathol. **34:**645, 1958.

359. Pai, M.P., and Hunt, T.K.: Effect of varying oxygen tensions on healing of open wounds, Surg. Gynecol. Obstet. **135:**756, 1972.

360. Paré, A.: The works of that famous chirurgion Ambrose Parey, London, 1634, Cates and Young. (Translated from Latin and compared with the French by T. Johnson.)

361. Paul, T.N.: Treatment by local application of insulin of an infected wound in a diabetic, Lancet **2:**574, 1966.

362. Peacock, E.E., Jr.: Production and polymerization of collagen in healing wounds of rats: some rate-regulating factors, Ann. Surg. **155:**251, 1962.

363. Peacock, E.E., Jr.: Some aspects of fibrogenesis during the healing of primary and secondary wounds, Surg. Gynecol. Obstet. **115:**408, 1962.

364. Peacock, E.E., Jr.: Control of wound healing and scar formation in surgical patients, Arch. Surg. **116:**1325, 1981.

365. Peacock, E.E., Jr.: Wound repair, Philadelphia, 1984, W.B. Saunders Co.

366. Peacock, E.E., Jr., and Biggers, P.W.: Measurement and significance of heat-labile and urea-sensitive cross-linking mechanisms in collagen of healing wounds, Surgery **54:**144, 1963.

367. Pearce, C.W., et al.: The effect and interrelation of testosterone, cortisone and protein nutrition on wound healing, Surg. Gynecol. Obstet. **111:**274, 1960.

368. Pearlstein, E.: Plasma membrane glycoprotein mediates adhesion of fibroblast to collagen, Nature **262:**497, 1976.

369. Perasalo, O., Wiljasalo, M.A., and Wiljasalo, S.: Some studies of hormonal influence on wound healing, Ann. Chir. Gyn. Fenn. **42:**168, 1953.

370. Perez-Tamayo, R., and Ihnen, M.: The effect of methionine in experimental wound healing: a morphologic study, Am. J. Pathol. **29:**233, 1953.

371. Persinger, M.A., et al.: Mast cell numbers in incisional wounds in rat skin as a function of distance, time and treatment, Br. J. Dermatol. **108:**179, 1983.

372. Phillips, J.L., and Peacock, E.E., Jr.: Importance of horizontal plane cell mass integrity in wound contraction, Proc. Soc. Exp. Biol. Med. **117:**534, 1964.

373. Picou, D., Halliday, D., and Garrow, J.S.: Total body protein, collagen, and non-collagen protein in infantile protein malnutrition, Clin. Sci. **30:**345, 1966.

374. Pinkus, H.: Examination of the epidermis by the strip method of removing horny layers. I. Observations on thickness of horny layer and on mitotic activity after stripping, J. Invest. Dermatol. **16:**383, 1951.

375. Pinnell, S.R., et al.: A heritable disorder of connective tissue: hydroxylysine-deficient collagen disease, N. Engl. J. Med. **286:**1013, 1972.

376. Pirani, C.L., and Levenson, S.M.: Effect of vitamin C deficiency on healed wounds, Proc. Soc. Exp. Biol. Med. **82:**95, 1953.

377. Pirani, C.L., Stepto, R.C., and Sutherland, K.: Desoxycorticosterone in wound healing, J. Exp. Med. **93:**217, 1951.

378. Polverini, P.J., et al.: Activated macrophages induce vascular proliferation, Nature **269:**804, 1977.

379. Pories, W.J., et al.: The measurement of human wound healing, Surgery **59:**821, 1966.

380. Pories, W.J., et al.: Acceleration of healing with zinc sulfate, Ann. Surg. **165:**432, 1967.

381. Postlethwaite, A.E., et al.: Induction of fibroblast chemotaxis by fibronectin: localization of the chemotactic region to a 140,000-molecular weight nongelatin-binding fragment, J. Exp. Med. **153:**494, 1981.

382. Powanda, M.C., and Moyer, E.D.: Plasma protein and wound healing, Surg. Gynecol. Obstet. **153:**749, 1981.

383. Prockop, D.J., et al.: The biosynthesis of collagen and its disorders, N. Engl. J.Med. **301:**13, 1979.

384. Radice, G.P.: The spreading of epithelial cells during wound closure in *Xenopus* larvae, Dev. Biol. **76:**26, 1980.

385. Ragan, C., et al.: Effect of cortisone on production of granulation tissue in rabbit, Proc. Soc. Exp. Biol. Med. **72:**718, 1949.

386. Ragnell, A.: The tensibility of the skin: an experimental investigation, Plast. Reconstr. Surg. **14:**317, 1954.

387. Rahmat, A., Norman, J.N., and Smith, G.: The effect of zinc deficiency on wound healing, Br. J. Surg. **61:**271, 1974.

388. Ramirez, A.T., et al.: Experimental wound healing in man, Surg. Gynecol. Obstet. **128:**283, 1969.

389. Rasmussen, D.M., Khalil, G.W., and Winkelmann, R.K.: Isotonic and isometric thermal contraction of human dermis. III. Scleroderma and cicatrizing lesions, J. Invest. Dermatol. **43:**349, 1964.

390. Rechler, M.M., and Podskalny, J.M.: Insulin receptors in cultured human fibroblasts, Diabetes **25:**250, 1976.

391. Remensnyder, J.P., and Majno, G.: Oxygen gradients in healing wounds, Am. J. Pathol. **52:**301, 1968.

392. Reynolds, B.L., and Buxton, R.W.: Aberrations produced in healing regenerating tissue by exogenously administered testosterone, hydrocortisone, and methandrostenolone, Am. Surg. **29:**859, 1963.

393. Rhoads, J.E., Fliegelman, M.T., and Panzer, L.M.: The mechanism of delayed wound healing in the presence of hypoproteinemia, J.A.M.A. **118:**21, 1942.

394. Riley, W.B., Jr., and Peacock, E.E., Jr.: Identification, distribution, and significance of a collagenolytic enzyme in human tissues, Proc. Soc. Exp. Biol. Med. **124:**207, 1967.

395. Robson, M.C., et al.: Quantitative bacteriology and delayed wound closure, Surg. Forum **19:**501, 1968.

396. Robson, M.C., et al.: The efficacy of systemic antibiotics in the treatment of granulating wounds, J. Surg. Res. **16:**299, 1974.

397. Rosenberg, B.F., and Caldwell, F.T., Jr.: Effect of single amino acid supplementation upon the rate of wound contraction and wound morphology in protein-depleted rats, Surg. Gynecol. Obstet. **121:**1021, 1965.

398. Rosenthal, S.P., and Enquist, I.F.: The effects of insulin on granulating wounds in normal animals, Surgery **64:**1096, 1968.

399. Ross, R.: The fibroblast and wound repair, Biol. Rev. **43:** 51, 1968.

400. Ross, R., and Benditt, E.P.: Wound healing and collagen formation. II. Fine structure in experimental scurvy, J. Cell. Biol. **12:**533, 1962.

401. Ross, R., Everett, N.B., and Tyler, R.: Wound healing and collagen formation. VI. The origin of the wound fibroblast studied in parabiosis, J. Cell. Biol. **44:**645, 1970.

402. Ross, R., and Odland, G.: Human wound repair. II. Inflammatory cells, epithelial-mesenchymal interrelations, and fibrogenesis, J. Cell. Biol. **39:**152, 1968.

403. Rovee, D.T., Kurowsky, C.A., and Labun, J.: Local wound environment and epidermal healing: mitotic response, Arch. Dermatol. **106:**330, 1972.

404. Rovee, D.T., and Miller, C.A.: Epidermal role in the breaking strength of wounds, Arch. Surg. **96:**43, 1968.

405. Rovin, S., and Gordon, H.A.: The influence of aging on wound healing in germfree and conventional mice, Gerontologia **14:**87, 1968.

406. Rudolph, R.: Location of the force of wound contraction, Surg. Gynecol. Obstet. **148:**547, 1979.

407. Rudolph, R., and Woodward, M.: Spatial orientation of microtubules in contractile fibroblasts in vivo, Anat. Rec. **191:** 169, 1978.

408. Rutherford, R.B., and Ross, R.: Platelet factors stimulate fibroblasts and smooth muscle cells quiescent in plasma serum to proliferate, J. Cell. Biol. **69:**196, 1976.

409. Ryan, G.B., et al.: Myofibroblasts in an avascular fibrous tissue, Lab. Invest. **29:**197, 1973.

410. Ryan, G.B., et al.: Myofibroblasts in human granulation tissue, Hum. Pathol. **5:**55, 1974.

411. Salmela, K., and Ahonen, J.: The effect of methylprednisolone and vitamin A on wound healing, Acta Chir. Scand. **147:**307 and 313, 1981.

412. Sandberg, N.: On the healing of wounds in rats during the period of cicatrization, Acta Chir. Scand. **126:**294, 1963.

413. Sandberg, N.: Time relationship between administration of cortisone and wound healing in rats, Acta Chir. Scand. **127:** 446, 1964.

414. Sandberg, N., and Zederfeldt, B.: Influence of acute hemorrhage on wound healing in the rabbit, Acta Chir. Scand. **118:**367, 1960.

415. Sandblom, P.: The tensile strength of healing wounds, Acta Chir. Scand. **90**(Suppl. 89), 1944.

416. Sandblom, P.: The effect of injury on wound healing, Ann. Surg. **129:**305, 1949.

417. Sandblom, P., Petersen, P., and Muren, A.: Determination of tensile strength of the healing wound as a clinical test, Acta Chir. Scand **105:**252, 1953.

418. Sandblom, P.: Wundheilungsprobleme, mit Reissfestigkeitsmethoden untersucht, Langenbeck. Arch. Klin. Chir. **287:** 469, 1957.

419. Sandblom, P., and Muren, A.: Differences between the rate of healing of wounds inflicted with short time interval, Ann. Surg. **140:**449, 1954.

420. Sandstead, H.H., and Shepard, G.H.: The effect of zinc deficiency on the tensile strength of healing surgical incisions in the integument of the rat, Proc. Soc. Exp. Biol. Med. **128:**687, 1968.

421. Santoro, S.A., and Cunningham, L.W.: Fibronectin and the multiple interaction model for platelet collagen adhesion, Proc. Natl. Acad. Sci. U.S.A. **76:**2644, 1979.

422. Savlov, E.D., and Dunphy, J.E.: The healing of the disrupted and resutured wound, Surgery **36:**362, 1954.

423. Savlov, E.D., and Dunphy, J.E.: Mechanisms of wound healing: comparison of preliminary local and distant incisions, N. Engl. J. Med. **250**:1062, 1954.

424. Schilling, J.A.: Wound healing, Surg. Clin. N. Am. **56**(4): 589, 1976.

425. Shepard, G.H.: The healing of wounds after delayed primary closure: an experimental study, Plast. Reconstr. Surg. **48**: 358, 1971.

426. Shepard, G.H.: Wounds treated by the healing of delayed primary closure: a clinical study, Milit. Med. **146**:473, 1981.

427. Shepherd, J.P., and Dawber, R.P.: Wound healing and scarring after cryosurgery, Cryobiology **21**:157, 1984.

428. Shulman, A.G., and Krohn, H.L.: Influence of hyperbaric oxygen and multiple skin allografts on the healing of skin wounds, Surgery **62**:1051, 1967.

429. Silver, I.A.: The measurement of oxygen tension in healing tissue, Prog. Resp. Res. **3**:124, 1969.

430. Silvetti, A.N.: An effective method of treating long-enduring wounds and ulcers by topical applications of nutrients, J. Dermatol. Surg. Oncol. **7**:501, 1981.

431. Simpson, D.M., and Ross, R.: The neutrophilic leukocyte in wound repair, J. Clin. Invest. **51**:2009, 1972.

432. Sisson, R., et al.: Comparison of wound healing in various nutritional deficiency states, Surgery **44**:613, 1958.

433. Smith, J.C., Jr., et al.: Zinc: a trace element essential in vitamin A metabolism, Science **181**:954, 1973.

434. Smythe, P.M., et al.: Thymolymphatic deficiency and depression of cell-mediated immunity in protein-calorie malnutrition, Lancet **2**:939, 1971.

435. Snowden, J.M., Kennedy, D.F., and Cliff, W.J.: Wound contraction: the effects of scab formation and the nature of the wound bed, Aust. J. Exp. Biol. Med. Sci. **60**:73, 1982.

436. Snowden, J.M., Kennedy, D.F., and Cliff, W.J.: The contractile properties of wound granulation tissue, J. Surg. Res. **36**:108, 1984.

437. Soderberg, T., and Hallmans, G.: Wound contraction and zinc absorption during treatment with zinc tape, Scand. J. Plast. Reconstr. Surg. **16**:255, 1982.

438. Southwood, W.F.W.: The thickness of the skin, Plast. Reconstr. Surg. **15**:423, 1955.

439. Spain, D.M., Molomut, N., and Haber, A.: The effect of cortisone on the formation of granulation tissue in mice, Am. J. Pathol. **26**:710, 1950.

440. Spain, K.C., and Loeb, L.: A quantitative analysis of the influence of the size of the defect on wound healing in the skin of guinea pig, J. Exp. Med. **23**:107, 1916.

441. Spector, W.G., and Lykke, A.W.J.: The cellular envolution of inflammatory granulomata, J. Pathol. Bact. **92**:163, 1966.

442. Sporn, M.B., et al.: Polypeptide transforming growth factors isolated from bovine sources used for wound healing in vivo, Science **219**:1329, 1983.

443. Squier, C.A., et al.: Electron microscopic immunochemical localization of action in fibroblasts in healing skin and palate wounds of beagle dog, Histochemistry **78**:513, 1983.

444. Staley, C.J., Trippel, O.H., and Preston, F.W.: Influence of 5-fluorouracil on wound healing, Surgery **49**:450, 1961.

445. Stankler, L., and Ewen, S.W.B.: The effects of corticosteroid injections at sites of skin damage, J. Invest. Dermatol. **59**:394, 1972.

446. Stearns, M.L.: Studies on the development of connective tissue in transparent chambers in the rabbit ear, Am. J. Anat. **67**:55, 1940.

447. Stein, H.D., and Keiser, H.R.: Collagen metabolism in granulating wounds, J. Surg. Res. **11**:277, 1971.

448. Stein, J.M., and Levenson, S.M.: Effect of the inflammatory reaction on subsequent wound healing, Surg. Forum **17**:484, 1966.

449. Stenn, K.S.: Epibolin: a protein of human plasma that supports epithelial cell movement, Proc. Natl. Acad. Sci. U.S.A. **78**:6907, 1981.

450. Stenn, K.S., Madri, J.A., and Roll, F.J.: Migrating epidermis produces AB_2 collagen and requires continual collagen synthesis for movement, Nature **277**:229, 1979.

451. Stephens, F.O., Dunphy, J.E., and Hunt, T.K.: Effect of delayed administration of corticosteroids on wound contraction, Ann. Surg. **173**:214, 1971.

452. Stephens, F.O., and Hunt, T.K.: Effect of changes in inspired oxygen and carbon dioxide tensions on wound tensile strength, Ann. Surg. **173**:515, 1971.

453. Stone, N., and Meister, A.: Function of ascorbic acid in the conversion of proline to collagen hydroxyproline, Nature **194**:555, 1962.

454. Straile, W.E.: The expansion and shrinkage of mammalian skin near contracting wounds, J. Exp. Zool. **141**:119, 1959.

455. Sullivan, D.J., and Epstein, W.S.: Mitotic activity of wounded human epidermis, J. Invest. Dermatol. **41**:39, 1963.

456. Sussman, M.D.: Aging of connective tissue: physical properties of healing wounds in young and old rats, Am. J. Physiol. **224**:1167, 1973.

457. Tanzer, M.L.: Crosslinking of collagen, Science **180**:561, 1973.

458. Tanzer, M.L., and Hunt, R.D.: Experimental lathyrism, J. Cell. Biol. **22**:623, 1962.

459. Taubenhaus, M., and Amromin, G.D.: The effects of the hypophysis, thyroid, sex steroids, and the adrenal cortex on granulation tissue, J. Lab. Clin. Med. **36**:7, 1950.

460. Taubenhaus, M., Taylor, B., and Morton, J.V.: Hormonal interaction in the regulation of granulation tissue formation, Endocrinology **51**:183, 1952.

461. Taylor, F.W., Dittmer, T.L., and Porter, D.O.: Wound healing and the steroids, Surgery **31**:683, 1952.

462. Taylor, H.E., and Saunders, A.M.: The association of metachromatic ground substance with fibroblastic activity in granulation tissue, Am. J. Pathol. **33**:525, 1957.

463. Taylor, T.V., et al.: Ascorbic acid supplementation in the treatment of pressure sores, Lancet **2**:544, 1974.

464. Thakral, K.K., Goodson, W.H., III, and Hunt, T.K.: Stimulation of wound blood vessel growth by wound macrophages, J. Surg. Res. **26**:430, 1979.

465. Thompson, J., and Van Furth, R.: The effect of glucocorticosteroids on the kinetics of mononuclear phagocytes, J. Exp. Med. **131**:429, 1970.

466. Thompson, W.D., Ravdin, I.S., and Frank, I.L.: Effect of hypoproteinemia on wound disruption, Arch. Surg. **36**:500, 1938.

467. Topol, B.M., Lewis, V.L., and Benveniste, K.: The use of antihistamine to retard the growth of fibroblasts derived from

human skin, scar, and keloid, Plast. Reconstr. Surg. **68:**227, 1981.

468. Torring, S.: Our routine in pressure treatment of hypertrophic scars, Scand. J. Plast. Reconstr. Surg. **18:**135, 1984.

469. Udupa, K.N., Woessner, J.F., and Dunphy, J.E.: The effect of methionine on the production of mucopolysaccharides and collagen in healing wounds of protein-depleted animals, Surg. Gynecol. Obstet. **102:**639, 1956.

470. Uitto, J.A.: A method for studying collagen biosynthesis in human skin biopsies in vitro, Biochim. Biophys. Acta **201:** 438, 1970.

471. Uitto, J., and Prockop, D.J.: Synthesis and secretion of underhydroxylated procollagen at various temperatures by cells subject to temporary anoxia, Biochem. Biophys. Res. Commun. **60:**414, 1974.

472. Vande Berg, J.S., Rudolph, R., and Woodward, M.: Comparative growth dynamics and morphology between cultured myofibroblasts from granulating wounds and dermal fibroblasts, Am. J. Pathol. **114:**187, 1984.

473. Van Winkle, W., Jr.,: The fibroblast in wound healing, Surg. Gynecol. Obstet. **124:**369, 1967.

474. Velasco, M., and Guaitero, E.: A comparative study of some antiinflammatory drugs in wound healing of the rat, Experientia **29:**1250, 1973.

475. Vihersaari, T., Kivisaari, J., and Niinikoski, J.: Effect of changes in inspired oxygen tension on wound metabolism, Ann. Surg. **179:**889, 1974.

476. Viljanto, J., Isomäki, H., and Kulonen, E.: Effect of an anabolic steroid on the tensile strength of granulation tissue in various nutritional states, Acta Endocrinol. **41:**395, 1962.

477. Viljanto, J., Penttinen, R., and Raekallio, J.: Fibronectin in early phases of wound healing in children, Acta Chir. Scand. **147:**7, 1981.

478. Wahl, S., Arend, W.P., and Ross, R.: The effect of complement depletion on wound healing, Am. J. Pathol. **75:**73, 1974.

479. Wald, H.I., et al.: Effect of intensive hyperbaric oxygen therapy on the survival of experimental skin flaps in rats, Surg. Forum **19:**497, 1968.

480. Watts, G.T.: Wound shape and tissue tension in healing, Br. J. Surg. **47:**555, 1960.

481. Watts, G.T., Grillo, H.C., and Gross, J.: Studies in wound healing. II. The role of granulation tissue in contraction, Ann. Surg. **148:**153, 1958.

482. Watts, G.T., et al.: Wound healing: biochemical methods for observation of the cellular and intercellular phases, Br. J. Clin. Pract. **16:**733, 1962.

483. Weiss, P.: Cell contact, Int. Rev. Cytol. **7:**391, 1958.

484. Weiss, P.: The biologic foundations of wound repair, Harvey Lecture Series **55:**13, 1959-60.

485. Wells, G.C.: The effect of hydrocortisone on standardized skin surface trauma, Br. J. Dermatol. **69:**11, 1957.

486. Wester, J., et al.: Morphology of the hemostatic plug in human skin wounds, Lab. Investigations **41:**182, 1979.

487. Westerhof, W., and Bos, J.D.: Trigeminal trophic syndrome: a successful treatment with transcutaneous electrical stimulation, Br. J. Dermatol. **108:**601, 1983.

488. White, B.N., Shetlar, M.R., and Schilling, J.A.: The glycoproteins and their relationship to the healing of wounds, Ann. N.Y. Acad. Sci. **94:**297, 1961.

489. Williams, G.: The late phases of wound healing: histological and ultrastructural studies of collagen and elastic-tissue formation, J. Pathol. **102:**61, 1970.

490. Williams, K.J., et al.: The effect of topically applied zinc on the healing of open wounds, J. Surg. Res. **27:**62, 1979.

491. Williams, P.L., and Warwick, R.: Gray's anatomy, ed. 36, Philadelphia, 1980, W.B. Saunders Co.

492. Williamson, M.B., and Fromm, H.J.: The incorporation of sulphur amino acids into the proteins of regenerating wound tissue, J. Biol. Chem. **212:**705, 1955.

493. Williamson, M.B., and Fromm, H.J.: Effect of cystine and methionine on healing of experimental wounds, Proc. Soc. Exp. Biol. Med. **80:**623, 1952.

494. Williamson, M.B., McCarthy, T.H., and Fromm, H.J.: Relation of protein nutrition to the healing of experimental wounds, Proc. Soc. Exp. Biol. Med. **77:**302, 1951.

495. Winter, G.D.: Formation of scab and the rate of epithelialization of superficial wounds in the skin of the young domestic pig, Nature **193:**293, 1962.

496. Winter, G.D.: Effect of air exposure and occlusions on experimental human skin wounds, Nature **200:**378, 1963.

497. Winter, G.D.: A note on wound healing under dressings with special reference to perforated film dressings, J. Invest. Dermatol. **45:**299, 1965.

498. Wolbach, S.B., and Howe, P.R.: Intercellular substances in experimental scorbutus, Arch. Pathol. **1:**1, 1926.

499. Wolman, M., and Gillman, T.: A polarized light study of collagen in dermal wound healing, Br. J. Exp. Pathol. **53:** 85, 1972.

500. Woodley, D.T., O'Keefe, E.J., and Prunieras, M.: Cutaneous wound healing: a model for cell-matrix interactions, J. Am. Acad. Dermatol. **12**(2):420, 1985.

501. Yaoita, H., Foidart, J.M., and Katz, S.I.: Localization of the collagenous component of skin basement membrane, J. Invest. Dermatol. **70:**191, 1978.

502. Zahir, M.: Contraction of wounds, Br. J. Surg. **51:**456, 1964.

503. Zederfeldt, B.: Studies on wound healing and trauma with special reference to intravascular aggregation of erythrocytes, Acta Chir. Scand. (Suppl.) 224, 1957.

504. Zika, J.M., and Klein, L.: Relative and absolute changes in skin collagen mass in the rat, Biochim. Biophys. Acta **229:** 509, 1971.

505. Zitelli, J.A.: Wound healing by secondary intention: a cosmetic appraisal, J. Am. Acad. Dermatol. **9:**407, 1983.

Anatomy for Cutaneous Surgery

Thorough knowledge and understanding of gross and microscopic anatomy are essential to any physician performing surgery, particularly on the cutaneous surfaces and underlying subcutaneous structures. The skin is an intricate organ, overlying and intimately associated with blood vessels, nerves, and muscles. Appreciation of these interrelationships aids in producing superior surgical results and minimizing problems associated with surgery.

Different regions of the body have anatomic similarities and differences. Familiarity with these peculiarities facilitates the rendering of effective local anesthesia and creating favorable lines of incision. In addition, fundamental knowledge of anatomy is helpful in explaining differences in wound healing, types of scars produced, and difficulties associated with surgery.

The study of gross anatomy is said to arouse "irrational hostility"[51] or even "retrograde amnesia"[9] in many physicians. In addition, gross anatomy is no longer considered fashionable, since it has been superseded by microscopic anatomy.[51] However, human anatomy is the language of medicine. The correlation between clinical knowledge and knowledge gained through dissection furthers the understanding of fundamental structures and helps in the development or refinement of surgical techniques.

This chapter emphasizes functional and practical anatomy essential to dermatologic surgery. It is not intended to replace the basic anatomy textbooks[28,36,58] or anatomic atlases[1,14] that should be consulted frequently when questions arise. Because much dermatologic surgery is performed on the head and neck and because this area is perhaps the most anatomically complex region of the body, its anatomy is emphasized. Other chapters discuss additional anatomy relevant to certain procedures.

ANATOMY OF THE HEAD AND NECK

Anatomy of the head and neck is important. Most skin cancers arise in this area; therefore cutaneous surgery is common here. Since the face is a difficult part of the anatomy to coverup or camouflage, it is essential to produce good cosmetic and functional results in this region.

Surface anatomy

The surface of skin on the head and neck is divided, somewhat artificially, into a number of different designated areas (Fig. 3-1). This allows the physician to specify more accurately the location of lesions and to communicate more precisely with other physicians. Although the boundaries of these areas are frequently apparent, they may also be indistinct and arbitrary. Pertinent to a discussion of these areas are the creases, elevations, depressions, and dimples of the face (Fig. 3-2). The so-called aesthetic zones of the face are actually composites of these various regions and, along with the creases, must be taken into account when planning incisions on the head and neck.

The hair-bearing scalp has four areas—frontal, parietal, temporal, and occipital. The frontal scalp extends from the forehead to approximately the interauricular line and is bounded by parietal and temporal scalp areas. These latter areas form the sides of scalp, with the parietal superior to the temporal. The occipital scalp is the most posterior and inferior. *Frontotemporal* or *frontoparietal* are sometimes used to designate areas common to both regions.

The forehead extends from the frontal scalp to the eyebrows and glabella. Crossing the forehead horizontally are the forehead creases, which run perpendicular to the underlying musculature. If the skin is particularly sun damaged, secondary crease lines may also run somewhat obliquely on the forehead. The glabella is the area between the eyebrows, but superior to the nasal root. The glabellar creases (frown lines) may be seen in this area. During a frown, deeper depressions (glabellar furrows) caused by muscle contraction become apparent (see Fig. 17-1, *A* and *B*). The temple is situated lateral to the eyebrows and eyes.

The cheek is divided into six different areas with rather

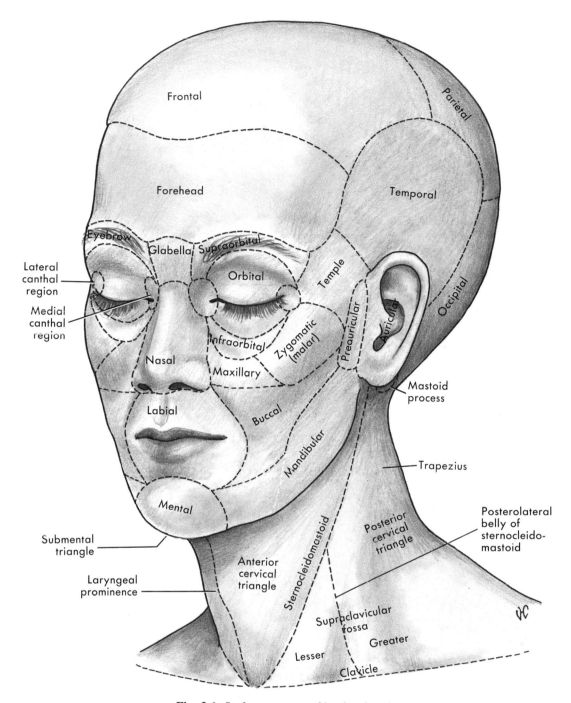

Fig. 3-1. Surface anatomy of head and neck.

indistinct boundaries. The mandibular cheek overlies the mandible and extends from the chin to the ear and preauricular area. The buccal cheek lies in the center of the cheek overlying the buccal fat pad. The maxillary and zygomatic (malar) areas overlie the maxillary and zygomatic bones, respectively. Immediately superior to these two areas is the infraorbital region, lying immediately below the lower eyelids. The final portion of cheek, the preauricular area, is situated in front of the ear. In a man this is easily apparent as the non–hair-bearing skin between the sideburn and ear.

The labial area is bounded by the mental (chin) region, the nose, and the buccal region of the cheeks. The lips are two mobile structures at the entrance to the mouth. The upper lip is separated from the cheek by the labial (melolabial) crease and is divided into two halves by the philtrum (Fig. 3-2). This latter structure consists of a depression in the central upper lip extending from the nasal septum inferiorly and is bounded by two prominences (philtral ridges) that blend into the vermilion border of the upper lip. It is thought that the philtrum is formed by the crossing over of

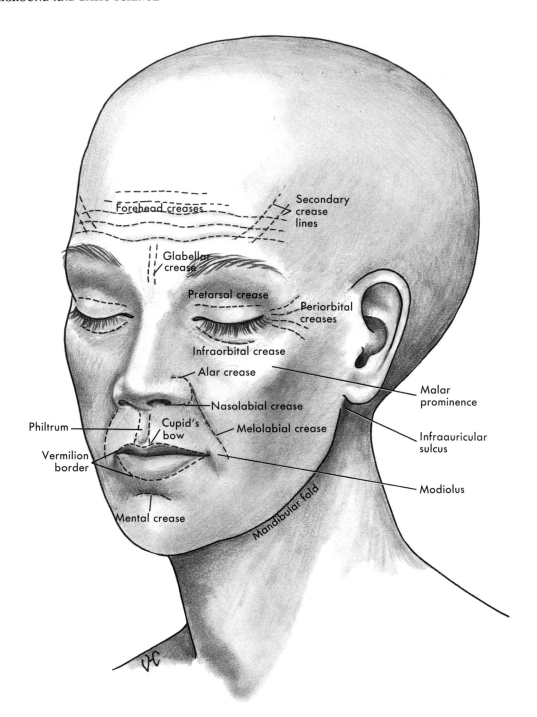

Fig. 3-2. Important landmarks and creases of face.

muscle insertions in the superficial portion of the orbicularis oris muscle.[42] On biopsy, the depression (philtrum) appears as denser connective tissue than that underlying the two paramedial philtral ridges.[39] Because of its resemblance to a bow, the raised contoured area of the vermilion border that extends across where the philtrum attaches is known as Cupid's bow. The lower lip is bounded by the mental crease inferiorly. The red portion of the lip, the vermilion zone, obtains such a color because of the rich vascular supply underneath a thin epithelium. The junction of the skin to the vermilion zone is the vermilion border. In the upper lip, just inferior to the philtrum in the vermilion zone, is the labial tubercle, a fleshy protuberance of varying size. The two lips are connected laterally by labial commissures. Lateral to the commissures on the cheeks is a slight protuberance, the modiolus, which represents the meeting place of many of the muscles surrounding the mouth.

The eye (Fig. 3-3) (excluding the orbit and its contents)

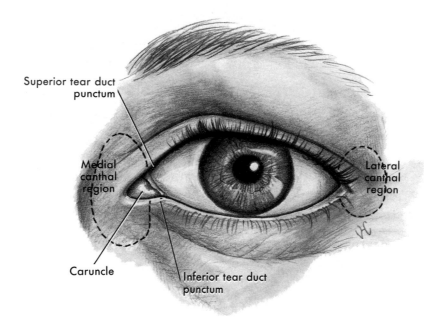

Fig. 3-3. Surface anatomy of eye.

includes the upper and lower eyelids that join in the medial and lateral canthal regions at the medial and lateral palpebral commissures. The skin of the eyelids is thin and loosely attached to the underlying muscles. Thus it is difficult to cut without crimping and tends to allow fluid accumulation. The upper lid is more mobile than the lower. When open, the aperture between the lids is known as the palpebral fissure. The medial commissure is separated from the eyeball by the lacrimal lake, in which a fleshy projection, the lacrimal caruncle, is situated. This small, reddish yellow island contains modified sebaceous and sweat glands that secrete a whitish substance.

The eyelashes (cilia) are arranged in two or three rows and are associated with sebaceous glands (of Zeis) and apocrine glands (of Moll). A stye is the result of blockage and inflammation of either of these ciliary glands. Underlying the distal eyelids is a fibrous structure, the tarsal plate, in which meibomian glands (modified sebaceous glands) are embedded. Blockage of these glands can result in a chalazion.

Medially, on both the upper and lower eyelids, are posteriorly directed elevations, the lacrimal papillae. Each papilla has a central opening, the tear duct (lacrimal) punctum, into which tears flow from the lacrimal lake. These puncta open into the lacrimal ducts, which run medially to connect with the lacrimal (tear) sac that in turn drains into the nose through the nasolacrimal duct. The location of the tear duct apparatus is shown in Fig. 3-4. The lacrimal gland is situated in the upper outer corner of the orbit underneath the orbicularis muscle and orbital septum.

Creases may be particularly prominent around the eyes (Fig. 3-2). The pretarsal crease is on the upper eyelid, but is usually hidden by overlying eyelid skin (the pretarsal fold) when the eye is open. The infraorbital crease in the lower eyelid may be particularly prominent in patients with atopic dermatitis. Periorbital creases, also known as crow's feet, extend laterally from the lateral canthal area of the eye. These creases are important when planning incisions around the eye.

The external nose (Fig. 3-5) is shaped like a pyramid and divided into the dorsum, tip, ala, and lateral side. The dorsum extends from the tip, the lower rounded portion of the nose, to the root. It should be emphasized that the skin overlying the dorsum is freely movable, whereas the skin over the tip adheres tightly to underlying cartilage and fibrous tissue. This contributes to difficulties in reconstruction in the area of the nasal tip. The portion of the dorsum overlying the nasal bones is known as the bridge. The lateral sides of the nose extend from the nasal dorsum to the cheeks. The indistinct area of blending of the lateral sides to the cheek is known as the margin of the nose (nasofacial angle).

The ala is separated from the lateral side of the nose by the alar crease and separated from the lip by the nasolabial crease or groove, which extends inferiorly as a continuation of the alar crease. The root of the nose is the uppermost attachment of the nose to the glabella. The nares (the openings into the anterior nasal vestibules) are separated by the nasal septum and bounded laterally by the nasal alae. The freely movable inferior portion of the nasal septum, which does not overlie cartilage, is known as the columella.

The external ear (the auricle or pinna) (Fig. 3-6) is bounded anteriorly by the preauricular area and posteriorly by the postauricular scalp. It is separated from the scalp by

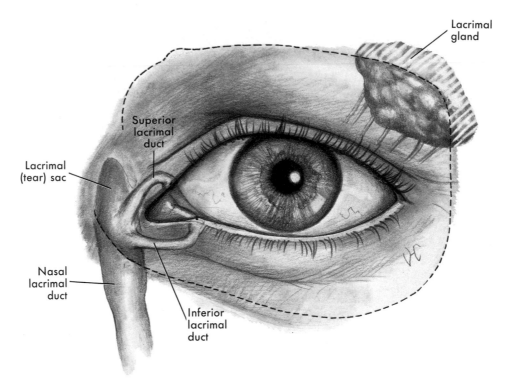

Fig. 3-4. Lacrimal drainage system of eye.

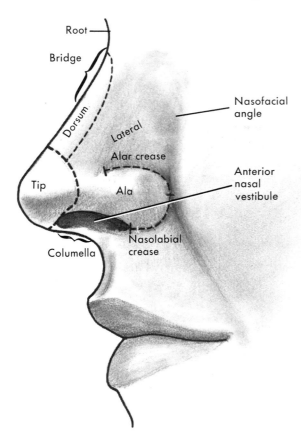

Fig. 3-5. Surface anatomy of nose.

the postauricular sulcus, the upper portion of which is known as the auriculotemporal sulcus. The mastoid process (prominence) is situated behind the ear at the inferior end of the postauricular scalp. Immediately anterior to this, but inferior to the ear, is the infraauricular sulcus (Fig. 3-2), deep to which is the exit for the facial nerve. The term *posterior auricular surface* refers to the posterior aspect of the ear and should not be confused with the term *post-auricular scalp*.

The ear itself is divided into several contoured areas of skin overlying elastic cartilage that serve as a framework. The skin is tightly attached on the lateral and anterior surfaces, whereas it is more loosely attached on the posterior surface. The tight attachment accounts for the marked pain on injection of anesthesia in this area. The cartilage of the auricle is continuous with that of the external auditory meatus. The auricle is attached to the skull by ligaments from the cartilage to the bone, by continuity of the cartilaginous framework with that of the external auditory meatus, and by the skin and extrinsic muscles. The helix stretches between the lobule (or lobe) and the crus of the helix. In some individuals a small prominence, the darwinian tubercle, may be seen on the medial rim of the helix. The antihelix extends from the antitragus to the crura of the antihelix. Between the latter is found the triangular fossa. The scaphoid fossa lies between the helix and the antihelix. The tragus lies anterior to the external ear canal. The area between the tragus and antitragus is the incisura intertragica (intertragic

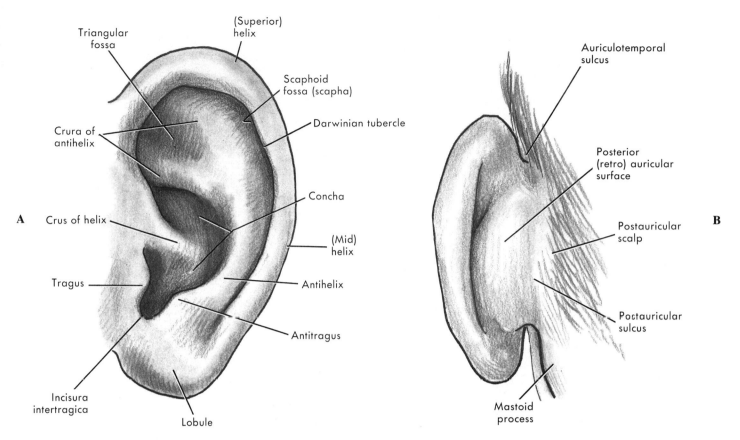

Fig. 3-6. Surface anatomy of ear. **A,** Lateral surface. **B,** Posterior surface.

notch). The concha is a fossa situated between the antihelix and crus of the helix. This is separated by the crus of the helix into a superior portion (cymba conchae) and inferior portion (cavum conchae).

The neck (Fig. 3-1) is divided into anterior and posterior cervical triangles, with the sternocleidomastoid muscle as the dividing line. In the anterior midline is the laryngeal prominence. The anterior triangle is bordered superiorly by the mandible, medially by the anterior midline, and laterally by the anterior border of the sternocleidomastoid muscle. The posterior triangle is bordered by the clavicle below, the posterior border of the sternocleidomastoid muscle, and the anterior border of the trapezius muscle. The supraclavicular fossae are immediately above the clavicle. The lesser supraclavicular fossa lies between the anterior and posterior origins of the sternocleidomastoid muscle. The greater supraclavicular fossa lies posterior to the posterior origin of the sternocleidomastoid. Immediately underneath the chin is the submental triangle, an area particularly prone to fat deposition and thus the double chin. Posterior to this and under the mandible on either side are the submandibular triangles. Both the submental and submandibular triangles are situated in the superior portion of the anterior cervical triangle.

Framework

Before describing the muscles, blood vessels, and nerves of the head and neck, it is necessary to review the bony and cartilaginous framework. This framework is perhaps the most complex part of the human skeleton, and knowledge of its structure helps to clarify the relationship of the different anatomic systems to each other.

The skull consists of upper calvaria enclosing the brain, and a lower facial skeleton (Fig. 3-7). Anteriorly, the frontal bone forms the forehead and passes back to the coronal suture. It is joined there by the two parietal bones, forming most of the calvaria's sides, which are joined together superiorly at the midline sagittal suture. These two bones extend back to meet the occipital bone to form the back of the skull. The lambdoid suture joins the parietal and occipital bones. The sides of the cranium are completed by the temporal and sphenoid bones. The cranial vault's arched configuration helps to withstand fractures.

The bones of the skull are covered by periosteum. With the exception of the temporal bone, the skull has little power of regeneration. The temporal bone usually heals better, because it is thinner and thus has a superficial blood supply. The thickness of the skull varies with individuals, but averages about 5 mm.[28] Furthermore, this thickness

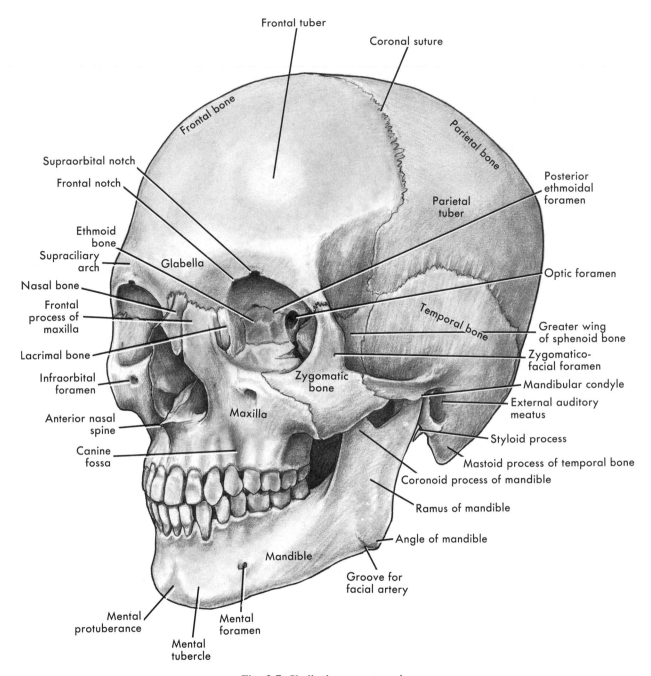

Fig. 3-7. Skull, three-quarters view.

varies with different bones in the skull and with age. The bones of the cranium have three layers: an inner table (or lamina), an outer table, and a middle layer (or diploë) (Fig. 3-12). This middle layer is cancellous bone and is supplied by numerous vessels from arteries on both the external and internal surfaces of the skull. The diploic veins drain either into the scalp veins or into the dural venous sinuses and may provide direct communication between these two venous channels.

The inferior portion of the frontal bone forms the superi-

or portion of the orbit (pars orbitalis) and connects with the nasal bones. The rounded elevation immediately above the medial orbit is known as the supraciliary arch. The arches from each orbit meet medially at the glabella, a slight medial elevation. About 3 cm above the supraciliary arch is the frontal tuber (tuberosity or boss) in the midforehead bilaterally. Inferior to the supraciliary arch is the supraorbital margin, which forms the upper border of the orbital openings. At the medial third of this margin lies an easily palpated structure, the supraorbital notch (which in some individuals may be a foramen). This notch contains the supraorbital vessels and nerve. Medial to the supraorbital notch is the frontal notch or foramen, present in 50% of skulls.[58] Laterally the supraorbital margin of the frontal bone ends with the zygomatic process, which extends to articulate with the zygomatic bone. Medially the frontal bone projection downward is the nasal part. Its rough surface articulates with the nasal bone medially and more laterally with the frontal process of the maxilla and lacrimal bone. The attachment of the frontal bone to the nasal bone is shingled under the latter. The point at which the internasal and frontonasal sutures meet is the nasion.

The parietal bones form the sides and roof of the cranium. Near the center of each is a slight elevation, the parietal tuber (tuberosity), which may be felt on the side of the head. Beneath this area are the superior and inferior temporal lines, which are the sites of attachment of the temporal fascia and muscle, respectively. The bone above these lines is covered by the galea aponeurotica.

The occipital bone forms much of the back and base of the skull. The midexternal portion superior to the foramen magnum has a protuberance, the external occipital protuberance, that may be easily felt in the midline. Also easily felt are two ridges extending laterally on either side. The highest protuberance is known as the highest nuchal line and the lowest is the superior nuchal line. To the former, the galea aponeurotica attaches and above this area is the occipital belly of the occipitofrontalis muscle. The superior nuchal line is the point of attachment of several neck muscles, including the trapezius medially and the sternocleidomastoid laterally.

The temporal bones help to form the sides and base of the skull. They are divided into four morphologically distinct parts: the squamous, the petromastoid, the tympanic parts, and the stylomastoid process. The squamous part, so called because it is thin (scalelike), forms the upper and anterior part of the bone. The zygomatic process, part of the zygoma, projects laterally. On the inferior border of this process is the mandibular fossa, the site of articulation of the mandible. It is bounded anteriorly by the articular tubercle and posteriorly by the postglenoid tubercle.

The most posterior part of the temporal bone is the petromastoid portion. It includes the mastoid process as an inverted conical projection on the inferior border. The outer surface of this portion of the temporal bone is roughened by attachments of the occipital belly of the occipitofrontalis. The petrous bone is the more medial part of the petromastoid portion. This bone forms the carotid canal and the anterior portion of the jugular foramen.

The tympanic part of the temporal bone lies below the squamous part but in front of the mastoid process. It forms the anterior wall, the floor, and a part of the posterior wall of the bony external auditory meatus. The superior wall is formed by the squamous portion of the temporal bone.

The styloid process is a small portion of bone that projects inferiorly and anteriorly from underneath the inferior border of the tympanic part of the temporal bone. This bone is approximately 2.5 cm in length. Immediately behind this process lies the stylomastoid foramen, from which emerge the facial nerve and stylomastoid artery. Lateral to the styloid process is a portion of the parotid gland, and the carotid artery passes its tip. This process is the site of attachment of certain muscles and ligaments. Although the styloid process is often cited as an important landmark for localization of the facial nerve, it is poorly developed or absent in approximately one third of individuals.[17]

The sphenoid bone is one of the central bones of the skull with a portion forming the side of the cranium. This bone houses the sphenoid sinus and the hypophysial fossa and helps to form the optic canal and posterior portion of the orbit. Laterally its greater wing articulates with the temporal bone posteriorly at the sphenosquamosal suture. The inferior projections of this bone are known as the pterygoid processes, to which the pterygoid muscles, important muscles of mastication, attach.

The nasal bones are two small bones that form the bridge of the nose. They are situated side by side between the frontal processes of the maxillae and articulate superiorly with the nasal part of the frontal bone. The internal surfaces is traversed by a groove in which runs the anterior ethmoidal nerve. Medially and inferiorly the nasal bone forms a small dorsal part of the nasal septum and articulates with the nasal spine of the frontal bone, perpendicular plate of the ethmoid bone, and cartilaginous nasal septum.

The lacrimal bone is the most fragile of the external cranial bones. One is situated in the medial portion of each orbit. The lateral surface is divided by a vertical ridge, the posterior lacrimal crest (Fig. 3-8). Anterior to this is a depression, the fossa for the lacrimal sac, which is formed partially by the lacrimal bone and partially by the maxillary bone. This fossa leads inferiorly to a bony canal, the nasolacrimal canal, which empties into the nose. The lacrimal bone articulates with four other bones: the anterior border articulates with the frontal process of the maxilla, the inferior border with the orbital surface of the maxilla, the posterior surface with the ethmoid bone, and the superior border with the frontal bone.

The maxillae are relatively large bones, which united form the whole of the upper jaw. In addition, they form the floor of the orbit, most of the roof of the mouth, and the lateral nasal wall. Each maxilla is generally divided into a body and four processes: the zygomatic, the frontal, the alveolar, and the palatine.

The anterior portion of the body contains the canine fossa above and slightly posterior to the canine teeth. Superior to this but inferior to the anterior end of the orbital rim is the infraorbital foramen. From this emerge the infraorbital vessels and nerves. Medially the anterior portion of the maxilla

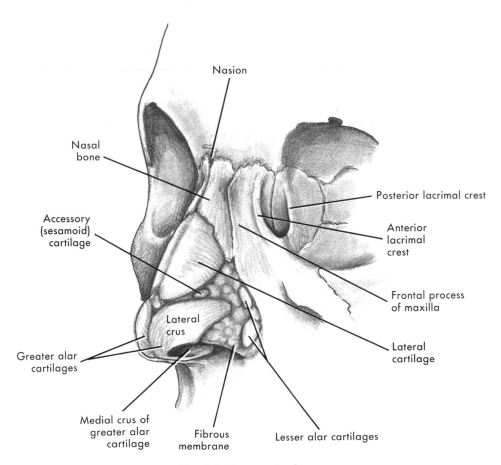

Nasion

Nasal
bone

Accessory
(sesamoid)
cartilage

Posterior lacrimal crest

Anterior
lacrimal
crest

Frontal process
of maxilla

Lateral
cartilage

Lateral
crus

Greater alar
cartilages

Medial crus of
greater alar
cartilage

Fibrous
membrane

Lesser alar cartilages

Fig. 3-8. Framework of nose.

ends with the nasal notch coming to a point, the anterior nasal spine. Inside the body of the maxilla is the maxillary sinus.

The zygomatic process of the maxilla helps form the anterior portion of the cheekbone and articulates posteriorly with the zygomatic bone. The frontal process projects superiorly between the nasal and lacrimal bones. On its lateral surface is a ridge, the anterior lacrimal crest, to which attaches the medial palpebral ligament. Between the anterior lacrimal crest of the maxillary bone and the posterior lacrimal crest of the lacrimal bone is the fossa for the lacrimal sac previously mentioned.

The alveolar process is the most inferior process of the maxilla. It is thick and arched and holds the teeth. The palatine process forms most of the hard palate. The posterior portion of the hard palate is formed by the palatine bones.

The zygomatic bone forms the malar prominence on the cheeks and contributes to the formation of the lateral wall and floor of the orbit. It articulates with the maxilla anteriorly, the temporal bone posteriorly, and the frontal bone superiorly. The zygomaticotemporal foramen pierces the upper lateral side. Anteriorly the zygomatic bone forms the anterior wall of the temporal fossa and more inferiorly

forms much of the lateral wall of the infratemporal fossa.

The mandible or jawbone is the only freely movable bone of the skull. It is also stated to be the largest and strongest bone of the face.[58] It consists of a horizontally placed, horseshoe-shaped body with a laterally situated ramus on each side of the body. The ramus projects upward and backward to end in two processes, the coronoid process anteriorly and the condylar process posteriorly. It is with this latter process that the mandible articulates with the rest of the skull at the temporal bone. The region where the ramus and body meet laterally is known as the angle of the mandible.

At the anterior portion of the mandible one may palpate the mental protuberance, which lies on the midline just above the lower edge of the bone. This represents the lower portion of the fusion line of the mandible, the mandibular symphysis. Lateral and slightly inferior to the mental protuberance bilaterally are two small bony projections, the mental tubercles. On the lateral surface of the mandible is found the mental foramen. This opening is directed posteriorly and is the site of exit for the mental nerve and vessels. It is situated in a line approximately between the first and second premolars, but its location can vary slightly.[53] In early adulthood it is situated slightly more toward the inferior edge of the body of the ramus. However, with advancing age and absorption of the alveolar ridge, it becomes relatively closer to the alveolar border.

The inferior lateral ramus is the site of attachment of the masseter muscle. Just anterior to this attachment on the lower border of the body of the mandible is a shallow groove, which is the groove for the facial artery. At this point, the facial artery may be palpated. The anterior projection from the ramus is a flattened triangular process called the coronoid process. It is the site of attachment of the temporalis muscle and can be felt beneath the zygomatic arch when the jaw is opened. The posterior condylar process, as mentioned previously, articulates with the mandibular fossa of the temporal bone. It has a flattened surface, which is covered by fibrocartilage. The lateral surface of the condylar process is blunt and can be palpated just anterior to the tragus when opening and closing the mouth. The area just inferior to the condyle is the neck of the mandible; onto this medial surface the lateral pterygoid muscles insert. The inverted arch between the coronoid process and the condylar processes is the mandibular notch, through which the masseteric nerve and vessels run to supply the masseter muscle.

Other important landmarks on the mandible include the retromolar triangle and the mandibular foramen. The retromolar triangle is a shallow, triangular depression just posterior to the third molar. This triangle becomes continuous with the lateral (buccal) alveolar crest and the medial alveolar crest. Posterior to the retromolar triangle on the medial surface of the ramus is the mandibular foramen, the site of entrance for the inferior alveolar nerve and vessels. The lingula, a small projection of bone, points posteriorly above and guards this foramen.

The framework of the nose is partly bony, partly cartilaginous, and partly membranous (Fig. 3-8). The piriform aperture is the anterior opening of the nose on the skull without the cartilaginous or cutaneous tissue. It is bounded superiorly by the nasal bones and laterally as well as inferiorly by the maxilla. The cartilages of the nose include the lateral nasal cartilages superiorly, the greater alar cartilages inferiorly, and the septal cartilage medially. The lateral nasal cartilages are continuous with each other and the septal cartilage. They are triangular in shape and articulate with the nasal bones and usually with the maxillary bones. The greater alar cartilages are thin and curved to hold open the nasal apertures. These cartilages are divided into a medial and a lateral crus that joins at the apex of the nose. The lateral crus gives shape to the ala and is joined to the maxilla by a fibrous membrane, in which are embedded several lesser alar cartilages. Sometimes between the lateral nasal cartilage and the greater alar cartilage, a few accessory (sesamoid) nasal cartilages are found. The medial crus runs posteriorly in the nose to form the movable lower portion of the nasal septum. The medial crura are joined to each other and the lower nasal septum.

The internal junction of the lateral cartilage and lateral crus of the greater alar cartilage produces a protrusion into the nasal vestibule. This protrusion, known as the limen vestibuli, acts as a nasal valve and an air baffle. This region is the smallest cross-sectional area of the respiratory tract and therefore provides the point of greatest resistance to airflow. Thus only a small decrease in the diameter and mobility (by scar tissue) produces nasal obstruction.

In a study by Dion et al.,[20] in which careful dissection and measurements of nasal cartilages were done, the relationship between the upper lateral and lower alar cartilages was shown to vary. In some specimens there was overlap between these two cartilages, whereas in others separation was apparent. Small sesamoid cartilages were observed in all noses studied. These same authors emphasize the function and importance of fibrofatty tissue (the fibrous membrane) on the lateral ala in supporting the cartilages of the nose. The variable relationship of the cartilages of the nose is explained by the embryonic development. A single nasal cartilage is cleaved into an upper lateral and lower greater alar cartilage by fibrous ingrowth.[57] The extent of this process and of cartilage resorption determines the distance separativity of the alar cartilages, as well as the presence or absence of cartilage remnants, such as the accessory and lesser alar cartilages.

The ear contains of a framework of a continuous, elastic cartilage except the lobe, which has no underlying cartilage. This cartilage roughly conforms to the shape of the ear and extends into the distal half of the external auditory meatus.

The cartilage of the ear, unlike that of the nose, has a yellowish appearance and is distinguished by an abundance of elastic fibers in its matrix. The cartilage of the nose is hyaline cartilage, which has a more glassy, pearly appearance. As pointed out by Williams and Warwick,[58] elastic cartilage is found in sites, such as the ear and larynx, where vibrational qualitites are important functional characteristics.

Skin, fascia, and muscles

The skin on the head and neck is unique in that it has a more intimate and direct relationship to the underlying muscles and other structures than skin elsewhere on the human body (see Fig. 2-2). This complex connection accounts for the wide range of facial expressions that separates humans from the lower animals. In addition, the skin on the face is continuous with the mucous membranes over the lips, nose, and margins of the eyelids. The thickness of the skin is also quite variable in this region, being extremely thin, for instance, over the eyelids (see Fig. 2-4).

It is important to understand that most of the superficial muscles of the scalp and face insert into the skin either directly through fibrous bands running in the subcutaneous

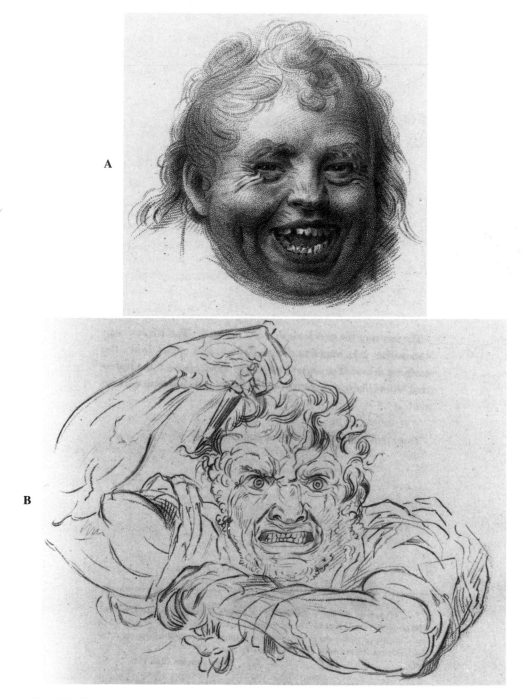

Fig. 3-9. Sketches showing extreme facial expressions. **A,** Smiling; **B,** rage. (From Bell, C.: Essays on the anatomy of the expression in painting, London, 1806, Longman, Hurst, Rees, and Orme.)

tissue (Fig. 2-2) or indirectly by attachment to the superficial musculoaponeurotic system (an organized fibrous tissue, described later, in the subcutaneous tissue), which in turn is attached to the skin (Fig. 3-10). These attachments account for wrinkle lines, dimples, and the enormous motility of the facial muscles, making numerous facial expressions possible (Fig. 3-9). When the skin is undermined during surgery in this area, these connections can be direct-

ly visualized, and in some areas they make separating the dermis from underlying fat or muscle fascia particularly difficult. One exception is the skin overlying the eyelid muscles. Here there is no tight attachment between skin and muscle, allowing edema to evolve much more easily in this area.

The term *fascia* is widely used but frequently misunderstood. Fascia usually means a sheet or band of connective

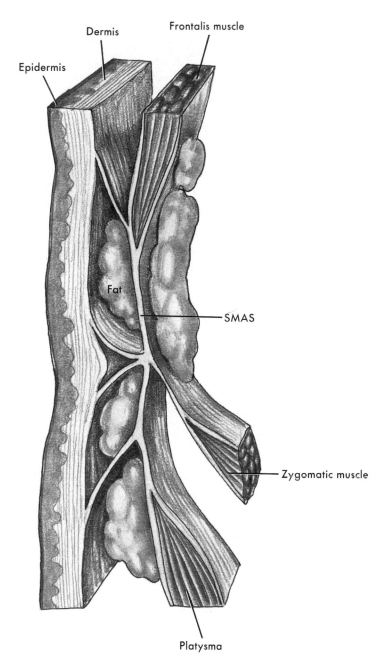

Fig. 3-10. Relationship of SMAS to skin and muscles. (Modified from Mitz, V., and Peyronie, M.: Plast. Reconstr. Surg. **58**:80, 1976).

tissue seen with the unaided eye. Spatially and because of differences in composition, it is convenient to divide fascia into superficial and deep. Superficial fascia is basically sub-cutaneous tissue and is situated immediately beneath the dermis of the skin. It contains both fibrous and fat tissue in various proportions and hence is described as fibroareolar. In some regions of the body (the abdomen, for example), a relatively large amount of fat accumulates. In other areas, like the scalp, a large amount of fibrous tissue predominates. The superficial fascia is thin over the dorsum of the hands and neck and almost absent over the ears.

Beneath the superficial fascia, the deep fascia may be present, which is composed of more compact and regularly arranged collagen fibers, and thus is more highly organized than the superficial fascia. Usually the deep fascia provides a compact cover for muscles, but in some areas it is more specialized, forming retinacula, coverings of tendon sheaths, or aponeuroses. An aponeurosis is a broad, sheet-like, tendinous attachment. Although most muscles in humans are situated deep to the deep fascia, the platysma muscle of the neck is an exception; it is in the superficial fascia of the neck.

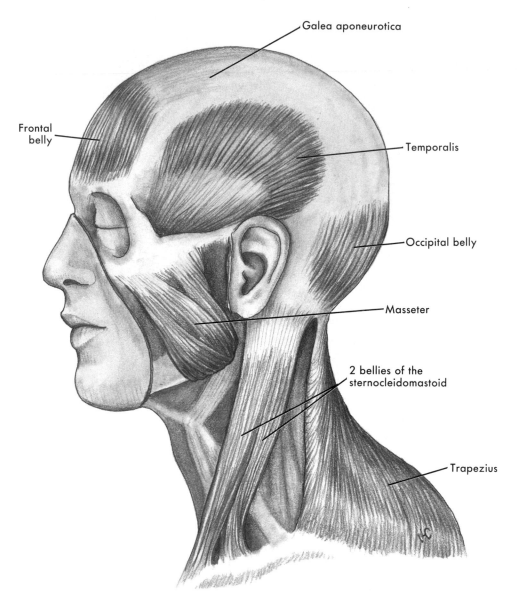

Fig. 3-11. Relationship of scalp muscles, masseter muscle, and sternocleidomastoid muscle.

As mentioned, the subcutaneous tissue on the head and neck is quite specialized and somewhat complex. In some areas the fibrous tissue in this layer is highly organized, for example, over the lateral cheeks, into a fibrous sheet sandwiched between the deep fascia and fat below and the fat above immediately beneath the dermis (Fig. 3-10). This sheet, with its fibrous attachments to the dermis on one side and the facial muscle fascia on the other, has been recently described and termed the *superficial musculoaponeurotic system* (SMAS).

The concept that the superficial fascia of the face is a highly organized and definable unit was set forth by Mitz in 1976.[38] According to Mitz, who dissected 14 facial halves, the superficial fascia of the lateral face is made up of a dense fibrous unit, which he termed *SMAS,* sandwiched between a deep and superficial layer of fat. This SMAS is stretched over the cheeks between the temporalis and frontalis muscles above and the platysma muscle below. Anteriorly it attaches to the orbicularis oculi muscles and posteriorly to the trapezius muscle. Over the area of the parotid and masseter muscle (the lateral cheek), SMAS is thick and attached to the parotid sheath beneath. In the buccal area, however, this thick fibrous layer becomes thin and even discontinuous. Its attachment at the nasolabial fold is thought to produce the cheek fold in this area.

The relationship of SMAS to the skin on one side and the muscles on the other is illustrated in Fig. 3-10. As can be seen, SMAS is in reality attached to both. Fibrous attach-

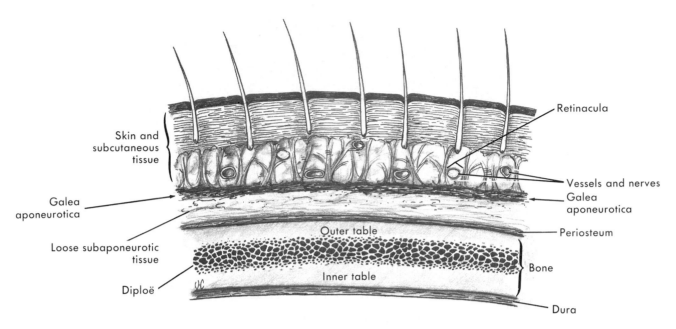

Fig. 3-12. Anatomy of skull bone scalp (superior).

ments run from SMAS to the skin on one side and to the muscles below on the other. In addition, some muscles attach at different angles to SMAS. The result is that SMAS helps to modulate and amplify contractions of facial muscles, yielding an enormous range of facial expressions.

With aging, SMAS becomes stretched and is less efficient in transmitting facial expressions. It has therefore been recommended, when performing rhytidectomies (face-lift procedures), that SMAS in particular be visualized, stretched, and partially resected.[44] Most major arteries and nerves run within or deep to SMAS.

The vascular network of the skin consists of a superficial plexus of blood vessels atop the dermis connected to a deeper plexus of vessels in the top of the superficial fascia buried in fat. A knowledge and appreciation of the variability in depth of the deeper plexus and its association with nerves is necessary for thoughtful dermatologic surgery.

One may consider the neck to be invested by a collar of fascia completely encircling it. On the top and bottom it is attached to bone. The superficial fascia splits to invest the major superficial neck muscles, the trapezius posteriorly, the sternocleidomastoid anteriorly, and the parotid gland superiorly. The anterior and posterior cervical triangles previously described are areas where the fasciae from both sides of these muscles have fused.

Scalp

The scalp is a structural unit consisting of the following five layers: (1) skin (epidermis and dermis), (2) subcutaneous tissue, (3) musculoaponeurotic layer, (4) loose subaponeurotic tissue, and (5) periosteum (Fig. 3-12). The skin contains many closely set hair follicles that project into the subcutaneous layer. The subcutaneous layer contains thick fibrous bands (retinacula), which help to unite skin to the fascia below. These bands, in addition, help to support the blood vessels, holding the latter open when cut and thus promoting profuse and continual bleeding. The third layer of the scalp, the musculoaponeurotic, consists of muscle between two layers of fascia in occipital or forehead regions. On the top of the skull, as shown in Fig. 3-11, the muscle is absent and the two layers of fascia fuse to form a fibrous sheet, the galea aponeurotica, which unites the frontal and occipital muscles over the superior scalp. These top layers of the scalp are intimately fused and move as a unit because of the fibrous bands between the galea and skin.

The fourth layer of the scalp is a loose subaponeurotic layer that attaches the top three layers of the scalp to the underlying fifth and final layer, the pericranium (periosteum). This final layer is loosely attached to the underlying bone except at the suture lines. The periosteum of the scalp differs from periosteum elsewhere on the body in that it provides little nourishment for the underlying bone and has limited bone-forming power. Therefore stripping the scalp of the layer and exposing the bone does not cause subsequent bone necrosis.[36] The looseness of the subaponeurotic tissue allows for the free movement of the overlying three layers over the cranium.

The space beneath the galea aponeurotica has been termed the *danger space* of the scalp.[28] Its loose arrangement allows for easy dissection. Large amounts of blood can form hematomas there after a blow to the head. Infections in this area can possibly spread to the meninges through the emissary veins that pass through the skull bones to the dura.

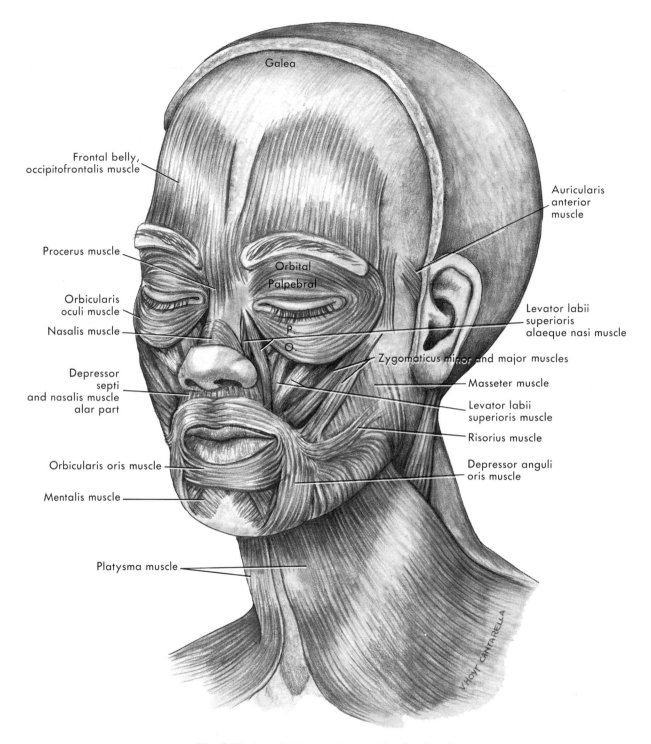

Fig. 3-13. Superficial musculature of head and neck.

Recently the subaponeurotic layer was studied and found to contain more fibrous tissue than previously thought.[13] This fibrous tissue, the subaponeurotic fascia, is thought to arise from the fascia deep to the muscles of the scalp. If this is true, the galea aponeurotica may not represent the fusion of the total fascia investing the muscles of the scalp. Further supporting evidence for this is the fact that the galea aponeurotica probably originates purely from fibroblasts without the presence of myoblasts.[24]

The nerves and blood vessels on the scalp are located above the galea aponeurotica. Therefore when an anesthetic is injected into the scalp, it should be placed above this layer to provide quicker onset of anesthesia (see Fig. 6-9). If the injection is made beneath the galea, it takes a long time before adequate diffusion occurs up through the galea aponeurotica into the overlying nerves. However, local anesthesia tends to dissect in the loose subaponeurotic area, which may on occasion be useful as a means of visualizing a plane for dissection. Any fluid or infection in the subaponeurotic space tends to dissect easily, for example, into the periorbital space.

Muscles

The muscles of facial expression are the most superficial on the face and insert into the skin. They arise from either bone or fascia and are all innervated by the facial nerve. Their main action is to move the overlying skin.

The muscles of the scalp consist of the occipitofrontalis muscles with their frontal and occipital bellies (Fig. 3-11). The two frontal bellies cover the forehead. The frontalis portion (also known as the frontalis muscle) has no bony attachments; it originates in the galea aponeurotica and inserts into the skin of the forehead at the eyebrows. The fact that the frontalis muscle is split in the midline helps to explain why midline vertical forehead scars often heal with minimal spread scarring. The occipital belly covers the occipital scalp and also inserts into the galea aponeurotica. It originates from the highest nuchal line of the occipital bone and the mastoid portion of the temporal bone. Unlike the frontal bellies, which lie relatively close together, the occipital bellies are separated by a larger space that is filled with an extension of the galea aponeurotica. The function of the occipitofrontalis muscle is to raise the eyebrows and wrinkle the forehead.

Although the occipitofrontalis muscle is described as if comprised of a single muscle, its two parts are formed separately, with the frontal belly developing last.[24] As already mentioned, the galea aponeurotica probably originates from fibroblasts without the presence of myoblasts.

The muscles of the ear include the anterior auricular muscle (Fig. 3-13), the superior auricular muscle, and the posterior auricular muscle. All three muscles insert onto the ear. The anterior and superior muscles originate in the galea aponeurotica, whereas the posterior auricular muscle originates on the mastoid process. These muscles are usually not moved by voluntary control.

The importance of the auricular muscles is that their proper development is necessary for a normal-appearing ear.[52] A protruding ear may be associated with lack of formation of the posterior auricular muscle. Such a deformity is seen in fetal alcohol syndrome, Down's syndrome, and fetal hydantoin syndrome. Lack of the superior auricular muscle leads to a lop-ear deformity. This muscle holds the top of the ear toward the head. Slanted auricles are thought to be related to developmental problems of the anterior auricular muscle.

Protruding auricles may also be a result of the lack of nerve supply to the auricular muscles. The ear muscles are innervated by the seventh cranial nerve (CN VII), and therefore in syndromes with involvement of this nerve, for example, in Möbius' syndrome, a protruding auricle is frequently present. Möbius' syndrome is bilateral facial paralysis resulting from neurologic developmental problems with the third (III), fifth (V), sixth (VI), seventh (VII), and twelfth (XII) cranial nerves. Children with this syndrome have a masklike facies, an open mouth that drools, paralysis of the soft palate, and atrophy of the tongue.

The ear also has six intrinsic ear muscles, which in humans are thought to be unimportant. However, their development may be related to the variability in ear folds.

The muscle surrounding the eye is the orbicularis oculi (Fig. 3-13). This is a circular muscle that is divided into two parts, an orbital and a palpebral portion. The orbital portion originates on both the medial palpebral ligament and the nasal portion of the frontal bone. Its fibers spread out superiorly and inferiorly, forming a ring around the orbit and extending beyond the orbital rim. Some of the fibers in this muscle are completely circular. The palpebral portion also originates from the medial palpebral ligament, as well as from the posterior nasal crest. The muscle fibers of this portion of the orbicularis oculi interdigitate at the lateral canthal raphe. The orbital portion of the orbicularis is more tightly bound to the overlying skin than the palpebral part and thus limits spread of fluid beyond the orbit. Underlying the palpebral portion of the orbicularis muscle in both upper and lower eyelids is the tarsal plate, a thick fibrous tissue in which meibomian glands are embedded. This plate is sandwiched between the mucosa on one side and muscle on the other.

The functions of the orbicularis oculi muscle are to close the eyelids and to compress the lacrimal sac. The palpebral portion alone is capable of closing the eyelids, but the whole orbicularis oculi muscle contracts on forced closure. Thus the orbital portion is mainly under voluntary control, whereas the palpebral portion is under both voluntary and involuntary (reflex) control. During eye closure not only does the upper lid come down, but the lower lid elevates as well. Also, on contraction of the eye muscles, the skin of the forehead, temple, and cheek is drawn and displaced medially. This throws the skin into folds that radiate from the lateral angle of the eye. These wrinkles may become permanent and are sometimes referred to as crow's feet.

Assisting in opening of the upper eyelid is the levator palpebrae superioris. This is a nonstriated muscle under sympathetic control. It originates deep in the orbit on the lesser wing of the sphenoid bone and attaches to both the superior tarsal plate and the skin of the upper eyelid. Contraction of this muscle helps to raise the upper eyelid.

Another muscle sometimes grouped with the orbital muscle is the corrugator supercilii (Fig. 3-14). This muscle

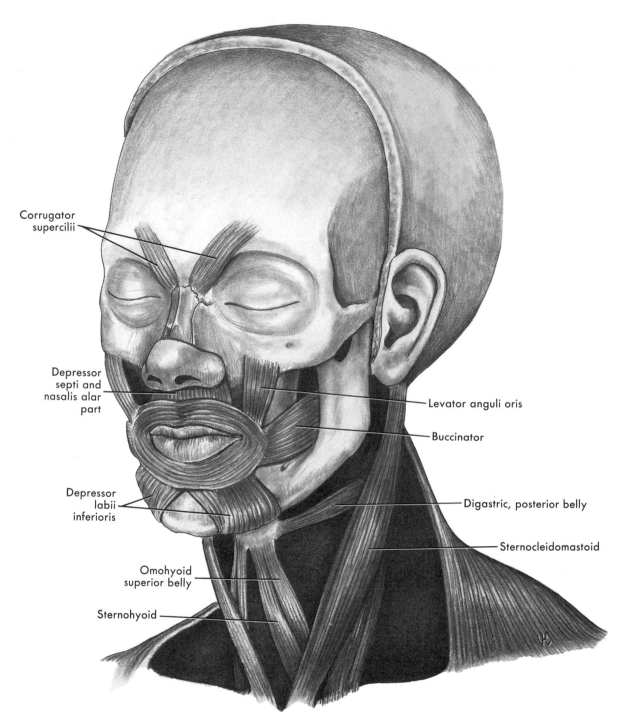

Fig. 3-14. Deep musculature of head and neck.

lies directly on the frontal bone, from which it originates close to the nasofrontal suture. It lies deep to the frontalis muscle from which it develops[24] and inserts into the skin of the medial portion of the eyebrow. Contraction of this muscle draws the eyebrows down, which medially produces a frown and vertical wrinkle lines in the glabellar area, the so-called frown lines of the face. The corrugator supercilii also helps to move the eyebrows medially toward each other. When the eyebrows are also at the same time raised by the frontalis muscle, arched eyebrows are produced giving a haughty ("supercilious") appearance.[34]

The muscles of the nose are poorly developed and often difficult to demonstrate. However, there are four muscles usually placed in this group (Fig. 3-13). The procerus arises from the upper portion of the lateral nasal cartilages, as well as the nasal bones, and inserts into the skin at the root of the nose. Contraction of this muscle draws the skin of the forehead down and produces transverse wrinkle lines over the root of the nose. The nasalis muscle stretches across the dorsum of the nose above the tip. It arises from the skin of the nasolabial sulcus and inserts into an aponeurosis that stretches across the nose to the nasalis muscle on the opposite side. Thus a sling is produced by the portion of the muscle that on contraction draws the alae toward the septum and depresses the cartilage. A smaller second portion of the nasalis muscle, the dilator naris, inserts onto the greater alar cartilage and dilates the naris. This latter second part of the nasalis muscle blends with the depressor septi, which is inferior to the nose. It arises on the maxilla and inserts onto the septum and posterior part of the ala. Its action is to narrow the nostrils. The last muscle of the nasal group is the levator labii superioris alaeque nasi, whose medial portion arises from the frontal process of the maxilla and passes inferiorly to insert onto the skin at the margin of the alar rim. Contraction of this muscle assists in dilation of the naris. The muscles in the nasal group are supplied by the zygomatic and superior buccal branches of the facial nerve.

The muscles concerned with movement of the lips and cheek are generally considered in four groups—the lower group, the upper group, the orbicularis oris, and the buccinator (Figs. 3-13 and 3-14). The central muscle is the orbicularis oris, around which the remaining muscles are grouped. The orbicularis oris is a circular muscle arranged around the mouth in a sphincterlike fashion. This is a complex muscle, much of which is intrinsic to the lips and arranged in layers. However, many of the seemingly circular fibers (Fig. 3-15) are in reality continuations (insertions) of surrounding muscles, which blend into the orbicularis oris. At the angles of the mouth the fibers cross each other to insert into the mucosa or skin rather than remaining continuous. The orbicularis oris draws the lips and the corners of the mouth together. In addition, it presses the lips to the teeth or protrudes the lips. The orbicularis oris is supplied by the lower buccal and the marginal mandibular branches of the facial nerve.

The lower group of oral muscles consists of the depressor anguli oris (triangularis), the depressor labii inferioris (quadratus labii inferioris), and the mentalis. The most superficial of this group, the depressor anguli oris, arises from the mandible and inserts into the skin and the upper part of the orbicularis muscle. The point at which its fibers insert and end in the medial upper lip helps form the philtrum.[42] In approximately 50% of individuals, its fibers continue underneath the chin to form a strap muscle.[56] These latter fibers are known as the transversus menti. Deep to the depressor anguli oris is the depressor labii inferioris, which also arises from the mandible, passes over the mental foramen, and inserts into the skin and mucosa of the lower lip and into the fibers of the inferior portion of the orbicularis

oris. Its fibers run medially so as to cross those on the other side. The action of the two depressors is to draw the corners of the mouth down and back. The depressors of the lower lip are supplied by the marginal mandibular branch of the facial nerve. The third and deepest muscle of this lower group is the mentalis. It arises in the mandible near the lip and inserts into the skin of the chin. Its fibers pass down and medially, with convergence of fibers from both sides of the chin at the insertion. The mentalis helps to raise the lower lip and assist in its protrusion.

The upper group of oral muscles consists of six muscles. The risorius begins in the subcutaneous tissue over the parotid and runs across the cheek to insert into the skin and mucosa at the corner of the mouth. This muscle is responsible for helping to retract the corner of the mouth. The zygomaticus major and the more medial zygomaticus minor originate from the lateral zygomatic bone and run medially downward, inserting into the upper lip near the corner of the mouth. The levator labii superioris and the more medial levator labii superioris alaeque nasi raise the upper lip and along with the zygomaticus muscle help to produce the nasolabial furrow seen when crying. The levator labii superioris originates from the maxilla at the infraorbital margin. It extends medially down and inserts into the orbicularis oris and skin of the lateral upper lip. The levator labii superioris alaeque nasi originates from the frontal process of the maxilla. It runs down and splits. The medial portion inserts into the skin and greater alar cartilage as previously described. The more lateral portion passes obliquely down to the skin and lateral orbicularis oris muscle. The deepest muscle of the upper group is the levator anguli oris, which arises from the maxilla and inserts into the corner of the mouth. Above this muscle run the facial artery and branches of the infraorbital nerve and vessels. The levators raise the lip, whereas the risorius and zygomaticus major and minor draw the corner of the mouth up and laterally. All six muscles in the upper group are supplied by the buccal branch of the facial nerve.

The last muscle of the oral group is the buccinator. This muscle forms the muscular substance of the cheek, arising from the alveolar processes of both the mandible and maxilla and passing forward to insert onto the orbicularis oris muscle and the skin of the lips and mucosa. Its central fibers at the angle of the mouth cross, so that those from below are continuous with the upper part of the orbicularis oris and those from above are continuous with the lower part. The highest and lowest fibers continue with the highest and lowest segments of the orbicularis oris muscle, respectively (Fig. 3-15). This muscle is important as a landmark for several important structures. The facial artery and vein pass over it, the parotid duct passes through it into the mouth (opposite the third upper molar tooth), and the buccal branch of the facial nerve emerges at its superior border. Its action is to compress the cheek against the gums and teeth

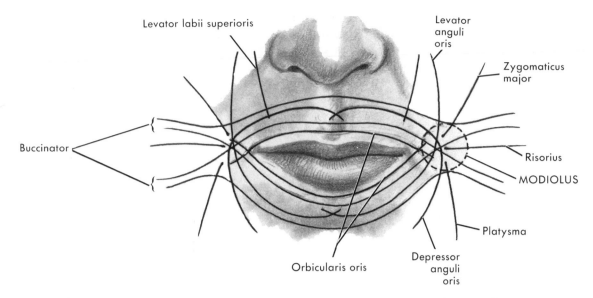

Fig. 3-15. Muscles comprising orbicularis oris and modiolus *(dashed circle).* Not shown are insertions of the depressor labii inferioris muscle into the orbicularis oris muscle of lower lip, and zygomaticus minor and levator labii superioris alaeque nasi muscles into the orbicularis oris of upper lip.

to aid in mastication and to compress the cheeks when distended by air. (Buccinator means trumpeter in Latin.) It is supplied by the lower buccal branches of the facial nerve.

The intermixture of the muscles surrounding the mouth thus produces a complex structure (Fig. 3-15). The meeting place of many of these muscles is just lateral to the angle of the mouth and produces a thickened mass, which is the modiolus. In Latin modiolus means the hub of a wheel. It can be seen clinically in many individuals as a rounded eminence on the check just lateral to the mouth[33] (Fig. 3-2).

There are seven muscles that meet at the modiolus: (1) the levator anguli oris, (2) the depressor anguli oris, (3) the buccinator, (4) the zygomaticus major, (5) the risorius, (6) the orbicular oris, and (7) the platysma. The orbicular oris uses the modiolus as a fixed area of origin. This knotty crossroads is fixed in a given position by the zygomaticus major, the levator anguli oris, and the depressor anguli oris.

The physiognomy of a smile has been studied by Rubin.[48] He classified smiles into the following three types: (1) the Mona Lisa smile (67%), (2) the canine smile (31%), and (3) the full-denture smile (2%). The Mona Lisa smile is a result of the pull at the corners of the mouth (at the modiolus). The canine smile expose the canine teeth and results from contraction of both the elevators at the corner of the mouth and the lip elevator muscles. In the full-denture smile, both upper and lower teeth are seen with increased contraction of the lower lip depressors. Rubin also dissected six cadavers and found that insertions of the levator labii superioris insert into the vermilion and vermilion border rather than into the orbicular oris muscle. He hypothesizes this helps produce the canine smile. The important contribu-

tion of the platysma muscle in depressing the angles of the mouth and helping to produce a full-denture smile was emphasized by Ellenbogen, who pointed out that damage to the cervical branch of the facial nerve, which supplies the platysma, would convert a full-denture smile into one of the other two types.[21]

The anatomy of the lips is also important to understand not only from a functional point of view, but also from an overall structural standpoint. The concept that the orbicularis oris muscle is a circular muscle surrounding the mouth is obviously fallacious (Fig. 3-15). Basically there are three separate muscle groups whose spatial relationships are of importance in repairing the lip. In cross section, the deeper orbicular oris muscles, which surround the mouth at the vermilion, help to evert the mucosa. More superficially there are two groups of muscles. One group is situated more proximal to the oral opening and is composed of fibers from those muscle fibers passing through the modiolus. A more distal group is also present and composed of the elevators or depressors of the lips. When repairing the upper or lower lip, these three muscle groups should be identified and sutured independently.[42]

The muscles concerned with the movement of the mandible (known also as the muscles of mastication) include the masseter, the temporalis, and the lateral and medial pterygoids. All these muscles insert onto the mandible and are involved with biting and chewing. The masseter muscle (Fig. 3-11) originates from the anterior and lateral zygomatic arch and passes backward to insert onto the lateral surface of the ramus of the mandible. Because it is superficial, the masseter muscle may be easily palpated when one clenches the jaws and thus contracts the muscle. The temporalis muscle has a large site of origin, the temporal fossa and temporal fascia. It inserts onto the medial ramus and coronoid process. This muscle passes underneath the zygomatic arch. Both the temporalis and masseter function to close the mouth. Two other deeper muscles, the medial and lateral pterygoids, originate from the pterygoid processes and insert onto the medial surface of the mandible. The medial pterygoid inserts on the mandible on the opposite side from the masseter muscle, so the two together form a sling. The muscles of mastication are innervated by the fifth facial nerve.

The buccal fat pad is a collection of fat limited by fascia that is situated in the cheek between the masseter and the buccinator muscle and then more posteriorly between the bend of the ramus and the insertion of the temporalis muscle. Its importance is that it represents a potential anatomic space that may be conducive to potentiating infection.[31]

The anatomy of the neck is characterized and complicated by numerous fascial spaces, which are beyond the scope of this text. The more superficial muscles important in dermatologic surgery are described here, however. The platysma muscle (Fig. 3-13) is a broad sheet that extends from the thorax over the clavicle and across the anterolateral neck and mandible toward the mouth. It inserts on the inferior mandible and skin. The platysma is extremely thin and pliable. This muscle is innervated by the cervical branch of the seventh nerve, which lies deep to the muscle. The platysma helps to open the jaw, draw down the lower lip, and depress the angles of the mouth. Although some consider this muscle in humans to be a vestigial remnant of the panniculus carnosus,[40] it is more properly classified as one of the muscles of facial expression.[2] This is evidenced by the common nerve innervation (VII) for the platysma muscle and the muscles of facial expression.

The presence and configuration of the platysma can be somewhat variable. In a study of 50 cadaver dissections, Cardoso de Castro[12] showed that the medial fibers from each side meet at the mandible beneath the chin without crossing in 10% of the cases. In most cases (75%) there was some interlacing of fibers in this area, usually extending 1 to 2 cm posteriorly. In the remaining 15% of cadavers, the opposite platysma muscle fibers interdigitated from the thyroid cartilage to the chin. These findings are somewhat at variance with those of Vistnes,[55] who dissected 18 cadavers. This latter study showed the noncrossing pattern of insertion in 61% of cases and the crossed pattern from thyroid to chin in the remaining 39%. With age, the individuals with the non-crossing pattern will develop two bands in the anterior neck representing the medial aspects of the paired platysma muscle. The submental fat pad herniates easily through these bands.

Deep to the platysma is the sternocleidomastoid muscle,

BRANCHES OF THE FACIAL NERVE (VII) AND MUSCLES INNERVATED

Posterior auricular
  Occipitalis
  Auricularis posterior
  Sensory to mastoid region

Temporal
  Frontalis
  Corrugator supercilii
  Orbicularis oculi
  Auricular muscles (anterior and superior)

Zygomatic (infraorbital)
  Orbicularis oculi
  Upper lip muscles
  Buccinator
  Ala muscles

Buccal
  Buccinator
  Upper lip muscles
  Lower lip muscles

Marginal mandibular (supramandibular)
  Lower lip muscles

Cervical (inframandibular)
  Platysma

---

which arises from the sternum and clavicle (Figs. 3-11 and 3-14). It travels superiorly and posteriorly to attach onto the mastoid process behind the ear and acts to turn down and rotate the head to the side. Posteriorly the most superficial muscle on the neck is the trapezius, which begins at the occipital bone, ligamentum nuchae, and spinous processes of C7 and T1 through T12 and inserts onto the lateral clavicle and scapula. This muscle moves the scapula and head.

Motor nerves

Most of the muscles of the face are innervated by the facial cranial nerve (VII). During embryonic development the facial muscles develop in conjunction with this nerve that develops deep to them.[24] Thus a trophic influence is established early on. The extracranial branches of the facial nerve are listed in the box on this page and illustrated in Fig. 3-16.

Injury to the facial nerve or its branches is of great concern to all physicians performing surgery on the face. It has been stated to be the "major anatomic obstacle between the surgeon and his equanimity."[23] The physical appearance of

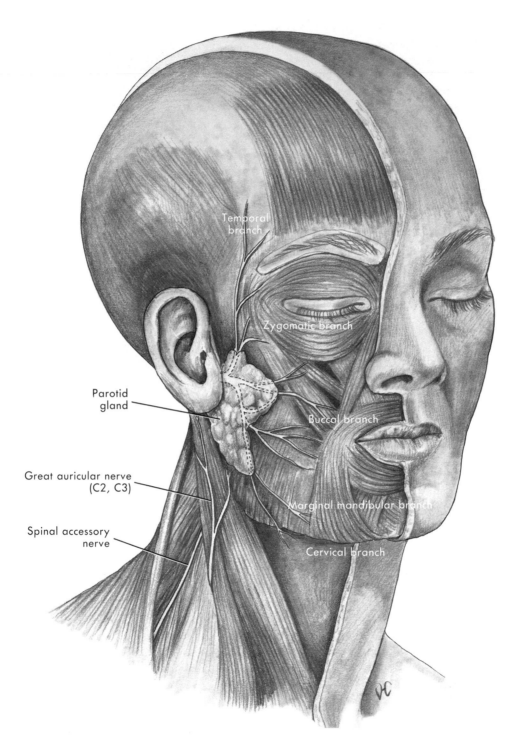

Fig. 3-16. Distribution of branches of facial nerve.

a patient with an injured facial nerve is changed markedly. This was graphically described by Bunnell in 1927[11]:

> The eye cannot close and constantly weeps. The mouth dribbles, the speech is interfered with, and mastication is impaired. The delicate shades of continence are lost. Joy, happiness, sorrow, shock, surprise, all the emotions have for their common expression the same blank stare.

The facial nerve exits the skull through the stylomastoid foramen, which is slightly posterior and lateral to the styloid process. This is anterior but medial to the mastoid process. In some individuals the nerve may be aberrant and more superficial, exiting directly in front of the mastoid process. In children the nerve tends to lie more superficially in this location than in adults.[23] Rarely, the facial nerve may be exposed in the ear canal itself.[26] After exiting, the nerve

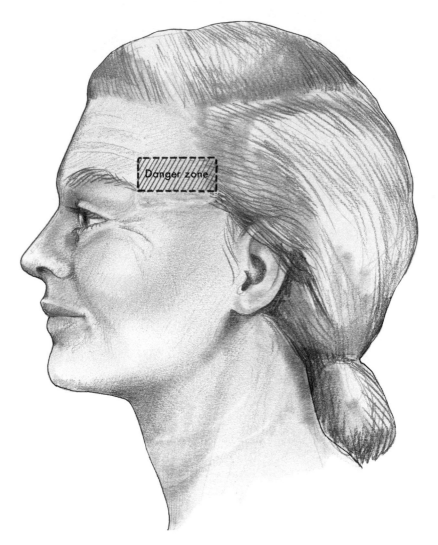

Fig. 3-17. Danger zone in which temporal branch of facial nerve courses superficially.

crosses in front of the stylomastoid process and enters the substance of the parotid gland, in which it divides into its main branches.

As the facial nerve emerges from the stylomastoid foramen, it gives off its first branch, the posterior auricular, which runs posteriorly between the external acoustic meatus and the mastoid process. This branch divides to supply the most posterior facial muscles. The occipital branch innervates the occipital muscle and the auricular branch goes to the auricularis posterior, part of the auricularis superior, and the intrinsic muscles of the auricle. In addition, it contains sensory fibers that supply the skin overlying the mastoid process and posterior ear. The posterior auricular nerve communicates with other nerves in the neck, the auricular branch of the vagus, the great auricular, and lesser occipital nerves.

The relationship between the facial nerve and the parotid gland is somewhat complex. The older concept that there are two lobes of the parotid gland, a deep and a superficial, has been disputed. It is now felt that "lobe" is an inappro-

priate term and that *portions* is preferable.[25] This is based on the fact that no cleavage planes are observed in gland primordium as are observed in other structures, for example, the liver. Therefore the facial nerve may be at different levels within the parotid gland.

The facial nerve enters the parotid gland at about the level of the intertragic notch. Its main trunk usually does not descend any lower than the earlobe, and its bifurcation occurs posteromedially to the mandibular ramus at a distance two thirds of the way from the angle of the mandible to the temporomandibular joint.[23] Within the substance of the parotid gland, the facial nerve is usually divided into an upper and lower branch, sometimes referred to as the temporofacial and cervicofacial divisions. These may give off other branches that have multiple anastomoses forming a nerve plexus (the parotid plexus), or these branches simply pass through the parotid without anastomoses. In a recent study 100 parotidectomies were performed and the course of the facial nerve traced out. The investigators found that in 50% of cases, no anastomoses existed between the differ-

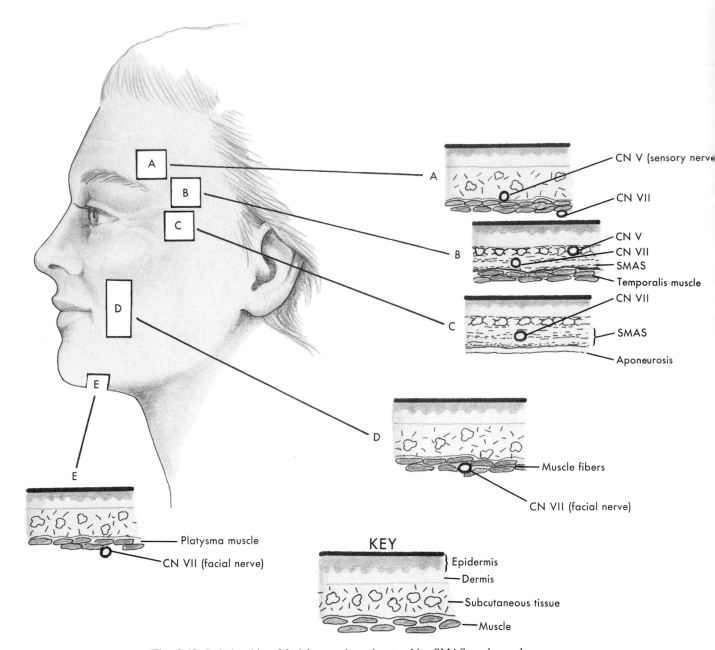

Fig. 3-18. Relationship of facial nerve branches to skin, SMAS, and muscle.

ent branches after exit from the temporal bone.[37] Other investigators,[17,35] however, mapped out various patterns of branching and anastomoses. Another interesting finding was that in 18% of individuals, anastomoses occurred between the upper and lower main divisions.[37] The result of the branching within the parotid gland is a variable number of branches that emerge to innervate the face. Traditionally, these are divided into the following five main branches: (1) temporal, (2) zygomatic, (3) buccal, (4) marginal mandibular, and (5) cervical. One may minimize injury to these nerves by knowing their course, relative depth, and distribution.

The temporal branch of the facial nerve courses superior-

ly across the temple to supply the frontalis muscle, the orbicularis oculi, and the anterior and superior muscles of the ear. Damage to this nerve results in an inability to elevate the eyebrows or close the eyelids. In an attempt to delineate the course of this nerve precisely, several investigators[18,32,45,47] have mapped out its course and outlined a danger zone (Fig. 3-17). This zone forms a rectangular box, which is 2 cm in height and extends from above the lateral eyebrow posteriorly to the anterior hairline. This is an area in which incision or dissection could compromise or in some way injure the nerve. The temporal branch crosses the zygomatic arch at a point approximately intersected by a line drawn downwards from the anterolateral hairline. The nerve then continues on a gentle, inclining curve across the temporal region, passing superior and lateral to the eyebrow. The depth of the nerve (Fig. 3-18) is in the organized superficial fascia (SMAS) until it reaches the muscle, at which point it is deep to the muscle. Therefore above the eyebrow the temporal nerve is deep to the frontalis muscle, but lateral to the eyebrow it is in the SMAS just above the temporalis fascia and muscle. When undermining in this area, it is a good idea to stay in the superficial subcutaneous fat layer above the SMAS to keep from causing any injury to the nerve.

The zygomatic branch of the facial nerve, which usually runs initially with the temporal branch, innervates the orbicularis oculi, the nasal muscles, the lip elevators, and the buccinator. The buccal branch also innervates the bucinnator. In addition, this nerve supplies the upper and lower lip muscle. In the area of the nasolabial fold, the branches of the facial nerve are deep in the muscle and so less danger of injury exists there. In the medial third of the cheek the buccal and zygomatic branches interconnect, so that surgical damage to small areas does not result in persistent motor weakness.

The marginal mandibular branch of the facial nerve runs along the lower border of the mandible to supply the muscles of the lower lip. It is situated beneath the platysma muscle, so there is little danger of injuring this nerve if one dissects superficial to the muscle. Some have found the point at which this nerve branch crosses the facial artery to be of importance in determining its course. Dingman[19] states that anterior to this point branches of the marginal mandibular nerve are above the mandibular border in 100% of cases. This was disputed by Nelson et al.[41] who found nerve branches below the mandible running to innervate the mentalis and depressor labii inferioris muscles. Posterior to the facial artery, the marginal mandibular nerve is below the lower border of the mandible in 20% of cases.[19] Injury to this nerve branch results in marked facial deformity manifested by drooping of the corner of the mouth. The marginal mandibular nerve may be damaged during a face-lift operation while the surgeon undermines along the margin of the mandibular ramus.

The cervical branch of the facial nerve usually receives little attention. This is because it innervates the platysma muscle, which is regarded as insignificant. However, as previously mentioned, this muscle helps to create a downward and lateral pull on the corner of the mouth. When the cervical branch is injured, therefore, a pseudoparalysis of the marginal mandibular branch may occur.[21] The cervical nerve branch may run beneath the platysma.

Ziarah et al.[60] studied the course of the cervical branch of the facial nerve in 110 facial cadaver halves. These investigators found that the cervical and mandibular nerves emerged together along the lower border of the parotid. At a variable distance from the gland, but always by the time they reached the angle of the mandible, the two nerves diverged. The cervical branch was always posterior to the mandibular branch. In 80% of the specimens examined, the cervical branch was single, whereas in the remaining 20% it was double. Interestingly, in several specimens the cervical branch also anastomosed with the transverse cervical and great auricular nerves of the cervical plexus.

The facial nerve is mainly a motor nerve; however, there is evidence of sensory (pain) and proprioceptive fibers traveling with this nerve beyond its exit from the stylomastoid foramen. In a classic 1915 study patients who had facial *motor* nerve weakness caused by herpes zoster infection of the seventh cranial nerve were studied.[29] Interestingly, several of these patients developed cutaneous herpes zoster of the anterior ear and inferior posterior auricular sulcus, leading to the conclusion that the cutaneous eruption was a result of the cutaneous *sensory* component of the seventh nerve. In addition, these patients complained of deep-seated pain on the side of the face.

The fibers of the facial nerve are interconnected with fibers of several other cranial and spinal nerves, including the auriculotemporal nerve of CN V and the auricular branch of the vagus. The functional significance of the communications between the facial and trigeminal nerve was reviewed by Baumel.[6] Although uncertainties exist, it is felt that the sensory fibers from the seventh nerve are the ones that join with the fifth nerve. In addition, sensory muscle spindles are present in facial muscles and are important for optional functioning of several muscles.[54]

On severing the facial nerve or a major branch of this nerve, obvious motor function is lost. In addition, there may also be facial spasm, contractures, and associated movements. Sometimes denervated muscle may be reinnervated by spontaneous regeneration of the affected nerve or perhaps by alternative routes via other nerves, such as the trigeminal nerve.[6] In an analysis of the literature on branches of the facial nerve damaged during rhytidectomies, Baker found overall an 86% recovery within 6 months to 1 year from the time of surgery.[5]

Large severed nerves may be anastomosed if the ends can be localized or, if the intervening defect is large, a nerve graft could be used. Using grafts from the greater auricular nerve or sural nerve, Baker[4] reported good return of function in 79% of patients. Part of the reason that nerve grafting works fairly well in a situation where there are complex innervations is that the spatial arrangement of fibers within the nerve trunk itself is not very precise.[15,30] Also, the rich blood supply to the facial nerve helps to preclude permanent injury[8] and encourage healing.

Motor nerves of the neck

The platysma muscle, as already mentioned, is supplied by the cervical branch of the facial nerve. The other important superficial muscles of the neck, the sternocleidomastoid

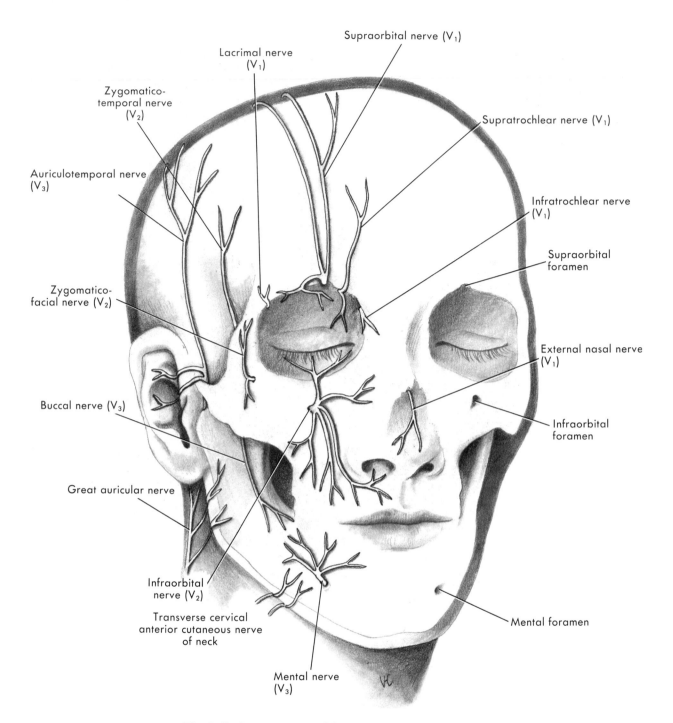

Lacrimal nerve (V₁)

Supraorbital nerve (V₁)

Zygomatico-temporal nerve (V₂)

Supratrochlear nerve (V₁)

Auriculotemporal nerve (V₃)

Infratrochlear nerve (V₁)

Supraorbital foramen

Zygomatico-facial nerve (V₂)

External nasal nerve (V₁)

Buccal nerve (V₃)

Infraorbital foramen

Great auricular nerve

Infraorbital nerve (V₂)

Mental foramen

Transverse cervical anterior cutaneous nerve of neck

Mental nerve (V₃)

Fig. 3-19. Sensory nerves of face and scalp (anterior view).

and trapezius, are supplied by CN XI, the spinal accessory (Fig. 3-16). It emerges from the jugular foramen and crosses the internal jugular vein running down and back of the sternocleidomastoid muscle. It gives off branches to the sternocleidomastoid muscle and then appears at the upper middle posterior edge of this muscle. It then passes inferiorly, crossing the posterior triangle to disappear beneath the anterior border of the trapezius muscle. During its course in the posterior triangle, the spinal accessory nerve is covered only by skin and subcutaneous fascia. Before entering the trapezius muscle, the spinal accessory nerve receives sensory branches from the third and fourth cervical nerves. Denervation of the trapezius muscle may lead to shoulder syndrome, in which the patient's shoulder droops and is

---

**CUTANEOUS BRANCHES OF THE
TRIGEMINAL NERVE (V)**

V_1 *Ophthalmic division*
   Supraorbital nerve
   Supratrochlear nerve
   Infratrochlear nerve
   External nasal branch nerve
   Lacrimal nerve

V_2 *Maxillary division*
   Infraorbital nerve
   Zygomaticofacial nerve
   Zygomaticotemporal nerve

V_3 *Mandibular division*
   Mental nerve
   Buccal nerve
   Auriculotemporal nerve

---

painful. If muscular activity is slight, a frozen shoulder may follow with periarthritis of the shoulder joint. The patient will be unable to abduct the arm. Therefore, surgery in the posterior triangle, for example, radical neck dissections, should be performed to preserve, if possible, function of the spinal accessory nerve.[10]

Sensory supply to the face

The majority of the face is supplied by the trigeminal nerve, the largest sensory nerve, which separates into three primary divisions before exiting from the skull. Each division in turn sends several cutaneous branches to the face. These branches supply not only the cutaneous surface, but the whole thickness of tissue from bone or mucous membrane to skin. The major sensory branches from the trigeminal nerve are listed in the box on this page and illustrated in Fig. 3-19. In addition, the trigeminal nerve is the motor nerve for the muscles of mastication.

The supraorbital nerve exits from the supraorbital foramen or notch, which is palpable on the superior medial orbital rim. This is the largest extracranial branch of the ophthalmic division (V_1). This nerve supplies the skin of the forehead and anterior scalp. Medial to the supraorbital nerve is the supratrochlear nerve, which supplies the medial forehead. This exists from a smaller notch (the frontal notch), which may be felt medial to the supraorbital notch (Fig. 3-7). Both of these nerves initially run deep in the frontal belly of the occipitofrontalis muscle. However, the medial branch of the supraorbital nerve pierces the muscle in the midforehead. Both the supraorbital nerve and the supratrochlear nerve are branches of the frontal nerve, the largest branch of the ophthalmic division of the fifth cranial nerve.

The infratrochlear nerve exits in the superior medial canthus, and the lacrimal nerve at the lateral canthus. These four nerves (supraorbital, supratrochlear, infratrochlear, and lacrimal) supply the skin of the upper lids, the medial and lateral canthi, and the bridge and part of the sides of the nose. The external nasal branch of the anterior ethmoidal branch of the nasociliary nerve exists bilaterally between the frontal bone and lateral nasal cartilages to supply the skin of the dorsum of the nose to the nasal tip.

The maxillary division (V_2) of the trigeminal nerve supplies the lower eyelids, a portion of the side of the nose, the malar cheek, the upper lip, and part of the temple. Its largest branch, the infraorbital nerve, exits through the infraorbital foramen. The infraorbital foramen is located in the maxilla in a line approximately between the supraorbital notch and the mental foramen. This nerve anastomoses with branches of the zygomatic branches of the facial nerve. It supplies the lower lid, the lower side of the nose, the malar cheek, and the upper lip. The infraorbital foramen is very close to the oral cavity, so anesthesia can be administered through the mouth.

The cutaneous innervation of the nose is shown in Fig. 3-20. The nose is innervated by four different nerves: the infraorbital nerve, the external nasal branch of the anterior ethmoidal nerve, and the supratrochlear and infratrochlear nerves. Because of these different nerve distributions, the tip of the nose is spared in the trigeminal trophic syndrome, a condition in which ulceration occurs in the nasolabial area usually after surgery (for instance, for trigeminal neuralgia) that injures the maxillary (V_2) division spares the ophthalmic (V_1) division.

The zygomatic branch of the maxillary division (V_2) divides into two branches. The most inferior, the zygomaticofacial nerve, exits through the lateral zygomatic bone and supplies a small area of skin in the lateral canthal area. The other branch, the zygomaticotemporal nerve, emerges from the anterior temporal fossa and supplies the skin over the anterior portion of the temporal region.

The third major division of the trigeminal nerve is the mandibular (V_3). This nerve supplies the skin of the chin, cheek, lower lip, and temporal scalp. The mental branch, a continuation of the inferior alveolar nerve, exits through the mental foramen. It supplies the chin and lower lip to the angle to the mouth. A block of the mental nerve can anesthetize the lower lip and adjacent chin. A topical anesthetic, such as lidocaine (2% to 4%) may first be applied between the gingiva and the oral mucosa of the lip, after which lidocaine may be injected through this topically anesthetized area into the area around the mental foramen. The buccal branch passes through the lower temporal is muscle and buccal fat pad and supplies both the skin and mucosa between the upper and lower jaws. The auriculotemporal branch emerges anterior to the temporomandibular joint and inferior to the zygomatic arch and supplies the most anterior

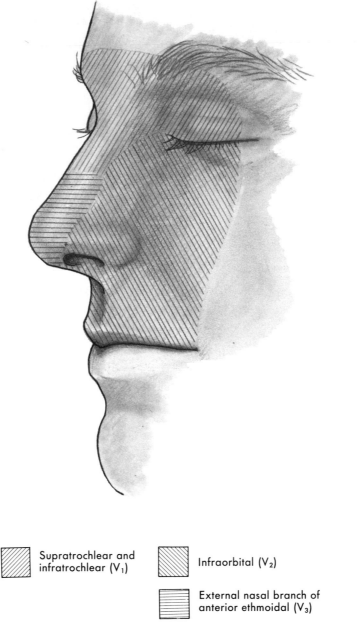

Supratrochlear and
infratrochlear (V₁)

Infraorbital (V₂)

External nasal branch of
anterior ethmoidal (V₃)

Fig. 3-20. Sensory nerve distribution of nose. (Modified from Hollinshead, W.H.: Anatomy for surgeons. Vol. 1: The head and neck, Philadelphia, 1982, Harper & Rowe.)

portion of the auricle and the temporal region. This branch also supplies both the external ear canal and the tympanic membrane and anastomoses with the facial nerve just proximal to the latter nerve's exit from the parotid gland.

Tic douloureux, or trigeminal neuralgia, is a condition characterized by paroxysmal attacks of severe pain over the distribution of one or more branches of the trigeminal nerve. Although the cause of this condition is unknown, over the years various surgeries have been developed to transect the nerve to relieve the pain. These procedures have

demonstrated many important facts about the trigeminal nerve and its distribution. When only part of the trigeminal nerve is severed, there is some unpredictability as to which areas will be relieved. Therefore nerve fibers to the three main divisions interlace or cross somewhere within the main nerve trunk.[49]

Cushing[16] published a classic study in which he mapped anesthetic areas of the face after trigeminal nerve disruption surgically. Although most of the classic patterns of anesthesia were found, as shown in Fig. 3-21, Cushing showed

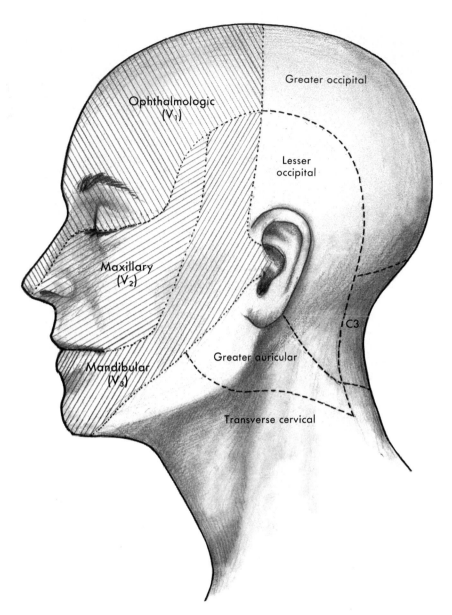

Fig. 3-21. Sensory nerve distribution of head and neck. Note that area overlying lateral mandible is not innervated by V_3.

that near the posterior border of the V_1 and V_3 zones there was an intermediate area in which pressure could be felt, but not pain. In addition, he was one of the first to point out that the concha and the posterior wall of the auditory canal retained their sensitivity because they were supplied by a peculiar aberrant cutaneous branch from the vagus nerve, the auricular branch. The presence of this nerve helps to explain the cough reflex seen on manipulation of the external auditory canal and also the results with acupuncture in this area.

There is some discrepancy between the nerve supply to the ear described by anatomists and that commonly recognized by clinicians. Possibly the only sensory supply from the fifth nerve to the ear is the tragus and anterior auditory meatus.[59]

The peculiar cutaneous sensory distribution of the ear is illustrated in Fig. 3-22. Although the cervical and trigeminal nerves account for most of the surface, there are contributions from CN VII, IX, and X as well. This accounts for the difficulties in producing complete nerve blocks of the external ear.

The autonomic nervous system has a complex interrelationship with the facial nerve, as well as the trigeminal nerve, mainly through the mandibular division (V_3). Parasympathetic fibers of the facial nerve travel to the glands of the nose and palate in the pterygopalatine ganglion, and to

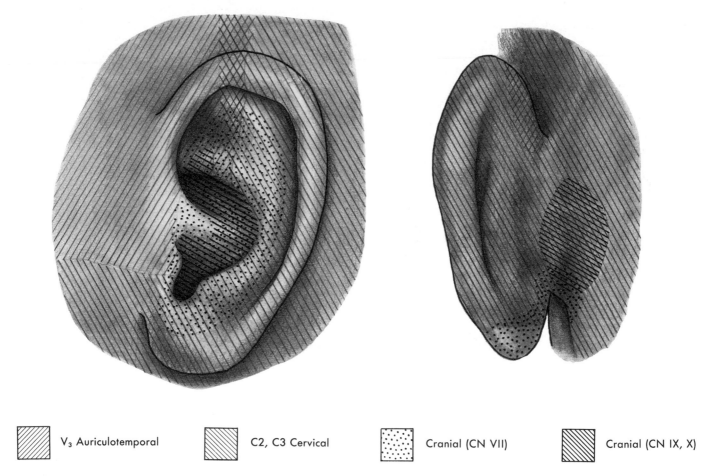

| | V₃ Auriculotemporal | | C2, C3 Cervical | | Cranial (CN VII) | | Cranial (CN IX, X) |

Fig. 3-22. Sensory nerve distribution of ear. (Modified from Hollinshead, W.H.: Anatomy for surgeons. Vol. 1: The head and neck, Philadelphia, 1982, Harper & Rowe.)

the salivary glands via the chorda tympani, through the otic ganglion to the parotid and submandibular ganglion, and on to the remaining glands. Sympathetic fibers pass to the parotid via the superior cervical ganglion and the carotid plexus. Other sympathetic fibers to the face come from the ciliary, sphenopalatine, otic, and submaxillary ganglia. Sometimes after the trigeminal nerve is severed, certain sensory functions return. Helson[27] feels this is the result of an unmasking of sympathetic function. He believes that sympathetic fibers have both an afferent and an efferent function. To support this hypothesis, there is a further loss of sensation when both sympathetic and trigeminal function are lost simultaneously.

Frey's syndrome (auriculotemporal syndrome) is a condition characterized by pain, vasodilation, and hyperhidrosis of the cheeks when eating (gustatory sweating). Usually this occurs following parotid gland surgery and is thought to be a consequence of haphazard nerve regeneration, so that the parasympathetic fibers instead of the sympathetic fibers mistakenly innervate the sweat glands and blood vessels of the skin.

Sensory nerves of the neck and posterior scalp

The nerve supply to the lateral neck and posterior scalp is from the cervical plexus, formed by the union of the anterior rami of the second, third, and fourth cervical nerves. The cutaneous branches from this plexus include the lesser occipital, the great auricular, the transverse cervical, and the supraclavicular nerves (Fig. 3-23). The lesser occipital nerve (C2) passes along the posterior portion of the sternocleidomastoid muscle after exiting near the spinal accessory nerve (CN XI) and follows the muscle superiorly to supply the scalp posterior to the ear and the superior portion of the posterior auricle. The great auricular nerve (C2, C3) also passes around the posterior border of the sternocleidomastoid muscle more inferiorly than the spinal accessory nerve. It then runs superiorly toward the lower border of the ear (Fig. 3-16). It supplies the skin over the parotid gland, the lower anterior ear, the lower posterior ear, and the mastoid process. The transverse cervical nerve (C2, C3) arises with the great auricular but turns sharply over the midposterior border of the sternocleidomastoid muscle and passes first transversely, then dividing into branches that

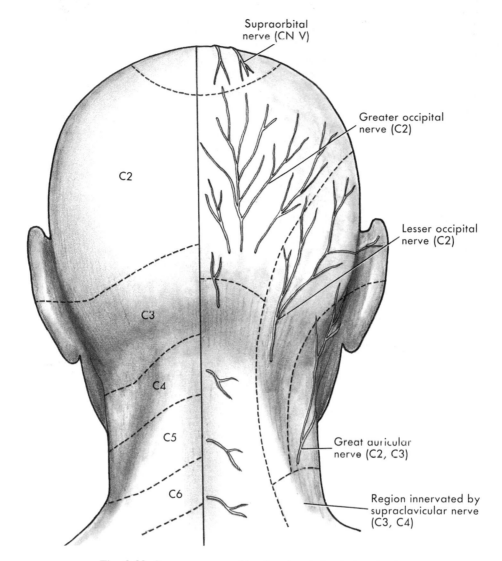

Fig. 3-23. Sensory nerves of head and neck (posterior view).

supply the anterior portion of the neck. Some upper branches anastomose with the cervical branch of CN VII. The supraclavicular nerve (C3, C4) supplies the skin of the lower neck, clavicle, and shoulder.

The greater occipital nerve (C2) is formed from the posterior ramus of the second cervical nerve and supplies the skin on the occipital scalp. It appears in the suboccipital region at the lateral border of the trapezius and then courses superiorly from between the trapezius and sternocleidomastoid attachments. The first cervical nerve has no cutaneous branches. On the midposterior scalp the posterior divisions of the cervical nerves (C2 through C6) supply the skin. Careful planning of incisions on the scalp minimizes denervation. Incisions that are midline or follow the superior aspect of the temporal bone generally minimize sensory nerve loss.

Blood vessels

The scalp is richly supplied by blood vessels that in general run upwards. Because of the frequent anastomoses of these vessels, it is difficult to reduce the blood supply to any one area. Therefore large flaps with relatively small pedicles may survive in this area. These anastomoses promote free bleeding in this area with profuse blood flow from both cut surfaces of an artery.

Anteriorly the supraorbital artery exits from the supraorbital foramen with the supraorbital nerve. More medially the supratrochlear (frontal) artery emerges. These arteries supply the forehead. They are branches of the ophthalmic artery that come off the internal carotid artery. The rest of the scalp is supplied by the branches of the external carotid artery: the occipital artery, the posterior auricular artery, and the superficial temporal artery.

The occipital artery branches off the posterior surface of the external carotid at about the same level as the facial artery. The occipital artery then runs backward and superiorly onto the occipital scalp under cover of the sternocleidomastoid muscle. Superior to the origin of the facial artery on the external carotid, the posterior auricular artery arises. It sends branches to the posterior portion of the ear and ascends to supply the scalp above and behind the ear. Within the parotid, the superficial temporal and maxillary arteries arise from the external carotid as terminal branches. The superficial temporal artery continues superiorly, while the maxillary artery passes inside the ramus of the mandible. A branch of the maxillary artery, the buccal artery, enters the cheek to supply the buccinator muscle. The transverse facial artery arises from the base of the superficial temporal artery and passes across the face just below the zygomatic arch. The superficial temporal artery begins deep to or in the parotid gland immediately in front of the ear, where it is crossed above by the temporal and zygomatic branches of the facial nerve. Its course can usually be palpated as it passes superiorly with and anterior to the auriculotemporal branch of the mandibular nerve. This artery courses over the zygomatic process and divides into an anterior frontal branch and a posterior parietal branch.

The facial artery is a branch of the external carotid artery. It runs anteriorly under the mandible and across the lower border of the mandible near the anterior border of the masseter muscle. The artery then runs superiorly to the side of the nose. Its continuation along the side of the nose is known as the angular artery, which anastomoses with the supratrochlear artery in the medial canthal region. The labial arteries are branches from the facial artery. The labial arteries lie deep in the lips, either deep in the muscles or between the muscle and the mucosa. When the mucosa is undermined for lip shaves for superficial carcinoma of the lower lip, these arteries may be uncovered. As the facial artery continues alongside the nose and becomes the angular artery, it gives off the lateral nasal artery to supply the lateral side of the nose. This latter artery may anastomose with the dorsal nasal artery superiorly.

The infraorbital artery emerges from the infraorbital foramen and supplies the skin and muscles in the infraorbital region, including the lower eyelid. It arises from the maxillary artery. The dorsal nasal artery, a branch of the ophthalmic artery, penetrates the upper eyelid septum and courses inferiorly in the nose. It may anastomose with the angular artery of the nose or the lateral nasal artery.

As seen in Fig. 3-24, the venous drainage of the face roughly parallels that of the arterial supply. The main vein of the face is the facial vein, which begins as the angular vein in the inner canthal area. At this point it communicates freely with the ophthalmic vein. In addition, it also communicates superiorly with the veins of the forehead, as well as with those of the other surrounding structures, the eyelids and the nose. As the facial vein runs inferiorly, it connects with the infraorbital vein through the infraorbital foramen, which in turn empties into the deep pterygoid plexus. The facial vein courses behind the facial artery and is deep to most of the facial muscles. After crossing the mandible, the facial vein runs over the surface of the submandibular gland and drains into the internal jugular vein.

The veins of the face, unlike those on the trunk and extremities, do not have valves. Therefore blood may flow in either direction in this area. The communications of the facial vein with the ophthalmic vein, the infraorbital vein, and the deep facial vein are thus relatively direct avenues into the deeper pterygoid plexus and cavernous sinus. Infections of the face, particularly in the central area where these interconnections lie, may spread through this route. Because of these anastomoses, some physicians advise against surgically evacuating infections in this area. It is felt that manipulation of infectious tissue possibly promotes the transmission of infections through the branches of these veins. Fortunately, since the advent of antibiotics, we do not often see serious infections in this area.

The vascular supply of the neck is quite complex; it is not discussed in great detail here. The common carotid artery bifurcates into the internal and external carotid arteries approximately at the level of the junction of the hyoid bone and the thyroid cartilage. The internal carotid continues on into the carotid canal as the main vascular supply for the brain. The external carotid arises slightly anterior and medial to the internal carotid and runs superiorly across the ramus of the mandible. It gives off several branches superiorly, many of which have already been mentioned, including the facial artery and temporal artery. The occipital artery arises from its posterior border and runs up and back to supply the posterior scalp, trapezius muscle, and sternocleidomastoid muscle.

The external jugular vein is the most superficial large vein in the neck. It arises in the substance of the parotid gland and runs superficially across the surface of the sternocleidomastoid muscle. The external jugular vein empties into the subclavian veins or, in approximately one third of individuals, into the internal jugular.

Lymphatic system

Excess tissue fluid along with proteins, fats, cells, and large particulate matter are absorbed into the lymphatic vessels that drain into lymph nodes along their course. These lymph nodes filter the lymph drainage and trap foreign material. The lymph nodes are fixed in location and become swollen because of infection or proliferating tumor metastases. The physician should always be aware of the location of the principal lymph nodes of the head and neck and their areas of drainage so that the location of cancer or infection may be more easily deduced. However, it should be emphasized that with tumors the metastatic patterns

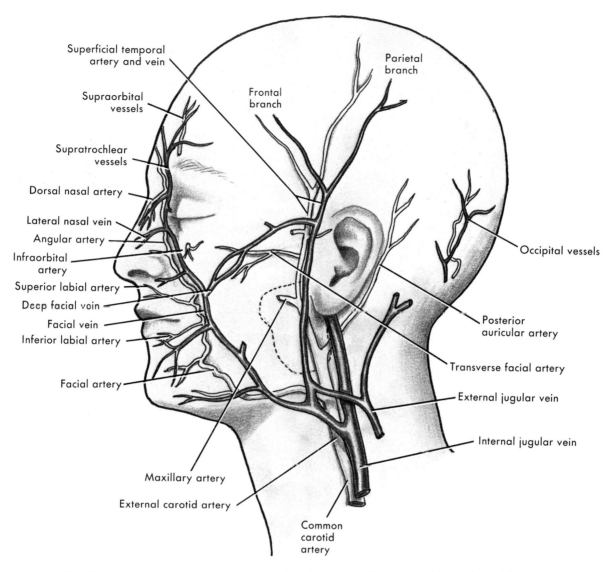

Fig. 3-24. Arterial and venous distribution of head and neck. Branching of internal carotid artery from common carotid artery is not shown, but occurs just inferior to point at which external carotid artery is indicated.

within lymphatics do not always adhere to textbook descriptions.[43] Because early detection of metastatic disease probably leads to increased chances of survival, proper examination of the lymph nodes in patients at high risk for metastases is essential. These methods have been well described by Sage.[50]

The major lymph nodes and lymphatic drainage are shown in Fig. 3-25. In general the lymphatic vessels on the face drain inferiorly and laterally. The major nodes of the face include the buccal, mandibular, and parotid nodes. The buccal nodes are located over the buccinator muscle, whereas the mandibular nodes overlie the anterior surface of the mandible. The parotid nodes are in the superficial parotid fascia, as well as deep within the substance of the gland itself. A few preauricular nodes anterior to the tragus are more properly classified as superficial parotid nodes.

The lymphatics of the scalp also drain inferiorly. The posterior auricular lymph nodes are situated over the mastoid process just above the insertion of the sternocleidomastoid muscle. Two or three small nodes, the occipital lymph nodes, lie in the posterior scalp at the apex of the posterior triangle between the insertions of the trapezius and sternocleidomastoid muscles.

The lymph nodes in the head and neck eventually all drain into a terminal series of lymph nodes known as the deep cervical group. This series of nodes lies deep to the sternocleidomastoid muscle and is associated with the internal jugular vein. These are somewhat artificially divided into two groups, a superior and an inferior group. Occasionally, when enlarged, a few of the superior deep group may be felt

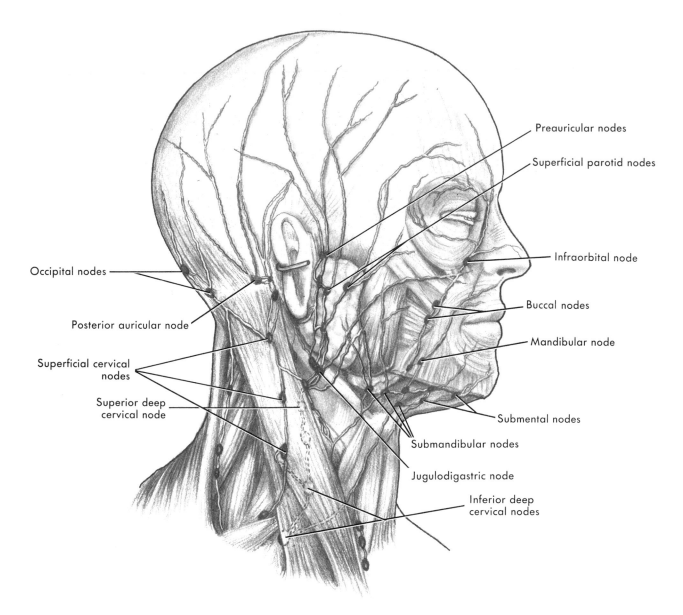

Fig. 3-25. Lymphatic drainage of head and neck.

along the anterosuperior border of the sternocleidomastoid muscle. In addition, a few of the inferior deep cervical lymph nodes extend posteriorly to this muscle. These are the transverse cervical lymph nodes.[3]

The more superficial lymph nodes in the neck include the submental nodes, submandibular nodes, and superficial cervical nodes. The submental nodes are located just under the anterior border of the chin medial to the mandible. The submandibular nodes are in close proximity to the submandibular glands and intimately associated with their fascia. The superficial cervical nodes are associated with the external jugular vein as it courses over the surface of the sternocleidomastoid muscle.

The lymphatic drainage from the forehead, in general, empties into the superficial parotid nodes as does that from the eyelids. Drainage from the nodes in the medial canthal area courses through the buccal and mandibular nodes. Lymphatics from the lower lip drain into the submental nodes underneath the chin or into the submandibular nodes via the mandibular nodes. The submental and submandibular nodes then drain commonly into the superior or inferior deep cervical nodes anterior or deep to the sternocleidomastoid muscle. Besides drawing into the submandibular nodes, the submental lymph nodes may drain directly into the lower deep cervical group.

The lymph vessels from the parietal and temporal scalp pass in front of and behind the ear and drain into either the superficial parotid nodes or the posteriorauricular lymph

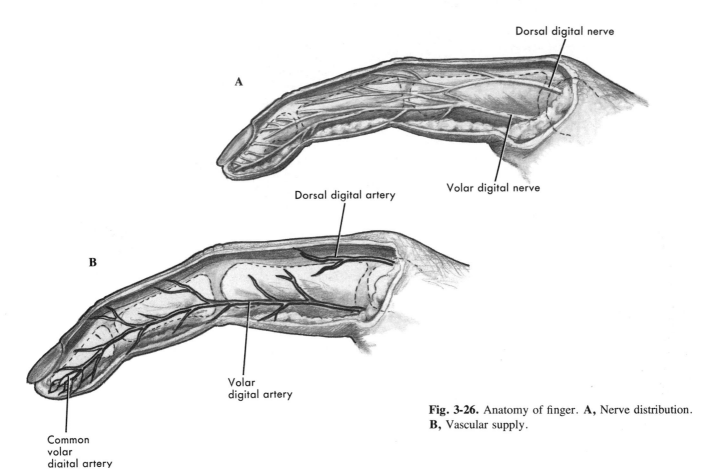

Dorsal digital nerve

A

Dorsal digital artery

Volar digital nerve

B

Volar digital nerve

Fig. 3-26. Anatomy of finger. **A,** Nerve distribution. **B,** Vascular supply.

Volar
digital artery

Common
volar
diaital artery

nodes and then into the superficial cervical nodes or superior deep cervical nodes. Drainage from the occipital region goes into the occipital nodes and then into the superficial cervical nodes.[22] In addition, the occipital nodes may have a connection along the posterior border of the sternocleido-mastoid muscle to reach the inferior deep cervical nodes.[28]

In summary, the nodes from the posterior head generally drain to the superficial cervical lymph nodes and then to the inferior deep cervical lymph nodes. Lymph drainage in the anterior face flows to the superior deep cervical nodes and then to the inferior deep cervical nodes. The parotid nodes drain to either the superficial cervical nodes or to the superior deep cervical nodes and then to the inferior deep cervical nodes.[22] In addition, this inferior group of cervical nodes receives drainage from the axilla and tracheal nodes. The efferent vessels from the inferior cervical nodes form the jugular trunk. On the left side this joins the thoracic duct, whereas on the right it empties at the junction of the internal jugular and subclavian veins.

Development

An appreciation of embryonic development is important in understanding anatomic relationships and developmental problems. The face forms from a fusion of a number of processes—the nasofrontal process, the maxillary pro-

cess, the mandibular process, and the hyoid arches. This creates planes of fusion in which the subcutaneous fascia is not continuous. The fusion areas include the ear, the side of the nose, and the inner canthal areas. Skin tumors may descend in depth in these areas as they follow the path of least resistance, and therefore excisions for cancers in these areas should be deep and wide.

The bones of the cranium and face develop at completely different times and at different rates. At birth the bones of the face are less developed than those of the cranial vault, being one eighth the size of the latter. In adults the proportion increases to about half.[58] After birth, the cranial vault grows quickly during the first year, but then slowly to the seventh year at which time it has reached adult dimensions. The growth of the face continues into puberty and even later. In old age the skull becomes thinner and the mandible and maxilla decrease in size with absorption of the alveolar ridge.

The timetable of these developmental stages is important for suggesting when extensive procedures should be undertaken. For instance, it may be best to delay an extensive serial resection of a giant nevus sebaceus in the newborn scalp until after 6 or 7 years of age when the cranial bones are set. Absorption of the alveolar ridge changes the relationship of the mental foramen to the edge of the mandible.

This must be taken into account when injecting local anesthetics to block the mental nerve.

ANATOMY OF THE FINGER

The main superficial anatomic structures to be concerned with on the fingers are the arteries and the nerves. The tendons and joint capsules are situated more deeply, except over the ventral creases that closely overlie the tendons. The fingers (Fig. 3-26, *A*) have a dorsal and a ventral (volar) nerve. These are situated on both the ulnar and radial sides of all the fingers.

The finger is supplied by both dorsal and ventral (volar) arteries, each of which has an ulnar and radial branch (Fig. 3-26, *B*). These arteries run longitudinally. The dorsal digital arteries are branches off the dorsal metacarpal artery, which originates in the dorsal carpal arch. It supplies the more proximal portion of the finger. The main arterial supply to the finger is the volar digital arteries in the ventral surface. These are direct branches of the superficial palmar arch and supply the volar surface of the fingers. The volar arteries send branches dorsally to supply the distal dorsal surface of the fingers and in pulp of the finger anastomoses with the artery on the other side. On the thumb, however, there may be a lack of direct bilateral blood supply because of aberrant arterial connections. Therefore one needs to be careful when performing surgery in this area.[46] Longitudinal incisions in the fingers minimize damage to nerves and arteries.

REFERENCES

1. Anderson, J.E.: Grant's atlas of anatomy, Baltimore, 1983, Williams & Wilkins.
2. Andrew, E.J., and Huber, E.: Evolution of facial expression: two accounts. New York, 1972, Arno Press.
3. Asarch, R.G.: A review of the lymphatic drainage of the head and neck: use in evaluation of potential metastases, J. Dermatol. Surg. Oncol. **8**:869, 1982.
4. Baker, D.C.: Facial nerve grafting: a thirty-year retrospective review, Clin. Plast. Surg. **6**(3):343, 1979.
5. Baker, D.C., and Conley, J.: Avoiding facial nerve injuries in rhytidectomy: anatomical variations and pitfalls, Plast. Reconstr. Surg. **64**:781, 1979.
6. Baumel, J.J.: Trigeminal-facial nerve communications: their function in facial muscle innervation and reinnervation, Arch. Otolaryngol. **99**:34, 1974.
7. Bell, C.: Essays on the anatomy of the expression in painting, London, 1806, Longman, Hurst, Rees, and Orme.
8. Blunt, M.J.: The blood supply of the facial nerve, J. Anat. **88**:520, 1954.
9. Bowsher, D.: What should be taught in anatomy? Med. Ed. **10**:132, 1976.
10. Brandenburg, J.H., and Lee, C.Y.S.: The eleventh nerve in radical neck surgery, Laryngoscope **91**:1851, 1981.
11. Bunnell, S.: Suture of the facial nerve within the temporal bone, Surg. Gynecol. Obstet. **45**:7, 1927.
12. Cardoso de Castro, C.: The anatomy of the platysma muscle, Plast. Reconstr. Surg. **66**:680 (1980).
13. Chayen, D., and Nathan H.: Anatomical observations of the subgaleotic fascia of the scalp, Acta Anat. **87**:427, 1974.
14. Clemente, C.D.: Anatomy: a regional atlas of the human body, Philadelphia, 1975, Lea & Febiger.
15. Crumley, R.L.: Interfascicular nerve repair: is it applicable in facial injuries? Arch. Otolaryngol. **106**:313, 1980.
16. Cushing, H.: The sensory distribution of the fifth cranial nerve, Bull. Johns Hopkins Hosp. **15**:213, 1904.
17. Davis, R.A., et al.: Surgical anatomy of the facial nerve and parotid gland based upon a study of 350 cervicofacial halves, Surg. Gynecol. Obstet. **102**:385, 1956.
18. de Castro Correia, P., and Zani, R.: Surgical anatomy of the facial nerve as related to ancillary operations in rhytidoplasty, Plast. Reconstr. Surg. **52**:549, 1973.
19. Dingman, R., and Grabb, W.: Surgical anatomy of the mandibular ramus of the facial nerve based on a dissection of 100 facial halves, Plast. Reconstr. Surg. **29**:266, 1962.
20. Dion, M.C., Jajek, B.W., and Tubin, C.E.: The anatomy of the nose: external support, Arch. Otolaryngol. **104**:145, 1978.
21. Ellenbogen, R.: Pseudo-paralysis of the mandibular branch of the facial nerve after platysmal face-lift operation, Plast. Reconstr. Surg. **63**:364, 1979.
22. Friedman, S.M.: Visual anatomy. I. Head and Neck, New York, 1970, Harper & Row.
23. Furnas, D.W.: Landmarks for the trunk and the temporofacial division of the facial nerve, Br. J. Surg. **52**:694, 1965.
24. Gasser, R.F.: The development of the facial muscles in man, Am. J. Anat. **120**:357, 1967.
25. Gasser, R.F.: The early development of the parotid gland around the facial nerve and its branches in man, Anat. Rec. **167**:63, 1970.
26. Greisen, O.: Aberrant course of the facial nerve, Arch. Otolaryngol. **101**:327, 1975.
27. Helson, H.: The part played by the sympathetic system as an afferent mechanism in the region of the trigeminus, Brain **55**:114, 1932.
28. Hollinshead, W.H.: Anatomy for surgeons: vol. 1, The head and neck, Philadelphia, 1982, Harper & Row.
29. Hunt, J.R.: The sensory field of the facial nerve: a further contribution to the symptomatology of the geniculate ganglion, Brain **38**:418, 1915.
30. Kempe, L.G.: Topical organization of the distal portion of the facial nerve, J. Neurosurg. **52**:671, 1980.
31. Kostrubala, J.G.: Potential anatomical spaces in the face, Am. J. Surg. **68**:28, 1945.
32. Liebman, E.P., et al.: The frontalis nerve in the temporal brow lift, Arch. Otolaryngol. **108**:232, 1982.
33. Lightoller, G.H.S.: Facial muscles: the modiolus and muscles surrounding the rima oris with some remarks about the panniculus adiposus, J. Anat. **60**:1, 1925.
34. Loudon, I.S.: Sir Charles Bell and the anatomy of expression, Brit. Med. J. **285**(6357):1794, 1982.
35. McCormack, L.J., Cauldwell, E.W., and Anson, B.J.: The surgical anatomy of the facial nerve with special reference to the parotid gland, Surg. Gynecol. Obstet. **80**:620, 1945.
36. McVay, C.B.: Anson and McVay surgical anatomy, ed. 2, Philadelphia, 1984, W.B. Saunders Co.

37. Miehlke, A., Stennert, E., and Chilla, R.: New aspects in facial nerve surgery, Clin. Plast. Surg. **6:**451, 1979.

38. Mitz, V., Peyronie, M.: The superficial musculo-aponeurotic system (SMAS) in the parotid and cheek area, Plast. Reconstr. Surg. **58:**80, 1976.

39. Monie, I.W., Cacciatore, A.: The development of the philtrum, Plast. Reconstr. Surg. **30:**313, 1962.

40. Montagna, W., and Parakkal, P.F.: The structure and function of skin, New York, 1974, Academic Press.

41. Nelson, D.W., et al.: Anatomy of the mandibular branches of the facial nerve, Plast. Reconstr. Surg. **64:**479, 1979.

42. Nicolau, P.J.: The orbicularis oris muscle: a functional approach to its repair in the cleft lip, Br. J. Plast. Surg. **36:**141, 1983.

43. Ossoff, R.H., et al.: Lymphatics of the floor of the mouth and neck: anatomical studies related to contralateral drainage pathways, Laryngoscope **91:**1847, 1981.

44. Owsley, J.Q., Jr.: SMAS—plastysma face lift, Plast. Reconstr. Surg. **71:**573, 1983.

45. Ozersky, D., Baek, S., and Biller, H.F.: Percutaneous identification of the temporal branch of the facial nerve, Ann. Plast. Surg. **4:**276, 1980.

46. Parks, B.J., et al.: Medical and surgical importance of the arterial blood supply of the thumb, J. Hand Surg. **3:**383, 1978.

47. Pitanguy, I., Ramos, S.: The frontal branch of the facial nerve, the importance of its variations in face lifting, Plast. Reconstr. Surg. **38:**352, 1966.

48. Rubin, L.R.: The anatomy of a smile, its importance in the treatment of facial paralysis, Plast. Reconstr. Surg. **53:**384, 1974.

49. Sachs, E., and Wilkins, H.: Variations in skin anesthesia following subtotal resection of the posterior root, Arch. Neurol. Psychiatr. **29:**19, 1933.

50. Sage, N.: Palpable cervical lymph nodes, J.A.M.A. **168:**496, 1958.

51. Sinclair, D.: The two anatomies, Lancet **1:**875, 1975.

52. Smith, D.W., et al.: Ear muscles and ear form, Birth Defects **16**(4):299, 1980.

53. Tebo, H.G., Telford, I.R.: An analysis of the variations in position of the mental foramen, Anat. Rec. **107:**61, 1950.

54. Vidic, B.: The anatomy and development of the facial nerve, Ear Nose Throat J. **57:**236, 1978.

55. Vistnes, L.M., et al.: The anatomical basis for common cosmetic anterior neck deformities, Ann. Plast. Surg. **2:**381, 1979.

56. Weaver, C.: Frequency of occurrence of the transversus menti muscle, Plast. Reconstr. Surg. **61:**231, 1978.

57. Wen, C.I.: Ontogeny and phylogeny of the nasal cartilages in primates, Carnegie Contributions to Embryology **22:**109, 1930.

58. Williams, P.L., and Warwick, R.: Gray's anatomy, ed. 36, Philadelphia, 1980, W.B. Saunders Co.

59. Wood-Jones, F., and I-Chuan, W.: The development of the external ear, J. Anat. **68:**525, 1934.

60. Ziarah, H.A., et al.: The surgical anatomy of the cervical distribution of the facial nerve, Br. J. Oral Surg. **19**(3):171, 1981.

4

Microbiologic Considerations in Cutaneous Surgery

Perhaps no facet of the surgical wound is as emotionally discussed by surgeons as infection. It is disheartening for patient and physician to see the success of a surgical procedure reversed by infection. Such infections, besides damaging tissues and interfering with wound healing, are expensive and uncomfortable. Convalescence is prolonged, and the ultimate cosmetic result may be jeopardized.

Equally important but perhaps discussed less is the infection of the surgical team by the patient. Surgical wounds are sources of bacteria, viruses, and fungi. Although this source of infection has been ignored in the past, there is reason for increasing concern and investigation in this area.

Almost 100 years ago, A.T. Cabot remarked that "every surgical operation is an experiment in bacteriology."[45] All wounds are contaminated by bacteria from the time of incision until healing is complete. The questions are how to minimize contamination and how to limit a variety of infection-potentiating factors in the wound and the patient.

The voluminous literature on wound infection and its prevention is heavily biased in favor of history and tradition and based more on conjecture and hypothesis than on fact. Conclusions are all too frequently drawn from experiments on contamination rather than infection and on animals rather than humans.

This chapter explores the basis of current surgical thought regarding wound infection and traces its evolution. Many questions regarding wound infection may never be answered and may remain forever philosophic. Other questions can be answered, although the facts are deeply buried in the medical literature. Only with a firm historical foundation can cutaneous surgeons understand the basis for current surgical techniques. It is hoped that this background will minimize infection and ensure the best possible functional and cosmetic results for the patient.

HISTORY

Wangensteen recently reviewed the advances of surgical cleanliness and concluded that "since the beginning of the twentieth century, there have been essentially no original surgical innovations to protect the patient during operation."[296] Although this statement may seem somewhat extreme, we shall see that many so-called innovations are without foundation and lacking in scientific merit. Wound infection rates, particularly for clean surgical wounds, are currently about the same as they were almost 80 years ago.

An exploration of the past, particularly the recent past, helps illuminate present problems and questions. The problems confronting our predecessors in surgery are similar to the problems we see daily. This is especially true regarding wound infection.

Physicians have always concerned themselves with cleanliness and somehow sensed that purification was good. In the Bible there are references to pouring wine on wounds, and even in Homer[146] we find mention of sulfur being used to purify rooms.

. . . Odysseus spoke to the dear nursemaid Eurycleia: "Bring sulfur, madame, that cleanses pollution and bring me fire, so that I will be able to fumigate the great hall. . . ."

However, it was not until the 1840s Ignaz Semmelweis in Europe in and Oliver Wendell Holmes in the United States advocated the washing of hands that progress in wound infections was made. Although there was bitter resentment in the medical establishment, Semmelweis lowered the incidence of childbed fever from 8.3% to 2.3%. Interestingly, even such a simple infection control measure as hand washing is still not uniformly practiced by many physicians. This is explored in greater detail later. It is also interesting to note that this "advance" in surgery predated by decades the

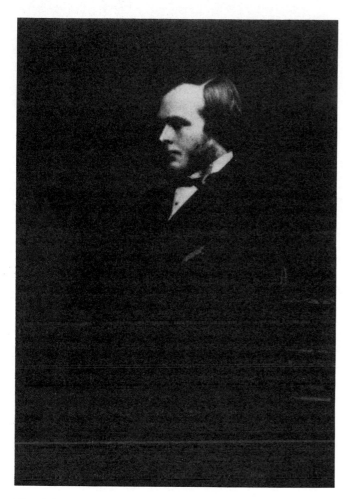

Fig. 4-1. Joseph Lister. (From The Collected Papers of Joseph Baron Lister, Oxford 1909, Clarendon Press. Courtesy of The Classics of Medicine Library.)

establishment of bacteria as the source of wound infection and suppuration.

In 1867 Joseph Lister recognized the importance of Pasteur's research, which suggested that minute organisms floating in the atmosphere caused destruction of exposed protein (Fig. 4-1). Lister reasoned that perhaps decomposition of exposed tissue could be prevented by applying some substance capable of killing the floating particles and protecting the wounds. Initially the substance he chose was carbolic acid (phenol) because it did such a good job cleaning up the sewage in the town of Carlisle.[181] Not only was the carbolic acid used directly on wounds, but it was also used as a aerosol in an attempt to destroy the microbes floating in the air around wounds or surgical incisions. This was the beginning of chemical antisepsis. This term means a method of combating bacteria or other living organisms. Antisepsis (also known as listerism) implies the existence, already present, of microbes in the area in which they are to be destroyed by the antiseptic.

The results of using carbolic acid compresses were dramatic, reducing the incidence of hospital suppuration, gangrene, and erysipelas.[182] Interestingly, 12 years previously Nélaton had recognized that alcohol-soaked sponges applied to wounds also decreased the infection rate[6]; that work is now almost forgotten.

With time Lister came to recognize that the "floating particles" in the atmosphere were not in themselves as important as protecting the wound from them was, wherever they could be found. Instead of spraying the atmosphere around the wound with carbolic acid, the emphasis was changed to disinfection of instruments, sponges, and other surgical supplies. Thus began the ritual of surgical asepsis. This term means techniques or procedures that prevent or minimize the introduction of organisms into surgical wounds. The early success of asepsis led the majority of surgeons in the first part of the twentieth century to disregard the airborne route of bacterial contamination. It is still controversial whether reduction of airborne bacteria in the surgical room results in a lower wound infection rate.

Further refinements in aseptic techniques occurred in the 1890s and included steam sterilization, masks, sterile gloves, gowns, and drapes. However, the basis for modern antiseptic and aseptic surgical technique is largely the result of Lister's research and his dogged persistence in popularizing his experience in the face of much resistance.

Another name associated with asepsis is William Halsted, who was a professor of surgery at Johns Hopkins University during the 1890s and early twentieth century. Halsted formed the basic curriculum for surgical residencies in the United States. His insistence on refinement of aseptic technique led to its wide acceptance around the world. For example, one of his proteges, J.C. Bloodgood, reported a series of herniorrhaphies without a single postoperative infection if gloves were worn, compared to an earlier series where wound infection was common without gloves.[29]

Other names connected with early developments in microbiology include Robert Koch and Elie Metchnikoff. Between 1876 and 1881 Koch cultured and isolated many bacteria pathogenic for humans. He is considered the father of bacteriology. In 1883, Metchnikoff described phagocytes and their ability to digest microbes.

Many early studies on wound infection in the United States were carried out by W.H. Welch, affectionately called "Papa Welch," at Johns Hopkins in collaboration with Halsted in the 1890s.[300] Welch recognized the importance of *Staphylococcus aureus* as a major pathogen in wounds and was instrumental in establishing the scientific basis of the aseptic surgical technique. Welch found that the skin had its own unique bacterial flora and that *S. aureus* could be found floating on dust particles in hospital wards.

DEFINITION OF TERMS

Before beginning a discussion of surgical infection, it is necessary to define a few terms.[227]

antisepsis   Technique or measure directed against potentially pathogenic microbes, including degerming the skin before surgery, washing the hands with antiseptics (disinfectants), or using antimicrobial agents on wounds that are assumed to be colonized by microorganisms. Antiseptics are substances applied to living tissue to kill or prevent the growth of microbes.

asepsis   Techniques or measures to prevent the entrance of microbes into wounds. Asepsis includes use of sterile gloves, masks, gowns, drapes, instruments, and the so-called sterile technique.

cleanse   To remove dirt or grease; this term does not necessarily imply removal or killing of microbes, although this might occur secondarily by removal of bacteria-laden organic debris. Cleansing is usually done with soaps that have little if any direct effect on bacteria.

degerm   To reduce the number of microbes. This may be applied to both inanimate and animate objects, although it is perhaps more applicable to animate.

disinfect   To get rid of pathogenic organisms; usually applied to inanimate objects, but may be applied to animate objects as well. A *disinfectant* prevents infection by destruction of pathogenic organisms.

germicide   An agent that destroys microbes and includes bactericides, fungicides, virucides, or amebicides.

sterile technique   Used synonymously with *aseptic technique.* However, no surgical procedure is absolutely sterile, but only relatively so. Therefore this term is a misnomer.

sterilization   To destroy completely all living microbes by chemical or physical means. This applies to both inanimate and animate objects, although it is virtually impossible to sterilize the human skin. Mechanical cleansing of the hands with a disinfectant may degerm the hands, but it is not possible to sterilize them, however vigorously one continues to scrub.

superasepsis   Refers to techniques or measures over and above those routinely employed in surgical rooms to prevent bacterial colonization of wounds. Superasepsis includes special operative rooms with complex ventilation facilities and special ventilated gowns for the operative team.

ultraasepsis   Synonymous with superasepsis.

In reality, most surgical procedures involve a combination of antisepsis (cleansing of the operative site with antiseptics) and asepsis (sterile instruments, sterile sutures, and so on).[60] Some authorities further subdivide asepsis into medical or surgical asepsis. Medical asepsis does not involve sterile gowns for patient or physician and refers to procedures performed outside the rigid constraints of the surgical room. Surgical asepsis refers to asepsis in the surgical room where the greatest attempt possible is made to prevent colonization of wounds by bacteria. However, such distinctions are somewhat arbitrary and confusing.

MICROBIOLOGY OF THE CUTANEOUS SURFACES
Normal flora

Humans are not germ free, but have a normal flora inhabiting the external and internal surfaces of the body. Pasteur hypothesized that this normal flora was essential to life.[187] This flora comprises bacteria, fungi, and protozoa. Normal viral flora probably does not exist in human beings.

Our environment is characterized by the ubiquitous presence of bacteria. Therefore humans live in a balance with a wide variety of microorganisms; some are harmful, but most innocuous. Factors such as immunosuppression upset this balance. The greatest protection against this bacterial environment is an intact epidermal barrier.

Shortly after the discovery and identification of bacteria, it was appreciated that the skin had its own unique bacterial flora.[300] This population of microbes is as follows:

I. Resident flora
  A. Gram-positive bacteria
    1. Aerobes
      a. *Bacillus* spp.*
      b. *Crynebacterium* spp.
        (1) Lipophilic diphtheroids
        (2) *C. minutissimum*
      c. *Micrococcus* spp.
      d. *Staphylococcus epidermidis*†
      e. *Staphylococcus aureus**
    2. Anaerobes
      a. *Propionibacterium acnes* (formerly *Corynebacterium acnes*)
      b. *Peptococcus* spp.*
  B. Gram-negative bacteria
    1. Aerobes
      a. *Acinetobacter calcoaceticus*
        (1) *var. anitratus (Herellea vaginicola)*
        (2) *var. lwoffii (Mima polymorpha)*
      b. *Klebsiella* sp.
      c. *Enterobacter* sp.*
      d. *Proteus* sp.*
  C. Fungi
    1. *Candida* spp.
    2. Dermatophytic spp.
    3. *Pitysporum ovale*
    4. *Pitysporum orbiculare (Malassezia furfur)*
II. Transient flora
  A. Gram-positive bacteria
    1. Aerobes
      a. *Bacillus* spp.
      b. *Staphylococcus aureus*
      c. *Streptococcus* spp.
        (1) β-hemolytic Group A
        (2) *Streptococcus viridans*
    2. Anaerobes
      a. *Clostridium perfringens*
      b. *Peptococcus* spp.
      c. *Peptostreptococcus* spp.

---

*Not present in all individuals.

†*Staphylococcus epidermidis* was formerly included within the *S. albus* group. The latter term is no longer used.

B. Gram-negative bacteria
1. Aerobes
   a. *Escherichia coli*
   b. *Klebsiella* spp.
   c. *Enterobacter* spp. *(Aerobactor)*
   d. *Proteus* spp.
   e. *Pseudomonas* spp.
2. Anaerobes: *Bacteroides fragilis* group
C. Fungi: dermatophytic spp.

This population is customarily divided into *residents* and *transients* (Table 4-1).[185,237] Residents are specific bacteria that include aerobic and anaerobic corynebacteria (especially *Propionibacterium acnes*), aerobic staphylococci, some Gram-negative flora, and fungi. Most residents are nonpathogenic and are anaerobes, which could be predicted by their deeper location, mostly in hair follicles.[207] However, given the right set of circumstances, each member of the resident flora is capable of becoming harmful to the host. These residents are present in all patients at all times and have relatively stable population densities.

The transients, on the other hand, include any organism that comes into contact with the skin. Frequently these are pathogenic and include staphylococci, streptococci, and gram-negative flora. The number and types of transients depend on the cleanliness of the individual and his exposure to sources of contamination. Hospital workers, for example, are frequently contaminated by pathogenic transients.[283] Certain transient bacteria like *S. aureus* may overstay their welcome and change their status, becoming permanent residents.

The difference between *pathogens* and *nonpathogens* is that nonpathogens are bacteria that are saprophytes and that do not normally cause a reaction in the host; pathogens, on the other hand, are organisms that, when allowed to multiply, result in injury and elicit a host response. Some organisms are less likely to produce injury except in large numbers. These less pathogenic bacteria have been termed *amphibionts*.

The residents are microbes that live on the surface of the skin, as well as deeper in the follicles. Complete removal even by mechanical means is difficult, if not impossible. Transients are superficially located, usually on exposed surfaces and loosely attached along with dirt. They are more easily removed by soaps alone. Factors making it difficult for microorganisms to colonize the cutaneous surfaces include epidermal cell turnover with shedding of scales, local immune defenses, and indigenous microbial inhibitors, which are discussed later.

The resident flora forms a relatively stable population size and composition. This size depends on multiplication versus loss because of shedding, washing, or death. The transient organisms are inconstant and usually do not multiply in healthy skin. Their population depends on contact.

TABLE 4-1

Comparison of resident and transient cutaneous flora

	Residents	Transients
Location	Surface, deep	Surface, exposed skin
Attachment	Firm	Loose
Type	Specific bacteria (Table 2-1)	Any microbe
Removal	Difficult	Easy
Population size	Stable	Variable
Population composition	Constant	Inconstant
Pathogenicity	Usually harmless	Acquired by contact

After degerming or thorough washing by mechanical means, the resident population reestablishes itself.

Location of flora

The normal bacterial flora changes in density and composition from one cutaneous location to another; thus it is difficult to generalize. For example, the relatively arid area of the back is sparsely populated compared with the more humid environment of the axilla or groin, which is teeming with bacteria.[9] The creases, cracks, and crevices are also heavily populated compared to the hillocks and elevations.[237] The total number of organisms per square centimeter varies from fewer than 10 to more than 800,000.[101]

The location of the resident flora is both superficial and deep. The deep location is mainly in the hair follicles, as demonstrated by light and electron microscopy[207] (Fig. 4-2). In this location, bacteria, particularly the anaerobes, find an ideal environment for growth and development. It has been estimated that approximately 20% of the bacteria live in inaccessible locations and are unaffected by disinfection scrubs. Bacteria do not appear in sweat glands under normal circumstances.[185]

Modifying effects on flora

The skin is said to have a self-sterilizing capacity against a number of pathogenic bacteria. This occurs in a number of ways. First, the pH of the skin surface is slightly acid (the acid-mantle), which is somewhat protective. Second, a number of fatty acids (produced by breakdown of triglycerides) are secreted by the sebaceous glands and have some antibacterial activity.[243] Third, the normal skin flora exerts a territorial imperative that is hostile to invaders. Certain bacteria of the skin actively inhibit other bacteria, and there is an antagonism between certain species of bacteria.[101] The protection afforded by the resident flora is demonstrated by the effects of antibiotic suppression, which creates an ecologic vacuum that is filled by opportunistic bacteria.[163]

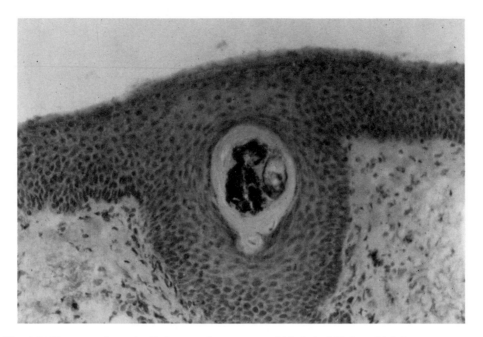

Fig. 4-2. Numerous bacteria (dark amorphous mass) within hair follicle, which is most common location of resident bacterial flora of skin. Stain is toluidine blue. ($\times$ 100.)

Some of the resident flora are capable of producing antibiotic substances. Selwyn estimated that such substances were produced by approximately 23% of the normal cutaneous population.[269] Fourth, invading organisms find it difficult to gain a foothold because of shedding of the stratum corneum and the relatively arid conditions on the exposed skin surfaces.

Moisture tends to promote growth of pathogenic and nonpathogenic bacteria.[241] Occlusion hydrates the skin and alters pH and skin surface lipids. Thus population densities are expected to increase. Aly et al.[10] found that occlusion raised the pH from 4.38 to 7.05 and increased the population density 10,000-fold.

Age also influences the population density of organisms probably because of increased dryness of the skin and a decrease in the sebaceous gland secretion.

Dermatitis promotes the growth of pathogenic organisms as the moisture of the skin is increased. This has been found not only in eczematous conditions but also in dry skin disease, such as psoriasis, as well.[196] These patients are more likely to have staphylococcal wound infection.[167]

Carriage of pathogens

Some normal individuals chronically carry organisms considered to be pathogens. Since these pathogens do not produce an inflammatory reaction in the host, they are considered part of the normal flora in those individuals. The most widely studied of such pathogens is *S. aureus*.

Humans are probably the principal reservoir of staphylococci; thus its elimination from the flora of humans will probably not occur. *S. aureus* is a common cause of subclinical, asymptomatic, or latent infections that may become serious in the young, the elderly, or those with lower-than-normal host resistance. Infection with *S. aureus* is of epidemiologic importance, as it can colonize those susceptible by way of asymptomatic carriers.

Staphylococcus aureus is frequently carried in the nose, although other important sites include the perineum[244] or scalp can be hair.[285] Summers et al. found that 20% of hair carriers were not nasal carriers; they then suggested that *S. aureus* was more common in the hair than in the nose.[285] The importance of this organism in this location is that there appear to be more postoperative wound infections in the hair carriers.

The perineum is another frequently overlooked but important location where *S. aureus* infection is carried and from which it may be disseminated.[138] Ridley[244] cultured 50 male medical students and determined that 48% were *S. aureus* carriers. However, only 26% were nasal carriers only. The other 22% had *S. aureus* in the perineum. Of these, 12% had *S. aureus* in both the nose and perineum, so that if just the nose were cultured, some perineal carriers (about 10%) would be missed. Thus the perineum can be an important source of bacteria from the physician or patient during a surgical procedure.

Other sites where individuals may carry *S. aureus* or other pathogens include the axillae, umbilicus, and exposed skin. Davies et al. remark that in their experience *S. aureus* and gram-negative flora are more frequently isolated from the skin of the elderly than from that of students.[75]

Transmission of pathogens

There are four basic ways by which microbes may be transmitted: contact, airborne, vehicle, or vector route. The *contact route* may be direct, indirect (through inanimate objects, such as instruments), or by droplets. Droplets (usually <100 μm in diameter) travel only 3 feet or less and then settle immediately to the floor. These are infectious when they come into contact with mucous membranes.

The *airborne route* includes microbes on droplet nuclei (about 2 to 10 μm in diameter and defined as residue of evaporated droplets) or dust particles (about 10 to 100 μm in diameter). Droplet nuclei remain suspended for long periods of time and may be inhaled. This is the common means of tuberculosis transmission. *S. aureus* was found to be floating on dust particles on surgical wards as early as 1891.[300] Dust particles settle to the floor.

The vehicle route includes contaminated vehicles, such as food, drugs, or blood. Flies and mosquitoes are important in the vector route, which is usually not common in developed countries, but should be kept in mind.

During or after surgical procedures, the contact route is the most important means of transmission. Organisms may be transmitted to a surgical wound by direct contact from the patient (endogenously) or from some exogenous source. *S. aureus,* for example, contaminates the skin or clothing from carriage sites and may be shed into the environment by cutaneous scales. Nasal carriers frequently contaminate the environment by such circuitous routes rather than by direct droplet spread.[138]

WOUND INFECTION

Surgical wounds may become infected. Should this occur, the cosmetic result can be compromised. An infected surgical wound is also inconvenient and expensive for the patient, requiring extra postoperative care, which prolongs recuperation from surgery. Under unusual circumstances wound infections, such as in decubitus ulcers, can result in bacteremia and death.[39]

Not every surgical wound that is contaminated becomes infected. Indeed, all surgical wounds are colonized (contaminated) by bacteria. Whether infection results depends on a somewhat delicate balance between the host (humans) and the parasite (microbes). Host factors, such as general resistance to infection and local wound resistance, are as important as the quantity and pathogenicity of the contaminating organisms.

Definition of wound infection

Although it would seem that wound infection needs no definition, for statistical purposes and for understanding the voluminous surgical literature on this subject, it is necessary to define what is meant by wound infection. Unfortunately, Celsus' definition (redness, heat, pain, swelling) is insufficient for modern science.

TABLE 4-2

Clinically useful surgical definition of wound infection

	Drainage	Inflamed	Culture
Noninfected	0	0	0
Possibly infected	0 or + (nonpurulent)	+	0 or +
Definitely infected	+ (purulent)	+	0 or +

The most popular surgical definition of an infected wound is any wound that discharges pus, even if the culture is negative or not taken.[70,235,277] *The surgical definition of wound infection is not based on culture.* A positive culture does not necessarily indicate infection, since a wound may be colonized by pathogenic bacteria without being infected. Conversely, obviously infected wounds may not yield pathogens by culture. This latter situation can result from inadequate culture techniques or systemic antibiotics. A wound may be considered possibly infected if it is inflamed with or without a serous discharge. If such a reaction resolves, the wound is considered to have been noninfected. However, should such a wound go on to suppurate, it is classified as infected (Table 4-2).

An exception to this definition is a suture abscess that is not normally considered to represent a wound infection unless the incision is involved. This is because such abscesses are frequently a result of *Staphylococcus epidermidis* and resolve without further treatment with removal of the suture.[300] However, should such abscesses persist beyond 72 hours after suture removal and result in wound drainage, the wound should be considered infected.

The time during which a wound infection may occur (for statistical purposes) has arbitrarily been set at 1-month postoperatively. It is appreciated that rarely infections may be delayed sometimes by months or years, and therefore such time restrictions may result in misleading information.[77] Nevertheless, such definitions need to be understood to appreciate the medical literature and its applicability.

The method of culture of a possibly infected wound is important. A swab culture of a wound surface may detect qualitatively only superficial contaminants, including pathogens. More exact are quantitative measurements of the surface bacteria that measure the level of bacterial growth.

Another perhaps better approach to defining wound infection has been to quantify the level of bacterial contamination within a tissue sample. This approach is predicated on the fact that the mere presence of bacteria in a wound is less important than the quantity of bacterial growth. Generally a wound that contains greater than 10^5 bacteria per gram of tissue is considered to be infected. The practical implications of such a definition are that wounds having this critical number of bacteria cannot be closed side-to-side without becoming purulent, or, if grafted, grafts will not take.[252] Open granulating wounds have a slow rate of healing if infected.[49] This quantitative approach, however, is impractical with sutured wounds that have a purulent exudate from around a suture, since one cannot easily quantitate the number of bacteria. Wound healing without infection depends on successful control of a critical quantitative growth of bacteria and is not the result of preventing the bacterial presence altogether.

Anaerobic cultures require special transport media and should be performed so that air is minimized or eliminated in the collection of the specimen. When an abscess is drained, pus should be withdrawn into an airless syringe. The contents may either be placed into anaerobic media or the syringe may be corked with a rubber stopper to prohibit air from entering it.

Classification of wounds

To enable the calculation of wound infection rates, it is necessary to differentiate wounds that are probably heavily contaminated and more likely to become infected from those that are unlikely to be contaminated heavily. Clean wounds are less likely to become infected than grossly dirty ones.

The American College of Surgeons has established a classification of wounds that is listed in the box on this page. Although many of these wounds obviously do not apply to dermatologic surgery, wounds from all categories can involve the cutaneous surfaces. All operations should be categorized according to this scheme.[234] Such a classification is useful, since it allows valid comparisons of wound infection rates that can be correlated with different techniques, surgeons, or clinical settings.[277]

Most wounds in dermatologic surgery are *clean wounds*. These are elective excisions made under aseptic conditions in which no purulence or inflammation is encountered. If the excision is performed with minor degrees of contamination (as from instruments), the wound is considered *clean-contaminated*. *Contaminated* wounds include traumatic wounds as found in an emergency room or inflamed nonpurulent wounds. When frank pus is found, as in a draining abscess, the wound is classified as *dirty*.

Incidence of wound infection

The surgeon's percentage of infection in clean wounds is an index of his or her entire surgical philosophy and reflects a knowledge of the principles of wound healing, as well as good surgical technique. The first reported incidence of wound infection using aseptic technique in 1899 was 2.3% by Kocher.[171] That low incidence of wound infection has been difficult to improve on even with modern techniques and antibiotics.

CLASSIFICATION OF WOUNDS BASED ON DEGREE OF CONTAMINATION

I. Clean
   A. Refined
      1. Nontraumatic
      2. Elective
      3. Primary closure
      4. No entry into gastrointestinal (GI), respiratory, or genitourinary (GU) tract
      5. No break in technique (performed under aseptic circumstances)
      6. No infection encountered
   B. Other
      1. Not elective
      2. Not closed primarily
      3. Drains used
II. Clean-contaminated
   A. Operations on GI or respiratory tract
   B. Entry into biliary or urinary tract (in absence of infected bile or urine)
   C. Break in technique (minor)
III. Contaminated
   A. Acute inflammation (without pus) encountered
   B. All fresh, traumatic wounds
   C. Spillage from GI tract
   D. Major break in aseptic technique
IV. Dirty
   A. Pus
   B. Perforated viscus
   C. Old or dirty traumatic wounds
   D. Fecal, urinary discharge

Modified from Ad Hoc Committee of the Committee on Trauma, Division of Medical Sciences, National Research Council Report: Ann. Surg. **160**(suppl.):1, 1964 and American College of Surgeons, Committee on Control of Infection in Surgical Infections: Manual on control of infection in surgical patients, Philadelphia, 1984, J.B. Lippincott Co.

Most clean surgical procedures carry an infection rate ranging between 1% and 5%,[1,78,220] although rates as high as 5.9%[172] to 8.1%[139] are reported. The reported incidence of wound infection for removal of superficial tumors of the skin and other procedures performed by plastic surgeons has been reported to be less than 1%.[70,274] Since most procedures on the cutaneous surfaces are elective and can be performed under controlled conditions, infection rates as low as 0.08% have been reported.[92] Infection rates also vary with the clinical setting, perhaps being higher in the office (2.3%)[194] or higher in certain anatomic locations, such as the extremities (1.3%).[197] The infection rate for lacerations sutured in emergency rooms was 1.33% in one series, even though many of these wounds were contaminated.[193]

Surveillance of wound infection

A determination and recording of every wound infection should be made so that precise infection rates can be calculated. Precise knowledge of the clean wound infection rate is helpful in assessing adherence to standards of aseptic technique. Also, because surgical technique influences wound infection rate, it can become a means of assessing the ability of different physicians.[70] This knowledge is otherwise difficult to obtain. Surveillance of infection rates also alerts physicians to the presence of mini-epidemics within clinics or offices and thus leads to their proper investigation and elimination.

Brewer[35] in 1915 and Meleney[201] in 1935 were two of the early champions of careful recording of wound infection rates. Both of these physicians realized that when careful statistics were not kept, the number of infections was grossly underestimated, since impressions can be quite misleading.

It is recommended that one unbiased individual, either physician or nurse, assess all wounds up to 1-month postoperatively for wound infection and keep track of the infection rate.[78,234] This designated individual should know the definitions of surgical wound infection, perform the appropriate cultures, establish and maintain adequate follow-up records, and calculate wound infection rates for the office or clinic as a whole and for the individual physicians.

The work of Brewer[35] is particularly interesting regarding the correlation of clean wound infection rates with the implementation of various aseptic techniques. His careful record keeping and recording of statistics of wound infection helped to establish the value of aseptic technique. As seen in Table 4-3, there was a dramatic decrease in the infection rate from 39% in 1895 to 9% in 1897 due largely to the implementation of a sterilizer. The further fall of infection rates between 1898 and 1914 to under 1% was a result of adherence to aseptic procedure and better operative technique. Brewer gave a prize to the resident on his service who had the lowest number of infections in clean wounds.

The maintenance of careful statistics of clean wound infection rates can help to decrease the infection rates with time.[70,220] Cruse and Foord[70] particularly make a point of announcing the infection rates of all surgeons publicly at their hospital and find that doing so leads to a decrease in infection rates. Physicians, being goal-oriented, are quick to take up the challenge and try to attain better rates by more careful techniques. Certainly residents-in-training should have some knowledge of their clean wound infection rates so that they can more objectively assess their surgical ability.

Another benefit of surveillance of wound infection rate is the knowledge of which organisms are causing infection.

TABLE 4-3

Correlation of implementation of aseptic techniques with fall in clean wound infection rate

Year	Infection rate (%)	Change
1895	39	—
1897	9	Sterilizer used; new operating rooms
1898	7	Rubber gloves used; disinfection of patient
1900	3.2	Refined operative techniques
1912	2.4	Refined operative techniques
1913	1.2	Refined operative techniques
1914	0.2	Refined operative techniques

From Brewer, G.E.: J.A.M.A. **64:**1369, 1915.

This allows one to track down the sources of infection and institute measures for prevention. For instance, it was demonstrated that in the 1960s there was a rise in the incidence of gram-negative infections (from 29% to 45.4%) and a fall in staphylococcal infections (from 44.4% to 18.1%) on surgical wards in hospitals.[163] This was ascribed to the vigorous and indiscriminate use of broad-spectrum antibiotics. Only by careful culturing and calculation of infection rates could one obtain such statistical information.

Clean wound infection rates will probably never be zero, but one hopes that some day they will approach what Meleney[201] calls the "irreducible minimum." By this he means that as with many other biologic phenomena, such a sterilization, it is impossible to reduce the number of organisms to zero, and thus some wounds will become infected no matter how careful one may be. However, this should not deter one from trying to be as careful as possible. Individual patients are not statistics, and everything possible within reason should be done to eliminate the likelihood of infection.

EXPERIMENTS IN BACTERIAL CONTAMINATION

The current concepts of wound infection, its cause, potentiating factors, and prevention are based not only on years of clinical experience, but on experimentation in human subjects and animals. An understanding of these experiments helps one to appreciate the use of certain techniques in surgery.

Soon after the discovery of bacteria as the cause of wound infection, investigators turned toward uncovering the types of organisms involved. The initial experiments were on human volunteers or the investigators themselves.

S. aureus was recognized early as the cause of extensive wound suppuration[219] and thus became the organism most

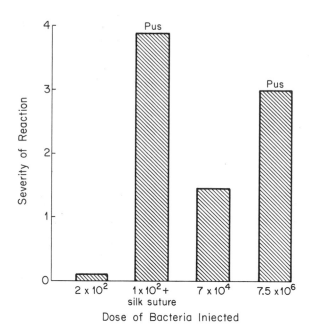

Fig. 4-3. Increasing inoculum size of *S. aureus* is necessary to produce purulent reaction. With silk suture many fewer bacteria are necessary to produce infection. (Data from Elek, S.D.: Ann. N.Y. Acad. Sci. **65**:85, 1956.)

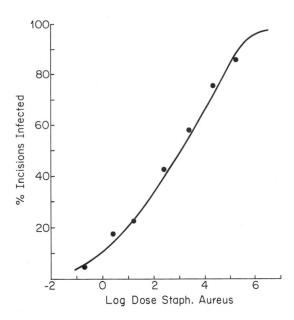

Fig. 4-4. Dose-response curve of increasing infection rate of wounds in guinea pigs by increasing inoculation size of *S. aureus*. (From Morris, P.J.: Arch. Surg. **92**:367, 1966. (Copyright 1966, American Medical Association.)

frequently studied in wounds even to the present time. In 1891 Welch[300] described this bacterium as the most common organism in suppurating surgical wounds. *S. aureus* was also recognized early as a frequent cause of carbuncles, furuncles, and other suppurative cutaneous lesions. In 1885 Garré rubbed *S. aureus* onto the skin of his forearm.[112] This resulted in small pustules around hairs. These pustules soon enlarged and coalesced into a large carbuncle that took 3 weeks to heal. In 1887 Bockhart confirmed Garré's work and showed that *S. aureus* caused impetigo by similar experiments in humans.[31] Bockhart's name subsequently became associated with staphylococcal follicular impetigo (Bockhart's impetigo).

Inoculum size

With the ubiquitous presence of *S. aureus* (even being carried by the patients themselves) and the frequent inoculation of wounds, what is suprising is not that staphylococcal wound infection occurs, but that it does not occur more frequently than reported. The size of the inoculum was discovered to be of importance in this regard. Elek performed the critical experiments by *injection* of human volunteers and calculated that 7.5×10^6 bacteria *(S aureus)* were necessary to produce pus[99] (Fig. 4-3). He called this the "minimum pus-forming dose," but noted that lower numbers of bacteria caused redness and swelling. This latter fact should be kept in mind when reviewing wound infection rates based only on the formation of pus.

Factors other than just the size of the inoculum, how-

ever, have been shown to be important in producing wound infection. Some wounds appear to be more susceptible than others to small inocula of bacteria.[153] Morris et al. inoculated wounds of guinea pigs with increasing numbers of bacteria.[209] Although the rate of wound infections was proportional to the dose of organisms (Fig. 4-4), lower dosages (below 1000 organisms) also caused infection in some wounds. Therefore local wound and individual host resistance factors undoubtedly play a role in the production of wound infection.

A surgical wound is a break in the defense system of the host. Therefore it could be predicted that it would take many fewer bacteria to infect a surgical wound than it would if bacteria were injected into unwounded skin. This was shown by Taylor et al.[289] who found that it took a thousand times fewer bacteria to produce wound suppuration in guinea pigs if the bacteria were inoculated into an open wound than if injected into normal skin.

The inoculum size necessary to induce wound infection may be reduced greatly by means of foreign bodies, such as suture material (Fig. 4-3). Elek found that he could induce a purulent infection in a human with as few as 100 *S. aureus* on a silk suture thread.[99] This represented a 10,000-fold reduction in the number of bacteria necessary to induce infection in the presence of suture. Therefore foreign bodies, for example, devitalized tissue or sutures, appear to affect greatly whether infection will occur by lowering the minimum pus-forming dose.

Another approach to the problem of critical dosage of

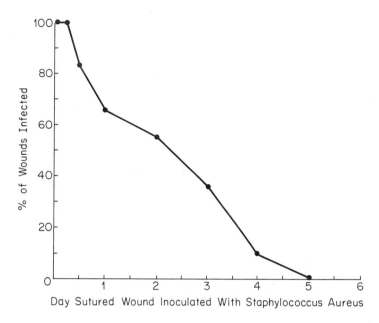

Fig. 4-5. Curve demonstrating susceptibility to infection of sutured wound that is inoculated. Susceptibility depends on time after closure when inoculation occurs. (From DuMortier, J.J.: Surg. Gynecol. Obstet. **56:**762, 1933.)

bacteria has been to analyze quantitatively the number of bacteria in wounds and to correlate this with the development of subsequent wound infections. Krizek, Robson, and co-workers in the late 1960s determined through both animal and human investigations that the critical number of bacteria in a wound was 10^5 organisms *per gram of tissue*.[175,252] When wounds had more than this number, they suppurated if closed secondarily or grafted. For example, with lacerations in an emergency room that are examined for the number of bacteria, it has been found that wounds less than 1½ hours old do not have more than 10^5 bacteria/g tissue. If these wounds are sutured, all heal without any signs of infection. However, of wounds that are more than 3 hours old, 20% have more than 10^5 bacteria/g tissue. If these latter wounds with excessive numbers of bacteria are sutured 50% go on to become infected, causing delayed wound healing.[87] Presumably this extra time before treatment gives the bacteria in the initial inoculum time to proliferate. It should be emphasized that the critical number of 10^5 organisms/g tissue applies mainly to *S. aureus*. Streptococcus may be clinically significant at lower levels.

Time of inoculation

Wounds become progressively more difficult to infect experimentally with time. This fact was appreciated almost a century ago as physicians recognized that open granulating wounds were more difficult to infect.[28] Thus if infection is to gain a foothold easily it must do so before granulation.

There is a surgical axiom that "open wounds are safe wounds." This dogma does have some basis in fact.

Halley and co-workers studied 11- to 16-day-old granulating rabbit wounds that were inoculated with a number of different organisms.[134] They found that although such wounds acted as barriers to bacterial dissemination in general, degree of shielding depends on the type of infecting bacteria. For example, streptococci were prevented from dissemination by granulation tissue. Staphylococci also were prevented from dissemination but survived on the granulation tissue, although not for any great length of time. Some organisms on the other hand, like the fowl cholera bacillus *(Pasteurella multocida)* were able to pass through the granulation tissue and cause the death of the animals. It was thus concluded that granulating wounds offered some local mechanism that limited infection and generally prevented invasion by bacteria. But because there was a difference in the behavior of granulation tissue in the rabbit to different kinds of pathogens, one finds that it is difficult to make generalizations.

In 1933 DuMortier[88] studied the effects of inoculating bacteria *(S. aureus)* onto wounds that had been previously sutured in guinea pigs. He found that after 6 hours until the fifth day after inoculation the rate of infection steadily decreased (Fig. 4-5). After the fifth day, the resistance of the sutured wound to infection was comparable to that of intact tissue. This study has been the object of criticism by others because the size of the bacterial inoculum was not calculated.[2] Nevertheless, the general principles dis-

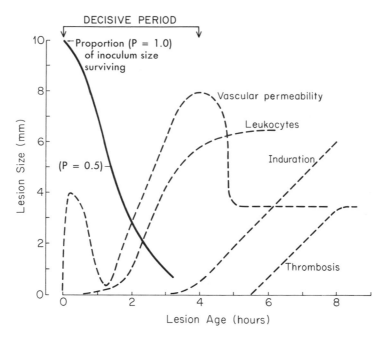

Fig. 4-6. Relationship of "decisive period" of defense against infection to events in wound healing. Ordinate represents lesion size judged by induration or necrosis (thrombosis). No ordinates are given for leukocytosis or vascular permeability. The curve representing portion of inoculum size surviving is the ratio of the inoculum size surviving to the inoculum size applied to the tissue. (Modified from Miles, A.A.: Ann. N.Y. Acad. Sci. **66:**356, 1956.)

covered in that study have been confirmed by others.[2,206]

The sequence of inflammatory events that occurs in a wound after inoculation of bacteria was studied in the guinea pig by Miles.[206] He defined what is known as the decisive period. During this period, which he found to be about 3 hours after a wound was created, the animals were most susceptible to development of infection with survival of bacteria. If inoculation occurred *after* that period of time, infection was less likely.

The relationship of the decisive period to events that occur during inflammation are shown in Fig. 4-6. As one can see when the inflammatory events, such as vascular permeability and diapedesis of leukocytes, are minimal, bacteria are more likely to gain a foothold. During this period of time, a greater number of colonizing bacteria survive. Note that the initial increase in vascular permeability is soon followed by a decrease in permeability that slowly increases with time. During this time other factors, such as shock or epinephrine, that further compromise the decreased vascular permeability have been shown to potentiate wound infection.[102,206]

Factors enhancing infection

Besides the size of the inoculum, the type of bacterium, and the time of infection, other factors experimentally determine whether clinical wound infection will take place. These factors are related to host resistance and wound resis-

tance. Although many of these variables have been studied and are discussed elsewhere, a few are discussed here.

The effect of foreign material, such as suture, has already been mentioned as potentiating infection by decreasing the inoculum size.[99] Other foreign material, such as drains[190] or glove powder[157] and devitalized tissue that is produced by the electrocoagulation apparatus,[189] can also lead to an increase in infection rate.

Local decrease in vascular supply has been shown to promote wound infection. Miles injected *S. aureus* into guinea pig wounds and showed that infection was enhanced by epinephrine and by shocking the animals.[206]

Period of antibiotic activity

Antibiotics treat wound infections and aid in their resolution. But how soon before or after inoculation must they be given to prevent infection from occurring? Most investigators have concluded that to prevent or modify clinical infection antibiotics must be given within 2 to 3 hours after inoculation.[2,42,206] This concept was effectively shown by Burke in 1961 in experiments with *S. aureus* in guinea pigs.[42] Since that time "Burke's law" has been widely quoted; it states that antibiotics give maximal suppression of infection if given before bacteria colonize tissue. This concept is shown in Fig. 4-7. Note that at 3 hours, the antibiotic used had little effect on prevention of clinical infection. Therefore antibiotic therapy should be instituted before the

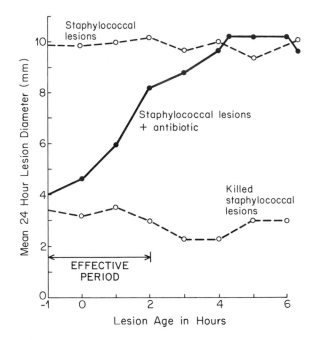

Fig. 4-7. Decreasing effect of penicillin in preventing clinical infection (induration) with age of inoculated wound. (Modified from Burke, J.F.: Surgery **50:**161, 1961.)

time of surgery in situations in which there is a high likelihood of bacterial inoculation.

It should be noted that most of the experiments performed to define the period of antibiotic activity following wound inoculation have used *S. aureus* and penicillin. Experiments with other antibiotics, for instance, streptomycin, indicate a longer period, up to 5 hours, when the antibiotic may prevent *S. aureus* infection.[206]

As Miles pointed out, it is interesting to note that the decisive period of efficacy of antibiotics coincides with the decisive period of defense.[206] This may be a result of the increased vascular permeability initially that allows antibiotics to enter the wound and ends with the sealing off of the wound by vascular thrombosis.

Effect of infection on wound healing

Any physician who has taken care of infected sutured wounds knows that wound healing is prolonged. If such wounds are tested early, they are weaker and have less collagen than noninfected wounds of the same age.[281] Infection in granulating wounds also prolongs the time of wound healing as shown by Carrel and Hartmann[49] and Marks et al.[195]

Paradoxically, any wounds infected with *S. aureus* have a greater ultimate tensile strength than noninfected wounds.[127,160] This acceleration of gain in wound strength may be related to the prolonged inflammatory response induced by the infection. Although the initial wound strength may not be as great, the ultimate result is a stronger wound.

These results were based on animal experiments. In humans the same result may be true; however, this may be the result of a broader, thicker, and inelastic scar that forms in infected tissue.

USUAL MICROBIAL INFECTIONS

Wound infections subsequent to cutaneous surgery are usually caused by *S. aureus*. More unusual are infections resulting from β-hemolytic streptococcus (Group A). Staphylococcus produces a purulent infection, frequently characterized by an abscess. An abscess is a localized collection of necrotic tissue, white blood cells, and bacteria. Streptococcus, on the other hand, produces a cellulitis. Cellulitis is an erythematous, tender swelling of tissue indicating spread of bacterial infection within tissue planes.

The treatment of an abscess is drainage, since it reduces the bacterial number and pressure within the abscess. Then the body's defense mechanisms will operate more efficiently. Antibiotics may be less effective than drainage in the treatment of abscesses (Fig. 4-8).

Cellulitis, on the other hand, is managed differently: antibiotics are important, as is rest. Muscle exertion tends to spread bacteria, perhaps even into veins or lymphatic vessels.

Appropriate cultures and sensitivities should be performed even for routine infections. Unusual patterns of drug susceptibility may be present, especially for bacteria in teaching hospitals; unusual sensitivity patterns may need to be defined for effective antibiotic therapy.

UNUSUAL MICROBIAL INFECTIONS

Although *S. aureus* undoubtedly is the most frequent cause of suppurative cutaneous wound infections, occasionally unusual infections may occur under seemingly normal circumstances or during periods of decreased host resistance. Such events should keep the physician always alert to the possibility of unusual infections.

Bacteremia

Bacteremia is the invasion of the vascular spaces by bacteria and their subsequent dissemination by means of the blood. This event with cutaneous infection probably occurs more frequently than is commonly appreciated. Bryan et al.[39] reported 104 episodes of bacteremia in 102 patients with decubitus ulcers. Many of these cases had an underlying osteomyelitis, and the bacteremia had an exceedingly high mortality rate (55%). Bacteremia associated with boils has been reported to be as high as 38.5% and to be increased with massage or other manipulation.[242] Such bacteremia may be higher after surgery is performed on infected areas of the face than it is after surgery that is performed elsewhere.[267] Acute glomerulonephritis has been reported from presumed bacteremia that occurred after piercing of the ears.

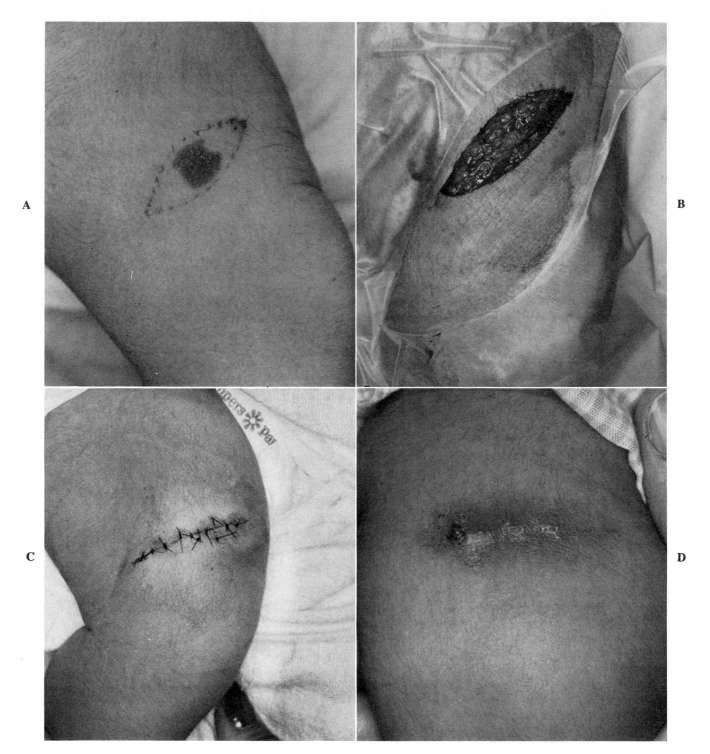

Fig. 4-8. A, Congenital cell nevus on leg of newborn infant. **B,** Excision performed under aseptic conditions using sterile technique while infant is still in newborn nursery. **C,** Sutured incision immediately after operation. **D,** Abscessed suture line 4 weeks postoperatively. Despite systemic antibiotics begun 2 weeks postoperatively for wound infection, suture line abscess failed to resolve. Simple drainage at this point resulted in rapid healing. It was thought that patient's young age and inpatient procedure may have contributed to increased likelihood of infection.

Delayed infection

The use of antibiotics may result in delay of expression of infection.[77] Bacteria may persist in wounds for years and for some unknown reason, perhaps a decrease in host resistance, become activated. Delayed infection is also more characteristic of some bacteria of low pathogenicity, such as *S. epidermidis*.

Antibiotic-resistant *Staphylococcus aureus*

With widespread, often indiscriminate use of antibiotics, resistant bacteria tend to emerge. Over the years, *S. aureus* has been particularly successful in this regard. Initially gaining resistance to penicillin, *S. aureus* has shown increasing resistance to erythromycin and most recently to methicillin.[132] This latter resistance is perhaps more frequent in bacteria found in large teaching hospitals where the house staff themselves tend to harbor and disseminate these resistant organisms. Therefore it is wise to obtain a culture and sensitivity to antibiotics before instituting therapy, because of the increasing trend of resistance.

Toxic shock syndrome

Toxic shock syndrome has been reported to occur in association with *S. aureus* wound infections.[34,210] This syndrome is characterized by erythema, peeling palms, fever, and a falling blood pressure, presumably a result of a circulating bacterial toxin. An *S. aureus* wound abscess may not be apparent at the time of the syndrome. Certainly this constellation of symptoms and signs in the postoperative period should suggest an occult abscess associated with the surgical wound.[34]

Coagulase-negative *Staphylococcus epidermidis*

S. epidermidis is usually harmless, but does have pathogenic potential, particularly after insertion of foreign bodies, such as pacemakers. Under these circumstances, its presence in culture should not be discounted as spurious. *S. epidermidis* occurs commonly on the skin, as well as inside the nose, mouth, nasopharynx, and vagina, so that infection, are possible from any of these sources. The potential of subacute bacterial endocarditis is always present from a focus of infection or inoculation with *S. epidermidis*.

Gas gangrene

Gas gangrene has been reported to occur following foot surgery involving bone.[203] Usually the patient is the source of the bacteria (autogenous infection). Typical surgical scrub preparations are inadequate for the removal of clostridial spores. Such infections should be kept in mind on the lower extremities where the vascular supply is poor and seeding from the lower bowel is more likely.

Pseudomonas

Pseudomonas aeruginosa has been termed an *amphibiont* bacterium because it is unlikely to cause disease in the host under normal conditions but is capable of doing so if it reaches a sufficient population level.[174] Such organisms are not particularly pathogenic.[206] However, when colonization has occurred in the right setting, infection has occurred. Amphibionts are opportunistic nonpathogens that kill when they are allowed to become dominant because of an altered bacterial ecology.

Pseudomonas spp. have caused serious infections from contaminated solutions of hexachlorophene (*Pseudomonas pyocyanea*),[12] iodophor (*Pseudomonas aeruginosa*),[226] benzalkonium chloride (*Pseumomonas cepacia*),[111] or aqueous chlorhexidine (*Pseudomonas maltophilia* or *Pseudomonas aeruginosa*).[13,304] Thus almost no antiseptic seems to be immune to this gram-negative organism. Contamination of antiseptics has led to "pseudobacteremias" or false positive blood cultures because of skin preparation with such solutions before obtaining the cultures.[22,69]

Chromobacterium violaceum

Chromobacterium violaceum is a gram-negative organism that produces a violet pigment in culture and is normally a saprophyte in soil or water. It has, however, been reported to have caused chronic abscesses with breast prostheses.[292]

Fungal infection

Candidal growth on wounds is probably more common than previously appreciated[274] (see Plate 1-A). Growth of this fungus may also promote hypergranulation tissue.

Unusual fungal infections may occasionally occur in surgical wounds, particularly in immunocompromised hosts.[63] Rhizopus has been reported to have been associated with wound infections by contamination of Elastoplast used as a dressing.[168]

Mycobacterium

Breast prostheses have also been reported to be associated with *Mycobacterium fortuitum* and *Mycobacterium chelonei* infection.[62] Although such infections are rare, they should always be remembered and cultured for. The mean incubation period for the study's infections was 28 days, longer than for a bacterial suppurative abscess. Although the source of the Mycobacterium infections was unclear, there have been reported cases after venous stripping in which the source of infection was an antiseptic solution.[110]

Legionella pneumophilia

Legionella pneumophilia has been reported to have colonized wounds from a Hubbard tank.[33] These authors point out that povidone-iodine may not be effective at low concentrations against *Legionella* organisms.

UNUSUAL SOURCES OF INFECTIONS

Antiseptic solutions can be a source of *Pseudomonas* organisms.[226,304] Hospital whirlpool tubs can be a source of

Pseudomonas organisms as well, in addition to more exotic organisms, which may colonize wounds *(L. pneumophilia).*[33] Topical solutions prepared in the pharmacy, for example, cocaine, have been reported to be contaminated with *Pseudomonas* organisms if prepared with tap water.[264] Use of such solutions has resulted in infection.

Taplin and Mertz[287] reported flower vases in hospitals to be contaminated by *P. aeruginosa* with antibiotic sensitivities similar to those of the same nearby patients. Skin cream preparations may also harbor bacteria.[225] There are documented cases of septicemia resulting from *Klebsiella pneumoniae* originating from a hand-cream dispenser.[211] Bar soap without added antibacterials frequently is surrounded by sludge in soap receptacles. This sludge may contain gram-negative organisms that may be spread to patients if the soap is used.[159]

CAUSES OF WOUND INFECTION

Every cutaneous surgical procedure breaches the epithelial barrier that invests humans, which then allows the ubiquitous environmental microbes access to tissue and the potential opportunity for survival and multiplication. Usually surgical wound infection is not the result of any single cause, but of a combination of circumstances. Basically the following factors determine the emergence of infection in a surgical wound: operative factors, wound factors, patient factors, and drugs. In the following section each of these is examined separately.

Prevention is the best treatment of wound infection. It is felt by some, with a reasonable amount of scientific evidence, that the best method of preventing wound infections is good operative technique. Good technique is a habit taught during the physician's medical education (medical school, internship, and residency). At the completion of training and with increasing age, surgical habits are difficult to change. Much of surgical ritual is meant to prevent wound infection, but is based on tradition and taboo rather than on objective scientific data.[234] Excellent discussions of the standards applicable to the prevention of surgical wound infection can be found in the *Manual of Control of Infection in Surgical Patients* written by the American College of Surgeons.[11] Furthermore, the Centers for Disease Control (CDC) have recently published *The CDC Guidelines for Prevention of Surgical Wound Infection,* which has been reproduced and discussed in some detail by Polk[234] and Simmons.[276,277] Although many of these guidelines were developed for general surgery, many are applicable to cutaneous surgery and are discussed here. In addition, this chapter attempts to present the applicable objective evidence in favor of these guidelines. Our highly motivated colleagues in either basic science or other surgical subspecialties should not be allowed to set arbitrary standards that deter our own efficiency and have an adverse impact upon our patients.

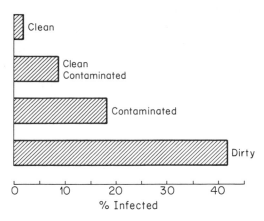

Fig. 4-9. Types of surgical wounds. Increasing percentage of infected wounds correlates with wounds classified as increasingly more contaminated. (Modified from Cruse, P.J.E., and Foord, R.: Surg. Clin. North Am. **80:**29, 1980.)

Operative factors

The evolution of aseptic operative techniques emerged at the beginning of the twentieth century and contributed greatly to the lowering of operative wound infection rates. In 1899 Kocher[171] stressed adherence to sterility, whereas Halsted[136] emphasized good surgical techniques around the same time. Physicians who currently perform surgery should become, as they did in the past, models of adherence to accepted standards and take the lead in instituting preventative measures. Our goal is to achieve the irreducible minimal number of bacteria in every surgical wound. Since all surgical wounds are contaminated,[43] the problem is to minimize the contamination as much as possible.

The type of surgery influences the likelihood of infection. Cutting through purulent tissue may seed organisms. When possible, infections in skin lesions should be brought under control before surgery is performed.

As discussed previously, surgical wounds are categorized into one of four different types: clean, clean-contaminated, contaminated, and dirty. Although most cutaneous surgical wounds resulting from elective procedures are clean, occasionally a surgical procedure must be done on infected lesions, such as cysts, and doing so produces a dirty wound. These wounds have an increased likelihood of becoming infected (Fig. 4-9).

The duration of the surgery can be correlated with the likelihood of subsequent wound infections. This is based on the concept that the longer an incision is open, the more numerous the bacteria are found to be. Sompolinsky et al.[282] estimate that every hour approximately 8000 to 26,500 infected particles fall into a 1 m² sterile field of a major surgical procedure. Although the main colonization of wounds is during the first 2 hours,[43] statistically procedures lasting longer than 2 hours have an increased rate of infection.[1,38,64] Cruse and Foord[70] estimate that for clean surgical

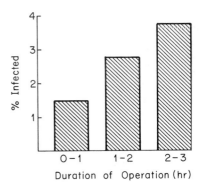

Fig. 4-10. Increasing percentage of infected wounds with greater length of surgery. (Modified from Cruse, P.J.E., and Foord, R.: Surg. Clin. North Am. **80:**29, 1980.)

procedures the infection rate roughly doubles for every hour the surgery lasts (Fig. 4-10).

Wounds that are seen in patients in an emergency room, besides being contaminated, are often open for a considerable period of time before treatment. It has been found that when lacerations were sutured within 4 hours, 5.4% became infected, but when sutured after that period of time 8.5% became infected.[290]

The place of surgery and recuperation have an influence on infection rate. A long preoperative stay in a hospital increases the likelihood of infection.[1,70,140] Although it could be argued that patients requiring longer hospitalization before surgery are more ill and therefore more prone to infection, there is more evidence incriminating the hospital environment as a source of wound contamination. Surgery performed in an outpatient setting has a lower incidence of infection than similar operations performed in the hospital.[216] Patients operated on in the hospital but allowed to recuperate at home also have lower wound infection rates.[297]

It was known in the 1890s that dust in the hospital environment, particularly on surgical wards, carried *S. aureus*.[300] Some authorities have incriminated the "ward staphylococci" as the culprit in the majority of staphylococci infections.[74] These organisms usually arise from and persist in human sources—whether patients or hospital personnel. Surgical wounds are good sources of cross infection, particularly in secluded hospital wards.[41] Inanimate objects, however, are thought to be negligible sources of microorganisms.[191] Some authorities argue that patients are the sources of bacteria for their own wound infections[139]; however, some of these patients may have been colonized in the hospital environment. It seems wise therefore to keep patients out of the hospital before, during, or after surgery. If this is not possible, hospitalization should be shortened as much as is medically safe for the patient.

The surgical room environment is thought by some to be important in minimizing wound infection. However, where newer, more modern surgical rooms were used, the infection rates were not lowered when compared with those from surgery performed in older facilities.[270] The floors in surgical rooms have been emphasized as a source of bacteria and actually used as an index of the environment's infectivity.[295] Patients and physicians continually shed organisms, and these settle to the floor on droplets, droplet nuclei, or dust particles. Particularly high bacterial counts, reaching astronomic proportions, have been found around weighted but movable surgical tables without wheels. These tables are infrequently moved and cleaned under. Unfortunately, these are the types of tables most commonly used in office surgery. Although more attention should be paid to disinfection of the floor in this setting, excessive cleaning of the floor between surgical cases, as practiced in hospital surgical rooms, does not lower the wound infection rate.[297]

The airborne bacteria in surgical rooms are frequently discussed in the medical literature as a cause of wound infection.[58] Lister actually tried to degerm the air over the patient in the surgical room with a carbolic acid spray.[179]

During surgery, bacteria may colonize a wound from several sources (Fig. 4-11). These sources include the patient, the surgical team, casual onlookers, air from corridors adjacent to the surgical room through open doors, and inanimate objects, such as instruments or the floor. In addition, movement during surgery tends to stir the atmosphere and raise the bacteria in the air. As previously mentioned, it has been estimated that every hour the bacterial fallout is approximately 8000 to 26,500 potentially infectious particles that settle into a 1 m² surgical field.[282]

The origins of surgical wound infections have been traced to members of the surgical team carrying *S. aureus* in the nasopharynx,[282] perineum,[138] or infected dermatologic lesions.[186,273] Those carrying *S. aureus* frequently infect their own skin. Some *S. aureus* carriers shed more staphylococci than do others; men appear to be greater dispersers than women.[27]

Bacteria are not merely suspended in air but are attached to cutaneous scales.[76] In humans, a complete layer of skin (one cell layer of stratum corneum) is shed every 1 to 2 days.[259] With viral infections, an increased number of cells are shed from the upper respiratory tract, which probably leads to increased bacterial dispersal. The scales with bacteria that are shed go through cotton gowns, clothing, and masks (or around masks) and make their way into the air. The floor also contains large numbers of bacteria, and the levels found on the floor appear to parallel those in the air.[295]

Some authorities, however, place little importance on the presence of bacteria in the air as a source of wound infection.[83,305] These investigators feel that the patient is the most likely source of bacteria that produce infection or that bacteria may pass directly through glove punctures. Although there is no doubt that these are important sources of

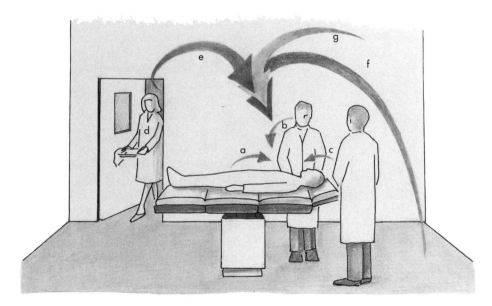

Fig. 4-11. Sources of bacterial contamination of a surgical wound during surgery. *a,* Patient; *b,* physician; *c,* surgical assistants; *d,* casual onlookers; *e,* air from corridors through open doors; *f,* inanimate objects and floor; and *g,* air particles in surgery room.

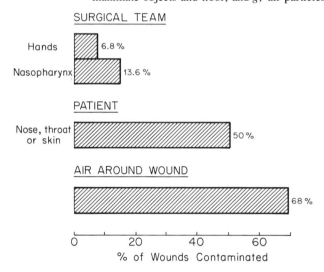

Fig. 4-12. Sources of typable *S. aureus* found in wounds at end of surgical procedures in surgical room. Apparent importance of contamination from air is shown. Only small percentage (8.6%) of all contaminated wounds subsequently become infected. (Modified from Burke, J.F.: Ann. Surg. **158:**898, 1963.)

infection, bacteria in the air are still potentially harmful, particularly to the compromised host. Burke[43] studied *S. aureus* in wounds at the completion of surgical procedures and found that 68% of the time it was the same phage type as that in the air in contact with the wound (Fig. 4-12). However, only a small percentage of these contaminated wounds subsequently became clinically infected.

The number of bacteria in the air in the surgical room is a function of shedding from patients, physicians, and other personnel in the vicinity, as well as removal of this shedding by the ventilation system in the facility. Sophisticated laminar air flow units that quickly carry away bacteria-carrying particles are expensive and have not consistently been shown to lower the clean wound infection rates,[70,169,277] although they may lower the actual bacteriologic counts in the air or on instruments.[248,249] There is some evidence in the literature as to the value of these ventilation systems, particularly in hip replacement surgery or other orthopedic prosthetic surgery.[58]

The best method to minimize the bacteria in the air of surgical facilities is to keep the doors closed and the traffic to a minimum (traffic control).[234,247] The number of persons in the surgical room, particularly the unscrubbed personnel, should be minimal, since they may be the main source of contamination.[43,247] Individuals in motion contribute the largest share of pathogenic bacteria to the environment. The use of tightly woven or disposable gowns also reduces the shedding of bacteria into the air.

One method used successfully to reduce the bacteria in the surgical room that was demonstrated to decrease the infection rate was the use of ultraviolet lights.[1,36,277] However, this method has not met with full acceptance and has not been well studied.

Patient preparation. The manner in which patients are prepared for surgery can eliminate potential sources of bacterial contamination. Important factors include hair removal near the operative site, preoperative bathing, gowns worn to surgery by the patient, the preoperative scrubbing of the wound site, and the proper draping of the operative site.

Hair removal, if this must be done, is best accomplished with a depilatory or by clipping. Use of a safety razor tends to nick the skin and produce crevices that provide havens for bacterial proliferation.[137] Wound infection rates have been demonstrated to be higher with shaving than with either a depilatory or merely clipping the hair.[3,70,220,238,271] Although this has been known for over 20 years, its acceptance has been slow. In one study the infection rate was much higher (20%) if shaving was done 24 hours preoperatively compared with immediately before surgery (3.1%).[271] Clipped hair, although not as short as hair removed by a depilatory or shaver, has been shown not to increase the infection rate with clean wounds.[17] Although hair can be a source of *S. aureus,* not shaving or clipping the hair results in the lowest wound infection rates.[70]

Preoperative bathing, particularly with an antibacterial soap, has had its proponents.[70] However, there is evidence that bathing does not help prevent postoperative infections in clean wounds.[15] Some cutaneous surgeons recommend a shampoo before a hair transplant. Whether doing this actually decreases the wound infection rate is questionable. Certainly prolonged use of antibacterial soaps reduces the gram-positive organisms, but in their place allows colonization by gram-negative organisms, especially *Pseudomonas* organisms, that are capable of invasion.[98] In addition, it has been shown that bathing immediately before surgery actually increased dissemination of *S. aureus,* so if this is done, it is best done the preceding night.[27]

Patient gowning. In outpatient surgery, particularly in office settings, some physicians prefer to have patients in surgical gowns. However, it has been shown that the usual surgical cotton gowns are ineffective barriers to bacteria and do not decrease bacterial shedding any more than street clothes do[27]; therefore street clothes are probably acceptable for most outpatient office surgery. Although paper or closely woven cotton gowns reduce bacterial shedding, during office surgery the patient is not fully draped and therefore shedding can still be expected from the uncovered areas.

Preoperative scrubbing of site. Careful skin preparation of and around the operative site before incision is an essential part of the surgical ritual. The purpose of this procedure is to lower the immediate bacterial level to a level that the natural host resistance will be able to overcome. However, certain basic concepts must be borne in mind. First, many of the bacteria that reside on the skin do so beneath the surface within the follicular apparatus. Although in certain areas, such as the abdomen, pathogens may be infrequent and can be easily removed, scrubbing the skin, no matter how vigorously or for how long, does not sterilize it.[237] Therefore, the weakest link in the sterile field is considered to be the skin. Bacteria that remain after a surgical scrub may colonize an incision and produce wound infection. It has been estimated that approximately 20% of cutaneous bacteria remain inaccessible to disinfection.[268] However, preoperative skin preparation is valuable and should not be abandoned. Davidson et al.[74] found 6% of

patients had *S. aureus* in their skin near the operative site before surgery, but after skin preparation, this pathogen was not cultured.

A second concept regarding surgical skin preparation is that scrubbing is more important than the solution used as a disinfectant.[237] Appropriate scrubbing rids the skin of loosely attached pathogens and, if certain antiseptic agents are used, they continue to exert their effects on the skin during the time of surgery.

An interesting study was performed by Cole in 1964.[65] This investigator cultured the operative sites in 100 patients brought to surgery before and after skin preparation and correlated his results with the subsequent development of wound infection. Fourteen of the 100 patients had positive cultures on the skin for *S. aureus.* After shaving and a 10-minute scrub with hexachlorophene followed by iodophor, seven of these fourteen patients still had positive cultures for *S. aureus.* Four of these seven patients subsequently developed wound infections. Since three of the four patients with infections had had clean procedures, this suggests contamination from the skin.

The current recommendations on preparation of operative sites include a detergent scrub to remove loose dirt followed by an antiseptic solution.[234] A detergent reduces the surface tension between soil and oil on the skin, solubilizes these substances, and facilitates their removal. Antiseptics kill the viable microbes. However, detergents and antiseptics may be toxic to tissues and should be used cautiously on open wounds. The recommended antiseptic solutions include tincture of chlorhexidine, iodophors, and tincture of iodine. Plain soap, alcohol, and hexachlorophene are not currently recommended as antiseptics. There does not appear to be an antiseptic solution that is clearly superior to all others under all circumstances.[64]

The ideal antiseptic would be effective against all resident and transient bacteria and other microbes. Its effect would be sustained throughout the surgical procedure. In addition, the antiseptic would be nontoxic, nonirritating, and nonsensitizing so that it would be capable of being used on any part of the body. Finally, the ideal antiseptic would not be rendered ineffective by blood, serum, soap, or alcohol.

The length of time of scrubbing the skin before surgery has not been correlated with subsequent infection rates, but only with the decrease in the resident flora. Price found that there was a 50% reduction in the bacteria for each 6 minutes of scrubbing.[237]

Almost any antiseptic solution can be contaminated by bacteria capable of causing infection. This has been reported to have occurred with *Pseudomonas* organisms in solutions of hexachlorophene,[12] iodophors,[22,69] chlorhexidine,[13,304] and benzalkonium.[111] Single-use prepackaged swabs help to eliminate the problem. If possible, it may be best not to use multiuse containers of antiseptics.

TABLE 4-4

Antiseptic surgical scrub and skin preparation solutions

Group	Available preparations	Class	Spectrum activity	Onset activity	Sustained activity	Comments
Alcohol	Ethanol (ethyl alcohol 40%-70%) Isopropanol (Isopropyl alcohol 70%-100%)	Alcohol	Gram-positive	Fast	None	75% reduction with wipe No killing spores, fungi, viruses
Iodine	Iodine tincture (2% I_2, 2.4% NaI, 50% ethanol) Lugol's solution (5% I_2, 10% KI, aqueous) Iodine topical solution (5% I_2, 2.4% NaI, aqueous)	Halogen	Gram-positive (cidal) Gram-negative	Fast	None	May sensitize patient
Iodophor	Betadine, Isodine (povidone-iodine) applicator (10%), solution (2%) Preptodyne, Septodyne (poloxomer-iodine), scrub (.75% + detergent), solution (1%)	Halogen	Gram-positive (cidal) Gram-negative	Moderate Fast	Yes Up to 1 hour	Absorbed through skin Activity enhanced if not removed after application
Hexachlorophene	pHisoHex (3% hexachlorophene + pHisoDerm)	Phenol	Gram-positive (static)	Slow	Yes (hours)	May be teratogenic Not sporicidal
Chlorhexidine	Hibiclens (4% aqueous chlorhexidine in detergent base) Hibitane (1% tincture of chlorhexidine)	Biguanide	Gram-positive (static) Gram-negative	Fast	Yes (hours)	Low skin absorption, irritates eyes
Benzalkonium chloride	Zephiran (1% benzalkonium chloride)	Cationic Surfactant	Gram-positive (cidal and static) Gram-negative	Slow	No	Frequently contaminated Inactivated by detergents Nonirritating to tissues

The most useful preoperative antiseptic scrub solutions are compared in Table 4-4. There are distinct advantages and disadvantages to all of these antiseptics. It would seem that the selection of which antiseptic to use, given the fact that none are completely effective, should be predicated more on which one has the potential for doing the least harm rather than the most good.

At this time, tincture of chlorhexidine (Hibitane) appears to offer theoretic advantages over the other agents listed, because it has a broad spectrum of activity, is fast acting, and has a good duration of activity.[200,229] In one study in which tincture of chlorhexidine was compared to povidone-iodine with respect to incidence of wound infection in clean wounds, chlorhexidine was superior.[25] Compared with hexachlorophene, there is little skin absorption with chlorhexidine.

Since chlorhexidine may irritate the eyes, another antiseptic should be chosen for surgery in this area, for example, an iodophor. Another disadvantage is that some *Pseudomonas* spp. may develop resistance to it.[239]

The iodophors, povidone (polyvinylpyrrolidone)-iodine and poloxomer-iodine, are commonly used for both preoperative wound preparation and hand scrubbing. Iodine is normally poorly water soluble, but when complexed with a surface active agent it is solubilized to form an iodophor. The iodine in the iodophor is in dynamic equilibrium between the complexed form and the free form. The free iodine governs the antibacterial activity of the iodophor. Free iodine is slowly released from the carrier, which accounts for the prolonged activity of the iodophor solutions. However, complexing iodine to produce an iodophor severely limits the quantity of free iodine available. Early studies that compared Betadine scrub to pHisoHex found Betadine superior in eliminating bacteria on the skin surface[164]; however, other studies showed no difference in surgical infection rate between these two scrub solutions.[301] By comparison, noncomplexed iodine solutions do not have prolonged activity, but are inactivated rapidly during application. Tincture of iodine may provide a rapid bacterial kill, but does not protect the wound against further inevitable contamination.

The reduced amount of free iodine in iodophor solutions also eliminates the adverse properties of free iodine solutions such as staining, irritation, instability, and sensitizing properties (iodine tincture may sensitize up to 15% of patients on whom it is used[164]). Iodophors may act slightly slower, but do provide sustained protection. This prolonged protection is limited, however, to about 1 hour after application and only if the iodophor is not wiped off after application. This is because the free iodine is slowly released over time providing protection. There is no bacteriostatic film produced. In comparison, hexachlorophene and chlorhexidine both produce a bacteriostatic film that results in protection from bacterial growth for hours after application.[224] In addition, blood or serum protein may adversely affect the bacteriostatic activity of iodophors.[37] Repeated use of povidone-iodine over a long period of time has been reported to produce an acquired goiter in neonates as a result of cutaneous absorption.[57] When povidone-iodine scrub (which contains an anionic detergent) was used on broken skin, it produced tissue damage and reduced the wound's ability to resist infection.[254] Polymorphonuclear leukocytes may also be inhibited by povidone-iodine.[307]

Alcohol has been used for many years as a convenient skin disinfectant, particularly before injections. Usually 70% ethyl alcohol (rubbing alcohol, U.S.P.) is used for this purpose, as more concentrated solutions are found to be less efficient antibacterials. With a wipe, ethanol kills approximately 75% of organisms. Davies et al. compared ethanol to tincture of chlorhexidine and povidone-iodine and concluded that for most operations, 70% ethyl alcohol is adequate for preoperative skin preparation.[75] Only during operations lasting longer than 3 hours is chlorhexidine or povidone-iodine useful. Further substantiation for the adequacy of alcohol as a preoperative skin antiseptic was the extensive study performed by Cruse and Foord in 1980.[70] They compared green soap and alcohol to povidone-iodine followed by chlorhexidine and did not note a difference in the surgical wound infection rate. If alcohol is used, it should be carefully wiped off, since it may be ignited by a spark from the electrosurgical apparatus if one is used.

Hexachlorophene (3,4,6-trichlorophenol) is a polychlorinated bisphenol that has a rather interesting history. It was developed initially in 1939 in the United States. Hexachlorophene is bacteriostatic against gram-positive organisms and is characterized by substantivity, which is a tendency to remain on the skin after rinsing. This ability allows it to act as a sustained-release bacteriostatic agent.[198] Not only is the activity of hexachlorophene sustained after a simple exposure, it is also cumulative and persistent, because with repeat applications, a film is produced that penetrates into the deeper layers of the stratum corneum. However, this film may be removed by some soaps or alcohol. In contrast, chlorhexidine also produces a bacteriostatic film that does not need repeat application for its production.[37]

The onset of activity in killing microbes with hexachlorophene is not instantaneous, as it is with tincture of iodine.

After its discovery, hexachlorophene was used routinely in hospitals for handwashing, particularly in newborn nurseries where it was recognized as an effective agent in the control of *S. aureus* infections.[105] It was used widely in surgical rooms and on surgical wards during the 1960s. In a study by Shepherd and Kinmonth in 1959, the addition of a 5-minute hexachlorophene scrub after application of a surgical skin preparation (2% tincture of iodine) caused a fall in wound infection rates following removal of superficial tumors from 3.3% to 0.7%.[24] However, also instituted at the same time were hand dips in chlorhexidine rather than the previously used saline.

The commonly used preparation, pHisoHex, is 3% hexachlorophene with an anionic detergent, pHisoDerm. Like Betadine scrub, pHisoHex has been demonstrated to be toxic to tissues and to increase the likelihood of infection in open wounds.[72,104]

Hexachlorophene does have one major drawback, however: it is absorbed through the skin, even with just handwashing. Butcher et al.[44] showed that hexachlorophene could be detected in the blood of surgical team personnel who scrubbed with it. Subsequently, it was reported from Scandinavia that excessive use of hexachlorophene for handwashing by women hospital personnel who were pregnant led to an unexpectedly high incidence of teratogenic effects in fetuses.[59]

In newborns, hexachlorophene is also absorbed and crosses the blood-brain barrier. Hexachlorophene possesses a relatively high lipid/water partition coefficient that favors skin penetration and retention. This same property also enables this substance to cross the blood-brain barrier, particularly in premature infants. If high enough concentrations are reached, vacuolization of the white matter of the brain may be produced—a condition known as status spongiosis. One of the most bizarre and unfortunate incidents with hexachlorophene occurred in France in the 1970s. There occurred 224 episodes of hexachlorophene poisoning among 204 babies, 36 of whom died. All of the children had a diaper dermatitis to which a talc had been applied. Unfortunately, the manufacturer of the talc had added too much hexachlorophene to the cannisters, producing a powder with 6.3% hexachlorophene. Autopsy on the children revealed status spongiosus. Therefore antiseptics should not be considered innocuous, even though applied to the skin surface, particularly if the skin is broken.

Benzalkonium chloride (Zephiran) belongs to the quaternary ammonium detergents ("quats") and is little used anymore because its solution is more prone to becoming contaminated than are the other antiseptics. However, its degerming activity is comparable to that of liquid soap plus ethyl alcohol and therefore is effective.[164] The single-use towlettes may be useful as these would not be contaminated. Zephiran is not irritating to the mucous membranes and may be useful around the eye.

Wound draping. Like the use of skin degerming agents, draping wounds with various materials is an accepted part of the surgical ritual. This is based on protection of the wound from contamination by nearby organisms during the surgical procedure, and ensures that sutures, instruments, and other materials are not contaminated by the surrounding skin. Drapes are considered an important theoretic factor in preventing bacterial migration and are a logical part of the aseptic technique.

In the past, muslin cotton was acceptable as a drape. However, because the large pore size of this material allowed bacterial passage, bacteria-proof materials, such as tightly woven cotton, paper, or plastic sheets have become commonplace. It should be mentioned that the use of towel clips with any material produces holes that are a possible entry point of bacteria. Because such holes are rarely repaired on towels that are reused, the towels' effectivity in reducing bacterial contamination is lessened.

In 1952 Beck and Colette were the first to point out the "wicking effect" of wet drapes.[19] A dry cloth drape loses its property as an aseptic barrier when it becomes wet, since bacteria is drawn through a wet cloth. Actually bacteria could travel in both directions.

Drapes can be categorized as woven or nonwoven. The woven drapes are either muslin (linen cotton with 140 threads/in^2) or pima cotton (270 threads/in^2). This latter material may be treated with Quarpel to ensure water proofing. Treated pima cotton is impermeable to moist bacteria, but only up to 75 to 100 washings. Ordinary muslin is readily permeable to bacteria.

There are several types of nonwoven disposable drapes available. Some of these are made from polyester and wood pulp fibers, whereas others are made from plastic drapes. All offer the theoretic advantage of being impermeable to bacteria. In addition, they are less expensive, more water repellent, and do not shed lint into the wound. A further advantage of synthetic drapes is that they are treated with fire-retardant chemicals so that they meet the current National Fire Protection Association standards. Despite this, fires have occurred with these materials and resulted in second- and third-degree burns for the patient.[115,222] This may occur because a flammable substance, such as alcohol on the drape is ignited by a spark from the electrocogulation apparatus, or the spark may ignite the drape directly.

The newer nonwoven drapes have been compared to more conventional woven drapes and have been found to have lowered the incidence of wound infection where used. Moylan et al. reported a decrease in wound infection rate with spun-bonded olefin (Tyvek), compared with cotton, drapes and gowns.[214] Baldwin et al. also showed a reduction in infection rates for all surgery from 1.11% to 0.43% using Basic Fabric Sontara by Dupont.[16] This fabric is 40%

polyester and 60% wood pulp. However, these studies can be criticized because they do not differentiate between drapes and gowns, with the latter being used at the same time as the drapes. The impervious gowns may have contributed more to the drop in infection rate.

Ha'eri and Wiley studied the migration of radioactively tagged particles through drapes at the time of surgery.[131] The particles used were roughly the same size as most particles that carry bacteria in surgical rooms. They found that these particles did not move through nonwoven drapes, but did through conventionally woven fabrics. Both wetting the woven fabrics and prolonging the surgery increased the penetration of the woven draping materials. This study suggests that nonwoven materials offer good protection against bacterial migration. Ha'eri also repeated his study with plastic adhesive drapes and found no tagged particles in the surgical wounds.[130]

The question remains, however, as to whether the use of newer adhesive plastic drapes, even right up to the wound margin, actually decreases the number of bacteria in a wound. Lilley et al.[180] and Raahave[240] found no difference in bacterial counts in wounds whether or not adhesive plastic drapes were used. Additional evidence in favor of the futility of using these drapes is the incidence of wound infections, which did not decrease significantly with their use.[70,156] Although adhesive drapes may prevent bacterial migration into the wound, the overall bacterial count in wounds probably has less to do with this migration than with contamination from other sources during surgery. Skin bacteria usually constitute only a small portion of the background contamination present in a surgical room. Plastic drapes are an unnecessary expense.[70]

Operative clothing. Does wearing surgical gowns instead of street clothing lower the clean wound infection rate? What is the value of surgical scrub suits in preventing dissemination of bacteria?

Clothing, particularly street clothes, may be a source of bacteria. Dust from clothing is more likely to shed *S. aureus* than sneezing is.[86] These staphylococci may remain alive for 1 month when dried in clothing, and routine laundering does not eliminate these pathogenic bacteria.[213] Air contamination is reduced by half if a sterile, loose cotton gown is placed over clothing. If an impermeable nonwoven gown or a tightly woven gown is used instead, the air contamination is reduced further to only one tenth or one twentieth of control levels.[23,86]

Cotton gown scrub suits without an overlying gown are not an effective means to stop dispersal of bacteria during surgery. In fact simply wearing a surgical scrub top with an open neck without an overlying gown may actually disseminate great numbers of bacteria. Interestingly, wearing an overlying cotton gown in addition may cut down on the dispersed bacteria by only one third, because bacteria are smaller than the holes in woven cotton.[302]

Much of the bacterial contamination in surgical rooms is a result of shedding below the waist[27,138]; therefore a gown alone is of limited value. One of the prime carriage locations for *S. aureus* is the perineum, and open ends of trouser legs are particularly good sources of falling scales. In addition, commonly used surgical scrub are not efficient barriers to bacteria. It has been shown that closing the trouser leg openings at the ankles reduces bacterial dissemination, whereas closing the neck or arm openings produces no such reduction.[30]

Use of cotton gowns and scrub suits results in only a modest fall in bacterial air contamination in surgical rooms. Newer disposable gowns do result in further reduction of bacterial counts. However, the evidence is lacking as to whether the use of such gowns actually decreases wound infection rates for clean surgical wounds and for relatively uncomplicated procedures, such as cutaneous skin flaps. Cotton scrub suits may be more comfortable, however and, should soiling occur during surgery, are preferable to street clothes.

Disposable gowns that prohibit bacterial transgressions also help to protect the operating room staff. When gowns become wet, bacteria may be drawn in either direction. The disposable waterproof gowns therefore theoretically protect both patient and physician to some degree.

Handwashing and scrubbing. Although washing and scrubbing the hands is artfully practiced in surgical room environments, simple washing of hands is neglected in outpatient clinics and hospital wards. Hands are an important, if not the most important, means of transport of pathogens from one patient to another.[97,120] If hands are not washed after handling contaminated dressings, pathogens may become part of one's permanent resident flora and become difficult to eradicate.[237] Hands with a dermatitis or damaged by trauma may be more prone to pick up such organisms. The hands are also the means by which nasal carriers of *S. aureus* transfer these bacteria to their own skin.[202] It is recommended that all personnel wash their hands before and after taking care of a surgical wound.

Open wounds should not be touched (no-touch technique). If open wounds must be touched, sterile gloves should be worn.[234,277] One should still wash one's hands before and after taking care of such patients, since the skin immediately around a wound or elsewhere on the patient is possibly colonized by pathogenic organisms.[237]

Routine quick handwashing, even with just tap water and a towel, is sufficient to remove recently acquired bacteria.[283] Some bacteria, such as streptococci or coliforms, appear to be more easily removed than others—for example, staphylococci. Although plain bar soap removes the majority of contaminating organisms from the hands by mechanical means, the use of antiseptics, such as chlorhexidine, may be preferable because of its broad spectrum of degerming activity and relatively fast onset of action.[50]

In 1938 Price performed a series of classic experiments to determine the effectiveness of mechanical cleansing before surgery.[237] He found that scrubbing degermed the hands and arms at a regular logarithmic rate. This rate was constant and did not vary regardless of the size of the original flora. Price calculated the rate of fall of the flora to be one half for each 6 minutes of scrubbing. Also of interest in this study was the fact that scrubbing and the vigor used in brushing were more important determinants in ensuring the fall in the level of bacteria than whether soap was used at all. Rubbing the hands together was far less effective than scrubbing with a brush. Because the fall was logarithmic, Price also showed that it was impossible to sterilize the hands. He ended his study recommending a 7-minute scrub.

Another more recent study done by Gross et al. demonstrated that the routine 5-minute surgical scrub did not reduce the quantity of bacteria underneath fingernails of most persons to low levels.[125] Previous studies had showed decreases in the bacterial population only at various sites other than underneath the nails.

When gloves are put on after scrubbing the hands, the bacterial population rises as the generation time of bacteria is lowered.[237] Cultures done on the inside of gloves of surgical teams have demonstrated *S. aureus* in 27% to 52% of individuals.[43,260] Scrubbing the hands and wearing gloves are not by any means a sure way to eliminate bacteria.

There is a tendency in general surgery to shorten the length of the surgical scrub, partly because of the problem just mentioned. For example, Cruse and Foord[70] decreased the scrub time to 3 minutes without an increase in the wound infection rate. Decreasing the scrub time still further has not been studied, although Dineen suggests that a 1-minute scrub may be adequate.[85] It is also recommended that rings be removed before the surgical scrub.[277] This is because of the fact that the skin underneath the ring is difficult to degerm, and the ring itself may harbor pathogens.

The scrub solutions recommended at this time for preoperative hand scrubs include the iodophors, hexachlorophene, or chlorhexidine.[234] The type of solution used does not affect the infection rate.[70] However, as mentioned previously, routine use of pHisoHex probably should be avoided because of the possibility of teratogenic effects. Chlorhexidine offers the advantages of broad-spectrum activity and forms a film with a sustained activity.[229] Betadine offers similar advantages, but its sustained activity is not as long as with chlorhexidine.

What is the recommendation for minor outpatient surgery? Probably a surgical scrub should be done with an antiseptic solution. The value of the length of the scrub is questionable, but the scrub should probably last for at least 1 minute. Scrubbing with a brush undoubtedly is more efficacious than simple handwashing. Another factor is how many times per day the hands are scrubbed. Each time hands are scrubbed, the bacterial population is lowered further so that at the end of the day it is at a low point. However, the length of the surgeries in between scrubs also affects the bacterial population on the hands; the population levels rise with the increasing length of surgery.

Gloves. Gloves have become an accepted part of surgery, but this was not always the case. Halsted at Johns Hopkins and one of his first residents, Bloodgood, were the first to use rubber gloves routinely in surgery; they confirmed that the gloves helped to lower wound infection rates. In 1899 Bloodgood[29] reported a series of hernia repairs in which no infection occurred when the surgeons wore gloves compared to a previous series of procedures without them in which infection had occurred. However, it was still many years before surgeons fully accepted the use of gloves in surgery. Even today there are physicians who do not wear gloves for minor surgery in outpatient clinics or emergency rooms.[32,280] This is not to be condoned for two reasons— protection of the patient and protection of the physician.

It has been stated that the 11 most common causes of wound infection are the 10 fingers and the nasopharynx.[33] Certainly this is true where the surgical personnel are carriers of pathogens like *S. aureus*. Although the patient may also be a source of pathogens much of the time, Burke[43] identified the hands of physicians, even though gloved, as a source of wound contamination 6.8% of the time and the nasopharynx 13.6% of the time.

The fact that few or no wound infections occur even though hands in gloves have pathogens is evidence demonstrating the effectiveness of gloves.[43] For example, Howe[150] showed that use of gloves did not result in one infection, despite the fact that bacteria could be cultured from them in 82% of operations.

There is some evidence that does support the idea that not wearing gloves does not increase the infection rate for minor procedures. Bodiwala and George studied 418 wounds sutured in an emergency room.[32] Subsequent infection rates were analyzed on the basis of whether gloves were worn during suturing or not. There was no difference in the wound infection rates between these two groups. They emphasized that the gentle handling of tissues contributed to their low infection rates without use of gloves. However, despite this study, wherever personnel or patients are carriers of pathogens, gloves are protective of both patient and physician.

Perforations in gloves may occasionally occur but are not usually associated with an increased wound infection rate. Cruse and Foord[70] found 11.6% of gloves to be punctured at the end of surgical procedures, but not one wound infection occurred in any glove puncture case. Nakazawa et al. showed that puncture holes in gloves are a function of the type of surgery and the length of the procedure.[215] For short ophthalmic surgery, puncture rates of 4% could be expected, but for more prolonged procedures, 9.3% of the

gloves were perforated. Older surgical literature reports glove punctures to be as high as 24%. However, gloves at that time were frequently reused after sterilization.

The presumption that gloves that have holes have lost their barrier function would seem logical and obvious. A finger as it moves in a glove with a hole acts as a piston pumping blood (from the wound) into the glove and bacteria (from the finger) out into the wound. Physicians who were staphylococci carriers have been reported to cause high infection rates through punctured gloves.[83]

One could make the point that physicians who are carriers of pathogens should take extreme precaution in adhering to aseptic and antiseptic technique. However, there is also good evidence that physicians secondarily infected with hand eczema or other dermatologic conditions should not operate or if they do must be rendered as pathogen free as possible (Fig. 4-13). For instance, Shanson et al. report a case of a surgeon who had chronic eczema of the hands who infected many of his patients.[273] After washing with povidone-iodine he continued to infect his patients. It was not until he began routine hexachlorophene washings that infections in his patients stopped.

Glove powder can be a cause of wound granulomas, but this is seldom a problem in superficial cutaneous surgery. However, glove powder has been shown experimentally in rats to increase the likelihood of producing staphylococcal abscesses by a factor of 10.[157] Whether this is important clinically in dermatologic surgery remains to be seen.

Gloves may also be a source of allergic reactions for the wearer. Both contact dermatitis and contact urticaria have been reported to occur.[109] Interestingly, only a very small percentage (less than 10%) of patients allergic to rubber react to latex gloves. In individuals with contact allergy to rubber or latex gloves, hypoallergenic gloves are available; for instance, Elastyren hypoallergenic surgical gloves may be purchased from Allerderm Laboratories, Mill Valley, California.

The concept that gloves protect the physician from possible infection seems obvious. This fact has been recently reemphasized to physicians, as well as dentists, particularly regarding hepatitis B virus (HBV) and acquired immune deficiency syndrome (AIDS).[53,280]

Masks. Someone facetiously remarked once that the reason physicians wear masks in surgery is so that the patient will not recognize them afterward. The necessity of this part of the surgical ritual is currently undergoing reevaluation.

The use of face masks came about during the late 1920s as a result of serious wound infections that were traced to hemolytic streptococcus cultured from the throats of operating room personnel.[202,294] Since none of the infected personnel were wearing masks during the surgery, it was presumed that wearing masks would have prevented the infectious episodes. In addition, it was also noted that at that time the increased incidence of surgical wound infections in

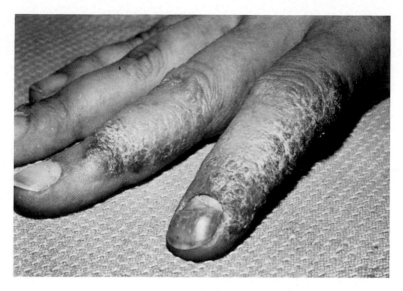

Fig. 4-13. Chronic hand eczema in surgeon frequently is colonized by *S. aureus* and may be source of surgical wound infections despite proper antiseptic washing of hands and wearing sterile gloves.

hospitals correlated with a similar increased incidence of epidemic infections in the community. However, it should be pointed out that these investigations were done in the preantibiotic era, when there was probably a much higher incidence of streptococcal carriers. In 1930 Walker found that 50% of all operating room personnel were carriers of β-hemolytic streptococcus.[294] Undoubtedly this figure is much lower today.

The principal role of face masks is to protect the patient against microbes discharged from the mouth and upper respiratory tract of attendants. Also, face masks may protect the attendants from possible infectious discharges from the patient that could be inhaled. Face masks alter the projectile effect that occurs during talking, breathing, or sneezing and redirects the flow of bacteria out the sides of the masks. However, masks may not be totally effective in this regard unless lined with waterproof material, such as rubber. Bacteria also may be discharged into the atmosphere around the sides of the mask as a result of coughing or sneezing. The natural inclination to turn the head away from the patient when sneezing may thereby actually redirect bacteria right over the wound if a mask is worn. Masks may also present somewhat of a hazard, because by rubbing the skin on the face they may dislodge skin scales that are a known source of *S. aureus*.

It is interesting to note that some surgeons wear a mask over the mouth, but not the nose. Since pathogens mainly reside in the nose rather than the mouth, this does not appear to be logical. However, this is probably predicated on the premise that performing surgery in silence lowers bacterial counts. Whether or not this is true is debatable.

There have been several recent challenges to the value of wearing face masks. For instance, there appears to be no difference in the total number of airborne bacteria in surgical rooms whether face masks are worn or not.[247] For simple suturing in emergency rooms, Caliendo[47] compared the infection rate between 44 lacerations repaired by physicians without face masks with that of 47 repairs in which face masks were worn. Only one wound infection occurred and that was in a laceration sutured while the physician wore a mask.

In 1981 Orr reported that the incidence of wound infection in a hospital surgical room was not altered by discontinuing the use of face masks for a 6-month period of time.[221] He advises that the routine use of face masks be abandoned.

Certainly, use of face masks is the most questionable part of the surgical aseptic ritual. For minor procedures performed in an office or clinic setting, use of face masks is probably unnecessary unless the attendants are pathogen carriers with upper respiratory infections. Under this circumstance there is increased shedding from the mucosa of the nasopharynx and the possibility of increased bacterial contamination. Also, should a physician or dentist be a known carrier of HBV, it is recommended by some that a mask be worn.[73] This is of unproven value, however, in preventing the spread of HBV under such circumstances.

Operative technique. Regardless of what other factors may contribute to surgical wound infection rates, most authorities seem to agree that good surgical technique and judgment are probably the most important factors in preventing infection.[234,277] Although these qualities are well recognized, they are difficult to measure. Cruse and Foord[70] observed that physicians with a "punctilious surgical style" had lower clean wound infection rates. Another study comparing wound infections of lacerations sutured by emergency room physicians found higher infection rates if less experienced medical students did the suturing.[250] Pollock, however, showed that there was no difference in wound infection rates between surgical residents in training and older, more experienced consultant physicians.[235]

The often quoted remark of John Halle summarizes the gentleness of good surgical technique[133]:

> A chirurgien should have three dyvers properties in his person. That is to saie, a harte as the harte of a lyon, his eyes like the eyes of an hawke, and his handes the handes of a woman.

Halsted was the pioneer in stressing good surgical technique, careful control of bleeding, gentle handling of tissues, and minimization of devitalized tissue or foreign material in the wound.[136]

An experiment cited by Dunphy illustrates the value of careful technique. Two parallel incisions were made in experimental animals. In one wound, bleeding points were tied with a mass of catgut, the fascia was closed tightly, and dead space was left in the subcutaneous tissue. In the other incision atraumatic technique was used, bleeding points were tied off with fine suture, and the tissue was closed in layers. Before closure of this carefully closed wound, feces were thrown in. The results were startling. Only 8% of the nontraumatized feces-infected wounds broke down, whereas 50% of the traumatized noninfected wounds suppurated.[90]

The following factors during experimental surgery are associated with increased wound infection rates: devitalized tissue, presence of dead space, hematoma, and poor suture selection and technique. Good control of hemostasis with the least tissue destruction possible minimizes tissue trauma and subsequent problems with bleeding. Devitalized tissue produced by electrosurgery[189] crushed tissue,[199] dried-out wound edges,[279] or strangulation[149] has been shown experimentally to result in wound infection. The presence of dead space also promotes wound infection,[67,81] but attempting to suture dead space with excessive suture or sutures pulled too tight may do more harm than good.[81,106,135,136,300] The formation of hematomas is also thought to promote infection,[173] although this has not been uniformly substantiated.[64,300] Poor suturing techniques include pulling sutures too tight, burying excessive amounts of suture, or making excessive numbers of puncture holes with surgical needles.[48,96] Poor selection of suture includes using suture of greater diameter than necessary[96] or suture more prone to cause infection, such as braided suture.[4,158] These and other facets of good surgical technique are explored in subsequent chapters.

A final comment to this section is the finding of Russel et al. that excessive overtime employment of personnel led to an increase in the surgical wound infection rate.[262] These authors speculated that fatigue coupled with hasty action led to breaks in aseptic technique. When personnel, including physicians, are tired, surgery may become sloppy. When possible, patients should be scheduled to minimize the fatigue factor. Usually morning surgery tends to be performed faster and more carefully because everyone is fresher and (it is hoped) well rested.

Local wound factors

As mentioned previously, by the end of surgery all wounds are colonized by bacteria.[43] However, whether infection occurs or not depends on the level of bacterial contamination in a wound, the local wound defenses, and the general resistance of the patient. Local resistance of the wound is usually more important than the general resistance of the patient. This was demonstrated by Kocher[171] and Halsted,[136] who achieved low wound infection rates with gentle meticulous surgical technique that avoided damage to tissue.

A surgical wound may be viewed as a "locus minoris resistentiae," that is, a site of lesser resistance. Because of this fact, bacteria that colonize a wound do so in a privileged area where the patient's defenses against infection are weakened. Therefore they have a better chance of survival and an opportunity for proliferation.

There are numerous local factors that tend to lower resistance of a wound to infection. These include the location of the wound, the vascularity of the tissue, the local immune response, and the state of the wound with respect to devitalized tissue. These factors, in addition to other factors in the patient, are balanced against the level and type of bacterial contamination to determine the inevitability of infection (Fig. 4-14).

Wound location. Wounds that are located in more highly vascular areas are much less likely to be infected. It was noted in World War II that scalp wounds healed well and were resistant to infection.[14] In emergency rooms where infection rates of lacerations are compared in various parts of the body, wounds of the head and neck consistently heal with lower infection rates than wounds of the lower extremities.[32,154,263] Lacerations on the hands also had high infections rates, but not as high as the lower extremities.[154,263]

Other evidence pointing up the importance of regional differences in susceptibility to infection comes from experiments on human volunteers. Duncan et al. applied a mixture of staphylococci and streptococci to skin that had had stab incisions made with a lancet.[89] The inoculum was then occluded with microporous tape. Different sites were inoculated and the percentage of successful infections calculated. The back was infected in 15% of attempts and the arm in 13%, whereas the leg had more than double these rates, 38%. They speculated that the significantly higher rate of infection induced on the lower extremities was a result of the lower dermal blood flow that perhaps adversely influenced the initiation or continuance of the host's natural

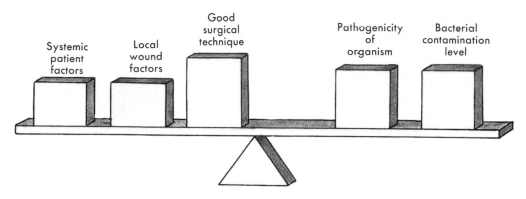

Fig. 4-14. Whether wound infection occurs is determined by surgical technique, local factors and systemic (patient) factors balanced against level and type of bacterial contamination.

defense mechanisms, allowing bacteria to establish themselves.

For the sake of completeness it should be pointed out that in guinea pig experiments, Roettinger et al.[258] did not find regional or tissue differences to make a significant difference with respect to the development of wound infections. Nevertheless, the clinical and experimental human evidence presented above is overwhelming in this regard and therefore the animal evidence is difficult to extrapolate.

Vascular supply. The vascularity of the tissue is partially determined by location, but if wounds are compared in similar locations, other factors influencing vascularity must be considered if differences are found. Irradiation of tissue is known to decrease the vascularity and cause scar tissue to form. Wounds in irradiated tissue are therefore more commonly infected. Occlusive vascular disease also decreases blood supply to wound sites, making infection more likely.

Certain drugs locally injected may influence the local vascular response. Epinephrine, for example, has been shown experimentally to increase wound infection rates in animals probably on the basis of a temporary decrease in vascularity of tissue.[100,206] This substance probably interferes with local removal of bacteria by decreasing the infiltration with inflammatory cells.

The surgery itself may modify blood supply to tissue. For example, a poorly designed skin flap may impede blood supply on the distal part of the flap leading to necrosis and infection.

Increased wound infection rates have also been associated with congestive heart failure and hypotension during surgery.[64] This may be related to poor tissue perfusion.

Oxygenation. The oxygenation of tissue influences the growth of microorganisms[155] and the response of polymorphonuclear leukocytes.[192] Hyperoxygenation is bacteriostatic, and oxygen is necessary for polymorphonuclear leukocytes to kill certain microorganisms effectively.[170] Under conditions of decreased tissue perfusion, because of poor vascularity or low blood oxygen concentration, oxygen supply might theoretically become a factor in wound infection. Hyperbaric oxygenation reputedly helps increase the oxygen content of tissue.

Local immune response. The local defenses against bacterial survival are related to systemic immune response and may also be influenced by the vascularity of the tissue and the level of bacterial contamination.

Devitalized tissue. Devitalized tissue provides a nidus for bacterial proliferation. In addition, once tissue is dead, local inflammatory infiltrates must dispose of it. If the amount of devitalized tissue is great, it provides a greater haven for bacterial growth. Moreover, a large amount of dead tissue may overwhelm the body's mechanism for eliminating it because it is farther removed from the vascular channels. As already discussed, devitalized tissue may be produced by poor operative techniques, such as clamping tissue, strangulation of blood vessels, or excessive electrocoagulation.

Foreign bodies. Foreign bodies may also be a nidus for the production of infection. Soil,[257] suture material,[265] or prostheses are all associated with increased infection rates.

Hematoma. Although many surgeons have a fear of the presence of blood in wounds, there is conflicting evidence that its presence predisposes to wound infection. Welch[300] reported experiments in dogs in which wounds were allowed to fill with blood and were than inoculated with *S. aureus*. These blood-filled wounds did not suppurate. Therefore perhaps when hematomas are associated with infection, it may have more to do with sutures employed to obliterate dead space, which in turn tend to strangulate tissue, than with the blood itself. Thus the tissue vascular supply, which otherwise is able to handle a significant level of microorganisms, is impaired. This supposition was also echoed by Halsted.[135,136]

Other evidence suggests that blood alone enhances bacterial survival. Iron, which is found in red blood cells, is important for sustaining the growth of many bacterial pathogens.[233,298] Injection of *E. coli* and red blood cells subcutaneously in rats led to an increased likelihood of bacteremia than if either *E. coli* or the red blood cells were injected alone.[173]

Dead space. The presence of dead space, like hematomas, also is somewhat controversial. Ferguson found that comparing general surgical wounds closed with layered closures with wounds in which no subcutaneous sutures were used, there was an increase in infection, but a decrease in hematoma formation in wounds with layered closures.[106] This tends to support the suggestions of Halsted[135] and Welch[300] that the increased amount of suture material used in attempting to close dead space actually promotes infection.

In studies on rabbits, de Holl et al. created wounds with dead space and inoculated the wounds with bacteria.[81] Wounds in which the dead space was closed were compared to wounds in which the dead space was not closed. Although the presence of unclosed dead space compared with no dead space resulted in a greater infection rate, closing the dead space did not lower the infection rate and in some instances actually increased it. Therefore it is best to avoid dead space with excision. But when it does occur, probably no great effort should be made to obliterate it totally. Careful and meticulous technique should be emphasized, and one should avoid burying as much suture as possible.

Drains. The use of drains in cutaneous surgery probably should be avoided except to drain purulent material. Drains certainly should not be used as a substitute for careful control of hemostasis or meticulous surgical technique. Although a drain provides a conduit for blood from a wound, it may also become a two-way street allowing bacteria to travel into a wound.[190]

Level of wound contamination. As previously emphasized, all wounds are contaminated by bacteria at the end of surgery.[43] There are several ways in which to limit this contamination during surgery. However, some operations, especially through a purulent field, result in wounds that are dirty and therefore more likely to become infected. The classification of wounds into clean, clean-contaminated, contaminated, and dirty has been discussed. Increased infection rates occur with increasing degrees of contamination.

Wounds that are contaminated may be closed after 2 to 4 days with less likelihood of becoming infected,[94,143] because wounds with time become more resistant to infection.[2] Granulating wounds are particularly resistant to invasion of bacteria.[93]

Dressings. Proper dressings help to protect a wound from bacteria during the critical period of time when it is most acceptible to infection—the first 48 hours. Dressings should be changed when wet, since wet dressings may become conduits for bacteria.[66] After 48 hours, wounds can probably be safely exposed without increasing the infection rate[70]; however, in certain areas prone to infection, such as the extremities, prolonged use of dressings may be essential in decreasing the likelihood of infection.[306] Dressings also influence the rate of wound healing. Dressings are further discussed in Chapter 9.

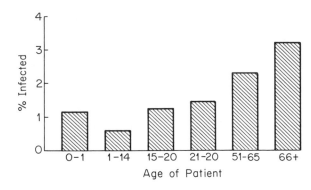

Fig. 4-15. Age factor. Patients who are elderly or very young (less than 1 year) are more likely to have infection of clean surgical wounds than children. (Modified from Cruse, P.J.E., and Foord, R.: Surg. Clin. North Am. **80:**29, 1980.)

Skin grafts could be considered as an ideal type of dressing that covers a wound, closes dead space, and in so doing decreases the number of viable organisms.[93,252] This is true whether the skin graft is an autograft, homograft, or even a xenograft.

Wound care. Many antiseptic solutions are more toxic to white blood cells than they are to bacteria. Although some investigators[229] have shown that scrubbing wounds with detergents or even Dial soap is beneficial, not all detergents are innocuous. Rodeheaver et al.[254] showed that when a povidone-iodine antiseptic or saline solution was used to clean wounds, the infection rates were similar, but if povidone-iodine scrub solution (containing a detergent) was used, wound infection rates actually were increased. Therefore local wound care, particularly on open wounds, may be important in modifying local resistance to infection.

Patient factors

"Every surgeon knows that wounds in some persons do better than in others."[300] This statement by Welch is still as true as it was almost 100 years ago. There are obviously variations in the susceptibility of different people to infections, which under certain circumstances may be more important than any local factors or other factors under the control of the physician.

Age. Age has definitely been demonstrated to influence the probability of a patient developing wound infection.[1,64,70,272] It is a common observation that children older than 1 year of age heal better than adults. In one study,[1] infection rates rose steadily after the age of 24 and in infants less than 1 year of age. Cruse and Foord[70] found that patients who are 66 years old are six times more likely to develop infection compared to patients of 1 to 14 years. Their data are presented in Fig. 4-15. Interestingly, these rates parallel those for susceptibility to staphylococcal disease in general.[167]

There are probably several factors to account for the

susceptibility to wound infection in various age groups. Very young and very old patients have immunologic deficiencies that may result in impaired host response. Also, vascular problems are more common in the elderly, as well as a plethora of other medical ailments as is discussed later (Fig. 4-16).

Obesity. Obesity has been observed in some studies to be associated with an increased rate of wound infection.[1] It is thought that perhaps there is relatively less vascular supply to excessive fat tissue, making it more susceptible to infection should a significant number of bacteria lodge there.

Remote infection. The presence of remote infection is associated with an increased infection rate.[1] Altemeier et al.[7] found, for example, an 18.7% incidence of wound infection if the patients had active infection elsewhere compared with a 6.7% rate if there was no infection elsewhere. The authors speculated that this might be caused by the patient's general increased susceptibility to infection, or a bacteremia, or heavy skin colonization by bacteria. Studies performed on animals confirm the association of remote infection to wound infection.[80]

One often overlooked, remote source of infection is dermatitis. Skin diseases, especially those that are eczematous, as well as even "dry" dermatoses, like psoriasis, may be associated with secondary bacterial colonization by *S. aureus*.[196] Noble[218] has shown that greater than 50% of patients hospitalized for skin disease carried *S. aureus*, whereas only 10% of inpatients without skin disease carried

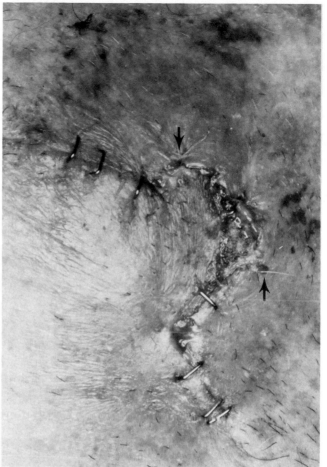

A

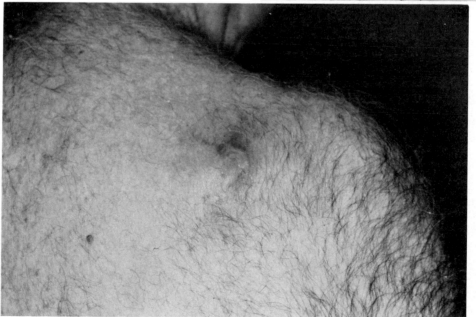

B

Fig. 4-16. A, *S. aureus* infection of skin flap. Note use of Vicryl sutures *(arrows)* as cutaneous wound sutures in addition to staples. It was thought that poor vascular supply of area, patient's advanced age (84), and percutaneous use of braided sutures contributed to development of wound infection here. **B,** Healed surgical wound 6 weeks later. Infection delayed union of wound and made daily dressing changes by a visiting nurse necessary (because of wound's location and patient's old age) during the 6-week healing period.

such pathogens. In patients with eczema, 82% carried *S. aureus* in the nose.[303] Therefore patients with certain skin problems may be more likely to carry pathogens.

Remote trauma. Injury, for example, muscle contusion, some distance from a surgical wound may increase the likelihood of wound infection. This was shown experimentally in rabbits.[68]

Carriers of pathogens. Pathogens, particularly *S. aureus,* are commonly carried in the anterior nares, skin, and hair. Miles[205] found a 22% to 45% carrier rate for *S. aureus* in the nose and a 5% to 24% carrier rate for the skin. These rates were on hospital staff. Patients were found to have even higher carrier rates, approaching 40% to 50%. Since the nose is a site with a higher carriage rate, it is considered to be the primary source of the bacteria. Also, the skin carriage is associated with nasal carriage but not vice versa, so this also implicates the nose as the primary focus for carriage. Persons who harbor *S. aureus* tend to do so chronically.

Carriers of pathogens, especially of *S. aureus,* are more likely to develop postoperative wound infections.[38,91,177,299] However, where the infecting bacteria is *S. aureus,* the phage type causing the wound infection is not usually the same type as that carried by the patient.[74,78] When patients are hospitalized, usually the endemic "ward staphylococci" are found to be the culprit.[74] Most ward infections are exogenous rather than endogenous or autogenous.

Skin carriers of *S. aureus* are even more likely to develop wound infections than nasopharyngeal carriers.[46] Kune et al. found an infection rate of 27.5% for skin carriers compared with 4.8% for nasopharyngeal carriers.[177] The infection rate for noncarriers was 2.3%. Although Dyas et al.[91] emphasized that this usually is not the same phage type, patients who are carriers are perhaps somehow more suceptible to *S. aureus* infection in general.

Severe protein deficiency. Although it seems logical that severe protein deficiency predisposes to an increase in wound infection rates, definitive evidence is lacking.[234] However, protein deficiency may result in poor production of serum antibodies or transferrin, both of which are theoretically associated with greater susceptibility to infection.[298] Short-term (1 day) starvation of guinea pigs did not result in an increased infection rate.[289]

Vitamin C deficiency. Although the incidence of wound infection may not be greater in vitamin-deficient animals, the infections produced experimentally are more severe. In guinea pigs made vitamin-C deficient and inoculated with *S. aureus,* there were more bacteria cultured from abscesses that formed. The necrotic centers of the abscesses were not walled off, and the abscesses were not well defined.[204] It is difficult to know if these effects are the indirect result of poor wound healing that has been caused by vitamin C deficiency or a more direct effect of the lack of vitamin C itself.

Diabetes mellitus. It is a commonly held belief that diabetic patients are more susceptible to infections and poor wound healing. Diabetic patients have been shown to have an increased susceptibility to staphylococcal disease,[167] but larger studies of surgical wound infection rates usually do not find any greater incidence in diabetic patients.[64] Experimentally, Krizek and Davis were unable to show a greater incidence of wound infections in diabetic rats compared with normal rats.[172]

The state of control of the diabetes appears to be crucial to the development of wound infection. Uncontrolled diabetic patients have five times the wound infection rate as controlled diabetic patients. In addition, controlled diabetic patients have the same incidence of infection that nondiabetic patients have.[119,151]

Miscellaneous medical problems. Congestive heart failure and episodes of hypotension have been associated with an increased incidence of wound infection, probably based on poor tissue perfusion.[64] Other medical problems, such as anemia, chronic lung disease, renal failure, systemic cancer, or liver disease, are not shown by themselves to predispose to wound infection.

Immunologic defense. The immunologic defense against microbes is complex and beyond the scope of this chapter. An excellent discussion of this subject has been written by Hohn.[145] However, a few key relevant areas are briefly discussed here.

Antibody defense has been shown to play a role in due to infection *S. aureus.* For example, if mice that are infected with *S. aureus* are given human gamma globulin injections, the infection rate is lessened.[288] Other studies have shown that in rabbits, recovery from *S. aureus*–infected burns is associated with the development of serum antibody titers to staphylococcal hemolysin.[121] Patients who are severely protein depleted (starved) are undoubtedly less able to manufacture serum antibodies and are less able to mount a defense against some organisms.

Generalized anergy has also been correlated with severe wound infection.[188] Lack of cell-mediated immunity can occur in extensive burns and protein malnutrition. Buffone[40] studied patients who developed sepsis, some of whom died on a surgical intensive-care ward. He found that either anergy or relative anergy (reaction to one antigen) was associated with a much increased rate of sepsis and death. Although it is difficult to say whether the surgery or trauma had induced the anergy or whether the patient was unable to mount a sufficient reaction, the bottom-line result was the same.

Specific problems with polymorphonuclear leukocytes (PMNLs) have also been detected in patients developing sepsis after surgery. The patients with a decreased neutrophil chemotaxis are much more likely to develop sepsis and death than patients whose chemotaxis was normal.[40] Chemotactic defects also have been detected in patients who are malnourished or who have infections other than in surgical wounds. This may help to explain why patients with infection elsewhere are more likely to develop infection after surgery.

Foreign bodies, for example, dirt, are known to potentiate wound infection. Haury et al.[141] studied the effect of clay particles found in soil on leukocyte function in vitro. They found that clay particles interacted with leukocytes to impair their capacity to phagocytize and kill *S. aureus*. Clay particles also inactivated natural antibodies.

Drugs

Many, if not most or even all surgical patients take some medication that may directly or indirectly influence the probability of wound infection. It is commonly believed that cytotoxic agents may interfere with wound defense, anticoagulants may promote hematoma formation, and steroids may interfere with wound healing. However, generalizations may not hold true for the individual patient and these effects cannot be considered inevitable. For instance, in a large study of surgical wound infections, patients on steroids were no more likely to become infected than those not on steroids.[64] But the reasons why the patients were on steroids must be taken into account along with doses given and length of treatment. Such parameters were not analyzed. The effects of drugs on infection are difficult to distinguish from the effects of the patient's problem for which he or she is given the drug.

Drug effects are also dose related. In addition, multiple drugs may be given to patients, which interact and result in effects that neither drug alone would produce.

Antibiotics rather than decreasing the likelihood of infection may actually increase it.[7] Tetracycline may increase the likelihood of a patient to be colonized by *S. aureus*.[24] Certain antibiotics may also promote emergence of gram-negative organisms or fungi, such as *C. albicans*. The relationship of antibiotics to wound infection is discussed in the next section.

ANTIBACTERIALS, ANTIBIOTICS, AND INFECTION

With the acceptance of the germ theory of disease, use of various chemicals (antibacterials) topically to rid wounds of bacteria was enthusiastically employed by physicians. However, their use was never scientifically established and compared to other methods of treatment. Because systemic antibiotics were developed, this further obscured the value or possible deleterious effects of antiseptics.

With the discovery of antibiotics, it was hoped that surgical wound infection rates would be diminished and bacterial sepsis eradicated. However, antibiotics brought their own special set of problems and have not been found to be a substitute for good surgical technique.

The indiscriminate use of antibiotics in the early 1950s led to a rise in postoperative infection rates, especially with penicillin-resistant *S. aureus*.[147] However, with more education and judicious use of these drugs, wound infection rates dropped to one half.[148]

The use of an antibiotic, although seemingly eliminating one organism, creates an ecologic void that is quickly filled by other sometimes more deadly organisms. For instance, when broad-spectrum antibiotics were developed, a fall in the gram-positive infection rate concomitantly occurred with a rise in gram-negative infections.[163] As mentioned previously, tetracycline administration, by altering the nasal flora, may be associated with the increased ability of individuals to become nasal carriers of staphylococcus.[97,98]

Since most surgical procedures, especially on the cutaneous surfaces, are clean procedures, the need for antibiotics applied either topically or systemically is unusual. Certainly antibiotics should not be used to cover up poor surgical technique. The physicians should weigh the risk of antibiotic use, which is always underestimated, against the risk of wound infection. Problems, such as superinfection, development of antibiotic-resistant organisms, and patient sensitization, should be kept in mind.

Topical antibacterial agents and wound care

Every wound is undoubtedly contaminated by bacteria, both at the time of surgery and later if left open to heal by granulation, so it seems logical that wounds should be cleansed to rid them of bacteria and that an antibacterial substance would be useful. However, scrubbing itself has been shown to be harmful to wounds,[256] and antibacterial agents are not always innocuous. Fleming, the discoverer of penicillin evaluated many antiseptic agents and concluded that most were more toxic to white blood cells than to bacteria.[108] If used, antibacterial agents should not decrease the body's normal defense mechanisms.

Saline is used as a time-honored method of irrigation of contaminated wounds or as a soak for debriding open wounds. Its value is that it is probably more innocuous than other substances that might be used. However, its ability in ridding wounds of bacteria is doubtful.[72,117] For instance, Rodeheaver et al.[255] found that saline-soaked gauze removed only 0.6% of bacteria from wounds. Scrubbing with saline may further decrease the bacteria in wounds but may lead to a decrease in the wound's ability to resist infection.[256] However, saline removes blood clots and other debris in the gentlest manner possible.

Some chemicals are astringents—that is, they precipitate protein and have mild antiseptic activity when applied topically. Precipitation of protein helps to dry oozing wounds, thereby promoting desiccation that is antithetical to bacterial proliferation. One such agent useful on open wounds is Burrow's solution, which contains about 5% aluminum acetate. This solution, which yields aluminum oxide and acetic acid, is diluted 1:10 to 1:40, depending on how much drying effect is desired. Aluminum subacetate solution contains about 8% aluminum diacetate (which also yields aluminum oxide and acetic acid, but in higher concentrations) and thus is stronger than Burow's solution at equivalent dilutions. Unlike other astringents, such as potassium permanganate, aluminum acetate or subacetate does not stain. A convenient form of aluminum astringent is Domeboro packets or tablets (aluminum sulfate and calcium acetate). One tablet or packet in 1 quart of water yields a 1:80 dilution, but it must be used immediately because evaporation tends to concentrate this solution and make it too irritating to use. Other astringents include Epsom salts (hydrated magnesium sulfate), potassium permanganate, and silver nitrate.

Soaps and detergents are useful in solubilizing debris in wounds and may remove bacteria. However, some soaps may actually increase inflammation and perhaps the incidence of wound infection.[230] Experimentally, scrubbing staphylococcal-contaminated wounds in guinea pigs with pHisoHex or Betadine scrub solutions leads to an increased infection rate, compared to no treatment. This seeming paradox has been ascribed to the detergent in these solutions being toxic to tissue.[72,104] Therefore one should be cautious about using very caustic substances. However, mild soaps or baby shampoos have not in my experience been deleterious to wound healing or promoted infection.

A major reason why most topical methods are not more useful in ridding wounds of bacteria is that these microbes are trapped in the fibrinous wound exudate and are shielded from physical or chemical debriding methods.

In an effort to increase the effectiveness of wound debridement by scrubbing or with antibacterial substances, various so-called wound-debriding agents were developed in the 1970s. These were composed of proteolytic enzymes that chemically help breakdown debris on open wounds and render bacteria more accessible to irrigation. For example, trypsin, which is a debriding agent, increased the removal of bacteria from wounds 16-fold over normal saline.[255]

Proteolytic enzymes also were said to make bacteria more accessible to antibiotics, whether the latter are given topically or systemically. It was felt that in an open wound, bacteria are protected from systemic antibiotics by granulation tissue and that the fibrin layer on the wound also protects organisms from the environment.

Two topical enzymatic debriding agents used to debride ulcerations are Elase and Travase. Elase is a combination of two hydrolytic enzymes, fibrinolysin (derived from bovine plasma) and deoxyribonuclease (from bovine pancreas). The fibrinolysin acts on the fibrin of blood clots, breaking it down so that bacteria are more accessible. The deoxyribonuclease hydrolyzes deoxyribonucleic acid (DNA). Travase contains a proteolytic enzyme made by *Bacillus subtilis*.

Although early experimental work in animals with wound-debriding agents was encouraging, the reality of the situation is that these agents probably have added little to standard methods of wound care.

Antiseptics may be useful on open wounds, particularly if specific bacteria have been cultured from the wounds. For instance, acetic acid is excellent for *Pseudomonas* spp., and silver nitrate has a broad-spectrum activity. Hydrogen peroxide is particularly excellent in debriding wounds and promoting wound healing, probably because it produces effervescence that mechanically cleans the crevices of wounds.[128] Therefore it is valuable in ridding the wound of bacteria. However, large amounts of hydrogen peroxide should not be poured into deep wounds or forced into wounds under pressure. Cases have been reported of oxygen embolisms or local tissue crepitation associated with hydrogen peroxide used in this manner.[279]

The value of topical antibiotics on surgical wounds is a subject of controversy. Their use must be qualified by assessing the type of wound on which they are used, the level of bacterial contamination (usually not known), and the sensitivities of the organisms. It is also difficult to differentiate the antibacterial effects of the base ointment in which many antibiotics are placed from the effects of the antibiotic itself.

Irrigation of potentially contaminated wounds before closure in the emergency room with antibiotic solutions has not lowered the wound infection rate[79]; however, the level of contamination was not taken into account. If inoculum sizes were very large (10^{10} staphylococci), topical antibiotics in such wounds before closure were found to be useful experimentally.[21] In practice such degrees of contamination are unusual in wounds for which closure is contemplated.

On open wounds that are allowed to heal by granulation, if the wound healing is prolonged, use of topical antibiotics may result in the emergence of resistant bacteria or fungi. For instance, *Candida* overgrowth is not infrequent in such situations.

Another problem associated with the use of antibacterials on wounds is sensitization to the antibiotics themselves. Although it is commonly held that Polysporin ointment (polymyxin B sulfate and bacitracin zinc) is less sensitizing than Neosporin ointment (neosporin, bacitracin), I have seen a significant number of allergic reactions to Polysporin ointment. Probably any antibiotic is capable of sensitization. Some of the more common topical antibiotics and antibacterial agents with their antibacterial spectra are as follows:

Bacitracin	*Staphylococcus, Streptococcus*
Gramicidin	*Staphylococcus, Streptococcus*
Neomycin	*Proteus, E. coli*, gram-negative rods except *Pseudomonas*
Polymyxin B	*Pseudomonas, E. Coli*, Gram-negative rods except *Proteus*

Gentamycin (Gara-mycin)	*Staphylococcus, E. coli, Proetus, Pseudomonas,* other gram-negative rods
Mafenide (Sulfa-mylon)	Broad spectrum, but some *Streptococcus, Proteus, E. coli* resistant
Silver sulfadiazine (Silvadene)	Broad spectrum, very effective against *Pseudomonas,* effective against yeasts
Nitrofurazone (Furacin)	Broad spectrum
Silver nitrate .5% aqueous solution	Broad spectrum, but some *Staphylococcus* and gram-negative rods resistant; astringent
Acetic acid 1% to 5% solution	*Pseudomonas*
Potassium permanganate 1:10,000	Broad spectrum, antifungal, astringent

Some topical antibiotic preparations may be valuable in promoting wound healing. In an evaluation of various topical antibiotic preparations used on superficial wounds in pigs, some (Neosporin ointment and Silvadene) were found to increase the epithelialization rate of wounds, whereas one (Furacin) appeared to decrease the rate of epithelialization.[114] These effects appeared to be independent of the antimicrobial effects of the topical antibiotics and were possibly related to the vehicle in which the antibiotic was placed. A more detailed discussion of these topical antibacterial products is found in Chapter 9.

Systemic antibiotics

Physicians performing surgery on the cutaneous surfaces administer systemic antibiotics under two sets of circumstances, either therapeutically or prophylactically. Therapeutic antibiotics imply the presence of infection. Here appropriate cultures should be performed, and the choice of antibiotic should be predicated on the organism involved, its antibiotic sensitivities, and the mechanism of action of the antibiotic. Prophylactic antibiotics, on the other hand, are given before an organism proliferates in tissue and produces an infection. Here the choice of antibiotic is based on a guess as to which microbe would be the most likely to be involved.

The need for obtaining a culture if infection is present or suspected cannot be too greatly emphasized. Sometimes special cultures that require extra effort need to be done, in addition to routine cultures. For instance, if anaerobic infection is suspected, as in hidradenitis suppurativa, anaerobic cultures and sensitivities should be taken. Sometimes it is necessary to culture for fungi or *Mycobacterium* organisms as well.

Based on the organism's sensitivities to various antibiotics, a careful and thoughtful treatment should be instituted. In reality, physicians often must make decisions on

institution of an antibiotic without benefit of culture, because it is some time before culture results are known. However, this should not in any way discourage the physician from performing a culture.

If antibiotics are used, whether therapeutically or prophylactically, the hazards of allergic reactions, idiosyncrasy, toxicity, and unpleasant untoward effects, such as nausea, vomiting, or diarrhea, must be accepted. In addition, as sensitive bacteria are killed, an ecologic alteration occurs in the microbial environment, and resistant populations of organisms may supervene. Such potential alterations of the normal flora are frequently overlooked or ignored.

The choice of antibiotics for infection is beyond the scope of this chapter. New antibiotics with purported advantages appear each year, but these are not reviewed here.

Prophylactic use. The use of antibiotics to prevent infection is known as prophylactic use. This is based on the concept that the microorganism is attacked at the time of tissue contamination, before colonization, or, if colonization has occurred, at least before tissue invasion and massive proliferation (infection). Employment of antibiotics in this way whether topically or systemically is considered by many to be ill advised and perhaps a poorly disguised attempt to provide protection for poor surgery.[152] Still, there is evidence that under some circumstances prophylactic antibiotics are valuable.

Early clinical studies of the relationship of prophylactic antibiotics to the subsequent development of wound infection in clean wounds found either no relationship[64,122,236] or an actual increase in wound infections.[7,79,100,147,162] However, these studies tend to lump all types of surgical procedures together and do not specify types of antibiotics given, dosage, or timing in relationship to the surgery.

Indications. The indications for prophylactic antibiotics include situations in which moderate or gross wound contamination is likely, such as procedures on infected cysts or closure of wounds left open for a long period of time (greater than 3 or 4 hours). Traumatic wounds are also considered to be contaminated. Some patients are also more prone to infection and may be candidates for prophylactic antibiotics. Such patients include those with poor host defenses, poor vascular supply, poor nutrition, or remote preexisting infections elsewhere.

Several studies have been made of lacerations sutured in emergency rooms, which compared the infection rates with and without prophylactic antibiotics. The weight of the evidence favors the uselessness of antibiotics in this situation,[79,122] even when wounds were greater than 4 hours old[290] or on the hand (a site of increased wound infection following lacerations).[126,250] However, if wounds were older than 12 hours, treatment with antibiotics did decrease the infection rate significantly.[208]

Some studies suggest that prophylactic antibiotics are

useful in clean surgical wounds. Hoffman[144] claims a 0% clean wound infection rate with the use of neomycin sulfate 0.5% solution irrigation of wounds during surgery combined with systemic antibiotics in the immediate postoperative period. However, 1.7% of his patients developed a drug-related dermatitis and 0.9% a drug fever. Johnson[161] found that there was a lower incidence of infection using prophylactic antibiotics if surgery involved the respiratory tract.

Despite all this, there have been no published data establishing the value or lack of value of prophylactic systemic antibiotics in purely cutaneous surgery within the confines of a dermatology clinic. Therefore summary articles do not specifically address prophylactic antibiotic use in dermatologic surgery.[116] Recommendations can be extrapolated only from evidence produced in experimental studies of animals or from data on other surgical specialties.

Experimentally in animals, the combined use of topical and systemic antibiotics has been found to be more efficacious in reducing wound infection rates compared to either alone.[117] Bergamini et al.[21] showed a reduction of infection rates in guinea pig wounds inoculated with *S. aureus* when topical neomycin was used on wounds combined with systemic antibiotics. The reduction was greater than that induced with either topical or systemic antibiotics alone. These investigators showed that the size of the inoculum was important in determining the value of the prophylactic antibiotics. If the inoculum size was small, topical or systemic antibiotics lowered wound infection rates. On the other hand, if the inoculum was large, systemic antibiotics lowered the wound infection rates and systemic with topical antibiotics lowered the infection rates even more. This suggests that topical antibiotic solutions at the time of surgery may be valuable in cutaneous surgery. There is some evidence to suggest that for clean surgical wounds there was a decrease in infection rates when some topical antibacterials were used alone, prophylactically.[107,192]

Timing. Most physicians agree that the time at which the antibiotic is given in relationship to the surgery determines the likelihood of the antibiotic being effective in preventing infection.[232,284] In 1965 Burke demonstrated in guinea pigs that if antibiotics were given within the first few hours (up to 3) after the arrival of bacteria in tissue, the degree of wound infection was greatly reduced.[42] This became known as "Burke's Law." Miles showed that the decisive period differed with different organisms and antibiotics.[206] Although overall it lasted for approximately 3 hours with penicillin for *S. aureus*, it lasted up to 5 hours with streptomycin for *S. aureus*, and up to 8 hours using streptomycin for *Streptococcus* spp.

The current trend is that, if used, prophylactic antibiotics should be given before surgery or at least within a short time thereafter. Antibiotics that are present in tissue when the bacteria arrive render the maximum benefit in preventing wound infection.[2,152] In addition, there is a difference in the ability of an antibiotic to perfuse a wound after it is made. As time goes on, this ability becomes less and less as bacteria become relatively protected within a fibrous exudate.

The duration of prophylactic antibiotics also should be considered. Most people do not recommend that these be continued for more than a few days postoperatively, perhaps for as short a time as 24 hours,[284] because the incidence of untoward reactions is lessened, as is the cost involved. Ironically, if a short course of prophylactic antibiotics indeed reduces the incidence of postoperative infections, it also reduces the total antibiotic use and minimizes the evolution of bacterial resistance by eliminating the need for prolonged treatment of postoperative infections.

Patients with valvular heart disease. Although there might be controversy over whether prophylactic antibiotics are of value in clean surgery, there appears to be agreement about the treatment of patients with valvular heart disease or permanent protheses. Transient bacteremia in these patients may lead to endocarditis with potentially grave consequences.

Asymptomatic bacteremia may occur during many different medical procedures and during daily functions, such as tooth brushing or bowel movements.[103] This is particularly true with mucous membrane trauma. Indeed, the first association of endocarditis with bacteremia occurred after extraction of teeth.[261] Therefore dentists are well aware of the dangers of oral surgery in high-risk patients.

Procedures on the cutaneous surfaces that may lead to bacteremia include manipulation or drainage of infected abscesses or ulcers.[39] For instance, Richards[242] found the incidence of bacteremia following massage of infected boils to be 38.5%. Bacteremia seems to be more common following procedures on the soft tissues of the face.[267]

Although clinical evidence is lacking that administration of prophylactic antibiotics to those at risk prevents endocarditis, there is experimental evidence on rabbits to support this recommendation.[103] Therefore for procedures on septic foci, particularly associated with the mucous membranes or nasopharynx, it seems advisable to give patients at risk prophylaxis as recommended by the Committee of the American Heart Association (Table 4-5).[166] If organisms are present for which these antibiotics are not useful, one may wish to substitute other suitable antibiotics. For example, infected cutaneous lesions are most often associated with *S. aureus*, so a penicillinase-resistant penicillin or cephalosporin antibiotic seems best.

Therapeutic use. Antibiotics should be considered therapeutic rather than prophylactic when given to patients with wounds that are dirty or obviously infected. Under these conditions, the choice of the antibiotic and how long it is used should be determined by several factors that include the pathogens most likely to be involved, the site, and the clinical response.

TABLE 4-5

Recommendation for prophylactic antibiotics in patients with valvular heart disease, prosthetic heart disease, and congenital heart disease

Antibiotic	Dosage	Schedule
Parenteral*		
Aqueous penicillin G	1 million u IM or IV	30-60 min before procedure
Plus procaine penicillin G	600,000 u IM	
Then penicillin V	500 mgm by mouth	q6h × 8 doses
Parenteral with penicillin allergy		
Vancomycin	1 gm IV	30-60 min before procedure; infuse over 30 min
Then erythromycin	500 mgm by mouth	q6h × 8 doses
Oral		
Penicillin V	2 gm by mouth	30-60 min before procedure
Then penicillin V	500 mgm by mouth	q6h × 8 doses
Oral with penicillin allergy		
Erythromycin	1 gm by mouth	1½ to 2 hours before procedure
Then erythromycin	500 mgm by mouth	q6h × 8 doses

Modified from the Report of the Committee on Prevention of Rheumatic Fever and Bacterial Endocarditis of the American Heart Association and Johnson, J.T.: Am. J. Otolaryngol. **4:**433, 1983.

*Parenteral regimens recommended for those at very high risk, for example, prosthetic valves. May also add streptomycin (1 gram IM, 30 to 60 minutes before procedure) for those particularly at risk if not allergic to penicillin.

A surgical wound presents a unique environment in which an antibiotic may act. Not only is it important to know the sensitivities and types of organisms in a wound infection, it is also essential to know how well an antibiotic reaches bacteria in the wound. For example, in a study by Johnstone of 401 patients given prophylactic antibiotics with surgery, staphylococcal wound infection occurred in 48 patients, 13 of whom were being treated by antibiotics to which the bacteria in vitro were sensitive.[162]

Other factors that might influence how efficiently an antibiotic reaches an infection site include foreign bodies or the presence of an abscess. Foreign bodies may prevent the antibiotic from reaching the organism. Walled-off abscesses are impediments to antibiotic perfusions. The use of antibiotics here is considered adjunctive rather than therapeutic.

Surgical drainage is more beneficial in hastening a resolution of such infections. On the other hand, inflammation in wounds may aid in concentrating antibiotics into a wound site. The use of hot soaks also theoretically aids in bringing the antibiotic into the area of infection by increasing vasodilation.

Antibiotics go into wounds from plasma by passive diffusion. The higher the plasma level, the more antibiotic diffuses into a wound. The highest plasma levels of antibiotics are attained if the antibiotics are given by IV push. Serum half-life and other pharmacokinetic factors help determine antibiotic selection, dosage, and route of administration.[142] In addition, some antibiotics are relatively poor getting into wounds compared to others. For instance, Alexander et al.[5] found that erythromycin did not pass into wounds nearly as easily as penicillin, cephalosporins, or tetracycline.

Wounds that are left open to granulate in general contraindicate the use of systemic antibiotics.[95,253] These wounds tend to have a large fibrinous exudate as fluid from the extravascular space fills the surgical defect. This fibrinous exudate surrounds bacteria and thus shields them from antibiotics, whether systemic or topical. When infection is present in this type of wound, proteolytic enzymes have been used with some success, at least experimentally.[255] It is thought that these substances chemically debride the fibrin and allow antibiotics to enter the wound environment.

The choice of antibiotic for any infection should ideally be predicated on the type of bacteria and known sensitivities. Practically speaking, antibiotics are given before culture results are known. One may guess which antibiotics will be useful based on the clinical situation and information in the literature. For instance, hand infections are usually infected with penicillin-resistant *S. aureus*.[217,224] Since these staphylococci are found to be frequently sensitive to tetracycline, this antibiotic appears to be a wise choice for "blind" treatment.[217] Alternately, a penicillinase-resistant penicillin can be used.

VIRAL HEPATITIS
Types

Although hepatitis may be caused by several different viruses, the most common types of hepatitis include those caused by the hepatitis A virus (HAV), previously known as infectious hepatitis, with an incubation period of about 30 days and acquired by contact; hepatitis B virus (HBV), previously known as serum hepatitis, with an incubation period of 70 to 80 days and acquired parenterally; and non-A, non-B (NANB) hepatitis with an incubation period of 50 days and probably caused by several different viruses. This latter hepatitis is a diagnosis of exclusion.[184] HBV infection produces a form of hepatitis that is more serious than the other types, sometimes producing liver failure or chronic hepatitis. Of the 200,000 new cases of HBV each year in the United States, approximately 1000 patients die (0.5%) and

10,000 to 20,000 (5% to 10%) patients develop chronic hepatitis.[176] HBV infection is also associated with the development of liver carcinomas.

Following infection with HBV, many patients (approximately 5% to 10%) become chronic asymptomatic carriers.[223] They are infectious to others. Many people are infected without symptoms; in fact as few as 25% of infected adults develop clinical hepatitis. There are an estimated 400,000 to 800,000 HBV carriers in the United States.[52] In a recent study by Berry 20% of anesthesiologists who were seropositive for hepatitis B surface antigen (HB$_s$Ag) had a negative history for hepatitis.

Infectivity

The concept that small amounts of serum, saliva, or wound exudate of chronic asymptomatic carriers of HBV can be infective is based on experimental evidence,[18] as well as on the fact that needlesticks can transmit hepatitis. It has been estimated that 1 ml of serum contains 10^8 infective doses of HBV.[118] In addition, HB$_s$Ag has been found on exudate from impetiginous cutaneous lesions.[231] Dermatologists in particular should take note that perhaps the handling of skin lesions may transmit infection. Either wearing gloves or washing hands should be considered when examining oozing lesions. However, it should be stressed that gloves by themselves do not prevent transmission of the virus if the blood or the saliva from a patient is splashed directly onto the eye, oral mucosa, or broken skin of a physician.

Incidence among physicians

Anyone involved in surgery is at great risk to develop hepatitis. In fact, hepatitis has been known since the early 1950s to be an occupational hazard to physicians, particularly to those exposed to blood or blood products.[291] Almost 40% of all reported cases of HBV are found among hospital or dental workers.[8] The incidence of antibodies to HB$_s$Ag (anti-HB$_s$Ag) among all physicians is approximately 18.5%, with increasing rates among pathologists (27%) and surgeons (28%).[82] The rate of infection is also increased among oriental physicians and those with an increasing number of years in practice.[82,212] This high prevalence among health care workers has been confirmed by several other studies and is approximately five to eight times that of the general population.[26,123,165]

The problem of physicians who are carriers of HBV infecting their patients has not been studied. This event is probably rare, because physicians in general wear gloves during all surgical procedures, even skin biopsies. However, dentists, who do not routinely wear gloves, have been found to be a source of HBV outbreaks.[129,178,246] In one study 55 cases of HBV were traced to a single oral surgeon during a 4-year period of practice.[246] In another interesting case a dentist who had HBV infected six patients when he

was not wearing gloves, but after he began wearing gloves no patients became infected.[129]

Many dermatologists, as well as other physicians, routinely perform minor surgical procedures, such as incision and drainage of furuncles or abscesses, acne surgery, or skin biopsies, without gloves.[280] Since gloves are a simple, practical means to prevent the spread of HBV, they should be worn for these procedures.

Even though gloves are worn, tears or holes may theoretically lead to infection with HBV. This problem has not been studied. Rigel et al.[245] recommend reinforcing the fingertips of gloves with surgical tape (Dermaclear) to preclude tears in gloves and prevent exposure to hepatitis.

The concept of "having gotten this far without hepatitis" appears to be false security for those who still do not wear gloves. As has already been pointed out, the incidence of seropositivity for HBV increases with the age of physician and the number of years in practice.

It may be possible that previous exposure to HBV renders some individuals immune to further infection in the same way as the new hepatitis vaccine.[26,84,228] These nonvaccine recipients have serum antibody patterns suggestive of recent vaccination (anti-HB$_s$Ag positive, but negative anti-HB$_c$Ag).

It has also been suggested that face masks should be worn to prevent spread of hepatitis from physician or dentist carriers to the patient.[73] There are no data to substantiate this recommendation.

Some physicians have suggested that perhaps all patients undergoing elective surgical procedures should be screened for serologic markers of HBV. Although this may seem logical, it is an ineffective means of reducing the risk of hepatitis. Routine testing of blood donors for HB$_s$Ag did not decrease the frequency of posttransfusion hepatitis.[266] Positive serologic characterizations can be stigmatizing and provoke anxiety in patients and should not be routinely performed.

Vaccine

A vaccine (Heptavax-B manufactured by Merck, Sharp, Dohme) available since 1982 for HBV is recommended for all medical personnel. The vaccine is composed of chemically inactivated HB$_s$Ag that has been pooled from chronic carriers and put through several processes that inactivate all known virus types.[113] It contains no nucleic acid and is thus considered to be noninfectious.

The efficacy of the hepatitis B vaccine was evaluated in 865 members of 43 hemodialysis units.[286] The investigators found an incidence of HBV infection in 9.9% of a placebo group compared to a 2.2% incidence among vaccine recipients. The surface antibody (anti-HB$_s$Ag) developed in 92.6% of subjects after two doses and in 96% after a third injection, a 6-month booster. Therefore three doses are recommended. The protective antibody lasts for at least 3 years. After this period of time, an additional booster dose may be necessary. For the best response, the vaccine should be given as an injection into the deltoid and not into the buttock.

It is felt that the safety of the HBV vaccine is extremely high. After 200,000 health care workers were vaccinated, only 6 developed serious illnesses possibly related to the vaccine. These included one case of Guillain-Barré syndrome. It seems that the possible risk of vaccine-induced complications is low and is far outweighed by the potential benefit to those at risk.

Issue has been raised about the possible transmission of AIDS to vaccine recipients.[56] This fear is based on the fact that the vaccine is made from pooled plasma from donors, many of whom are at high risk for AIDS. Although there were two cases of AIDS among the original vaccine recipients that developed after the vaccine was given, this is not significantly different from the incidence of AIDS among those screened for participation in the original trial but not vaccinated.[54] In addition, the HBV vaccine has been checked for the presence of the human retrovirus, human immunodeficiency virus (HIV) which is associated with AIDS. These tests showed no evidence of this virus contaminating the HBV vaccine.[56]

The current recommendation of the Immunization Practices Advisory Committee of the CDC is that all persons at high risk for HBV who are serologically negative for hepatitis B antigen or antibody should receive HBV vaccine.[52] This recommendaton is based on two facts. First the risk of HBV infection for the groups at high risk far exceeds any vaccine-related infection or other conceivable complications. Second, incidence of HBV infection would be lowered by as much as one half if all high-risk groups, especially health care workers, received the vaccine.[176] It is hoped that by immunizing dental and medical workers, the chain of transmission and acquisition of HBV will ultimately be broken.

Before the vaccine is received, the appropriate laboratory tests should be performed to determine if the patient has evidence of prior infection and thus already has acquired immunization to HBV. This eliminates the risk of any possible untoward effects from the vaccine. The HB_sAg should be checked, as well as the antibody to the core antigen (anti-HB_cAg) and the antibody to the surface antigen (anti-HB_sAg). Individuals who carry HBV (HB_sAg positive) or who have evidence of previous infection (anti-HB_cAg positive) do not benefit from the vaccine. As previously mentioned, positivity for anti-HB_sAg alone is unusual, but may indicate prior exposure rendering immunity.[76] In addition, a check to see if seroconversion has occurred following vaccination should be done, since a small percentage (5%) of individuals do not convert.

It is currently unclear whether spouses of HBV carriers should be vaccinated, although the weight of the evidence shows that doing so would do little good. In a study by Perrillo et al., 34 spouses of HBV carriers were tested serologically.[228] All were negative for HB_sAg, but all were positive for both anti-HB_sAg and anti-HB_cAg. None of the 34 spouses had had symptoms of viral hepatitis. This again demonstrates the high infectivity of HBV and the frequent lack of symptoms with infection.

ACQUIRED IMMUNODEFICIENCY SYNDROME

AIDS is a newly recognized, fatal condition that is caused by a transmissable virus. Those who are performing surgery on AIDS patients therefore need to take special precautions.

AIDS is manifested clinically by either Kaposi's sarcoma or opportunistic infections (or both) in previously healthy individuals.[51,293] Before the development of AIDS, many patients have prodromal symptoms of weight loss, lymphadenopathy, fever, and diarrhea, which may last weeks to months. About 80% of cases in the United States have occurred in homosexual or bisexual men; the remainder of the cases have occurred in heterosexual men and women, frequently drug addicts.

The cause of AIDS is currently thought to be a newly recognized retrovirus, called HIV (human immunodeficiency virus; formerly known as HTLV-III/LAV, or human T-lymphocyte virus type III [lymphadenopathy virus]).[55] Current clinical observations are consistent with the theory that transmission requires inoculation with the blood or blood products of infected individuals, or intimate sexual contact with such individuals.

The CDC currently recommends that great caution be exerted in handling specimens (secretions, excretions, and biopsies) of AIDS patients.[53] Specifically, the following suggestions have been made:

1. Extreme care should be taken to avoid accidental wounds from sharp instruments.
2. Gloves should be worn for blood specimen handling or surgery. Masks are also recommended during surgery and protective eyewear should be considered for any procedures that aerosolize body fluids. This is particularly important when working on the mucosal surfaces, which have an increased amount of body secretions.
3. Gowns should be worn.
4. Hands should be washed after removing gowns and gloves.
5. Tissue or blood should be labeled "AIDS PRECAUTIONS."
6. Needles used should be placed in puncture-resistant containers.
7. Only disposable needles and syringes should be used.

The patients who are considered at high risk to transmit AIDS include known AIDS patients, sexual partners of AIDS patients, sexually active homosexual men, drug abusers, hemophiliacs, and sexual partners of those at increased risk. In addition, patients with chronic generalized lymphadenopathy, unexplained weight loss or prolonged fever should also be considered as possible AIDS carriers.

There has been one reported case of AIDS developing in a hospital worker 14 months after an accidental needle stick.[20] In this case, pooled gamma globulin for hepatitis was given and apparently had no protective effect. Whether this case is anecdotal or truly represents transmission of AIDS through inoculation is unknown.

REFERENCES

1. Ad Hoc Committee of the Committee on Trauma, Division of Medical Sciences, National Research Council Report: Postoperative wound infection: the influence of ultraviolet irradiation of the operating room and the influence of various other factors, Ann. Surg. **160**(suppl.):1, 1964.
2. Alexander, J.W., and Altemeier, W.A.: Penicillin prophylaxis in experimental staphylococcal wound infections, Surg. Gynecol. Obstet. **120**:243, 1965.
3. Alexander, J.W., et al.: The influence of hair-removal methods on wound infection, Arch. Surg. **118**:347, 1983.
4. Alexander, J.W., Kaplan, J.Z., and Altemeier, W.A.: Role of suture materials in the development of wound infection, Ann. Surg. **165**:192, 1967.
5. Alexander, J.W., et al.: Concentration of selected intravenously administered antibiotics in experimental surgical wounds, J. Trauma **13**:423, 1973.
6. Altee, W.F.: Clinical lectures on surgery by M. Nélaton, Philadelphia, 1855, J.B. Lippincott Co.
7. Altemeier, W.A., Culbertson, W.R., and Hummel, R.P.: Surgical considerations of endogenous infections: sources, types and methods of control, Surg. Clin. North Am. **48**: 227, 1968.
8. Alter, M.: National surveillance of viral hepatitis: 1981, MMWR **32**:23SS, 1983.
9. Aly, R., and Maibach, H.I.: Aerobic microbial flora of intertriginous skin, Appl. Environ. Microbiol. **33**:97, 1977.
10. Aly, R., et al.: Effect of prolonged occlusion on the microbial flora, pH, carbon dioxide, and transepidermal water loss on human skin, J. Invest. Dermatol. **71**:378, 1978.
11. American College of Surgeons, Committee on Control of Surgical Infections: Manual on control of infection in surgical patients, Philadelphia, 1984, J.B. Lippincott Co.
12. Anderson, K.: The contamination of hexachlorophene soap with *Pseudomonas pyocyanea,* Med. J. Aust. **2**:463, 1962.
13. Anyiwo, C.E., et al.: *Pseudomonas aeruginosa* in postoperative wounds from chlorhexidine solutions, J. Hosp. Infect. **3**:189, 1982.
14. Ascroft, P.B.: Treatment of head wounds due to missiles, Lancet **2**:211, 1943.
15. Ayliffe, G.A., et al.: A comparison of preoperative bathing with chlorhexidine-detergent and non-medicated soap in the prevention of wound infection, J. Hosp. Infect. **4**:237, 1983.
16. Baldwin, B.C., et al.: Affect of disposable draping on wound infection rate, Va. Med. **108**:477, 1981.
17. Balthazar, E.R., et al.: Preoperative hair removal: a randomized prospective study of shaving versus clipping, South. Med. J. **75**:799, 1982.
18. Barker, L.F., et al.: Hepatitis B virus infection in chimpanzees: titration of subtypes, J. Infect. Dis. **132**:451, 1975.
19. Beck, W.C., and Collette, T.S.: False faith in the surgeon's gown and surgical drape, Am. J. Surg. **83**:125, 1952.
20. Belani, A., et al.: AIDS in a hospital worker, Lancet **1**:676, 1984.
21. Bergamini, T.M., et al.: Combined topical and systemic antibiotic prophylaxis in experimental wound infection, Am. J. Surg. **147**:753, 1984.
22. Berkelman, R.L., et al.: Pseudobacteremia attributed to contamination of povidone-iodine with *Pseudomonas cepacia,* Ann. Intern. Med. **95**:32, 1981.
23. Bernard, H.R., Cole, W.R., and Gravens, D.J.: Reduction of iatrogenic bacterial contamination in operating rooms, Ann. Surg. **165**:609, 1967.
24. Berntsen, C., and McDermott, W.: Increased transmissibility of staphylococci to patients receiving an antimicrobial drug, N. Engl. J. Med. **262**:637, 1960.
25. Berry, A.R., et al.: A comparison of the use of povidone-iodine and chlorhexidine in the prophylaxis of postoperative wound infection, J. Hosp. Infect. **3**:55, 1982.
26. Berry, A.J., et al.: The prevalence of hepatitis B viral markers in anesthesia personnel, Anesthesiology **60**:6, 1984.
27. Bethune, D.W., et al.: Dispersal of *Staphylococcus aureus* by patients and surgical staff, Lancet **1**:480, 1965.
28. Billroth, T.: Beobachtungs-Studien ueber Wundfieber und accidentelle Wundbrankheiten, Arch. Klin. Chir. **6**:443, 1865.
29. Bloodgood, J.C.: Operations on 459 cases of hernia, Johns Hopkins Hosp. Rep. **7**:223, 1899.
30. Blowers, R., and McCluskey, M.: Design of operating room dress for surgeons, Lancet **2**:681, 1965.
31. Bockhart, M.: Über die Ätiologie und Therapie der Impetigo, des Furunkels, und der Sykosis, Monatsh. Prakt. Dermatol. **6**:450, 1887.
32. Bodiwala, G.G., and George, T.K.: Surgical gloves during wound repair in the accident-and-emergency department, Lancet **2**:91, 1982.
33. Brabender, W., et al.: *Legionella pneumophila* wound infection, J.A.M.A. **250**:3091, 1983.
34. Bresler, M.J.: Toxic shock syndrome due to occult postoperative wound infection, West. J. Med. **139**:710, 1983.
35. Brewer, G.E.: Studies in aseptic technic with a report of some recent observations at the Roosevelt Hospital, J.A.M.A. **64**:1369, 1915.
36. Brown, I.W.: Discussion on Culbertson, W.R., Altemeier, W.A., and Gonzalez, L.: Studies on the epidemiology of postoperative infection of clean operative wounds, Ann. Surg. **154**:599, 1961.
37. Brown, T.R., et al.: A clinical evaluation of chlorhexidine gluconate spray as compared with iodophor scrub for preoperative skin preparation, Surg. Gynecol. Obstet. **158**:363, 1984.
38. Bruun, J.N.: Postoperative wound infection: predisposing factors and the effect of a reduction in the dissemination of staphylococci, Acta Med. Scand. (Suppl.) **514**:3, 1970.
39. Bryan, C.S., Dew, C.E., and Reynolds, K.L.: Bacteremia associated with decubitus ulcers, Arch. Intern. Med. **143**: 2093, 1983.

40. Buffone, U., et al.: Neutrophil function in surgical patients: relationship to adequate bacterial defenses, Arch. Surg. **119:** 39, 1984.
41. Burke, J.E., and Corrigan, E.A.: Staphylococcal epidemiology on a surgical ward: fluctuations in ward staphylococcal content, its effect on hospitalized patients and extent of endemic hospital strains, N. Engl. J. Med. **264:**321, 1961.
42. Burke, J.F.: The effective period of preventive antibiotic action in experimental incisions and dermal lesions, Surgery **50:**161, 1961.
43. Burke, J.F.: Identification of the sources of *Staphylococcus* contaminating the surgical wound during operation, Ann. Surg. **158:**898, 1963.
44. Butcher, H.R., et al.: Hexachlorophene concentrations in the blood of operating room personnel, Arch. Surg. **107:**70, 1973.
45. Cabot, A.T.: Discussion. In Gerster, A.G.: Aseptic and antiseptic details in operative surgery, Tr. Congr. Am. Phys. Surg. **2:**51, 1891.
46. Calia, F.M., et al.: Importance of the carrier state as a source of *Staphylococcus aureus* in wound sepsis, J. Hyg. (Lond) **67:**49, 1969.
47. Caliendo, J.E.: Surgical masks during laceration repair (letter), JACEP **5:**278, 1976.
48. Carpendale, M.T.F., and Sereda, W.: The role of the percutaneous suture in surgical wound infection, Surgery **58:**672, 1965.
49. Carrel, A., and Hartmann, A.: Cicatrization of wounds: the relation between the size of the wound and the rate of its cicatrization, J. Exp. Med. **24:**429, 1916.
50. Casewell, M.W., and Phillips, I.: Hands as route of transmission for *Klebsiella* species, Br. Med. J. **2:**1315, 1977.
51. CDC Special Report: Epidemiologic aspects of the current outbreak of Kaposi's sarcoma and opportunistic infection, N. Engl. J. Med. **306:**248, 1981.
52. CDC: Inactivated hepatitis B. virus vaccine, MMWR **31:** 318, 1982.
53. CDC: Acquired immune deficiency syndrome (AIDS): precautions for clinical and laboratory staffs, MMWR **31:**577, 1982.
54. CDC: The safety of hepatitis B virus vaccine, MMWR **32:** 134, 1983.
55. CDC: Human T-cell leukemia virus infection in patients with acquired immune deficiency syndrome: preliminary observations, MMWR **32:**233, 1983.
56. CDC: Hepatitis B vaccine: evidence confirming lack of AIDS transmission, MMWR **33**(49):685, 1984.
57. Chabrolle, J.P., and Rossier, A.: Danger of iodine skin absorption in the neonate (letter), J. Pediatr. **93:**158, 1978.
58. Charnley, J.: A clean-air operating enclosure, Br. J. Surg. **51:**202, 1964.
59. Check, W.: New study shows hexachlorophene is teratogenic in humans, J.A.M.A. **240:**513, 1978.
60. Cheyne, W.W.: An address on asceptic and antiseptic surgery, Lancet **1:**347, 1903.
61. Chirife, J., et al.: In vitro study of bacterial growth inhibition in concentrated sugar solutions: microbiological basis for the use of sugar in treating infected wounds, Antimicrob. Agents Chemother. **23:**766, 1983.
62. Clegg, H.W., et al.: Infection due to organisms of the *Mycobacterium fortuitum* complex after augmentation mammoplasty: clinical and epidemiologic features, J. Infect. Dis. **147:**427, 1983.
63. Codish, S.D., Sheridan, I.D., and Monaco, A.D.: Mycotic wound infections: a new challenge for the surgeon, Arch. Surg. **114:**831, 1979.
64. Cohen, L.S., Fekety, F., and Cluff, L.E.: Studies of the epidemiology of staphylococcal infection. VI. Infections in the surgical patient, Ann. Surg. **159:**321, 1964.
65. Cole, W.R.: Relationship of skin carriage to postoperative staphylococcal wound infection, Surg. Forum **15:**52, 1964.
66. Colebrook, L., and Hook, A.M.: Infection through soaked dressings, Lancet **2:**682, 1948.
67. Condie, J.D., and Ferguson, D.J.: Experimental wound infections: contamination versus surgical technique, Surgery **50:**367, 1961.
68. Conolly, W.B., et al.: Influence of distant trauma on local wound infection, Surg. Gynecol. Obstet. **128:**713, 1969.
69. Craven, D.E., et al.: Pseudobacteremia caused by povidone-iodine solution contaminated with *Pseudomonas cepacia*, N. Engl. J. Med. **305:**621, 1981.
70. Cruse, P.J.E., and Foord, R.: The epidemiology of wound infection: a ten-year prospective study of 62,939 wounds, Surg. Clin. North Am. **60:**27, 1980.
71. Culbertson, W., et al.: Studies on the epidemiology of postoperative infection of clean operative wounds, Ann. Surg. **154:**599, 1961.
72. Custer, J., et al.: Studies in the management of the contaminated wound. V. An assessment of the effectiveness of pHisoHex and Betadine surgical scrub solutions, Am. J. Surg. **121:**572, 1971.
73. Czaja, A.J.: Hepatitis and the dentist, Mayo Clin. Proc. **58:**550, 1983.
74. Davidson, A.I.G., Smith, G., and Smylie, H.G.: A bacteriological study of the immediate environment of a surgical wound, Br. J. Surg. **58:**326, 1971.
75. Davies, J., et al.: Disinfection of the skin of the abdomen, Br. J. Surg. **65:**855, 1978.
76. Davies, R.R., and Noble, W.C.: Dispersal of bacteria and desquamated skin, Lancet **2:**1295, 1962.
77. Davis, J.M., et al.: Delayed wound infection: an 11-year study, Arch. Surg. **117:**113, 1982.
78. Davis, N.C., Cohen, J., and Rao, A.: The incidence of surgical wound infection: a prospective study of 20,822 operations, Aust. N.Z. J. Surg. **43:**75, 1973.
79. Day, T.K.: Controlled trial of prophylactic antibiotics in minor wounds requiring suture, Lancet **2:**1174, 1975.
80. DeHaan, B.B., Ellis, H., and Wilks, M.: The role of infection in wound healing, Surg. Gynecol. Obstet. **138:**693, 1974.
81. deHoll, D., et al.: Potentiation of infection by suture closure of dead space, Am. J. Surg. **127:**716, 1974.
82. Denes, A.E., et al.: Hepatitis B infection in physicians: results of a nationwide seroepidemiological survey, J.A.M.A. **239:**210, 1979.
83. Devenish, R.A., and Miles, A.A.: Control of *Staphylococcus aureus* in an operating theatre, Lancet **1:**1088, 1939.
84. Dienstag, J.L., and Ryan, D.M.: Occupational exposure to

hepatitis B virus in hospital personnel: infection or immunization? Am. J. Epidemiol. **115:**26, 1982.

85. Dineen, P.: An evaluation of the duration of the surgical scrub, Surg. Gynecol. Obstet. **129:**1181, 1969.

86. Duguid, J.P., and Wallace, A.T.: Air infection with dust liberated from clothing, Lancet **2:**845, 1948.

87. Duke, W.F., Robson, M.C., and Krizek, T.J.: Civilian wounds, their bacterial flora and rate of infection, Surg. Forum **23:**518, 1972.

88. DuMortier, J.J.: The resistance of healing wounds to infection, Surg. Gynecol. Obstet. **56:**762, 1933.

89. Duncan, W.C., McBride, M.E., and Knox, J.M.: Experimental production of infections in humans, J. Invest. Dermatol. **54:**319, 1970.

90. Dunphy, J.E.: On the nature and care of wounds, Ann. R. Coll. Surg. Engl. **26:**69, 1960.

91. Dyas, A.C., et al.: Sources of staphylococcal wound sepsis in surgical patients, J. Hosp. Infect. **3:**345, 1982.

92. Dykes, E.R., and Anderson, R.: Atraumatic technic—the sine qua non of operative wound infection prophylaxis, Cleve. Clin. Q. **28:**157, 1961.

93. Eade, G.G.: The relationship between granulation tissue, bacteria, and skin grafts in burned patients, Plast. Reconstr. Surg. **22:**42, 1958.

94. Edlich, R.F., et al.: Studies in the management of the contaminated wound, Am. J. Surg. **117:**323, 1969.

95. Edlich, R.F., Smith, Q.T., and Edgerton, M.T.: Resistance of the surgical wound to antimicrobial prophylaxis and its mechanisms of development, Am. J. Surg. **126:**583, 1973.

96. Edlich, R.F., et al.: Studies in the management of the contaminated wound. I. Technique of closure of such wounds together with a note on a reproducible experimental model, J. Surg. Res. **8:**585, 1968.

97. Ehrenkranz, N.J.: Person-to-person transmission of *Staphylococcus aureus:* quantitative characteristics of nasal carriers spreading infection, N. Engl. J. Med. **271:**225, 1964.

98. Ehrenkranz, N.J., Taplin, D., and Butt, P.: Antibiotic-resistant bacteria on the nose and skin: colonization and cross infection, Antimicrob. Agents Chemother. p. 255, 1966.

99. Elek, S.D.: Experimental staphylococcal infections in the skin of man, Ann. N.Y. Acad. Sci. **65:**85, 1956.

100. Evans, C., and Pollock, A.V.: The reduction of surgical wound infections by prophylactic parenteral cephaloridine: controlled clinical trial, Br. J. Surg. **60:**434, 1973.

101. Evans, C.A., et al.: Bacterial flora of the normal human skin, J. Invest. Dermatol. **15:**305, 1950.

102. Evans, D.G., Miles, A.A., and Niven, J.S.F.: The enhancement of bacterial infections by adrenaline, Br. J. Exp. Path. **29:**20, 1948.

103. Everett, E.D., and Hirschmann, J.V.: Transient bacteremia and endocarditis prophylaxis: a review, Medicine **56:**61, 1977.

104. Faddis, D., Boyer, J., and Daniel, B.: Tissue toxicity of antiseptic solutions: study of rabbit articular and periarticular tissues, J. Trauma **17:**895, 1977.

105. Farquharson, C.D., et al.: The control of staphylococcal skin infections in the nursery, Can. Med. Assoc. J. **67:**247, 1952.

106. Ferguson, D.J.: Clinical application of experimental relations between technique and wound infection, Surgery **63:**377, (1968).

107. Fielding, G., et al.: Prophylactic topical use of antibiotics in surgical wounds: a controlled trial using polybactrin, Med. J. Aust. **2:**159, 1965.

108. Fleming, A.: The action of chemical and physiological antiseptics in a septic wound, Br. J. Surg. **7:**99, 1919-20.

109. Forstrom, L.: Contract urticaria from latex surgical gloves, Contact Dermatitis **6:**33, 1980.

110. Foz, A., et al.: *Mycobacterium chelonei* iatroenic infections, J. Clin. Microbiol. **7:**319, 1978.

111. Frank, M.J., and Schaffner, W.: Contaminated aqueous benzalkonium chloride: an unnecessary hospital infection hazard, J.A.M.A. **236:**2418, 1976.

112. Garré, C.: Zur Aetiologie acut eitriger Entzundungen (Osteomyelitis, Furunkel und Panaritium), Fortschr. Med. **3:**165, 1885.

113. Gerety, R.J., and Tabor E.: Newly licensed hepatitis B vaccine: known safety and unknown risks, J.A.M.A. **249:**745, 1983.

114. Geronemus, R.G., Mertz, P.M., and Eaglstein, W.H.: Wound healing effects of topical antimicrobial agents, Arch. Dermatol. **115:**1311, 1979.

115. Gibbs, J.M.: Combustible plastic drape, Anaesth. Intensive Care **11:**176, 1983.

116. Gilbert, D.N.: Current status of antibiotic prophylaxis in surgical patients, Bull. N.Y. Acad. Med. **60:**340, 1984.

117. Gingrass, R.P., Close, A.S., and Ellison, E.H.: The effect of various topical and parenteral agents on the prevention of infection in experimental contaminated wounds, J. Trauma **4:**763, 1964.

118. Gmelin, K., et al.: Follow-up of needlesticks in medical staff, Dev. Biol. Stand. **54:**357, 1983.

119. Goodson, W.H., and Hunt, T.K.: Wound healing and the diabetic patient, Surg. Gynecol. Obstet. **149:**600, 1979.

120. Gorshevikova, E.V.: Routes of staphylococcal infection spread in the surgical clinic, Klin. Khir. (4)**:**51, 1979.

121. Goshi, K., Cluff, L.E., and Johnson, J.E., III: Studies in the pathogenesis of Staphylococcal infection, III. The effect of tissue necrosis and antitoxic immunity, J. Exp. Med. **113:**259, 1961.

122. Gosnold, J.K.: Infection rate of sutured wounds, Practitioner **218:**584, 1977.

123. Grady, G.F.: Hepatitis B immunity in hospital staff targeted for vaccination: role of screening tests in immunization programs, J.A.M.A. **248:**2266, 1982.

124. Gray, F.J., and Kipp, E.E.: Topical chemotherapy in prevention of wound infection, Surgery **54:**891, 1963.

125. Gross, A., Cutright, D., and D'Alessandro, S.M.: Effect of surgical scrub on microbial population under the fingernails, Am. J. Surg. **138:**463, 1979.

126. Grossman, J.A.I., Adams, J.P., and Kunec, J.: Prophylactic antibiotics in simple hand lacerations, J.A.M.A. **245:**1055, 1981.

127. Gruber, D.K., et al.: Acceleration of wound healing by *Staphylococcus aureus,* Surg. Forum **32:**76, 1981.

128. Gruber, R.P., Vistres, L., and Pardoe, R.: The effect of commonly used antiseptics on wound healing, Plast. Reconstr. Surg. **55:**472, 1975.

129. Hadler, S.C., et al.: An outbreak of hepatitis B in dental practice, Ann. Intern. Med. **95:**133, 1981.

130. Ha'eri, G.B.: The efficacy of adhesive plastic incise drapes in preventing wound contamination, Int. Surg. **68:**31, 1983.

131. Ha'eri, G.B., and Wiley, A.M.: Wound contamination through drapes and gowns: a study using tracer particles, Clin. Orthop. **154:**181, 1981.

132. Haley, R.W., et al.: The emergence of methicillin-resistant *Staphylococcus aureus* infections in United States hospitals: possible role of the house staff-patient transfer circuit, Ann. Intern. Med. **97:**297, 1982.

133. Halle, J.: Familiar medical quotations, Cited by Strauss, M.B., ed., Boston, 1968, Little Brown & Co.

134. Halley, C.R.L., Chesney, A.M., and Dresel, I.: On the behavior of granulating wounds of the rabbit to various types of infection, Bull. Johns Hopkins Hosp. **41:**191, 1927.

135. Halsted, W.S.: The treatment of wounds with especial reference to the value of blood clot in the management of dead spaces, Johns Hopkins Hosp. Rep. **2:**255, 1891.

136. Halsted, W.S.: Ligature and suture material: the employment of fine silk in preference to catgut and the advantages of transfixing tissues and vessels in control of hemorrhage; also an account of the introduction of gloves, gutta-percha tissue, and silver foil, J.A.M.A. **60:**1119, 1913.

137. Hamilton, H.W., Hamilton, K.R., and Lone, F.J.: Preoperative hair removal, Can. J. Surg. **20:**269, 1971.

138. Hare, R., and Ridley, M.: Further studies on the transmission of *Staphylococcus aureus*, Br. Med. J. **1:**69, 1958.

139. Hasselgren, P.O., et al.: Sources and routes in postoperative wound infections, Acta Chir. Scand. **147:**99, 1981.

140. Hasselgren, P.O., et al.: Postoperative wound infections in patients with long preoperative hospital stay, Acta Chir. Scand. **148:**473, 1982.

141. Haury, B.B., et al.: Inhibition of nonspecific defenses by soil infection-potentiating factors, Surg. Gynecol. Obstet. **144:**19, 1977.

142. Henness, D.M., and Gordon, W.E.: Effective once daily or twice-daily treatment of skin and skin structure infections with a new cephalosporin (Cefadroxil), Infection **8**(55): S633, 1980.

143. Hepburn, H.H.: Delayed primary closure of wounds, Br. Med. J. **1:**181, 1919.

144. Hoffman, E.: Prophylactic antibiotic usage in clean surgical procedures, Am. Surg. **50:**161, 1984.

145. Hohn, D.C.: Host resistance to infection: established and emerging concepts. In Hunt, T.K., editor: Wound healing and wound infection, New York, 1980, Appleton-Century-Crofts.

146. Homer: Homerii opera: Odysseae, London, Oxford, 1954, Book XXII. (Translated by R.G. Bennett, M.D.)

147. Howe, C.W.: Postoperative wound infections due to *Staphylococcus aureus*, N. Engl. J. Med. **251:**411, 1954

148. Howe, C.W.: Prevention and control of postoperative wound infection owing to *Staphylococcus aureus*, N. Engl. J. Med. **255:**787, 1956.

149. Howe, C.W.: Experimental studies on determinants of wound infection, Surg. Gynecol. Obstet. **123:**507, 1966.

150. Howe, C.W., and Marston, A.T.: A study on sources of postoperative staphylococcal infection, Surg. Gynecol. Obstet. **115:**266, 1962.

151. Hunt, T.K.: Surgical wound infections: an overview, Am. J. Med. **70:**712, 1981.

152. Hunt, T.K., et al.: Antibiotics in surgery, Arch. Surg. **110:** 148, 1975.

153. Hunt, T.K., et al.: A new model for the study of wound infection, J. Trauma **7:**298, 1967.

154. Hutton, P.A.N., Jones, B.M., and Law, D.J.W.: Depot penicillin as prophylaxis in accidental wounds, Br. J. Surg. **65:** 549, 1978.

155. Irvin, T.T., et al.: Hyperbaric oxygen in the treatment of infections by aerobic micro-organisms, Lancet **1:**392, 1966.

156. Jackson, D.W., Pollock, A.V., and Tindal, D.S.: The value of a plastic adhesive drape in the prevention of wound infection, Br. J. Surg. **58:**340, 1971.

157. Jaffray, D.C., et al.: Does surgical glove powder decrease the inoculum of bacteria required to produce an abscess? J. R. Coll. Surg. Edinb. **28:**219, 1983.

158. James, R.C., and MacLeod, C.J.: Induction of staphylococcal infections in mice with small inocula introduced on sutures, Br. J. Exp. Path. **42:**266, 1961.

159. Jarvis, J.D., et al.: Handwashing and antiseptic-containing soaps in the hospital, J. Clin. Pathol. **32:**732, 1979.

160. Johnson, B.W., et al.: Primary and secondary healing in infected wounds: an experimental study, Arch. Surg. **117:** 1189, 1982.

161. Johnson, J.T.: Prophylaxis in surgical procedures, Am. J. Otolaryngol. **4:**433, 1983.

162. Johnstone, F.R.C.: An assessment of prophylactic antibiotics in general surgery, Surg. Gynecol. Obstet. **116:**1, 1963.

163. Johnstone, F.R.C.: Infection on a surgical service: present incidence compared with that of 1957, Am. J. Surg. **120:** 192, 1970.

164. Joress, S.M.: A study of disinfection of the skin: a comparison of povidone-iodine with other agents used for surgical scrubs, Ann. Surg. **155:**296, 1962.

165. Jovanovich, J.F., et al.: The risk of hepatitis B among select employee groups in an urban hospital, J.A.M.A. **250:**1893, 1983.

166. Kaplan, E.L., et al.: Prevention of bacterial endocarditis, Circulation **56:**139A, 1977.

167. Keene, W., Minchew, B., and Cluff, L.: Studies of the epidemiology of staphylococcal infection. III. Clinical factors in susceptibility to staphylococcal disease, N. Engl. J. Med. **265:**1128, 1961.

168. Keys, T.F., et al.: Nosocomial outbreak of *Rhizopus* infections associated with Elastoplast wound dressings, MMWR **27:**33, 1978.

169. Kimmonth, J.B., et al.: Studies on theatre ventilation and surgical wound infection, Br. Med. J. **2:**407, 1958.

170. Knighton, D.R., et al.: Oxygen as an antibiotic: the effect of inspired oxygen on infection, Arch. Surg. **119:**199, 1984.

171. Kocher, T.: On some conditions of healing by first intention with special reference to disinfection of hands, Trans. Am. Surg. Ass. **17:**116, 1899.

172. Krizek, T.J., and Davis, J.H.: Effect of diabetes on experimental infection, Surg. Forum **15:**60, 1964.

173. Krizek, T.J., and Davis, J.H.: The role of the red cell in subcutaneous infection, J. Trauma **5:**85, 1965.

174. Krizek, T.J., and Robson, M.C.: Biology of surgical infection, Surg. Clin. North Am. **55:**1261, 1975.

175. Krizek, T.J., Robson, M.C., and Kho, E.: Bacterial growth and skin graft survival, Surg. Forum **18:**518, 1967.

176. Krugman, S.: The newly licensed hepatitis B vaccine: characteristics and indications for use, J.A.M.A. **247:**2012, 1982.

177. Kune, G.A., et al.: Postoperative wound infections: a study of bacteriology and pathogenesis, Aust. N.Z. J. Surg. **53:** 245, 1983.

178. Levin, M.L., et al.: Hepatitis B transmission by dentists, J.A.M.A. **228:**1139, 1974.

179. Lidwell, O.M.: Airborne bacteria and surgical infection, Am. J. Med. **70:**693, 1981.

180. Lilly, H.A., et al.: Effects of adhesive drapes on contamination of operation wounds, Lancet **2:**431, 1970.

181. Lister, J.: New method of treating compound fractures, abscess, etc., with observations on the conditions of suppuration, Lancet **1:**326, 1867.

182. Lister, J.: On the antiseptic principle in the practice of surgery, Lancet **2:**353, 1867.

183. Loomis, A.L.: Fibroid processes: (chronic interstitial) inflammation, sclerosis): their pathology and aetiology, with special reference to the influence of diathesis and heredity, Tr. Congr. Am. Phys. Surg. **2:**121, 1891.

184. Losowsky, M.S.: The clinical course of viral-hepatitis (review), Clin. Gastroenterol. **9:**3, 1980.

185. Lovell, D.L.: Skin bacteria: their location with reference to skin sterilization, Surg. Gynecol. Obstet. **80:**174, 1945.

186. MacDonald, S., and Timbury, M.C.: Unusual outbreak of staphylococcal postoperative wound infection, Lancet **2:** 863, 1957.

187. MacKowiak, P.A.: The normal microbial-flora (review), N. Engl. J. Med. **307:**83, 1982.

188. Mac Lean, L.D., et al.: Host resistance in sepsis and trauma, Ann. Surg. **182:**207, 1975.

189. Madden, J.E., et al. Studies in the management of the contaminated wound. IV. Resistance to infection of surgical wounds made by knife, electrosurgery, and laser, Am. J. Surg. **119:**222, 1970.

190. Magee, C., et al.: Potentiation of wound infection by surgical drains, Am. J. Surg. **131:**547, 1976.

191. Maki, D.G., et al.: Relation of the inanimate hospital environment to endemic nosocomial infection, N. Engl. J. Med. **307:**1562, 1982.

192. Mandell, G.L.: Bactericidal activity of aerobic and anaerobic polymorphonuclear neutrophils, Infec. Immun. **9:**337, 1974.

193. Marburg, K.C., et al.: Reasonable infection rate of simple suturing (letter), JACEP **5:**714, 1976.

194. Markle, G.B., IV: The case for doing more office surgery, Med. Econ. **51:**75, 1974.

195. Marks, J., et al.: Prediction of healing time as an aid to the management of open granulating wounds, World J. Surg. **7:**641, 1983.

196. Marples, R.R., Heaton, C.L., and Kligman, A.M.: *Staphylococcus aureus* in psoriasis, Arch. Dermatol. **107:**568, 1973.

197. Martin, W.J., Mandracchia, V.J., and Beckett, D.E.: The incidence of postoperative infection in outpatient podiatric surgery, J. Am. Podiatry Assoc. **74:**89, 1984.

198. Martin-Bouyer, G., et al.: Outbreak of accidental hexachlorophene poisoning in France, Lancet **1:**91, 1982.

199. McDowell, A.J.: Wound infections resulting from the use of hot wet sponges, Plast. Reconstr. Surg. **23:**168, 1959.

200. Medical Letter Drugs Therapeutics: Chlorhexidine and other antiseptics, Med. Lett. Drugs Ther. **18**(21):85, 1976.

201. Meleney, F.L.: Infection in clean operative wounds, Surg. Gynecol. Obstet. **60:**264, 1935.

202. Meleney, F.L., and Stevens, F.A.: Postoperative haemolytic streptococcus wound infections and their relation to haemolytic streptococcus carriers among operating personnel, Surg. Gynecol. Obstet. **43:**338, 1926.

203. Meltzer, R.M., et al.: Postoperative gas gangrene, J. Foot Surg. **22:**126, 1983.

204. Meyer, E., and Meyer, M.B.: The pathology of staphylococcus abscesses in vitamin C-deficient guinea pigs, Bull. Johns Hopkins Hosp. **74:**98, 1944.

205. Miles, A.A.: The carriage of *Staphylococcus (pyogenes) aureus* in man and its relation to wound infection, J. Pathol. Bacteriol. **56:**513, 1944.

206. Miles, A.A., Williams, R.E.O., and Clayton-Cooper, B.: Nonspecific defense reactions in bacterial infections, Ann. N.Y. Acad. Sci. **66:**356, 1956.

207. Montes, L.F., and Wilborn, W.H.: Anatomical location of normal skin flora, Arch. Dermatol. **101:**145, 1970.

208. Morgan, W.J., Hutchinson, D., and Johnson, H.M.: The delayed treatment of wounds of the hand and forearm under antibiotic cover, Br. J. Surg. **67:**140, 1980.

209. Morris, P.J., Barnes, B.A., and Burke, J.F.: The nature of the "irreducible minimum" rate of incisional sepsis, Arch. Surg. **92:**367, 1966.

210. Morrison, V.A., and Oldfield, E.C.: Postoperative toxic shock syndrome, Arch. Surg. **118:**791, 1983.

211. Morse, L.J., et al.: Septicemia due to *Klebsiella pneumoniae* originating from a hand-cream dispenser, N. Engl. J. Med. **277:**472, 1967.

212. Moseley, J.W., et al.: Hepatitis B virus infection in dentists, N. Engl. J. Med. **293:**729, 1975.

213. Moylan, J.A., Balish, E., and Chan, J.: Intraoperative bacterial transmission, Surg. Gynecol. Obstet. **141:**731, 1975.

214. Moylan, J.A., et al.: The importance of gown and drape barriers in the prevention of wound infection, Surg. Gynecol. Obstet. **151:**465, 1980.

215. Nakazawa, M., Sato, K., and Mizuno, K.: Incidence of perforations on rubber gloves during ophthalmic surgery, Ophthalmic Surg. **15:**236, 1984.

216. Natof, H.E.: Complications associated with ambulatory surgery, J.A.M.A. **244:**1116, 1980.

217. Nicholls, R.J.: Initial choice of antibiotic treatment for pyogenic hand infections, Lancet **1:**225, 1973.

218. Noble, W.C.: *Staphylococcus aureus* on the skin, J. Clin. Pathol. **19:**570, 1966.

219. Ogston, A.: Report upon microorganisms in surgical diseases, Br. Med. J. **1:**369, 1881.

220. Olson, M., et al.: Surgical wound infections: a 5-year prospective study of 20,193 wounds at the Minneapolis VA Medical Center, Ann. Surg. **199:**253, 1984.

221. Orr, N.W.: Is a mask necessary in the operating theatre? Ann. R. Coll. Surg. Engl. **63:**390, 1981.

222. Ott, A.E.: Disposable surgical drapes—a potential fire hazard, Obstet. Gynecol. **61:**667, 1983.

223. Oxman, M.N.: Hepatitis B vaccination of high-risk hospital personnel, Anesthesiology **60:**1, 1984.

224. Page, R.E., and Freeman, R.: Superficial sepsis: antibiotic of choice for blind treatment, Br. J. Surg. **64:**281, 1977.

225. Parker, M.T.: The clinical significance of the presense of microorganisms in pharmaceutical and cosmetic preparations, J. Soc. Cosmetic Chem. **23:**415, 1972.

226. Parrott, P.L., et al.: *Pseudomonas aeruginosa* peritonitis associated with contaminated poloxamer-iodine solution, Lancet **2:**683, 1982.

227. Perkins, J.J.: Principles and methods of sterilization in health sciences, Springfield, Ill., 1969, Charles C Thomas.

228. Perrillo, R.P., et al.: Should spouses of heptitis B surface antigen carriers receive hepatitis vaccine? N. Engl. J. Med. **308:**280, 1983.

229. Peterson, A.F., Rosenberg, A., and Alatary, S.D.: Comparative evaluation of surgical scrub preparations, Surg. Gynecol. Obstet. **146:**63, 1978.

230. Peterson, L.W.: Prophylaxis of wound infection, Arch. Surg. **50:**177, 1945.

231. Peterson, N.J., et al.: Hepatitis B surface antigen in saliva, impetiginous lesions, and the environment in two remote Alaskan villages, Appl. Environ. Microbiol. **32:**572, 1976.

232. Polk, H.C., Jr., and Lopez-Mayor, J.F.: Postoperative wound infection: a prospective study of determinant factors and prevention, Surgery **66:**97, 1969.

233. Polk, H.C., Jr., and Miles, A.A.: Enhancement of bacterial infection by ferric iron, kintics, mechanisms and surgical significance, Surgery **70:**71, 1971.

234. Polk, H.C., Jr., et al.: Guidelines for preventions of surgical wound infection, Arch. Surg. **118:**1213, 1983.

235. Pollock, A.V.: Surgical wound sepsis, Lancet **1:**1283, 1979.

236. Pollock, A.V., and Tindall, D.S.: The effect of a single dose of parenteral antibiotic in the prevention of wound infection: a controlled trial, Br. J. Surg. **59:**98, 1972.

237. Price, P.B.: The bacteriology of normal skin: a new quantitative test applied to a study of the bacterial flora and the disinfectant action of mechanical cleansing, J.Infect. Dis. **63:**301, 1938.

238. Prigot, A., Garnes, A.L., and Nwagbo, U.: Evaluation of a chemical depilatory for pre-operative preparation of 515 surgical patients, Am. J. Surg. **104:**900, 1962.

239. Prince, H.N., et al.: Drug resistance studies with topical antiseptics, J. Pharm. Sci. **67:**1629, 1978.

240. Raahave, D.: Effect of plastic skin and wound drapes on the density of bacteria in operation wounds, Br. J. Surg. **63:**421, 1976.

241. Rebell, G., et al.: Factors affecting the rapid disappearance of bacteria on normal skin, J. Invest. Dermatol. **14:**247, 1950.

242. Richards, J.H.: Bacteremia following irritation of foci of infection, J.A.M.A. **99:**1496, 1932.

243. Rickells, L.R., et al.: Human skin lipids with particular reference to the self-sterilizing power of the skin, Clin. Sci. **10:**89, 1951.

244. Ridley, M.: Perineal carriage of *Staphylococcus aureus,* Br. Med. J. **1:**270, 1959.

245. Rigel, D.S., et al.: Surgical gem: modification of surgical gloves to prevent exposure to hepatitis during hair transplant surgery, J. Dermatol. Surg. Oncol. **9:**114, 1983.

246. Rimland, D., et al.: Hepatitis B outbreak traced to an oral surgeon, N. Engl. J. Med. **296:**953, 1977.

247. Ritter, M.A., et al.: The operating room environment as affected by people and the surgical face mask, Clin. Orthop. **111:**147, 1975.

248. Ritter, M.A., et al.: The effect that time, touch, and environment have upon bacterial contamination of instruments during surgery, Ann. Surg. **184:**642, 1976.

249. Ritter, M.A., French, M.L.V., and Eitzen, H.E.: Bacterial contamination of the surgical knife, Clin. Orthop. **108:**158, 1975.

250. Roberts, A.H.N., and Teddy, P.J.: A prospective trial of prophylactic antibiotics in hand lacerations, Br. J. Surg. **64:**394, 1977.

251. Robson, M.C., and Krizek, T.J.: The effect of human amniotic membranes on the bacterial population of infection rat burns, Ann. Surg. **177:**144, 1973.

252. Robson, M.C., et al.: Quantitative bacteriology and delayed wound closure, Surg. Forum **19:**501, 1968.

253. Robson, M.C., et al.: The efficacy of systemic antibiotics in the treatment of granulating wounds, J. Surg. Res. **16:**299, 1974.

254. Rodeheaver, G., et al.: Bactericidal activity and toxicity of iodine-containing solutions in wounds, Arch. Surg. **117:**181, 1982.

255. Rodeheaver, G., et al.: Proteolytic enzymes as adjuncts to antibiotic prophlaxis of surgical wounds, Am. J. Surg. **127:**564, 1974.

256. Rodeheaver, G.T., et al.: Mechanical cleansing of contaminated wounds with a surfactant, Am. J. Surg. **129:**241, 1975.

257. Rodeheaver, G., et al.: Identification of the wound infection-potentiating factors in soil, Am. J. Surg. **128:**8, 1974.

258. Roettinger, W., et al.: Role of inoculation site as a determinant of infection in soft tissue wounds, Am. J. Surg. **126:**354, 1973.

259. Rothman, S.: Physiology and biochemistry of the skin, Chicago, 1954, University of Chicago Press.

260. Roundtree, P.M., et al.: Staphylococcal wound infection in a surgical unit, Lancet **2:**1, 1960.

261. Rushton, M.A.: Subacute bacterial endocarditis following the extraction of teeth, Guys. Hosp. Rep. **80:**39, 1930.

262. Russell, B., et al.: An outbreak of *Staphylococcus aureus* surgical wound infection associated with excess overtime employment of operating room personnel, Am. J. Infect. Control **11:**63, 1983.

263. Rutherford, W.H., and Spence, R.A.J.: Infection in wounds in the accident and emergency department, Ann. Emerg. Med. **9:**350, 1980.

264. Schaffner, W., Reisig, G., and Verrall, R.A.: Outbreaks of *Pseudomonas cepacia* infection due to contaminated anaesthetics, Lancet **1:**1050, 1973.

265. Schauerhamer, R.A., et al.: Studies in the management of the contaminated wound. II. Susceptibility of surgical wounds to postoperative surface contamination, Am. J. Surg. **122:**74, 1971.

266. Seeff, L.B., et al.: Cooperative study of post-transfusion hepatitis 1969-1974: incidence and characteristics of hepatitis and responsible risk factors, Am. J. Med. Sci. **270:**355, 1975.

267. Seifert, E.: Ueber Bakterienbefunde im Blut nach Operationen, Arch. Klin. Chir. **138:**565, 1925.

268. Selwyn, S.: Skin bacteria and skin disinfection reconsidered, Br. Med. J. **1:**136, 1972.

269. Selwyn, S.: Natural antibiosis among skin bacteria as a primary defense against infection, Br. J. Dermatol. **93:**487, 1975.

270. Seropian, R., and Reynolds, B.M.: Importance of airborne contamination as a factor in postoperative wound infection, Arch. Surg. **98:**654, 1969.

271. Seropian, R., and Reynolds, B.M.: Wound infections after preoperative depilatory versus razor preparation, Am. J. Surg. **121:**251, 1971.

272. Shambaugh, P.: Postoperative wound complications, Surg. Gynecol. Obstet. **64:**765, 1937.

273. Shanson, D.C., et al.: Operating theatre acquired infection with a gentamicin-resistant strain of *Staphylococcus aureus:* outbreaks in two hospitals attributable to one surgeon (letter), J. Hosp. Infect. **1:**171, 1980.

274. Shepherd, R.C., and Kinmonth, J.B.: Skin preparation and towelling in prevention of wound infection, Br. Med. J. **1962**(5298):151, 1962.

275. Siegle, R.J., et al.: Cutaneous candidosis as a complication of facial dermabrasion, J. Dermatol. Surg. Oncol. **10:**891, 1984.

276. Simmonds, B.P.: CDC guidelines on infection control, Infect. Control 3(suppl. 2):187, 1982.

277. Simmons, B.P.: Guideline for prevention of surgical wound infections, Am. J. Infect. Control **11:**133, 1983.

278. Singleton, A.O., Jr., and Julian, J.: An experimental evaluation of methods used to prevent infection in wounds which have been contaminated with feces, Ann. Surg. **151:**912, 1960.

279. Sleigh, J.W., and Linter, S.P.K.: Hazards of hydrogen peroxide, Br. Med. J. **291:**1706, 1985.

280. Smith, J.G., and Chalker, D.K.: A glove upon that hand (editorial), South Med. J. **75:**129, 1982.

281. Smith, M., and Enguist, I.F.: A quantitative study of impaired healing resulting from infection, Surg. Gynecol. Obstet. **125:**965, 1967.

282. Sompolinsky, D., et al.: A series of postoperative infections, J. Infect. Dis. **100:**1, 1957.

283. Sprunt, K., Redman, W., and Leidy, G.: Antibacterial effectiveness of routine hand washing, Pediatrics **52:**264, 1973.

284. Stone, H.H., et al.: Prophylactic and preventive antibiotic therapy: timing, duration, and economics, Ann. Surg. **189:** 691, 1979.

285. Summers, M.M., Lynch, P.F., and Black, T.: Hair as a reservoir of staphylococci, J. Clin. Pathol. **18:**13, 1965.

286. Szmuness, W., et al.: Hepatitis B vaccine in medical staff of hemodialysis units: efficacy and subtype cross-protection, N. Engl. J. Med. **307:**1481, 1982.

287. Taplin, D., and Mertz, P.M.: Flower vases in hospitals as reservoirs of pathogens, Lancet 2(7841):1279, 1973.

288. Taubler, J.H., Mudd, S., and Sall, T.: Partial protection of mice by human gamma-globulin against *Staphylococcus aureus* on subcutaneous sutures, Proc. Soc. Exp. Biol. Med. **109:**20, 1962.

289. Taylor, G.W., et al.: Staphylococcal wound infection: an experimental study in guinea pigs, Br. J. Surg. **49:**569, 1962.

290. Thirlby, R.C., et al.: The value of prophylactic antibiotics for simple lacerations, Surg. Gynecol. Obstet. **156:**212, 1983.

291. Trumbull, M.L., and Greiner, D.J.: Homologous serum jaundice: an occupational hazard to medical personnel, J.A.M.A. **145:**965, 1951.

292. Victoria, B., Baer, H., and Ayoub, E.M.: Successful treatment of systemic *Chromobacterium violaceum* infection, J.A.M.A. **230:**578, 1974.

293. Vieira, J., et al.: Acquired immune deficiency in Haitians: opportunistic infections in previously healthy Haitian immigrants, N. Engl. J. Med. **308:**125, 1983.

294. Walker, I.J.: The efficiency of the face mask, Surg. Gynecol. Obstet. **50:**266, 1930.

295. Walter, C.W., and Kundsin, R.B.: The floor as a reservoir of hospital infections, Surg. Gynecol. Obstet. **111:**412, 1960.

296. Wangensteen, O.H., Wangensteen, S.D., and Klinger, C.F.: Surgical cleanliness, hospital salubrity, and surgical statistics, historically considered, Surgery **71:**477, 1972.

297. Weber, D.O., et al.: Influence of operating-room surface contamination on surgical wounds: a prospective study, Arch. Surg. **111:**484, 1976.

298. Weinberg, E.D.: Iron and susceptibility to infectious disease, Science **184:**952, 1974.

299. Weinstein, H.J.: The relation between the nasal-staphylococcal-carrier state and the incidence of postoperative complications, N. Engl. J. Med. **260:**1303, 1959.

300. Welch, W.H.: Conditions underlying the infection of wounds, Tr. Congr. Am. Phys. Surg. **2:**1, 1891.

301. White, J.J., and Duncan, A.: Comparative effectiveness of iodophor and hexachlorophene surgical scrub solutions, Surg. Gynecol. Obstet. **135:**890, 1972.

302. Whyte, W., Vesley, D., and Hodgson, R.: Bacterial dispersion in relation to operating-room clothing, J. Hyg. (Cambridge) **76:**367, 1976.

303. Wilson, P.E., White, P.M., and Noble, W.C.: Infections in a hospital for patients with diseases of the skin, J. Hyg. (Lond) **69:**125, 1971.

304. Wishart, M.M., and Riley, T.V.: Infection with *Pseudomonas maltophilia:* hospital outbreak due to contaminated disinfectant, Med. J. Aust. **2:**710, 1976.

305. Wood, D.D.B., et al.: Relationship of operating room carriers of *Staphylococcus aureus* to wound infections, Surg. Forum **12:**40, 1961.

306. Wood, P.B.: Wound infection in undressed sutured wounds of the hand, Br. J. Surg. **58:**543, 1971.

307. Zamora, J.L., and Feldtman, R.W.: Povidone-iodine strikes back (letter), Arch. Surg. **118:**367, 1983.

MATERIALS FOR CUTANEOUS SURGERY

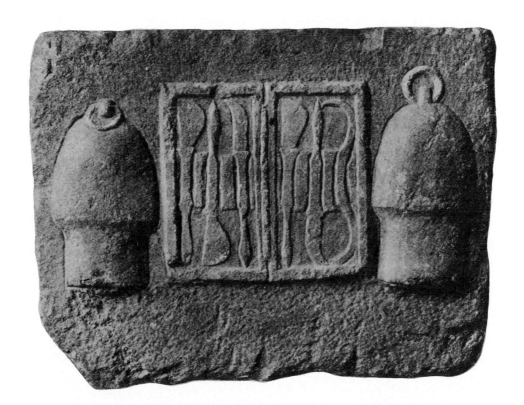

Bas-relief from Temple of Ascelipius ('Ασκληπιειον) depicting
Greek surgical tools and cupping vials. Note that these instruments
had dual purpose, with different surgical device at each end. (National Archaeological Museum, Athens.)

5

Office Surgical
Facility

The dermatologist performing surgery usually does so within the confines of an office or clinic. The widespread use of office-based surgery in dermatology has been essential for professional development and teaching, both within medical centers and within the community. Because dermatologists have traditionally performed and developed surgery in this setting, other specialists (particularly those who are hospital based) do not envision or comprehend the scope of dermatologic surgery. A lack of them in hospital operating rooms has led to the widespread erroneous belief that dermatologists have little to offer surgically. This is far from the truth. Dermatologists have performed surgery in their offices for years because long ago they realized that this is less expensive, provides better care, and is more convenient for both physician and patient without jeopardizing the safety and welfare of the latter. It is interesting to note that other specialists have recently come to realize the advantages of office-based surgery. During the last 10 years plastic surgeons, otolaryngologists, and ophthalmologists have shifted much of their surgery, previously performed within the confines of the hospital operating room, to their offices. This has led to the concept of "office-based surgery," which is currently undergoing definition and regulation, as well as the promulgation of certain standards. Dermatologists must familiarize themselves with these standards because they are integral to the goals of the overall health care team. Moreover, dermatologists must help establish these standards and demonstrate their qualifications to do so by showing the wide range of surgery they can perform in the office.

DEFINITIONS

Ambulatory surgery is surgery that does not require the patient to stay overnight in the hospital. Its procedures are relatively brief and require little assistance. Such surgery may be provided in one of three different facilities: an outpatient surgical center within a hospital, a "freestanding" surgical center (physically separate from a hospital), or a physician's office. Usually in the hospital or freestanding surgical center an anesthesiologist or anesthetist is present at all times to administer anesthesia or to provide help in event of an emergency. Indeed it was the anesthesiologists themselves who first established the concept of successful outpatient surgery under their control and jurisdiction.[6,16] One legal definition of an outpatient surgery center (in Arkansas) is "a facility in which surgical services are offered which require the use of general or intravenous anesthetics . . . ."[11] Usually the surgical procedures performed in these facilities are more complex than procedures in offices are, which are usually performed with local anesthetics. The widespread acceptance of such outpatient surgical facilities is underscored by the fact that 70% of all hospitals currently offer ambulatory surgical services.[3]

The pros and cons of hospitals versus freestanding surgical centers are discussed by Stetson.[44] Basically the major advantages of the hospital-based units are the emergency backup facilities and the availability of immediate admission to the hospital if necessary. Both types of facilities are well organized for obtaining financial remuneration from medical insurance companies and for marketing themselves to the public and physicians alike.[3,36]

Office-based surgery, on the other hand, is performed within a physician's office or clinic. It usually does not rely on the presence of an anesthesiologist, although some physicians advocate this.[2] Instead, the operating physician administers and maintains the anesthesia as well as performs the surgery. The safe administration of certain anesthetics may be performed by graduates of medical schools.[31] This dual role for the physician has resulted in greater responsibility and greater liability than that attached to performing surgery in the hospital, not only in terms of the surgery itself but also with respect to planning, staffing, and equipping the outpatient operating facility.[16] In addition to this, office surgical facilities frequently are not reimbursed by medical insurance carriers for the facility's overhead.[33]

HISTORY OF OFFICE-BASED SURGERY

In antiquity and during wars outpatient surgery was the norm. Hospital operating rooms were nonexistent, and common sense prevailed. During the earlier part of the twentieth century, extensive outpatient surgery was routinely performed outside the confines of hospitals.[22,35] Occasionally offices were set up and run by anesthesiologists, in which general anesthesia was given for surgical procedures.[50] The surgery performed was then termed "minor surgery,"[5,21,28] a term which has since fallen out of vogue.[23] With the emergence of hospital structures and the proliferation of teaching institutions associated with them, surgery was performed more and more in operating rooms. Both patients and physicians came to accept this as the norm, not necessarily liking it. However, because costs for hospitalization have climbed steadily since 1960, more and more surgery is performed in an outpatient environment. Initially, early reports of such surgery were from teaching institutions that adapted themselves for extensive outpatient surgery.[6,29] Then freestanding surgical centers arose in the early seventies.[16,38] Finally, extensive office-based surgery was reported and recommended, particularly for the cutaneous surfaces.* There is little doubt that office surgery will continue to grow in the future.

Literature on office surgery is scarce. The types of surgery appropriate for an office or clinic surgical facility versus the other types of ambulatory surgical facilities (hospital-based or freestanding) have not been well defined or established. Factors such as patient selection and extent of procedures are reported but are unclear and too few in number and type for a proper assessment of outcome in terms of patient satisfaction, complications, or costs.[10,48] For instance, should extensive full-thickness skin grafts be done in the office? Many cutaneous surgeons perform this procedure in the office setting without reporting any problems, but the data are lacking to assess fully the merits of such surgery. Some argue strongly against these grafts being performed in an outpatient setting,[8] whereas others feel comfortable with this approach.[51,52,53] Obviously interdisciplinary vested interests ("turf") are at stake. With a lack of firm data, however, no opinions can be confirmed.

Davis[9] discussed the current confusion over defining the types of surgical cases that are best performed in the office or outpatient ambulatory surgical unit (whether in the hospital or freestanding). He proposed that the distinction be made on the basis of necessity for postoperative care or observation. He defines operations not requiring such care as *minor ambulatory surgery.* These procedures can probably be performed safely in an office or clinic setting. *Major ambulatory surgery,* on the other hand, requires more extensive recovery room facilities such as those found in an ambulatory surgical unit. This categorization is in keeping with my concepts of performing surgery—for instance, small skin grafts or flaps—in the office, since these procedures usually do not require a recovery room.

RATIONALE OF OFFICE-BASED SURGERY
Personalized service

Office-based surgery offers personalized service and is tailored to the needs of the patients and the type of surgery performed. A physician's assistants can be trained exclusively for that physician's particular techniques and types of patients. The noninstitutional atmosphere fosters the concept of treating patients with compassion and ensuring their self-respect as well as privacy. Because such a unit is small, it allows those in charge to function freely and efficiently and thus become more effective in providing good patient care.

Office procedures commonly are taught in an institutional clinic setting with residents, interns, or medical students in attendance. Although this may entail more red tape for the patients, the physician performing and supervising the surgery should make every effort to provide the same service as that found within the community. Only by direct exposure to surgery in such a setting can tomorrow's practicing physicians be taught.

The rationale of office-based surgery is simple: to serve the patients and the community as well as possible. Patients are people and not items of medical merchandise. Their time is important, and their medical expenses should always be minimized, provided that their safety and welfare are not compromised.

Convenience

Performing surgery in the office is more convenient for patient and physician alike. This saves the physician the time it takes to go to the hospital and fill out unnecessary paperwork. Most patients, in my experience, do not wish to be in the hospital unless it is absolutely necessary; they prefer to be operated on as an outpatient and return home the same day. Therefore patient acceptance of this approach is high.

Cost

The high cost of performing surgery in the hospital has been the subject of national inquiry and debate. This is particularly true of minor procedures. It has been estimated that 40% of elective nonemergency surgery currently performed in the hospital operating room could just as easily and safely be performed in an outpatient setting.[40] Hospitals continue to make money by "overhead shifting," whereby the less expensive medical or surgical conditions help to pay for the most expensive procedures. Such accounting policies should become a device of the past, as more and more surgery is performed away from the hospital.

Cost is an important factor to health insurance carriers.

---

*References 23, 27, 32, 40, 41, 52.

In fact many private companies, as well as Medicare, currently encourage patients to have appropriate surgical procedures performed on an outpatient basis.[12] It is interesting to note that these same companies have been reluctant to reimburse physicians specifically for surgical office expenses, which otherwise would not be incurred by the physicians if the surgery were performed in the hospital or even in a freestanding surgical center.[33] Thus the cost savings to the insurance company is borne by the physician, who may in turn pass the added expense on to the patient. The insurance company—not the patient—is the big winner.

Cost by itself should not be a major consideration for performing surgery in the office or clinic. First, there is some doubt as to whether a properly equipped surgical facility is more cost effective than a hospital operating room.[1,45] However, no one doubts that the physicians in charge have more control over minimizing the costs for the patient. Most physicians report that costs are significantly less (up to 70% less) when surgery is performed in the office rather than a hospital operating room.[39,41] The second reason for minimizing the emphasis on potential cost savings is that this is probably of less importance to patients than previously emphasized. To quote Gurdin, "I have had many patients thank me for a good result, but no patient ever thanked me for saving him money."[8] Part of the reason for this is that the cost savings is really not to the patients but to the insurance carriers. A third reason for minimizing the cost factor is that the costs of office surgery are frequently borne by the physician as part of his all-inclusive fee. Therefore performing surgery in the office may actually cost the physician money by decreasing the amount realized from his fees when the increased overhead factor is taken into account.

Safety

The safe record of office surgery is attested to by a lack of recorded serious complications and by a number of reports showing no greater problems than if similar surgery is performed on an inpatient basis.[26,46] In fact, Natof[34] reported a low incidence of infection in outpatient surgery, which may be of extreme importance for the elderly, who are more susceptible to pneumonia and cross infection.

A low infection rate in outpatient surgery requires self-discipline, adherence to accepted standards of sterile technique, and common sense.[23,34] Reducing the problems with bleeding also requires meticulous control of small bleeding vessels.[46] Recuperation may also be faster and more pleasant for the patient in the familiar confines of his home. In addition, the continuous close contact between physician and patient in the office during and immediately after the procedure helps in the recognition of problems sooner and thus leads to faster attendance to them.

Most authorities attribute the low morbidity associated with outpatient surgery to careful patient selection and the type of procedure being performed.[6,37] Certainly if a patient is seriously ill, elective surgery is unwise. The presence of heart disease is not, however, a contraindication for a small amount of local anesthesia and a minor procedure. If the surgery will be extensive but necessary and the patient is elderly or medically in poor health, surgery is best provided on an inpatient basis in the hospital. I have rendered such services for patients in a hospital clinic setting while they remained inpatients. Such patients are more comfortable, are less stressed, and can be watched closely.

STANDARDS AND LIABILITY

The standards for office-based surgical facilities should include four broad areas: structural and equipment, personnel, patient selection and processing, and outcome. These broad areas are dealt with separately later in this chapter. The American Society for Dermatologic Surgery (ASDS) and the American Academy of Dermatology (AAD) currently do not address the issues of standards in office surgery. Other groups do, however, and include the Joint Commission on Accreditation of Hospitals (JCAH), the Accreditation Association for Ambulatory Health Care (AAAHC), and the American Association for Accreditation of Ambulatory Plastic Surgery Facilities (AAAAPSF).[3,36,49] The latter two groups arose in response to the proliferation of surgery being performed on an outpatient basis and the lack of standards that existed as late as 1976.[19] None of the three groups have any legal status. Furthermore, being accredited by one of these groups does not increase or decrease one's liability in an office surgical unit.[16] For those practicing dermatologic surgery in clinics within medical centers, the rules laid down by the JCAH may be brought to bear and should be reviewed and adapted as much as feasible. There are obvious differences among specialties which should, however, be taken into account, as should the community's standards of care.

The standards among surgeons for outpatient surgery were initiated by anesthesiologists.[6,16] Lund[31] proposed in 1963 that standard facilities include adequate sterilization equipment, a recovery room, adequate personnel (at least one R.N.), and resuscitation equipment. Williams[52] suggested the addition of equipment for monitoring heart rate and rhythm, such as a continuous ECG, and a cardiac defibrillator. In *Christopher's Minor Surgery* (1959),[35] a minor surgical room is depicted without CPR equipment but with a gooseneck lamp and an autoclave in the same room. Obviously the standard of care has evolved quickly and somewhat quietly over the last 25 years.

It is recommended that an informed consent be signed by the patient or a person legally responsible for the patient. This consent form should acknowledge some element of risk. In addition, the physician should provide a standard of care that is "reasonably prudent." Guidelines for preoperative and postoperative care should be developed. Pa-

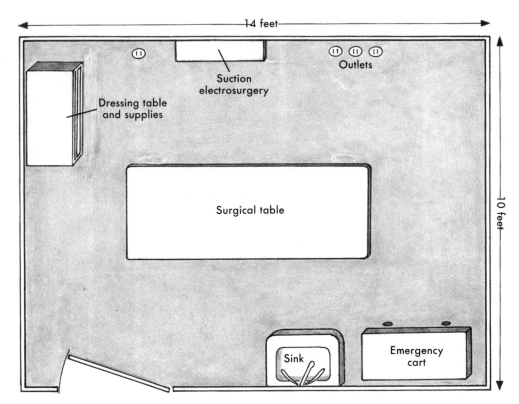

Fig. 5-1. Suggested floor plan for office operating room. Planning must be done in advance for proper number and placement of designated electrical outlets.

tients should be screened to make sure that the procedure is appropriate. History and physical examination forms should be individualized, and the responsible physicians should make certain that the patient is discharged in good condition. The interested reader may find it useful to review the legal issues involved.[4,15]

OFFICE SURGICAL FACILITY DESIGN

Cutaneous surgery requires special equipment and facilities so that both the patient and the physicians are more comfortable during the surgery. This contributes to a better surgical result. When planning an outpatient surgical facility, some forethought is therefore desirable. I have found that a well-chosen interior designer with an architectural background is worth the added expense for achieving a warm and friendly decor in which to provide surgical services. The office staff should be consulted on this subject; it frequently is of great assistance.

It is extremely helpful to visit other physicians' offices in which outpatient surgery is performed. Not only does this give one ideas from which to begin planning, but one can learn by others' mistakes as well as their successes. There are a few good sources of information. I highly recommend the *Symposium on Office Surgery,* edited by Courtiss,[7] as well as *Outpatient Surgery* edited by Schultz.[40] *Outpatient Surgery,* edited by Hill,[24] may also be useful but concerns

itself more with outpatient surgery units associated with emergency departments or hospitals.

If one contemplates performing only minor procedures in the office or clinic, then a simple operating room may be all that is needed. However, for longer procedures of a more complex nature (such as large skin flaps), it may be necessary to consider incorporating a recovery room, a nurse's station, a separate clean-up and sterilization area, and a storage room.

Operating room

The minimal size of a room in which one may adequately and comfortably perform cutaneous surgery is 10 by 14 feet (Fig. 5-1). Smaller examination rooms (the standard size is 8 by 10 feet) tend to become rather cramped. When one considers that there will be at least one assistant, the heat generated from 3 bodies (patient, physician, and assistant) over a period of time will become noticeable. Add medical students or residents to this, and the atmosphere becomes stuffy, overcrowded, and unpleasant for all concerned. Also, as one becomes more sophisticated surgically, more equipment may be moved in, so that having a large room will be useful.

The JCAH specifies that operating rooms in hospital facilities should be at least 18 by 18 feet, in part because general anesthesia is rendered, which usually is not done in most dermatologic surgical procedures. Elliot[13] recommends an operating room of at least 250 square feet for larger procedures and a minor operating room size of 160 square feet. However, in his diagram of the latter, if one subtracts the nurses' station, the usable floor space becomes approximately 120 square feet. In a later paper[14] Elliot suggests a larger operating room: 316 to 324 square feet. Other authors suggest room sizes as small as 72 square feet,[28] 150 square feet,[46] 207 square feet,[41] 270 square feet,[47] and 361 square feet.[37] Obviously the issue of space is far from settled and should in part depend on the type of surgery contemplated, the type of anesthesia used, and the availability of space.

One of the main considerations when planning operating room size is easy access to the patient. Therefore the table should be situated roughly in the middle of the room with adequate space on all sides to perform surgery easily or to take care of any unforeseen emergency. Should an extreme emergency arise, the room should be large enough to accommodate a stretcher (not a walker-style stretcher). The doorway needs to be at least 36 inches wide to accommodate a stretcher or wheelchair comfortably. The exit route of a stretcher should be considered, as should emergency exits. The hallways should be wide enough (probably 5 feet) to accomodate such traffic.

The operating room ideally should be situated in an isolated low-traffic area of the office or clinic. There should be only one doorway to the room, to enhance sterility and eliminate patient exposure to threatening sights and sounds, thus enhancing a feeling of warmth and reassurance. The presence of noise and busy office congestion is disturbing to patient and physician alike. Solid doors and music help eliminate extraneous noise. I prefer a portable radio for selecting music that both patient and physician can enjoy.

The floors should be smooth linoleum tile, and the walls covered by vinyl, since this is easiest to clean. Ceramic tile is expensive and more difficult to maintain. Electrical outlets should be plentiful and situated by taking into account the type and placement of electrical equipment one uses at any one time. I have found it useful to have at least one electrical outlet at waist height to plug in a camera flash (to eliminate stooping). Also, floor outlets may be installed for power tables, but such outlets are somewhat expensive. Power tables themselves frequently are manufactured with outlets that can be useful. All outlets should be three-pronged and self-grounded. Most surgical equipment is 110 V, 60 cps (cycles per second). Many buildings have electrical codes that regulate the number of outlets allowed to accommodate equipment. A good space planner or architect can be very helpful in designing a functional operating room that conforms to these requirements.

Fig. 5-2 shows our surgical operating room. Note that an overhead track light is mounted on the ceiling and that custom-designed storage space and instrument racks are built in. This helps to maximize the available floor space.

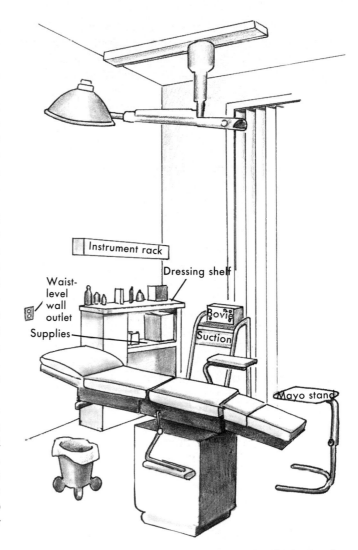

Fig. 5-2. Dermatologic surgical room. One wall socket is placed at waist level for plug from camera flash unit. Not shown in this illustration are emergency cart, monitoring equipment, and scrub sink.

Storage cabinets should be covered with Formica (laminated plastic), which is cheaper than steel and easier to clean. My storage space is open shelving, to which some may object. However, it eliminates the need to keep opening cabinets and allows readier access to materials; because of the rapid turnover of supplies it does not, in my opinion, compromise sterility. The top of our storage space doubles as a dressing table.

The cabinetry should be placed in a readily accessible position. Note that I have placed the dressing table, instrument rack, and suture rack all within an arm's length of the patient. This enhances efficiency. The instrument rack particularly has been of great benefit. I have this rack divided into six separate compartments. In each compartment the different types of instruments are placed standing straight up in individual sterilization bags.

The ceiling construction and background lighting in the ceiling should be considered. Usually building codes take care of these details. Fire-resistant materials are recommended. Fluorescent lighting is usually standard, but "more natural daylight" fluorescent lights may be specially ordered. The light in the surgery room may be further enhanced by additional banks of fluorescent lighting beyond the standard lighting of the building. A sprinkler system and smoke detector can also be added to the ceiling.

It is desirable to have a separate temperature control in the operating room, so that one may keep the temperature at about 68° F in all seasons—comfortable for both patient and surgeon during lengthy procedures. In addition, an exhaust system is advisable, particularly where the smoke odor from extensive use of the electrosurgical apparatus is offensive. Laminar air-flow systems are not of proven value in an office surgery setting and therefore are not necessary.

A sink should be installed in the surgical room so that physicians can wash their hands before and perhaps after surgery. A wall-mounted soap dispenser with a foot control and foot controls on the sink are ideal. The hand-washing sink may also be placed immediately outside the surgical room if the room has a swinging door.

A phone should be placed not in the operating room but immediately adjacent to it for convenience. This promotes privacy for all concerned and a relaxed, nondisruptive atmosphere for the patient. Dictating equipment is also necessary and is most conveniently placed near the operating room.

A fire extinguisher should be kept outside the operating room and be easily accessible.

Nurse's station

One may wish to add a nurse's station to an office if the office is used mainly for surgical practice. I find it convenient to use the check-in counter of the office to double as a nurse's station. From this vantage point the nurse has full view of all operating rooms. This point is the hub of the surgical facilities and is essential for patient surveillance and communication. In addition, patient records are maintained in this area, and all important forms, including the surgical log, are kept here. This space may also have a full view of the waiting room should any problems arise there. It is also best that a double-locked box for narcotic storage be kept out of view in the nurse's station.

Recovery room

Although a designated recovery room is not usually necessary, on occasion it is useful. A recovery room becomes a necessity if one uses intravenous sedation or general anesthesia. If one has a separate designated recovery room, there must be some form of communication device, such as a call button, to enable the patient to reach the nursing or physician staff.

Bathroom facilities

Convenient bathroom facilities should be available in the office for patients, preferably close to the operating facility or recovery area.

Preparation and clean-up room

A separate room for cleaning, packing, and sterilizing instruments or other surgical materials is desirable. It should be situated in an isolated area of the office or clinic. Such a room should have a stainless steel double sink for washing materials and ample storage cabinets as well as counterspace. It is desirable to have custom-built cabinets in this preparation area with recessed lighting over the countertops for easier visibility. The built-in cabinets can be used to store sterile equipment and supplies.

One may consider purchasing a washer-dryer unit for washing surgical scrub suits and towels. Although this is said to save money, my experience has been that inexpensive laundry services are available and that the nurse's primary responsibility is patient care rather than the laundry.

Storage room

A separate storage room with liberal cabinet space is also good to have, since this allows one to buy in bulk, which saves money for expensive surgical items such as gauze, gloves, and suture material. The last is extremely important to stock because when one orders it on an emergency basis, the price goes up markedly.

SURGICAL OFFICE EQUIPMENT

Surgical office equipment is a significant monetary investment. Efficient equipment, however, makes life easier, so initial cost should not deter one from purchasing top-quality merchandise. All equipment should be well-designed and made from materials that are stain resistant and easy to clean. Stainless steel is desirable, when possible, because it resists corrosion.

On delivery one should thoroughly test the surgical equipment to make sure it is in proper working order. Any brochures, operation manuals, maintenance instructions, and warranty agreements should be filed for future reference. One should follow the manufacturers' suggestions regarding routine maintenance, testing, and calibration.

Surgical lights

Surgical lights are extremely important; one should buy the best lights available, depending on the extent of one's surgical practice. The many variables to consider when purchasing lights are listed as follows, and are shown schematically in Fig. 5-3.

Considerations	*Related factors*
Intensity of light	Type of bulb
	Filter

Heat produced	Type of bulb
	Filter
	Venting
	Reflective lighting
Shadows, glare	Reflective lighting
Color correction	Filter
Field size, focused depth of field, focal point	Reflective dish diameter and shape (concavity)
	Ability to focus
Maneuverability, range of motion	Mounting
	Track or nontrack
	Counterbalancing
	Handles
Cost	Dish size
	New or used

The intensity of the light, usually expressed in footcandles, is related to the type of bulb and any filters the light passes through. Small operating lights are in the range of 3000 footcandles, whereas larger lights approach 8000 footcandles.

The *heat* produced is related not only to the type of bulb but also to the filters and ventilation provided; also, reflected light is not as hot as direct light. Some companies incorporate heat-absorbing materials into the reflective sur-

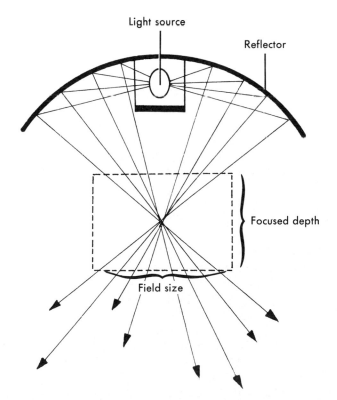

Fig. 5-3. Production of light from a surgical lamp. Note that width of field depends on reflective dish diameter.

faces. Heat can be an important factor in lengthy procedures. Smaller lights (those with a dish diameter of 12 inches or less) produce considerable heat compared with larger lights (with 18- to 24-inch dish diameters).

Shadows are minimized by reflective lighting, which also cuts down on glare. Usually filters are added for color correction, giving tissues a more natural appearance and allowing one to record on film a more natural appearance.

Perhaps the most important considerations are the field size and the focused depth of field provided by any light source. Both of these factors are related to the reflective dish diameter and shape. As can be seen in Fig. 5-3, as the dish diameter is decreased (assuming that the same concavity is maintained), the field size also decreases. The focused depth of field and focal point, on the other hand, are mostly related to the degree of the dish's concavity. Some lights have a focusing knob whereby one may sharpen the intensity of light within the depth of field by bringing (with convergence) more rays together into one area.

The range of motion for a light is related to its mounting (floor, wall, or ceiling) and, if on the ceiling, whether it is track or nontrack mounted. Track lighting offers the greatest range of motion (360 degrees) and is the more useful. However, it requires special structural steel supports (beams) to accommodate the weight and to provide stability. The installation of these supports alone may be expensive. Mobile floor lighting takes up precious floor space and is thus inconvenient and not very efficient. Wall-mounted lights in general do not allow easy access to patients. A ceiling-mounted light without a track is acceptable but offers a range of motion of only about 300 degrees; moreover, nontrack lights are poorly maneuverable. Most maneuverable are the track lights, because they are counterbalanced. Handles, which may be sterilized, may also be purchased for many types of ceiling lights.

Some companies offer ceiling-mounted lights in pairs. I have not found this to be useful in dermatologic surgery, particularly when working around the face. One of the two lights may shine in the patient's eyes, and there is double the trouble with maneuverability.

Cost may be an overriding consideration. A market exists for used medical equipment, particularly surgical lights, tables, and sterilizers. Bargains can be found for a fraction of their list price. If cost is a major consideration, contact should be made with a broker in used medical equipment.

I have found it most convenient to have a rheostat mounted on the wall for turning the surgical light on and off. Be sure the rheostat can be turned on and off by a push of the knob as well as by rotation.

Under some circumstances—during work on deep recesses, such as the ear canal or nasal vestibule—a fiberoptic headlight may be extremely useful. For everyday use I have found them to be heavy.

Surgical tables

The best way to discover the value of a surgical table one wishes to purchase is to lie on it. This gives some idea of the comfort of the surface pads and their contour, which are important to the patient under local anesthesia during longer procedures. Basic considerations other than cost are the overall dimensions of the table, the ease of adjustability, and the probability of breakdown.

The dimensions of the table should be taken into account during the planning of a surgery room. The wider the table is, the less usable floor space there will be in the room. The patient is less accessible on a wider table. Some argue that large patients are more comfortable on wider tables and that it is easier to operate on their hands on such tables; I have found that the narrower tables are adequate and the saving of floor space they allow is crucial. Some power tables move not simply straight up and down but also forward while going up (Dextra Corp.). These tables cut down on the available floor space and make it inconvenient to work around the head of the patient.

One should consider the positioning of the surgical table within the room and where the outlet should be placed if one is using a power table. Although it is more expensive, an electrical outlet on the floor may be installed to keep the table's electrical cords out of the way during surgery.

The base of the table should be weighted to prevent slipping during surgery. Instead of a stationary base, a base with rollers may be ordered, which helps the staff to clean underneath the table. One can also more easily change the table's position—to accommodate a stretcher for instance. However, rollers raise the height of the table and thus may inconvenience elderly patients. I have not found the addition of rollers to be a necessity. A swivel base is a good modification if rollers are not present. It allows one more easily to bring parts of the patient's anatomy closer to any fixed equipment, such as a light or electrosurgical apparatus. Like the rollers, this feature also helps to make more room to accommodate a stretcher.

Adjustability is probably the most important consideration when one buys a surgical table. The physician should try operating the table. Tables of a fixed height are inadequate for dermatologic surgery; power tables with foot-operated controls are the most desirable. Although most tables are fully electric, some are hydraulic. The latter are smoother in operation and faster moving up and down. When operating a table, note the speed and smoothness with which it moves up and down (these vary between brands of surgical tables). If one continually uses the table—several times a day in a busy practice—speed becomes an important factor.

The highest and lowest positions to which a power table moves should be considered but are fairly standard. The lowest position is important for ease of the patient getting onto the table. The highest position is important to the surgeon. Factors such as the height of the surgeon and the surgeon's usual position during surgery should be taken into account. Obviously tables of a fixed height are less convenient for patient and surgeon alike.

Adjustability of the backrest and tilt are important considerations also. Occasionally patients with cardiopulmonary disease or orthopedic problems have a problem lying flat. One should therefore easily be able to elevate separately the head of the table with the patient lying flat. It is a good idea to have a few pillows on which patients may elevate their heads while lying flat. The table should be capable of easy adjustment into the Trendelenburg position in case a patient becomes faint.

Headrest size may or may not be specially ordered with certain surgical tables. However, the headrest size should be considered. For working around the head I recommend a relatively small headrest (but not an occipital headrest) that gives all members of the surgical team good accessibility to the patient.

Surgical tables can be ordered with various accessories. Cushion color may be selected to blend with the overall decor of the operating room. Armrests are very useful; they may be locked in the upright position when the patient lies flat. This helps patients to orient themselves to the edge of the table and keeps the senile patient from rolling off onto the floor. Straps may also be used for this purpose. Other accessories that can be ordered include attachable Mayo stands, arm boards, and stirrups.

Cost is a factor for surgical tables as well as surgical lights. The same rules apply: buy good quality equipment and save your back.

Hemostasis equipment

A fuller discussion of equipment to stop bleeding is found in Chapter 16. The main consideration in judging which equipment to buy is to know what procedures will be performed. Electrosurgical apparatuses vary with respect to power output and therefore with respect to their ability to stop bleeding. Most machines made for dermatologists (Hyfrecator) do not generate enough heat in tissue quickly to stop bleeding and tend to be destructive. Solid-state units tend to require less maintenance than the spark-gap equipment. I find it more useful to have this equipment mobile rather than fixed to the wall, although the latter saves space. Disposable electrode tips (Concept Corp., Clearwater, Fla.) and handpieces may be useful in aseptic procedures.

Suction machine

A good suction machine is indispensible during cutaneous surgery. There are many reliable models on the market, all of which do an adequate job. The suction unit should be an adjustable electrical vacuum pump capable of producing a negative suction of 40 to 60 cm Hg and have an easily cleanable trap. The suction machine may be mobile so that it can be easily brought to the patient. Flexible disposable tubing with a glass eyedropper tip is useful in cutaneous surgery. Wall-mounted suction outlets connected to a central suction unit will conserve floor space, but this is quite costly. However, the remote location of the central suction unit eliminates noise, the most bothersome feature of portable suction machines.

Instrument table

When performing surgery, one needs a nearby table on which to place instruments and other surgical supplies. A mobile Mayo stand is most convenient for this purpose; one can position the table at various heights and positions to be suitable for the surgery being performed. Mayo stands can be ordered in various sizes; some have a convenient foot control. Alternatively, one can use a built-in table top near the head of the patient; however, unless one is operating mainly on the head and neck, this may prove to be inconvenient.

Dressing table

A cabinet should be specially designated as a dressing table (Fig. 5-2). This is very useful when putting the final dressing on patients. A stainless steel metal cart with a drawer is adequate, or one could have this space as part of built-in cabinetry. The contents of the dressing table are listed on p. 340.

Anesthetic equipment

Most cutaneous surgery is performed on an outpatient basis with local anesthetics; general anesthetics are rarely used. However, nitrous oxide or methoxyflurane (pentrane) may be administered safely by the nonanesthesiologist and is becoming more widely used. Those who contemplate using nitrous oxide frequently may wish to modify the surgical facility to accommodate the special lines that need to be installed (see Chapter 6).

Monitoring equipment

Some physicians emphasize the need for monitoring equipment, even when local anesthesia is being used,[20,52] and particularly if the patient is given diazepam (Valium) intravenously or meperidine (Demerol).[42] Such equipment monitors the heart rate, respiratory rate, and blood pressure and provides a continuous ECG. These data can be provided in a digital mode, and the ECG can be visualized on an oscilloscope with a built-in recorder. The necessity of such equipment depends on the types of medical and surgical procedures one is doing, the amount of medications one uses, and the type of anesthesia one employs. Certainly for minor procedures on young patients, such monitoring equipment is unnecessary. For heavily premedicated elderly patients in poor health undergoing a lengthy operation, however, such equipment is desirable.

Monitoring equipment is costly, and most data that can be recorded or seen on it can be ascertained by routine methods; nevertheless, monitoring equipment is more convenient and less subject to human error.

Resuscitation equipment

A properly equipped emergency cart or kit should be available in case a patient has a cardiopulmonary arrest or life-threatening drug reaction. The fact that office emergencies happen so infrequently makes it very difficult to prepare for them. It is prudent for all office personnel to take a course in cardiopulmonary resuscitation (CPR) Advanced Life Support Systems course and to have a clear idea of the procedure to follow in case of emergency.[30] One needs not only the equipment but a staff properly drilled in its use. Each office should have a plan to get patients to the hospital should the need arise. The guidelines for cardiopulmonary resuscitation (CPR) and emergency cardiac care (ECC) should be reviewed on a yearly basis.[43] Although older textbooks, for instance *Christopher's Minor Surgery,*[35] do not discuss emergency care or equipment, the modern standard of care mandates the availability of such equipment.

A list of suggested emergency equipment is found in Appendix F. Emergency equipment kits can be purchased commercially and have an adequate number of drugs. However, some of these kits have only one ampule of sodium bicarbonate and may not have any IV solutions or oxygen. Additional supplies may therefore need to be purchased to supplement the basic unit.

Some physicians purchase a red tool cart, which works well as an emergency cart. It is sturdy, inexpensive, mobile, and easily visible. The basic components of this cart should be emergency drugs, an Ambu bag with intubation equipment, oxygen, and cardioversion equipment (defibrillator). The latter may be bought in conjunction with the monitoring equipment mentioned previously.

Sterilizing equipment

Sterilizing equipment should be kept in an area separate from the surgical operating room. It should be of sufficient capacity and quality for the anticipated needs. Table-top models are available, which are adequate for small packs and individually packed instruments. The reliability and servicing of this equipment are important. I do not recommend a used steam sterilizer, since the steam lines may be corroded from misuse, leading to instruments' damage. Steam sterilizers and ultrasonic machines are discussed more fully in Chapter 7. Cold sterilizing solutions are inappropriate for modern office surgical facilities.

Newer table-top gas sterilizers are also available, which are good for plastics or rubber. An inexpensive, convenient method of gas sterilization for the office is the Anprolene Sterilizer System (H.W. Anderson Products Inc., Oyster Bay, N.Y. 11771) described by Glogau.[18]

Miscellaneous equipment

Waste containers may be ordered to match the decor. A kick wastebucket with wheels is particularly useful (Fig. 5-2) for surgery because it is easily moved and convenient. Other accessories that may be useful are stools and platforms for members of the surgical team. For possible electrical power failures a back-up portable power source may be worth considering, particularly if the surgical facility has no outside source of light. A wheelchair and stretcher should also be accessible. A hand mirror kept in a drawer is useful for showing patients their wounds and demonstrating how to apply dressings. I prefer this to a mirror on the wall, which the patient may glance at while the nurse or physician is absent and find upsetting.

SURGICAL SUPPLIES

A checklist of surgical supplies is given in Appendix C. An inventory catalogue should be developed that lists the manufacturer, the supplier, the quantity per case, and the unit cost per item. Comparison of unit costs is necessary to lower the overall cost of surgical supplies, which may be considerable, and to justify adjustment of charges. The inventory list should be looked at on a weekly basis.

Most of the surgical supplies are discussed in other chapters. One item worthy of mention here pertains to laundry. Usually an inexpensive laundry service is obtainable in larger cities for surgical drapes, pillow cases, and other surgical apparel. If this is not available, disposable items should be considered. Some physicians recommend a small washer-dryer unit in the office for doing one's own laundry.

PERSONNEL

The staff in an office or clinic is extremely important when surgery is to be performed. The person scheduling patients for surgery should know the basic surgery to be performed to allay the patient's fears and answer any questions. The completeness and manner with which the staff communicates with the patient and family regarding treatment and the patient's condition are important.

A procedure manual that describes the functions and job descriptions of all office or clinic personnel as well as office or clinic policies should be compiled. Also included would be instructions in case of emergencies such as fire or cardiopulmonary arrest.[17] This manual should be updated yearly.

The professional staff members should be encouraged to attend postgraduate educational programs of relevance to their jobs. It is essential that all office personnel have at least biannual CPR instruction, which is offered by most hospitals. If possible, hospital privileges for nursing personnel are desirable so that continuity of the patients' care is facilitated. Physicians in an office setting are less and less inclined to hire registered nurses to perform nursing duties during surgery because their salaries are relatively high.

Instead, licensed practical nurses, operating room technicians, and even partially trained unlicensed individuals are used. When these latter are employed it is wise to remember that the physician's liability increases if injury occurs caused by negligence, because a defense citing professional standards of the R.N. cannot be used.[15]

OTHER CONSIDERATIONS
Emergency situations

The office or clinic staff should be drilled for emergency situations; these should be covered in the procedure manual. Phone numbers of the fire and police departments and the hospital emergency room should be nearby. Routes and equipment (stretchers) for rapid evacuation of patients and personnel should be worked out in advance.

Safety precautions

Smoking should not be permitted in the outpatient operating facility or clinic. Electrical outlets should be grounded and not overloaded. If gases such as nitrous oxide are used, the safety precautions regarding their use should be discussed among the personnel and observed. Special containers for sharp needles or surgical blades should be present to minimize injury to the staff or clean-up personnel. Fire extinguishers and other emergency equipment should be present; the staff should know their locations and be drilled in their use.

Waste disposal

Contaminated supplies and tissues should be kept in closed containers (plastic bags) and removed from the office daily. Red disposable bags are particularly visible and will alert the clean-up personnel that the contents include tissue or other potential contaminants.

Medications

All controlled substances should be kept in an inconspicuous place—preferably in a wall-mounted double-locked medication box. There should also be an accounting of all medications dispensed, which should include the date, patient's name, amount dispensed or amount destroyed, and signature of the staff member. Prescriptions for controlled substances should be locked up.

RECORDS

Records for surgery include the patient chart as well as the surgery log (see Appendix E). The patient chart should include a history and physical examination, consent for surgery and photographs, operative reports, and evaluation of the surgery performed. The history and physical examination form should be individualized as much as possible. Specific, written preoperative and postoperative instructions are desirable, and if they are given to the patient, they should be noted in the patient's record.

The surgery log is a frequently overlooked but extremely important item. At the very least this log should list the date of surgery, patient's name and age, pre- and postoperative diagnoses, names of the surgical team members, length of time the procedure took, anesthetic used, condition of the patient on discharge, and finally any drains or complications. The log is a good source for the office or clinic personnel to assess operative reports and billings as well as to follow up on the patients. It also serves as an official legal document should problems occur in the future. An additional reason for the surgical log is that it allows one to keep accurate records of the type and number of procedures being performed. This may be useful in future renovations or justifications for renovation of the surgical facility.

Short-term follow-up examinations

At the time of discharge from the office or clinic, written instructions should be given to the patient regarding care of the surgical wound. These instructions should include a telephone number for reaching the physician or a staff member in the event of an emergency. It is also good for the nurse or physician to contact the patient the day after surgery to see how he or she is feeling. Such concern is appreciated by patients and adds to the quality of care provided.

Long-term follow-up examinations

Each office or clinic performing surgery should have a recall system to assess the long-term results of surgery. This becomes particularly important if the surgery was performed on a cutaneous neoplasm. Many patients deny the recurrence of skin cancers, so all patients treated for skin cancers should be evaluated yearly for 5 to 10 years after treatment. Recall cards are very useful and should be sent to the patient who does not return for a follow-up examination.

ECONOMICS OF OFFICE SURGERY

Performing many surgical procedures in the office or out-patient clinic increases the overhead expenses. However, since one increases the billings as a result of the surgery performed, the overall profit should increase as well (Profit = Collection − Expenses).

The reimbursement from insurance companies for the overhead costs of performing surgery in the office has been the subject of recent discussion, particularly in the field of plastic surgery.[3,12,25,33] It is interesting to note that the various formulas proposed for estimating the overhead costs do not take into account such factors as the savings of physician's time and the actual ownership of equipment. The consensus among physicians is that the increased costs of performing surgery in the office should not be borne by the physician, but rather the patient[1,25] or insurance company.[12] Physicians argue that since they are saving the insurance companies money, the savings should be passed back to the physicians.

Although it is generally believed that performing surgery in the office saves money for all concerned,[2] this has not been confirmed by all physicians critically looking at this issue.[1,45] Probably the simpler the procedure that is done in the office and which might have been done in the hospital operating room, the larger are the savings. As one does more complex procedures requiring more personnel, supplies, and equipment, the savings decrease. Insurance carriers have been reluctant to pay a facility fee for office surgery,[33] although if one fulfills certain guidelines and requirements one may be able to get such payment.[3,12] Certainly the increased costs to meet these rules may in themselves be prohibitive. One should inquire about such payment from the larger insurance companies with whom one does business. The reimbursement rules vary widely from state to state and even, in some states, from city to city.

The charges for use of an office surgical facility vary widely among physicians but average around $35 to $40 for a simple, small procedure and $60 to $75 for a more difficult operation.[32,45,47] As a rule of thumb, a dollar a minute was a reasonable charge in 1978. This fee includes surgical supplies, use of the operating facility, and personnel costs.

Kaye and Kaye[25] have extensively and meticulously estimated the cost of performing surgery in the office. They point out that the total cost is actually the sum of three factors: direct costs, labor, and overhead. Direct costs are the supplies actually used for the surgery. Labor costs are the salaries necessary for nursing personnel and other assistants. Overhead is calculated by multiplying the indirect costs of running the office (rent, office supplies, and so on) by the operating room area expressed as a percentage of the total floor space for the office divided by the number of hours of use of the operating room per year as expressed a percentage of the total office hours per year. Thus

$$\text{Total cost} = \text{Direct cost} + \text{Labor cost} + \text{Indirect cost}$$
$$\times \frac{\% \text{ Operating room area (sq. ft.)}}{\% \text{ Operating room use (hrs/yr)}}$$

Based on this formula* a simple lesion excision in 1981 resulted in a facility charge of $92.00, whereas a hair transplant was $256.00.

Dermatologic surgeons would do well to review the assessment of charges for an outpatient surgical facility in the plastic surgery literature. However, since most dermatologists often perform procedures much less extensive than those performed by the plastic surgeons, such comparisons are of limited usefulness. Still, there is much overlap in the types of procedures performed.

---

*This formula assumes that the operating room is not used for other (nonsurgical) purposes, such as follow-up visits or suture removal. If the room is used for these other purposes, the indirect cost is multiplied by both the operating room area (% total office floor space) and the operating room use for surgery (% total use for surgery) and nonsurgery.

Personally I feel that a reasonable charge should be made for sterile surgical supplies if the surgery is more extensive than a skin biopsy. One may wish to adjust the tray and supply charge to suit the operation. Many insurances do not pay this charge specifically but include it in the all-inclusive fee.[38] In other words, if one charges less than the allowable charge for a procedure and adds in addition a charge for surgery tray and supplies, the insurance company will pay up to the allowable amount, including payment for the surgical tray and supply charge. If the charge for surgery alone is more than the allowable amount, however, no tray and supply charge will be paid.

SUMMARY

The surgery being performed by dermatologists in both office and clinic settings is increasing in volume and extent. This development has brought with it the need for standards in this area to provide cost-effective care without compromising the safety or welfare of the patient.

Dermatologists perform many types of surgery that differ from those of other surgical subspecialists although much overlap exists. This has given rise to specific instrumentation, equipment, and facilities most suitable for this specialty. The rules governing dermatologists thus must arise from within their own specialty, yet be reasonably compatible with those of other surgical specialties.

As more experience is gained in surgery, dermatology will undoubtedly make its mark in the growing area of office surgery and contribute its share of research to surgical knowledge. The result will undoubtedly be better patient care.

REFERENCES

1. Barker, D.E.: Costs and charges for use of office operating, Plast. Reconstr. Surg. **57**:7, 1976.
2. Bloomenstein, R., et al.: Cost containment and safety for office surgery, J. Med. Soc. N.J. **78**(3):213, 1981.
3. Burns, L.A.: Ambulatory surgery: developing and managing successful programs, Rockville, Md., 1984, Aspen Systems Corp.
4. Caniff, C.E., Jr.: Legal aspects. In Schultz, R.C., editor: outpatient surgery, Philadelphia, 1979, Lea & Febiger.
5. Christopher, F.: Minor surgery, ed. 6, Philadelphia, 1948, W.B. Saunders Co.
6. Cohen, D., and Dillon, J.B.: Anesthesia for outpatient surgery, J.A.M.A. **196**:1114, 1966.
7. Courtiss, E.H., editor: Symposium on office surgery, Clin. Plast. Surg. **10**(2):221, 1983.
8. Davis, G.M.: Office surgery and the pursuit of excellence (editorial), Plast. Reconstr. Surg. **54**:345, 1974.
9. Davis, J.E.: The need to redefine levels of surgical care, J.A.M.A. **251**:2527, 1984.
10. Detmer, D.E., and Buchanan-Davidson, D.J.: Ambulatory surgery, Surg. Clin. North Am. **62**:685, 1982.
11. Division of Hospitals and Nursing Home Act, Arkansas Statutes Annotated Title 82§328(p.), 1975.
12. Edwards, B.J.: Insurers' policies for reimbursement boost day surgery, AORN J. **38**:582, 1983.
13. Elliot, R.A., Jr.: Organization and efficient function of office surgery. In Schultz, R.C., editor: Outpatient surgery, Philadelphia, 1979, Lea & Febiger.
14. Elliot, R.A., Jr., and Hoehn, J.G.: The office surgery suite: the physical plant and equipment, Clin. Plast. Surg. **10**(2): 225, 1983.
15. Epstein, L.I.: The surgeon's liability in office surgery, Clin. Plast. Surg. **10**(2):247, 1983.
16. Ford, J., and Reed, W.: The surgicenter, Ariz. Med. **26**:801, 1969.
17. Gilbert, D.A., and Adamson, J.E.: Procedure manuals in office surgery, Clin. Plast. Surg. **10**(2):269, 1983.
18. Glogau, R.G.: New office equipment. In Callen, J.P., editor: Current issues in dermatology, vol. 1, Boston, 1984, G.K. Hall Medical Publications.
19. Goran, M.J., and Donaldson, M.C.: Ambulatory surgery standards needed, Hosp. Prog. **57**(8):47, 1976.
20. Grande, D., Koranda, F.C., and Guthrie, D.: Monitoring respirations for outpatient surgery, J. Dermatol. Surg. Oncol. **9**:338, 1983.
21. Heath, C.: A manual of minor surgery and bandaging for the use of house surgeons, dressers and junior practitioners, eds. 1-20, Philadelphia, 1861-1930, Blakiston and F.A. Owens Co. (Late editions by G. Williams.)
22. Hertzler, A.E., and Chesky, V.E.: Surgery of a general practice, St. Louis, 1934, The C.V. Mosby Co.
23. Hill, G.J., II: Outpatient surgery—what are the indications for it? (editorial) Surgery **77**:333, 1975.
24. Hill, G.J., II, editor: Outpatient surgery, Philadelphia, 1980, W.B. Saunders Co.
25. Kaye, J.B., and Kaye, B.L.: The economics of office surgical practice, Clin. Plast. Surg. **10**(2):257, 1983.
26. Klein, D.R., and Rosenberg, A.: A comparison of complications between in-hospital patients and outpatients for aesthetic surgical procedures: a ten-year study, Plast. Reconstr. Surg. **67**:17, 1981.
27. Kopf, A., and Baer, R.: Yearbook of dermatology: dermatologic office surgery, Chicago, 1964, Yearbook Medical Publishers.
28. Kyle, D.: Minor surgery, London, 1968, Butterworths.
29. Levy, M., and Coakley, C.S.: Survey of in and out surgery: first year, South. Med. J. **61**:995, 1968.
30. Lewis, C.M.: For your peace of mind (letter), Plast. Reconstr. Surg. **65**:696, 1980.
31. Lund, P.C.: Anesthesia for minor surgery in the office or outpatient department, Ariz. Med. **20**:103, 1963.
32. Markle, G.B., IV: The case for doing more office surgery, Med. Econ. **51**:75, 1974.
33. Markovits, A.S.: Health insurers won't let us save them money, Med. Econ. **54**(1):227, 1977.
34. Natof, H.E.: Complications associated with ambulatory surgery, J.A.M.A. **224**:1116, 1980.
35. Ochsner, A., DeBakey, M.E., editors: Christopher's minor surgery, ed. 8, Philadelphia, 1959, W.B. Saunders Co.
36. Palmer, P.N.: Ambulatory surgery means business, AORN J. **38**:470, 1983.
37. Porterfield, H.W., et al.: Ten year's experience with outpatient office surgery, Ohio State Med. J. **73**(2):63, 1977.

38. Reed, W.A., and Williams, R.C: Unique financial considerations. In Schultz, R.C., editor: Outpatient surgery, Philadelphia, 1979, Lea & Febiger.

39. Saltzstein, E.C., et al.: Ambulatory surgical unit: alternative to hospitalization, Arch. Surg. **108:**143, 1974.

40. Schultz, R.C., editor: Outpatient surgery, Philadelphia, 1979, Lea & Febiger.

41. Simons, R.L.: The office surgical suite: pros and cons, Otolaryngol. Clin. North Am. **13:**391, 1980.

42. Singer, R., et al.: Rhytidectomies in office operating rooms, Plast. Reconstr. Surg. **63**(2):173, 1979.

43. Standards and guidelines for cardiopulmonary resuscitation (CPR) and emergency cardiac care (ECC), J.A.M.A. **244:** 453, 1980.

44. Stetson, P.A.: Ambulatory surgery: hospital affiliated or free-standing units—which are best? AORN J. **38:**1049, 1983.

45. Terino, E.O.: A cost analysis of office plastic surgery, Plast. Reconstr. Surg. **63:**355, 1978.

46. Tipton, J.B.: Office plastic surgery, Plast. Reconstr. Surg. **54:**660, 1974.

47. Tobin, H.A.: Office surgery in otolaryngology, Otolaryngol. **86**(2):176, 1978.

48. Trivedi, V.M., et al.: Planning and decision making for ambulatory surgery, J. Med. Syst. **4:**327, 1980.

49. Truppman, E.S.: Accreditation of ambulatory plastic surgery facilities, Clin. Plast. Surg. **10**(2):223, 1983.

50. Waters, R.M.: The down-town anesthesia clinic, Am. J. Surg. [Suppl.] **33:**71, 1919.

51. Weatherly, R.C.A., and Mayer, A.W.: Skin grafting in the emergency room and outpatient department, Surg. Clin. North Am. **49**(6):1461, 1969.

52. Williams, J.E.: Plastic surgery in an office surgical unit, Plast. Reconstr. Surg. **52:**513, 1973.

53. Wood, W.A., and Wayne, J.: Office-based surgery in podiatry, J. Am. Podiatry Assoc. **71:**591, 1981.

CHAPTER

6

Anesthesia

Surgery of the cutaneous surfaces usually necessitates the use of anesthesia to minimize pain. Successful use of the available anesthetic agents requires a knowledge of their biochemistry, metabolism, physiology of action, and side effects. This chapter provides background for a thoughtful approach to their use.

All surgical procedures carry with them a risk. This risk is affected not only by the type of surgery and the medical condition of the patient but also by the type of anesthesia. Although most operations performed on the cutaneous surfaces are easily and safely performed with local anesthetics, general anesthesia can alternatively be used under some circumstances. The type of anesthesia to select should be the safest method possible for the patient. Unfortunately greater weight is frequently given to other considerations, such as the physician's previous training and experience, the availability of appropriate operative facilities, or the patient's previous experiences.

SELECTION OF ANESTHESIA
Risk of general versus local anesthesia

General anesthesia, compared to local anesthesia, carries a much increased risk of morbidity and mortality. Because of this fact, operations that were routinely performed with general anesthetics a decade ago are currently often performed under local regional anesthesia. This includes not only operations on the cutaneous surfaces, such as extensive resections and repairs for skin cancers, but also inguinal hernia repairs,[281] breast biopsies,[64] and even endarterectomies.[175]

The true incidence of mortality caused by general anesthesia alone is unknown,[137] but has been estimated to be approximately 1 in every 10,000 operations.[183] This is partially caused by a lack of reporting and bias on the part of the anesthesiologist in rendering the true cause of death.[161] Human error does occur with general anesthesia and may be a significant factor,[76] as well as drug reactions or interactions.

Dentists come into daily contact with pain, and therefore they have been instrumental over the years in the development of both general and local anesthesia. Dentists who even today use both types of anesthesia know that death rates are much increased with general anesthesia.[176] The estimated general anesthesia mortality is about 1 in 15,000 dental operations, compared to approximately 1 in 2,500,000 operations using local anesthesia.[284]

For nondentistry operative procedures, general anesthesia still carries a significantly higher risk for the patient. Abortions performed with general anesthesia are associated with two to four times the overall death rates of abortions performed under local anesthesia.[227] Cardiac arrest occurs in patients in seemingly good health under general anesthesia,[280] although a history of previous myocardial infarctions substantially increases this risk.[128,270] If the previous myocardial infarction was recent (within 6 months of the surgery), the risk of reinfarction under general anesthesia is high: from 11% to 27%.[270] Use of local anesthesia on this high-risk group decreased the incidence of reinfarction dramatically: 0% for ophthalmic surgery patients.[30] Cardiovascular collapse can even be associated with so-called innocuous nitrous oxide analgesia.[191]

The advantages of local anesthesia, besides the decreased mortality, are that the cardiovascular and respiratory systems are not disturbed. In addition, patients with ischemic heart disease can communicate they are having pain in the chest in the event of myocardial insufficiency. Studies have compared local versus general anesthesia for breast biopsies[64] and inguinal hernia repairs[281]; there is less morbidity with local anesthesia and similar patient acceptance. It seems prudent, then, to perform surgical operations with local anesthesia if feasible, to avoid the inherent risks of general anesthesia.

Preoperative evaluation related to anesthesia

The type of anesthesia to use for a patient is selected at the preoperative evaluation. Among the factors to consider when choosing an anesthetic agent are the type and duration of the operation and the physical state of the patient. Before

TABLE 6-1

Drug interactions with local anesthetics and epinephrine

Drug	Reacts with	Untoward reaction
MAO inhibitors	Epinephrine	↑ BP (mild)*
Tricyclic antidepressants	Epinephrine	↑ BP, hyperthermia, cerebrovascular accident, death
Amphetamines	Epinephrine,	↑ BP, tachycardia,
	Local anesthetics	↑ central nervous system irritability
Cocaine	Epinephrine	↑ BP, vasoconstriction
Chlorpromazine	Epinephrine,	↓ BP (paradoxical vasodilation)
	Local anesthetics	↑ Vasodilation, ↓ BP
Propranolol	Epinephrine	↑ Vasoconstriction, ↑BP
Antihypertensives	Epinephrine,	↑ BP (with reserpine)
	Local anesthetics	↑ Vasodilation, ↓BP
Digitalis	Epinephrine	Automaticity enhanced
Phenytoin	Local anesthetics	↑ Toxicity (competes for plasma protein-binding sites)[125,157]
Diazepam	Local anesthetics	↓ Toxicity (central nervous system)
Cimetidine	Lidocaine	↑ Serum lidocaine[166]

From Smith, N.T., Miller, R D., and Corbascio, A.N., editors: Drug interactions in anesthesia, Philadelphia, 1981, Lea & Febiger.
*BP, Blood pressure.

performing a surgical procedure it is essential to take a medical history and perform a physical examination. Various medical conditions modify how anesthetics—either general or local—are handled by the body. In addition, a number of medications that the patient may be taking may interact unfavorably with anesthetics. The preoperative evaluation also gives the surgeon an opportunity to examine the surgical site, so that the type and duration of the operation can be determined.

Many of the medical problems to question patients about are listed in Table 9-1. Patients who are hyperthyroid or on a thyroid medication may be particularly sensitive to epinephrine.[50] Certainly anesthetics diffuse across the placenta in pregnant patients and have some effect on the fetus. Therefore elective surgery during pregnancy is best postponed until after the patient has given birth. Many anesthetics are metabolized in the liver and excreted by the kidneys; one should inquire specifically about these organ systems.

Cardiac problems are very important to determine before surgery. The anxiety of surgery alone increases the heart rate (in addition to the plasma epinephrine), and may even lead to extrasystoles.[97] However, most patients with significant well-documented cardiovascular disease handle local anesthesia well. In a study in which 40 cardiac patients underwent an oral surgical procedure that required 1.8 ml of 2% lidocaine with 1:50,000 epinephrine, the investigators found no significant changes in the ECG, blood pressure, and heart rate.[100] However, extensive surgery requires higher dosages than those used in this particular study. As mentioned previously, recent history of a myocardial infarc-

tion adds significantly to the risk of general anesthesia but much less to that of local anesthesia.[30] An additional reason for preferring local anesthesia for patients with cardiovascular disease is that the patients can communicate to the physician if they feel any pain. Such communication is impossible if the patient is under general anesthesia.[194]

Patients also have a decreased tolerance to local anesthetics if they are febrile or in poor physical condition.[13] In addition, acidosis, either respiratory or metabolic, is associated with decreased tolerance to local anesthetics.

Perhaps the most important questions to ask patients concern the drugs they are currently taking and allergies to previous drugs and particularly anesthestics.[263] Many of the known drug interactions with local anesthetics and with epinephrine are listed in Table 6-1. The most important ones concern the MAO inhibitors, the tricyclic antidepressants, and chlorpromazine. The first two drugs combined with epinephrine lead to a rise in blood pressure. Chlorpromazine with epinephrine, on the other hand, leads to a paradoxic vasodilation. An awareness of any allergy to anesthetics is important so that the particular agent or any cross-reacting substances can be avoided. Allergies and other drug interactions are discussed more fully later.

PREOPERATIVE MEDICATION

Some patients are particularly anxious before surgery and may benefit from preoperative medications. These medications should decrease anxiety without making the patient unduly drowsy, relieve pain, and produce some degree of amnesia. Frequently to produce these effects, more than one medication is necessary. This has given rise to a number of drug regimens and a general lack of agreement on the optional combinations.

There are three basic categories of preoperative medications (Table 6-2). In general the hypnotics produce drowsiness, the tranquilizers have a calming effect, and the opioids relieve pain. These effects are not necessarily clear cut;

TABLE 6-2

Preanesthetic medications

Hypnotics (drowsiness)
Barbiturate 100-200 mg IM or po
Antihistamine 50-150 mg IM

Tranquilizers (anxiety)
Benzodiazepine 5-10 mg IV
Phenothiazine 20-50 mg IM

Opioids (pain)
Morphine 8-12 mg IM
Meperidine 50-100 mg IM
Fentanyl 0.05-0.1 mg IM

Data from Smith, T.C., Cooper, L.H., and Wollman, H.: In Gilman, A.G., Goodman, L.S., and Gilman, A., editors: The pharmacological basis of therapeutics, ed. 6, 6th Edition, New York, 1980, Macmillan Co.

---

for instance, some tranquilizers also produce drowsiness. The important medications that may interact with preanesthetic medications are given in Table 6-3.

Hypnotics

The hypnotics include barbiturates and antihistamines. The barbiturates include phenobarbitol, which produces a slight depressant action on the respiratory and circulatory system but does not give good relief of pain during or after a surgical procedure. Physiologically phenobarbitol causes an increase in the systolic blood pressure and heart rate.[27] In addition, patients already on a barbiturate for other reasons, or who take aspirin, anticoagulants, or drink heavily may be somewhat tolerant of these drugs. The antihistamines are useful, especially in children, for sedation. Promethazine (Phenergan) is available for this purpose in both tablet and syrup forms. Antihistamines have in addition an antiemetic and bronchodilatory effect. Therefore they are frequently used in combination with opioids to counteract the bronchoconstrictive effects of the latter and provide sedation in addition to relief of pain. Hydroxyzine (Vistaril) causes a decrease in heart rate and cardiac output along with an increase in total peripheral resistance.[27]

Tranquilizers

The tranquilizers include both phenothiazines and benzodiazepines. The phenothiazines may produce a greater respiratory depression than the benzodiazepines. The most commonly used drug in the latter category is diazepam (Valium). Valium may be administered orally (PO), intramuscularly (IM), or intravenously (IV). Preoperatively only

---

TABLE 6-3

Drug interactions with preanesthetic medications

Drug	Reacts with	Untoward reaction
MAO inhibitors	Meperidine	Hyperpyrexia ↑ Respiratory depression
Tricyclic antidepressants	Meperidine Central nervous system (CNS) depressants	↑ Ventilatory depression ↑ CNS depression
Chlorpromazine	Narcotics CNS depressants	↓ BP ↑ CNS depression ↑ Sleep time
Propranolol, antihypertensives	Morphine CNS depressants	↑ Airway resistance ↑ Sleep time ↓ BP
Alcohol	CNS depressants Narcotics	↑ CNS depression ↑ CNS depression
Barbiturates	Barbiturates Meperidine	↑ Tolerance to barbiturates CNS depression
Aspirin	Barbiturates	↑ Tolerance to barbiturates
Anticoagulants	Barbiturates	↑ Tolerance to barbiturates
Cimetidine	Diazepam	↓ Plasma clearance of diazepam[165]

From Smith, N.T., Miller, R.D., and Corbascio, A.N., editors: Drug interactions in anesthesia, Philadelphia, 1981, Lea & Febiger.

the IV route appears to have predictably good results in decreasing anxiety[269] and producing amnesia.[145] Significant blood levels are easily obtained intravenously but poorly obtained by the intramuscular route. Oral administration is also superior to intramuscular administration in obtaining good blood levels. In one study 10 mg of diazepam was given IV to 15 patients with anxiety.[79] In 11 of these patients anxiety was decreased, in 8 there was a decrease in the systolic blood pressure, and in all patients hypoventilation occurred within 10 minutes. This last effect was mostly caused by a decrease in tidal volume but was associated with a decreased PaO_2. The hypoventilation effect did not require any therapy. This respiratory depression may be partially caused by hypotonia of the inspiratory muscles and is potentiated by other premedications, especially opiates.[93] Other studies have not seen respiratory rate depression with diazepam by any route of administration[145]—or, if it is seen, it is lost in 9 to 12 minutes following intravenous infusion.[29] Perhaps some of the confusion in the literature is caused by the types of patients studied. It is well known that elderly patients are more prone to develop hypoxia with heavy sedation. Under such circumstances the PaO_2 may drop as low as 45 mm Hg.[1]

A unique feature of diazepam is the amnesia produced by IV administration.[145] This amnesia has been described as anterograde (that is, for events after trauma, such as the beginning of surgery) and lasts for 10 minutes after infusion, with a lesser effect for 30 minutes. The memory problems are probably less related to recall than consolidation of events[67] and occur in most (60%) patients.[265] Therefore many patients given diazepam IV do not remember the surgical procedure or, at least, its details.

The recovery period after IV diazepam has also been studied. After IM administration of 10 mg in 11 volunteers, Korttila and Linnoila found coordination to be impaired at 5 hours but not at 7 hours.[168] They compared this with meperidine (Demerol), which still impaired reactive skills at 12 hours and then recommended against the use of meperidine in an outpatient surgery practice because of the prolonged impairment of psychomotor skills.

Occasionally a patient has an idiosyncratic reaction to IV diazepam, characterized by apnea and cyanosis.[59] The frequency of such reactions, however, must be rare, judging by the paucity of such reports in the medical literature.

The plasma clearance of diazepam may be affected by cimetidine because of the latter drug's ability to inhibit microsomal metabolism in the liver.[165] In addition, diazepam raises the seizure threshold and therefore, if given to a patient who would have a seizure reaction to a high dose of local anesthetic, this reaction may be prevented.[84]

Opioids

The third category of premedication is comprised by the opioids. This group includes both meperidine (Demerol) and morphine. Morphine given IM frequently produces nausea, vomiting, and hypotension. Similar reactions may occur with meperidine, with a respiratory depression lasting as long as 2 to 3 hours.[92] One problem with meperidine is its long time of onset (1 hour). Fentanyl is another opioid sometimes successfully used for outpatient surgery and successfully combined with diazepam.[123] Like diazepam, it also produces some respiratory depression but of shorter duration (1 to 2 hours).[92]

Problems

Some patients are very sensitive to preoperative medications. Asiatic persons appear to tolerate these medications less well than caucasians do, so lower dosages should be used.[91] Moreover, patients with underlying medical problems may also be prone to reactions. Barbiturates may cause an attack of acute intermittent porphyria. Patients with myxedema are particularly prone to excessive depressive effects of sedatives. Thyrotoxicosis may require heavier premedication. Patients who have had preoperative medication should not be allowed to leave the office unless accompanied by a responsible adult. Driving an automobile on the day of surgery should be prohibited. Full recovery to "street fitness," the ability to resume normal daily activities, may take 12 hours or even a full day, depending on the type of premedication and the stress of the surgery. If no preoperative medication but only local anesthesia is given, there appears to be no impairment of perceptual function after minor dental surgery.[123] This has not been studied with extensive cutaneous surgery, however.

Children

Children should be treated differently than adults with respect to premedication. Anxious children are frequently the product of anxious parents, so every attempt should be made to lessen anxiety in the parents. A calm mother helps to calm the child.

In some cases premedication makes a simple office procedure less traumatic for children. This is particularly true if the procedure promises to be painful or prolonged. Dosages on all medications need to be adjusted to the weight of the child. Some medications, promethazine, for instance, come in a syrup for ease of administration.

Chloral hydrate is one of the easiest and safest sedatives to prescribe to infants and small children. It is well tolerated by children of all ages, even neonates. The dose is 20 to 40 mg/kg given either by mouth or p.r., with a peak activity 30 to 60 minutes after administration. Caution should be exercised, however, when prescribing it to patients with liver disease.

A particularly successful preoperative combination of medications for children is "DPT" or the "lytic cocktail." It consists of meperidine (Demerol) 25 mg, promethazine (Phenergan) 6.25 mg, and chlorpromazine (Thorazine) 6.25

mg, mixed to 1 ml. The dose is 1 ml/15 kg IM but not more than 2 ml. It is not used for children below 1 year of age. The advantage of the lytic cocktail is that it provides both sedation and analgesia. The disadvantage is that the response can be variable; sometimes hyperactive children manifest a hyperactive response. The onset of action is from 15 to 45 minutes after administration. If the lytic cocktail does not work well, it may be supplemented by a low dose of chloral hydrate.

For children older than 10 years, diazepam may be used. The dose is 2.5 to 5 mg by mouth 20 to 30 minutes preoperatively. It should not be used for younger children because of the potential for respiratory depression.

Another sedative that may be useful in children is alcohol. It is administered by mouth as 10 ml of brandy in 30 ml of water. It can be used in infants weighing more than 5 kg.

Music

In addition to medication, music has also been recommended to help sedate patients.[192,210] Certainly for lengthy procedures this helps to divert the patient's attention from the procedure and has a calming effect on the mood of the office. I have found that head phones attached to a radio are particularly soothing for patients to use during surgery.

GENERAL ANESTHESIA

General anesthesia is not frequently used in performing dermatologic surgery, since local anesthesia is usually sufficient and safer. However, under some circumstances—for instance an overly anxious patient—it may be preferable.

General anesthesia has effects on many tissues of the body from which it takes some time for the patient to recover. This fact was appreciated by Bernard[42] over a century ago when discussing chloroform:

> . . . let us remember that chloroform does not act solely on the nerve tissues. Far from that, it has an action on all the tissues and attacks each one at time which is a function of its susceptibility . . . An anesthetic is not a special poison for the nervous system. It anesthetizes all the cells, benumbing all the tissues, and stopping temporarily this irritability.

General anesthetics are not as specific as local anesthetics with respect to the tissues they affect (Table 6-4). General anesthetics are inhaled or injected into the blood stream and result in unconsciousness. Their site of action is the central nervous system, whereas local anesthetics act on the peripheral nervous system. Because general anesthetics act to depress the central nervous system, their action in decreasing pain is not specific. Local anesthetics depress impulse conduction in axons, whereas general anesthetics depress synaptic transmission. These distinctions are not completely clear-cut, however, since local anesthetics also gain access to the blood stream and thus affect distant organs. The word *anesthesia* was reputedly coined in 1846 by the jurist and physician, Oliver Wendell Holmes, who prefixed

TABLE 6-4

Comparison of general and local anesthesia

	Local anesthesia	General anesthesia
Consciousness	Yes	No
Intermediate carrier	None	Blood
Target tissue	Peripheral nervous system	Central nervous system
Loss of sensation	Local	General
Selectivity	Yes	No
Reversible	Yes	Yes
Mode of action	Depresses impulse conduction in axons	Depresses synaptic transmission

$\grave{\alpha}\nu$-(without) to the Greek $\alpha\check{\iota}\sigma\theta\eta\sigma\iota\varsigma$ (perception) to signify the absence of perception by the senses.

General anesthesia is properly administered by anesthesiologists who have special training in those particular drugs. Recommendations for its use should be predicated on the extensiveness of the procedure and the medical condition of the patient.

Nitrous oxide

Recently there has been a resurgence of interest in the use of 30% to 60% nitrous oxide combined with oxygen (N_2O-O_2) in the outpatient setting for use not only by dentists but also by pediatricians, podiatrists, emergency room physicians, and dermatologists. Correctly used, N_2O-O_2 is said to be safe,[24,126,247] providing a wide margin of safety.[187] Proper administration requires little special training or equipment. N_2O-O_2 is reasonably free of serious untoward reactions or toxic side effects. Its proponents emphasize that such usage is *not* to provide general anesthesia (which requires greater than 65% nitrous oxide) in the sense of unconsciousness and loss of all sensation but rather sedative analgesia.[133,189] Communication between the patient and the physician is always maintained, and the patient's vital functions, such as spontaneous respiration and normal protective airway reflexes, are preserved. When used in this fashion, nitrous oxide is safe[126,133]; when used for general anesthesia, it carries much more risk of problems.

Sedative analgesia can be defined as sedation with less perception of pain. Anxiety is lessened, and the pain threshold is lifted but not eliminated—so local anesthetics might be required with N_2O-O_2.[187] N_2O-O_2 does make local anesthesia more tolerable when it is required. The need for supplemental local anesthesia depends on the magnitude and extensiveness of the surgical procedure and the patient's threshold for pain. Simple suturing of lacerations in children might not require additional local anesthesia.[133]

TABLE 6-5

Stages of nitrous oxide-oxygen analgesia-anesthesia

	N$_2$O concentration	Clinical state	Subjective feelings
Stage 1	6%-25%	Moderate analgesia	Relaxation
Stage 2	26%-45%	Dissociation analgesia	Detachment
Stage 3	46%-65%	Analgesic anesthesia	Amnesia
Stage 4	66%-85%	Light anesthesia	None (unconsciousness)

Data from Parbrook, G.: Br. J. Anaesth. **39**:974, 1967.

In 1772, shortly after he discovered oxygen, Priestley discovered nitrous oxide. Its initial medical usage was pioneered by dentists, who have used this "laughing gas" for almost 150 years. Morton, a dentist and medical student, knew of nitrous oxide from Wells, who had one of his own teeth extracted while breathing nitrous oxide in 1844; however, Wells's first public demonstration of nitrous oxide for anesthesia was a failure. This is interesting in view of its somewhat variable results even today in providing less perception of pain. Morton successfully demonstrated another general anesthetic subsequently: diethyl ether.[265]

Nitrous oxide is an inert, inorganic gas. Although it is considered noninflammable and nonexplosive, it nevertheless supports combustion. This gas has a pleasant fruity odor and is colorless; it is nonsensitizing and nonirritating.[189] It is nonaddicting but frequently abused.

On administration N$_2$O-O$_2$ is absorbed through the lungs and carried in solution in plasma. It is preferentially distributed to the body lipids, large amounts of which are taken up by the brain.[187] N$_2$O-O$_2$ has a short equilibration time. Within 10 minutes a plateau concentration is achieved in arterial blood. The initial gas concentration correlates closely with plasma and brain levels.[189] Therefore a rapid onset and offset of analgesia is provided. This allows the physician to titrate the patient's depth of analgesia closely.

Factors that influence alveolar concentration include concentration of the N$_2$O-O$_2$ mixture, rapidity of plasma uptake, and tension of the gas. At higher altitudes an increased O$_2$ concentration may thus be required for safe administration.[133] N$_2$O depresses the hyperventilatory response to hypoxia but not to hypercarbia; it should therefore be administered with oxygen.[298]

The effects of the N$_2$O-O$_2$ gas mixture on inhalation have been described as "sedation,"[133] "analgesia,"[187,223] "disorientation analgesia,"[223] "analgesic anesthesia,"[223] and "anxiolytic."[274] This profusion of names shows that at the recommended concentrations (30% to 65% N$_2$O), a patient experiences sedation, some relief from anxiety, and elevation of the pain threshold. The amount that any of these effects is produced is a function not only of N$_2$O concentration but also of individual patient response. Children tend to

be more susceptible than adults, and the patients who are highly suggestible seem to respond more positively.

The use of N$_2$O-O$_2$ for outpatient surgery was recently reviewed.[133] After 3000 administrations, there were very few problems: 9 patients who vomited and 1 who disliked the experience. An additional 2 patients reported unpleasant experiences with previous doses. A distinct advantage of this form of analgesia and sedation is that it may be used conveniently and safely in children as young as 16 months. In addition, since it is inhaled through a mask, the use of needles is prevented, which greatly diminishes anxiety in children.

With N$_2$O-O$_2$ administration, the vital signs and skin color remain normal. Patients are able to talk, follow instructions, and maintain a gag reflex. They appear sleepy, are less aware of their surroundings, and respond less to painful stimuli.

Administration technique

Before administration the physician should inform the patient of the effects of inhaling N$_2$O-O$_2$ gas, emphasizing relaxation and pain relief. The patient should be allowed to accommodate to the mask or mouthpiece by breathing pure oxygen for a minute or two. The physician then adds N$_2$O and increases the concentration while allowing the patient to describe his or her feelings. The recommended flow rates for N$_2$O and O$_2$ are 1 to 2 L/minute.[132]

The effects of N$_2$O are a function of its concentration[223] (Table 6-5). Moderate analgesia is produced by 6% to 25% N$_2$O. This is the equivalent of 15 mg of morphine. The patient feels relaxed and is free of any serious side effects. At a concentration of 26% to 45% N$_2$O, dissociation analgesia occurs. The patient feels detached from the environment, although full verbal contact between patient and physician is maintained; the patient appears drunken or dreamy. Although complete analgesia is probably not present, the patient is relatively free from anxiety.[274] Some patients are particularly sensitive to nitrous oxide and may become unresponsive with concentrations as low as 40%. The sense of detachment may be scary for some patients, who describe it as a bad experience.

As the concentration of N_2O is raised still higher, between 40% and 65%, analgesic anesthesia occurs. At this stage the patient experiences marked amnesia. At concentrations of 60% to 65% many patients become unresponsive. From 66% to 85% N_2O, contact with the patient is no longer possible. At this point, complete amnesia and analgesia occur.

As stated previously, the required concentrations of N_2O and O_2 vary with atmospheric pressure (higher concentrations are needed for higher altitudes).[133] In addition, individual patient responses vary,[223] underscoring the importance of maintaining communication with the patient so as to adjust the concentration of N_2O for the desired level of sedation and analgesia.

Usually after 3 to 4 minutes of breathing N_2O-O_2 mixture of 30% to 60%, the desired level of analgesia is produced.[189] Because it is critical to maintain patient contact during the procedure, lesser concentrations of nitrous oxide not exceeding 50% are safer, especially in children. Usually few adjustments are necessary in the flow rates during surgical procedures. Maloney recommends lowering the concentration of N_2O once the desired states of analgesia is produced.[187,189]

On completion of the surgical procedure, the patient is allowed to breath pure O_2 for a few minutes. This helps to flush out N_2O and prevents diffusion hypoxia (explained later). In addition, severe light-headedness and dizziness are prevented.[133]

The concurrent usage of other medications, such as barbiturates, sedatives, narcotics, modifies the effect of N_2O on patients.[223] Because the effects are unpredictable and difficult to control, such combinations should be avoided in an office or clinic. The use of local anesthesia may be necessary even with N_2O[189,274]; however, N_2O makes the pain of local anesthesia more tolerable. As previously mentioned, for simple suturing of lacerations in children N_2O may preclude the need for local anesthesia completely.[133] Lidocaine in the blood also interacts with nitrous oxide and lowers the general anesthetic requirements.[146]

Equipment

The equipment necessary for nitrous oxide administration should be obtained and installed by experts. There are systems designed specifically for office use with various safety features and so-called fail-safe devices. The tanks should be different colors for different gases (green for oxygen, blue for nitrous oxide). Different sizes and shapes of connectors for different gases will prevent mistakes in mixing gases. The tubing should be tested and free of leaks; proper venting should exist to prevent contamination of the office atmosphere with nitrous oxide. Some systems are installed with an alarm that sounds if the flow of oxygen drops below a certain level. It should be emphasized that "fail-safe" devices, like any mechanical device, are falli-

ble; they must be constantly checked and monitored.[300]

The patient inhales the N_2O-O_2 mixture by means of a nasal mask[133] or an oral airway (Puritan-Bennett Corporation, 401 East 13th Street, Kansas City, Mo., 64106).[189] When operations are performed on the central face, the nasal mask is an obstruction, and the oral airway may be used. Maloney recommends using cotton in the nostrils when using the oral airway to prevent nasal breathing.[189] The disadvantage of using the oral airway is that patients have difficulty holding it in place for long procedures (greater than 30 or 40 minutes), and without a firm hold on the mouthpiece, leaks develop, polluting the office atmosphere with nitrous oxide. The nasal mask is a more open system, which, when attached to a reservoir bag, mixes atmospheric gases with N_2O and O_2.[133] Scavenging systems to remove stray nitrous oxide in masks are necessary to minimize atmospheric pollution,[268] but because the patients may exhale N_2O around the mask, some pollution will occur. This pollution is, of course, increased during procedures that take more time.

The cost of N_2O-O_2 equipment and installation is roughly $2500 to $3000; however, after the initial investment, the maintenance cost is negligible. The Mapleson D with a Bain circuit allows inhaled and exhaled gases to move separately in a double-lumen tube. A scavenger valve is also attached, to minimize atmospheric pollution. Manufacturers of office units include Fraser-Harlake, Inc. (145 Midcounty Drive, Orchard Park, N.Y., 14127) and Porter Instrument Co. (PO Box 326, Township Line Road, Hatfield, Penn., 19440).

Advantages

The lack of toxicity and safety of nitrous oxide are well documented.[24,126,247] Compared to systemic medications, nitrous oxide has a rapid onset and can be modulated more easily to achieve the desired effects.[187] This is caused by the rapid equilibration of N_2O between plasma and brain. In contrast, systemic medications are slow in onset, more unpredictable in effect, and relatively slow in wearing off. Therefore with nitrous oxide the physician can titrate the depth and duration of analgesia. Should side effects occur, the concentration can be rapidly lowered. An inhaled analgesic also offers distinct advantages over inherently painful injectable sedatives and local anesthetics. Thus nitrous oxide is of particular benefit in children. Patients who are particularly anxious or who have low pain thresholds are good candidates for this type of sedative analgesia.

Untoward effects

When nitrous oxide pollutes the atmosphere, it may be harmful to all exposed, which includes not only patients but office personnel. Some of the effects of nitrous oxide are immediate, whereas others take a much longer time to become observed.

While inhaling nitrous oxide, patients may become light-headed and drowsy. In addition, nausea and vomiting may occur.[133,282] Because of the dissociative analgesia produced some patients may have an unpleasant experience. When the patient shows signs of irritability, such as restlessness or hypermobility, the level of anesthesia is probably becoming too deep. Usually these side effects can be partially controlled by lowering the concentration of the gas being administered. Having the patient breathe pure oxygen at the end of the procedure also helps to minimize dizziness and light-headedness.

Nitrous oxide replaces gaseous nitrogen in the enclosed air spaces within the body. Because N_2O diffuses into these spaces faster than gaseous nitrogen diffuses out, the pressure within these spaces increases.[62] Abdominal distension may occur, and air embolism is possible.[223] Patients with middle ear disease, eustachian tube malfunction, or previous rupture of tympanic membranes are at great risk for rupture of tympanic membranes with nitrous oxide.[80,225]

Patients with lung disease are particularly susceptible to lowered or elevated oxygen concentrations in administered gases. If patients are accustomed to retaining CO_2, a high oxygen concentration may produce hypoventilation. When N_2O administration is discontinued, the N_2O tends to diffuse out to fill the lungs. When this occurs in the absence of oxygen administration, a phenomenon known as diffusion hypoxia occurs and results in an increased inert gas concentration and a lowered arterial oxygen concentration. This normally results in hyperventilation in response to hypoxemia. However, N_2O may itself depress this respiratory response.[298] It is therefore essential to administer pure oxygen for a few minutes at the end of N_2O-O_2 analgesia to wash out the nitrous oxide.

It is preferable that patients be able to communicate with their physicians to prevent reaching a greater depth of anesthesia than is necessary or safe. Obviously, very young children are not able to verbalize their feelings and therefore should be watched closely. Patients who have taken sedatives or alcohol or are unconscious are not suitable candidates for N_2O-O_2 analgesia. This form of analgesia may also be contraindicated in those with myocardial ischemia.[133] A study has associated a 50% nitrous oxide and 50% oxygen mixture with a slight (12%) decrease in cardiac output.[283]

There has been one reported case of cardiovascular collapse associated with N_2O administration for analgesia in a child.[191] N_2O increases the pulmonary arterial pressure, and the child in that case report had pulmonary arterial hypertension. Therefore, in an already compromised patient, right ventricular failure and arrest may occur under such circumstances.

Long-term exposure (greater than 6 hours)[26] or multiple short-term exposures[217] to nitrous oxide may interfere with proper B_{12} function. This is thought to be caused by inactivation of B_{12} by nitrous oxide, possibly by oxidation. B_{12} is necessary for the production of tetrahydrofolate, which in turn is required for the conversion of deoxyuridine to thymidine and ultimately to DNA.[88] The immediate effects are megaloblastic changes in the bone marrow[215] and megaloblastic anemia.[261] These effects have been confirmed in human cell lines in vitro.[155]

The untoward effects of nitrous oxide caused by occupational exposure are controversial but worthy of mention. Spontaneous abortion but not fetotoxicity has been linked to nitrous oxide exposure to personnel working in environments in which nitrous oxide is commonly used for anesthesia.[70,293] It is therefore recommended that women wishing to be pregnant or who are pregnant should not work in an atmosphere possibly polluted with anesthetic gases. Fetotoxicity has been demonstrated with nitrous oxide in animals[172]; however, N_2O was found to be neither mutagenic nor carcinogenic in Ames testing.[31]

Another effect associated with occupational exposure to nitrous oxide is a neuropathy in the form of numbness, tingling, and muscle weakness. The neuropathy resembles the combined degeneration of the cord caused by B_{12} deficiency and thus may be caused by the known effects of nitrous oxide on B_{12}, already discussed. This neuropathy has been reported in dentists[70] and in those habituated to repeated inhalation of N_2O.[174] Other studies, however, dispute the effect of chronic nitrous oxide exposure in the production of neuropathy.[95,108]

Unfortunately, safe exposure levels to N_2O are not well defined.[293] Screening devices and proper equipment reduce but do not eliminate atmospheric pollution. It has been estimated that nitrous oxide administration at 3 L/minute for a 20-minute procedure leads to 780 parts per million (ppm) nitrous oxide in a treatment room. This is 30 times the acceptable level of 25 ppm established by the National Institute of Occupational Safety and Health (NIOSH).[268] This level can be reduced by scavenging masks. Still, a critical review of the effects of trace concentrations of anesthetic gases concluded that statistical evidence proving that tract concentrations N_2O exert harmful effects was lacking.[108]

Summary

N_2O-O_2 analgesia is a possibly effective alternative to injectable sedatives for short surgical procedures performed in an outpatient setting. It is too soon to assess its value and untoward reactions properly, since it has not been in widespread use by dermatologists for a long enough period of time. However, based on the experience of dentists and physicians, those who employ N_2O-O_2 should be well versed in its use, abuse, and possible untoward reactions. Precautions concerning proper equipment, scavenging masks, and low-level exposure to personnel should be of utmost concern.

Methoxyflurane

Methoxyflurane (Penthrane) is an alternative to nitrous oxide and may be inhaled by the patient in an office setting.[127] Like nitrous oxide, it may be insufficient to mask the pain of a surgical procedure completely, so a supplemental local anesthetic must be given.

Methoxyflurane is a fluorinated ether and is the most potent of the inhaled anesthetics in common use. It is a clear, colorless liquid with an innocuous odor and is noninflammable and nonexplosive in air or oxygen. Patients can breathe Penthrane by means of a hand-held inhaler, the analgizer (available through Abbott Laboratories, Chicago, 60064), a lightweight cylinder of high-density polyethylene, which has a nasal mouthpiece for inhaling. A felt wick is saturated with methoxyflurane and placed in the cylinder. The patient is allowed to breathe it (usually it is self-administered) until feeling lightheaded.

Methoxyflurane induces analgesia slowly. The analgesia is also slowly reversed, leaving no hangover. Patients can develop hepatic toxicity, which may be idiosyncratic or allergic. Nephrotoxicity is also possible, but this usually occurs only if the patient breathes methoxyflurane for a long time; thus it should not be given to patients with liver or kidney disease or those on nephrotoxic medications or hepatic enzyme inducers (such as phenobarbital). Self-administration by the patient produces discontinuous anesthesia, which lowers the probability of untoward problems.

Another potential problem with methoxyflurane is that general anesthesia may inadvertently cause a loss of the gag reflex. Should the patient vomit under such circumstances, aspiration could occur.

LOCAL ANESTHESIA

For most procedures in cutaneous surgery, local anesthesia is ideal. It is easy to administer, rapidly effective, and relatively inexpensive. In addition, local anesthetics are relatively free of side effects and do not affect the patient's coordination or ability to think.[153] For patients with ischemic heart disease, local anesthesia is far preferable to general anesthesia.[194]

Local anesthesia results in the temporary absence of the sensation of pain and is limited in location, so that surgical operations can be performed without the necessity of rendering the patient unconscious. Central control of vital functions is not impaired. Localized anesthesia may be produced not only by drugs or chemicals but also by physical means, such as pressure or low temperature.

Local anesthetics are drugs that slow or stop nerve conduction when applied close to nerve tissue in sufficient concentrations. Every type of nerve fiber is affected by local anesthetics, and complete recovery of nerve function without damage to nerve fibers is the usual course of events. Local anesthetics can cause both sensory loss and motor paralysis in the distribution of the anesthetized nerves. Lo-

cal anesthetics can also affect other cells capable of excitation, for instance, in the myocardium.

Selection of a local anesthetic is based on the type of surgical procedure, the clinical needs, and the pharmacologic properties of various anesthetic drugs. Since no one local anesthetic is an ideal agent for all clinical situations, a background knowledge of the chemistry and biologic behavior of local anesthetics is necessary to make a logical choice of which agent to use. Although generally safe, local anesthetics can produce harmful side effects locally and systemically. These effects are determined by the type of anesthetic used and the method of its use. Therefore knowledge of the pharmacology and effects of local anesthetics is necessary to prevent problems. The following true case report illustrates the potential seriousness of injection of local anesthetics[276]:

> After preparation of A.B. the surgeon, unassisted, infiltrated the right side of the face, head and neck with a 2% lidocaine solution. The volume used was not noted, but found at the scene were three 2% lidocaine bottles of 50 ml. capacity. Two were empty, but one still contained 25 ml. After the injections were completed the patient requested some orange juice. Upon his return to the surgery room the surgeon found her on the table unconscious, with no detectable pulse rate. He injected 1 ml. of epinephrine, to no avail.
>
> Since this solution had been in the surgery room for a long time, a fresh bottle was obtained. The injection of 1 ml. of this fresh solution was also of no value, nor were cardiac massage and artificial respiration by massage of the heart cage.
>
> Autopsy . . . revealed the following as the only abnormal pathological changes: partial pulmonary peripheral atelectasis, cardiac dilatation, and visceral congestion.

History and development

General anesthetics were developed before local anesthetics, in part because of the easy route of administration of general anesthetics and the lack of proper equipment (hollow needles) for administering local anesthetics. It was not until 1845 that Rynd (in Ireland) and 1853 that Wood (in England) introduced the first hollow metallic needle.[130] Pravez introduced a similar device in France in 1853.

Although the Indians in South America had probably used cocaine for centuries as a topical anesthesia, von Annep in 1880 was one of the first to report that subcutaneously infiltrated cocaine produced lack of sensation to a pinprick.[294] In 1884 Koller, at the suggestion of Freud, reported on the successful use of topical cocaine for anesthesia in the eye.[167] Halsted, the renowned surgeon at Johns Hopkins, reported in 1885 over a thousand cases of successful cocaine-induced nerve conduction block in man; unfortunately, he himself became a cocaine addict. It is interesting to note that this general surgeon pioneered the use of local anesthesia, which is used extensively in dentistry,

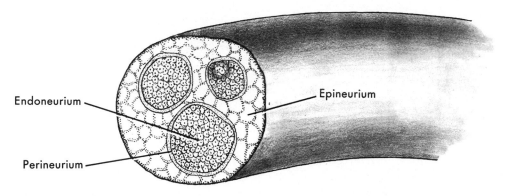

Fig. 6-1. Cross section of large peripheral nerve demonstrating connective tissue barriers (epineurium, perineurium, and endoneurium) to local anesthetics. (Modified from Covino, B.G., and Vassalo, H.G.: Local anesthetics: mechanism of action and clinical use, New York, 1976, Grune & Stratton, Inc.)

whereas dentists developed the use of general anesthesia. Procaine was synthesized in 1904 and lidocaine in 1948.[81]

Before widespread use of local anesthetics, both pressure and cold were used to produce anesthesia.[178] Pressure blocks tactile sensations first, and pain is affected last. Cold, on the other hand, affects pain sensations first, then thermal stimuli, and finally tactile stimuli. These alternative physical methods were not nearly as successful as drug-induced local anesthesia and therefore fell into disuse.

Nerve anatomy

To understand the mechanism of action of local anesthetics fully, one must review the microscopic anatomy of nerve fibers (Figs. 6-1 and 6-2). Peripheral nerves contain both sensory afferent fibers and motor efferent fibers and are therefore mixed nerves. The cell body of the afferent sensory nerve lies in the dorsal root ganglion. The axon is comprised of axoplasm (neural cytoplasm), which is bounded by a nerve membrane (axolemma) composed of a bimolecular phospholipid with a protein coat. The axolemma is the key to nerve excitability. All peripheral nerves are further surrounded by Schwann cells, described later, and by two or three membranes.

Nerve axons are individually surrounded by a thin connective tissue sheath, the endoneurium. Several axons with their endoneuriums are bound together into a bundle by the perineurium, a fibroelastic membrane. This membrane is the main diffusion barrier for local anesthetics. Several bundles may be bound together by a third outermost membrane, the epineurium. This latter structure is formed by loose areolar tissue and is not a significant barrier to anesthetic diffusion. Therefore, to get to the nerve fiber, an anesthetic may need to diffuse across a number of membranes. The ability of different anesthetics to diffuse across these membranes is related to their chemical structures.[75]

Peripheral nerves fibers are classified as myelinated or unmyelinated (Table 6-6). The main difference between these two types of fibers is the manner in which they are encased by the Schwann cell covering, which encases all peripheral nerves. The Schwann cell wraps around some nerve fibers, producing a laminated fatty (lipoprotein) covering (myelin sheath) and thus a myelinated nerve. Between the Schwann cells are gaps, Ranvier's nodes, where there is a lack of this covering around the nerve fibers (Fig. 6-2). In small myelinated nerves the Ranvier's nodes occur every 0.2 or 0.3 mm. When the nerve fibers are simply enmeshed in Schwann cells as an indentation of their membrane, these nerves are considered unmyelinated. Both myelinated and unmyelinated nerves are surrounded by Schwann cells.[81]

In the afferent nerves of the skin the unmyelinated fibers far outnumber the myelinated fibers.[43] It has been suggested that many of these unmyelinated fibers are continuations or branches of myelinated fibers that have lost their myelin more proximately; however, "naked" nerve filaments, which were described by light microscopists, probably do not exist.[260] Both myelinated and unmyelinated fibers carry pain impulses.[57]

Conduction of an impulse in a unmyelinated nerve is a relatively slow process. Myelinated nerve cells, on the other hand, allow for a much more energy-efficient and faster (50 times faster) conduction of impulses because of the Ranvier's nodes. The current leaps from node to node (known as saltatory conduction) instead of progressing by sequential depolarization of adjacent membrane patches. Conduction of impulses is also increased by an increase of the diameter of nerve fibers. As the thickness of myelinated axon increases, the thickness of the myelin sheath increases proportionally. The internodal distance similarly increases, as does the conduction velocity.[81]

Peripheral nerve fibers have been categorized into three different types: A fibers, B fibers, and C fibers[122] (Table 6-6 and Fig. 6-2). In man, pain is carried by two types of fibers, the δ fibers (a type of A fiber) and the C fibers. Therefore

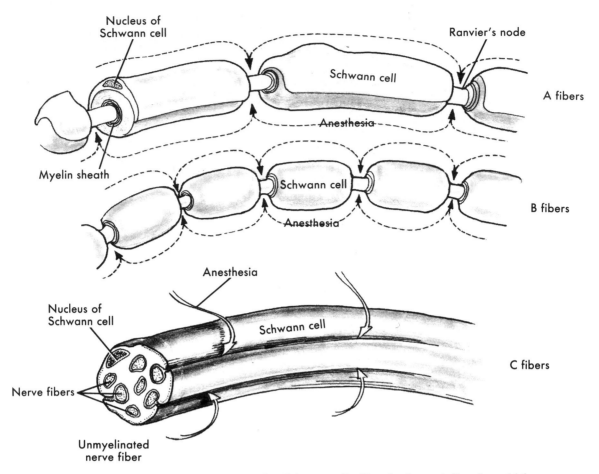

Fig. 6-2. A, B, and C fibers with surrounding Schwann cells. Note that larger A fibers have thicker Schwann cells and greater distance between the Ranvier's nodes. More anesthetic is therefore required for larger fibers. Anesthetic enters between Ranvier's nodes for A and B fibers but along course of nerves for C fibers.

TABLE 6-6

Comparison of myelinated and unmyelinated nerves

	Myelinated nerves	**Unmyelinated nerves**
Myelin sheath	+	−
Schwann cell covering	+	+
Ranvier's nodes	+	−
Conduction	Saltatory	Nonsaltatory
Relative conduction velocity	Fast	Slow
↑ Conduction velocity	↑ ∝ diameter	$\uparrow \propto \sqrt{\text{diameter}}$
Types of fibers	A fibers	C fibers
	α proprioceptive 20 μm	pain 1 μm
	β touch, pressure	postganglionic, autonomic
	γ muscle spindle	
	δ pain 3 μm	
	B fibers	
	preganglionic autonomic	

pain impulses may be conveyed by both the myelinated (Aδ fibers) and unmyelinated (C) fibers.[57] The sizes of these two pain fibers differ, as does the speed at which pain impulses are conducted. For practical purposes both types of fibers are blocked by similar, clinically useful concentrations of local anesthetic, despite the fact that the A fibers are larger than the C fibers and the latter are unmyelinated; however, at very low concentrations the myelinated Aδ fibers are blocked completely, whereas the C unmyelinated fibers are not.[212] The Aδ fibers are thought to be responsible for sharp pain, and the C fibers convey dull pain.[81]

Generation of a nerve impulse

Following a stimulus to a nerve an impulse is generated. This impulse is known as an action potential (Fig. 6-3) and results from the movement of sodium and potassium ions.[148] These action potentials move down or up a nerve as a wave of depolarization. Since local anesthetics block the generation and propagation of action potentials in nerves, it is necessary to review this phenomenon to understand the mechanism of action of these drugs.

Nerves have inner and outer concentrations of both sodium and potassium ions. During inactivity the inner concentration of sodium ions is low, whereas the inner concentration of potassium ions is high, compared to the surrounding medium. The resting potential across the cell membrane is about −70 mV due to the potassium concentration gradient, since the unstimulated nerve membrane is fully permeable to potassium ions but not to sodium ions. With excitation a predictable chain of events takes place. Channels on the nerve membrane allow inward movement of sodium ions and an outward flow of potassium ions. The overall charge within the cell becomes less negative (slow depolarization) until the firing threshold is reached (usually −50 mV), at which point rapid depolarization occurs. K^+ diffuses back out of the cell down its concentration gradient, and Na^+ rapidly diffuses in. Usually this depolarization reaches +40 mV before rapid repolarization occurs. At the peak of the action potential, which occurs at the end of depolarization, sodium ion concentration determines the membrane potential. On repolarization a small hyperpolarization occurs. The difference between the resting potential and the peak depolarization potential is known as the action potential. Depolarization and repolarization together occur within 1 msec. A voltage difference occurs between adjacent resting and depolarized membranes, and it sets in motion local currents. The current reduces the transmembrane potential of the resting nerve and results in depolarization and a propagated impulse.[75,81]

Mechanism of action of local anesthetics

Local anesthetics interfere with the excitation-conduction process of nerve fibers. These drugs directly block the

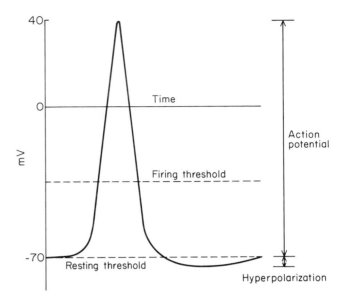

Fig. 6-3. An action potential.

membrane action potential without significantly affecting the resting potential, and thus result in a nondepolarization block. Local anesthetics are therefore not metabolic inhibitors in nerves. When exposed to local anesthetics, nerve membranes remain polarized. However, impulses are blocked because depolarization is impaired and a propagated action potential fails to develop. One sees a progressive decrease in the amplitude of action potentials, a retardation in their rate of rise, and an elevation of the firing thresholds.[141] In addition, there is a slowing in the velocity of impulse conduction and a lengthening of the refractory period. These events are best interpreted as being the result of a diminished sodium current.

Local anesthetics somehow prevent the active influx of Na^+ ions associated with the generation of action potentials—evidenced by the fact that local anesthetic agents have no effect on the resting membrane potential but rather on depolarization, which is directly related to the sodium current.[141] When depolarization does not occur to the point of the threshold level, a propagated action potential does not occur, and conduction blockage ensues. The literature supports four main mechanisms[237] (depicted schematically in Fig. 6-4): (1) anesthetics interact with receptors near or inside of the sodium channels and thereby block sodium ions, (2) anesthetics cause swelling of the nerve membrane and thus blockage of the sodium channels, (3) anesthetics change the membrane surface charge, or (4) anesthetics physically block the other mouth of the sodium channel.

Some local anesthetics actually physically block the sodium channel (*4* in Fig. 6-4). Marine toxins such as tetrodotoxin (TTX) and saxitoxin (STX) act in such a way and wedge themselves into the external aperture of the sodium channel.[144] Interestingly, a combination of saxitoxin and certain other local anesthetics produces nerve

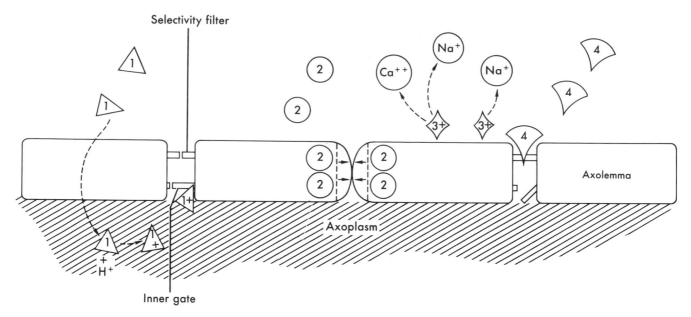

Fig. 6-4. Schematic concept of possible mechanisms of action for local anesthetics. (1) Ionization within axoplasm and subsequent intercalation within inner gate in sodium channel, locking it in closed position. (2) Membrane expansion with subsequent plugging of sodium channel. (3) Changing of surface charge. (4) Plugging of outer sodium channel.

blocks of longer duration than does either agent alone.

Another mechanism by which some anesthetics may work is to cause a conformational change in the sodium channels by protein-lipid expansion within the axolemma[286] (*2* in Fig. 6-4). Local anesthetics are interspersed among lipid membrane components, causing a spatial realignment. This disordering is thought to be caused by fluidizing. The result is a conformational change in the ion-conducting channels, which is reflected in the decreased sodium permeability. Swelling of the neural membrane thus effectively produces a gating effect.

Local anesthetics such as benzyl alcohol or lidocaine are known to cause structural changes of expansion in biologic membranes such as red blood cell membranes.[195] The undissociated anesthetic benzocaine probably acts primarily by such a mechanism.[239] The local anesthetic penetrates into a lipid-containing membrane and produces physical changes.[262] This mechanism has less to do with concentration of local anesthetics than with the volume of hydrophobic space disturbed or occupied by anesthetic molecules.[256]

Another possible mechanism of local anesthetic action involves the positively charged local anesthetic cation changing the nerve-membrane surface charge (*3* in Fig. 6-4). This raises the transmembrane voltage profile, which makes it more difficult to draw the membrane potential to the firing level. In addition, the cationic tails of local anesthetics repel positively charged sodium ions. Calcium ions, which are also positively charged, may be displaced as well.[6]

Although different local anesthetics probably act in sev-

eral different ways to block the nerve impulses, most local anesthetics (including lidocaine) mainly act by the first mechanism depicted in Fig. 6-4. The lipid-soluble base form of an anesthetic diffuses through the nerve membrane[211] or through the sodium channels themselves. The acidic environment within the nerve promotes formation of the catonic form of the local anesthetic, which then occupies a receptor in the sodium channel.[143] It was shown that quaternary lidocaine externally applied had little effect on membrane currents, but when placed inside the axoplasm inhibited sodium currents by more than 90%.[211,273] Strichartz concluded that lidocaine enters the sodium channels from the axoplasmic (inside) side of the nerve membrane and probably binds within the channels about half way down the electrical gradient from inside to outside.[273] More specifically, the positively charged anesthetic cation attaches by electrostatic forces to the negatively charged anionic phosphate tails of the phospholipids of the nerve membrane.[106]

The sodium channel has been schematically thought to contain two separate barriers or gates[273] (Fig. 6-4). An outer gate, the "selectivity filter," is fixed and determines which ions can pass through the open channels based on the size of the ions (usually no larger than 3×5 Å[142,266]). A second barrier, the inner gate or m-gate, is located on the inner side of the sodium channel. It opens and closes in response to different membrane potentials. When open, sodium ions flow inward, producing an action potential. It is this latter gate to which some anesthetics attach (intercalate) and in so doing lock it in the closed position, preventing the inward flow of sodium ions and thus the production of an action potential. Evidence for this site as the receptor for local anesthetics is that inactivation of the sodium channels by local anesthetic could be reversed by perfusion of the axoplasmic spaced with the proteolytic enzyme pronase.[242]

Another piece of evidence placing the usual site of local anesthetic action in the sodium channel's internal mouth is the fact that if the nerve is fired off with prepulses, opening up the sodium channels, the onset of block is faster.[72] This may help explain why when the needle injection site is closer to the nerve to be anesthetized, the onset of block is faster.

Physiochemistry

Local anesthetics are divided into two major categories with different chemical structures: the esters and the amides (Table 6-7). The basic structure of these drugs is as follows:

$$COOR_1N\diagdown^{R_2}_{R_3} \qquad NHCOR_1N\diagdown^{R_2}_{R_3}$$

Ester type   **Amide type**

Both groups have an aromatic portion, an amide portion, and an intermediate (R_1) portion. The aromatic portion is responsible for the lipid solubility, whereas the amide portion is responsible for the hydrophilic properties. Note that the major difference between the ester and the amide local anesthetics is the linkage of the aromatic portion of the molecule to the intermediate chain (R_1). One group has an ester link and the other an amide link.

Local anesthetics are weak bases (usually tertiary amines) that are prepared as solutions of a salt (RNH^+Cl^-) because by themselves they are poorly soluble in water. In aqueous solutions the salts of these local anesthetics exist in both an uncharged tertiary amine base (RN) and a positively charged quaternary amine cation (RNH+). The total concentration *(C)* of local anesthetic could thus be expressed as follows:

$$C = RN + RNH^+$$

The relative proportions of RN and RNH^+ depend on the hydrogen ion concentration (pH) of the solution as well as the dissociative constant (pKa) of each local anesthetic. The more acid the solution (lower pH), the more cation and less base are present. The pKa is constant for each anesthetic and reflects the strength or weakness of the base characteristics of the anesthetic. The higher the pKa, the stronger the base, and the more ionized cation exists, compared to local anesthetics with a lower pKa at any given pH.

As has been discussed previously, it is thought that the uncharged anesthetic base, being lipid soluble, diffuses through the nerve membrane into the axoplasm. On entering the axoplasm, the base becomes a positively charged cation, which attaches to the phospholipid membrane at a receptor

in the internal orifice of the sodium channel. The entrance of sodium is thus denied and depolarization does not take place.

The hydrogen ion concentration is a very important determinant of how well an anesthetic works (Table 6-8). If the pH of an anesthetic solution is raised, more un-ionized base becomes available, which more easily diffuses across nerve membranes, thus increasing the rapidity of onset and depth of anesthesia. Conversely, if the pH is lowered, less base but more ionized cation is present. This makes it difficult for diffusion across nerve membrane. The pH of anesthetic solutions is lowered by the addition of sodium bisulfite, sodium metabisulfite (sodium pyrosulfite), or other antioxidants added to prevent oxidation of epinephrine in commercially prepared local anesthetic-epinephrine solutions.[84]

The environment into which an anesthetic is injected may also affect its activity, depending on the pH of the tissue. The more alkaline the environment, the lower the hydrogen ion concentration and the more base available for diffusion. The more acid the environment, the greater the hydrogen ion concentration and the weaker the block. Because most commercially prepared anesthetics with epinephrine are acidic, reinjection into an anesthetized site after a period of waiting or surgery of 45 minutes or 1 hour may result in observed tolerance, or tachyphylaxis, to the local anesthetic.[69] Infected tissues such as acute abscesses are known to have a lower pH than that of noninfected tissue. It has been observed clinically that anesthetics work less well in infected tissue.[45] Mucous membranes—in the mouth, for instance—have a low pH and therefore work against the potency of topical local anesthetics. Higher concentrations of local anesthetics (for instance, 4% lidocaine) are therefore used on mucous membranes. Of interest is the fact that benzocaine with a pKa of 3.5 exists with significant amounts of un-ionized base even at a low pH; consequently, it is an excellent topical anesthetic on mucous membranes. However, there is some experimental evidence to suggest that lidocaine may work better at a lower pH level.[3,238]

Chemical modification may influence the activity of local anesthetic solutions. The importance of the pH has already been discussed. Potassium,[22] dextran,[4] and even carbon dioxide[55] have been added to improve performance of local anesthetics. Potassium, when added to 2% lidocaine, prolongs nerve blocks, probably because the increased extraneural concentration of potassium delays repolarization. Dextran forms molecular complexes with local anesthetics and favors increased onset and prolongation of nerve blocks by delaying their absorption. Improved nerve blocks may also be obtained by carbonation of local anesthetic solutions. Carbon dioxide diffuses across nerve membranes and lowers the intraneural pH. As local anesthetics diffuse into this acidic intraneural space, there is greater production of positive ions, leading to an enhanced nerve block.[63] Wheth-

TABLE 6-7

Structure-activity relationship of local anesthetics

Generic and proprietary name	Aromatic (lipophilic)	Chemical structure Intermediate chain	Amide (hydrophilic)

A. Esters
  Cocaine

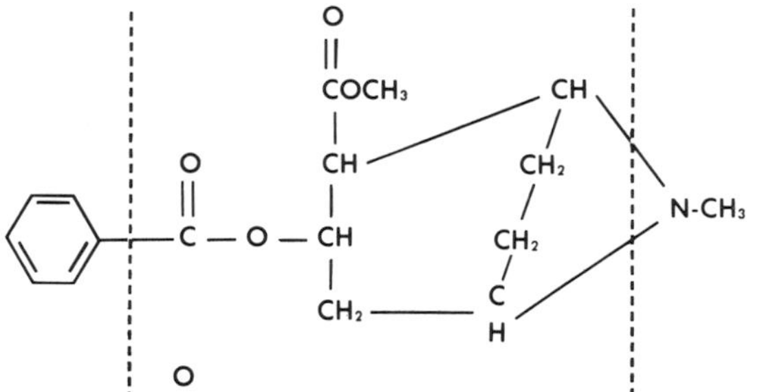

  Procaine
    (Novocain)

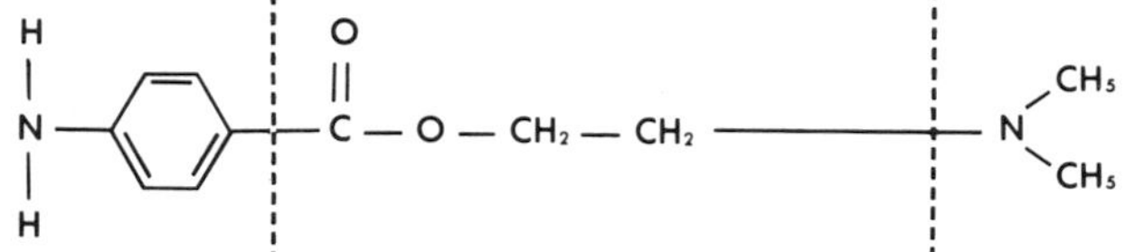

  Tetracaine
    (Pontocaine)

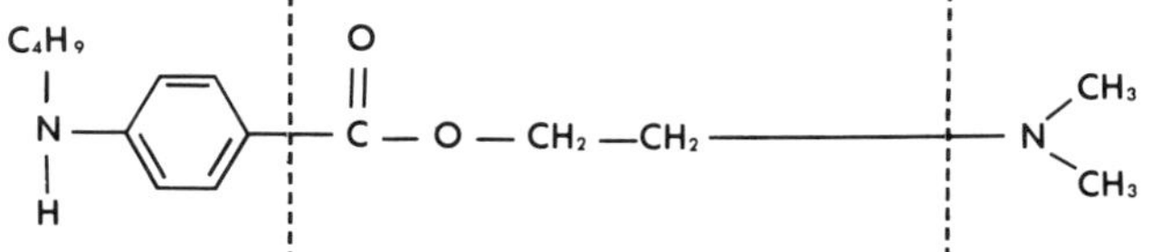

B. Amides
  Lidocaine
    (Xylocaine)

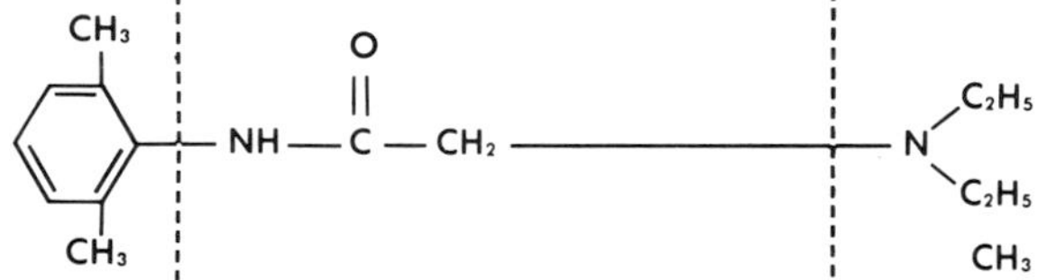

  Mepivacaine
    (Carbocaine)

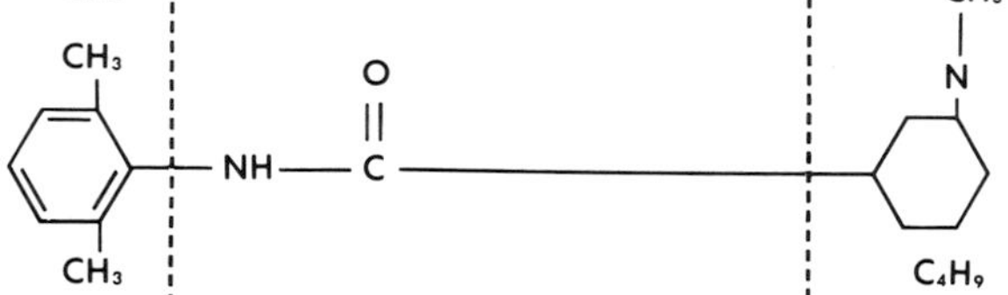

  Bupivacaine
    (Marcaine)

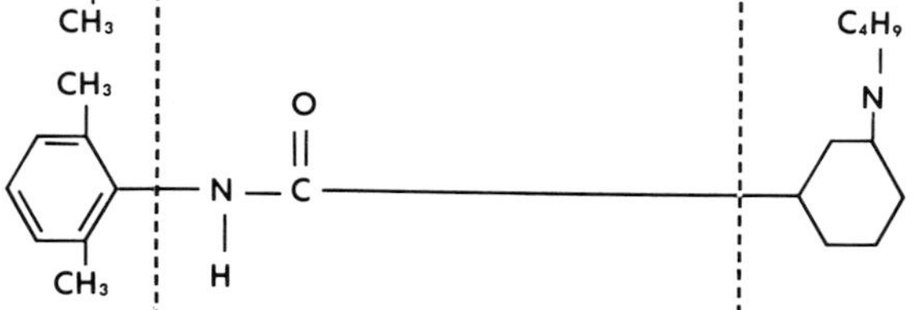

  Etidocaine
    (Duranest)

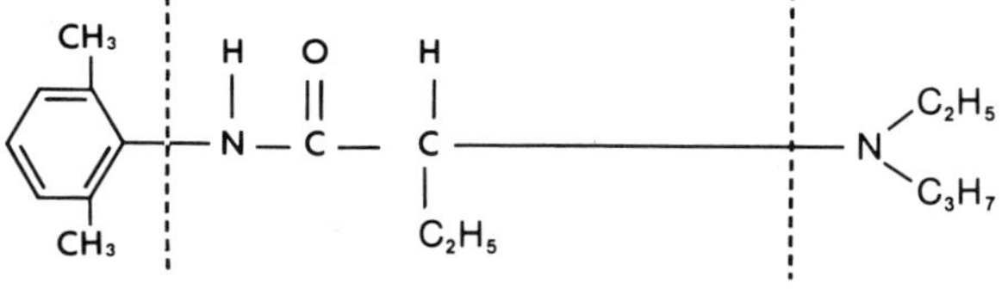

Modified from Covino, B.G., and Vassalo, H.G.: Local anesthetics: mechanisms of action and clinical use,
*Data from rat sciatic nerve blocking procedure.
1. Oleyl alcohol/pH 7.2 buffer; 2. N-heptane/pH 7.4 buffer; 3. Nerve homogenate binding; 4. Plasma protein

Partition coefficient	Physiochemical properties Protein binding (%)	Site of metabolism	Biologic properties Approximate anesthetic duration (min)*	Equi-effective anesthetic concentration*
		Plasma	45	
0.6[1]	5.8[3]	Plasma	50	2
80[1]	75.6[3]	Plasma	175	0.25
2.9[2]	64.3[4]	Liver	100	1
0.8[2]	77.5[4]	Liver	100	1
27.5[2]	95.6[4]	Liver	175	0.25
141[2]	94[4]	Liver	200	0.25

New York, 1976, Grune & Stratton, Inc.

binding 2 μg/ml

TABLE 6-8

Factors influencing local anesthetic behavior

	Onset time	Duration	Potency
↑ Dosage (concentration × volume)	↓	↑	↑
Vasoconstrictor added	↓	↑	↑
↑ Lipid solubility	↓	—	—
↑ Percentage of protein binding	—	↑	↑
↓ pH (tissue)	↑	—	↓
↓ pH (solution)	↑	—	—
↑ K^+ (solution)	↓	↑	—
CO_2 gas added	↓	—	↑
Dextran added	—	↑	—
Scleroderma	—	↑	—

er such chemical manipulation of local anesthetics is of value in cutaneous surgery remains to be seen. Most of the time adequate infiltrative and nerve-block anesthesia is produced by the available local anesthetics.

The two main factors that influence the ultimate action of a local anesthetic are its ability to diffuse through nerve sheaths and its degree of binding at the receptor sites in the cell membrane. The chemical structures of local anesthetics have some relationship to these types of biologic behavior. As mentioned earlier, local anesthetic molecules are divided into three parts, (1) the aromatic portion, (2) the intermediate chain, and (3) the amine portion. The aromatic portion is responsible for the lipophilic properties and the amine portion for the hydrophilic properties. Alterations in any one of these three parts modify an anesthetic's potency, time of onset, and duration of action. Increasing the molecular weight by lengthening the intermediate chain tends to increase anesthetic potency up to a point. The lipophilic properties are reflected by the time required for onset of activity, since the anesthetic must first diffuse through a lipid membrane (the myelin sheath that surrounds many nerves). This time is roughly correlated with the partition coefficient between oil and water. The percentage of protein binding reflects how tightly local anesthetics are bound to nerves and thus reflects the duration of anesthesia[288] (Tables 6-7 and 6-8).

An example of the modification of the chemical structure that causes a change in biologic activity is seen if one compares lidocaine to etidocaine. Etidocaine is formed by substitution of a propyl group for an ethyl group at the amine end of lidocaine and by the addition of an ethyl group in the intermediate chain. These changes result in a 50 times greater solubility in oil compared to water (expressed as partition coefficient) and a 50% increase in the attachment

to proteins (measured as the percentage of protein binding).[75] The biologic behavior of this compound is changed commensurate with these chemical alterations. Etidocaine is approximately four times as potent as lidocaine. Moreover, the duration of action is twice as long. These biologic results are consistent with a greater lipid solubility of etidocaine, which implies that it should pass through the lipid myelin sheath and axolemma more easily than lidocaine does and thus have a shorter onset of activity. The increased protein binding suggests that etidocaine attaches more tightly to the protein component of the membrane. This results in increased anesthetic potency and longer duration of action.

The anatomic location is very important in determining the absorption rate of local anesthetics. Highly vascular areas, such as the scalp, predispose to more rapid absorption of local anesthetics. The poor vascularity of the lower extremities favors slower absorption and longer-lasting anesthesia. It has been observed in patients with scleroderma that local anesthesia tends to last longer in the sclerodermatous tissue, probably because of the decreased vascularity.[99,177] This may be true even in areas not obviously affected by scleroderma,[159] but it has been my observation that such an effect is not clinically significant.

The chemical structure of each local anesthetic affects its toxicity. Drugs that are metabolized rapidly and whose metabolites are relatively nontoxic are safer than those metabolized slowly or those with toxic metabolites. In general the more potent a local anesthetic is, the more toxic it is.

A major difference between the amides and the esters is the site of metabolism. The esters are hydrolyzed in the plasma by pseudocholinesterase. Amides, on the other hand, are degraded in the liver. Some patients have a deficiency of pseudocholinesterase and demonstrate a reduced tolerance to the ester type of local anesthetics. Patients with liver disease, on the other hand, may show a reduced tolerance to amide local anesthetics.

Another difference between these two broad categories of anesthetics is their allergenic potential. One of the metabolites of the ester agents is paraaminobenzoic acid, which is a common sensitizing agent. Patients who have been sensitized to this somewhat ubiquitous compound may develop alarming allergic reactions to the ester local anesthetics, such as procaine. The amides, on the other hand, do not often induce sensitization and thus allergic reactions occur rarely. There does not appear to be any cross-sensitivity between the amide and ester local anesthetics.

Local anesthetic agents

The injectable local anesthetics may be categorized by duration of activity or relative potency, as shown in Table 6-9. The recommended maximal safe doses are also given. In general the longer-acting local anesthetics are more toxic, resulting in lower maximal safe dosages.

Esters. Most drugs in this category are derivatives of paraaminobenzoic acid (PABA); individuals who are allergic to PABA therefore may react to the ester local anesthetics.

Procaine was synthesized in 1905 by Einhorn and was the first widely used local anesthetic. It is the prototypic ester local anesthetic; its trade name (Novocain), is still synonymous with local anesthetic agents in the minds of many patients. It has a very low toxicity, compared to the amides, and thus in the past large amounts of it were given for regional anesthesia. It is nonirritating to tissues on injection[279] and is hydrolyzed in the plasma to PABA and diethylaminoethanol (DEAE).[52] The hydrolysis occurs via a plasma enzyme, pseudocholinesterase. Some individuals are deficient in this enzyme, and this anesthetic should not be given to them. As already pointed out, it is very sensitizing, and many individuals become allergic to it. Procaine also has the ability to conjugate with other drugs—for instance, penicillin—and prolong their action as well as provide some measure of anesthesia on injection.

Tetracaine is a powerful ester type of local anesthetic. It is ten times more potent than procaine but also ten times more toxic. Therefore it is not used for infiltration anesthesia because safer agents are available. Part of the reason for the extreme toxicity of tetracaine is the slow hydrolysis that occurs in plasma.[114]

Cocaine and benzocaine are both useful topical ester anesthetics. They are discussed in the section on surface anesthetic agents.

Amides. The first amide local anesthetics were synthesized in Sweden in 1943 and represented a significant advance in local anesthesia. Unlike the esters the amides are apparently not associated with the allergic reactions common with the ester local anesthetics. The first synthesized amide local anesthetic was lidocaine, and it soon replaced procaine as the standard local anesthetic.

Lidocaine is the most common local anesthetic currently in use. It was the first amide synthesized (in 1943) and commercially is known as Xylocaine. It is useful not only for infiltration anesthesia but for topical anesthesia as well. It can be purchased in multi-use vials from 0.5% to 2% with or without epinephrine 1:100,000 or 1:200,000 for infiltration. For most procedures in cutaneous surgery 1% lidocaine with epinephrine 1:100,000 or 1:200,000 is the preferred solution. Lidocaine may also be purchased as a 2% solution, which is very useful for nerve blocks. Topical preparations include ointments (from 2.5% to 5%), a jelly (2%), and a topical solution (4%).

On absorption from the site of infiltration, lidocaine distributes first in the vascular compartment and is then distributed to tissues. The distribution time from the vascular space to the peripheral tissue is rather short: approximately 8 minutes. The drug is then almost entirely metabolized in the liver by microsomal oxidases by dealkylation.[275] The

TABLE 6-9

Injectable local anesthetics

Potency	Duration (min)	Agent	Suggested maximal safe dose (in mg)*	
			Without epinephrine	With epinephrine
Low	20-45	Procaine	1000	—
Intermediate	60-120	Lidocaine	200	500
		Mepivacaine	350	350
High	200-400	Tetracaine	100	—
		Bupivacaine	150	150
		Etidocaine	300	400

Based on Swedish figures assuming 70 kg body weight. Data from Ericksson, E.: Illustrated handbook in local anesthesia, Philadelphia, 1980, W.B. Saunders Co.
*These doses are not necessarily safe, since severe reactions may occur with smaller doses.

resultant metabolites, monoethylglycinexylidide (MEGX) and glycinexylidide (GX), are then excreted by the kidneys. Unfortunately, the metabolites of lidocaine have some toxic and antiarrhythmic properties. The half-life of lidocaine from a bolus injection is 90 to 108 minutes.[47,246]

Mepivacaine (Carbocaine) is another amide with approximately the same onset and duration of action (seen experimentally) as that of lidocaine. However, in my experience the potency is not as great for infiltrative anesthesia. I have also noted a slower onset of action clinically, which may reflect a lower partition coefficient (lipid solubility).[288] Because its toxicity is less than for either lidocaine or even procaine,[289] it is considered by some to be useful when the toxic side effects of anesthetics must be considered. Mepivacaine is metabolized in the liver slightly differently from lidocaine, since CO_2 is produced. Also in contrast to lidocaine, mepivacaine is poorly metabolized by newborns, although it is excreted well by way of the kidneys. It was one of the first anesthetics to be shown to be excreted in the urine. Although some elimination by bile may also occur in man, not only with mepivacaine but with lidocaine, it is unknown to what extent bile is a pathway for excretion.[138]

Bupivacaine (Marcaine) is a long-acting anesthetic that is more potent but also more toxic than lidocaine or mepivacaine.[140,201] Its duration of action is much longer than lidocaine, but its onset of action is also much longer. This latter feature makes it difficult to use in a busy office practice. The maximal safe dose for an adult is 200 mg without epinephrine and 250 mg with epinephrine,[96] although lower dosages have been recommended by some (Table 6-9). It is degraded in the liver, like lidocaine. Its plasma half-life is 3.5 hours, compared to about 1.5 hours for lidocaine.[287]

Etidocaine (Duranest) is the newest amide local anesthetic first introduced clinically in 1973.[182] Although structurally it is similar to lidocaine, it is four times as potent and lasts twice as long.[51,173,255] However, unlike bupivacaine, etidocaine has a relatively short onset time, similar to that of lidocaine.[173] Therefore for procedures in which one does not wish to use epinephrine—for instance, digital nerve blocks—etidocaine is an excellent alternative to plain lidocaine.[38] The toxicity of etidocaine is probably greater than that of lidocaine,[7,54,204] although some authorities think it is lower.[51,181] It is certainly less toxic than the other long-acting anesthetic, bupivacaine, particularly when given subcutaneously.[7,204] Maximal safe dosages have been reported to be 300 mg without epinephrine and 400 mg with epinephrine.[181] The pharmacokinetics of etidocaine are similar to those of lidocaine, with a serum half-life of 114 minutes.[255]

Mixing local anesthetics

Local anesthetics are sometimes mixed to take advantage of the useful properties of each drug. Such mixtures may be less toxic than the sum total of the toxicities of the component drugs.[86] Some authorities, though, feel such mixtures are unpredictable and the proposed advantages only theoretic.[120]

When local anesthetics are mixed, the pH of the resultant solution may be important. The importance of pH on modifying the efficacy of local anesthetics has been discussed. Bupivacaine added to lidocaine results in a pH of 6.5. If bupivacaine is added to chloroprocaine, however, the resultant pH is 3.7.[53] Although this lower pH will probably be buffered to a more favorable pH by the tissue, repeated injections could theoretically overwhelm the tissue's buffering capacity.

Bupivacaine is an excellent long-acting local anesthetic, but its onset time may be quite prolonged. Therefore it has been suggested that mixing another local anesthetic with a shorter onset time—for instance, lidocaine—with bupivacaine would produce a more efficacious solution. In a study that evaluated this solution by pinprick, both the onset and duration of anesthesia were no different than those of plain bupivacaine.[278] This supports the contention that mixtures of local anesthetics are usually dominated by the properties of one drug and therefore offer no real advantages.[120]

The mixing of epinephrine with local anesthetics is covered in the section on vasoconstrictors.

Other agents. Antihistamines may be used for local infiltrative anesthesia when other local anesthetics are contraindicated. In a ranking of the antihistamines for this purpose, promethazine (Phenergan) was found to be most efficacious, followed by tripelennamine (Pyribenzamine), pyrilamine maleate (Neo-Antergan), and diphenhydramine (Benadryl).[160] Pyribenzamine in particular has been reported to provide excellent anesthesia.[44] Prochlorperazine (Compazine) has been shown experimentally to decrease the sodium current in nerves, as does lidocaine.[141] When used for local anesthesia, the antihistamines may be combined with epinephrine (1:100,000 or 1:200,000), which enhances the anesthetic potency and decreases bleeding. Although they are considered very safe, antihistamines may on occasion cross-react with local anesthetics in persons with an allergy to the latter drugs.[37] It should be remembered that injections of antihistamines (unlike local anesthetics) also have a sedative effect, particularly when doses exceeding 50 mg are given.

Both water and saline have been reported to provide local anesthesia, at least for superficial surgery,[190,267,296] and—like antihistamines—offer an alternative for individuals who claim to be allergic to all standard local anesthetics. These agents are discussed in the section on allergy to anesthetics.

Newer agents that are currently being investigated for local infiltrative anesthesia include the quinolone derivatives, particularly centbucridine.[250] Because every local anesthetic occasionally causes some problem, the quest for alternative local anesthetics continues.

Addition of vasoconstrictor agents

The addition of vasoconstrictors, usually epinephrine, helps to increase the activity of anesthetic agents. However, problems may occur with vasoconstrictors of which the physician should be aware.

Effects on anesthesia. Vasoconstrictors shorten the time of onset, prolong the duration,[45] and increase the depth of anesthesia. These effects are partly caused by the vasoconstrictor activity on blood vessels, which helps to localize the anesthetic to the area in which it is placed and thereby minimizes systemic absorption and precludes possible toxic side effects of anesthetics.[275] Experimentally epinephrine has been shown to increase the intraneural concentration of local anesthetics.[110] Such an increase is more than can be accomplished by merely increasing the anesthetic concentration alone. One possible explanation for this may be that epinephrine, by decreasing the local blood flow, causes a slowing of tissue metabolism and an increase in local tissue anoxia.[3] The result is a rise in pCO_2 and a fall in the tissue pH. This favors formation of the active (ionized) form of the local anesthetic within the nerve itself.

The addition of vasoconstrictors affects the nerve blocks of some anesthetics more than others. In general, long-acting anesthetics such as bupivacaine and etidocaine show little benefit with the addition of epinephrine, whereas the shorter-acting anesthetics benefit greatly by the addition of vasoconstrictors.

Effects on bleeding. An added benefit from the addition of vasoconstrictors is that there is less bleeding at the time of surgery. However, as the anesthetic wears off and the epinephrine effect diminishes, a patient may experience bleeding, which would not have been apparent at the time of surgery.

Concentration. In general the concentration of epinephrine should be kept to the minimal effective level. The optimal concentration of epinephrine enhancing anesthetic activity appears to be approximately 5 μg/ml or 1 mg/200 ml (1:200,000). A concentration of 1:400,000 is of little value and has no more vasoconstrictive effect than saline has. A concentration of 1:80,000 adds little more vasoconstrictive activity than a concentration of 1:200,000, but the higher concentration is associated with frequent side effects.[202] Therefore the commercially prepared solutions of 1:100,000 (1 mg/100 ml, or 10 μg/ml) concentration probably are unnecessarily high under some circumstances and result in greater side effects, depending on the dose.

pH. Epinephrine rapidly deteriorates on exposure to air and turns brown. This brownish color is caused by quinones, which are oxidation products of epinephrine. These discolored solutions should be discarded. To prevent such oxidation, commercially prepared solutions contain sodium bisulfite and/or sodium metabisulfite (sodium pyrosulfite). Unfortunately these compounds significantly lower the pH of the anesthetic solution, frequently to as low as 3.75.[200] Because such acid solutions result in relatively less free anesthetic base for diffusion across nerve membranes, they are theoretically not as effective as personally mixing one's own epinephrine-containing solutions, which will be free of acid-producing antioxidants and will thus have a higher pH. In addition, solutions of lower pH have been found to cause more pain for the patients[220]; therefore Moore recommends mixing an epinephrine-containing solution of 1:200,000 by taking 0.1 ml of 1:1000 epinephrine and placing it in 20 ml of anesthetic solution.[200] The pH of this mixture is about 6.3. However, whether such effort—to mix fresh lidocaine-epinephrine solutions—is of true clinical value remains to be proven. When actual measurements of the tissue pH have been performed in rabbits, the excess acidity of commercial preparations is quickly buffered by the extracellular tissue fluid.[295]

Untoward effects. Vasoconstrictors may be absorbed systemically, resulting in restlessness, an increase in the heart rate, palpitations, pounding in the head, and even chest pain. These symptoms are frequently misinterpreted by the patient or physician as an allergy or intolerance to the local anesthetic rather than a normal reaction to epinephrine. Such symptoms should alert the physician to the fact that significant amounts of local anesthetic have been absorbed from the injection site and that central nervous system toxicity may occur on further injection.

The cardiovascular effects of epinephrine in local anesthetic solutions are those of β-adrenergic stimulation. In a study of dental patients an increase in heart rate of up to 40 beats/minute was found in two thirds of the patients using 1:80,000 epinephrine.[14] However, this was not confirmed

in a more recent study on 40 patients with documented atherosclerotic heart disease.[100] In this study 1:50,000 epinephrine was used and no changes were seen in the ECG, blood pressure, or heart rate; however, the overall dose of epinephrine was less.

Epinephrine is particularly more prone to affect the heart rate and blood pressure in hyperthyroid patients. Also, patients who are extremely nervous may become more so with epinephrine solutions. Cardiac arrhythmias are not seen if the dose is kept to less than 50 ml of 1:100,000 dilution of epinephrine.[158] Tachycardia also is less likely to occur if phenylephrine (a pure α-adrenergic agonist and therefore a noncardiac stimulant) is used as a substitute for epinephrine[14]; still, phenylephrine is not as good a vasoconstrictor as epinephrine is.

On injection of anesthetic solutions with epinephrine the overlying skin becomes pale. This may be followed at a later time by cyanosis. The cyanosis has been explained as caused by blood pooling and the high content of deoxygenated hemoglobin.[164] This results in tissue hypoxia, which may adversely affect wound healing but, practically speaking, probably does not.

Necrosis of the skin with slough or even gangrene may occur subsequent to injection of epinephrine-containing solutions[198,248] (Fig. 6-5). Although such cases were much more frequently reported in the first half of this century[121,159,170,224,259] (when physicians were forced to mix their own concentrations of epinephrine-containing solutions), there are occasional recent case reports.[61,245] A hazard for those who mix their own anesthetic solutions is that incorrect amounts of epinephrine may be added to anesthetic solutions.[291] Many of the earlier cases were possibly the result of inordinately high epinephrine concentrations or unstable solutions. The necrosis from anesthetics containing vasoconstrictors is in tissues with restricted circulation to begin with. In the earlier reported cases patient selection probably did not take into account the vascular status of the digits. Several of the patients were anesthetized for infectious problems in the days before antibiotics.[159] Patients with peripheral vascular disease (such as diabetic patients) appear to be particularly prone to necrosis.[11] (Fig. 6-5). Vascular impairment may be further compounded by injection of large quantities of local anesthetic into closed anatomic spaces, impeding blood flow. The use of narrow tourniquets may also be a factor in restriction of blood flow.[18] In an interesting 1944 study, 30 rat tails were injected with procaine and epinephrine of varying concentrations.[224] One third of the rats developed necrosis in the injected tails, some with as small an epinephrine concentration as 1:100,000. Control animals injected either with saline or plain procaine did not develop necrosis.

The local ischemic problems in the literature associated with epinephrine-containing local anesthetic solutions almost invariably involve the digits. This has been my per-

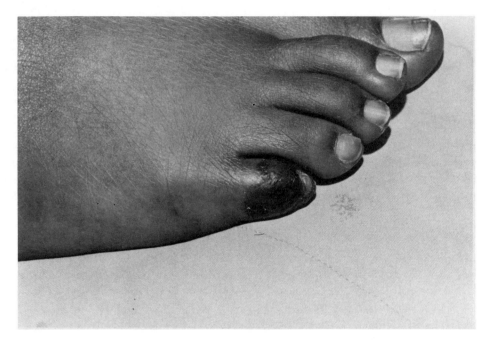

Fig. 6-5. Tissue necrosis in diabetic patient 2 days after removal of corn with use of local anesthetic with epinephrine (1:100,000) solution. Injection was given by corpsman in U.S. Navy.

ADVERSE REACTIONS ASSOCIATED WITH LOCAL ANESTHETIC SOLUTIONS

I. Generalized reactions
   A. Normal (expected)
      1. Toxic
         a. Central nervous system
         b. Cardiovascular
      2. Sympathetic stimulation
      3. Drug interactions
   B. Abnormal (unexpected)
      1. Vasovagal
      2. Sympathetic stimulation
      3. Allergy
      4. Idiosyncracy
      5. Intolerance
II. Localized reactions
   A. Normal (expected)
      1. Neurotoxicity
      2. Myotoxicity
      3. Vasodilation, or vasoconstriction
   B. Abnormal (unexpected)
      1. Allergy
      2. Necrosis

---

sonal experience as well (Fig. 6-5). Therefore *for anesthesia on the digits I do not use epinephrine-containing solutions.* Nevertheless, some authorities condone the use of weak (1:200,000) epinephrine solutions in these areas.[102,152,156] Certainly in young healthy individuals lidocaine with epinephrine 1:200,000 does not lead experimentally to prolonged ischemia in the toes.[129] However, for practical purposes one cannot always be certain that one is not dealing with a patient who is diabetic or who has a local vascular insufficiency at the time of surgery.

The ear lobes and nose have an adequate blood supply, and I do not feel epinephrine is contraindicated in those areas. Some authorities recommend against infiltration of skin flaps with epinephrine-containing solutions.[217] Certain medications (such as antihypertensives that block the uptake of catecholamines by nerve endings) may also potentiate the sympathomimetic action of epinephrine and lead to necrosis of the injected tissue.[119]

Adverse reactions to local anesthetics. Reactions to local anesthetics, like those to all drugs, may be classified as either generalized or localized, and further subclassified as normal (expected) or abnormal (unexpected) (see box). Normal, expected reactions are dose related and are seen when enough drug is present to alter the physiology. Such normal effects include toxic reactions. Drug interactions are usually normal reactions. Abnormal, unexpected reactions include allergy or individual idiosyncracies.

Any drug can potentially cause other reactions than are intended. The physician therefore should be familiar with both the toxic and allergic potential of all drugs used, as well as any miscellaneous reactions that might ensue.

The toxic effects of local anesthetics occur both systemically and locally. Symptoms and signs of central nervous system (CNS) toxicity appear rarely. More often, systemic sympathomimetic responses are caused by the epinephrine in anesthetic solutions, which on absorption results in anxiety, tremor, tachycardia, and diaphoresis. Vasovagal reactions are varied; one may see hyperventilation, apprehension, and syncope. Local reactions include swelling, erythema, and even abscess formation with necrosis of tissue caused by local toxic effects or the addition of epinephrine.

True allergic reactions include pruritis, rhinorrhea, urticaria, and angioedema with bronchospasm manifested as coughing or wheezing. In a study of untoward reactions to local anesthetics in 1978, 25% of patients had localized swelling, 15% had immediate urticaria or facial swelling, and 60% had other systemic or local reactions.[151] Death caused by anaphylactic reactions to lidocaine has also been reported.[206]

In addition to the preceding types of reactions to local anesthetics, Adriani and Naraghi add two more: intolerance and idiosyncrasy.[11] Intolerance implies a toxic reaction at a lower dose than normal, that is, a quantitatively abnormal response. Idiosyncrasy, on the other hand, is a qualitatively unanticipated response to a drug that differs entirely from its usual pharmacologic action. One must distinguish intolerance and idiosyncrasy from true allergic reactions, which are caused by immune responses.

Drug responses, like other biologic variables, can be described only statistically, and not be too surprised at occasional great variations from the mean. Basic resuscitative equipment should therefore be available whenever local anesthetics are given.[12] (See Appendix F.)

Toxicity. All local anesthetics are toxic agents. Maximal safe dosages are stated in Table 6-9. Toxic reactions can occur after routine infiltrative anesthesia or nerve blocks. Whatever the route of administration, local anesthetics eventually make their way to the blood stream. These toxic reactions may either be local, giving rise to inflammation or gangrene, or systemic. The systemic reactions are discussed here. Specific drug therapy for toxic reactions is described in Appendix F.

The extent of systemic toxicity depends on the concentration of local anesthetic in the blood. With lidocaine subjective symptoms appear at plasma concentrations of 3 to 5 μg/ml and objective signs appear at higher concentrations—6 to 10 μg/ml.[41] Plasma concentration is the result of a balance between the rate of absorption of a local anesthetic and its rate of elimination and depends on certain factors: total dosage,[188] speed of the injection, vascularity of the injection site, presence of a vasoconstrictor in the anesthetic solution, physicochemical characteristics of the local anesthetic, inadvertent intravascular injection, and decreased metabolism of the local anesthetic. Anesthetic over-

dose may occur in the elderly or sick, for whom a toxic dose is less than for healthy adults. Patients who are acidotic (for instance, by hypoventilation) cause a greater amount of ionized local anesthetic base to be present; this enhances toxicity.[58] Moreover, preexisting renal, hepatic,[258] or cardiac failure[232] also contributes to an elevated plasma concentration of local anesthetics. Drugs such as phenytoin, which is metabolized in the liver, may also potentiate the CNS side effects of local anesthetics such as lidocaine.[157]

Toxic blood levels of local anesthetics are usually caused by either inadvertent intravenous injection (into an artery or a vein), injection into a highly vascular area, or extravascular deposition of a large amount of anesthetic.[74] It is wise to remember that the perineural concentration of a local anesthetic is several times greater than that tolerated systemically—thus the smallest volume of the lowest concentration of local anesthetic that provides effective anesthesia is least likely to result in toxic side effects.

The site of injection has been shown to contribute to the blood levels attained, since the rate of absorption from various extravascular anatomic sites is markedly different. Injection into the deltoid area (of the arm), for instance, results in a higher blood level than injection into the vastus lateralis muscle (of the leg).[253] Injection into highly vascular areas, such as the scalp, may raise the plasma levels of anesthetics, which results in minor signs of CNS toxicity.[189] On the other hand, injection into areas of low vascularity, such as fat tissue of the buttock, results in slow absorption and low plasma levels. In highly vascular areas the total dose (volume X concentration) will therefore more closely reflect subsequent blood levels.

Probably the most common reason for toxic blood levels of local anesthetics is inadvertent intravascular injection.[16] In a retrospective study of 13,287 nerve blocks or local infiltrations, there were 7 instances of seizures, all thought to be caused by unintentional intravascular injection.[202] In this case use of higher concentrations of local anesthetic solutions are more likely to result in toxic side effects.

Aldrete et al.[23] emphasize that inadvertent injection of local anesthetics into an artery in the scalp may more easily reach the cerebral circulation and produce a CNS toxic response. They estimated that as little as 1 mg of lidocaine can produce a toxic concentration in the cerebral circulation if introduced into the carotid artery.

For local infiltrative anesthesia of the skin, 1% lidocaine with 1:100,000 epinephrine works very well. Some physicians recommend a lower concentration (0.5% lidocaine with 1:200,000 epinephrine) on the basis that there is less likelihood of toxic side effects.[36,75] However, successful anesthesia may not be as easily obtained with lower concentrations, and the duration of anesthesia is not as long. This latter factor may be important for larger and more prolonged procedures. Nerve blocks are also better (earlier onset, longer duration, greater potency) with even higher concentrations of local anesthetics (2% lidocaine).[111]

On intravenous infusion, a local anesthetic is distributed within two compartments in two phases, followed by an elimination phase. The drug is initially dispersed in the small central compartment, comprised of the vascular spaces and highly perfused tissue. Then a slower distribution phase occurs from the small central compartment to the much larger compartment of peripheral tissues. Finally an elimination phase occurs during which the anesthetic and its metabolites are cleared from the circulation by way of the kidneys. For lidocaine the total distribution phase lasts about 8 minutes, and the half-life in plasma is 90 to 108 minutes.[47,246]

The systemic toxic reactions of local anesthetics mainly involve the central nervous system and the cardiovascular system. Both of these systems are involved in the conduction and transmission of impulses. The CNS effects, however, mirror the local anesthetic's concentration in the blood. The higher the blood level, the more effect on the brain. In general the toxic reactions first are expressed by signs of CNS excitation, followed by CNS depression and then respiratory arrest.

CNS toxicity is first manifested by light-headedness, disorientation, muscle twitching, slurred speech, irritability, nystagmus, restlessness, and tremor. Just before these appear the patient may complain of circumoral numbness and tingling as the local anesthetic concentrates in this highly vascular area. The stimulation of the CNS is thought to be caused by selective depression of the inhibitory neurons in the cerebral cortex.[116,271] Convulsions may occur and are tonic and clonic in type. With further depression of the CNS, the medulla and pons are affected, resulting in decreased respirations and eventually death.[272]

Convulsions occur when the blood level of a local anesthetic reaches a certain threshold level. The best way to prevent such a blood level is to limit the total dosage, to add a vasoconstrictor, and to take precaution against intravascular injection. Some authorities suggest, perhaps unwisely that it may be useful to premedicate the patient with diazepam (0.1 mg/kg) should large amounts of local anesthetic be used.[18] It has been found that diazepam helps to prevent CNS seizures induced by local anesthetics[82]; however, it may also cause respiratory depression and mask the CNS signs of irritability, allowing the patient to slip into respiratory depression. In addition, diazepam also does not prevent the adverse circulatory effects of local anesthetics.[81,85]

Different local anesthetics have different threshold levels at which toxic effects are seen. In general, however, for lidocaine, subjective symptoms of toxicity occur at plasma concentrations of 3 to 5 μg/ml and objective signs at 6 to 10 μg/ml.[41,114] Minor toxicity of the CNS (such as light-headedness, circumoral numbness, slurred speech, or spots in front of the eyes) has even been reported at lower levels of 1 to 2 μg/ml,[188,254] which may occur with procedures such as hair transplantation or even local anesthesia for

cardiac catheterization.[213] A dose of 50 mg of lidocaine IV results in a blood level of about 1 μg/ml.[139]

In a study by Maloney et al., serum concentrations of lidocaine were monitored during hair transplantation.[188] Lidocaine 2% was used, some of which contained epinephrine 1:100,000. These investigators found that the peak serum concentration in μm/ml roughly correlated with the total dose in milligrams (injected intradermally or subcutaneously) and could be calculated by multiplying the total dose in milligrams by 0.0025. An infiltrated dose of 400 mg into the scalp thus results in a peak serum concentration of 1 μg/ml (400 mg $\times$ 0.0025 = 1 μg/ml).

Lidocaine is better tolerated milligram for milligram with respect to CNS toxicity than etidocaine, which is better tolerated than bupivacaine.[254] That is, the CNS toxicity is proportionate to the relative anesthetic potency.[7,179] Although there is no evidence that these agents differ in their cardiotoxic properties,[203] there have been reports of refractory cardiac arrest caused by bupivacaine used for obstetric purposes.

Parenthetically it should be mentioned that on injection of procaine penicillin, a patient may occasionally experience symptoms and signs (dizziness, twitching, shaking, or even convulsions) similar to those resulting from CNS toxicity from other local anesthetics. Such symptoms may be associated with an increased plasma concentration of procaine and are probably the result of increased absorption rate or inadvertent intravascular injection.[131]

Should signs of CNS toxicity develop, one should protect the patient from physical injury and place him or her in the Trendelenberg position. The patient should also be hyperventilated with oxygen to lower the CO_2 tension. This increases the plasma pH, making less anesthetic cation available within nervous tissue, and raises the cortical seizure threshold.[82,101,271] Diazepam is the drug of choice should seizures occur.[81] Convulsions caused by local anesthetics may be a threat to life.[83]

The toxic cardiovascular effects of local anesthetics include effects on both the heart and peripheral arteries. However, the cardiovascular system is more resistant to the toxic actions of local anesthetics than the CNS is. All local anesthetics except cocaine are vasodilators; that is, they can cause vasodilation. The blood pressure may fall, and the patient may be pale with nausea and cold sweating. Since these symptoms occur more frequently if the head is raised, it is preferable to inject local anesthetics with the patient lying flat. Should the patient become faint, lower the head and administer oxygen.

Some of the decrease in blood pressure may be caused by the direct effect of local anesthetics on the heart itself. Decreases in the rate of conduction and the force of contraction may occur. It has been stated that on occasion small amounts of anesthetic employed for simple infiltrative anesthesia can cause cardiovascular collapse and death.[240] Although such cases are rare, they have been documented in the medical literature.[49,162,284] There appears to be more of an effect on patients with known conduction disturbances or the sick sinus syndrome, particularly if the patient is taking antiarrhythmic medications.[49,162]

Allergy. A history of allergy to local anesthetics may lead to denial of the benefits of local anesthesia. Most of the time the history of allergy cannot be substantiated. However, general anesthesia is recommended, sometimes under hazardous conditions.

It has been estimated that less than 1% of all reactions to local anesthetics are truly allergic.[56,291] The majority of patients with a history of allergy to local anesthetic drugs are not truly allergic; most of the time the patient is describing the effect of epinephrine (which may be added to local anesthetic solutions) or a toxic drug overdose. Although allergy to the ester type of local anesthetics certainly occurs, allergy to the amide anesthetics is rare. Still, such reactions can occur, and resuscitative equipment and drugs should be available.[12]

Many patients with a demonstrated allergic reaction to local anesthetics have underlying immunologic problems. In one study of 27 patients with a history of allergies to local anesthetics, almost half the patients had a history of allergies to other medications, penicillin being the most frequent (perhaps the procaine portion of procaine penicillin).[21] In another study 6 out of 8 patients were atopic or had immunologic problems such as urticaria.[32] A positive antinuclear antibody (ANA) was reported in one patient with a true allergy to bupivacaine, an amide local anesthetic.[56] Of a series of patients with drug allergies, 40% had positive intracutaneous reactions to the ester local anesthetics.[19]

The esters are the main local anesthetics responsible for true allergic reactions. Procaine has fallen into disuse partially because of its sensitizing potential. Many dentists even became contact sensitized to procaine because of repeated exposure on a daily basis.[171] Procaine can cross-react with other anesthetics of the ester series as well as with the procaine portion of procaine penicillin. Procaine is a para-aminobenzoic acid (PABA) ester, and many individuals sensitized to PABA may react to procaine. Benzocaine, another ester type of local anesthetic, is currently in common use in every orifice: ear, mouth, vagina, and rectum.[112] Thus exposure to this substance is widespread.

Allergy to procaine is relatively simple to elicit. One study used 0.1 ml of various anesthetics intradermally and found procaine reactions in 20 of 27 patients with a history of allergy to local anesthetics.[21] In none of these patients was a reaction to lidocaine found. Several of these allergic reactions were confirmed by means of the Prausnitz-Küstner (P-K) reaction, which is perhaps the most sensitive indicator of true allergic reactions. In this test a nonallergic individual is intradermally inoculated with serum from someone who is allergic. The serum presumably contains antibodies

that fix to the skin. Injection of the antigen into the same area 2 days later leads to an allergic response if the antibody was present in the initial inoculation. This test is no longer used because of the danger of transmitting hepatitis or other viral diseases.

Allergy to the amide type of local anesthetics can occur, but lidocaine allergy is undoubtedly very rare. Although there have been a number of case reports of allergy to lidocaine* most of them have not been substantiated. Some of these cases had positive intradermal tests to lidocaine; however, a possible reaction to preservatives, especially parabens, was not always considered. Parabens (usually methyl- or butyl-paraben) are used as preservatives in multiple-dose vials of local anesthetics, of both amide and ester types. These chemicals, whose structures are similar to that of para-aminobenzoic acid, have been used since the 1930s as bacteriostatic and fungistatic agents in drugs, cosmetics, and even foods. Parabens in local anesthetics may act as sensitizers and cause systemic allergic reactions, including anaphylaxis.[73,209] Single-dose vials do not contain parabens and are safe for these paraben-sensitive individuals to use. However, the package inserts should be double-checked to make sure solutions are paraben free.

In a study of 10 patients with a history of allergy to lidocaine, none had a positive test with intracutaneous injection[20]; interestingly, 4 of the 5 tested gave a positive reaction to parabens. Similar negative results to testing several patients allegedly sensitive to lidocaine have been found by other investigators.[32,90] In one report, 8 patients with a history of allergy to lidocaine did not react on direct challenge with lidocaine.[32] The investigators concluded that true anaphylaxis to injected lidocaine has never been conclusively demonstrated, although case reports do occasionally appear.[206]

Topical sensitization to lidocaine appears to be more firmly substantiated[15,118,163] and is a risk with topical anesthetics. This may be related to the higher concentrations (4% to 5%) used topically compared with those used intradermally (1% to 2%). Anaphylaxis possibly may occur with topical lidocaine sensitization.[15]

A few rather unusual reactions to lidocaine reported in the literature include urticarial dermographism[65] and a generalized exfoliative dermatitis.[149] In both these cases no studies were done to substantiate lidocaine as the true cause and to exclude parabens.

Among the remaining amide anesthetics, bupivacaine,[56] mepivacaine,[21] and prilocaine[37] have been shown to cause positive reactions on skin testing in patients with a history of allergies to these local anesthetics. With the bupivacaine reaction, the patient was shown to have a decrease in C4 (fourth component of complement) in the plasma on chal-

---

*References 20, 32, 104, 150, 185, 206, 207, 216, 243.

lenge with a minute quantity of anesthetic solution, indicating that the reaction was immunologically mediated.[56]

The approach to the patient with a history of allergy to local anesthetics is confusing. Frequently such patients give a history of multiple allergies to several drugs or anesthetics, making selection of an alternative anesthetic difficult if not impossible. The patient's history is almost worthless.[151] In one large series of 90 patients who gave a history of allergy to local anesthetics, no patient tested had an allergy to local anesthetics.[90] Epicutaneous patch tests are of little value even where true allergy exists,[21] and intranasal testing, as recommended by some,[104] is unproven.[32]

Considerable disagreement exists regarding the validity of intradermal skin tests in either diagnosing or predicting immediate reactions to local anesthetics. However, such tests may be useful as a challenge technique.[68] Fisher et al. advocate intradermal testing with local anesthetics in high dilution (1:100,000) as well as testing drugs in both the amide and ester groups.[113] Testing should also be performed for preservatives, such as methylparaben. A positive reaction is seen as a wheal and flare. If no response is seen, it is probably safe to use that particular anesthetic.

It is also recommended that increasing amounts of local anesthetic should be given intradermally as a challenge technique to eliminate the possibility, although remote, of drug intolerance or idiosyncratic reaction.[11] One should test with a preservative-free solution (single-dose vial). Other investigators advocate using 0.1 ml of local anesthetic in usual concentrations intradermally for testing.[21] The Prausnitz-Küstner (P-K) reaction may also be used but is not currently recommended because the risk of transmitting hepatitis or other viruses is possible.[21]

In a study in which 19 patients were positive to local anesthetics by intradermal testing, the P-K reaction was positive in only 14.[21] Therefore a positive intradermal test is only presumptive evidence of allergy to a local anesthetic. A negative intradermal test is good evidence against a possible reaction but may also suggest tolerance. Tolerance may help explain the negative intradermal tests in case reports of lidocaine sensitivity.[185] Therefore one should still be cautious despite a negative intradermal test.

In another interesting study, 5 of 59 patients tested had positive intradermal skin tests to local anesthetics.[151] Although all 59 patients had given a history of reactions to local anesthetics, the 5 positive responses were positive to local anesthetics other than the one mentioned by each patient; 3 of the 5 patients with positive tests were subsequently given the local anesthetic to which they had had a positive response. In no patient was there a detectable adverse reaction. The authors conclude that skin testing is neither sufficient nor necessary.

When allergy testing is unavailable, inconvenient, or inconclusive, antihistamines, water, or saline may be used as a substitute for common local anesthetics. Antihistamines have the structural features that render local anesthetic activity without the antigenic determinant of the more conventional anesthetic agents. Diphenhydramine is readily available and has a weak anesthetic action; however, if more than 50 mg is given (5 ml of a 1% solution), the patient experiences sedation. The onset of anesthesia is very slow. Both water[267] and saline[190,296] have had their advocates for local anesthesia. However, commercially available sterile solutions of both these substances probably contain benzyl alcohol as a bacteriostatic agent, and therefore this agent itself may have local anesthetic properties.[235] Because benzyl alcohol may induce an irreversible effect on nerve conduction, its use should be discouraged.[105] Benzyl alcohol–free sodium chloride can be obtained. To be effective, sodium chloride must be injected to produce a wheal.[190] Although it may be used for small procedures, it is inadequate for larger surgery.[296] Distilled water can be used for local anesthesia, but it is very painful—probably caused in part by the tissue expansion that occurs on injection.[94,267]

Necrosis and gangrene. Tissue necrosis followed by slough and even gangrene caused by vascular impairment has been reported.[61] Usually this is caused by the addition of a vasoconstrictor, so, this topic is more fully dealt with in the section on vasoconstrictors. However, the hydrostatic pressure of large amounts of local anesthetic itself in confined anatomic spaces can contribute to vascular occlusion. This may occur in the digits or penis if the whole structure is ringed tightly with anesthesia[1]—so this practice should be discouraged. Certain drugs, such as antihypertensives, have also been reported to potentiate the action of epinephrine and result in necrosis at the site of injection of local anesthetic with epinephrine.[119]

Effects on fetus and newborn. Although there are reasons to believe that local anesthetics may be more toxic when used on pregnant women and newborn infants, reactions of clinical significance have not been described.[25] Lidocaine has been found to be metabolized in the immature liver of newborns,[169] so this probably accounts for a lack of untoward reactions. One word of caution, however. Parabens, which are used as preservatives in local anesthetics, competitively bind to albumin.[234] Therefore bilirubin, which also binds to albumin, may be displaced. Consequently, paraben-free local anesthetics should be used on jaundiced newborn infants if minor surgery becomes necessary.

Death. Death has been reported with local anesthesia.[87,276] This usually has been stated to be caused by excessive doses, far above what are regarded as maximal safe dosages. In one case, the patient probably received 125 ml of 2% lidocaine (2500 mg) resulting in a serum concentration at autopsy of 12 mg/ml.[276] Death may also occur by anaphylaxis.[206]

Drug interactions. Several types of drug interactions between local anesthetic agents (including epinephrine) and other medications being taken by patients are possible. The most important ones are listed in Table 6-1. The two most important drugs that might cause problems are the mono-amine oxidase (MAO) inhibitors and the tricyclic antidepressants. Patients on these drugs should be given local anesthetics with great caution. Some authorities recommend discontinuance of these medications for 1 to 2 weeks before elective surgery. The MAO inhibitors block the action of monoamine oxidase on naturally occurring amines, including epinephrine. Therefore cocaine, which is a vasoconstrictor, results in a slightly elevated blood pressure if given to patients on MAO inhibitors.

The tricyclic antidepressants probably act by blocking the re-uptake of norepinephrine at the nerve endings, enhancing epinephrine's effect and thus resulting in elevation of the blood pressure and tachycardia.[128,277] However, vasodilation and bleeding have also been reported. A case of profuse bleeding occurred when the nasal mucosa of a patient taking a tricyclic antidepressant was operated on.[252] The epinephrine in the local anesthetic solution may have stimulated the β-2 receptors locally, resulting in vasodilation. The α-1 receptors were probably blocked by the tricyclic antidepressant, leaving unopposed the action of epinephrine on the β receptor.

Chlorpromazine (Thorazine) and the other phenothiazines may interact with epinephrine, causing a paradoxical vasodilation and a fall in blood pressure. This effect is apparently not seen when phenylephrine is substituted for epinephrine.

The widely used β-blocker, propranolol (Inderal), may interact with epinephrine and cause a marked hypertensive episode followed by reflex bradycardia. This reaction is potentially fatal.[115] Basically it is thought that the propranolol blocks the peripheral β receptors (β-2), leaving unopposed the action of epinephrine in the α receptors. This leads to enhanced vasoconstriction and hypertension. The ensuing reflex bradycardia is made worse because the β receptors of the heart (β-1) are also blocked. This may lead to either hypertensive stroke or cardiac arrest. It is recommended that patients on propranolol discontinue this medication at least 3 days before surgery, or local anesthetics without epinephrine should be utilized. Should such a reaction occur, one should consider using intravenous chlorpromazine, which is an α blocker, or aminophylline, a β agonist.

Although Foster and Aston[115] reported several patients on β-blockers who had hypertensive episodes while receiving local anesthetics that contained epinephrine, it should be pointed out that these patients were also receiving multiple medications at the time of surgery. These additional medications in conjunction with the β-blocker may in some way modulate the response to epinephrine. I have seen no untoward reactions to small doses (5 to 10 ml of lidocaine 1% with epinephrine 1:100,000) in patients on β-blockers.

Some drugs displace the plasma binding of local anesthetics, resulting in higher levels of free local anesthetic in the blood and thus greater likelihood of toxic side effects. This has been shown to be true with patients taking phenytoin (Dilantin), who were given lidocaine[157] or bupivacaine.[125] Meperidine may also displace bupivacaine.

Another mechanism by which local anesthetic blood levels may be elevated is by inhibiting the metabolism of the drug. Cimetidine is known to inhibit microsomal metabolism and thus impairs elimination of anticoagulants and diazepam.[165] In perhaps the same way, it also interferes with the metabolism of lidocaine and results in higher lidocaine blood levels.[166]

Miscellaneous. Local anesthetics may influence the immune response. Lidocaine has been shown to bind to the cell membranes of lymphocytes and to inhibit the membrane-mediated events necessary for activation by polyclonal mitogens.[107] Both E (erythrocyte) rosette and EA (erythrocyte-antibody) rosette formation (the lining up of red blood cells around T and B cells, respectively) are also blocked by lidocaine.[249] These immunologic blocking reactions are dose related, and it is uncertain that they are significant at the lidocaine concentrations used in clinical practice. However, high concentrations can occur at sites of injection that are lethal in vitro to lymphocytes.[77]

Local anesthetics have been found to have profound effects on nerves. All local anesthetics are neurotoxic if the concentration is high enough. Neural damage probably occurs with intrafascicular injection and results in both axonal and myelin degeneration[124]—but such changes may disappear by 48 hours.[231] Neural damage was not substantiated by investigators who injected the trigeminal nerve with lidocaine without epinephrine,[60] suggesting that the presence of epinephrine in the anesthetic solution potentiates the axonal degeneration.[257] Other authorities dispute this.[124] Some local anesthetics of the ester type (particularly 2-chloroprocaine) are more neurotoxic than the amides.[35,124] However, neuropathy has been reported with lidocaine at a concentration of 1.5%.[199] Moreover, protein transport within nerves has been shown to be inhibited and oxygen uptake decreased.[109]

Local anesthetics have been demonstrated to be myotoxic as well.[214] Injection of 2% lidocaine into muscle fibers with epinephrine 1:100,000 produces myonecrosis with hyalinization and invasion of fibers by macrophages.[299] Although this effect is followed by regeneration of fibers, in some areas microscarring may occur.[39] This effect is related to the concentration of the local anesthetic, since no damage to muscle occurred with lidocaine 0.5% and significant damage occurred with 2%.[40] Epinephrine may also make the myonecrosis worse.[39]

Wound healing has been shown to be affected by local anesthetics.[66,205,214] Use of a local anesthetic (lidocaine) was found to decrease wound tensile strength.[205] This effect is enhanced by more concentrated solutions and by the addi-

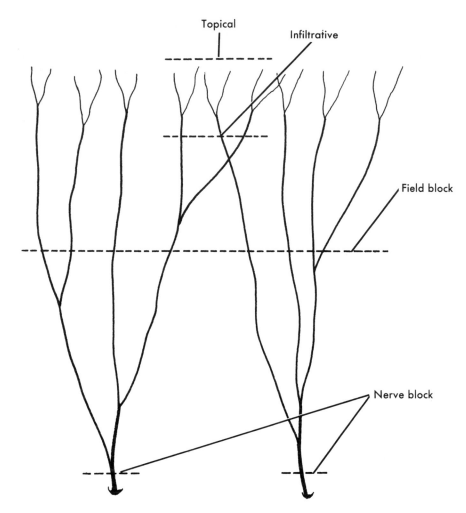

Fig. 6-6. Types of regional anesthesia. Note that with nerve block anesthesia, small volumes of anesthetic anesthetize large areas, whereas with field block larger amounts of anesthesia are required.

tion of epinephrine. Concentrations of local anesthetics of 1% or less probably do not adversely affect wound healing.[214]

Impotence has been reported following injection of the corpus cavernosum of the penis with lidocaine.[221] Both lidocaine[89] and prilocaine[147] have been associated with methemoglobinuria, a condition of little clinical significance unless the patient has poor oxygen reserves. Because local anesthetic solutions are slightly hypertonic, the water content of infiltrated tissue is increased, promoting edema.[251] Increased thrombosis of vessels is also noted if local anesthesia is used in conjunction with laser therapy.[184]

Increased bleeding from the operative site may occur in alcoholic patients with cirrhosis on whom local anesthetics are used. Such individuals often have vasodilation, particularly on the face. Local anesthetics, which are also vasodilators, thus enhance bleeding. Therefore epinephrine is very useful in local anesthetic solutions to counteract the vasodilation found in these circumstances.

Injection of local anesthetics

Successful use of local anesthetics to block peripheral nerves requires certain techniques based on a knowledge of anatomy and an understanding of the physiochemical properties of anesthetic agents. Regional anesthesia can be divided into four categories pertinent to cutaneous surgery (Fig. 6-6): topical, infiltrative, field block, and peripheral nerve block anesthesia. Infiltrative and topical anesthesia primarily affect nerve endings. The difference between these two techniques is the method of getting the anesthetic to the nerve endings. With infiltrative anesthesia the anesthetic is placed into the skin and subcutaneous tissue with a needle; with topical anesthesia the anesthetic diffuses across the skin or mucous membrane after being applied topically.

Peripheral nerve block requires deposition of an adequate amount of anesthetic in close proximity to the membrane of a nerve trunk. Field block occurs when a local anesthetic is infiltrated more distal to a major nerve trunk. It is less exacting than a nerve block, so relatively greater amounts of local anesthetic are used. It is used where the location of nerves cannot be precisely known; therefore one blocks a field through which such nerves traverse.

Equipment. Proper equipment helps to minimize pain of injection for the patient and to increase efficiency for the physician. Syringes should hold 1 ml, 3 ml, or 5 ml, depending on the amount of anesthetic necessary. The smaller the diameter size of the plunger in the syringe, the easier it is to inject an anesthetic solution (given the same needle size). This is based on the following formula:

$$P = \frac{F}{A}$$

P is the pressure of the anesthetic solution leaving the syringe, *F* is the force on the plunger, and *A* is the area of the bottom surface of the plunger.[301] Larger syringes (10 ml) make giving anesthesia difficult and require more pressure. All syringes should be the Luer-Lok type to prevent inadvertent slippage of the needles from the syringe. When this occurs, the patient and physician are embarrassingly doused with anesthetic.

Although it is probably preferable to use disposable syringes, a few specialized glass syringes may be useful on occasion. One type of glass syringe has rings for the first two fingers and the thumb. This allows one to withdraw the plunger easily with one hand to check to see if inadvertent entry has been made into a blood vessel. Another special type of syringe is the self-filling syringe (the Pitkin or Cornwell).[2] This type of syringe has a side attachment that can be placed in a basin of anesthetic solution. When the syringe plunger is withdrawn, the syringe fills with anesthetic solution. This may be useful when large amounts of anesthetic are necessary and saves the cost of syringes and needles as well as time.

The caliber of the needles is important in minimizing pain for patients. A small puncture in the skin hurts less and causes less trauma than a large one does. The use of the 30-gauge needle has become routine in cutaneous surgery. Smaller-gauge needles (which are larger in caliber) are usually unnecessary. An added benefit to the smaller needle size is that it limits the speed with which anesthetic is instilled and so lessens the pain of injection. A small 32-gauge needle is also available but is not useful for injection of local anesthetics because it is too flexible, too short, and too small for easy injection. Its main use is for injection into small veins of the skin. Needles also come in different lengths. The half-inch length is adequate for most cutaneous surgery. The longer 1-inch needles are more flexible and therefore more cumbersome to use; however, greater distances can be injected underneath the skin than with the half-inch needles. Specially ordered 2-inch, 25-gauge needles may also be ordered (Dermatologic Lab and Supply Co., 25 Ridge, Council Bluffs, Iowa 51501).

Local anesthesia may also be administered by means of a high-pressure device, such as the Dermajet or Madajet. However, the depth of penetration of the anesthetic is difficult to control, and histologic alterations of tissue can occur with such devices. Moreover, high-pressure jets are expensive and subject to mechanical problems. Nevertheless, some physicians use these devices to raise an initial wheal in the skin before injecting larger amounts of infiltrative anesthesia.

Minimizing pain. Injections of anesthetic solutions always cause some pain for the patient. The physician should be truthful about this. Honesty helps to establish and maintain good rapport between patient and physician. Patients appreciate the physician's concern regarding minimization of pain. Gentle technique and attitude are important. There are several other factors that are helpful, though, in decreasing the pain for the patient.

The rate of injection has been found to be related to the pain of local anesthesia.[28] A slowly injected anesthetic hurts less than a quick injection of the same solution. A smaller needle size certainly encourages slow injection, but the physician should also consciously inject slowly. The smallest readily available needle size (usually a 30-gauge needle) should be used to minimize pain.

Distension of tissue, whether by local anesthetic or plain water, causes pain. Therefore the deeper one injects an anesthetic, the less the pain. In a study of injection techniques on 11 patients, superficial injections hurt more than deep injections.[28] Wherever the dermis is bound tightly to the underlying tissue and there is little fat, such as on the nose or anterior aspect of the ear, there is more resistance to the instillation of a local anesthetic; injections in these areas are particularly painful. Distension of tissue is also related to the volume of anesthetic injected. The greater the volume, the more the distension, and the greater the pain for the patient. Therefore, one should aim at using the smallest possible volume to do the job.

The waiting time between injection of anesthetic and surgery is critical. Despite misconceptions, local anesthetics do not work instantaneously. Time is necessary for an adequate amount of anesthetic to diffuse across nerve membranes and impede action potentials. Waiting 5 or even 10 minutes between injections of the anesthetic and surgery allows a deeper block to ensue. Although it is sometimes difficult to wait in a busy office practice, a more complete block allows relatively painless surgery. The larger the anesthetized area, the more is gained by waiting.

Some physicians state that with very small needles (30 gauge) the pain of insertion may be minimized by directing the needle tip down hair follicles. I have tried this but have not been convinced that the pain of insertion is significantly reduced. One should remember that most of the pain of local anesthesia is not caused by the needle stick itself but by the inevitable expansion of tissue on injection and the speed with which it occurs.

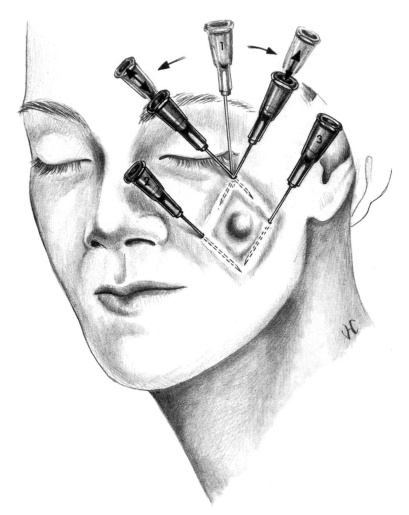

Fig. 6-7. Infiltrative anesthesia. One may "ring" small lesion with as few as 2 to 4 injections if one injects from points around lesion. For large lesions more injections may be necessary.

One factor occasionally mentioned by dentists as reducing the pain of anesthesia is the temperature of the anesthetic solution. Although it has been stated that anesthetic solutions at body temperature hurt less than solutions at room temperature, this has not been substantiated in the literature.[28,226] The temperature of anesthetic solutions is therefore probably not important.

Technique for infiltrative anesthesia. Local infiltrative anesthesia is the most frequently used regional anesthesia in cutaneous surgery. It is easily administered and rapidly effective. However, large amounts of drug must occasionally be used to anesthetize relatively small areas, and sometimes very large amounts of local anesthetic may be necessary for larger surgery, making toxic reactions possible. In general one should aim for the lowest possible dose by using the smallest volume of the lowest effective concentration.

The basic technique of injection is shown in Fig. 6-7. One injects the anesthetic around the lesion to be incised or excised. Before injection the needle should be checked for patency, and a small amount of anesthetic should be expressed from the needle tip to eliminate air in the syringe. The bevel of the needle should face up to ensure that the level of infiltration is at the level of the needle tip. A sharp thrust into the skin causes less pain than slow insertion of the needle causes, but the physician should still strive for gentleness and dexterity in technique. One can limit the number of times one needs to puncture the skin by trailing the needle, injecting as one goes. With subcutaneous injections the infiltrations should be steady and continuous. The needle should be withdrawn and advanced steadily, injecting the drug at a steady rate. It may be possible to inject around a whole lesion through only two or three puncture sites. The point of the needle should be withdrawn from the deeper areas of the subcutaneous tissue before any attempt is made to change its direction. This fan-shaped injection technique has been called ring block anesthesia. More points of injection and a longer needle (1 inch rather than a half inch) may be necessary for larger lesions. When the injec-

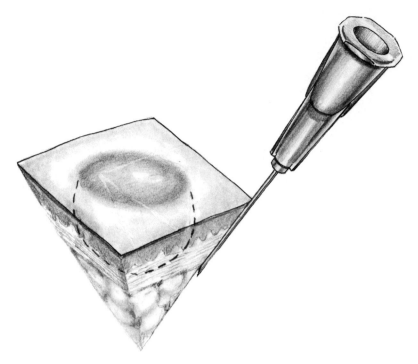

Fig. 6-8. Infiltrative anesthesia. When lesion is deep, one must inject in third dimension under neath, silhouetting inverted pyramid of tissue.

tions are complete, a 5- to 10-minute wait is suggested; the area supplied by the nerves to be blocked should be tested with the tip of the needle. If the field is still too sensitive to pain from the needle, additional injections may be required.

Some authorities recommend raising a small wheal with anesthetic before deeper injection; however, creation of small wheals is more painful because the superficial local anesthetic is more painful. Since one may inject in numerous directions without withdrawing the needle from the skin, such wheals are probably superfluous, unless one is performing a nerve block.

Another technique at the time of injection is to pull back on the plunger after instillation of the needle but before injection. If blood is seen, one presumably has inadvertently entered a small blood vessel—either an artery or a vein. Repositioning of the needle tip can then prevent inadvertent injection into the vascular system. This maneuver is particularly important in highly vascular areas, such as the scalp, where large amounts of local anesthetic are injected. An inadvertent injection of local anesthetic into the vascular spaces can give rise to toxic side effects. It should be noted that not seeing blood on withdrawal of the plunger does not necessarily mean that one is not in a vessel, since small veins collapse under negative pressure.

Although superficial ring block anesthesia may be adequate for small, shallow lesions, a pyramidal block is usually required in addition for larger, deeper lesions.[8] This type of block is illustrated in Fig. 6-8. Here the needle is introduced in a third dimension oblique to the surface of the skin, including the undersurface of the lesion to be incised or excised. This is the most common technique used in cutaneous surgery. It is less painful than more superficial injections and provides more adequate anesthesia for the base of the lesion. However, the onset of anesthesia is longer with this more deeply placed anesthetic.

Occasionally anatomic peculiarities are important factors in determining how effectively anesthetics work. The scalp is a case in point (Fig. 6-9). The nerves and vessels supplying the scalp are located above the thick fibrous tissue layer, the galea aponeurotica. If anesthetics are injected deep to the galea, the scalp balloons up and gives one the false impression that an adequate volume of anesthetic has been given. It takes some time before the anesthetic diffuses through the galea to the nerves above. Therefore injection in the scalp above the layer of the galea more quickly and more deeply blocks the nerves supplying the scalp. Anesthetic solution in this area should first be deposited in the subcutaneous tissue above the aponeurosis, followed by infiltration beneath the aponeurosis.

Although there may be several reasons for inadequate infiltration anesthesia, usually it is caused by not waiting long enough between the injection of local anesthetic and the skin incision. Some local anesthetics, such as mepivacaine, take a longer time than lidocaine to become effective.

Technique for nerve block and field block anesthesia. A nerve block is the injection of a local anesthetic close to a

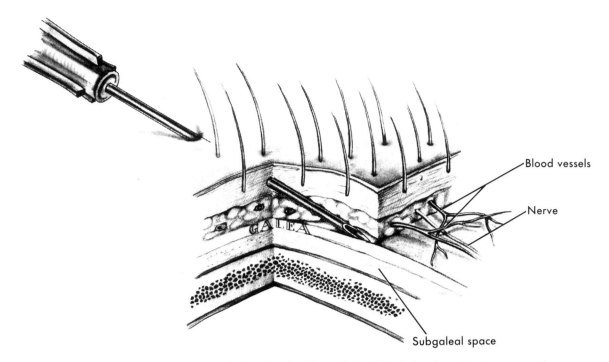

Fig. 6-9. Local infiltrative anesthesia of scalp. Note relationship of tip of needle to nerves and galea.

nerve of known location blocks the nerve supply to skin from this particular nerve. Nerve blocks are more exacting and require greater skill than simple infiltration anesthesia. Knowledge of the relevant neuroanatomy is a prerequisite to performing successful nerve blocks; less anesthetic solution is used and distortion of tissues may be prevented. Because neural damage can occur with nerve block anesthesia, it is advisable to perform a neurologic examination of the area that will be affected by the nerve block before injection of the local anesthetic.

Field block anesthesia refers to instillation of a local anesthetic to interrupt nerve transmission proximal to the site to be anesthetized. Unlike nerve block anesthesia, field block anesthesia numbs a particular area of the body by blocking more than one specific nerve. Esentially one encircles an operative field with walls of anesthetic. Knowing the location of major nerves is a necessary prerequisite to effecting this form of anesthesia. Like a nerve block, field block anesthesia may provide a greater area of anesthesia with less anesthetic than infiltrative anesthesia would. Another advantage of both nerve block and field block anesthesia is that the injection of anesthetic may be placed into tissues that are more distensible, thereby avoiding a more painful placement of anesthetic into tissues that are hardly distensible, such as the nose or ear.

Nerve blocks can be achieved in two ways. Either one places a large volume of anesthetic solution in the same fascial compartment that the nerve to be blocked lies in or one places the needle adjacent to the nerve. With the latter technique less anesthetic is used; however, one needs to elicit paresthesia. Some authorities feel that production of paresthesia is not associated with significant trauma to nerves, but this is disputed by others (Fig. 6-10). I feel it is best to avoid the possibility of intraneural injections. Therefore I do not try to elicit paresthesias.

The location of some of the major nerves of the face useful for nerve blocks is shown in Fig. 6-11. In addition, the major nerves to block for different areas of the head and neck are listed in the box on p. 226. The central forehead can be anesthetized by blocking the supratrochlear nerve. A wider area of anesthesia is provided by blocking in addition the supraorbital nerve as it exists from the supraorbital notch. This may be palpated as a depression in the supraorbital rim. The supratrochlear notch is sometimes felt more medially. If the whole forehead is to be blocked, one must also block the zygomaticotemporal nerve, which lies laterally and is not seen in Fig. 6-11.

The infraorbital nerve, a branch of the maxillary nerve, supplies the cheek and side of the nose, exiting through the infraorbital foramen, and the mental nerve supplying the central chin and lower lip exits from the mental foramen. Both the mental foramen and the infraorbital foramen are located approximately at points that intersect an imaginary line drawn straight down from the supraorbital foramen. This

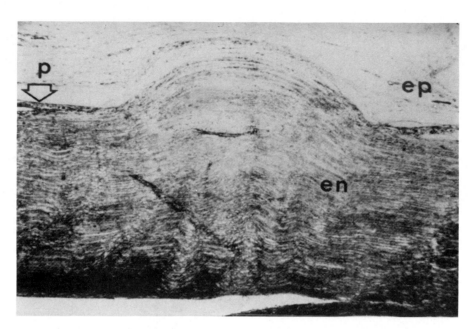

Fig. 6-10. Endoneurial herniation through punctured perineurium. *p,* Perineurium; *ep,* epineurium; *en,* endoneurium with nerve fibers (×50.) (From Selander, D., et al.: Acta Anaesthesiol. Scand. **23:**127, 1979.)

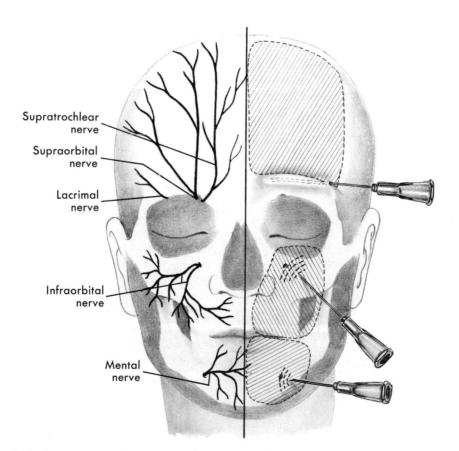

Fig. 6-11. Nerve blocks of face. Note location of supraorbital nerve, infraorbital nerve, and mental nerve and their exit from foramens that are approximately in straight line with each other.

NERVE BLOCKS ON HEAD AND NECK

Area to anesthetize	*Nerves to block*
Forehead	Supraorbital
	Supratrochlear
	Zygomaticotemporal
Temporal scalp	Auriculotemporal
Occipitoparietal scalp	Greater occipital
	Lesser occipital
Nose	Infraorbital
	Infratrochlear
	External nasal branch of anterior ethmoidal
Eyelids	Supraorbital
	Supratrochlear
	Infratrochlear
	Lacrimal
	Infraorbital
Upper lip	Infraorbital
Lower lip	Mental
Ear (external)	Greater auricular
	Auriculotemporal
Midcheek	Infraorbital
Chin	Mental
Neck	C2, C3, C4

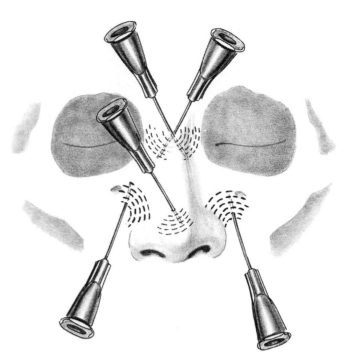

Fig. 6-12. Nerve block and field block of nose.

imaginary line also goes through the pupil with the eyes looking straight ahead. It may be more accurate to locate this line with the eyes looking up, since the pupils are thus locked in the central position. It should be emphasized that this gives only an estimate as to the location of these foramens. Individual variation does occur and is probably one reason for unsuccessful nerve blocks.

The external nose may be anesthetized by means of a combination of nerve blocks and field blocks, as shown in Fig. 6-12. The locations for injection are the infraorbital foramina and cheeks adjacent to the nose, the infratrochlear foramina, and the points on the paramedial dorsum of the nose between the lateral cartilages and nasal bones. These last points are the exits of the external nasal branches of the anterior ethmoidal nerve that supply the nasal tip. It should be stressed that to anesthetize the columella, an additional injection must be given at its base.

The digits are anesthetized by injection of anesthetic at the base, as shown in Fig. 6-13. Since there is overlap in the areas anesthetized by the four nerves at the tip of the finger, all four should be anesthetized. With one insertion of the needle one can inject an adequate amount of anesthetic into one side of a digit. Note that there are four points at which to inject the anesthetic: two superior and two inferior on each side. Also note that one must inject an adequate

amount of nerve length to provide anesthesia. One therefore injects lengthwise from point to point.

One should not inject a large anesthetic volume into the digit and "ring" the finger. Doing so may impede blood flow (venous return) and result in circulatory difficulties because the injection is into a closed space. Another point to stress on digital nerve blocks is that 2% lidocaine provides a more successful block. However, one should remember that the higher-concentration local anesthetic is also more vasodilatory, so the anesthesia does not last as long.

Three other useful nerve blocks that should be mentioned in cutaneous surgery are the ulnar and median nerve blocks at the wrist and the sural nerve block for the plantar surface of the foot. The ulnar nerve is found deep to the ulnar artery, which can be easily palpated and lies against the flexor carpi ulnaris tendon. The median nerve lies deep to the large palmaris longus tendon, which is seen when one flexes the wrist. Infiltration near these nerves results in anesthesia for the volar surface of the hand, precluding the use of more painful local anesthesia in this area.

The sural nerve supplies the volar surface of the foot in the heel. It arises as a union of branches of the tibial nerve and the peroneal nerve. It becomes superficial in the lower leg as it courses posterolateral to the lateral malleolus. Injection for block of this nerve is made between the Achilles tendon and the lateral malleolus.

Successful regional anesthesia

Successful regional anesthesia is related to several factors, which are listed in the box on p. 228 and are associated

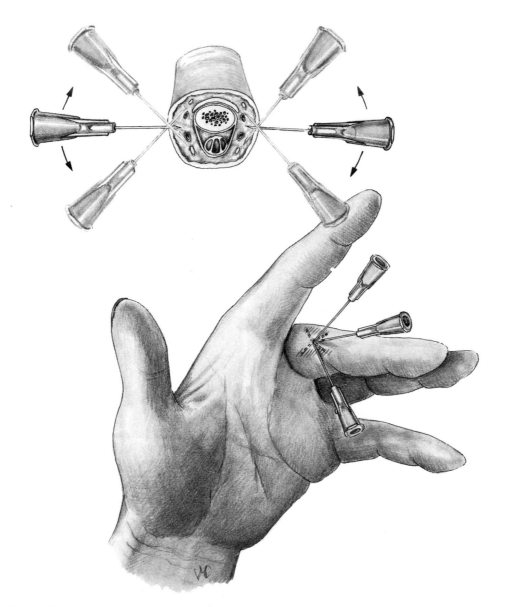

Fig. 6-13. Digital nerve block anesthesia. Note that with one insertion of the needle, one may anesthetize an adequate length of both superior and inferior digital nerves.

with peculiarities of anatomy, the anesthetic solution itself, or the technique of injection. Factors related to the anesthetic solution itself include the total dose of anesthetic, its concentration, its volume, the amount of anesthetic base available for diffusion (related to pH), the diffusion ability of the anesthetic, and the presence or absence of vasoconstrictors or other chemicals. Recovery from anesthesia is related to the concentration of the anesthetic and how tightly bound it is to the nerve (pharmacologic properties). Several of these variables were previously discussed and are listed in Table 6-8.

On infiltration the local anesthetic diffuses and penetrates the nerve. This takes place during a latency period that varies with the local anesthetic used and the conditions

under which it is used. When the critical concentration of local anesthetic is reached in the nerve, blockage of the nerve impulses occurs. This is divided into two phases. In the first phase the anesthetic concentration rises to a maximum. The addition of a vasoconstrictor maintains this concentration. The second phase represents the local anesthetic's diffusion out of the nerve. This is related to the drug's affinity for the nerve membrane and its concentration gradient across the cell membrane. A vasoconstrictor prolongs this phase.[110]

The total dose of an anesthetic agent may be calculated by multiplying the volume given by the concentration.

$$\text{Total dose} = \text{Volume} \times \text{Concentration}$$

FACTORS AFFECTING SUCCESSFUL REGIONAL ANESTHESIA

Anatomical factors

Distance for diffusion to nerve bundle
Barriers through which diffusion takes place
Size of nerve (differential diameter)
Myelination of nerve
Location of nerve within nerve bundles (differential diffusion)
Vascularity of tissue

Anesthetic factors

Concentration and volume
pH ambient tissue
pH anesthetic solution
Vasoconstrictor
Pharmacologic properties

Technical factors

Proper placement
Allowance of sufficient time for onset

As one increases the percentage of concentration or the volume of a local anesthetic, one increases the duration and the frequency of successful anesthesia. However, concentration itself appears to be more critical for successful anesthesia, whereas volume has more to do with its duration.[5,111] In other words, a small volume of a high concentration renders a better anesthetic effect than a large volume of low concentration. Neither volume nor concentration are related to the onset time of anesthesia experimentally.[5] Toxicity, on the other hand, is more commonly related to the total dose.

Successful nerve blocks. The major factor contributing to a unsuccessful nerve block is an inadequate amount of anesthetic at the site of the nerve. This may be caused by several factors, which are mainly related to the technique of injection and include improper site of deposition of the anesthetic, inadequate concentration of the anesthetic, inadequate length of the nerve anesthetized, and inadequate amount of time allowed for diffusion and the nerve block to occur.

Anatomic peculiarities sometimes make it difficult to locate nerves precisely. Some authorities recommend one to elicit tingling of the nerve (paresthesia) with the needle before injection to ascertain that one is near the nerve. For the nerve blocks already mentioned this is usually unnecessary, since their locations are relatively easy to determine. However, some areas are inherently more difficult to anesthetize because of the multitude of different nerves supplying the region, with variable and overlapping areas of innervation. For example, the ear is supplied by a number of nerves—all difficult to locate. It is my experience that ear blocks are usually unsuccessful, despite enthusiastic proponents.[222]

As mentioned previously, raising a wheal in the skin before instilling an anesthetic for a nerve block may be preferable because one may take some time to position the needle properly.

Nerve blocks are easier if a higher concentration of local anesthetic is used. The concentration and not the total dose appears to be more important in increasing the success of nerve block anesthesia.[5] Lidocaine 2% is therefore superior to lidocaine 1% when used for nerve blocks. Because of the problems encountered with increased concentrations, one should be careful to use small amounts. The 2% concentration is more efficacious because a larger number of molecules per milliliter is deposited and creates a steeper concentration gradient. In addition, an increased number of molecules is available to diffuse across the nerve membrane, providing more molecules per unit time and thus decreasing the time needed for adequate anesthesia. A lesser number of molecules (lower concentration) may mean waiting a longer time for adequate anesthesia to occur. Another point to stress, however, is that the higher-concentration local anesthetic results in more vasodilation, and therefore the duration of block is less than with a lower concentration of the same anesthetic.

Another reason for unsuccessful nerve blocks is that an inadequate length of the nerve has been exposed to local anesthetic. Since it is necessary to block at least three Ranvier's nodes (because impulses can jump over two nodes), theoretically one must block from 1.5 to 6 mm of nerve (each Ranvier's node is 0.5 to 2 mm apart).[71] Practically speaking, though, because of irregular diffusion, 8 to 20 mm of nerve may need to be exposed to ensure complete nerve block.[117] This is particularly important for digital blocks.

Other factors to consider include the size and type of nerves anesthetized. The onset time for a nerve block is longer for a large nerve than for a small nerve. Smaller myelinated nerves are blocked before larger myelinated nerves.[117] This is felt to be caused by an increased number of receptors on larger nerves for local anesthetics to block. In addition, a longer distance is necessary to block an adequate number of nodes in a larger nerve. Nonmyelinated nerves are more difficult to block than myelinated nerves of similar diameter,[214,244] since myelinated nerves are blocked more easily because of saltatory conduction.

Differential blockade. One important concept is differential blockade, that is, some nerves are more quickly or completely anesthetized than others.[81] As a corollary, some nerves return to normal after anesthesia more quickly. A nerve is not a homogeneous structure but rather a collection of a number of different fiber sizes with different functions (motor or sensory) and presence or absence of myelin. Different nerve fiber groups have distinctive thresholds of stimulation and durations of refractory periods.[103]

One clinical example of differential blockade is that on anesthetization of the skin a patient may not feel the prick of a needle or the scalpel blade but does perceive the sensation of pressure. Pain fibers are blocked before temperature fibers, which in turn are blocked before pressure fibers.[122] The patient who does not feel pain from the scalpel still complains of (misinterprets) the sensation of pressure as pain, and senses heat from the electrosurgical apparatus. As the nerve blocks deepen, sensations of heat and pressure disappear.

Another classic example of differential blockade is the difference between anesthesia rates of motor nerves and sensory nerves. Motor nerve fibers are blocked later than pain-conducting fibers, and their blocks are terminated sooner. This delayed onset of block to motor fibers is sometimes a source of anxiety for those performing surgery on the face, since the block was not apparent at the beginning of surgery when sensory block was present (Fig. 6-14). An explanation for this is that the larger motor nerves require more widespread diffusion of anesthetic (because of greater thickness and length), whereas the smaller pain fibers require less anesthetic.[117,122] Frequently the motor block lasts longer than the sensory block because of the location of the nerve fibers in the nerve bundle. It is thought that the sensory nerves are more central and thus in a better-vascularized area, whereas motor nerves are more peripheral and more poorly vascularized. Sometimes a motor block does not occur because the concentration of local anesthetic is insufficient to block the larger motor nerves but sufficient to block the smaller pain fibers.

Minimal blocking concentration. Another important concept for local anesthetics is the minimal blocking concentration (Cm).[78] This is the lowest concentration of local anesthetic necessary to block a nerve within a given period of time. The Cm can be calculated for different local anesthetics and thus serves as a gauge for comparing their relative potencies. Because a thick nerve fiber is blocked less readily than a thin one, the Cm is greater for a thick fiber than for a thin one. In addition, the Cm is increased with a decrease in pH. This is because at a higher pH there is more nonionized base available for diffusion across nerve membranes, which thus decreases the block time necessary to produce a nerve block.

Wedensky block. As the Cm of a local anesthetic is approached, an individual nerve fiber may be blocked to a single stimulus but not blocked to continuous stimuli. This transition block is known as the Wedensky block.[81] A clinical example of this phenomenon occurs when the skin is first anesthetized. The patient may not feel any sensation to the needle tip; however, when the skin is cut with the scalpel, the patient may complain of pain.[38] This is caused by the nerve being blocked to a single stimulus (pinprick) but not to a continuous stimulus (incision). One should simply wait a longer time to allow more anesthetic to diffuse into the nerves and provide a more solid block.

Surface anesthesia. The ability to anesthetize the epithelial surfaces of the body without infiltration by local anesthetics renders less pain to the patient and even allows patients to act as their own anesthetists. However, this method is not predictably successful in its production of anesthesia.

Cryoanesthesia

History. The idea of cold to cause anesthesia has probably been used for hundreds of years. In 1848 ice was mixed with salt to provide lower temperatures in a device for local anesthesia designed by Arnott.[46] The Arnott device was relegated to oblivion by the introduction of either spray in 1866 by Richardson. In 1891 ethyl chloride spray was introduced.

Effects. The effects of cold on nerves is to block pain fibers, then thermal fibers, and finally tactile fibers—similar to local anesthetic agents.

Agents. Topical freezing agents currently available include ethyl chloride, Frigiderm (dichlorotetrafluoroethane [Freon 114]), fluoroethyl (25% ethyl chloride and 75% dichlorotetrafluoroethane); cryOsthesia −30° C or Aerofreeze (dichlorodifluoromethane [Freon 12] mixed with trichlorofluoromethane [Freon 11]); and cryOsthesia −60° C, Cryokwik or MediFrig (dichlorodifluromethane [Freon 12]). Ethyl chloride is both inflammable and explosive; its boiling point is 12.2° C, and it produces a skin temperature of about −10° C. When used in any quantity—for dermabrasion, for instance—it must be blown away from the operator and the patient because of its general anesthetic effects. In 1955 Freon 114 was introduced for dermabrasions.[297] This agent (Frigiderm) has a lower boiling point of 3.6° C and chills the skin to between 0° and −32° C; this provides a slightly harder freeze and longer thaw time than that of ethyl chloride. In addition, it is noninflammable and nonexplosive. CryOsthesia is also noninflammable. It results in a skin temperature of from −20° to −30° C. However, clinical experience indicates that such low temperatures may result in excessive tissue damage, limiting the usefulness of such anesthetics. Liquid nitrogen may also be used for topical anesthesia for very small lesions. Because of the exquisite pain induced, this type of anesthesia also has limited usefulness.

Untoward effects. Cryoanesthesia is not without untoward effects. Nerve damage may result from extreme cold applied adjacent to a sizeable nerve, although the sensory loss that ensues usually returns in 3 months.[34] If local infiltration anesthesia with epinephrine is combined with cold, one gets greater tissue damage than with cold alone.[208] This

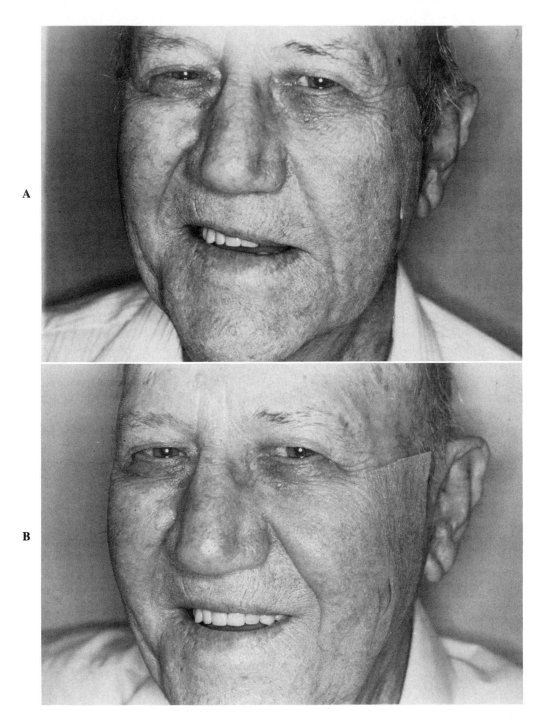

Fig. 6-14. Differential blockade. **A,** Immediately subsequent to surgery under local anesthesia. Note residual droop in left upper lip with loss of motor function. **B,** Return of motor function within 1 hour as local anesthesia wears off.

may be an advantage in the treatment of tumors, but for dermabrasion it may lead to more tissue damage than intended. An acute attack of cryofibrogenemia has also been reported with topical use of liquid nitrogen.[272]

Topical anesthetic drugs

Absorption. Skin, particularly the epidermis with its stratum corneum, offers an effective barrier to the diffusion of anesthetic agents. Stripping the stratum corneum allows for more effective penetration of topical anesthetics.[197] If these agents are simply placed on the unstripped skin, diffusion is very slow, resulting in anesthesia to pinprick in 3 to 4 hours. There is little detectable blood levels following application of topical anesthetics to the skin.[10] Cutaneous barriers are more easily crossed by the bases of local anesthetics than by the salt. Because the slight acid pH of the skin favors ionization of the anesthetic and less base, the pH provides yet another obstacle for diffusion. Some local anesthetics, particularly tetracaine, have been combined with dimethyl sulfoxide (DMSO) to enhance skin penetration,[48] but this combination induced pruritus and hyperesthesia.

Absorption of local anesthetics through the mucous membranes, on the other hand, occurs quickly, and the resultant blood levels almost parallel those with intravenous infusion.[10] Salts and bases are absorbed by the mucous membranes.

Agents. In a study of several topical local anesthetics, Adriani ranked the following agents in order of duration and degree of numbness: tetracaine (most potent), followed by cocaine, lidocaine, benzocaine, tripelennamine, and pramoxine (Tronothane). Tetracaine was found to have the longest latent period and benzocaine the shortest.[9]

Cocaine is found in the leaves of *Erythroxylon coca,* which is indigenous to Peru. It is chewed as a central nervous stimulant by the Indians in South America, resulting in circumoral numbness. Cocaine was the first topical anesthetic, initially used on the eye.[167] Its main use in modern times is for effective topical anesthesia for the mucous membranes of the nose. It is the only local anesthetic that is a vasoconstrictor, and thus is advantageous in a vascular area subject to bleeding, such as the nasal cavity. The vasoconstrictor activity results from the cocaine interfering with the uptake of norepinephrine at the adrenergic nerve terminals.[186] The maximal safe dosage in a 70 kg adult is 200 mg (10 ml of a 2% solution).[240] Usually one prepares a 1% to 2% solution from the bulk powder and soaks cotton balls in the solution. These are applied topically to the nasal mucosa with forceps. The peak anesthetic effect occurs in 2 to 5 minutes and lasts as long as 30 to 45 minutes. Cocaine is absorbed slowly from mucosa, possibly related to its vasoconstrictive properties. Elevated blood cocaine levels have been found 4 to 6 hours after nasal application, caused by this slow absorption[290] and by the slow metabolism of this drug

in man. Like procaine, cocaine is detoxified in the serum via hydrolysis by pseudocholinesterase.[292] It should be emphasized that in the nasal mucosa, topical application of cocaine renders anesthesia that is only superficial; it does not extend deeply. Therefore it may need to be supplemented by local anesthesia should one need to operate deeply; however, because cocaine is itself a vasoconstrictor, it may potentiate sympathomimetic amines infiltrated later to supplement the cocaine.

Benzocaine is perhaps the best topical anesthetic.[9] This was the first man-made local anesthetic, synthesized in 1890. It is poorly water soluble and therefore very poor as an injectable anesthetic. Being a very weak base (the pKa is 3.5), it performs well in an acid environment, such as the mouth of or the acid mantle of the skin. It was discovered to be quite efficacious as a topical local anesthetic; however, it is notorious as a sensitizer. Benzocaine is available commercially as a 20% gel or aerosol and a 2.5% to 20% solution.

Topical lidocaine has been used for both mucosal and skin anesthesia. A 30% lidocaine cream was recommended for minor operations on the skin of children.[180] The anesthetic took approximately 45 minutes after application to render successful anesthesia. Furthermore, an occlusive bandage was required to ensure close contact with the cutaneous surface and to enhance penetration of the chemical. With this method the authors were able to perform cyst excisions. Frequently patients were given the cream to apply before even coming to the office; however, the size of the procedure is probably a limiting factor with topical lidocaine. Concentrations in creams or ointments as high as 30% must be specially prepared; otherwise, lidocaine for topical use is available as a 2% jelly or viscous solution, or in ointments of 2.5% to 5%, or in a 4% nonviscous topical solution. Lidocaine 2.5% has also been combined with prilocaine 2.5% another amide local anesthetic, for superficial skin surgery[154]; however, with this mixture some physicians were often unable to perform even simple punch biopsies. This mixture has also been reported under the name EMLA (Eutectic Mixture of Local Anesthetics).[98,136]

On the already lacerated skin, a mixture of tetracaine 0.5%, adrenalin 1:2,000, and cocaine 11.8% in normal saline has been reported to be useful.[233] This solution (known as *TAC*), however, was later shown to promote infection in lacerations, possibly as a result of the vasoconstrictive activity of the added adrenalin or cocaine.[33] Tetracaine alone did not promote wound infection.

Several of the topical anesthetics already mentioned work best when applied to ulcerated surfaces of wounds in which the epithelial layer is broken, where they have a more profound and sustained anesthetic action. It should be emphasized, however, that topical anesthetics on denuded skin may result in significant blood levels caused by absorption and therefore, if used extensively, should be limited to the doses suggested for infiltrative anesthesia.[236]

Topical ketocaine, an aminoether local anesthetic, has had proponents recently in Europe. It has a very high partition coefficient and has been found to work well topically if mixed as a 10% solution in glycerol isopropanol and water.[134] As with other topical anesthetic agents, a long time is necessary for adequate anesthesia: up to 1 hour. Only pain fibers, not pressure fibers, appear to be blocked. The duration of anesthesia is several hours.[219] It has been used successfully for cutting split-thickness skin grafts[219] as well as for dermabrasion.[230] Its proponents claim no serious side effects. Experimentally, it has been shown to enhance skin flap survival[228] and to promote revascularization of skin grafts (based on increased iron content) compared to local infiltration anesthesia.[229] However, marked hyperemia may develop in the treated areas, probably the result of capillary venous congestion.[135] In addition, the solution is unstable, and local irritation may occur.[154]

Additional agents that provide some degree of topical anesthesia and thereby decrease the itch of some dermatoses include cyclomethycaine (Surfacaine), dimethisoquin (Quotane), and pramoxine (Tronothane). The latter two compounds are not benzoic acid esters; although they may therefore be less sensitizing than benzocaine, they may contain parabens.[285]

Technique for mucosal anesthesia. Anesthesia of the mucous membranes is specialized, in that anesthetics diffuse across mucous membranes much more easily than across skin. One can first apply a local anesthetic in the mouth that provides topical anesthesia. One may then inject less painfully into deeper tissues. Some physicians advocate using this technique (the intraoral route) for nerve blocks, particularly of the mental or infraorbital nerve, but this is probably of no great advantage and carries with it the potential introduction of oral flora into deep spaces of the face.

One should also remember that the mucosa of the eye, nose, and mouth is supplied by a separate nerve supply from the overlying skin and therefore needs to be anesthetized separately. For the eye 0.5% tetracaine (Pontocaine), 0.5% proparacaine (Ophthaine), or 0.4% benoxinate (Dorsacaine) can be used. Of these, tetracaine and benoxinate are derived from PABA and therefore cross-react with benzoic acid ester local anesthetics; proparacaine, on the other hand, is derived from a benzoate ester and does not chemically cross-react with the benzoic acid local anesthetics. For the nose, topical cocaine 1% to 2% is useful. The methods for its application and dosage have already been discussed. For a discussion of oral mucosal anesthesia, see the earlier section on topical anesthetic agents.

Untoward reactions. Even topical anesthetics are not without their problems. Tetracaine, perhaps the most potent topical local anesthetic, has caused fatalities when used topically on mucous membranes.[9,48] Therefore it is not recommended except for the eye, for which it is used in small amounts.

Topical lidocaine to the oral mucosa has been rarely associated with the development of methemoglobinemia[218] and seizures.[196] In the latter case viscous 2% lidocaine was used on an 11-month-old infant for teething.

Contact sensitization, as mentioned previously, can occur following use of topical anesthetics. The esters, especially benzocaine, and the amides, especially lidocaine, have been demonstrated to induce allergic reactions in patch testing.[21,241] Lidocaine may be more sensitizing when applied to the mucous membranes. Also, as pointed out earlier, parabens can be found with various formulations of topical anesthetics.

Other methods of reducing pain. The use of hypnoses and acupuncture[193] may be useful for relief of pain in cutaneous surgery. These methods require both specialized training and suggestible patients; therefore they probably have limited applicability. Investigations into their use and scientific basis are limited, and further research in these areas may prove fruitful in the future.

REFERENCES

1. Abadir, A.: Anesthesia for hand surgery, Orthop. Clin. North Am. **1**(2):205, 1970.
2. Abadir, D.M., et al.: Dermabrasion under regional anesthesia without refrigeration of the skin, J. Dermatol. Surg. Oncol. **6**:119, 1980.
3. Åberg, G.: Studies on the duration of local anesthesia: a possible mechanism for the prolonging effect of "vasoconstrictors" on the duration of infiltration anesthesia, Int. J. Oral Surg. **9**:144, 1980.
4. Åberg, G., Friberger, P., and Sydnes, G.: Studies on the duration of local anesthesia with a possible mechanism for the prolonged effect of dextran on the duration of infiltrative anesthesia, Acta Pharmacol. Toxicol. **42**:88, 1978.
5. Åberg, G., and Sydnes, G.: Studies on the duration of local anesthesia: effects of volume and concentration of a local anesthetic solution on a duration of dental infiltration anesthesia, Int. J. Oral Surg. **7**:141, 1978.
6. Aceves, J., and Machine, X.: The action of calcium and of local anesthetics on nerve cells, and their interaction during excitation, J. Pharmacol. Exp. Ther. **140**:138, 1963.
7. Adams, H.J., Kronberg, G.H., and Takman, B.H.: Local anesthetic activity and acute toxicity of (+/−)-2-N-ethyl-propylamino-2'-6' butyroxylidide, a new long-acting agent, J. Pharmacol. Sci. **61**:1829, 1972.
8. Adriani, J.: Labat's regional anesthesia: techniques and clinical applications, ed. 3, Philadelphia, 1967, W.B. Saunders Co.
9. Adriani, J., and Campbell, D.: Fatalities following topical applications of local anesthetics to mucous membranes, J.A.M.A. **162**:1527, 1956.
10. Adriani, J., and Dalili, H.: Penetration of local anesthetics through epithelial barriers, Anesth. Analg. **50**:834, 1971.
11. Adriani, J., and Naraghi, M.: Etiology and management of adverse reactions to local anesthetics, J. Am. Med. Wom. Assoc. **33**:365, 1978.
12. Adriani, J., and Zepernick, R.: Allergic reactions to local

anesthetics, South. Med. J. **74:**694, 1981.

13. Adriani, J., Zepernick, R., and Hyde, E.: Influence of the status of the patient on systemic effects of local anesthetic agents, Anesth. Analg. **45:**87, 1966.

14. Aellig, W.H., et al.: Cardiac effects of adrenaline and felypressin as vasoconstrictors in local anaesthesia for oral surgery under diazepam sedation, Br. J. Anaesth. **42:**174, 1970.

15. Agathos, M.: Anaphylactic reaction to framycetin (neomycin B) and lignocaine, Contact Dermatitis **6:**236, 1980.

16. Albright, G.A.: Cardiac arrest following regional anesthesia with etidocaine or bupivacaine, Anesthesiology **51:**285, 1979.

17. Aldrete, J.A.: An "allergic" reaction (letter), Anesthesiology **32:**176, 1970

18. Aldrete, J.A.: Neurotoxic reactions to local anesthetic drugs, J. Ky. Med. Assoc. **72:**543, 1974

19. Aldrete, J.A., and Johnson, D.A.: Allergy to local anesthetics, J.A.M.A. **207:**356, 1969.

20. Aldrete, J.A., and Johnson, D.A.: Evaluation of intracutaneous testing for investigation of allergy to local anesthetic agents, Anesth. Analg. **49:**173, 1970.

21. Aldrete, J.A., and O'Higgins, J.W.: Evaluation of patients with history of allergy to local anesthetic drugs, South Med. J. **64:**1118, 1971.

22. Aldrete, J.A., et al.: Studies on effects of addition of potassium chloride to lidocaine, Anesth. Analg. **48:**269, 1969.

23. Aldrete, J.A., et al.: Reverse arterial blood flow as a pathway for central nervous system toxic responses following injection of local anesthetics, Anesth. Analg. **57:**428, 1978.

24. Allen, G.D.: Nitrous oxide–oxygen sedation machines and devices, J. Am. Dent. Assoc. **88:**611, 1974.

25. Alper, M.H.: Agents in obstetrics: mother, fetus, and newborn. In Smith, N.T., Miller, R.D., and Corbascio, A.N., editors: Drug interactions in anesthesia, Philadelphia, 1981, Lea & Febiger.

26. Ames, J.A.L., et al.: Megaloblastic hematopoiesis in patients receiving nitrous oxide, Lancet **2:**339, 1978.

27. Andersen, T.W., and Gravenstein, J.S.: Cardiovascular effects of sedative doses of pentobarbital and hydroxyzine, Anesthesiology **27:**272, 1966.

28. Arndt, K.A., Burton, C., and Noe, J.M.: Minimizing the pain of local anesthesia, Plast. Reconstr. Surg. **72:**676, 1983.

29. Aukburg, S.J., Miller, J., and Smith, T.C.: Interaction between meperidine and diazepam on the ventilatory response to carbon dioxide, Clin. Res. **24:**506a, 1976.

30. Backer, C.L., et al.: Myocardial infarction following local anesthesia for ophthalmic surgery, Anesth. Analg. **59:**257, 1980.

31. Baden, J.M., and Monk, S.J.: Mutagenicity and toxicity studies with high-pressure nitrous oxide, Toxicol. Lett. **7:**259, 1981.

32. Barer, M.R., and McAllen, M.K.: Hypersensitivity to local anaesthetics: a direct challenge test with lignocaine for definitive diagnosis, Br. Med. J. **284:**1229, 1982.

33. Barker, W., et al.: Damage to tissue defenses by a topical anesthetic agent, Ann. Emerg. Med. **11:**307, 1982.

34. Barnard, D.: The effects of extreme cold on sensory nerves, Ann. R. Coll. Surg. Engl. **62:**182, 1980.

35. Barsa, J., et al.: A comparative in vivo study of local neurotoxicity of lidocaine, bupivacaine, 2-chloroprocaine, and a mixture of 2-chloroprocaine and bupivacaine, Anesth. Analg. **61**(12):961, 1982.

36. Bashein, G.: Use of excessive lidocaine concentrations for local anesthesia (letter), N. Engl. J. Med. **302:**122, 1980.

37. Bateman, P.P.: Multiple allergy to local anesthetics including prilocaine, Med. J. Aust. **2:**449, 1974.

38. Bennett, R.G., and Robins, P.: Etidocaine, a new local anesthetic, J. Dermatol. Surg. Oncol. **5:**551, 1979.

39. Benoit, P.W.: Microscarring in skeletal muscle after repeated exposure to lidocaine with epinephrine, J. Oral Surg. **36:**530, 1978.

40. Benoit, P.W., and Belt, W.D.: Some effects of local anesthetic agents on skeletal muscle, Exp. Neurol. **34:**264, 1972.

41. Benowitz, N.L., and Meister, W.: Clinical pharmacokinetics of lignocaine, Pharmacokinetics **3:**177, 1978.

42. Bernard, C.: Leçons sur les anesthésiques et sur l'asphyxie, Paris, 1875, J.B. Baillière.

43. Bessou, P., and Perl, E.R.: Responses of cutaneous sensory units with unmyelinated fibers to noxious stimuli, J. Neurophysiol. **32:**1025, 1969.

44. Betcher, A.M., and Tang, Z.T.: Pyribenzamine: evaluation of effectiveness as an analgesic agent in regional anesthesia, Anesthesiology **16:**214, 1955.

45. Bieter, R.N.: Applied pharmacology of local anesthetics, Am. J. Surg. **34:**500, 1936.

46. Bird, H.M.: James Arnott: a pioneer in refrigeration analgesia, Anaesthesia, **4:**10, 1949.

47. Boyes, R.N., et al.: Pharmacokinetics of lidocaine in man, Clin. Pharmacol. Ther. **12:**105, 1971.

48. Brechner, V.L., Cohen, D.D., and Pretsky, I.: Dermal anesthesia by the topical application of tetracaine base dissolved in dimethyl sulfoxide, Ann. N.Y. Acad. Sci. **141:**524, 1967.

49. Breithardt, G., et al.: Cerebral convulsions and cardiac arrest during local anesthesia on patient on antiarrhythmic treatment, Chest **67:**375, 1975.

50. Brewster, W.R., et al.: The hemodynamic and metabolic interrelationships in the activity of epinephrine, norepinephrine and the thyroid hormones, Circulation **13:**1, 1956.

51. Bridenbaugh, P.O., et al.: Preliminary clinical evaluation of etidocaine (Duranest) a new long-acting local anesthetic agent, Acta Anaesthesiol. Scand. **18:**165, 1974.

52. Brodie, B.B., Lief, P.A., and Poet, R.: The fate of procaine in man following its intravenous administration and methods for the estimation of procaine and diethylaminoethanol, J. Pharmacol. Exp. Ther. **94:**359, 1948.

53. Brodsky, J.B., and Brock-Utne, J.G.: Mixing local anaesthetics, Br. J. Anaesth. **50:**1269, 1978.

54. Bromage, P.R., Datta, S., and Dunford, L.A.: An evaluation of etidocaine in epidural analgesia for obstetrics, Can. Anaesth. Soc. J. **21:**535, 1974.

55. Bromage, P.R., et al.: Quality of epidural blockade. III. Carbonated local anaesthetic solutions, Br. J. Anaesth. **39:**197, 1967.

56. Brown, D.T., Beamish, D., and Wildsmith, J.A.W.: Allergic reaction to an amide local anaesthetic, Br. J. Anaesth. **53:**435, 1981.

57. Burgess, P.R., and Perl, E.R.: Myelinated afferent fibres responding specifically to noxious stimulation of the skin, J. Physiol. **190:**541, 1967.

58. Burney, R.G., DiFazio, C.A., and Foster, J.: Effects of pH on protein binding of lidocaine, Anesth. Analg. **57:**478, 1978.

59. Buskop, J.J., Price, M., and Molnar, I.: Untoward effect of diazepam, N. Engl. J. Med. **277:**316, 1967.

60. Byers, M.R., O'Neil, P.C., and Fink, B.R.: Lidocaine (without epinephrine) does not affect the fine structure or microtubules of the trigeminal nerve in vivo, Anesthesiology **51:**55, 1979.

61. Carroll, M.J.: Tissue necrosis following a buccal infiltration, Br. Dent. J. **149:**209, 1980.

62. Casey, W.F.: Nitrous oxide and middle ear pressure: a study of induction methods in children, Anaesthesia **37**(9):869, 1982.

63. Catchlove, R.F.H.: The influence of CO_2 and pH on local anaesthetic action, J. Pharmacol. Exp. Ther. **181:**298, 1972.

64. Chetty, U.: Comparison of general and local anesthesia for biopsy of breast lumps, J. R. Coll. Surg. Edinb. **28**(1):14, 1983.

65. Chin, T.M., and Fellner, M.J.: Allergic hypersensitivity to lidocaine hydrochloride, Int. J. Dermatol. **19:**147, 1980.

66. Chvapil, M., et al.: Local anesthetics and wound healing, J. Surg. Res. **27:**367, 1979.

67. Clarke, P.R.F., et al.: The amnesic effect of diazepam (Valium), Br. J. Anaesth. **42:**690, 1970.

68. Cloninger, P.: Reactions to local anesthetic agents, West. J. Med. **131:**316, 1979.

69. Cohen, E.N., et al.: The role of pH in the development of tachyphylaxis to local anaesthetic agents, Anesthesiology, **29:**994, 1968.

70. Cohen, E.N., et al.: Occupational disease in dentistry and chronic exposure to trace anesthetic gases, J. Am. Dent. Assoc. **101:**21, 1980.

71. Condouris, G.A., Goebel, R.H., and Brady, T.: Computer simulation of local anesthetic effects using a mathematical model of myelinated nerve, J. Pharmacol. Exp. Ther. **196:**737, 1976.

72. Courtney, K.R.: Mechanism of frequency-dependent inhibition of sodium currents in frog myelinated nerve by the lidocaine derivative GEA 968, J. Pharmacol. Exp. Ther. **195:**225, 1975.

73. Covino, B.G.: Local anesthesia, Part I, Engl. J. Med. **286:**975, 1972.

74. Covino, B.G.: Systemic toxicity of local anesthetic agents (editorial), Anesth. Analg. **57:**387, 1978.

75. Covino, B.G., and Vassallo, H.G.: Local anesthetics: mechanisms of action and clinical use, New York, 1976, Grune & Stratton, Inc.

76. Craig, J., et al.: A survey of anaesthetic misadventures, Anaesthesia **36:**933, 1981.

77. Cullen, B.F., Chretien, P.B., and Leventhal, B.G.: The effect of lignocaine on PHA-stimulated human lymphocyte transformation, Br. J. Anaesth. **44:**1247, 1972.

78. Daily, W.W.: Local anesthesia of the head and neck, Ear Nose Throat J. **60:**19, 1981.

79. Dalen, J.E., and Dexter, L.: The hemodynamic and respiratory effects of diazepam (Valium), Anesthesiology **30:**259, 1969.

80. Davis, I., Moore, J.R.M., and Lahiri, S.K.: Nitrous oxide and the middle ear, Anaesthesia **34:**147, 1979.

81. de Jong, R.H.: Local anesthetics, Springfield, Ill., 1977, Charles C Thomas, Publisher.

82. de Jong, R.H.: Toxic effects of local anesthetics, J.A.M.A. **239:**1166, 1978.

83. de Jong, R.H., and Bonin, J.D.: Deaths from local anesthetic-induced convulsions in mice, Anesth. Analg. **59:**401, 1980.

84. de Jong, R.H., and Cullen, S.C.: Buffer demand and pH of local anesthetic solutions containing epinephrine, Anesthesiology **24:**801, 1963.

85. de Jong, R.H., and Heavner, J.E.: Convulsions induced by local anaesthetic: time course of diazepam prophylaxis, Can. Anaesth. Soc. J. **21:**153, 1974.

86. de Jong, R.H., et al.: Toxicity of local anesthetic mixtures, Toxicol. Appl. Pharmacol. **54:**501, 1980.

87. Deacock, A.R.D., and Simpson, W.T.: Fatal reactions to lignocaine, Anaesthesia **19:**217, 1964.

88. Deacon, R., et al.: Selective inactivation of vitamin B_{12} in rats by nitrous oxide, Lancet **2:**1023, 1978.

89. Deas, T.C.: Severe methemoglobinemia following dental extractions under lidocaine anesthesia, Anesthesiology **17:**204, 1956.

90. DeShazo, R.D., and Nelson, H.S.: An approach to the patient with a history of local anesthetic hypersensitivity: experience with 90 patients, J. Allergy Clin. Immunol. **63:**387, 1979.

91. Dicker, R.L., and Syracuse, V.R.: Local anesthesia in facial plastic surgery, Otol. ORL **86:**461, 1978.

92. Downes, J.J., Kemp, R.A., and Lambertsen, C.J.: The magnitude and duration of respiratory depression due to fentanyl and meperidine in man, J. Pharmacol. Exp. Ther. **158:**416, 1967.

93. Dundee, J.W., and Haslett, W.H.K.: The benzodiazepines: a review of their actions and uses relative to anesthetic practice, Br. J. Anaesth. **42:**217, 1970.

94. Duhring, L.A.: Cutaneous medicine, Philadelphia, 1905, J.B. Lippincott Co.

95. Dyck, P.J., Grina, L.A., and Lambert, E.H.: Nitrous oxide neurotoxicity studies in man and rat, Anesthesiology **53:**205, 1980.

96. Dykes, M.H.M.: Evaluation of a local anesthetic agent, bupivacaine hydrochloride (Marcaine), J.A.M.A. **224:**1035, 1973.

97. Edmondson, H.D., Roscoe, B., and Vickers, M.D.: Biochemical evidence of anxiety in dental patients, Br. Med. J. **4:**7, 1972.

98. Ehrenström Reiz, G.M.E., and Reiz, S.L.: EMLA—a eutectic mixture of local anaesthetics for topical anaesthesia, Acta Anaesth. Scand. **26**(6):596, 1982.

99. Eisele, J.H., and Reitan, J.A.: Scleroderma, Raynaud's phenomenon, and local anesthetics, Anesthesiology **34:**386, 1971.

100. Elliott, G.D., and Stein, E.: Oral surgery in patients with atherosclerotic heart disease: benign effect of epinephrine in local anesthesia, J.A.M.A. **227:**1403, 1974.

101. Englesson, S.: The influence of acid-base changes on central nervous system toxicity of local anaesthetic agents, Acta Anaesthesiol. Scand. **18**:79, 1974.

102. Eriksson, E.: Illustrated handbook in local anesthesia. I. Experimental study in cats, Philadelphia, 1980, W.B. Saunders Co.

103. Erlanger, J., and Gasser, H.S.: The compound nature of the action current of nerve as disclosed by the cathode ray oscillography, Am. J. Physiol. **70**:624, 1924.

104. Eyre, J., and Nally, F.: Nasal test for hypersensitivity: including a positive reaction to lignocaine, Lancet **1**:264, 1971.

105. Feasby, T.E., Hahn, A.F., and Gilbert, J.J.: Neurotoxicity of bacteriostatic water, N. Engl. J. Med. **308**:966, 1983.

106. Feinstein, M.B.: Reaction of local anesthetics with phospholipids: a possible chemical basis for anesthesia, J. Gen. Physiol. **48**:357, 1964.

107. Ferguson, R.M., Schmidtke, J.R., and Simmonds, R.L.: Inhibition of mitogen-induced lymphocyte transformation by local anesthetics, J. Immunol. **116**:627, 1976.

108. Ferstandig, L.L.: Trace concentrations of anesthetic gases: a critical review of their disease potential, Anesth. Analg. **57**:328, 1978.

109. Fink, B.R.: Acute and chronic toxicity of local anesthetics, Can. Anaesth. Soc. J. **20**:5, 1973.

110. Fink, B.R., Ansheim, G.M., and Levy, B.A.: Neural pharmacokinetics of epinephrine, Anesthesiology **48**:263, 1978.

111. Fink, B.R., et al.: Neurokinetics of lidocaine in the infraorbital nerve of the rat in vivo: relation to sensory block, Anesthesiology **42**:731, 1975.

112. Fisher, A.A.: Allergic reactions to topical (surface) anesthetics with reference to the safety of Tronothane (pramoxine hydrochloride), Cutis **25**:584, 1980.

113. Fisher, M.M., and Pennington, J.C.: Allergy to local anaesthesia, Br. J. Anaesth. **54**:893, 1982.

114. Foldes, F.F., et al.: Comparison of toxicity of intravenously given local anesthetic agents in man, J.A.M.A. **172**:1493, 1960.

115. Foster, C.A., and Aston, S.J.: Propranolol-epinephrine interaction: a potential disaster, Plast. Reconstr. Surg. **72**:74, 1983.

116. Frank, G.B., and Sanders, H.D.: A proposed common mechanism of action for general and local anesthetics in the central nervous system, Br. J. Pharmacol. **21**:1, 1963.

117. Franz, D.N., and Perry, R.S.: Mechanisms for differential block among single myelinated and non-myelinated axons by procaine, J. Physiol. **236**:193, 1974.

118. Fregert, S., Tegner, E., and Thelin, I.: Contact allergy to lidocaine, Contact Dermatitis **5**:185, 1979.

119. French, A.J., and Patel, Y.V.: Total ischemia at the site of local anaesthesia in patient on debrisoquine (letter), Lancet **2**:484, 1980.

120. Galindo, A., et al.: Mixtures of local anesthetics: bupivacaine-chloroprocaine, Anesth. Analg. **59**:683, 1980.

121. Garlock, J.H.: Gangrene of the finger following digital nerve block anesthesia, Ann. Surg. **94**:1103, 1931.

122. Gasser, H.S., and Erlanger, J.: The role of fiber size in the establishment of a nerve block by pressure or cocaine, Am. J. Physiol. **88**:581, 1929.

123. Gelfman, S.S., et al.: Recovery following intravenous sedation during dental surgery performed under local anesthesia, Anesth. Analg. **59**:775, 1980.

124. Gentili, F., et al.: Nerve injection injury with local anaesthetic agents: a light and electron microscopic, fluorescent microscopic and horseradish peroxidase study, Neurosurgery **6**:263, 1980.

125. Ghoneim, M.M., and Pandya, H.: Plasma protein binding of bupivacaine and its interaction with other drugs in man, Br. J. Anaesth. **46**:435, 1974.

126. Gillman, M.A.: Safety of nitrous oxide (letter), Lancet **2**:1397, 1982.

127. Glogau, R.G.: New office equipment. In Callen, J.P., editor: Current issues in dermatology, vol. I. Boston, 1984, G.K. Hall Medical Publishers.

128. Goldman, L., et al.: Multifactorial index of cardiac risk in noncardiac surgical procedures, N. Engl. J. Med. **297**:845, 1977.

129. Green, D., et al.: The effects of local anesthetics containing epinephrine on digital blood perfusion, J. Am. Podiatry Assoc. **69**:397, 1979.

130. Greene, N.M.: A consideration of factors in the discovery of anesthesia and their effects on its development, Anesthesiology **35**:515, 1971.

131. Green, R.L., et al.: Elevated plasma procaine concentrations after administration of procaine penicillin G, N. Engl. J. Med. **291**:223, 1974.

132. Griffin, G.C.: Nitrous oxide–oxygen sedation (letter), J.A.M.A. **247**:302, 1982.

133. Griffin, G.C., Campbell, V.D., and Jones, R.: Nitrous oxide-oxygen sedation for minor surgery: experience in a pediatric setting, J.A.M.A. **245**:2411, 1981.

134. Haegerstam, G., Evers, H., and Broberg, F.: Local effect produced on intact skin by epicutaneously applied anaesthetic formulations, Arzneimittel-Forschung. Drug. Res. **29**:1177, 1979.

135. Haegerstam, G., Evers, H., and Jublin, L.: Hyperemia induced by topical application of anaesthetic formulations containing ketocaine, Scand. J. Plast. Reconstr. Surg. **13**:469, 1979.

136. Hallen, B., and Uppfeldt, A.: Does lidocaine-prilocaine cream permit painfree insertion of IV catheters on children? Anesthesiology **57**:340, 1982.

137. Hamilton, W.K.: Unexpected deaths during anesthesia, wherein lies the cause (editorial), Anesthesiology **50**:381, 1979.

138. Hansson, E., Hoffman, P., and Kristerson, L.: Fate of mepivacaine in the body. II. Excretion and biotransformation, Acta Pharmacol. Toxicol. **22**:213, 1965.

139. Hargrove, R.L., et al.: Blood lignocaine levels following intravenous regional analgesia, Anesthesia **21**:37, 1966.

140. Henn, F., and Brattsand, R.: Some pharmacological and toxicological properties of a new long-acting local analgesic, LAC-43 (marcaine), in comparison with mepivacaine and tetracaine. Acta Anaesthesiol. Scand. **21**(suppl.):9, 1966.

141. Hille, B.: Common mode of action of three agents that decrease the transient change in sodium permeability in nerves, Nature **210**:1220, 1966.

142. Hille, B.: The permeability of the sodium channels to organ-

ic cations in myelinated nerve, J. Gen. Physiol. **58**:599, 1971.

143. Hille, B.: Local anesthetics: hydrophilic and hydrophobic pathways for the drug-receptor reaction, J. Gen. Physiol. **69**:497, 1977.

144. Hille, B., Courtney, K., and Dum, R.: Rate and site of action of local anesthetics in myelinated nerve fibers. In Fink, B.R., editor: Molecular mechanisms of anesthesia, New York, 1974, Raven Press.

145. Hillestad, L., et al.: Diazepam metabolism in normal man. I. Serum concentrations, intramuscular and oral—administration, Clin. Pharmacol. Ther. **16**:479, 1974.

146. Himes, R.S., Jr., Difazio, C., and Burney, R.G.: Effect of lidocaine on the anesthetic requirements for nitrous oxide and halothane, Anesthesiology **47**:437, 1977.

147. Hjelm, M., and Holmdahl, M.H.: Biochemical effects of aromatic amines. II. Cyanosis, methaemoglobinaemia and Heinz-body formation induced by a local anesthetic agent (Prilocaine), Acta Anaesthesiol. Scand. **9**:99, 1965.

148. Hodgkin, A.L., and Huxley, A.F.: Currents carried by sodium and potassium ions through the membrane of the giant axon of Loligo, J. Physiol. (Lond.) **116**:449, 1952.

149. Hofmann, H., et al.: Presumed generalized exfoliative dermatitis to lidocaine (letter), Arch. Dermatol. **111**:266, 1975.

150. Holti, G., and Hood, F.J.: An anaphylactoid reaction to lidocaine, Dent. Pract. **15**:294, 1965.

151. Incaudo, G., et al.: Administration of local anesthetics to patients with a history of prior adverse reaction, J. Allergy Clin. Immunol. **61**:339, 1978.

152. Johnson, H.A.: Infiltration with epinephrine and local anesthetic mixture in the hand, J.A.M.A. **200**:990, 1967.

153. Johnstone, R.E., Prevoznik, S.J., and Ominsky, A.J.: Local anesthesia for minor dermatologic surgical procedures, Int. J. Dermatol. **14**:146, 1975.

154. Juhlin, L., et al.: A lidocaine-prilocaine cream for superficial skin surgery and painful lesions, Acta Derm. Venereol. (Stockh.) **60**:544, 1980.

155. Kano, Y., et al.: Effects of nitrous oxide on human cell lines, Cancer Res. **43**:1493, 1983.

156. Kaplan, E.G., and Kashuk, K.: Disclaiming the myth of use of epinephrine local anesthesia in feet, J. Am. Podiatry Assoc. **61**:335, 1971.

157. Karlsson, E., Collste, R., and Rawlins, M.D.: Plasma levels of lidocaine during combined treatment with phenytoin and procainamide, Eur. J. Clin. Pharmacol. **7**:455, 1974.

158. Katz, R.L.: Epinephrine and PLV-2: cardiac rhythm and local vasoconstrictor effects, Anesthesiology **26**:619, 1964.

159. Kaufman, P.A.: Gangrene following digital nerve block anesthesia, Arch. Surg. **42**:929, 1941.

160. Keating, J.U., and Code, C.F.: Anesthetic and antihistaminic action of a series of antihistaminic drugs in human skin (abstract), J. Lab. Clin. Med. **33**:1609, 1948.

161. Keats, A.S.: What do we know about anesthetic mortality? Anesthesiology **50**:387, 1979.

162. Keidar, S., Grenadie, E., and Palant, A.: Sinoatrial arrest due to lidocaine injection in sick sinus syndrome during amiodarone administration, Am. Heart J. **104**(6):1384, 1982.

163. Kernekamp, A.S., et al.: Contact allergy to lidocaine (Xylo-caine, Lignocaine), Contact Dermatitis **5**:403, 1979.

164. Klingenström, P., and Westermark, L.: Local effects of adrenaline and phenylalanyl-lysyl-vasopressin in local anaesthesia, Acta Anaesthesiol. Scand. **7**:131, 1963.

165. Klotz, U., and Reimann, I.: Delayed clearance of diazepam due to cimetidine, N. Engl. J. Med. **302**:1012, 1980.

166. Knapp, A.B., et al.: The cimetidine-lidocaine interaction, Ann. Intern. Med. **98**:174, 1983.

167. Koller, C.: On the use of cocaine for producing anesthesia on the eye, Lancet **2**:990, 1884.

168. Korttila, K., and Linnoila, M.: Psychomotor skills related to driving after intramuscular administration of diazepam and meperidine, Anesthesiology **42**:685, 1975.

169. Kuhnert, B.R., et al.: Maternal, fetal and neonatal metabolism of lidocaine, Clin. Pharmacol. Ther. **26**:213, 1979.

170. La Rossa, B., and Riccio, R.: Epinephrine in local anesthesia, Paris Med. **2**:341, 1925.

171. Lane, C.G., and Luikart, R., II.: Dermatitis from local anesthetics, J.A.M.A. **146**:717, 1951.

172. Lane, G.A., et al.: Anesthetics as teratogens: nitrous oxide is fetotoxic, xenon is not, Science **210**:899, 1980.

173. Laskin, J.: Use of etidocaine hydrochloride in oral surgery: a clinical study, J. Oral Surg. **36**:863, 1978.

174. Layzer, R.B.: Myeloneuropathy after prolonged exposure to nitrous oxide, Lancet **2**:1227, 1978.

175. Levin, B.H., and Schanno, J.F.: Local anesthesia: serious consideration for extracranial carotid artery surgery, Am. Surg. **46**:174, 1980.

176. Lewis, B.: Deaths and dental anesthetics, Br. Med. J. **286**:3, 1983.

177. Lewis, G.B.H.: Prolonged regional analgesia on scleroderma, Can. Anaesth. Soc. J. **21**:495, 1974.

178. Liljestrand, G.: The historical development of local anesthesia. In Local anesthetic, International Encyclopedia of Pharmacology and Therapeutics, Sect. 8, Vol. 1, New York, 1971, Pergamon Press.

179. Liu, P.L., et al.: Comparative CNS toxicity of lidocaine, etidocaine, bupivacaine and tetracaine in awake dogs following rapid intravenous administration, Anesth. Analg. **62**:375, 1983.

180. Lubens, H.M., et al.: Anesthetic patch for painful procedures such as minor operations, Am. J. Dis. Child. **128**:192, 1974.

181. Lund, P.C., Cwik, J.C., and Gannon, R.T.: Etidocaine (Duranest): a clinical and laboratory evaluation, Acta Anaesthesiol. Scand. **18**:176, 1974.

182. Lund, P.C., Cwik, J.C., and Pagdanganan, R.T.: Etidocaine—a new long acting local anesthetic agent: a clinical evaluation, Anaesth. Analg. **52**:482, 1973.

183. Lunn, J.N., and Mushin, W.W.: Mortality associated with anesthesia, Anaesthesia **37**:856, 1982.

184. Luostarinen, V., et al.: Antithrombotic effects of lidocaine and related compounds on laser-induced microvascular injury, Acta Anaesthesiol. Scand. **25**:9, 1981.

185. Lynas, R.F.A.: A suspected allergic reaction to lidocaine, Anesthesiology **31**:380, 1969.

186. MacMillan, W.H.: A hypothesis concerning the effect of cocaine on the action of sympathomimetic amines, Br. J. Pharmacol. **14**:385, 1959.

187. Maloney, J.M., III: Nitrous oxide–oxygen analgesia in

dermatologic surgery, J. Dermatol. Surg. Oncol. **6:**447, 1980.

188. Maloney, J.M., III, et al.: Plasma concentrations of lidocaine during hair transplantation, J. Dermatol. Surg. Oncol. **8:**950, 1982.
189. Maloney, J.M., III, et al.: Preoperative preparations and anesthesia. In Coleman, W.P., Colon, G.A., and Davis, R.S., editors: Outpatient surgery of the skin, New Hyde Park, N.Y., 1983, Medical Examination Publishing Co., Inc.
190. Mark, L.C.: Avoiding the pain of venipuncture (letter), N. Engl. J. Med. **294:**614, 1976.
191. Mayhew, J.: Cardiovascular collapse associated with nitrous oxide administration, Can. Anaesth. Soc. J. **30:**226, 1983.
192. McGlinn, J.A.: Music in the operating room, Am. J. Obstet. Gynecol. **20:**678, 1930.
193. Melzack, R., Stillwell, D.M., and Rox, E.J.: Trigger points and acupuncture points for pain: correlations and implications, Pain **3:**23, 1977.
194. Merin, R.G.: Local and regional anesthetic techniques for the patient with ischemic heart disease, Cleve. Clin. Q. **48:**72, 1981.
195. Metcalfe, J.C., and Burgen, A.S.V.: Relaxation of anaesthetics in the presence of cyto-membranes, Nature **220:**587, 1968.
196. Mofenson, H.C., et al.: Lidocaine toxicity from topical mucosal application, with a review of the clinical pharmacology of lidocaine, Clin. Pediatr. **22:**190, 1983.
197. Monash, S.: Location of the superficial epithelial barrier to skin penetration, J. Invest. Dermatol. **29:**367, 1957.
198. Moore, D.C.: Complications of regional anesthesia, Springfield, Ill., 1955, Charles C Thomas, Publisher.
199. Moore, D.C.: Local anesthetic drugs: tissue and systemic toxicity, Acta Anaesthesiol. Belg. **32:**283, 1981.
200. Moore, D.C.: The pH of local anesthetic solutions, Anesth. Analg. **60:**833, 1981.
201. Moore, D.C., et al.: Bupivacaine: a review of 2,077 cases, J.A.M.A. **214:**713, 1970.
202. Moore, D.C., et al.: Factors determining dosage of amidetype local anesthetic drugs, Anesthesiology **47:**263, 1977.
203. Moore, D.C., Thompson, G.E., and Crawford, R.D.: Longacting local anesthetic drugs and convulsions with hypoxia and acidosis, Anesthesiology **56:**230, 1982.
204. Morgan, M., and Russell, W.J.: An investigation in man into the relative potency of lignocaine, bupivacaine and etidocaine, Br. J. Anaesth. **47:**586, 1975.
205. Morris, T., and Tracey, J.: Lignocaine: its effects on wound healing, Br. J. Surg. **64:**902, 1977.
206. Morrisset, L.M.: Fatal anaphylactic reaction to lidocaine, Armed Forces Med. J. **8:**740, 1957.
207. Mulvey, P.M.: Allergy to local anaesthetics, Med. J. Aust. **1:**386, 1980.
208. Myers, B., et al.: The effect of local anesthesia and epinephrine on the size of cryolesions in the experimental animal, Plast. Reconstr. Surg. **68:**415, 1981.
209. Nagel, J.E., Fuscaldo, J.T., and Fireman, P.: Paraben allergy, J.A.M.A. **237:**1594, 1977.
210. Naidu, K.R.: Music sedation for local analgesia, Anaesthesia **37:**354, 1982.
211. Narahashi, T., and Frazier, D.T.: Site of action and active form of procaine in squid giant axons, J. Pharmacol. Exp. Ther. **194:**506, 1975.
212. Nathan, P.W., and Sears, T.A.: Some factors concerned in differential nerve block by local anaesthetics, J. Physiol. (Lond.) **157:**565, 1961.
213. Nattel, S., et al.: Therapeutic blood lidocaine concentrations after local anesthesia for cardiac electrophysiologic studies, N. Engl. J. Med. **301:**418, 1979.
214. Nilsson, E., and Wendeberg, B.: Effects of local anaesthetics on wound healing, Acta Anaesth. Scand. **1:**87, 1957.
215. Nitrous oxide and acute marrow failure (editorial), Lancet **2:**856, 1982.
216. Noble, D.S., and Pierce, G.F.M.: Allergy to lidocaine: a case history, Lancet **2:**1436, 1961.
217. Nunn, J.F., et al.: Megaloblastic haemopoiesis after multiple short-term exposure to nitrous oxide, Lancet **1:**1379, 1982.
218. O'Donohue, W.J., Jr., et al.: Acute methemoglobinemia induced by topical benzocaine and lidocaine, Arch. Intern. Med. **140:**1508, 1980.
219. Ohlsén, L., and Englesson, S.: New anaesthetic formulation for epicutaneous application tested for cutting split skin grafts, Br. J. Anaesth. **52:**413, 1980.
220. Oikarinen, V.J., Ylipaavalniemi, P., and Evers, H.: Pain and temperature sensations related to local analgesia, Int. J. Oral Surg. **4:**151, 1975.
221. Palmer, J.M., and Link, D.: Impotence following anesthesia for elective circumcision J.A.M.A. **241:**2635, 1979.
222. Panje, W.R.: Local anesthesia of the face, J. Dermatol. Surg. Oncol. **5:**311, 1979.
223. Parbrook, G.: The levels of nitrous oxide analgesia, Br. J. Anaesth. **39:**974, 1967.
224. Pelner, L.: Gangrene of the toe following local anesthesia with procaine-epinephrine solution, N.Y. State J. Med. **42:**544, 1944.
225. Perreault, L., et al.: Middle ear pressure variations during nitrous oxide anesthesia, Can. Anaesth. Soc. J. **29**(5):428, 1982.
226. Peterson, D.S., and Kein, D.R.: Pain sensation related to local anesthesia injected at varying temperatures, Anesth. Prog. **25:**164, 1978.
227. Peterson, H.B., et al.: Comparative risk of death from induced abortion at less than or equal to 12 weeks gestation performed with local versus general anesthesia, Am. J. Obstet. Gynecol. **141:**763, 1981.
228. Pettersson, L.O., and Akerman, B.: Effects of different types of anesthesia including percutaneous local anesthesia on survival of experimental skin flaps, Scand. J. Plast. Reconstr. Surg. **13:**237, 1979.
229. Pettersson, L.O., and Havu, N.: The iron content of split skin grafts after general infiltration and percutaneous anaesthesia, Scand. J. Plast. Reconstr. Surg. **13:**473, 1979.
230. Pettersson, L.O., and Strömbeck, J.O.: Percutaneous anaesthesia for dermabrasion, Scand. J. Plast. Reconstr. Surg. **12:**287, 1978.
231. Pizzolato, P., and Renegar, O.J.: Histopathologic effects of long term exposure to local anesthetics on peripheral nerves, Anesth. Analg. **38:**138, 1959.
232. Prescott, L.F., Adjepon-Yamoah, K.K., and Talbot, R.G.: Impaired lignocaine metabolism in patients with myocardial infarction and cardiac failure, Br. Med. J. **1:**939, 1976.

233. Pryor, G.J., et al.: Local anesthesia in minor lacerations: topical TAC vs. lidocaine infiltration, Ann. Emerg. Med. **9:**568, 1980.

234. Rasmussen, L.F., Ahlfors, C.E., and Wennberg, R.P.: The effect of paraben preservatives on albumin binding of bilirubin, J. Pediatr. **89:**475, 1976.

235. Rattenborg, C.C., Lichtor, J.L., and Lorincz, A.L.: Stellate-ganglion blockade after "placebo" injection (letter), N. Engl. J. Med. **309:**433, 1983.

236. Read, J.M., et al.: Sterile topical lignocaine jelly in plastic surgery: an assessment of its systemic toxicity, S. Afr. Med. J. **57:**704, 1980.

237. Reiser, G., Gunther, A., and Hamprecht, B.: Strychnine and local anesthetics block ion channels activated by veratridine in neuro-blastoma by glioma hybrid cells, FEBS Lett. **143** (2):306, 1982.

238. Ritchie, J.M., and Ritchie, B.R.: Local anesthetics: effect of pH on activity, Science **162:**1394, 1968.

239. Ritchie, J.M.: Mechanism of action of local anesthetic agents and biotoxins, Br. J. Anaesth. **47:**191, 1975.

240. Ritchie, J.M., and Greene, N.M.: Local anesthetics. In Gilman, A.G., Goodman, L.S., and Gilman, A., editors: The pharmacological basis of therapeutics, ed. 6, New York, 1980, MacMillan Publishing Co.

241. Roed-Petersen, J.: Contact sensitivity to metaoxedrine, Contact Dermatitis **2:**235, 1976.

242. Rojas, E., and Armstrong, C.M.: Sodium conductance activation without inactivations in pronase-perfused axons, Nature (New Biol.) **229:**177, 1971.

243. Rood, J.P.: A case of lignocaine hypersensitivity, Br. Dent. J. **135:**411, 1973.

244. Rosenberg, P.H.: Differential sensitivity of A nerve & C nerve fibers to long acting amide local anesthetics, Br. J. Anaesth. **55**(2):163, 1983.

245. Roser-Maass, E.: Fingertip necrosis after local anesthesia for nail extraction, Hautarzt **32:**39, 1981.

246. Rowland, M., et al.: Disposition kinetics of lidocaine in normal subjects, Ann. N.Y., Acad. Sci. **179:**383, 1971.

247. Ruben, H.: Nitrous oxide analgesia in dentistry: its use during 15 years in Denmark, Br. Dent. J. **132:**195, 1972.

248. Ruben, J.A.: Sloughing in local anesthetics—its causes and prevention, Penn. Med. **23:**713, 1920.

249. Ryhänen, P.: Lidocaine inhibition of rosette formation, Med. Biol. **57:**196, 1979.

250. Samsi, A.B., et al.: Evaluation of centbucridine as a local anesthetic, Anesth. Analg. **62**(1):109, 1983.

251. Sawinski, V.J., and Loiselle, R.J.: Osmolality of local anesthetics and associated injection site edema, J. Oral Ther. Pharmacol. **3:**44, 1966.

252. Schechter, G.L., Brase, D.A., and Powell, J.: Adverse effects of tricyclic antidepressants during nasal surgery, Otolaryngol. Head Neck Surg. **90:**233, 1982.

253. Schwartz, M., et al.: Antiarrhythmic effectiveness of intramuscular lidocaine: influence of different injection sites, J. Clin. Pharmacol. **14:**77, 1974.

254. Scott, D.B.: Evaluation of the toxicity of local anesthetic agents in man, Br. J. Anaesthesiol. **47:**56, 1975.

255. Scott, D.B., et al.: Factors affecting plasma levels of lignocaine and prilocaine, Br. J. Anaesth. **44:**1040, 1972.

256. Seeman, P.: Anesthetics and pressure reversal of anesthesia: expansion and recompression of membrane proteins, lipids, and water (editorial), Anesthesiology **47:**1, 1977.

257. Selander, D., et al.: Local anesthetics: importance of mode of application, concentration, and adrenalin for the appearance of nerve lesions—experimental study of axonal degeneration and barrier damage after intrafascicular injection or topical application of bupivacaine (Marcain), Acta Anaesthesiol. Scand. **23:**127, 1979.

258. Selden, R., and Sasahara, A.A.: Central nervous system toxicity induced by lidocaine: report of a case in a patient with liver disease, J.A.M.A. **202:**908, 1967.

259. Serafin, F.J.: A precaution in the uses of procaine-epinephrine for regional anesthesia, J.A.M.A. **91:**43, 1928.

260. Sinclair, D.: Normal anatomy of sensory nerves and receptors. In Jarrett, A., editor: The physiology and pathophysiology of the skin, vol. 2, New York, 1973, Academic Press, Inc.

261. Skacel, P.O., et al.: Studies on the haemopoietic toxicity of nitrous oxide on man, Br. J. Haematol. **53:**189, 1983.

262. Skou, J.C.: The effect of drugs on cell membranes with special reference to local anaesthetics, J. Pharm. Pharmacol. **13:**204, 1961.

263. Smith, N.T.: Dangers and opportunities. In Smith, N.T., Miller, R.D., and Corbascio, A.N., editors: Drug interactions in anesthesia, Philadelphia, 1981, Lea & Febiger.

264. Smith, N.T., Miller, R.D., and Corbascio, A.N., editors: Drug interactions in anesthesia, Philadelphia, 1981, Lea & Febiger.

265. Smith, T.C., Cooper, L.H., and Wollman, H.: History and principles of anesthesiology. In Gilman, A.G., Goodman, L.S., and Gilman, A., editors: The pharmacological basis of therapeutics, ed. 6, New York, 1980, MacMillan Publishing Co.

266. Smythies, J.R., et al.: The molecular structure of the sodium channel, J. Theor. Biol. **43:**29, 1974.

267. Sperling, L.C., et al.: Toward less painful anesthesia: water, saline, and lidocaine, J. Dermatol. Surg. Oncol. **7:**730, 1981.

268. Spooner, R.B.: Nitrous oxide–oxygen sedation (letter), J.A.M.A. **247:**302, 1982.

269. Steen, S.N., and Hahl, D.: Controlled evaluation of parenteral diazepam as preanesthetic medication: a statistical study, Anesth. Analg. **48:**549, 1969.

270. Steen, P.A., Tinker, J.H., and Tarhan, S.: Myocardial reinfarction after anesthesia and surgery, J.A.M.A. **239:**2566, 1978.

271. Steinhaus, J.E.: Local anesthetic toxicity: a pharmacological reevaluation, Anesthesiology **18:**275, 1957.

272. Stewart, R.H., and Graham, G.F.: A complication of cryosurgery in a patient with cryofibrinogenemia, J. Dermatol. Surg. Oncol. **4:**743, 1978.

273. Strichartz, G.R.: The inhibition of sodium currents in myelinated nerve by quaternary derivatives of lidocaine, J. Gen. Physiol. **62:**37, 1973.

274. Sundin, R.H., et al.: Anxiolytic effects of low dosage nitrous-oxygen mixtures administered continuously in apprehensive subjects, South. Med. J. **74:**1489, 1981.

275. Sung, C.Y., and Truant, A.P.: The physiological disposition of lidocaine and its comparison in some respects with pro-

caine, J. Pharmacol. Exp. Ther. **112**:432, 1954.

276. Sunshine, I., and Fike, W.W.: Value of thin-layer chromatography in two fatal cases of intoxication due to lidocaine and mepivacaine, N. Engl. J. Med. **271**:487, 1964.

277. Svedmyr, N.: The influence of a tricyclic antidepressive agent (protriptyline) on some of the circulatory effects of noradrenaline and adrenaline in man, Life Sci. **7**(1):77, 1968.

278. Sweet, P.T., Magee, D.A., and Holland, A.J.C.: Duration of intradermal anesthesia with mixtures of bupivacaine and lidocaine, Can. Anaesth. Soc. J. **29**(5):481, 1982.

279. Tait, C., Reese, N.O., and Davis, D.A.: A comparative study of hexylcaine, procaine and lidocaine with specific attention to tissue irritation, South. Med. J. **51**:358, 1958.

280. Taylor, G., Larson, C.P., Jr., and Prestwich, R.: Unexpected cardiac arrest during anesthesia and surgery: an environmental study, J.A.M.A. **236**:2758, 1976.

281. Teasdale, C., et al.: A randomized controlled trial to compare local with general anesthesia for short-stay inguinal hernia repair, Ann. R. Coll. Surg. Engl. **64**:238, 1982.

282. Thal, E.R., Montgomery, S.J., and Atkins, J.M.: Self-administered analgesia with nitrous oxide: adjunctive aid for emergency medical care systems, J.A.M.A. **242**:2418, 1979.

283. Thornton, J.A., et al.: Cardiovascular effects of 50% nitrous oxide and 50% oxygen mixture, Anesthesia **28**:484, 1973.

284. Tomlin, P.J.: Death in outpatient dental anaesthetic practice, Anaesthesia **29**:551, 1974.

285. Tronolane (pramoxine), Med. Lett. Drug Ther. **23**(23):100, 1981.

286. Trudell, J.R.: A unitary theory of anesthesia based on lateral phase separations in nerve membranes, Anesthesiology **46**:5, 1977.

287. Tucker, G.T., and Mather, L.E.: Clinical pharmacokinetics of local anesthetics, Clin. Pharmacokinet. **4**:241, 1979.

288. Tucker, G.T., et al.: Binding of anilide-type local anesthetics in human plasma. I. Relationships between binding, physicochemical properties, and anesthetic activity, Anesthesiology **33**:287, 1970.

289. Ulfendahl, H.R.: Some pharmacological and toxicological properties of a new local anesthetic, Carbocain, Acta Anaesthesiol. Scand. **1**:81, 1957.

290. Van Dyke, C., et al.: Cocaine: plasma concentrations after intranasal application in man, Science **191**:859, 1976.

291. Verrill, P.J.: Adverse reaction to local anesthetics and vasoconstrictor drugs, Practitioner **214**:380, 1975.

292. Verlander, J.M., Jr., et al.: The clinical use of cocaine, Otolaryngol. Clin. North Am. **14**:521, 1981.

293. Vessey, M.P., and Nunn, J.F.: Occupational hazards of anesthesia, Br. Med. J. **281**:696, 1980.

294. von Annep, B.: Ueber die physiologische Wirbung des Cocain, Archiv fur die gesammte Physiologie des menschen und der thiere **21**:38, 1880.

295. Wennberg, E., et al.: Effects of commercial (pH approximately 3.5) and freshly prepared (pH approximately 6.5) lidocaine-adrenaline solutions on tissue pH, Acta Anaesthesiol. Scand. **26**:524, 1982.

296. Wiener, S.G.: Injectable sodium chloride as a local anesthetic for skin surgery, Cutis **23**:342, 1979.

297. Wilson, J.W., Luikart, R., and Ayres, S.: Dichlorotetrafluoroethane for surgical skin planing: a safe anesthetic refrigerant, Arch. Derm. Syph. (Chic.) **71**:523, 1955.

298. Yacoub, O., et al.: Depression of hypoxic ventilatory response by nitrous oxide, Anesthesiology **45**:385, 1976.

299. Yagiela, J.A., et al.: Comparison of myotoxic effects of lidocaine with epinephrine in rats and humans, Anesth. Analg. **60**:471, 1981.

300. Young, M.G.: N_2O use by podiatrists—a good prescription? Tex. Med. **78**:64, 1982.

301. Zoltan, J.: Cicatrix optima, Baltimore, 1977, University Park Press.

7

Instruments and Their Care

The instruments used in cutaneous surgery are more than just tools of the trade. Knowing the best instrument to use at the appropriate moment may mean the difference between a good result and a great result cosmetically. As one gains experience in surgery, one favors certain instruments over others and gradually learns their benefits and limitations.

Cutaneous surgery requires manual skill and dexterity. The derivation of the word *surgery* is the Greek χείρ (hand) plus ἔργω (to work); together they mean "work by hand." As in handicrafts, instruments have evolved to facilitate movements and to ensure accomplishment of tasks for which human fingers by themselves are too clumsy. It has been said that the surgeon's hands would be of little service to him if not supplied with a variety of instruments.[84]

The evolution of surgical instruments has taken place over many centuries. During the Paleolithic period, the cutting knife was first fashioned from flaked flint or obsidian. This was probably the surgeon's first tool. It is interesting to note that as late as the 1880s, flint lancets were still used for bloodletting.[47] Hippocrates, realizing the great importance of good instruments, stated, "All instruments ought to be well suited for the purpose in hand as regards their size, weight, and delicacy"[84]—a statement as true today as it was in the fifth century BC. In ancient Rome instruments were made of bronze, although iron and steel were used to make blades.

Operative techniques were revolutionized in the mid nineteenth century with the introduction of the ratchet catch to lock pivot forceps by controlled compression; thus the modern hemostat and forceps were born. Physicians of that era were proud of their instruments, frequently fashioning handles on their knives from ivory, ebony, or tortoise shell. However, with the introduction of sterilization after 1885 instruments were all metal. Initially these instruments were nickel- or chrome-plated to prevent corrosion with heat and moisture, but these were gradually replaced, after 1925, by stainless steel.[46]

This chapter describes many of the instruments used in cutaneous surgery, especially excisional surgery. Other chapters dealing with more specialized techniques describe other instruments and equipment. The physician should be acquainted with how instruments are made and maintained to be able to purchase the tools of the trade wisely and use them to their fullest.

MANUFACTURE OF SURGICAL INSTRUMENTS

Variability in quality exists between instruments made by different instrument manufacturers because different formulas for steel are used. Moreover, tempering and workmanship are extremely important in the production of high-quality instruments. For these reasons the physician should consider purchasing only reliable brands of instruments and buying from suppliers of the highest integrity and reputation.

An instrument is no better than the steel from which it is made.[64] Steel by definition is iron that contains carbon in any amount up to 1.7% as an essential alloying element; the carbon is necessary to produce hardness. The carbon content is of extreme importance; the lower the percentage, the softer the steel. If the percentage is too high, the steel will be very brittle and hard to forge. Surgical stainless steel also has chromium (usually 12% to 18%) and nickel (8%), which are added as alloying constituents to produce a metal practically immune from rusting and corrosion. In general, the more chromium present in an alloy, the more resistant it is to corrosion. Unfortunately, the carbon that is added for hardness reduces the corrosion-resistant effect of chromium. The most satisfactory percentages of alloy constituents for surgical stainless steel are 12% to 14% chromium and 0.2% carbon.[64] For surgical instruments that require extremely sharp edges, fine points, or accurate jaw approximation, it is more desirable to have proper hardness and elasticity than absolute corrosion resistance.[36]

The two types of stainless steel are *martensitic* and *austenitic*. Martensitic stainless steel is magnetic and can be hardened. It is used for most surgical instruments, in which hardness and sharpness are essential. Austenitic stainless steel cannot be hardened and may therefore bend easily. It is nonmagnetic and has a greater tendency to corrode. Austenitic stainless steel is sometimes referred to as "eighteen and eight" because it contains 18% chromium and 8% nickel. It is used for trays and pans in surgical operating rooms.

"Stainless" is a misnomer because there is no steel in existence that is entirely stainproof under all conditions.[64] The production of a stainless steel instrument requires a number of different and somewhat tedious steps. It has been estimated that it takes 2.5 hours of work to produce 4 ounces of steel instruments.[47] The metal is first heated above the critical point (820° C for stainless steel) to soften it and then cooled slowly as it is hammered against standard shapes. The surface oxides are descaled in 50% HCl. The metal is subsequently filed into its final shape and the joints fitted. This is followed by hardening and tempering by quenching in oil, degreasing, and tempering in molten sodium nitrate. Finally the metal instruments are buffed and polished.

The surface of stainless steel is described as active or passive. An active surface is highly susceptible to corrosion, whereas a passive surface is resistant to corrosion. Passivity is accomplished by exposing the instruments to a dilute solution of nitric acid, a process known as passivation. The resultant passive surface is formed by a thin, inert, and impervious chromium oxide film and, any particles of carbon steel that may have been ground in during processing are dissolved away. Only stainless steel instruments containing at least 12% chromium develop passivity, since the chromium oxide coating is probably the mechanism by which chromium produces corrosion resistance in stainless steel. Instruments from reliable manufacturers are always passivated in the production process. As an alternative, instruments with a low chromium content may be chrome plated to prevent corrosion. However, the plating chips with time, inevitably leading to corrosion. One should not purchase such instruments when given a choice.

Polishing is another processing step that reduces corrosion. Polishing removes impurities from the surface and allows for a smooth surface with which the layer of chromium oxide (formed later) is continuous. Highly polished instruments are less prone to corrosion than those with dull satinlike finishes.[82]

The forging of stainless steel instruments induces built-in stresses. If these stresses are not "stress relieved," stress corrosion may result with acid detergents. In addition, instruments may break at points of high mechanical stress, such as the pivot or fulcrum, as will be seen in Fig. 7-40. This may be partially caused by excessive peening of rivets at the fulcrum, which produces invisible cracks.[64]

The introduction of homemade medical devices—from spoons[59] to glass cutters[13,92]—for the sake of convenience may produce problems. Quality control and high engineering standards are imposed on reputable manufacturers but do not apply to these homemade "medical" instruments.[94] Although this may result in a higher price paid for surgical instruments than for "homemade medical devices," malfunctions are probably less likely.

PURCHASE OF INSTRUMENTS

The choice of instruments is an individual decision but certain guidelines should be observed. First, one should have a clear idea of the types of instruments one needs. (See Appendix H for a list of suggested instruments to purchase for cutaneous surgery.) This protects the physician from the purchase of instruments he or she will never need. It is a good idea to request copies of instrument catalogues yearly and to peruse them carefully to make sure that all one's surgical needs are being met adequately. We suggest ordering the instrument catalogues of Miltex, Robbins, Storz, and Tiemann for the highest quality of instruments.* Different manufacturers may have different names for the same instrument and different codes for different sizes of the same instrument.

Second, it is a good idea to handle the instruments personally. No two physicians have the same dexterity or finger size; hence, many variations are possible when ordering instruments, such as ring sizes on scissors or left-handed instruments. Hold the instrument as it is meant to be used. In general, instruments for fine cutaneous surgery should be small or delicate. Standard instruments for abdominal surgery are too large both for handling tissue gently and for holding the small needles used in cutaneous surgery. Instruments may be demonstrated at national meetings, or the vendors themselves may come to the physician's office for a demonstration.

Third, compare prices when possible. Although quality may vary slightly among some instruments, particularly delicate or unusual ones, many commonly used and frequently replaced instruments are not subject to such nuances in manufacture. Identifying the manufacturers of less expensive quality instruments will result in significant cost savings over many years. Occasionally one may desire to pay more for one instrument from a given manufacturer because of superior workmanship, but in general this is the exception. Avoid chrome-plated instruments.

Finally, purchase of instruments should be supervised by the physician and not delegated to those who do not directly use the instruments. When receiving the instruments in the office, a physician should be responsible for checking the purchase order to ensure that the instruments ordered are the ones received and that they are in good working condition without defects in the metal or workmanship. *Caveat*

---

*Miltex Instrument Co., 6 Ohio Drive, Lake Success, N.Y. 11042; Robbins Instruments Inc., 2 North Passaic Ave., Chatham, N.J. 07928; Storz Instrument Co., 3365 Tree Court Industrial Blvd., St. Louis 63122; George Tiemann & Co., 84 Newtown Plaza, Plainview, N.Y. 11803.

emptor. One should look closely to see that the jaws close properly on all forceps and needle holders and that the teeth mesh properly on the former. There should be no roughness or tarnish on the surfaces. Scissors should close smoothly, and all box locks should work easily. The shanks on all instruments should be springy and yet allow closing to the last ratchet without undue effort. Pickups should be tested for proper tension. Save the boxing in which the instruments were sent in case they need to be returned immediately or in the future for repairs or reconditioning.

Instruments can be ordered from the manufacturer with a number of special features: left-handed design, larger rings for larger fingers, overlapping shanks on scissors for less twisting of the wrist, and gold handles for easier visibility on a cluttered instrument stand. Many instruments can be ordered as *delicate,* meaning smaller and lighter. These are particularly useful in dermatologic surgery. The finish on instruments may be shiny and highly polished or dull with a satin finish, which has non-glare characteristics.

The cost of instruments and their tendency to get lost was the subject of an interesting article by Anthony.[2] In one hospital large numbers of lost instruments were traced to the laundry. Salvaging instruments in this one area saved the hospital $47,000 in replacement costs in 3 years. Certainly in clinic situations instrument losses can be considerable. In such situations instruments should be either labeled with colored tape (Surg-I-Band) or engraved. Instrument manufacturers are happy to engrave instruments for identification purposes at the time of purchase. Although one can buy an inexpensive engraver, amateur use of it may damage an instrument (for instance, engraving over the box locks); therefore I prefer that engraving be left to the manufacturer.

Manufacturers of surgical instruments want every physician to be pleased with every purchase because they want a customer for a lifetime. Therefore the manufacturer should be consulted about any problems with the instruments as well as about care of the instruments for maximal benefit. The relationship between physician and manufacturer should be beneficial for both parties.

INSTRUMENTS
Scalpel handles and blades

Most dermatologic surgeons prefer a flat No. 3 scalpel handle with a No. 15 scalpel blade (Fig. 7-1). The scalpel handle may be purchased with or without a centimeter scale. They are ideally weighted and handle easily. A few surgeons prefer octagonal handles, claiming that they afford greater fingertip control,[6] but under most circumstances they are unnecessary in dermatologic surgery. No. 11 blades with a pointed tip are also useful for stab incisions into abscesses or for suture removal.

Scalpel blades may be made of carbon steel or stainless steel. The former are sharper but hold an edge less well than

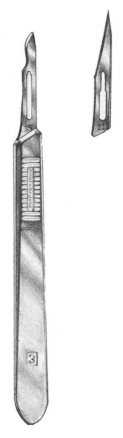

Fig. 7-1. No. 3 scalpel handle with No. 15 scalpel blade. Shown to the right for comparison is No. 11 scalpel blade.

stainless steel does. In general I prefer the carbon steel blades. The sharpest part of the blade edge is the belly and not the tip, so most cutting should be done with this part of the blade.

One of the greatest annoyances in a busy practice is removing the scalpel blades from the handles. Not only is this a clumsy procedure but it may result in unnecessary injury to the personnel involved. There is a strong likelihood of a slipped tool or snapped blade—and hence a cut finger. Therefore I recommend purchase of a blade extractor (Gramfield [No. 4135], New Hyde Park, N.Y.) (Fig. 7-2), which safely and quickly removes scalpel blades from handles. An English variety is also available.[57] Interestingly, at the Royal Infirmary in Glasgow the second most reported injury among personnel was cuts while discarding scalpel blades or scratches from used hypodermic needles.[57] Disposable scalpel blades on plastic handles may also be purchased, but in my experience the handles are not weighted properly and therefore are less than desirable for fine excisional surgery. In addition, the scalpel blade, being stainless steel, is not as sharp as carbon steel.

A unique addition to the dermatologic surgeon's armamentarium is the heated scalpel blade available with the Shaw scalpel. This is a Teflon-coated blade covering a

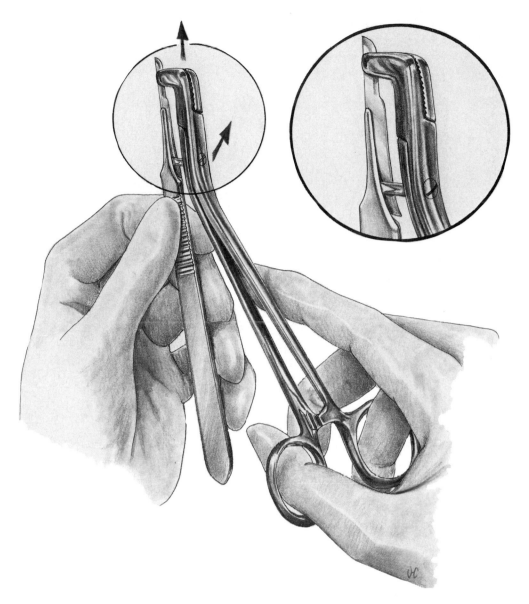

Fig. 7-2. Proper method of using scalpel blade extractor.

copper wire, which heats from 120° to 270° C. This instrument is discussed at greater length in the chapter dealing with electrosurgical apparatus (Chapter 16).

An alternative scalpel handle and blade for fine work is the Beaver handle and blade. Shown in Fig. 7-3 is the pencil-like, round, knurled 4-inch Beaver handle with a No. 67 Beaver blade (a smaller equivalent to the No. 15 blade). The Beaver equivalent of the No. 11 surgical blade is the No. 65 Beaver blade. Beaver blades are made of stainless steel, which I have found to be less sharp than the regular carbon steel blades. In addition, the thickness of the blades is not commensurate with the smallness. However, Beaver blades may still be desirable for small excisions, where larger blades produce larger incisions because of their size. Some physicians prefer a longer, heavier-weighted scalpel for the

Beaver system[32] or the hexagonal Beaver handle for better fingertip control.

Blade breaker and holder

The sharpest edge easily available for cutting is found on safety razor blades, especially the Gillette Super Blue Blade. This blade is made of steel with a high carbon content (1.25%) and has a cutting edge $\frac{1}{1,000,000}$ inch thick. In addition, it is coated with a fluorocarbon telomer (Vydax) to enhance its cutting capabilities and zinc naphthenate, a bacteriostat, in an anticorrosive oil.[76] Individually wrapped blades may be purchased from the Gillette Co.[28] or from surgical instrument companies.

The Castroviejo blade breaker and holder is illustrated in Fig. 7-4. Its special latch feature allows one to hold a

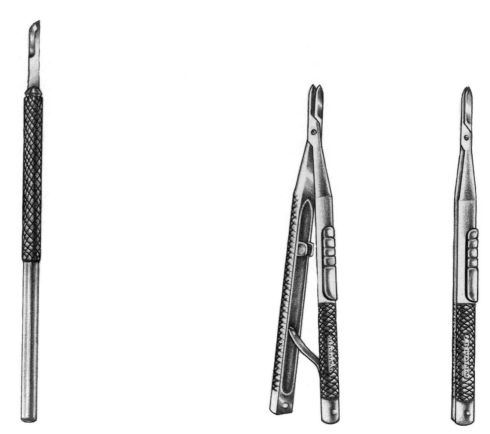

Fig. 7-3. Round, knurled Beaver handle with No. 67 Beaver blade.

Fig. 7-4. Castroviejo blade breaker and holder, in open and closed positions.

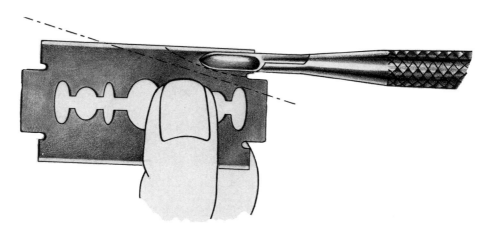

Fig. 7-5. Proper angle for breaking piece from razor blade with blade breaker and holder.

broken blade securely for maximal control when cutting. Holding a blade in forceps is to be avoided, because it does not provide a secure grip on the blade. Fig. 7-5 demonstrates the proper techniques for breaking a razor blade with the blade breaker. Note that the angle of bending relative to the edge of the blade determines the size and shape of the piece broken from the blade. Razor blades may also be used by themselves without a blade breaker and holder (see Fig. 14-11). Shelley[76] described manually breaking the safety razor blade in half longitudinally for this purpose. Although such a broken blade may be useful, one must be careful not to cut oneself while breaking the blade.

Prepackaged small razor blade edges are made and were initially pioneered in 1958 by Goldman and Preston,[37] but

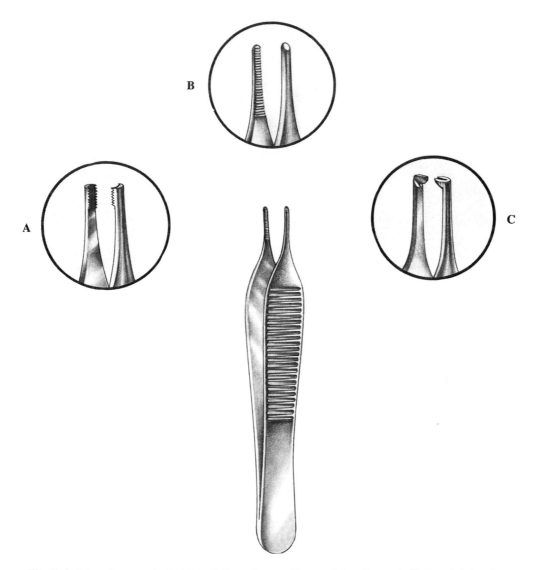

Fig. 7-6. Adson forceps. **A,** 7 × 7 teeth tissue forceps (Brown-Adson forceps). **B,** Serrated dressing forceps. **C,** 1 × 2 teeth (tissue forceps).

have not enjoyed much popularity in dermatologic surgery. The advantage of these blades is that they are packaged sterile (unlike razor blades), but whether they have the same sharp cutting edge is undetermined. Also packaged sterile are specially manufactured microblades for use with blade holders with specially designed handles.

One interesting supersharp blade is the obsidian blade made from volcanic molten lava, described by Scott et al.[74] This blade is said to have the sharpest edge of any blade naturally or humanly produced. However, it may be susceptible to splintering and leaving fragments of glass in the tissue. The advantage of extreme sharpness may thus not necessarily be as important as the possible consequences of its use. No studies have been performed to confirm if wound healing is superior with such a supersharp instrument.

The sharp edges provided by razor blades or microblades permit precise removal of superficial lesions and avoidance of deep cuts in the dermis[76]; the less tissue removed, the better the possible cosmetic results will be for the patient. A razor blade is of use for fine shave biopsies[1] (see Fig. 14-11). It is also useful when the skin is loose and thus more difficult to cut through without crimping except with a very sharp instrument. This type of tissue is found, for instance, on the eyelids and penis.

Tissue forceps (pickups)

The most useful tissue forceps in cutaneous surgery are the Adson forceps. A number of different tips may be useful, some of which are pictured in Fig. 7-6. The most helpful tip in cutaneous surgery is the serrated tip (Fig. 7-6, *B*), which is found on forceps the manufacturers refer to as dressing forceps. The serrated tip may be ordered as

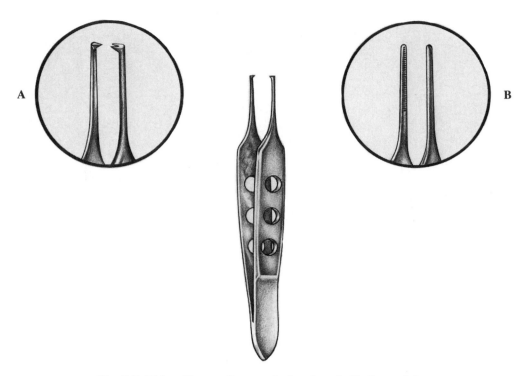

Fig. 7-7. Bishop-Harman forceps. **A,** 1 × 2 teeth. **B,** Serrated tips.

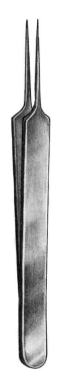

Fig. 7-8. Jeweler's forceps with very fine points.

regular or delicate, the latter meaning thin. These forceps allow one to handle tissue gently, minimizing trauma with adequate traction. When one requires more pulling force, for instance when removing a cyst with overlying skin, the toothed variety of Adson forceps (Fig. 7-6, *C*) may be useful. In general, toothed forceps should not be used to handle tissues to be sutured, since they tend to crush and tear, leading to poor cosmetic results (see Fig. 10-31, *B*). Even if the tissue is to be sent for biopsy, crush artifacts can be produced. The Brown-Adson forceps (Fig. 7-6, *A*) is said to distribute pressure evenly when grasping tissue. However, like the toothed Adson, this instrument still tends to bite into the tissue and should not be used in general. One can also order Adson forceps with absolutely smooth jaws—in my experience not adequate to hold tissue; or with diamond jaws—of no real advantage over serrated tips and three times as expensive. The diamond jaws may be made of tungsten-carbide inserts for longer wear.

The Bishop-Harman forceps (Fig. 7-7) is one of the most useful instruments for fine, delicate surgery. They may be purchased with serrated tips (Fig. 7-7, *B*) or cross-serrated tips, or they may be toothed (Fig. 7-7, *A*). As with the Adson forceps the serrated tips are most useful. This instrument is made with holes in the handles for a sure grasp and easier manipulation. It is particularly useful in working around the eyelid, where the skin is very thin.

One final type of forceps to mention is the jeweler's forceps (Fig. 7-8). They may be purchased with fine, extra-fine, or superfine tips and are most useful for spot coagula-

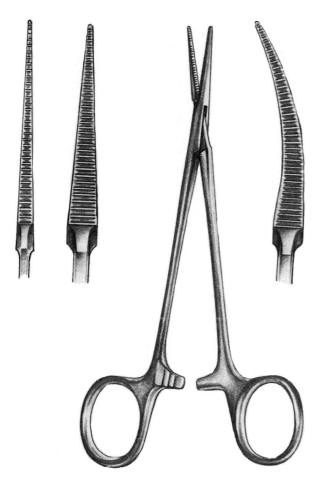

Fig. 7-9. Halsted mosquito hemostat, straight and curved, with delicate tips on far left.

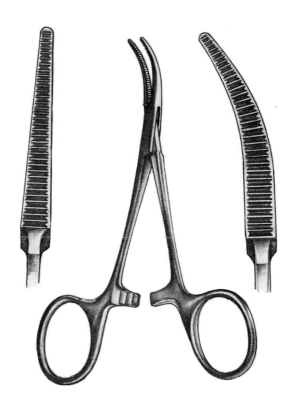

Fig. 7-10. Hartman hemostat straight and curved.

tion, to minimize tissue destruction when stopping bleeding. They may also be used to extract splinters and to remove sutures.

Hemostats (hemostatic forceps)

Occasionally one must clamp off the flow of blood in a vessel and individually place tie sutures securely to stop bleeding. For this purpose there are a number of different hemostats. The Halsted (Fig. 7-9), Hartmann (Fig. 7-10), and Kelly (Fig. 7-11) hemostats are most useful for this purpose in cutaneous surgery. For pinpoint accuracy, the Halsted and Hartmann hemostats are excellent. The Halsted hemostat (5 inch) is also known as the mosquito; the micromosquito is a smaller (4 to 4½ inches) model. I am particularly fond of the Halsted mosquito delicate pattern, both straight and curved. The Hartmann is similar to the Halsted but shorter (4 inches). The Kelly hemostat is broader at the tips and in length (5½ inches). The serrations on the face of the jaws exist only on the distal half rather than the entire surface, as with the Halsted or Hartmann. The Kelly forceps is used to clamp large vessels, for which a strong, secure hold strength is required. For most cutaneous surgery, its use should be discouraged because it tends to crush more tissue than the Halsted hemostat. Other hemostats comparable to the Kelly are the Crile, Lahey, or Providence. All the hemostats mentioned here may be purchased with either straight or curved tips. Both models are useful, although it may be easier under some circumstances to secure a tie under curved tips.

Scissors

There are four basic groups of scissors used in cutaneous surgery: tissue-cutting scissors, undermining scissors, suture-removal scissors, and bandage scissors.

Tissue-cutting scissors. Tissue-cutting scissors are used to cut tissue for excisions and therefore must be kept sharp. For this purpose I prefer the Stevens tenotomy scissors with blunt tips, either straight or curved (Fig. 7-12). The straight scissors provide a more precise straight-line cut than do the curved scissors. These scissors are ideal for most cutaneous surgery because they handle well and may also be useful in undermining. The tips can be ordered blunt, and the

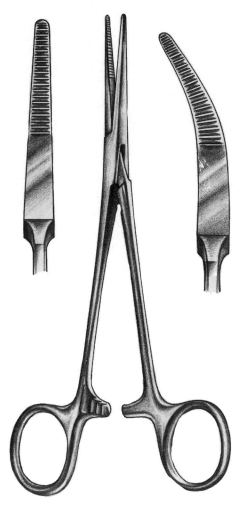

Fig. 7-11. Kelly hemostat, straight and curved.

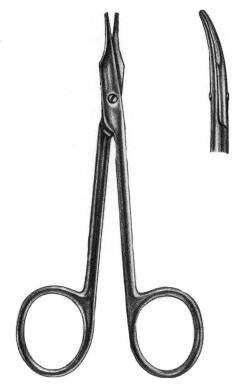

Fig. 7-12. Stevens scissors, straight and curved.

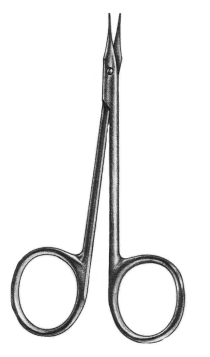

Fig. 7-13. Gradle stitch scissors.

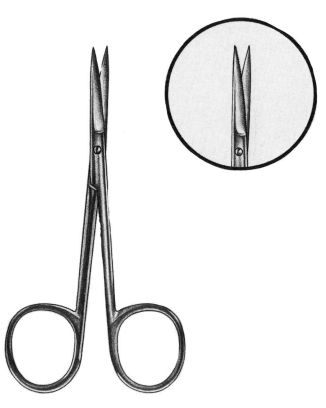

Fig. 7-14. Iris scissors. *Inset,* Serrated blade modification.

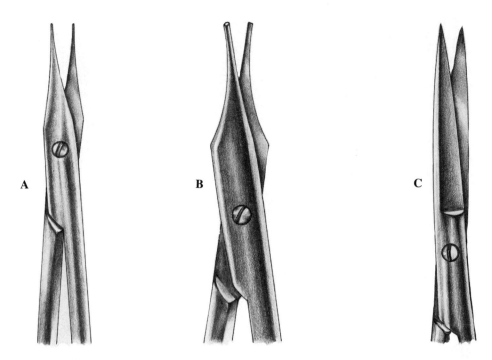

Fig. 7-15. Comparison of screw-to-tip distances (related to fulcrum power) of, **A,** Gradle, **B,** Stevens, and **C,** Iris scissors.

edges are relatively short, giving them greater power in cutting. Gradle stitch scissors (Fig. 7-13) are similar to the Stevens scissors except that the tips are slightly curved, smaller, and sharper; therefore they are not as versatile as the Stevens scissors, but may be useful for very small excisions or suture removal.[34]

The iris scissors, curved or straight (Fig. 7-14), belong to the third type of tissue-cutting scissors. Because the screw is placed relatively far back from the tips, the fulcrum power in cutting tissue is less than with the Gradle or Stevens scissors (Fig. 7-15). The Gradle scissors have by comparison the most fulcrum power for cutting tissue, the Stevens scissors less, and the iris scissors the least of those illustrated. However, the iris scissors may be modified so that serrations are placed along one or both cutting edges (see *inset,* Fig. 7-14). Serrations are useful in keeping tissue from slipping away from the blade,[52] thereby increasing the efficiency of cutting.[73] This is useful, for instance, in snipping off papillomas or acrochordons. Iris scissors may also be ordered with a "diamond" cutting edge (to enhance sharpness) and in a number of different sizes, ranging from 3½ to 4½ inches. The diamond cutting edges are produced by tungsten-carbide inserts, which are harder than stainless steel and thus hold a cutting edge longer. As with all instruments with tungsten-carbide inserts, however, the price is exorbitant for the convenience supposedly afforded by such a modification. The iris scissors labeled as delicate are of most value in cutaneous surgery. The straight 3½-inch very delicate iris scissors are excellent for suture removal.

Another excellent scissors for very fine work is the Castroviejo curved scissors (3½ inches with sharp tips). These have a spring action and are expensive.

Undermining scissors. As already mentioned, the Stevens tenotomy scissors with blunt tips are excellent for delicate undermining, particularly in critical areas on the face. The curved Stevens scissors have a 15- to 20-degree curve in the tips and are perhaps more ideal for undermining than the straight Stevens scissors are. The curve helps the plane of undermining to lie more parallel to the skin surface. However, one needs to make sure that the tips of the scissors are kept parallel to the surface, or they will puncture the overlying skin, especially if it is thin. When more extensive undermining is required for large areas, as in fibrous tissue, a larger instrument may be necessary. The Metzenbaum (Lahey) scissors (Fig. 7-16) is ideally suited for this. The longer shanks and wider, broader tips afford greater power with less effort. Other comparable undermining scissors to consider are the baby Metzenbaum (5 inches, curved, delicate) or the strabismus scissors (4 inches, curved). These scissors also have blunt tips and may be ordered curved or straight. Mayo scissors with wide, blunt tips are in general not useful in cutaneous surgery.

Modifications can be made on undermining scissors. The outer edge may be sharpened or beveled (Kaye fine dissecting scissors[44]) to aid in undermining. However, this has the effect of perhaps needlessly cutting through blood vessels and nerves instead of gently pushing such structures to the side. The blunt dissector of Luikart (Iconoclast) is an ex-

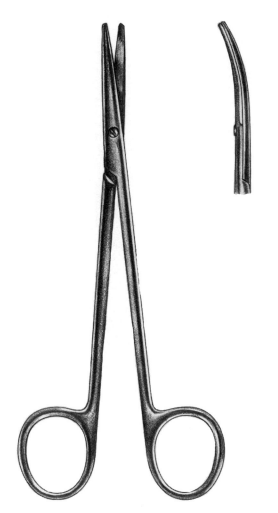

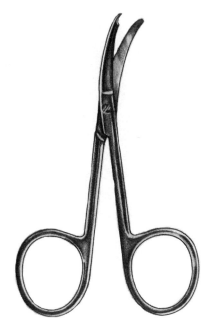

Fig. 7-17. Shortbent suture-removal scissors.

Fig. 7-16. Metzenbaum (Lahey) undermining scissors with curved blades.

ample of an instrument made with this latter principle in mind. This dissecting instrument, recommended by Webster,[91] has long, tapered ends without cutting edges. Another suggested modification of dissecting scissors is to change the angle of the rings of the handle to aid the hand in spreading the tips.[39]

Suture-removal scissors. Specially designed and manufactured scissors for the purpose of removing fine sutures are of great value. The Shortbent scissors (Fig. 7-17) have curved blades with a depression in one blade to grasp the suture loop more easily. The Spencer stitch scissors (3½ inches) is essentially the same scissors but with straight blades. A slightly larger variety with straight blades is the Littauer Junior stitch scissors with delicate blades (4½ inches). I have found that the Shortbent is generally the most adequate. However, with very fine sutures, even these specialized scissors may be too large, causing discomfort for the patient. Best for suture removal, as previously mentioned, are the short (3½ inch) delicate, straight iris scissors with sharp points. The sharp cutting points on these scissors

are smaller than those of the smallest suture-removal scissors. Another use for suture-removal scissors is to cut sutures at the time of surgery. Using them for this purpose prevents needless dulling of other tissue-cutting scissors.

Bandage scissors. The prototype of this type of scissors is the Lister bandage scissors (Fig. 7-18). These are made with angled blades, one of which has a large blunted tip to slip between the bandage and the skin without injuring the skin. The blades are thick for cutting gauze easily. Lister bandage scissors are readily available, either chrome plated or of stainless steel. As previously discussed, the chrome-plated instruments (sometimes called economy grade) should be avoided. Lister bandage scissors come in a variety of sizes; I use the 5½-inch model. A modified bandage scissors known as the Universal bandage and cloth scissors is illustrated in Fig. 7-19. These are heavy-duty scissors with a serrated edge and large ring sizes for greater power. They maintain their sharpness, unlike the Lister bandage scissors, and are capable of cutting metal without their cutting blades becoming significantly dulled. The large, thick, black plastic handles aid in visualizing the instrument on countertops. Their relative inexpensiveness and long-lasting qualities make this instrument a must for every office. The one disadvantage of the Universal scissors is that occasionally small pieces of gauze get caught in the pivot area, but they can be cleaned out.

Dermal curettes

The dermal curette, evolved from uterine curettes, is an instrument used almost exclusively by dermatologists. This instrument was popularized by such dermatologists as

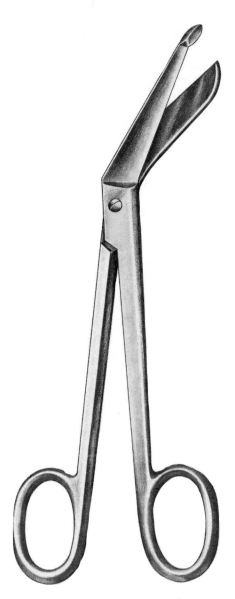

Fig. 7-18. Lister bandage scissors.

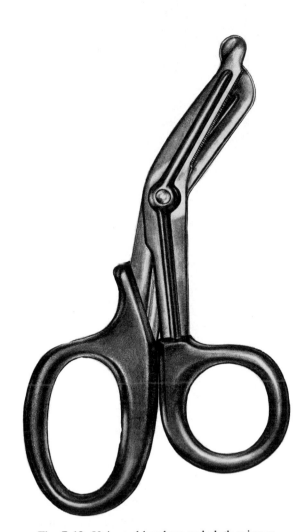

Fig. 7-19. Universal bandage and cloth scissors.

Wigglesworth[93] and initially used on almost any skin affliction. Over the years it has been found to be of extreme value in the treatment of superficial growths on the skin, both benign and malignant. The Fox curette (Fig. 7-20) has a slender handle that easily fits into the hand and a round cutting edge, which may be ordered straight or slightly angled to the handle to aid in scraping. The cutting edge is available in sizes from 1 mm to 7 mm. One should have a number of different sizes available in the office. I have found 3 mm and 4 mm to be the most useful sizes.

Another popular curette is the Piffard type, shown in Fig. 7-21. Compared to the Fox curette the cutting head of this instrument is oval and the handle much broader and heavier. In addition, it is routinely manufactured in only three sizes: small, medium, and large. In my experience this

currette does not handle as easily as the Fox curette does.

Other curettes of importance in cutaneous surgery are the little curettes[54] (Fig. 7-22): the Skeele, the Heath and the Meyhoefer curettes. The Skeele curette has a small, cupped head with little teeth (serrations) along the cutting edge. This is of value in curetting out small cyst walls. It is available in sizes from 0 (1.5 mm) to 2 (2.5 mm). The Heath curette (originally a chalazion curette) is a miniature Fox curette and is available in sizes 0 (0.5 mm), 1 (1 mm), 2 (2 mm), and 3 (3 mm). This is very useful in curetting the small pockets of tumor that the larger Fox or Piffard curette cannot dip into because of their larger size. Another curette well suited for this purpose is the Meyhoefer. This curette is available in sizes ranging from 000 (0.5 mm) to 4 (3.5 mm). The cutting head is cupped like the Skeele but unlike the

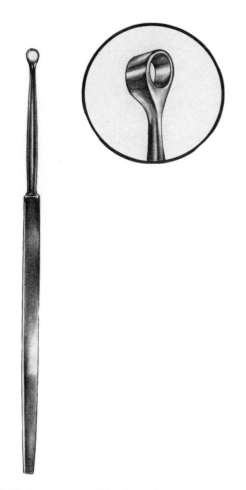

Fig. 7-20. Fox curette, with enlarged view of curette head.

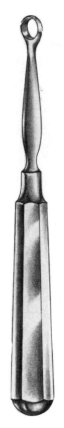

Fig. 7-21. Piffard curette. Note thick handle.

Heath. Therefore theoretically the Meyhoefer may not be as efficacious as the Heath curette in digging out small pockets of tumor because the open head of the Heath allows tissue to escape freely. On the other hand, the barrel-shaped Heath curette cannot get into small pockets of tumors as easily as the cup-shaped Meyhoefer can.

Curettes need to be sharpened; this is best done by the manufacturer. Homemade curettes have been described by Braun[13] and by White,[92] who bent razor blades to produce extrasharp curettes. However, such curettes may tend to dig inadvertently into normal skin and so are not as useful in separating normal from abnormal tissue. Very sharp is not always best.

Comedo expressors

There are many different comedo expressors available. My favorite is the Schamberg expressor (Fig. 7-23). The slightly curved ends make it easier to gain leverage when expressing comedones. The openings on each end allow easy passage of expressed contents and may be wiped clean easily. Other expressors tend to get clogged, mainly because their openings are too small. Moreover, the small ridges in the handle of this instrument aid in giving the operator a sure grasp.

Some comedo expressors are made with a lancet at one end, so that one can use that end to remove the top of the comedo and the other end to express the contents. Such extractors tend to be thrown into sterilizing solutions and used continuously during the day. Such practices should be a thing of the past. If one prefers such an instrument, the Zimmerman-Walton expressor (Fig. 7-24) has the advantage of being able to accept a sterile needle hub at one end.

Skin punch (trephine)

The skin punch is another instrument used almost exclusively by dermatologists. Although this instrument (a trephine) was originally used to cut through bone in the skull, in 1852 it was used successfully to remove an abscess in the

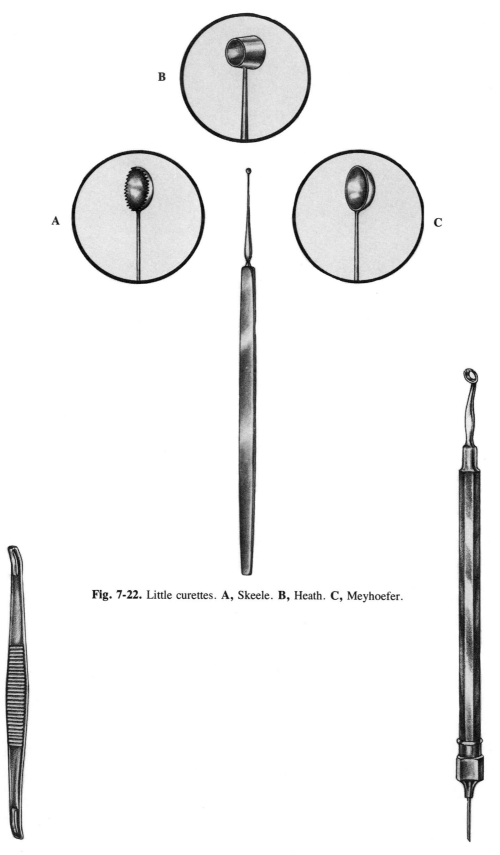

Fig. 7-22. Little curettes. **A,** Skeele. **B,** Heath. **C,** Meyhoefer.

Fig. 7-23. Schamberg comedo expressor.

Fig. 7-24. Zimmerman-Walton comedo expressor.

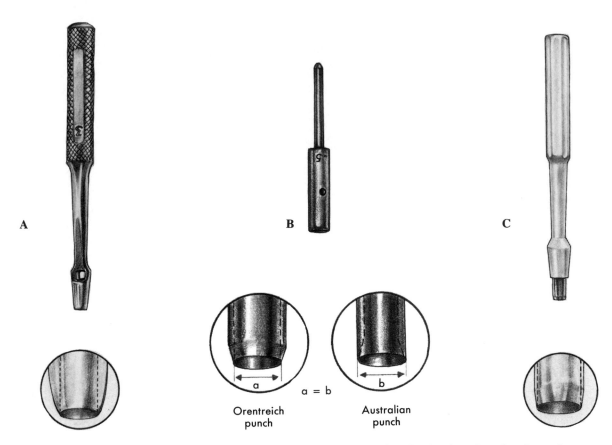

Fig. 7-25. Common cutaneous punches with cross section of cutting head to show locations of bevels. **A,** Keyes punch. **B,** Hair transplant punch with handle for power rotary machine. Orentreich punch has outward-beveled sides and straight inner surface, whereas Australian punch has straight outward sides and beveled inner surface. **C,** Disposable punch.

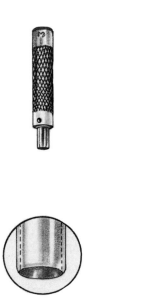

Fig. 7-26. Loo trephine. Note thin walls, compared with those of Keyes punch.

tibia.[85] In 1887 Keyes first reported its use in dermatology to remove tattooed gunpowder burns,[45] although this had been described earlier by Watson[90] in 1878.

The Keyes punch (Fig. 7-25) has been used for almost a century for skin biopsies. The rounded, sharp cutting end and thick handle make it well suited for small biopsies. Because of the thick walls with slanting sides above the cutting edge, tissue tends to be pushed away as the punch is made, causing less dermis to be cut through (in diameter) than overlying epidermis. This is also thought to be a function of the bevel, which is outside the barrel of the Keyes punch.[38] To surmount these difficulties, other punches have been modified.[80] The Loo trephine (Fig. 7-26) is one example in which the walls are thinner and less slanted than those of the Keyes punch, making it advantageous to use on depressed scars or minor autotransplants (where one wants to produce a straight perpendicular incision). This is difficult to do with a Keyes punch. The Keyes punch is routinely available, having sizes in 1 mm increments from 1 to 10 mm. A Keyes dermal punch set that includes a handle with several different size heads may also be purchased; each head

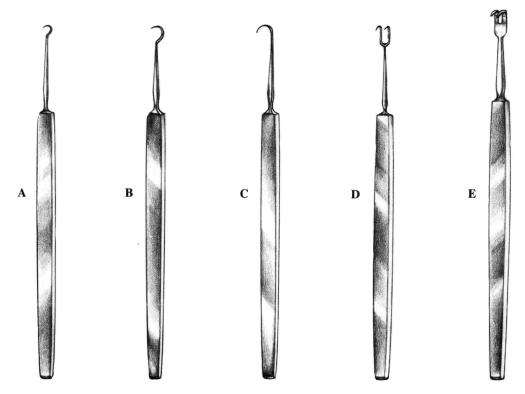

Fig. 7-27. Comparison of various types of skin hooks. Note subtle differences in size and radius of some hooks. **A,** Tyrell (iris). **B,** Frazier. **C,** Skin retractor. **D,** Guthrie. **E,** Double-prong retractor.

may be less expensive to replace than to resharpen. The Loo trephine is available in ½ mm sizes.

The newer disposable punches (Fig. 7-25, *C*) are excellent for punch biopsies or excisional work on cysts. The razor-sharp edge is a great advantage. This punch is made in a number of different sizes. It is not easy to keep many sizes in stock; moreover, a great variety of ½ mm increment sizes are not available, as with the Loo trephine. The specialized skin punches (Orentreich and so on) are discussed in more detail in other chapters.

Skin hooks

The gentle, nontraumatic handling of tissue at the time of excision or reconstructive work is facilitated greatly by the use of skin hooks.[67,68] These are retractors with relatively small heads, which are pictured for comparison in Fig. 7-27. Note that several different sizes (radii) of the hooks are shown. In addition, they may be ordered with heads that are blunt or sharp; single, double, or triple pronged; flexible or inflexible. The type of skin hook used is an individual decision. One should have both blunt and sharp skin hooks available, since there are instances in which each of these is of value (although the sharp skin hook is used more frequently). The single-pronged heads are used more frequently than the double-pronged heads are; however, the double-pronged skin hook allows one to visualize better the depth

of the wound. Double-pronged skin hooks may vary with respect to the space separating the hooks. If one works with a paucity of surgical assistants, one may consider using a weighted skin hook.[31]

Occasionally in emergency rooms or in clinic situations physicians may find themselves without a skin hook. One can easily be fashioned from a needle, hemostat, and cotton-tipped applicator, as described by Strauch[83] and shown in Fig. 7-28. One should use a 22-gauge or larger needle that is bent twice in right angles, as shown. Although this technique has been modified, using a hemostat instead of a cotton-tipped applicator to hold the bent needle,[3,62,81] I do not feel this is wise because it tends to damage a good hemostat. The cotton-tipped applicator is adequate and in my experience is not too wobbly or flexible, as claimed by some.[3] The use of two bent needles with one hemostat to make a double skin hook has been described.[63] Obviously the physicians who accomplished this were not paying for their own instruments.

Skin hooks may be added to the end of the Adson forceps for convenience, but this arrangement becomes inconvenient when one needs an Adson forceps without a skin hook. The ancient Greek arrangement—two instruments, one on each end of a handle—and other instrument combinations (see illustration on p. 179) did not survive the Middle Ages with good reason.

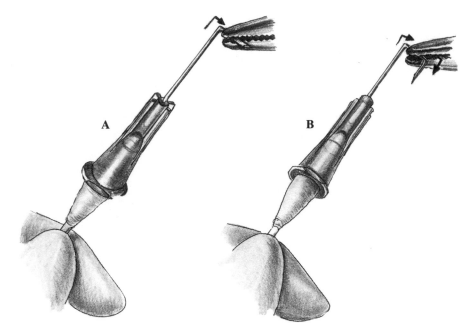

Fig. 7-28. Illustration of method to make skin hook under emergency situation. **A,** Grasping needle with hemostat and bending at right angle. **B,** Second right angle bend is made. Alternatively, one can make more rounded skin hook.

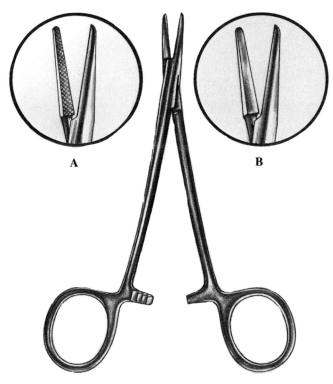

Fig. 7-29. Webster needle holder with smooth jaws. **A,** Diamond jaws. **B,** Smooth jaws.

Needle holders

The ideal needle holder for most cutaneous surgery is the Webster needle holder with smooth jaws (Fig. 7-29). The size (4½ inches) and tapered tips make it easy to use, especially with small suture and needle sizes. If purchased without special options (tungsten-carbide inserts and gold handles), this instrument is a bargain. The superhard tungsten-carbide inserts are placed in the jaws for greater strength and stability when holding the needle. My experience is that with time these inserts chip, and when they do, the instrument has a difficult time grasping even a suture. Although the manufacturer will replace the inserts, this is an inconvenience. The expense involved does not justify purchase of an instrument with these inserts.

Needle holders can also be purchased with cross striations in the tips for a more secure grasp on suture or needle. This feature is usually unnecessary and even undesirable, since it tends to enhance fraying of some types of suture (catgut or braided suture). If one is suturing with wire, cross striations may be necessary.

Other needle holders are made in combination with scissors, such as the Olsen-Hegar. Unfortunately, one may inadvertently cut a suture with the scissors, so I do not recommend such instruments. Other modifications in needle holders, such as bent finger rings,[61] are probably unnecessary.

For very fine suturing with small, delicate needles, some physicians prefer the Castroviejo needle holder (Fig. 7-30). This needle holder has very small tips, which are unlikely to bend small needles. In addition, it opens with a spring action, a feature that is helpful if many small sutures are to

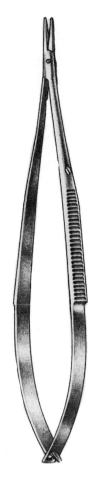

Fig. 7-30. Castroviejo needle holder without catch.

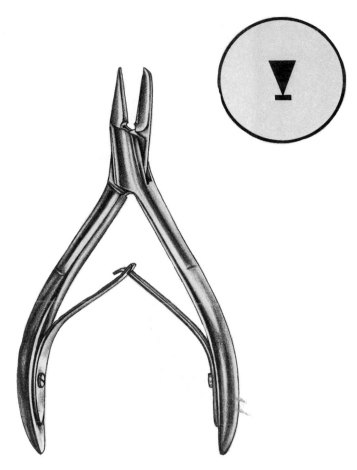

Fig. 7-31. Nail splitter, with diagram of cross-section through tip.

be placed. This needle holder also may be ordered with or without a catch, which takes practice to operate. The Castroviejo needle holder is held like a pencil and rotated on its axis by the thumb and index finger.

Nail splitter

The nail splitter is a very versatile instrument when removing nails (Fig. 7-31). One cutting edge is flat and tapered to fit easily underneath the nail without injury to the nailbed, while the other edge is thicker and curved, thereby slipping easily underneath the posterior nail fold. Its spring action and fulcrum design allow it to cut through the thickest of nails with ease. This instrument makes other nail instruments obsolete, and no dermatology office should be without one.

Chalazion clamp

Occasionally when working around the eyelids, nose, or lips, one desires hemostasis with a firm, immobilized, and sheltered surface on which to work. The chalazion clamp can be a great help in this regard.[7] The Desmarres chalazion clamp is shown in Fig. 7-32. The solid surface on

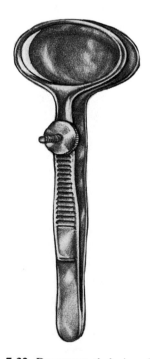

Fig. 7-32. Desmarres chalazion clamp.

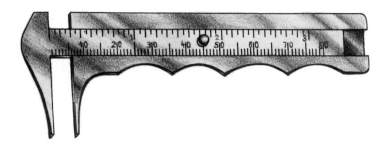

Fig. 7-33. Jameson caliper.

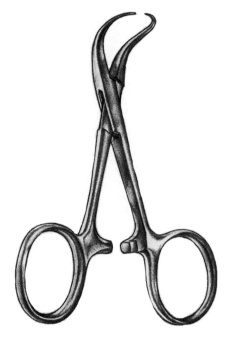

Fig. 7-34. Backhaus towel forceps.

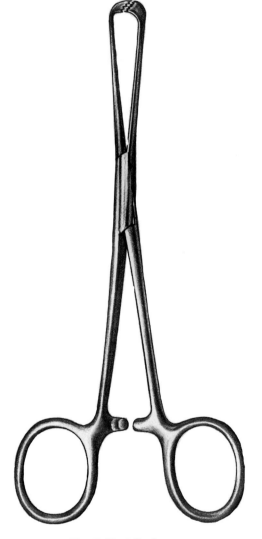

Fig. 7-35. Allis forceps.

should the insulation become defective, the patient could develop an unnecessary burn. Therefore I avoid using the insulated models. Many other types of chalazion clamps (forceps) are available with rounded instead of oval rings, but they are in general less useful in cutaneous surgery.

Caliper

For fine reconstructive surgery, a caliper is necessary. Although I have used crude methods of measurement in the past, my results have been much improved by the use of a caliper. The Jameson caliper (Fig. 7-33) is ideal because its centimeter scale is longer than that of most other calipers. The tips help to measure distance more accurately than do rulers, which are more subjective.

Towel clips

When draping a patient for skin surgery, sterile towels with towel clips (or forceps) are used. The Backhaus towel forceps (Fig. 7-34) is ideally suited for this purpose. Other, smaller towel clips are made but are of limited use on larger cases. Also, the ratchet of the Backhaus forceps holds the towels more securely.

Allis forceps

Occasionally when removing cysts or lipomas it is convenient to have a good grasping forceps. The Allis forceps (Fig. 7-35) is ideal for this purpose. The delicate model with 4 by 5 teeth is most useful.

one side and ring on the other side provides hemostasis when screwed tight. Traction is also easily obtained should it be desirable. The Desmarres clamp is made in three sizes: small (20 mm), medium (26 mm), and large (31 mm). These clamps may be specially insulated so that one may electrocoagulate without conducting a current; however,

Sponge forceps

When additional gauze is required at the time of surgery, it can be transferred by sponge forceps kept in disinfectant solution in a forceps jar. The Foerster sponge forceps is well suited for this purpose.

CARE OF INSTRUMENTS

To ensure a long lifetime and good function for one's instruments, special handling and care are essential. Instruments are expensive and if well cared for will last many years. Although office or hospital personnel are charged with the cleaning, wrapping, and storage of instruments, it is important for surgeons to understand the dangers and advantages of various methods, so that they can make suitable recommendations for the care of their instruments.

Cleaning

A special area should be designated for the cleaning and sterilization of surgical instruments and designed to minimize exposure of patients to infection. Ideally this area should be situated so that the instruments move from dirty to clean to sterile zones. Before being transferred to the cleaning area, many instruments are lost, so personnel should be alert to stray instruments in the trash and laundry baskets or on the floor.[2]

As soon as possible after use, instruments should be thoroughly rinsed with cold water to remove surgical debris before it hardens by drying.[58] Instruments are then soaked in a detergent solution with warm water. This is followed by vigorous and thorough cleaning with a brush, a hot water rinse, and drying (Fig. 7-36).

The most important step in sterilization or disinfection is a thorough physical hand-cleaning of all instruments. Besides removing infectious material, thorough cleaning prevents corrosion and results in smoothly working instruments. It has been established that the greater the number of organisms exist on an instrument, the greater the length of time is necessary to destroy them.[78] In addition, organisms may survive under oil films in autoclaves.[25] The sterilization process cannot be considered a substitute for adequate manual cleaning. We recommend a handbrush, such as a denture brush, with fairly stiff nylon bristles.

The personnel cleaning the instruments should wear gloves for protection. The uninformed person does not appreciate the potential hazards associated with the cleaning of instruments. In a study by Darmady et al.[24] recently used surgical instruments were cultured before cleaning. Pathogenic organisms were found on 9.5% of instruments. An infinitesimal amount of serum (0.0004 ml) is enough to spread hepatitis virus through an inadvertent cut.[26,33]

Some instruments, such as forceps or needle holders, are intrinsically difficult to clean, so greater attention should be paid to them, particularly to crevices such as box locks and ridges in the tips. Sharp instruments or those with delicate tips are more easily damaged than others, so greater care should be exercised in handling them.

Cleaning is affected by the kind of surface being cleaned, nature and amount of "dirt," composition and concentration of the detergent, time of exposure to the cleaning agent, hardness of the water, pH of the cleaning solution, mechanical factor of scrubbing, and heat (which enhances separation of debris).[64] Selection of a detergent for cleaning instruments is best left to the manufacturer, who should be consulted. Surgical instruments are delicate, easily damaged, and susceptible to corrosion. Obviously one should choose a detergent that cleans most effectively while least damaging the instrument. Perkins[64] recommends low-sudsing, moderately alkaline detergents, such as Edisonite (Colgate Palmolive Co., New York). Super Edisonite contains phosphates and an anionic detergent, which on dissolving in water yield a solution with a pH of about 8. Tiemann and Co. recommends Nutra-pH (Parke, Davis and Co.), which has a neutral pH and no phosphates. Harsh detergents with a very low or high pH should be avoided. The detergent lowers the surface tension of water, which allows intimate contact between water and the instrument and which also solubilizes proteins and greases, suspending particles in solution. Besides wetting agents, detergents for instruments have sequestering or chelating agents (for example, sodium metaphosphate) to prevent precipitation of hard water salts and corrosion inhibitors. In addition, most holding solutions have bacteriostatic agents, which offer some protection to the personnel. Such disinfectants may increase or decrease the effectiveness of the detergent solutions, depending on whether the lowered surface tension allows for a greater or lesser contact of the disinfectant with the bacterial cell wall or instrument being cleaned.[69]

Some authorities feel that washing instruments by hand is always inadequate because surgical contaminants are frequently lodged in inaccessible areas in some instruments. The ultrasonic cleaner is thought to be advantageous in such instances because it cleans in areas that are difficult to reach even by bristles of a brush. Ultrasonic cleaners are metallic tanks in which the instruments are placed in a cleaning solution. By means of a transducer, vibrations of discrete frequencies are produced, usually 20,600 to 38,000 vibrations per second (kc). These frequencies are well above the level perceivable by the human ear. The sound waves compress or rarify the medium through which they pass.

The effect of such sound waves on liquid medium is to produce minute bubbles. These tiny pockets of air, ranging in size from submicroscopic to very large, expand and then violently collapse (implode) because of hydrostatic pressure, generating temperature and pressure vacuums, a process known as cavitation. This process is thought to be responsible for cleaning (Fig. 7-37). The forces that occur at the time of implosion dislodge adherent soil on instru-

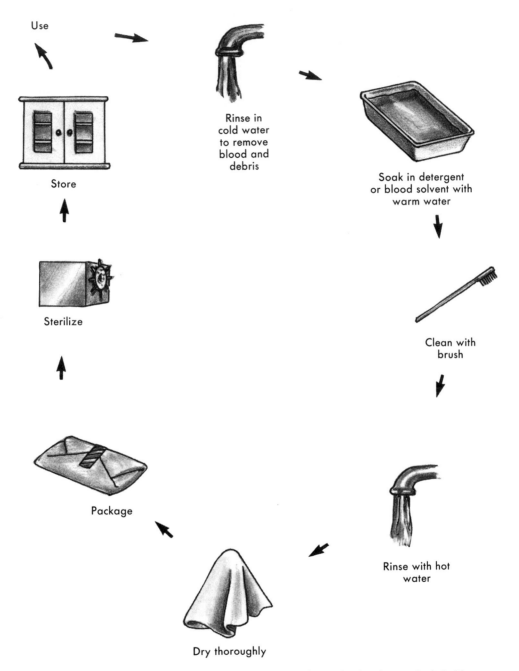

Fig. 7-36. Steps in instrument cleaning and sterilization. Ultrasonic cleaning not included but may be done after cleaning with brush.

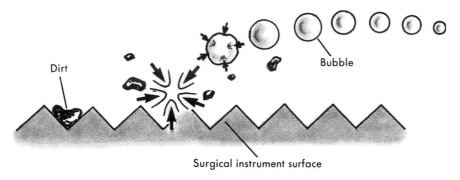

Fig. 7-37. Cavitation induced by sonic energy in ultrasonic machine.

ments. It is also thought that the shearing motion associated with bubble-induced eddying may play a role in ultrasonic cleaning.[42] Larger dense particles fall to the bottom of the tank, whereas other, soluble particles go into the solution. Nevertheless, some particulate matter may still remain on the instruments, although loosened, and must be washed off.

Other authorities state that ultrasonic cleaning of instruments is inadequate,[24,81] especially for tubular instruments.[58] Perkins,[64] on the other hand, states that when ultrasonics do not work, the personnel or equipment are at fault. It is his opinion that the quality of the cleaning by ultrasonics is vastly superior to hand cleaning alone. It is important when using ultrasonic cleaning that all instruments be opened wide for maximal exposure to and benefit from the ultrasonically generated forces.

Ultrasonic cleaning may be advantageous because of speed and completeness. An added advantage sometimes stated is that there is a decreased chance of injury and exposure of personnel to hepatitis.[75] However, no one knows the extent of hepatitis virus inactivation by this process. On the other hand, cavitation damages the cell walls of bacteria[42] and may cause increased sensitivity of pathogens to disinfectants.[86]

The main disadvantage of ultrasonic cleaning is the aerosolization that inevitably takes place.[86] As implosion occurs near the air-liquid interface, an aerosol is produced, which may be a source of contamination. For instance, ultrasonic cleaning solutions can be contaminated with *Pseudomonas* species; therefore the cover should always be on the tank. In addition, the ultrasonic detergents should be changed daily. Contaminated aerosols are a problem when ultrasonic tanks are used, and it is difficult to eliminate contamination of the surrounding work area. Ultrasonic cleaning may also promote the flaking of chrome on instruments, if corrosion has begun at the interface between the chrome plate and the parent metal. Furthermore, if different types of metals are mixed in an ultrasonic solution, galvanic currents may be established, and electroplating may occur.

Lubrication

Instruments with moving parts need lubrication. Lubrication with oil is inadvisable if steam sterilization is performed, since bacterial spores are much more heat resistant in anhydrous oil or fat.[71] The oil film acts as a protective barrier to organisms underneath the film, preventing moisture from contact with the instrument surfaces. However, should lubrication with oil be necessary, sterilization with dry heat is effective.

Silicone oil compounds do not interfere with steam sterilization and may be used to lubricate instruments. Also, oil-in-water emulsions (e.g., Nutra pH Instruments-Milk from Parke-Davis & Co., Deseret Division, N. Hollywood, Calif. 91605) are available, which precoat the instruments before sterilization. Such lubricating solutions may contain, in addition to nonsilicone lubrications, ingredients said to be antimicrobial and anticorrosive. The coating is steam permeable. Such solutions are excellent for preventing corrosion of low-speed handpieces before steam sterilization.[16]

Occasionally instruments are stiff at the joints. This is probably caused by accumulated debris, which can be relieved by placing a small amount of lapping compound (Grit No. 180 [water soluble], Clover Manufacturing Co., Norwalk, Conn.) into the joint and working it in by opening and closing the instrument.

Packing

Before being placed in the sterilizer, instruments are usually packed, either in paper or cloth. It is important that the instruments be left in the open position when packaged to allow for complete sterilization and to prevent damage from heat expansion, such as sprung hinges. It may be advantageous to package instruments as a group—for example, as an excision set. Each physician should list the instruments he or she finds necessary in an attempt to standardize basic sets and constantly update the list to minimize their nonavailability. Instrument sets are best wrapped in a double layer of muslin cloth (cotton). The pack should be assembled to allow penetration of steam throughout the contents to ensure complete sterilization and drying in the auto-clave. Autoclave tape (OK Indicator Tape) should be placed around the pack.

An alternative to surgical packs is an instrument tray, such as the Aesculap Container system.[70] This is an aluminum container into which mesh instrument trays are placed. This container saves wrapping instruments either individually or as a group and may thus be cost effective. However, as with surgical packs, many instruments are stored together and may thus be inaccessible.

Instruments may be wrapped in coarse brown paper (30- to 40-pound Dennison or Kraft-type paper), crepe paper, paper instrument packaging, or muslin. Paper passes steam freely but not as readily as muslin. Although paper is relatively inexpensive, it is noisy and subject to contamination through inadvertent rupture in handling. In addition, when unwrapped it does not fall away as easily as cloth because of its higher intrinsic memory. Standard muslin is plain woven cotton and if of good quality is 140 thread count (68 warp, 72 woof). Double layers of standard muslin or paper should be used to wrap instruments, or other materials, so bacterial penetration will be less with storage[79] and contamination will be minimized when unwrapping.[30] A higher-grade muslin is also available, with a thread count of 288; it therefore has twice as many threads per square inch as standard muslin. The higher-grade cloth may be adequate as a single layer of wrapping for instruments, in contrast to the double layer necessary with standard muslin.

My preference is to package individually and label most instruments in all-paper instrument containers (sterilizer bags), such as Protexmor (Order No. 111, Central States Diversified, Inc., St. Louis). These bags are relatively small, handy, and easy to store and open. Other instrument bags (for example, Surgipeel, Surgicot, Inc., Smithtown, N.Y.) are available with plastic on one side and paper on the other. However, these are larger, crinkle easily, and are difficult to open. Their supposed advantage is that one may easily visualize the instrument in the bag, and therefore labeling the contents is unnecessary (saves nursing time). In addition, the peel-back opening mechanism is less likely to contaminate instruments than all-paper packing bags are when opening the sealed end because dust is less likely to settle on the contents.[30] All-plastic bags do not allow adequate steam sterilization.[29]

DISINFECTION AND STERILIZATION

In a modern office or clinic in which cutaneous surgery is performed, sterile instruments and supplies should be used. Infection control is just as important in such an environment as it is in hospital operating rooms. To provide the best possible patient care and to achieve excellent surgical results, the high standards of surgical sterility should be met. Aseptic technique can be achieved only with properly sterilized equipment and good technique.

The idea of sterilization as a means of eliminating bacteria or other organisms in surgery goes back over 100 years. Pasteur, who was not a physician, stated in his lecture on germ theory to the French Academy of Medicine:

> If I had the honor of being a surgeon, convinced as I am of the dangers caused by the germs of microbes scattered on the surface of every object, particularly in hospitals, not only would I use absolutely clean instruments, but, after cleansing my hands with the greatest care and putting them quickly through a flame (an easy thing to do with a little practice), I would only make use of charpie, bandages, and sponges which had been previously raised to a heat of 130° C to 150° C; I would employ water which had been heated to a temperature of 110° C to 120° C. All that is easy in practice, and, in that way, I should still have to fear the germs suspended in the atmosphere surrounding the bed of the patient, but observation shows us every day that the number of these germs is almost insignificant compared to that of those which lie scattered in the surface of objects, or in the clearest ordinary water.[87]

Sterilization is defined as the process of destroying completely all forms of microbial life—bacteria, fungi, and viruses. *Disinfection,* on the other hand, is a process of destroying infectious agents but not necessarily bacterial spores, tubercle bacilli, or hepatitis virus. Usually disinfection is performed by exposing inanimate objects to chemicals (chemical disinfection). When disinfectants are applied to living tissue to destroy microorganisms, such chemicals are *antiseptics. Germicides* are chemicals applied to either living tissue or to inanimate objects that kill microbes but, like disinfectants, not necessarily bacterial spores. *Sanitization* is the process of reducing to safe levels (25 organisms per square inch) bacteria on utensils or other materials handled by patients. Comparison of the varous methods of disinfection and sterilization is outlined in Table 7-1.

Boiling water

The techniques available to disinfect instruments include exposure to boiling water or chemicals. The preoperative boiling of instruments is not recommended except in an emergency. This is because boiling water does not kill spores even with prolonged exposure.[25] The highest temperature possible to obtain in boiling water is 212° F (100° C) at sea level in an open container. The minimal exposure period at this temperature should be 30 minutes if this method must be used. As recommended by Schimmelbush,[72] sodium carbonate may be added to the water to increase the bactericidal efficiency. As an added benefit, this alkali decreases the corrosive action of water on instruments.

It is interesting to note that Krugman reported in 1960 inactivation of hepatitis virus by heating diluted hepatitis B serum at 98° C for 1 minute.[53] However, more recently (in 1979) the same author reported that a similar heating did not totally inactivate the virus and resulted in

TABLE 7-1

Comparison of methods for disinfection and sterilization of instruments

	Organisms killed	Temperature	Pressure	Time required	Instrument dulling	Comments
Boiling water	Not spores; all others	100° C	Atmospheric	30 minutes	Maximal	Use only in emergency
Chemical disinfection ("cold sterilization")	Possibly not hepatitis; all others	Room	Atmospheric	15 minutes	None	Promotes instrument corrosion
Dry heat sterilization	All	121° C	Atmospheric	1-12 hours	Minimal	No good for paper, cloth, rubber
Steam autoclave	All	121° C	15 psi*	30-45 minutes	Maximal	Might sterilize liquids
Unsaturated chemical vapor sterilization	All	132° C	20 psi*	30 minutes	Moderate	Might not sterilize liquids
Gas sterilization (ethylene oxide)	All	55°-60° C	Atmospheric	1-8 hours	Minimal	Not readily available, expensive, requires aeration of 6-30 hours; mutagenic

*psi, Pounds per square inch

subclinical hepatitis infection in 3 of 29 recipients of the heated serum.[53]

Chemical disinfection

A number of disinfectants are available for disinfection of instruments and include quaternary ammonium compounds (quats), chlorine compounds, iodine and iodophor solutions, alcohols, phenols, formaldehyde, and glutaraldehyde. These agents are thought to act on different sites on microorganisms and result in cell death. The mechanism of action on cells includes coagulation of protein (formaldehyde), lysis of cell walls (quats), oxidation of essential enzymes (iodines), or a combination of the foregoing bacteriologic actions (phenols). In addition, some disinfectants kill viruses by denaturation of proteins.[64] The term "cold sterilization" is sometimes applied to the use of these disinfectants on instruments but is a misnomer. *Cold disinfection* is a more appropriate term.[77]

Glutaraldehyde is perhaps the most commonly used and recommended chemical disinfectant for instruments. This is chemically related to formaldehyde but does not have its offensive odor. A 2% aqueous alkaline concentration (Cidex) is equivalent to 8% formaldehyde in ethyl alcohol (Bard-Parker Germicide). Glutaraldehyde must be buffered to an alkaline pH for activation and greatest effectiveness.[56] Glutaraldehyde solutions kill vegetative bacteria and fungi within 15 minutes, spores are destroyed in 3 hours, and tubercule bacilli in a few minutes. Carbon steel instruments are corroded in these solutions after a 24-hour exposure, and some instruments may show a slight tarnish after many immersions; however, this may be caused by scratches or poor plating rather than the solution itself.[12] To prevent rusting of instruments, 0.2% sodium nitrate should be added to these solutions.

In a study by O'Brien et al.[60] using Cidex for urologic instruments, it was recommended that instruments be allowed to soak for 20 minutes between procedures. This was based on the fact that the RNA viruses (Coxsackie virus B1 and Poliomyelitis type 3) are inactivated in this solution in 20 minutes, whereas the DNA viruses (herpes simplex and adenovirus) require only 5 minutes of exposure. Cidex can be used for 2 weeks unless grossly contaminated. However, as pointed out by these authors but little emphasized elsewhere, sterile water (not tap water) should be used to rinse the instruments after soaking in chemical disinfectants.

Cidex may be purchased in a special formulation with a longer life of 28 days (Cidex Formula 7). This may be useful when use is sporadic and cost effectiveness a prime consideration.[56] In addition, acid-potentiated glutaraldehyde solutions are available for ultrasonic machines (Sonicide). It is felt that such acid-potentiated solutions act synergistically with ultrasonic energy to inactivate microbes.[12]

The quaternary ammonium compounds are chemical disinfectants of another very commonly used category. Benzalkonium chloride is the prototype of this class and is commonly available as Cetylcide solution. Although effective against gram-positive and gram-negative bacteria and some fungi, it is ineffective against spore-forming bacteria, *Pseudomonas aeruginosa, Mycobacterium tuberculosis,* and some viruses.[75] Moreover, sterilizing solutions with chloride ions are inherently corrosive[82] (Fig. 7-39) and may themselves harbor pathogenic bacteria.

All methods of instrument decontamination include a thorough cleaning. This is particularly important if disinfectants are subsequently used, since blood and tissue absorb germicidal molecules and inactivate them. Organic soil may also protect organisms from the action of disinfectants. It has also been established that the absolute number of organisms an inanimate object contains determines the length of time a germicide takes to destroy them.[78] Disinfection time is thus proportional to the number of organisms and quantity of surgical soil but inversely proportional to the concentration of the disinfectant. In addition, one may also decrease the disinfection time by increasing the temperature of the solution.[64]

The most problematic aspect of using chemical disinfectants is their unproven ability to inactivate hepatitis virus. In 1956 Foley and Gutheim documented the high incidence (68%) of exposure to injections in a dentist's office among cases of serum hepatitis.[33] They implied that such infections were associated with chemical disinfection of syringes and needles, a practice at that time. Even more alarming is the fact that the viral agent causing scrapie survives 10% formalin for one year.[43]

A relatively new device (Ster-O-Lizer MD-200, from the Ster-O-Lizer Manufacturing Corp., 375 W. 400 North, Salt Lake City 84103) for chemical sterilization uses chlorine and oxygen and their free radicals, liberated electrolytically in a salt solution. This method, however, is of unproven value and still has the disadvantage of requiring a rinsing of the ''sterile'' instruments after removal from the sterilizing solution.

Dry heat sterilization

A more effective but time-consuming method of sterilization is by means of dry heat. Basically this is performed in an oven type of apparatus. Perkins[64] recommends a temperature of 320° F (160° C) for 60 minutes for sharp instruments, assuming that they are free from grease and oil and placed on a metal tray in the dry heat sterilizer to enhance the rate of heating through the heat-conducting properties of the metal. It is important to note that the recommended temperature is that of the heated instrument or material and not of the sterilizing oven. Darmady et al.[23] studied the heating time of various instruments and concluded that with conduction of heat, different instruments took different lengths of time to heat to 180° C—for example, scissors in 23 minutes compared to a scalpel in 19 minutes. In addition, if one started from a cold oven temperature, it took 38 minutes to heat the scissors to the same temperature.

Although the presumed advantage of dry heat sterilization is less damage to sharp cutting edges of instruments, the prolonged heating time necessary for sterilization may cause other problems. The temper (hardness) of instruments may be lost, and solder joints may melt. Furthermore, if the instruments are not absolutely dry, rust or corrosion may still occur. The surrounding temperature of the office environment will also be raised, sometimes to an uncomfortable level.

Dry heat heats objects by conduction, penetrating slowly and unevenly. The exterior of objects is heated first and then the interior. Moisture is absent in dry heat; this is advantageous for instruments with sharp cutting edges since dry heat tends not to corrode such surfaces, as the moist heat steam does. Some substances are best sterilized in dry heat, such as oils and greases. Other substances—such as fabrics and rubber—are destroyed by dry heat. The time it takes dry heat to heat different materials to sterilization varies with the conductive properties of each material. Therefore the time required for adequate sterilization is more variable and less easily controlled than with steam sterilization.

Bacteria are destroyed in dry heat by oxidation or a slow burning-up process,[8] unlike steam sterilization, which kills microorganisms by coagulation of proteins. One of the most heat-resistant spores, *Bacillus stearothermophilus,* survives dry heat of 250° F (121° C) for 2 hours but is destroyed at 320° F (160° C) in 1 hour.[64] Spores in anhydrous oil may take much longer (160 minutes at 320° F [160° C]).[71]

Some autoclaves can be used as hot air sterilizers without moisture. However, this may not be efficient at a temperature of 250° to 254° F (121° to 123° C), which calls for 6 hours of exposure for safe sterilization. In addition, the temperature gauge of the sterilizer is usually placed to measure the temperature of the chamber discharge line and not the chamber temperature. These two temperatures vary.

The following are time-temperature recommendations[64] for dry heat sterilization:

350° F (180° C)	30 minutes
340° F (170° C)	1 hour
320° F (160° C)	2 hours
300° F (150° C)	2½ hours
285° F (140° C)	3 hours
250° F (121° C)	6 hours (preferably overnight)

These times are based on the temperature of the load and not on the temperature of the chamber. No adjustments have been made for warm-up time. These recommendations are based on thermal death time of spores in garden soil, rarely found on surgical instruments. When *Clostridium tetani* is used as the test spore, less time is required for adequate killing.[22] Instrument exposure for less time at very hot temperatures may result in less injury to cutting edges.

Steam sterilization

The steam-pressure autoclave is the most frequently used apparatus for sterilization by dermatologic surgeons in their offices. This apparatus provides excellent sterilization within a reasonable period of time and at an economical price.

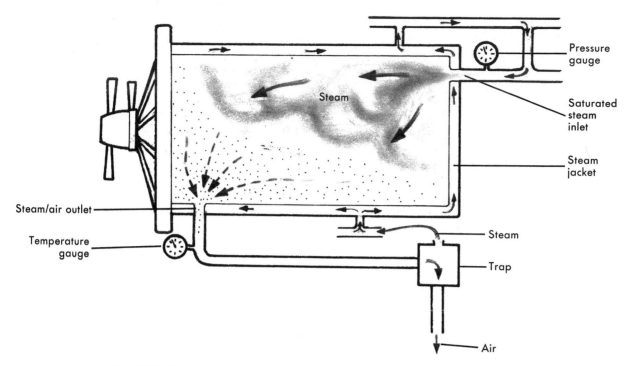

Fig. 7-38. Steam sterilizer. Trap passes air-steam mixture and retains pure steam.

The first pressure steam sterilizer was developed in 1880 by Charles Chamberland, a pupil of Pasteur. It resembled a modern pressure cooker, with a cover held in place by toggle bolts, and was able to obtain a temperature of 248° F (120° C). Until the 1930s autoclaves worked on the basis of pressure within the chamber rather than temperature. Since that time, temperature has been used as a guide to adequate sterilization. The term *autoclave* is synonymous with pressure steam sterilizer and literally means "self-closing," as in the case of a vessel closed by pressure of steam against the door or lid.

The basic design of a modern autoclave is shown in Fig. 7-38. Because of the pressure built up in the chamber, the door of the sterilizer has radial locking bars for safety. Distilled water is heated by means of a steam-producing heating coil. The heated water and steam help to heat the walls of the chamber. Some sterilizers are fitted with a complete steam jacket. Steam is first made to circulate in this jacket before entering the chamber. A steam jacket is more efficient in heating the walls of the chamber, drying sterilized items faster and also promoting superheated steam during sterilization.[9] When the surface of the chamber has acquired the temperature of the steam, steam is allowed into the chamber. The steam immediately moves upward because it is hotter and lighter than the cooler air. Eventually this steam heats the door of the chamber and forces air in the chamber out the bottom. This air is eliminated through a thermostatic trap, which closes when pure steam instead of air flows through it, recycling the steam into the chamber.

The thermometer is strategically located at the coolest portion of the chamber near or in the steam-discharge line. The pressure in the chamber is usually calibrated as a function of the temperature; as long as the temperature of the chamber is accurate, the pressure takes care of itself. Incidentally, the pressure gauge is set to read at 14.7 pounds/square inch above atmospheric pressure (that is, 0 on the gauge means 14.7 psi (pounds/square inch) or 1 atmosphere of pressure).

Besides the temperature control the timer is the other control to regulate on most sterilizers. Recommendations from each sterilizer manufacturer should be consulted regarding specifications for timing different loads. The size of the chamber may be of importance, particularly if one is sterilizing surgical packs, and should be considered before purchase of a steam sterilizer. I recommend a chamber diameter of at least 9 or 10 inches.

Steam sterilizers (autoclaves), like all mechanical devices, are subject to failure. Unfortunately, if this occurs, the temperature or pressure gauges may not reflect the malfunction.[41] Longer life of sterilizers is promoted by careful cleaning of the chamber and flushing of drainage lines. Because the same distilled water is reused several times and steam is recycled through the same pressure lines, additional exposure to surgical debris and corrosive chemicals is possible. Instructions from the manufacturer should be consulted. It is important to use distilled water in autoclaves because regular tap water contains more minerals, which corrode not only the autoclave but the instruments.

The early researchers in microbiology, in particular Koch and co-workers,[50,51] discovered that bacteria are more susceptible to moist heat than to dry hot air. Bacteria were destroyed at lower temperatures and in shorter periods of time when moisture was present.[71] The cause is thought to be the fact that cell death is based on coagulation of proteins, a phenomenon catalyzed by water. Pressure has little effect on sterilization; moist heat is what kills microbes.

It has been hypothesized that destruction of microbes in steam heat occurs by denaturation and coagulation of a critical protein site within the genetic structure of the cell.[27] Proteins are known to be more susceptible to heat coagulation in the presence of water than without it.[5] In the classic studies of Chick,[17,18] heat coagulation of proteins is shown to be caused by a reaction between water and the protein, a process deduced to be similar to the destruction of bacteria in the presence of water. The lack of water in spores may be a mechanism to protect bacteria from killing by moist heat.

The killing of microorganisms by disinfectants or sterilizers occurs gradually. There is no temperature at which all bacteria are killed instantaneously; the killing is at a rate proportional to the temperature but inversely related to time. Therefore if one increases the time of exposure to heat, the temperature may be lowered, or if one decreases the time, the temperature should be increased. At a given temperature, cell death rate (K) can be expressed as follows:

$$K = \frac{1}{t} \log 10 \frac{No}{Nt}$$

No is the initial number of organisms, *Nt* the surviving number of organisms, and *t* the time of exposure. The formula is important to understand because it implies two important concepts relative to sterilization. First, since bacterial cell death is a logarithmic function (that is a certain *percentage* of cells die each minute), complete sterilization (total absence of microorganisms) is never obtained, at least theoretically. Second, if more organisms contaminate an instrument, a longer period of time may be necessary to kill effectively the microbes and "sterilize" the instrument. This is because cell death rate at a given temperature is fixed but a function of time. Therefore, as mentioned earlier, careful removal of surgical debris (with microorganisms) by careful mechanical washing is essential to ensure efficient sterilization.

The standards for sterilization of surgical instruments or supplies are based on the killing of microorganisms in garden soil, which contains a variety of heat-resistant, aerobic and anaerobic, spore- and non–spore-bearing organisms. For instance, in a study done by Bang and Dalsgaard in 1948,[4] garden soil was autoclaved at 248° F (120° C). When heated for 20 minutes, effective sterilization took place, but when heated for 10 minutes, 200,000 organisms per gram of soil remained. The concept of using garden soil as a standard for sterilization could be challenged because garden soil rarely contaminates surgical instruments. In addition, none of the pathogenic organisms in humans have been shown to be resistant to 3 minutes of exposure to 250° F (121° C).

Viruses appear to be about as susceptible to heat as vegetative bacteria are and not nearly as resistant as spore-forming organisms. Although variations do exist, moist heat at 131° to 140° F (55° to 60° C) for 30 minutes is fatal for most viruses. Herpes is one of the most thermolabile viruses. Dry heat is not as effective as moist heat in the destruction of viruses. It is recommended that instruments potentially contaminated with the AIDS virus (HTLV-III) be washed and steam-sterilized for at least 10 minutes. For instruments used in patients with Jakob-Creutzfeldt disease, sodium hypochlorite cleaning is advisable, followed by steam-sterilization for 1 hour.

Hepatitis virus, especially hepatitis B virus, is difficult to study with respect to destruction by sterilization because of the lack of cell culture techniques. However, Kobayashi et al. studied inactivation of hepatitis B surface antigen by moist heat.[48,49] These researchers found that adequate inactivation occurs at 250° F (121° C) in less than 10 minutes. Other means of sterilization (ethylene oxide or formalin-steam) were not very effective. These studies have, however, been challenged on the grounds that the assumption that inactivation of hepatitis surface antigen is equivalent to inactivation of the live virus may not be true.[11]

Studies of uncommon microbes point out the limitations of standard sterilization procedures. For instance, the viral agent causing scrapie disease has been found to survive autoclaving for 1 hour.[43]

Effective steam sterilization requires direct contact of steam with all surfaces to be sterilized. All jointed instruments should be opened or unlocked to facilitate exposure of all surfaces to steam. Steam heats materials and passes through porous substances. The effect of steam on instruments is simply to heat the metal and thus sterilize the surface. Because of rapid heating of metal, instruments are sterilized faster than textiles, which require more time for heat permeation. Steam heat tends to dull sharp surfaces. In addition, the expansion of metal with heat tends to put stress on closed instruments at the box locks. Cloth-wrapped instruments or other materials should be wrapped in a double layer of muslin, autoclave-taped, and then loaded in the sterilizer to allow adequate exposure to the steam.

All fabrics and suture material may be adversely affected by heating, causing the loss of tensile strength and early disintegration. This is particularly a problem when the moisture content of the steam is low, approaching dry heat. Therefore suture material should be lightly moistened with water before being placed in the sterilizer. It is recommended that sterilization of suture materials, especially silk, be limited to three times.[64] It should be noted that swaged needles probably will be sterilized with suture material; should this occur, they will be more susceptible to dulling and rusting with moist heat.

The following are time recommendations for pressure steam autoclaving at 250° (121° C):[64]

Unwrapped metal instruments in metal tray	15 minutes
Paper-wrapped metal instruments	20 minutes
Muslin-wrapped (4-layer thickness) metal instruments	30 minutes
Dressings in cannisters	30 minutes

Because atmospheric pressure changes the pressure within the chamber, for each 1000-foot elevation above sea level, the pressure of the sterilizing chamber should be increased by approximately ½ pound/square inch. For instruments the usual time period should be 30 minutes at 250° F (121° C), followed by a drying period of 15 minutes with the sterilizer door slightly ajar. The period of exposure is measured from the time the thermometer shows the temperature of 250° F. This temperature should be measured from the coolest part of the chamber—the lower portion—or even better, from the steam-discharge line.

When one needs an instrument that is dirty immediately, so called flash sterilization may be performed. Basically this is steam sterilization at a higher temperature (270° F, or 132° C) for a shorter time (3 to 5 minutes), as described by Walter in 1938.[89] Specific recommendations for each sterilizer model should be consulted.

Unsaturated chemical vapor sterilization

An alternative type of pressure sterilizer is available, which uses a formaldehyde and alcohol mixture instead of water as the vaporized sterilizing medium. Thus this is an unsaturated chemical vapor–sterilization method. Because this type of sterlizer combines chemical and physical processes, the sterilization cycle is 20 minutes shorter than with a traditional pressure steam sterilizer. Although temperature and pressure are slightly higher than with steam autoclaves, less moisture occurs during the sterilization cycle. This low-water environment (less than 15% humidity) results in less dulling, rusting, and corrosion of metal instruments. The disadvantages of this system are that there is some doubt concerning the adequacy of killing of hepatitis B virus[49] or bacterial spores with such a low relative humidity.[14] In addition, formaldehyde is an alkylating agent (like nitrogen mustard) and is thus carcinogenic. Although the manufacturer claims that the chemicals in the sterilizing mixture do not contaminate the sterilized items, this must at least be considered a possibility. Atmospheric contamination with formaldehyde might also exceed safe levels, becoming a problem with these types of sterilizers. The Chemiclave (MDT Harvey Corp., Gardena, Calif. 90248) is an example of a chemical vapor sterilizer.

Gas sterilization

Gaseous sterilization is the treatment of objects or materials with a chemical in the gaseous state to kill all contaminating microorganisms. This method has been developed because many items cannot be subjected to heat.[14] Ethylene oxide, the simplest cyclic ether, is a low–molecular weight epoxy compound whose structural formula is the following:

$$\begin{array}{ccc} & H & H \\ & | & | \\ H - & C - C & - H \\ & \backslash \ / & \\ & O & \end{array}$$

It sterilizes by alkylating reactive groups on microorganisms, rendering them nonviable. It is inflammable in both gaseous and liquid states and is an ideal sterilant for heat-sensitive materials, but on use, trace amounts of derivatives (such as ethylene oxide, ethylene glycol, polyethylene glycol, ethylene chlorohydrin, and epichlorohydrin) remain.[66] The type of material being sterilized determines the amount of these chemicals remaining. Aeration for variable lengths of time subsequent to sterilization rids articles of the ethylene oxide or its derivatives and thus is considered essential.

As commonly used in hospitals, ethylene oxide 12% is usually mixed with Freon 88%. The techniques for use require proper integration of gases, a controlled humidity of 30% to 40%, a temperature of 130° to 140° F, and a minimal time of exposure: 1 hour (but usually much longer, up to 8 hours). In addition, the recommended aeration time is 6 to 30 hours—for most articles, 24 hours. However, some materials, such as polyvinylchloride, need to be aerated for as long as 7 days. The main advantages are that practically everything can be sterilized with ethylene oxide, including cameras and bone grafts. Moreover, corrosion of instruments is unlikely with ethylene oxide, since sterilization takes place at lower temperatures and humidity than with steam autoclaves. Ethylene oxide is about 20 times as expensive as steam pressure sterilization.[10]

There has been concern expressed about the hazards of ethylene oxide sterilization. However, a large Veterans Administration study in 1977 noted a very low injury rate.[20] Problems with use of ethylene oxide are usually caused by improper aeration.[35] Ethylene oxide can burn the skin on contact if such proper aeration has not taken place. In addition, an interesting reported case of anaphylaxis associated with hemodialysis was traced to the tubing, which had been sterilized with ethylene oxide. The patient was skin test positive to a solution prepared by flushing the tubing with a buffer, presumably producing a mixture with ethylene oxide or its derivatives.[66] Recent evidence suggests that ethylene oxide is both carcinogenic and teratogenic in laboratory animals. Because this gas is odorless, operators or other nursing personnel can unknowingly be exposed to hazardous concentrations.[40]

Another concern with the use of ethylene oxide is its inability to destroy certain microorganisms. Microbes do not seem to be killed uniformly with this method of sterilization; the rate of cell death is a function of the number of organisms present rather than the duration of exposure. In addition, some *Staphylococcus* species have been shown to survive 6 hours in ethylene oxide, and other microorganisms as long as 18 hours.[95] There is also evidence that destruction of hepatitis virus is not as effective with this sterilizing method as with pressure steam sterilization.[49]

Ethylene oxide sterilizers are manufactured for office use. However, because close control and supervision are necessary for their use and greater expense as well as hazard is incurred, this type of sterilization is not routinely recommended for office circumstances. Besides, such small table-model chambers are less reliable in killing spores than large pressurized gas sterilizers are. However, occasionally one has materials that cannot be sterilized in a pressure steam sterilizer. Under such circumstances, ethylene oxide should be considered. Usually personnel in a neighboring hospital are glad to be of assistance.

A reasonably priced compact gas-sterilizer system for office or clinic use is the Anprolene System (H.W. Andersen Products, Inc., Oyster Bay, N.Y. 11771). This system consists of a large stainless steel pan with a locking lid and gas-producing ampules placed within the pan. Instruments or other materials are placed in plastic liners with the ethylene oxide ampule. The ampule is broken, and the plastic liner is then placed in the steel pan with the top secured. The contents are left undisturbed for 12 hours.

Sterilization indicators

The proper functioning of sterilizers may be ascertained by specially made chemical or biologic indicators. Autoclave temperature and pressure gauges are not sufficient to monitor uniformity of processing, because they usually cannot detect leaks or air pockets that lower the temperature. Theoretically, small changes in temperature result in large changes in the time required for sterilization; however, sterility cannot be assumed by any indicator, since variables such as protective oils or microbial load are not taken into account. The most sensitive indicators are biologic, usually bacterial spores *(Bacillus stearothermophilus)* in glass tubes, which after exposure in a sterilizer must be cultured.[55] These types of indicators are required by hospitals.[65] Biologic indicators determine directly the level of sterility, whereas chemical indicators are indirect.[21] Biologic indicators are necessary for gas sterilizers.

Chemical indicators are used almost exclusively in office and clinic settings. They consist of chemically treated paper that turns a different color on exposure to proper sterilizing conditions in autoclaves (usually 121° C for 12 minutes with saturated steam). Some chemical indicators are also made for gas sterilizers. Unfortunately, these indicators are occasionally difficult to interpret because the color change end points are not clear enough to permit accurate interpretation. Autoclave tape may turn color sooner than the required amount of time.[64] In a study of 21 commercially available steam sterilizing indicators, only two appeared to change accurately with different times and temperatures between 240° and 270° F.[55] Some indicators were found to overestimate the sterilization effect and were in addition insensitive to the time-temperature relationship.

Despite the disadvantages mentioned, chemical indicators are useful and convenient if combined with many of the proper packaging systems available, such as Surgipeel or Protexmor.

STORAGE

After sterilization instruments and other materials are usually stored for various lengths of time before use. The length of time an article remains sterile depends on the type and condition of the packaging material, handling during storage, storage conditions, and the thickness of the wrapping material. All materials used to wrap instruments (muslin, paper, crepe) are susceptible to bacterial penetration with time. It has been determined that keeping wrapped instruments in closed shelving doubles the time it takes for penetration compared to storage in open shelving.[79] Time for penetration is also determined by the type and number of layers (single wrap versus double wrap) of material with which the instruments are wrapped. On open shelving, organisms penetrated single-wrapped muslin in two layers as early as 3 days but took 21 to 28 days if double-wrapped muslin was used and kept in open shelving. These times could be doubled if the same wrapping was used and the wrapped materials stored in closed cabinets.[79]

SHARPENING

Nondisposable instruments, such as scissors or curettes, need to be sharpened after considerable use. This is best done professionally by instrument manufacturers, although some physicians recommend personal sharpening.[19] Sharpening stones are available but are not a substitute for professional sharpening. Sharpening machines—such as the ℞ System II (℞ Honing Machine Corp., 1301 E. 5th St., Mishawaka, Ind. 46544)—can be purchased; they can sharpen instruments to a professional quality. Each time an instrument is sharpened, the width of the metal on which the cutting edge rests is shortened.

PROBLEMS WITH INSTRUMENTS

Having purchased high-quality instruments from reputable manufacturers, physicians are chagrined to see corrosion or breakage after a reasonable amount of care and handling (Fig. 7-39 and 7-40). The major causes and solu-

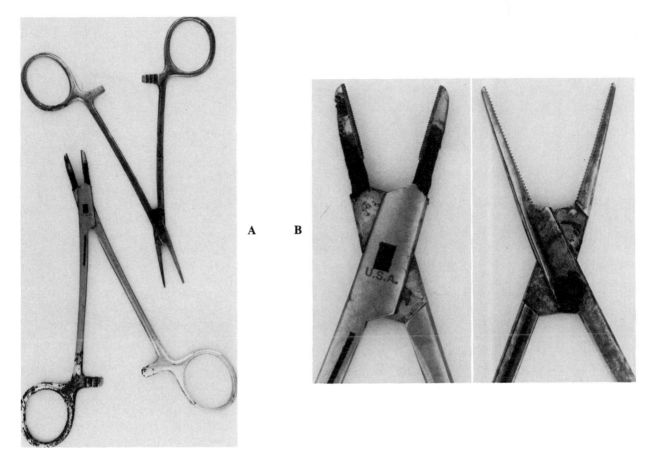

A   B

Fig. 7-39. Corrosion of instruments soaked for 3 hours in diluted sodium hypochlorite solution (Dakin's solution), which was recommended for initial cleaning after use of instruments on AIDS patients. **B,** Close-up of **A.** Immersion of instruments for prolonged periods of time with such agents leads to corrosion and is unnecessary.

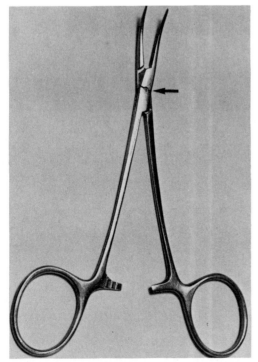

Fig. 7-40. Crack in instrument. Note this occurred adjacent to rivet, a common area of weakness in instruments.

TABLE 7-2

Problems with instruments

Problem	Cause	Solution
Corrosion (includes rust, pitting)	1. Nonpassivated instrument	Manufacturer should repassivate instrument.
	2. Improperly polished instrument	Manufacturer should repolish instrument.
	3. Inadequate cleaning and drying	Instruct personnel; do not rush the drying time.
	4. Corrosive sterilizing process	Change solutions or place rust inhibitors.
	5. Prolonged exposure to chemical sterilizing solutions	Change sterilizing method.
	6. Faulty autoclave	Use distilled water in autoclave; check autoclave for leaking valves; clean autoclave.
	7. Contaminated wrapping materials	Change wrapping materials.
	8. Damage on chrome-plated instruments	Replace instrument.
Stiffness in box locks	1. Corrosion	Soak instrument in equal parts of ethyl alcohol and aqueous ammonia for 12 hours; then rinse and brush.
	2. Accumulated debris	Clean thoroughly; may need to instill a water-soluble lapping compound.
	3. Shanks misaligned	Manufacturer should realign.
Spotting	1. Improperly treated boiler water leading to corrosion of autoclave steam lines	Use protective chemical of the filming type.
	2. Lack of proper cleaning or drying (deposition of mineral salt from tap water rinse)	Instruct personnel on proper cleaning and drying.
	3. Contaminated instrument wrapping	Instruct laundry to use pH between 6.8 and 7.2.
	4. Supersaturated steam	Consult sterilizer manufacturer.
	5. Improper drying times of sterilizer	Consult sterilizer manufacturer.
	6. Wrong detergent (low pH)	Change detergent.
	7. Electroplating (metallic staining)	Do not mix instruments of different metals in soaking solutions; remove with pencil eraser.
	8. Long exposure to sterilizing solutions (tarnish)	Change solutions or sterilizing methods.
Breakage	1. Instrument not properly stress relieved	Replace instrument.
	2. Excessive peening of rivets	Replace instrument.

tions of problems with instruments are outlined in Table 7-2.

In general the first place to look if problems are occurring with instruments is in their handling before sterilization. Sharp or delicate instruments are dulled, scratched, or bent by rough handling and being struck against hard objects. Immediate and thorough cleaning of instruments helps to protect against rusting and pitting. Tarnish may occur if instruments are allowed to lie around for hours before cleaning; this tarnish is difficult to clean. Mineral salts from tap water rinses may become deposited on metal, causing spotting that is usually dark blue in color. In some areas of the United States (California, Florida) excessive amounts of dissolved minerals are found in tap water. Rinsing instruments with distilled water is important in such places. Spotting may also occur when instruments have been improperly dried, and water with or without detergent dries on the instrument. Some detergents, especially those with a low pH, promote the deposition of mineral salts on instruments. Spotting has also been occasionally traced to detergents left in wrapping material.[15] Spotting usually does not affect the structure or function of instruments but may be viewed with annoyance by those who consider it unclean. Spots can usually be removed by a cloth buffing wheel or sometimes by a pencil eraser.

Different types of metals (such as stainless steel and metals that are chrome plated) should not be mixed in cleaning solutions or ultrasonic machines because electroplating may occur. Ferric ions from a chipped chrome-plated surface may break loose and be deposited on a stainless steel surface. These ions then oxidize and appear as rust. However, they may easily be removed with a pencil eraser, showing that they are only on the surface. Chemical sterilizing solutions are particularly hard on instruments, being prone to cause rust and tarnish.[12] Corrosion inhibitors should be added to such solutions, and the solutions themselves should be changed frequently.

Although stiffness in the box locks may be caused by corrosion—since such recesses are not properly polished and are thus corrosion susceptible—usually this is more likely to be caused by accumulated debris. Such instruments may be soaked for 12 hours in equal parts alcohol and aqueous ammonia and then rinsed.[82] This process removes most of the products of corrosion. Thorough cleaning with a brush is necessary. If stiffness still exists, a water-soluble lapping compound may be useful. This should be worked into the box locks by opening and closing the instrument.

The second place to look when having problems with instruments is the sterilizing process. Chemical sterilization, as already mentioned, can lead to corrosion or tarnishing. Steam sterilizers may be sources of corrosion, particularly if tap water is used instead of distilled water. Sources of corrosion also may be corrosive products of steam lines, improper drying cycles, or supersaturated steam. The sterilizer manufacturer should be consulted if the sterilizer itself is believed to be the source of the problem.

The third and last place to look is the instrument itself. Instrument defects can occur but are unusual. Chrome-plated instruments are especially prone to damage, with chipping of the plating and rust occurring at those points. Corrosion can occur at points of stress if the instrument has not been properly stress relieved, leading to breakage at points of high mechanical stress. If proper polishing or passivation has not been done, corrosion is more likely. Cracks may occur where there has been excessive peening of rivets at the fulcrum or if inappropriate engraving has been performed.

Proper selection, handling, care, and sterilization ensure a long life for surgical instruments, which affords the dermatologic surgeon the best means possible to achieve excellent cosmetic effects. Problems are, however, inevitable, and it is hoped that the background provided in this chapter will be of assistance in the solution of such problems.

REFERENCES

1. Albom, M.J.: Scalpel and scissors surgery. In Epstein, E., and Epstein, E., Jr., editors, Techniques in skin surgery, Philadelphia, 1979, Lea & Febiger.
2. Anthony, M.F., and Wilson, G.: Costly materials retrieved from laundry chutes, Hospitals **52**(10):119, 1978.
3. Ashbell, T.S.: The emergency skin and bone hook, J. Bone Joint Surg. **54**:1325, 1972.
4. Bang, O., and Dalsgaard, A.T.: Symposium on sterilization, Arch. Pharm. Chem. **25**:699, 1948.
5. Barker, H.A.: The effect of water content upon the rate of heat denaturation of crystallizable egg albumin, J. Gen. Physiol. **17**:21, 1933-34.
6. Barron, J.N.: Instruments for hand surgery, Hand **6**:211, 1974.
7. Bartlett, R.E.: Use of the Desmarres clamp in major eyelid surgery, Ann. Ophthalmol. **9**:360, 1977.
8. Bingel, K.F.: Absterbekurven gröberer Temperature: Zeitbereiche von vegetativen Keimen und Sporen unter Einwirkung feuchter oder trockener Hitze und ihre gegenseitigen Beziehungen, Arch. Hyg. Bakt. **142**:26, 1958.
9. Block, S.S.: Disinfection, sterilization and preservation, Philadelphia, 1977, Lea & Febiger.
10. Boger, W.: A better understanding of ethylene oxide sterilization: its advantages, disadvantages and costs, Hosp. Top. **54**:12, 1976.
11. Bond, W.W.: Can steam autoclaving be excessive? Med. Instrum. **13**:55, 1979.
12. Boucher, R.M.: Disinfection with glutaraldehyde (letter), Br. Med. J. **2**:444 1979.
13. Braun, M.: The razor curet, J. Derm. Surg. Oncol. **8**:830, 1982.
14. Bruch, C.W.: Gaseous sterilization, Ann. Rev. Microbiol. **15**:245, 1961.
15. Byrd, D.H., and McElmurry, M.: Prevent spotting of surgical instruments, AORN J. **17**(4):87, 1973.
16. Charbeneau, G.T., and Berry, G.C.: A simple and effective method of handpiece and instrument sterilization without corrosion, J. Am. Dent. Assoc. **59**:732, 1959.
17. Chick, H.: The process of disinfection by chemical agencies and hot water, J. Hygiene **10**:237, 1910.
18. Chick, H., and Martin, C.J.: On the "heat coagulation" of proteins, J. Physiol. **40**:404, 1910.
19. Cobey, M.C.: Sharp instruments, Clin. Orthop. **103**:101, 1974.
20. Cobis, J.: Should hospitals continue to use ethylene oxide for sterilization? Hospitals **51**:73, 1977.
21. Danielson, N.E.: Sterilization process indicators: biological vs. chemical, Med. Instrum. **16**:52, 1982.
22. Darmady, E.M., Hughes, K.E.A., and Jones, J.D.: Thermal death-time of spores in dry heat in relation to sterilization of instruments and syringes, Lancet **2**:766, 1958.
23. Darmady, E.M., et al.: Sterilization by conducted heat, Lancet **2**:769, 1958.
24. Darmady, E.M., et al.: The cleaning of instruments and syringes, J. Clin. Pathol. **18**:6, 1965.
25. Ecker, E.E., and Smith, R.: Sterilizing surgical instruments and utensils, Mod. Hosp. **48**:92, 1937.
26. Eichenwald, H.F., and Mosley, J.W.: Viral hepatitis, U.S. Dept. Health, Education and Welfare, Pub. No. 435, 1959, Washington, D.C.
27. El-Bisi, H., et al.: Chemical events during death of bacterial endospores by moist heat, J. Food Sci. **27**:219, 1962.
28. Epstein, L.I.: Obtaining razor blades suitable for use in plastic surgery, Plast. Reconstr. Surg. **59**:740, 1977.
29. Everall, P.H., et al.: Failure to sterilize in plastic bags, J. Clin. Pathol. **29**:1132, 1976.
30. Fallon, R.J.: Wrapping of sterilized articles (letter), Lancet **2**:785, 1963.
31. Field, L.M.: A weighed retraction hook, J. Dermatol. Surg. Oncol. **8**:531, 1982.
32. Field, L.M.: A new, rounded scalpel handle (surgical gem), J. Dermatol. Surg. Oncol. **8**:918, 1982.
33. Foley, F.E., and Gutheim, R.N.: Serum hepatitis following dental procedures: a presentation of 15 cases, including three fatalities, Ann. Intern. Med. **45**:369, 1956.
34. Gibbs, R.C.: A love affair with a gradle scissors, J. Dermatol. Surg. Oncol. **7**:771, 1981.
35. Gillespie, E.H., et al.: Ethylene oxide sterilization: is it safe? J. Clin. Pathol. **32**:1184, 1979.

36. Glassman, P.: Proper care enables longer trouble-free use of stainless steel instruments, Hosp. Top. **42**(8):107, 1964.

37. Goldman, L., and Preston, R.H.: Special small knives for minor dermatologic surgery: their value in the performance of small biopsies and in the removal of small milia, Arch. Dermatol. **78**:640, 1958.

38. Hagerman, D., and Wilson, H.: The skin biopsy punch: Evaluation and modification, Cutis **6**:1139, 1970.

39. Hartley, J.H., Jr.: A new face lift scissors, Br. J. Plast. Surg. **27**:365, 1974.

40. Hazard Alert No. 3: Ethylene oxide, California Department of Health Services, Sacramento, July, 1982, Hazard Evaluation System and Information Service.

41. Hoskins, H.T.: Sterile production and mechanical reliability of autoclaves, Med. Biol. Eng. **16**:330, 1978.

42. Hughes, D.E., and Nyborg, W.L.: Cell disruption by ultrasound, Science **138**:108, 1962.

43. Kast, R.E.: Introduction to the scrapie diseases: self-replicating agents surviving standard autoclaving for an hour and 10% formalin for a year, Mater. Med. Pol. **8**:3, 1976.

44. Kaye, B.L.: Useful scissors for fine dissecting, Br. J. Plast. Surg. **24**:319, 1971.

45. Keyes, E.L.: The cutaneous punch, J. Cutan. Geniturin. Dis. **5**:98, 1887.

46. Kirkup, J.R.: The history and evolution of surgical instruments, Ann. R. Coll. Surg. Engl. **63**:279, 1981.

47. Kirkup, J.R.: The history and evolution of surgical instruments. II. Origins: function—carriage manufacture, Ann. R. Coll. Surg. Engl. **64**:125, 1982.

48. Kobayashi, H.: What should be "practical" standard of treatment? Med. Instrum. **13**:56, 1979.

49. Kobayashi, H., et al.: Sterilization of hepatitis B surface antigen-contaminated materials, Med. Instrum. **12**:171, 1978.

50. Koch, R., Gaffky, G., and Loeffler, F.: Versuche über Verwerthbarkeit heisser Wasserclämpfe zu Desinfektionszwecken, Mitt Kaiserl Gesund **1**:322, 1881.

51. Koch, R., and Wolffhugel, G.: Untersuchungen über die Disinfection mit heisser Luft, Mitt Kaiserl Gesund **1**:301, 1881.

52. Koranda, F.C., et al.: Instruments and tips for dermatology surgery, J. Dermatol. Surg. Oncol. **8**:451, 1982.

53. Krugman, S., et al.: Viral hepatitis type B studies on natural history and prevention reexamined, New Engl. J. Med. **300**:101, 1979.

54. Krull, E.A.: Surgical gems: the little curet, J. Dermatol. Surg. Oncol. **4**:656, 1978.

55. Lee, C.H., et al.: Comparison of the efficacy of steam sterilization indicators, Appl. Environ. Microbiol. **37**:1113, 1979.

56. Mair, A.C.: Disinfection with glutaraldehyde (letter), Br. Med. J. **280**:403, 1980.

57. McKie, J., et al.: An extractor for scalpel blades, Lancet **2**:395, 1975.

58. Mostafa, A.B., et al.: Cleaning of surgical instruments: a preliminary assessment, Med. Biol. Engl. **14**:524, 1976.

59. Navarro-Gasparetto, C., et al.: The spoon as a surgical instrument, Plast. Reconstr. Surg. **63**:853, 1979.

60. O'Brien, H.A., et al.: The use of activated glutaraldehyde as a cold sterilizing agent for urological instruments, J. Urol. **95**:429, 1966.

61. Orlowski, T.M.: Modification of the needle holder, Am. J. Surg. **133**:768, 1977.

62. Peled, I., et al.: Improvised skin hook, Ann. Plast. Surg. **8**:263, 1982.

63. Peled, I.J., et al.: Improvised double skin hooks, Ann. Plast. Surg. **9**:516, 1982.

64. Perkins, J.J.: Principles and methods of sterilization in health sciences, Springfield, Ill., 1969, Charles C Thomas, Publishers, Inc.

65. Perkins, R.E., et al.: Monitoring steam sterilization of surgical instruments: a dilemma, Appl. Environ. Microbiol. **42**:383, 1981.

66. Poothullil, J., et al.: Anaphylaxis from the products of ethylene oxide gas, Ann. Intern. Med. **82**:58, 1975.

67. Popkin, G.L.: Surgical gems: another look at the skin hook, J. Dermatol. Surg. Oncol. **4**:366, 1978.

68. Popkin, G.L., and Brodie, S.J.: The versatile skin hook, Arch. Dermatol. **86**:343, 1962.

69. Rahn, O.: Physical methods of sterilization of microorganisms, Bact. Rev. **9**:1, 1945.

70. Reichert, M.C.: Innovations in sterilization technology for instrument processing, Med. Instrum. **17**:89, 1983.

71. Rodenbeck, H.: Ueber die thermische Sterilisation wasserfrier Stoffe und die Resisteng einiger Bakterien bei Erhitzung in solchen Stoffen, Arch. Hyg. Bakt. **109**:67, 1932.

72. Schimmelbusch, C.: A guide to the antiseptic treatment of wounds, New York, 1895, Putnam.

73. Schulman, J.: New fine pointed scissors with serrated edges for use in rhinoplasty, Br. J. Plast. Surg. **32**:147, 1979.

74. Scott, M.J., et al.: Obsidian surgical blades: modern use of a stone age implement, J. Dermatol. Surg. Oncol. **8**:1050, 1982.

75. Sebben, J.E.: Avoiding infection in office surgery, J. Dermatol. Surg. Oncol. **8**:455, 1982.

76. Shelley, W.B.: The razor blade in dermatologic practice, Cutis **16**:843, 1975.

77. Simmonds, W.L.: Sterilization, Cutis **25**:78, 1980.

78. Spaulding, E.H.: Principles of microbiology as applied to operating room nursing, Association of Operating Room Nurses Tenth Annual Congress, Washington, D.C., Feb. 18-21, 1963.

79. Standard, P.G., et al.: Microbial penetration of muslin and proper wrapped sterile packs stored on open shelves and in closed cabinets, Appl. Microbiol. **22**:432, 1971.

80. Stegman, S.J.: Commentary: the cutaneous punch, Arch. Dermatol. **118**:943, 1982.

81. Stegman, S.J., Tromovitch, T.A., ad Glogau, R.G.: Basics of dermatologic surgery, Chicago, 1982, Year Book Medical Publishers, Inc.

82. Storz instrument catalogue, ed. 13, St. Louis, 1977, Storz Instrument Co.

83. Strauch, B.: Immediate assembly of a disposable tissue hook, Plast. Reconstr. Surg. **42**:386, 1968.

84. Thompson, C.J.S.: The evolution and development of surgical instruments, Br. J. Surg. **25**:1, 1937.

85. Thompson, C.J.S.: The evolution and development of surgical instruments. IV. The trepan, Br. J. Surg. **25**:726, 1937.

86. Turner, A.G., et al.: Bacterial aerosolization from an ultrasonic cleaner, J. Clin. Microbiol. **1**:289, 1975.

87. Vallery-Radot, R.: The life of Pasteur, New York, 1926,

Doubleday. (Translation by R.L. Devonshire.)

88. Vecchione, T.R.: An effective tourniquet mechanism in surgery of the lip, Arch. Surg. **111**:918, 1976.

89. Walter, C.W.: Technique for the rapid and absolute sterilization of instruments, Surg. Gynecol. Obstet. **67**:244, 1938.

90. Watson, B.A.: Gunpowder disfigurements, St. Louis Med. Surg. J. **35**:145, 1878.

91. Webster, R.C., et al.: The iconoclast as an aid in blunt dissection of flaps of the scalp and forehead, J. Dermatol. Surg. Oncol. **8**:793, 1982.

92. White, S.W.: The razor curet (revisisted) and the twin-blade scalpel, J. Dermatol. Surg. Oncol. **9**:191, 1983.

93. Wigglesworth, E.: The curette in dermal therapeutics, Boston Med. Surg. J. **94**:143, 1876.

94. Zimmon, D.S., et al.: Homemade medical devices, N. Engl. J. Med. **297**:895, 1977.

95. Znamirowski, R., McDonald, S., and Roy, T.E.: The efficiency of an ethylene oxide sterilizer in hospital practice, Can. Med. Assoc. J. **83**:1004, 1960.

Materials for
Wound Closure

To achieve the best possible cosmetic and functional results in cutaneous surgery, discriminating use of wound closure materials is essential. Despite millenia of experience in wound apposition, there is general lack of agreement among those performing surgery about which suture material or even which suturing method is best. Apparently no one suture material is best under all circumstances for all patients at all times by all surgeons.

The choice of suture materials is too frequently arbitrary, based more on the subjective experiences or prejudices of one's teacher (or teaching institution) than on a thoughtful study of wound closure materials that takes objective scientific data into account. Although many of these prejudices have been disproved, others have stood the test of time. Some prejudices have been forgotten and perhaps need to be reexamined.

Since the beginning of surgery, the fastidiousness and strong feelings of surgeons have led them to swear by—or swear at—various types and kinds of sutures. For instance, Galen and Antyllus in the second century AD highly recommended a Celtic linen thread, which could be purchased at a certain shop along the Via Sacra near the temple of Rome.[74,128]

The choice of wound-closure materials should be predicated on secure approximation of wound edges during the necessary time and have minimal negative influence on wound healing.[32] The underlying scientific basis for use of these materials is a relatively recent development.

Proper surgical technique alone does not ensure the best surgical result if improper wound-closure materials are used. Conversely, proper wound-closure materials do not ensure a good result if used with poor surgical technique. With experience, one learns that there is some variation of suture quality among manufacturers and even by the same manufacturer. Furthermore, because cutaneous surgery is frequently performed in an office setting, the price of suture materials is an important consideration for the practicing physician.

Wound-closure materials are currently available in an ever-widening array of different materials and colors, with attached needles of different sizes and shapes. This has led to a perplexing array of choices for the dermatologic surgeon. In addition, the manufacturers do not use consistent nomenclature, so it is difficult to compare various items, such as needles.

Wound-closure materials are used for a number of different purposes. Most commonly they approximate wound edges. Ligation of blood vessels is also important, as is minimizing dead space. Correct placement of appropriate sutures results in minimization of connective tissue and scarring, yielding improved cosmetic results. Sutures may also be left buried for long periods of time (perhaps a lifetime) to impart lasting strength to a wound.

This chapter discusses the materials currently available to close wounds. These materials include not only sutures with attached needles, but staples, skin tapes, and even certain glues.

One definition to clarify at the outset is the difference between a ligature and a suture. A ligature is a thread used—without a needle—to tie or bind around a structure, such as a blood vessel. A suture is a thread with an attached needle used to bind one structure to another, such as one piece of skin to another. A ligature does not need a needle, whereas a suture does. If one ties a blood vessel to adjacent tissue to stop bleeding by passing a suture with a needle through this tissue, one is really suturing the blood vessel and ligating it.

HISTORY AND DEVELOPMENT

The historical development of wound-closure materials generally falls into three periods. The first begins in ancient times and lasts until the late nineteenth century. During this period of time little development of suture materials took place. The second period begins with Dr. William Halsted and Lord Lister in the 1890s and continues until after World War II. During this time the evolutions of modern scientific surgical thought began, and the choice of suture materials was given a scientific basis. Both surgical catgut and silk suture became standard, with few exceptions. The third period extends from the latter part of the 1940s to the present. This is the era of polymer science, during which newer, custom-made, synthetic sutures were produced, aiding greatly in the management of wounds and helping to ensure excellent cosmetic results.

The first recorded account of the use of sutures is the Edwin Smith surgical papyrus, which probably was written as early as 3000 BC. Interestingly, not only was suturing described but also supporting the wound with the earliest skin tapes (plaster with honey) if the sutures came loose.[28]

The Indian physician Susruta ca 600 BC described sutures in the Samhita using animal sinews, horse hair, leather strips, cotton, and tree bark fibers.[10] An interesting technique of using large black ants to bite the wound edges together and then twisting off the ant's body was also described in the ancient Indian literature[174] and was also used by the South American Indians.[116] This technique of wound closure is similar to stapling and is still used in the jungles of southern Bhutan in the Himalayas.

In AD 30 Celsus used wool and linen sutures and even small metal clips. In AD 165 Galen, the physician to the gladiators, suggested using ligatures to stop bleeding and referred to both catgut and silk.[10]

One method of suturing used by East African tribes was to push acacia thorns through the wound edges and then to wind vegetation around in a figure eight.[116] This technique of suturing—using metal pins instead of thorns—was used in the last century, particularly on cleft lip repairs.

In the latter part of the nineteenth century Lord Lister in England began treating catgut with carbolic acid to lessen the chance of infection.[111] He also suggested exposing catgut to chromic salts to delay absorption. Halsted in the latter 1890s taught that silk was an important suture and that it could be either buried or used percutaneously in the skin.[72]

During the first half of the twentieth century surgeons began to explore the use of other materials for wound closure and their possible consequences on wound healing. Ochsner became a great advocate of cotton,[124] whereas Babcock preferred stainless steel.[15] Disciples of Halsted continued to prefer silk. Many of these preferences depended on where one had trained, although all were claimed to have the scientific merit of producing excellent wound tensile strength.

An interesting story is related by MacKenzie regarding the beginning of the Ethicon Company.[116] In around 1900 surgical catgut was made almost exclusively in Europe by the Germans because of the use of sheep intestines in the sau-

sage industry. At the beginning of World War I, this left Britain without a source of catgut. Some Edinburgh surgeons convinced a local merchant, George Merson, to manufacture this material. Merson introduced to surgery the eyeless-needle sutures and patented them as "Mersutures." Such sutures caused less tissue damage because a single rather than double strand of suture was pulled through tissue. Merson's company eventually became Ethicon, Ltd., currently a major suture manufacturer.

The current modern era of suture materials began during the second World War with polymer science. Dupont laboratories produced the first nylons (polyamides) made for surgery, and this was followed by polyesters and polyolefins. In the 1960s and 1970s the synthetic biodegradable polymer sutures were developed. The first one introduced, Dexon, was a braided polyglycolic acid. In 1974 Vicryl, a braided copolymer of lactide and glycolide, came into the market. Both these sutures, being braided, are easy to tie. Compared to catgut these newer absorbable sutures are more uniform in terms of their tensile strength and absorption. The newest absorbable sutures, PDS (polydioxanone), is a monofilamentous suture that reputedly retains its tensile strength longer than the other absorbable sutures do. All these sutures are discussed in greater detail later.

SUTURE MATERIALS
Ideal suture

Currently no one suture material exists that is ideal under all circumstances. Several authors have attempted to define the characteristics of a perfect suture.[5,56,154,184] In general the hypothetical ideal suture can be used throughout any operation and will produce no adverse effects on wound healing; its tensile strength is adequate, and it remains stable as long as necessary and then disappears. The handling and knot tying are easy and secure; the suture will not promote infection and is easy to see. In addition such a suture can be reproduced at a reasonable cost, is capable of being sterilized and stored, and is noncarcinogenic, nontoxic, and nonallergic. As we shall see, no currently available suture materials conform to all these criteria.

Evaluation of suture materials

The three broad categories with which to evaluate suture materials include the physical characteristics, the handling characteristics, and the tissue interaction. Usually the physical characteristics are measured or visually determined by the material itself. The *United States Pharmacopeia (USP)*[185] is the official compendium providing definitions and descriptions of such physical characteristics as tensile strength, capillarity, and size. The *USP* also sets the standards and guidelines under which sutures are manufactured, packaged, sterilized, and labeled.

The handling characteristics of suture materials are more subjective, although the ability to hold knots can be measured. Tissue interaction and absorption rates are usually the result of animal studies and are rarely confirmed by studies on humans. As pointed out by Postlethwait,[151] sutures act differently on different animals, and therefore when critically assessing such studies it is important to know which animal is being used in each study. Also, different implantation sites even in the same animal render different results.

Two variables of extreme importance in comparative testing and evaluation of suture materials are the wetness and the size. Some sutures, such as catgut, swell when wet and thus lose tensile strength. Absorption rates for small-caliber sutures are generally faster than for larger material. One should be mindful of such variables whenever evaluating suture materials.

Physical characteristics

Configuration. The physical configuration of suture refers to whether it is a single strand (monofilament), such as nylon, or many strands (multifilament), such as silk. The multifilamentous sutures can be braided or twisted. Braiding increases the tensile strength and produces less fraying of cut ends than twisting produces. In addition, handling and knot tying are easier with braided sutures. Braiding, however, also increases a suture's ability to harbor organisms and decreases its tensile strength by producing shear forces between the filaments.

Suture material may be coated with various substances—for instance, Teflon or silicone—to provide a smoother passage through tissue and to make braided sutures more resistant bacteria. However, coating on suture material does not necessarily decrease a suture's ability to potentiate infection.[172] Such coatings can introduce additional foreign material (frequently causing more problems) into wounds.

Capillarity and fluid absorption ability. Capillarity of suture materials refers to its ability to draw fluid from the immersed wet end of the strand into the dry nonimmersed portion. This is distinguished from fluid-absorption ability, which is simply the ability of suture to soak up fluid when immersed.

A study of various suture materials showed that catgut had the greatest ability to absorb fluid, possibly caused by chemical binding between water molecules and protein molecules in the suture.[23] Nylon also absorbed some fluid. Polypropylene, on the other hand, had low fluid absorption caused by its known hydrophobic characteristics. Fluid absorption ability and capillarity both correlate with a suture's ability to take up and retain bacteria. Braided nylon, with greater capillarity, has three times monofilament nylon's ability to retain bacteria.[35] Apparently bacteria do not differentiate between the spaces in the tissue and those on the suture when choosing a habitat in which to reside.

Diameter. The diameter (caliber) of sutures is determined in millimeters and expressed in *USP* sizes with zeroes. For sutures that are 2-0 and smaller, the smaller the cross-sectional diameter of the suture, the more zeroes. It should be noted that not all *USP* sizes correspond to the same diameters for all suture materials. This is because the *USP* size is related to a specific diameter necessary to produce a specified tensile strength. The size listing is the diameter of the suture when a standard weight is applied under standard conditions. In general for each *USP* size, catgut is larger than the nonabsorbable sutures; Vicryl is also larger than Dexon at comparable sizes. Therefore 5-0 nylon is smaller than 5-0 catgut and 5-0 Vicryl (Fig. 8-1). Uniform diameters are consistently found in synthetic suture matrials. Catgut may vary in diameter somewhat due to processing.

Tensile strength. Tensile strength is an important suture characteristic. It is defined as the amount of weight (breaking load) necessary to break a suture divided by the cross-sectional area. It varies proportionally with the square of the suture diameter. Thus if one doubles the diameter, one quadruples the tensile strength.[156] The tensile strength also varies with the type of material being tested. In general, steel has the highest tensile strength, followed by the synthetics, and then by the natural materials. Stainless steel, for instance, is very strong compared with catgut. Tensile strength also may vary with the wetness of the material. Wet catgut is much weaker than dry catgut.

Variations in tensile strength can also be seen among different batches of suture materials after 1½ years of storage,[179] may be caused by variations in the manufacturing process, polymerizations of synthetic materials during prolonged storage, or the effects of the ionizing radiation used in the sterilization process. Tensile strength also depends on the configuration of the suture. Twisting or braiding sutures aligns fibers in such a way as to produce shear on extension—and thus a weaker strand than one which is not twisted or braided. In addition, a monofilamentous suture has a greater mass and therefore greater tensile strength than a comparably sized braided suture. The relative straight-pull tensile strength of several sutures is listed in the box below.

In surgery, one deals with tied loops of suture and not strands. This has led to the concept of "effective tensile strength," which takes into account the knot security and

---

RELATIVE TENSILE STRENGTH OF SUTURES

Greater ↑	Nonabsorbable	Absorbable
	Steel	
	Polyester	
	Nylon (monofilament)	Polyglycolic acid
	Nylon (braided)	Polyglactin 910
	Polypropylene	Polydioxanone
	Silk	Catgut

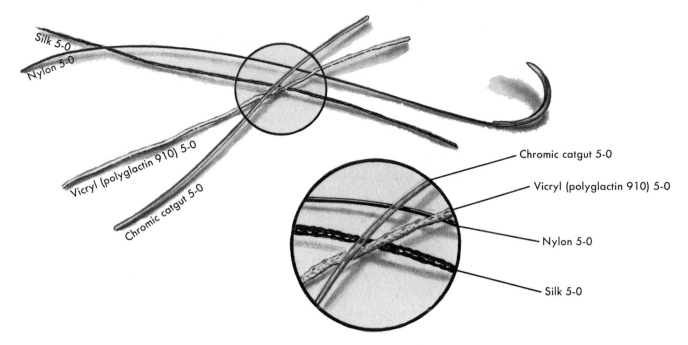

Fig. 8-1. Relative sizes of dry silk (5-0), nylon (5-0), polyglactin 910 Vicryl (5-0), and chromic catgut (5-0). Note that catgut is larger than nylon and that both are smaller than silk or Vicryl. When wet, catgut swells and becomes larger than comparably sized dry silk.

the fact that the knotted suture has about one third less tensile strength than the untied strand. Effective tensile strength is measured by breaking a loop of suture tied with a surgeon's knot; straight pull tensile strength measures the tensile strength of a strand of suture without a knot. In some instances the knot slips; in other instances, the suture ruptures adjacent to the knot because tying the knot weakens or cracks the suture material itself.

Knot strength. The knot strength is mainly determined by the coefficient of friction. In other words, the more slippery the suture material, the more likely it is that a given knot will slip. The tensile strength of a suture is greater than its knot-holding capacity, since the suture breaks or slips at the knot because it is weakened. The *USP* directs that the tensile strength of a suture thread is determined after a surgical knot (a two-turn throw followed by a one-turn throw tied square) has been tied over a thick rubber tube. In a study of tensile strengths of knotted sutures, the knotted tensile strength was only 5% to 99% of the tensile strength of the unknotted thread.[178] When testing further after implantation for 1 week in rabbits, the same investigators found a higher percentage of knot slippage.[180] Catgut was found most likely and Dexon least likely to slip of the materials tested.[180] Interestingly, when the same type of knot was used, thick threads were weaker than thin ones.

Elasticity and plasticity. Two other physical characteristics of suture materials frequently neglected in discussions are elasticity and plasticity. When a suture is stretched, the inherent ability to regain its original form and length is its elasticity. The ability to retain its new deformed length and

form is referred to as plasticity. Most sutures are elastic, but a few (polypropylene) are plastic also.[82] After wound swelling subsides, a plastic suture retains its larger size, and at that time its tied loop may be too wide to keep the wound edges together. Plasticity allows knots to be deformed, and thus they become more secure.

Memory and flexibility. Memory is related to both elasticity and plasticity and refers to a suture's capacity to return to its former shape on deformation, such as tying. Sutures that are stiff are thus said to have a high memory. A tied suture with a high memory, such as nylon, tends to untie as it tries to regain its former shape, whereas a suture with a low memory rarely becomes untied. One must be careful to tie knots in high-memory suture material more securely and in a greater number. Flexibility is the suture's resistance to being bent. It is expressed as the force required to bend a suture with a three-point bending procedure. Flexibility and memory are inversely related to each other.

Memory and flexibility are also related to handling and knot security (described later). Materials with a low memory, like silk, handle well and have excellent knot security.

$$\text{Knot security} \propto \frac{\text{Flexibility}}{\text{Memory}} \propto \text{Handling}$$

Handling characteristics

Pliability and coefficient of friction. The handling of a suture material is related to its pliability and its coefficient of friction. Pliability is a subjective term and refers to how easily one can handle the suture. The most pliable materi-

RELATIVE KNOT SECURITY OF SUTURES

	Nonabsorbable	Absorbable
	Steel	
	Polyester	Polyglycolic acid (Dexon "S")
Best	Silk	Polyglactin 910
	Nylon	Polyglycolic acid (Dexon Plus)
	Polypropylene	Catgut
	Polyethylene	

als, such as silk, are braided, whereas monofilamentous sutures are more difficult to handle.

The coefficient of friction determines how easily a suture slips through tissue and out of being tied; in other words, it is a measure of how slippery a material is. Some materials have a high coefficient of friction and tend to "drag" through tissue. These types of sutures are also difficult to tie, since the knots do not set easily. Vicryl used to behave in this manner, but the manufacturer subsequently coated the suture with calcium stearate and a copolymer to lower its coefficient of friction.[46] Materials used to coat other sutures include wax (silk), Teflon, silicone, and polybutilate.[45]

The coefficient of friction also affects the work it takes to remove a suture at the appropriate time. Prolene, for instance, has a very low coefficient of friction and therefore slides easily through tissue. Even after 1 or 2 weeks it still easily slips out of tissue, making it ideal for a running intradermal suture.[67]

Knot tying and knot security. Knot tying and knot security are also affected by the coefficient of friction. The more slippery the suture material, the easier it is to slip a knot into place. However, the knot is also less secure because it may more easily become undone. In general, braided, uncoated materials such as silk or polyester have good knot security, whereas monofilamentous sutures have poor knot security. The relative knot security of several sutures is listed in the box above.

Knot security is affected not only by the coefficient of friction but by the type of knot and the number of throws used.[180] In general, 2 × 2 knots (two turns tied on two turns) were strong with every material tested by Tera and Aberg.[179] Knot security increases with each throw, but the percentage of increase lessens with each tie. This is important because one wishes to bury as little foreign material as possible in a wound. Steel sutures are said not to slip with only two throws, whereas Teflon-coated Dacron still slips after six throws.

Static electricity. When suture material is removed from the package, static electricity may be generated by the friction created in pulling it against the cardboard container.[139] This is particularly true of suture material that is packaged dry rather than wet. The static electrical charge on the suture material draws it to objects with an opposite charge. The hair of the forearms is such a charged object. Wetting the material will result in added weight and decreased net charge and therefore will lessen its static electrical attractiveness. Suture manufacturers currently produce some suture materials that are packaged wet rather than dry. Catgut used to be the only suture packaged in fluid (alcohol).

Another factor enhancing the attraction between the suture material and the arm is the curl produced in packaging. To decrease this curling tendency, one should stretch the suture material on unpackaging it, holding it with two hands and not putting stress on the junction of the needle to the thread. This junction is much weaker than the suture material itself.

Tissue interactions

All suture material regardless of composition is a foreign substance to the body and therefore evokes a tissue reaction. The degree and type of reaction vary from one type of suture to another but become important in the selection of the material best suited for the particular task. As a general rule, the more suture material that is implanted, the greater the tissue reaction; therefore the least suture material that can do the job should be chosen, and the least number of knots that can adequately secure the sutures should be thrown.

Cellular reaction (tissue reactivity). Tissue reaction to the suture material is at least partially the result of injury inflicted by passage of the suture and needle. However, beyond these there is additional tissue reactivity to the suture material itself, which peaks 2 to 7 days after implantation. Experimental and clinical studies have shown that the more intense and prolonged the tissue reaction is to sutures, the greater is the chance of prolonged and disturbed wound healing, infection, and inadequate maintenance of wound approximation.[32]

The normal sequence of tissue reaction to suture material is in three stages, like wound healing.[117] In the first 4 days polymorphonuclear leukocytes, lymphocytes, and monocytes predominate. This is followed by a second stage from the fourth to the seventh day, in which macrophages and fibroblasts appear. After the seventh day fibrous tissue with chronic inflammation persists. Around persistent nonabsorbable sutures a thin fibrous capsule usually forms, and the inflammatory reaction is minimal. Around absorbable sutures the inflammatory reaction persists until the suture is absorbed or extruded. As a generalization, monofilamentous sutures produce less reaction than multifilamentous strands do. Also, the greater the amount of suture material embedded

```
┌─────────────────────────────────────────────┐
│                                               │
│   RELATIVE TISSUE REACTIVITY TO SUTURES       │
│        Nonabsorbable        Absorbable        │
│  ↑    Cotton, silk          Catgut            │
│  ↑    Polyester coated      Polyglactin 910   │
│ Most  Polyester uncoated    Polyglycolic acid │
│       Nylon                                   │
│       Polypropylene                           │
│                                               │
└─────────────────────────────────────────────┘
```

within a wound, the greater the tissue reaction is. This was a principle well known by Halsted, who advocated using the finest-gauge suture available to perform the job.[72]

Nylon and polypropylene produce the least cellular reaction. Silk, on the other hand, produces a marked inflammatory reaction, but less so than catgut. Polyester is intermediate between nylon and silk. Teflon, which is used as a coating on some suture materials, is shed off and evokes a giant cell response.[153] The relative tissue reactivity to several suture matrials is listed in the box above.

In general the nonabsorbable sutures, if buried in tissue, are encapsulated in time, whereas the absorbable sutures are absorbed over a period of time. The fibrous capsule around nonabsorbable sutures is usually formed by 28 days.

Absorption. The absorption of sutures is not synonymous with the loss of tensile strength in vivo. Tensile strength is lost long before absorption is complete for most sutures. For instance, uncoated Vicryl absorbs completely in approximately 70 to 90 days, but its tensile strength, which holds the wound together, may be effective for only 7 to 21 days.

The division of suture materials into absorbable and nonabsorbable is somewhat arbitrary. Absorbable sutures may be defined as those losing most of their tensile strength within 60 days after implantation. Polyglactin 910 (Vicryl), polyglycolic acid (Dexon), catgut, and polydioxanone (PDS) all are classified as absorbable by this definition. Yet catgut has been reported to persist in tissue years after implantation.[153] Silk and even nylon are classified as nonabsorbable but are also absorbed, more slowly, over many months; these sutures should more properly be categorized as slowly-absorbable sutures.

Catgut is absorbed through the action of cellular enzymes and is somewhat unpredictable. Its absorption is markedly increased in the presence of infection.[92] In contrast, the synthetic absorbable sutures, which include Vicryl and Dexon, are more reliable in their absorption rates. Absorption of these sutures takes place by hydrolysis.

In considering studies of absorption rates of suture materials, careful attention should be paid to the size of the sutures studied, the animals used, and the sites of implantation. All these variables affect the rate of absorption and

frequently make comparison between various studies difficult if not frankly impossible.

Wound healing. Suture material not only induces its own tissue reaction but also secondarily influences wound healing in the wound on which it is being used. When a wound occurs in the skin subsequent wound healing occurs in three stages. The initial inflammatory phase lasts for the first 3 to 5 days, characterized by numerous polymorphonuclear leukocytes and a decrease in the tensile strength of the wound. The proliferative phase follows, during which capillary buds grow and fibroplasia occurs. At this point the wound begins to gain tensile strength. The proliferative phase lasts from day 4 or 5 to 2 weeks. Afterwards, the wound gains strength slowly, in what is called the maturation phase. In general an increased inflammatory reaction to suture material results in a delay in wound healing but ultimately may lead to a stronger wound. The delay in gain of tensile strength in wounds sutured with catgut, which produces marked inflammation, was noted in 1943.[112] Catgut sutures are said to prolong the inflammatory phase of wound healing by increasing the already-present inflammatory reaction.[112] Nylon, on the other hand, shortens the inflammatory phase and thus leads to an earlier proliferative phase and often a more secure wound earlier. However, Van Winkle et al. examined the collagen synthesis of dog wounds and found no differences with a variety of suture materials tested.[187] Interestingly, in tensile strength tests of the same wounds the wound strength was greater at 70 days for the absorbable than for the nonabsorbable sutures. The investigators speculated that these results might have been caused by the greater rate of infection seen with nonabsorbable sutures. Stainless steel was not tested in this study, but at least one author claims that it results in the greatest tensile strength at 2 weeks.[155]

Cutting out. Some sutures are stiff and have more of a tendency to cut through some tissues than others. This is particularly a problem with sutures that have a low elasticity and a high tensile strength, such as Vicryl or Dexon. Inflammatory reaction around a suture may lead to softening of the sutured tissue. Cutting out of sutures is more likely within such weakened tissues, leading to initially weaker wounds.

Cutting out is also affected by suture size. The larger the suture caliber, the greater is the force required to cut through the tissue.[191] This is because a large-caliber suture generates less force per unit area on tissue than a small-caliber suture of equal tension does. There appears to be no significant difference in the cutting out tendency between silk and nylon of comparable *USP* sizes, possibly because silk is only slightly larger than nylon at each *USP* size.

Infection induction. In the classic experiment by Elek and Conen in 1957,[58] it was shown that silk suture material greatly aided in the production of infection. They found that an inoculum of only 3×10^2 organisms (*Staphylococ-*

POTENTIATION OF INFECTION BY SUTURES

	Nonabsorbable	Absorbable
↑	Cotton	Catgut
Highest	Silk	
	Stainless Steel	
	Polyester	Polyglycolic acid
		Polyglactin 910
	Nylon (multifilament)	
	Nylon (monofilament)	
	Polypropylene	
	Tape	

---

cus aureus) produced infection when introduced into the skin on a silk suture. Without this suture the same infection required 2 to 8 million organisms; therefore the silk suture multiplied the effective virulence by approximately 10,000.

The physical configuration of the suture has also been demonstrated to enhance infection. In general, suture materials that are twisted or braided have been shown to potentiate infection.[3,93,172] The tighter the braid was, the less the infection-enhancing qualities of suture turned out to be. Apparently bacteria become entrapped within the interstices of suture material.[35] Bacteria that become entrapped in the interstices of the braided or twisted suture are probably in the privileged position of being protected from the action of leukocytes; they can thus support and prolong infection as they leak into the surrounding tissue.[141,142] Monofilamentous suture material, such as nylon, is not likely to enhance infection.

It is generally felt that knots in suture material offer a harbor for bacteria and therefore the number of throws should be minimized, particularly on buried sutures. However, Greaney induced no difference in infection between knotted and unknotted polypropylene (Prolene).[71]

Some think that the chemical structure of the suture material also contributes to its ability to potentiate infection.[55] For instance, among the nonabsorbable monofilamentous sutures, polypropylene resulted in less infection than nylon. Stainless steel, as either monofilament or multifilament, resulted in a high incidence of infection. This may be caused by the metal's stiffness, which does not allow the metal suture to conform tightly to its pathway, leading to tissue damage and infection. The relative ability of several suture types to potentiate infection is listed in the box above.

It is important to emphasize that all suture materials, regardless of composition or configuration, enhance infection. When sutures have been compared with the taping of wounds, the rate of infection is increased three times in potentially contaminated wounds.[47] In one study the infection rate of nylon monofilament–sutured contaminated wounds in mice was higher than that in unsutured tissue with needle tracts contaminated with bacteria.[54]

Bactericidal properties. It has been suggested that some suture materials or suture-degradation products, in particular polyglycolic acid, are themselves antibacterial or at least inhibit bacterial penetration.[54,108] This is based on the lower-than-expected infection rates with this material, which is braided.

Interesting new suture products that are themselves impregnated with antibacterial substances, for instance neomycin, have been successfully tested.[162] Actually this idea is not new: catgut was used in the early twentieth century impregnated with iodine or silver. The latter has been reported recently to have produced a localized argyria in the skin.[198]

Allergy. Allergy to suture material, particularly catgut, is discussed in the medical literature.[87,88] Circulating antibodies to catgut have been found in patients subsequent to surgery.[110] Chromic salts added to catgut may also be a source of allergy in those who are chromate sensitive. A possible allergic reaction to polyglactin 910 (Vicryl) has also been reported but is poorly documented as such.[121] Further evidence of an allergy to sutures is the occasional presence in tissue of the Splendore-Hoeppli phenomenon, amorphous eosinophilic deposits that are PAS positive but disastase resistant. Such deposits are thought to represent an antigen-antibody reaction and are occasionally found around parasites or fungi. Liber found a few cases of such deposits around silk sutures.[106]

Thrombogenicity. The ability of sutures to induce clotting of blood differs among suture materials. Polypropylene is the least thrombogenic of all suture materials by a wide margin, probably related to its extremely smooth surface, which also has a very low coefficient of friction.[50]

Work of withdrawal. On placement of a suture through the cutaneous surface, a downgrowth of epidermis forms along the suture path.[140] This perisutural cuff accounts for 70% to 85% of the work of suture withdrawal.[88] In addition, the tissue near the suture shows some growth into the suture. Those sutures with the greatest interaction with tissue have the most resistance. Silk tends to require greater work when withdrawn because of fibrous ingrowth into the braids of material. Polypropylene requires little work when withdrawn because such ingrowth and tissue interaction are minimal.

PREPARATION OF SUTURES

Modern surgical sutures are packaged under minimal handling conditions and sterilized with either ethylene oxide or ionizing radiation, usually gamma rays from cobalt-60 or gamma and x-rays from a linear accelerator. Sutures are packed within an inner foil suture packet which is in turn packaged within an exterior foil-and-plastic packet, called the overwrap, to help ensure sterility.

Ethicon, Inc. introduced around 1956 gamma- and electron-induced radiation as an industrial method for sterilizing surgical sutures in the final package.[81] It is thought that such radiation damages bacteria by ionization of vital cell components, especially DNA. Although this form of sterilization is capable of killing even bacterial spores, which formerly were a problem with catgut, a few organisms may be resistant to the recommended sterilizing dosage used (2.5 megarad). Therefore a high degree of hygiene must be used in production.[135,144] Viruses in particular may be radiation resistant.

Dosages for ionizing radiation must be carefully controlled or loss of tensile strength of suture material may result.[144] In fact a few suture materials (Vicryl, Dexon, PDS, Prolene, cotton) are very susceptible to radiation damage and must be sterilized by ethylene oxide for this reason. However, at the recommended radiation dosages, there appear to be no substantive differences between gas and radiation sterilization for most suture materials with respect to either tensile strength or tissue reaction.[148]

TYPES OF SUTURES
Absorbable sutures

Sutures are somewhat arbitrarily divided into absorbable and nonabsorbable sutures. All sutures except stainless steel, polypropylene, and perhaps polyester are absorbable with time. The question is how fast and how completely a suture is absorbed.

At the beginning of the twentieth century Halsted astutely recognized the variation in absorption of suture when he stated "Catgut . . . No. 2 Chromaticized . . . was guaranteed by America's most reliable firm 'not to absorb' for twenty-six days, but not guaranteed 'to absorb' within as many weeks."[72] Absorbable sutures, mainly catgut, were recommended in infected wounds, and nonabsorbable sutures were preferred in clean wounds.[72,174]

The modern definition of an absorbable suture is one that loses most of its tensile strength by 60 days after implantation. Note that this definition does not say absorbs completely. There have been documented cases of catgut persisting in tissue for years.[153] Nylon, mistakenly thought by some to persist indefinitely in tissue, is actually partially degraded and begins to lose strength within 3 weeks after implantation.[138] At 6 months very thin nylon (5-0 or 6-0) may have almost no tensile strength left.[55]

Absorbable sutures are listed and compared in Table 8-1. They are either of animal origin (collagen) or synthetic. The synthetic sutures include polyglycolic acid (Dexon), polyglactin 910 (Vicryl), and polydioxanone (PDS).

Catgut. The origin of the name "catgut" is obscure, but may be a bastardization of "kitgut," referring to the string of a small violin called the kit. Although catgut is used hardly at all in this modern age of synthetic absorbable sutures, it is worthwhile to review its history and development, since many surgical principles came to be developed in association with it. Moreover, catgut represents a standard against which modern surgical sutures are compared.

History. Catgut suture was used in the second century AD by both Galen and Antyllus the Greek. However, it fell into disuse until Dr. P. Syng Physick reintroduced it in 1816. Physick demonstrated that catgut was absorbed by placing it in purulent secretions of ulcers and observing it to disappear.[101] Because absorbable suture was believed to be advantageous, various methods were used to improve catgut. Lister in 1869 introduced the idea of antiseptic catgut sutures, which were subjected to antiseptics. Lister was also instrumental in the development of tanning catgut sutures with chromic salts, which increased the strength of the sutures and helped to delay their absorption.[111]

Catgut, however, was fraught with problems. It provoked large tissue reactions and was associated with infections. Kocher recognized this problem in 1881 and abandoned its use saying "Fort mit den Catgut [Away with the catgut]."[133] Halsted also tended to abandon its use, preferring silk sutures; he realized that absorbability of sutures was not the sine qua non of suture performance.

Surgeons during the twentieth century, however, continued their fascination with catgut. It was pliable, absorbable, and had the requisite tensile strength. Catgut is collagen, and therefore other sources of collagen were sought besides intestine. These included extruded collagen made from the flexor tendons of cattle[131] or even from tendons of the tail of the kangaroo (especially the wallaby).[119] Extruded collagen sutures are currently used in ophthalmology.[197] Impregnation of catgut with various antibacterial substances, such as iodine, was tried. Still, with the emergence of synthetic absorbable sutures in 1970, catgut sutures have fallen mostly into disuse in cutaneous surgery.

Preparation. Catgut, also called surgical gut, is derived from the intestinal submucosa of sheep or the intestinal serosa of cattle.[177] The gut is removed from the animal, stripped of its contents, and slit. After the submucosa is stripped free, the collagen is washed, and scraped free of fat and other adherent particles; it is twisted into strands of required sizes and sanded to a uniform caliber.[133] Surgical gut is packaged wet in alcohol and is damaged if allowed to dry out.

It should be emphasized that catgut is only 95% pure collagen. It may also contain other adherent substances that can be a source of irritant or allergic reactions, discussed later. These substances include muscle fibers, lipoproteins, mucoproteins, blood vessels, and glandular tissue.[6] Flaws and foreign bodies have also been detected in catgut, but perhaps they were caused by older manufacturing techniques.[97]

The "pure collagen" catgut may be subjected to chromic salts, which react with the collagen of catgut to produce a tougher, harder substance (tanning). This chromic catgut is

TABLE 8-1

Comparison between absorbable sutures

Name	Company	Material	Configuration	Tensile strength	Tissue reactivity	Handling
Collagen (plain)	Davis & Geck	Beef flexor tendon	Twisted	Poor (0% at 2-3 weeks)	Moderate	Fair
Collagen (chromic)	Davis & Geck	Beef flexor tendon	Twisted	Poor (0% at 2-3 weeks)	Moderate	Fair
Surgical gut (plain)	Ethicon Davis & Geck	Animal collagen	Twisted	Poor (0% at 2-3 weeks)	High	Fair
Surgical gut (chromic)	Ethicon Davis & Geck	Animal collagen	Twisted	Moderately poor (0% in 2-3 weeks)	Moderately high	Fair
Coated Vicryl	Ethicon	Polyglactin 910–coated	Braided	Good (50% at 2-3 weeks)	Low	Good
Dexon "S"	Davis & Geck	Polyglycolic acid	Braided	Good (50% at 2-3 weeks)	Low	Fair
Dexon Plus	Davis & Geck	Polyglycolic acid–coated	Braided	Good (50% at 2-3 weeks)	Low	Good
PDS	Ethicon	Polydioxanone	Monofilament	Good (50% at 4 weeks)	Low	Poor

stronger and more resistant to tissue degradation than plain (nonchromic) catgut is.

The chromium concentration to which the suture is exposed determines the absorbability of chromic catgut.[94,117] Formerly three different types of chromic catgut were thus produced: mild (10 day), medium (20 day), and extra (40 day). The mild chromic catgut was theoretically supposed to maintain its tensile strength for 10 days, the medium for 10 to 20 days, and the extra for 30 to 40 days. However, there is great variation in absorption rates between different batches of the same chromic catgut and between different manufacturers, so these distinctions are not as important as formerly thought.[94]

Catgut used to be impregnated with various antibacterial substances, including iodine and silver, to minimize infection and fend off absorption of the suture.[117] Recently there was one interesting case report of localized argyria from silver-impregnated sutures.[198]

Tissue reaction and absorption. Catgut acts as a foreign body in tissue and thus may act as a detriment to wound healing. On implantation a specific and orderly sequence of events occurs. First, the suture is hydrated by the tissue fluid, which results in loss of tensile strength. This in effect makes catgut a larger foreign body; moreover, the swelling of catgut loosens the knots, so knot security is relatively poor with this suture material. In comparison, the synthetic absorbable sutures—Dexon, for instance—are not subject to such swelling.

The second event is the enzymatic degradation of catgut. Lysosomal proteolytic enzymes, probably from polymorphonuclear leukocytes, are released and digest catgut beginning 12 hours after implantation and reaching a maximum in 3 days. This is followed by giant cells and other phagocytes invading and removing the debris, which occurs in the next 7 to 10 days. The absorbing cells remain primarily at the periphery of the suture but may appear within clefts in the suture itself.[153] Finally, fibroblasts appear, producing a fibrous scar.[102,186] Although catgut is usually completely absorbed in a short period of time, fragments of it have been detected 8 months and even years later.[153]

Plain and chromic catgut evoke different degrees of an inflammatory reaction. Plain catgut is a much more violent irritant than chromic catgut. Therefore, one sees a larger, more dense, and prolonged infiltrate around plain catgut. This results in slower wound healing but faster absorption with plain versus chromic catgut.[117] Plain catgut loses tensile strength much faster, in as little as 3 days.[91]

Catgut-sutured wounds also show edema for longer periods of time than do wounds sutured with synthetic absorbable sutures. However, the early collagen metabolism as measured by hydroxyproline content is nearly identical in wounds sutured with either silk or plain catgut.[2] Therefore the inflammatory reaction to catgut does not adversely affect wound healing, as one might expect, measured by collagen synthesis.

Knot security	Memory	Absorption	Degradation	Comments
Poor	Low	Unpredictable (12 weeks)	Proteolytic	Less impure than surgical gut
Poor	Low	Unpredictable (12 weeks)	Proteolytic	Less impure than surgical gut
Poor	Low	Unpredictable (12 weeks)	Proteolytic	May be ordered as "fast-absorbing gut" (Ethicon) for percutaneous sutures
Fair	Low	Unpredictable (14-80 days)	Proteolytic	Darker, more visible (Davis & Geck) Mild or extra chromatization (Davis & Geck)
Fair	Low	Predictable (80 days)	Hydrolytic	Coated with polyglactin 370 Clear, violet
Good	Low	Predictable (90 days)	Hydrolytic	Uncoated
Fair	Low	Predictable (90 days)	Hydrolytic	Coated with poloxamer 188 Clear, green
Poor	High	Predictable (180 days)	Hydrolytic	Clear, violet

The degree of chromatization and its relationship to the speed of loss of tensile strength and thus absorption of catgut have already been discussed. It is thought that the chromium prevents digestion, and that when this disappears, absorption (digestion) begins. The greater the chromium concentration on the suture material, the slower the absorption. Interestingly, the large chromic sutures are not necessarily degraded more slowly than the small chromic sutures.[17]

Other factors exist that may also influence absorption of catgut. Wound infection is known to speed its absorption.[186] Species differences also occur, pointing up the difficulties of extrapolating animal studies to man. The uniformity of catgut, both plain and chromic, also varies from manufacturer to manufacturer and even between similar batches from the same manufacturer.

Advantages and current usage. The absorbability of catgut and its relative inexpensiveness are sometimes of value, particularly in open wounds. Complete negativism about its use is premature but exists. For instance, according to Laufman, "Catgut [will be] relegated to limbo—with a fond farewell—to join other historically important surgical devices of their day, such as *bec de corbin,* the flaxen threads, and gutta percha"[100]; however, catgut may still have a place under certain circumstances.

Webster et al. recommended the use of 6-0 mild chromic suture for cutaneous interrupted sutures (not buried).[189] The authors found that the mild chromic catgut made by Davis & Geck is particularly prone to early absorption and therefore ideal for this purpose. The sutures dissolve away by 3 to 4 days, making suture cross-hatching unlikely. This technique is also mentioned by other authors for use on the eyelids, where wound healing is quick and early suture removal can be performed.[84] My own experience is that the technique of using mild chromic suture for percutaneous sutures has unpredictable results. As pointed out by others, the less the chromium content of catgut, the less reliable the suture is.[117] Some batches of suture dissolve faster or slower than others; moreover, some patients tend to develop a reaction to the suture material itself.

Recently Ethicon has introduced a new catgut suture named "Fast-Absorbing Gut." This catgut is nonchromatized but is heat treated twice. The extra heat treatment lessens the catgut tensile strength and makes it more susceptible to tissue degradation. The fast-absorbing catgut suture is available on a fine, extra-sharp needle, the PC-1. Whether it performs better than the mild chromic catgut suture made by Davis & Geck has not yet been demonstrated satisfactorily. Both suture materials theoretically have similar disadvantages if used for percutaneous sutures.

Another reported use of catgut sutures is in children, to avoid suture removal. In fact one orthopedic surgeon claims that plain catgut is an excellent choice for percutaneous suturing on the hands, especially of children, to obviate the need for suture removal.[166] I predict that this would be fraught with the same difficulties already mentioned, in

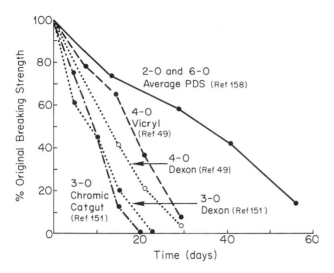

Fig. 8-2. Breaking strength loss of buried absorbable sutures.[151]

addition to which sutures on the hands need to be left a longer time than those on the face.

The Russians have recently found an interesting use of catgut on leg ulcers to stimulate wound healing.[169] Basically this takes advantage of the inflammatory reaction and subsequent granulation tissue stimulation that these sutures may provoke.

As mentioned earlier I use chromic catgut to ligate vessels of wounds that are left open to heal by granulation and epidermization. This may help to stimulate granulation, although my treatment is based more on the economy of the material.

Another use of catgut is in suturing of the nasal mucosa, where one wishes the sutures to fall (dissolve) out because of their inaccessibility at the time of suture removal. Vicryl or Dexon can be used for this purpose, but as discussed later, these sutures frequently take much longer to dissolve in this location.

Disadvantages. Some batches of catgut tend to have less tensile strength than others, which results in easier breaking of the suture material when tying. In addition to the problems with tissue reaction already mentioned, catgut does not maintain tensile strength in tissue as well as most synthetic nonabsorbable sutures do (Fig. 8-2). This is partially because knot slippage is great with catgut.[77,90,117] The wetting of catgut that occurs in tissue decreases its breaking strength.[197] As every string musician (or tennis aficionado) knows, wet catgut strings become soft and elastic; moreover, because catgut is twisted, it tends to fray when broken.

Sterility of catgut used to be a major problem before the advent of ionizing radiation for sterilization. In the first half of the twentieth century catgut was sterilized chemically, or by heating, or both. Unfortunately this was not totally successful in eradicating all pathogenic organisms; organisms

persisted in the center of the suture, and as the catgut dissolved, patients became infected. Stitch abscesses used to be commonplace when buried catgut was used. In one 1943 study, for instance, 20% of all catgut-sutured wounds became infected, compared to an infection incidence of only 4.7% to 7.8% in wounds sutured with nonabsorbable sutures (for instance, silk or nylon).[113] In an interesting 1931 study organisms responsible for gas gangrene were found in 12% of all catgut sutures examined.[127] The authors were prompted to perform this study by two cases of gas gangrene that had been traced to the catgut sutures used. Fortunately, since ionizing radiations (gamma rays from cobalt-60 or x-rays and gamma rays from a linear accelerator) are currently used to sterilize catgut, these problems are a thing of the past.

Allergy to catgut is discussed in the medical literature.[6,87,88] Although patients sensitized to chromic salts may react to chromic catgut, plain catgut may also be antigenic. It is possible to sensitize rabbits or guinea pigs to catgut.[87] In a study performed on patients who underwent eye surgery with catgut, 32% of the patients developed allergic reactions by 2 weeks to buried plain catgut in the forearm.[9]

Polyglycolic acid. In about 1970 the first synthetic absorbable suture, Dexon, was introduced.[5,150] This suture material is polyglycolic acid (PGA), a high molecular–weight linear chain polymer of glycolic acid (hydroxyacetic acid). The general chemical formula is the following:

$$\left(-\overset{\overset{\displaystyle O}{\|}}{C} - \overset{\overset{\displaystyle H}{|}}{\underset{\underset{\displaystyle H}{|}}{C}} - O - O \right)_n$$

The polymer is liquefied and then extruded through spinnerettes to form filaments, which are subsequently stretched and braided.[54] Because this material is recommended for total implantation in the human body, it was the first suture material to be categorized as a drug and thus subjected to the same testing and standards as other drugs, as well as requiring FDA approval for use.

Configuration and physical characteristics. The configuration of Dexon is braided, which allows easy handling and tying and thus does not fray like catgut. The uncoated surface is, however, not smooth, which causes drag through tissues. The cross-sectional area at each gauge is slightly smaller for Dexon than for nylon or silk and much smaller than for catgut.[78] It is manufactured both clear and, for easier visibility, green; the latter dye is drug and cosmetic green No. 6.[101]

The roughened surface of Dexon as initially manufactured made it difficult to tie and set the knot. This was referred to as "hanging up." There was the added disadvantage of increased drag as the material was pulled through tissue. The manufacturer (Davis & Geck) has since then

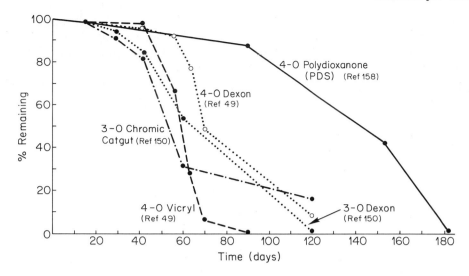

Fig. 8-3. Relative absorption rates of buried absorbable sutures.

made a coated Dexon suture (Dexon Plus) that slips through tissue and ties much more easily than the original Dexon (now called Dexon "S") did. The lubricant coating on Dexon Plus is Poloxamer 188, which is eliminated from the body within a few days. The manufacturer has continued to manufacture the uncoated Dexon "S" because it has greater knot security compared to the more slippery coated Dexon Plus.

Tissue reaction and absorption. The degradation of Dexon into CO_2 and H_2O occurs by hydrolysis, which is accelerated by enzymes released by macrophages or other cells in the inflammatory infiltrates.[194] Specifically, esterase and carboxypeptidase work best to facilitate the hydrolysis reaction. However, the primary biodegradation of Dexon sutures occurs independent of cellular activity and requires only an aqueous environment. The rate of this degradation is pH dependent, being slower in an acid pH (found in infections) and faster in an alkaline environment.[40] In contrast to catgut, Dexon stimulates a much reduced inflammatory reaction, and phagocytosis is not prominent.

The rate of Dexon absorption, like that of any suture, depends on the size used, its depth (subcutaneous tissue, muscle, fat), and its location (head and neck versus extremities). In animal studies Dexon was almost completely absorbed in 90 to 120 days,[49,150] whereas similarly sized chromic catgut was still present to a significant degree during the same time interval (Fig. 8-3). A small (4-0) Dexon suture was shown to disappear in 5 weeks.[159]

The loss of breaking strength of Dexon is similar to that of chromic catgut at 7 days (both lose about a third of their strength), but at 14 days the loss of strength of PGA (80%) is significantly greater than that of catgut (40%).[150] On the other hand, another study found that catgut and Dexon lost tensile strength at the same rate (90% in 15 days)[76] (Fig. 8-2). The absolute breaking strength of Dexon was superior to that of catgut at 5 to 10 days when implanted into dogs

and rats but not rabbits[151]; thus part of the reason for discrepancies in these studies are variations between the types of animals in which sutures were implanted.

Advantages. When Dexon was introduced,[4] it was compared with catgut, and several advantages were noted.[19] Unlike catgut, Dexon provoked minimal inflammatory infiltrate and little fibrous tissue reaction. In addition, Dexon could be easily standardized and sterilized, both of which were significant problems with catgut. Catgut, being of animal origin, also carried the potential of being antigenic, whereas Dexon, being synthetic, was nonantigenic. Most important was the fact that Dexon was predictably and completely absorbed at an earlier time than catgut.

One further advantage of Dexon is that it does not swell when wet as catgut does. Swelling results in a loss of knot strength for catgut as well as production of a larger foreign body. It is estimated that Dexon should therefore have 1.4 times as much wet knot strength as chromic catgut.[90] The rough surface of uncoated Dexon, already mentioned, adds to the knot security.

Compared to Vicryl, Dexon is slightly smaller at each *USP* gauge size. Theoretically this means that less suture is buried. Vicryl, unlike Dexon, is available only as a coated suture. Some feel that coated Dexon has less tissue drag and better knot security than coated Vicryl.[164]

Disadvantages. Because Dexon is braided, bacteria may become trapped in the interstices of the suture. Although an increased infection rate with this suture was reported early on in potentially contaminated wounds,[65] it is probably of no consequence in clean wounds.

Dexon has a high tensile strength and lack of elasticity, so it tends to cut through tissue. Moreover, if buried close to the wound surface, it may be extruded (spit).

Soon after its introduction Dexon was reported to be associated with hypertrophic scarring.[48,165] This was disputed by others and shown to be untrue when looked at critically in controlled studies.[7,95,145]

One might wonder if the dye used for colored Dexon leaves a tattoo. A study found no residual dye after absorption of the suture material.[159] A colored line seen during the month after suturing (if the green Dexon is used) is caused by incomplete absorption, but with complete absorption this disappears. I have noticed a similar phenomenon with colored Vicryl (see Fig. 10-66, *B*).

Uses. Dexon is useful as a buried suture to help maintain apposition of wound surfaces until healing is complete. Since it is absorbed with few problems, it is ideal for this purpose.

It has been suggested that Dexon may be used for interruptured percutaneous sutures. Since they are absorbable, these sutures fall out by themselves.[1] However, since there is some variation in absorption at different sites, these sutures may need to be removed anyway, sometimes 3 or 4 weeks after placement.[65]

In the mouth one cannot predict when Dexon will be absorbed and fall out, in part because of its slow degradation in the acidic environment and the lack of enzyme activity here on this suture material.[196] Therefore, if interrupted Dexon sutures are used in this area, they may need to be removed manually.

Dexon should not be used in infected or potentially infected wounds. The braided configuration may potentiate infection, which has been reported to be greater than that with nylon[65] but less than that with silk.[1] Additionally, the low pH found in infected areas slows the absorption of Dexon,[196] leading to persistence of foreign body material. Bacteria themselves may adhere to the suture and thus present a physical barrier to suture degradation.[194]

Polyglactin 910. This synthetic suture, similar to Dexon, was introduced in 1974 by Ethicon and called Vicryl.[44] Unlike Dexon, which is a homopolymer of glycolic acid, Vicryl is a copolymer formed by polymerization of a mixture of purified lactide and glycolide (cyclic intermediates derived from lactic and glycolic acids). The proportions of the mixture are 9 parts glycolide and 1 part lactide. The copolymer is converted into particles of uniform size, which are melted and extruded into fine fibers. The resultant filamentous extrudate is braided. To ensure tighter braids and more uniform fibers, the sutures are heat stretched. Finally the sutures are sterilized in ethylene oxide and packaged dry in an inert gas to prevent atmospheric moisture from degrading the suture material.[122]

Configuration and physical characteristics. Polyglactin 910 is braided and reported to be nonantigenic, nonpyrogenic, and noncarcinogenic. The thread itself has high fluid uptake but low capillarity. Vicryl's tensile strength is extremely high, second only (among absorbable sutures) to that of Dexon. However, this has led to Vicryl being smaller than catgut sutures at various sizes (suture sizes are determined by tensile strength), but slightly larger than Dexon.

Vicryl may be purchased as either undyed or colored. The colorant is drug and cosmetic violet No. 2 dye. Since 1980 all Vicryl has been manufactured with a coating that consists of a mixture of calcium stearate and a copolymer, polyglactin 370 (derived from 65% lactide and 35% glycolide). This allows smooth passage of the suture through tissue and smooth knot tying. The uncoated Vicryl had previously been described as "grabby" and thus difficult to handle[46]; however, the coated Vicryl has the disadvantage of holding knots less securely and therefore requiring more ties (four) than the uncoated Vicryl required (two) for adequate knot strength.[97]

Tissue reaction and absorption. Vicryl is an absorbable suture that like Dexon is broken down mainly by hydrolysis. The degradation is a two-step process.[168] Initially an aqueous environment adds water, which results in the breakdown of polyglactin 910 to lactic and glycolic acids. These acids are broken down, in the second step, to CO_2 and H_2O by oxidative enzyme systems in macrophages. In an interesting experiment polyglactin 910 was soaked in water for 14 days and then implanted in animals.[168] The suture was degraded two weeks later, as if it had been implanted for 28 days. In other words the hydrolysis depends solely on water. The degradation occurs faster in an alkaline than an acid environment.[41]

The histologically determined absorption of 4-0 Dexon is slower than that of 4-0 Vicryl (Fig. 8-3). In rats at 42 days, 99% of Vicryl and 97% of Dexon was still present. At 63 days, 26% of Vicryl was left, compared with 77% of Dexon.[49] At 90 days Vicryl had completely disappeared; Dexon, however, was still present at 120 days. In rabbits, on the other hand, 100% of 3-0 Vicryl remained at 5 days, 95% at 10 days, 60% at 30 days, and none at 60 days.[44] It is interesting to note the different rates of absorption between species. Vicryl was also compared with silk and chromic catgut.[44] At 30 days 60% of Vicryl remained whereas 75% of chromic catgut and 90% of silk were present.

Another method of assessing suture absorption is to test the breaking strength or tensile strength of the suture after various periods of implantation. Vicryl loses strength more slowly in tissue, even though catgut is more slowly absorbed.[122] Vicryl is also reported to retain breaking strength longer than Dexon (Fig. 8-2).[49] All strength is lost at 30 days for both 4-0 Vicryl and 4-0 Dexon.

Vicryl and Dexon were both developed so that complete absorption would be faster than with catgut and thus inflammatory reaction with subsequent foreign body reaction would be minimized. The inflammatory tissue response to Vicryl has been described as slight foreign-body reactive—certainly less than with catgut but similar to that with Dexon.[49] The cellular reactions are usually lymphohistiocytic (Fig. 8-4). In the oral mucosa the inflammatory reaction of Vicryl is similar to that of silk.[157]

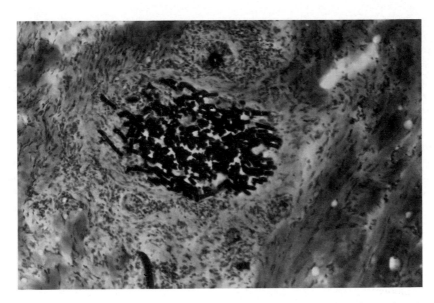

Fig. 8-4. Vicryl suture 4 weeks after implantation. Note mild lymphohistiocytic reaction. ($\times$ 100.)

Disadvantages. The high tensile strength and lack of elasticity of Vicryl cause some cutting through tissue, particularly if the tissue is pliable or soft. If Vicryl is placed too close to the surface of a cutaneous wound, the suture may be extruded (spit). In my experience newer coated Vicryl is more prone to be spit than the older, uncoated Vicryl. In addition I have found evidence of coated Vicryl 10 months after implantation, since absorption is slow. An initial reaction to Vicryl may also appear as a "lump" underneath an incision line that resolves with time. This again is more common with the new coated Vicryl.

Uses. Vicryl is most useful as a completely buried intradermal suture to approximate wound edges closely. Theoretically this suture does not lose significant tensile strength until the wound itself has gained enough tensile strength to keep the wound edges from spreading. When a fine scar is desirable, such as on the face, Vicryl, as either a subcutaneous or subcuticular buried suture, aids in taking tension off the epidermal wound edges. It handles like silk because it is braided. The purple Vicryl may be used for visibility, but I almost always use the white undyed suture, since the dyed suture may show through the skin, albeit temporarily, (see Fig. 10-66, *B*). Once the undyed Vicryl comes through the tissue, it becomes stained with blood, which increases its visibility anyway.

It should be stressed that Vicryl probably does not add much to the strength of a wound after 15 to 20 days.[49,137] This is because wound healing has progressed to a significant degree by that time. Furthermore, in individuals with poor wound-healing ability, its use (like that of other absorbable sutures) may not be as advantageous, since by the time significant tensile strength of the suture is lost, significant wound strength may not be present. Also, on wounds on the trunk or extremities (where spreading of

scars inevitably occurs) subcutaneous closure materials are of less value, despite claims to the contrary.

Sometimes Vicryl is used in the oral or nasal cavities for permucosal sutures because it is soft and therefore nonirritating. However, in these locations it does not dissolve out as soon as catgut. As previously pointed out, degradation of absorbable synthetic sutures (Vicryl or Dexon) in this environment is slower because of the lower pH. Therefore one should have the patient back to remove the sutures, just as one would do for a patient with silk sutures.

Occasionally physicians attempt to use Vicryl sutures as interrupted cutaneous sutures with the hope that they will dissolve out on their own. This should be discouraged because the capillarity of braided sutures, such as Vicryl, helps to induce bacterial infection of the wound (see Fig. 4-16).

Polydioxanone. A relatively new addition to the array of absorbable sutures is PDS (polydioxanone). This suture material was formulated to provide continuous wound support for an extended period of time. PDS is poly-p-dioxanone, a polymer made from paradioxanone in the presence of a catalyst. The final chemical formula is:

$$\left(-O - \overset{\overset{\displaystyle H}{|}}{\underset{\underset{\displaystyle H}{|}}{C}} - \overset{\overset{\displaystyle H}{|}}{\underset{\underset{\displaystyle H}{|}}{C}} - O - \overset{\overset{\displaystyle H}{|}}{\underset{\underset{\displaystyle H}{|}}{C}} - \overset{\overset{\displaystyle O}{\|}}{C} - \right)_n$$

The addition of the ether group in the backbone helps to make this suture flexible in the monofilamentous state—unlike Vicryl, which is much stiffer as a monofilament. The polymer is processed into small granules, which are dried and melted, extruded into monofilaments that are stretched and heat treated. The polymer is colorless and cystal-

TABLE 8-2

Comparison of nonabsorbable sutures

Generic or trade name	Company	Material	Configuration	Tensile strength	Tissue reactivity
Cotton	—	Cotton	Twisted	Good	High
Silk	Ethicon, Davis & Geck	Silk	Braided or twisted	Good	High
Ethilon	Ethicon	Polyamide (nylon)	Monofilament	High	Low
Dermalon	Davis & Geck	Polyamide (nylon)	Monofilament	High	Low
Nurolon	Ethicon	Polyamide (nylon)	Braided	High	Moderate
Surgilon	Davis & Geck	Polyamide (nylon) (coated with silicone)	Braided	High	Moderate
Prolene	Ethicon	Polyolefin (polypropylene)	Monofilament	Fair	Low
Surgilene	Davis & Geck	Polyolefin (polypropylene)	Monofilament	Fair	Low
Dermalene	Davis & Geck	Polyolefin (polyethylene)	Monofilament	Good	Low
Novafil	Davis & Geck	Polybutester	Monofilament	High	Low
Mersilene	Ethicon	Polyester	Braided	High	Moderate
Dacron	DeKnatel, Davis & Geck	Polyester	Braided	High	Moderate
Ethibond	Ethicon	Polyester (coated with poly- butilate)	Braided	High	Moderate
Ti-Cron	Davis & Geck	Polyester (coated with silicone)	Braided	High	Moderate
Polydek	DeKnatel	Polyester (coated with Teflon— light)	Braided	High	Moderate
Tevdek	DeKnatel	Polyester (coated with Teflon— heavy)	Braided	High	Moderate
Stainless steel	Ethicon	Stainless steel	Monofilament, twisted or braided	High	Low

line and manufactured as undyed and dyed. The added color is drug and cosmetic violet No. 2 dye. It is sterilized by ethylene oxide.[105,158]

Physical configuration. PDS is the only synthetic absorbable suture manufactured as a monofilament. It is somewhat flexible, compared with other synthetic absorbable sutures that are manufactured as monofilaments rather than braided multifilaments.

Tissue reactivity and absorption. PDS elicits a minimal tissue reaction. In studies performed on rats it was found to be totally absorbed in 180 days, compared with 60 to 90 days for Vicryl and 120 days for Dexon (Fig. 8-3). Absorption occurs mainly by hydrolysis, as with other synthetic absorbable sutures. PDS is said to retain significant breaking strength (58%) at 28 days compared to Vicryl or Dexon (1% to 5%)[158] (Fig. 8-2).

Advantages and uses. PDS is useful as a buried suture when one desires increased wound strength for a longer period of time. PDS loses tensile strength at a slower rate than catgut, Vicryl, or Dexon (Fig. 8-2). It does not tend to cut through tissue, nor does it tend to fray like the braided absorbable sutures. In addition, because of its low tissue reactivity, slow degradation rate, and monofilamentous state, it may also be useful as a "universal suture." Among the absorbable sutures, PDS was shown to have the least affinity for adherence of bacteria.[42] Not enough experience has been gained at this point to evaluate its usefulness properly.

Handling	Knot security	Memory	Comments
Good	Good	Poor	Obsolete
Good	Good	Poor	Predisposes to infection; does not tear tissue; D & G suture is silicone treated; Ethicon is waxed
Poor	Poor	High	Cuts tissues; black, clear, and green
Poor	Poor	High	
Good	Fair	Fair	May predispose to infection; black or white; waxed
Fair	Fair	Fair	
Poor	Poor	High	Very low coefficient of friction; blue and clear
Poor	Poor	High	
Poor	Poor	High	
Fair	Poor	Low	Blue or clear
Good	Good	Fair	Green or white
Good	Good	Fair	
Good	Good	Fair	Green and white
Poor	Poor	Fair	
Good	Good	Fair	
Poor	Poor	Fair	
Poor	Good	Poor	May kink

Disadvantages. PDS is in my experience somewhat stiff and difficult to handle and tie, despite claims to the contrary.[20]

Nonabsorbable sutures

The nonabsorbable sutures are listed and compared in Table 8-2. As mentioned previously, if buried, almost all these sutures are eventually degraded and absorbed, with the possible exceptions of polyester, polypropylene, and stainless steel sutures. For that reason the term "nonabsorbable" is useful only in the generic—not the literal—sense.

Silk. The use of silk sutures for clean wounds and even for buried sutures was advocated and taught by Halsted in the early twentieth century.[72] This led to its widespread use, which still has its proponents.

Silk is made from the natural protein (fibroin) fiber extruded by the silkworm larva as it fashions a cocoon. The new fibers are processed to remove natural waxes and gums. Surgical silk is further treated to decrease its capillarity. In "dermal silk," the fibers are encased by a tanned protein substance (such as gelatin) to prevent ingrowth of tissue along the suture tract.[177] Raw silk is white; surgical silk is dyed with black vegetable dye.

Configuration. Modern silk is braided rather than twisted, as it was in Halsted's time. Braided sutures have higher tensile strength than twisted sutures have.[124] There are minor braiding differences between different manufacturers:

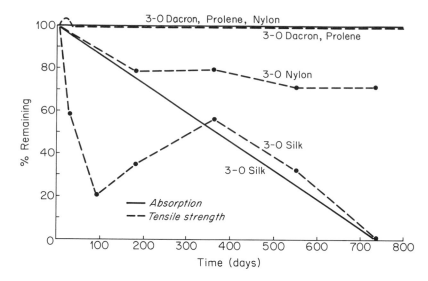

Fig. 8-5. Relative absorption rates and tensile strength loss of buried "nonabsorbable" sutures.[149]

Ethicon, for instance, produces a silk suture with a wide braiding angle, which results in a more flexible fiber. The caliber (cross-sectional area) of silk is slightly larger than that of comparable *USP*-sized nylon or Dexon, but smaller than that of wet catgut (Fig. 8-1).

Tissue reaction and absorption. Silk is classified as a nonabsorbable suture, but in reality it is slowly absorbed over many months (Fig. 8-5). Silk sutures implanted in rabbits were observed to absorb in 2 years, but the loss of tensile strength was somewhat variable.[149] Approximately 10% of the tensile strength was lost in 1 week, 20% at 2 weeks, and 50% at 1 year.[149,150] However, in some animals there was no tensile strength in 1 month.

The initial histologic reaction to silk is a leukocytic response within 24 hours, followed by a histiocytic response within 7 days.[39] By 3 weeks the suture is surrounded by a fibrous capsule, but occasionally invasion of the suture may be seen from fibrocytes or histiocytes. Rarely does a granuloma form. These reactions to silk show little change over time.[153]

Silk sutures are probably degraded by hydrolytic enzymes, especially acid phosphatase and leucine aminopeptidase, which are found at sites of silk fiber implantation.[167] These enzymes are usually associated with macrophage and giant cell populations.

Advantages and uses. Silk handles well, ties well, and is soft. This last quality makes it extremely useful for the oral mucosa, lips, intertriginous areas, and conjunctiva, where one wishes to avoid the bristle effect of stiffer sutures, such as nylon.

Silk is less likely to tear tissue than stiffer materials are. This quality makes silk useful as a temporary suture during surgery to elevate or retract tissue for greater visibility.

Silk ties well and results in excellent knot security. As pointed out by Holmlund, modern silk should be tied with three square throws.[83] When knot security is desirable because of tension—for instance, when tying a large exposed blood vessel or performing a tarsorrhaphy—silk is excellent. Under these circumstances the disadvantages of silk are overshadowed by more pressing considerations. Where wound healing is fast—for instance, on the eyelids—and sutures may be removed within 3 days, silk may be useful. Under these circumstances the silk may be removed before the intense inflammatory reaction. Another distinct advantage of silk is its low cost.

Disadvantages. Because silk has some capillary action, it tends to promote and even prolong infection in wounds. Furthermore, wound healing may be prolonged under such circumstances[89] and wound strength decreased.[30] When infection exists, a persistent sinus may develop that does not heal until the suture is removed or expelled.[124] It is interesting to note that there was a recent malpractice suit arising from a physician's ignorance that such an event could occur.[125] Even if infection is not induced dermal inflammatory reaction (including granuloma formation) to silk is much greater than with monofilamentous sutures,[107,149,153] although on a highly vascular area such as the scalp this might not be the case.[14]

Silk swells on implantation, increasing its diameter by 70% if left in place for as long as 14 days.[85] Moreover, silk becomes encrusted with and infiltrated by debris, which makes suture removal painful and more difficult.[67]

Cotton and linen. Cotton and linen sutures are little used in cutaneous surgery but are included here for historical interest. Cotton sutures are made from individual long cotton fibers, which are combed and twisted into a strand. Because it is twisted, cotton has less tensile strength than braided silk. Like silk, cotton evokes a significant tissue reaction.[149] Ochsner was a great proponent of cotton sutures in the 1930s and 1940s.[124] He claimed that compared to silk, cotton produced less tissue reaction and earlier wound healing with few problems. Surgeons preferring cotton were called "cotton men," as distinguished from the "silk men" who preferred silk. Cotton was a popular suture material during World War II when silk was relatively nonavailable.

Another suture material once used was linen, which dates back to Greco-Roman times. Linen is composed of twisted strands of flax fibers. Because it was difficult to control the cross-sectional diameter or tensile strength characteristics, these sutures are rarely used anymore. Both cotton and linen are referred to as "sutures of the field."

Nylon. Nylon was the first synthetic suture; it was introduced into surgery in 1940 as a result of polymer chemistry. The DuPont corporation was instrumental in its conception, inception, and surgical applications.

Surgical nylon (usually nylon 6,6) is a synthetic polyamide polymer fiber formed by condensation polymerization between adipic acid (an acid with more than one $-COOH$ group) and hexamethylenediamine (an amino with more than one $-NH_2$ group). The resultant polyamide is formed by elimination of water and may be extruded into monofilamentous, noncapillary single strands. Nylon fibers are long linear molecules that can be stretched and oriented along the axis of the fiber. The formula for nylon 6,6 is the following:

$$\left(-\underset{\underset{O}{\|}}{C}(CH_2)_4\,\underset{\underset{O}{\|}}{C}-\underset{\overset{|}{H}}{N}(CH_2)_6\,\underset{\overset{|}{H}}{N}- \right)_n + H_2O$$

Nylon is chemically inert and withstands repeated steam sterilizations without deterioration. It is unaffected by temperatures up to 455° F (235° C), at which point it melts.

Configuration and physical characteristics. Surgical nylon is manufactured in either monofilamentous or multifilamentous configurations. The monofilament is used most commonly. Ethilon is the monofilament manufactured by Ethicon; Dermalon is made by Davis & Geck. The multifilamentous nylon is braided with either a silicone coating (Surgilon) or a wax coating (Nurolon). The brading of nylon makes the suture more pliable and thus improves its handling characteristics; however, it also increases the capillarity of the suture, increasing the chance that bacteria may be drawn into a wound. Nevertheless, some believe the incidence of infection to be related more to the chemical structure of the suture than to its overall physical configuration; this is based on studies of the incidence of infection with various suture materials.[55] The investigators found a low incidence of infection with nylon whether it was braided or coated. Multifilamentous nylons are of little use in cutaneous surgery and are very expensive.

Monofilamentous nylon may be ordered black, green, or clear. The last is used when permanently burying suture underneath epidermis because it is not seen through the skin. Green nylon is useful for percutaneous sutures in hairbearing areas, where black sutures may be confused with black hairs. Although monofilamentous nylon is somewhat stiff and thus does not handle as easily as silk, it evokes much less tissue response. It has a high memory, so it requires more properly tied knots to be securely tied.

The dry (unburied) tensile strength of nylon is high and greater than that of silk[9] or Prolene.[136] However, in my experience nylon is stiffer, more inelastic, and less plastic than Prolene is. Nylon may be ordered in sizes 2 through 11-0, the smallest caliber suture made of any type.

Tissue reaction and absorption. Nylon is classified as nonabsorbable. This has led to the misconception that if it is buried, the loss in tensile strength is minimal and that most of the initial strength remains indefinitely.[84] In reality nylon is degraded if buried and loses significant tensile strength (Fig. 8-5). How quickly this occurs depends on the caliber of the suture and the site in which it is placed.[132]

The tissue degradation of nylon suture is caused by a slow hydrolysis of the polymer; the bonds break and the polymer chains shorten.

The importance of the caliber of nylon in determining absorption time was pointed out by Moloney.[132] This investigator found that very thick nylon (No. 2 or No. 5) retained two thirds of its initial strength after 11 years in human subjects, whereas the thinner nylon (2-0) used in cutaneous suturing retained no tensile strength after having been buried in tissues for 6 months. Moloney concluded that such thin nylon added no permanent strength to the wound. In another report nylon ruptured spontaneously in 3 patients 17 to 26 months after delicate ophthalmic surgery.[26] Obviously very thin nylon was used. In another study of various sutures implanted in rabbits, 3-0 nylon retained about 75% of its initial tensile strength at 2 years.[149]

How early degradation of nylon begins is unknown, but at least one investigator found a decrease in strength of buried 6-0 nylon as early as 3 weeks.[138] Burying nylon also appears to make it more stiff, which increases its tendency to cut through tissue.

Nylon evokes the least inflammatory response of the synthetic sutures, except for polypropylene (Prolene) or stainless steel.[152] As early as 1943 nylon was observed to shorten the initial inflammatory (lag) phase of wound healing, which resulted in earlier wound healing and initially stronger wounds than with silk or catgut.[112] If left buried, nylon is eventually encapsulated, as are the other "nonabsorbable" sutures, by a thin rim of fibrous tissue.[152]

Advantages. The low inflammatory reaction to nylon makes it an almost ideal suture for cutaneous surgery. This property outweighs any inconvenience of handling, since the patient ultimately benefits greatly with it.

Disadvantages. Monofilamentous nylon is somewhat stiff and difficult to tie. Its inherent high memory requires more care in knot tying and more throws to secure knots than with silk. In the mouth or lips it can be irritating, since the cut ends tend to bristle. In thin tissues the stiffness occasionally causes a cutting through the tissue, necessitating that it be handled gently (see Fig. 10-60). This is particularly a problem with very thin (6-0) nylon.

Uses. Monofilamentous nylon is excellent for cutaneous sutures, either interrupted or continuous. It is the workhorse of skin suturing. Its use as a permanently buried suture is of questionable value because the small-caliber sutures are eventually degraded. In studies comparing buried nylon with Vicryl, there was no difference seen in wound strength.[22] Because it is relatively inert, nylon may be used in infected tissues. Unlike silk it does not swell and thus results in less encroachment on the surrounding tissues.

Polypropylene. In 1962 polypropylene was introduced as a new suture material. Essentially a plastic, it is formed by the polymerization of propylene by means of a suitable catalyst. The plastic is extruded as monofilamentous fibers. Prolene (manufactured by Ethicon) and Surgilene (manufactured by Davis & Geck) are made of polypropylene. Dermalene (Davis & Greck) is made of polyethylene. Because of its chemical similarity to polypropylene it is included here.

Physical configuration and characteristics. Polypropylene is a flexible monofilament with fair tensile strength. It is the only synthetic suture produced only as a monofilament. Like nylon it evokes little tissue reactivity. It melts at 335° F (169° C), permitting autoclaving at lower temperatures. It may be ordered clear or blue. The suture is colored by copper phthalocyanine (pigment blue 15).[129,130]

One unique characteristic of polypropylene is its smooth surface. This results in a very low coefficient of friction, which allows one to pull this suture through tissue with very little drag. This makes for an ideal suture for a running intradermal (subcuticular) stitch, since it tends to slip out smoothly at the suture removal several days later. This is spoken of as "work of withdrawal" and has been calculated to be about one to two thirds that of nylon and a fourth to half that of silk.[67,85] The relatively smooth surface of polypropylene also makes it the least thrombogenic of suture materials.[50,84]

The low coefficient of friction also affects knot security. Being smoother, polypropylene knots tends to slip easily and should therefore be carefully set.

Another unique characteristic of polypropylene is its plasticity. By this one means that on relaxation, a stretched suture remains stretched, assuming a new length. There are differences in plasticity between various sizes of polypropylene sutures. The large 2-0 Prolene has been found to be more plastic than the small 6-0 size, for instance.[136] Plasticity allows knots to be deformed and thus more secure when set.

Tissue reaction and absorption. Like nylon, polypropylene has been found to evoke little tissue reaction.[129,167] At 21 days after implantation in rabbits no significant decrease was found in the tensile strength of polypropylene whereas it existed for nylon.[138] Polypropylene appears to persist in definitely in tissues.

Advantages and uses. Polypropylene is very useful, as already mentioned, for running intradermal sutures because they are easy to remove at the appropriate time (the work of withdrawal is less). Because of its elastic and plastic qualities, when a wound swells, this suture material is stretched and deformed with the wound, thus cutting less into the tissue. When wound swelling recedes, the suture is loose. This minimizes cross-hatch scarring.

Since polypropylene, like nylon, is unweakened by tissue enzymes, it is useful for suturing potentially infected wounds. Also, like nylon, polypropylene may be buried "permanently," but the long-term results of doing this in cutaneous surgery are of questionable value.

Disadvantages. Polypropylene has been reported to shed. Whether this results from rubbing one strand against the other when tying or is inherent in the material itself is unclear. However, because of this quality one should be careful while tying polypropylene to reduce abrasive contact between strands. Shedding or fragmentation of Prolene has been observed in vivo in 2% to 4% of cases.[129,149,152] In addition, bone and cartilage formation have been described in a small number of cases (2.5%) where this material was implanted in rabbits, but only after 29 months.[152] The causes of the fragmentation and bone formation are unknown and of little consequence clinically.

Polyethylene (Dermalene) has been noted in tissue to have minute cracks in its surface, which could be caused by stress.[67] This might lead to breaking and tissue ingrowth, making suture removal more difficult. Dermalene also has very poor knot-holding ability, compared with almost all other sutures.[180]

Polyester. Polyester fibers are polymers formed (like nylon) by condensation polymerization. Dacron, the basic suture material of this class, is formed in a condensation reaction from dimethyl terephthalate and ethylene glycol to yield the following:

$$\left(-\overset{\text{O}}{\underset{\|}{C}}-\bigcirc-\overset{\text{O}}{\underset{\|}{C}}-O-CH_2- \right)_n + CH_3OH$$

It should be stressed that methanol is lost in this condensation process, unlike nylon, from which water is eliminated. Since water is found on implantation in living tissue, nylon is more likely to be broken down by hydrolysis, whereas polyester is not. Dacron is dyed green to maximize visibility or may be purchased undyed for burying permanently.

Physical configuration and characteristics. All polyester sutures are multifilamentous and braided for better handling. The uncoated sutures are manufactured under the trade names of Mersilene (Ethicon) and Dacron (Davis & Greck). Because of the relatively rough surface, there is considerable drag through tissues and difficulty with knot tying. Lubricant coatings have been developed to overcome the grabby surface characteristics. Polyester may be coated either with Teflon (Ethiflex, Tevdek, Polydek), silicone (Ti-Cron), or polybutilate (Ethibond). Except for polybutilate, these coatings have no particular affinity for polyester fibers and are usually bonded to the suture filaments with an adhesive resin or are mechanically trapped in the braid.[45] The polybutilate coating is itself a polyester that has a natural affinity for the polyester suture strand. The problem with these coatings, except for polybutilate, is that pieces of coating may break off and cause tissue reactions described later. Moreover, lubricant coatings result in poor knot security.

Polyester fibers have high tensile strength, second only to that of metal sutures.[76] Still, if they are coated with the lubricants just mentioned, poor knot security results.

Tissue reactivity and absorption. Uncoated polyester, like nylon, usually causes little inflammatory reaction and if left buried over time evokes a few mononuclear cells and becomes surrounded by a fibrous tissue capsule.[149,152] In dogs, however, the inflammatory reaction and infection rate were great for Mersilene—similar to those for silk.[79] Furthermore, if polyester is coated by Teflon, fragments of the coating material may migrate into the tissues around the implanted sutures and elicit histiocytes, lymphocytes, or foreign body reactions.[45,152] On the other hand, polybutilate (the coating of Ethibond) has a natural affinity for polyester suture filaments and therefore does not migrate into surrounding tissue.[45]

Polyester sutures maintain their tensile strength longer and are less resorbable than even nylon sutures. Both polyester and polypropylene elicited less degradative enzyme activity on implantation than silk did.[167] Because nylon can be broken down in an aqueous environment, whereas polyester requires an alcohol, there is minimal degradation of polyester over time compared to nylon (Fig. 8-5).

Advantages and uses. Uncoated polyester sutures are difficult to pass through tissue and tie but theoretically are most useful if left buried for long lengths of time to preclude any widening of scars. Their high tensile strength makes them ideal to prevent this problem. There are, however, no studies to date that truly assess these sutures for this purpose. It should be pointed out that one may use smaller sutures of high tensile strength, like polyester, which result in less foreign body reaction.

The softness of braided polyester may be useful in the mouth and other mucous membrane sites, as well as in intertriginous areas. However, because it may produce the same degree of inflammation as silk and is much more expensive, it does not offer much advantage.

Disadvantages. The uncoated polyester sutures are difficult to work with, as just mentioned, and may act like silk in

promoting infection.[187] Moreover, Mersilene and Dacron tend to be spit when buried.[13] The high tensile strength of polyester results in a tendency for the suture to saw or tear through tissue. The coated polyesters tend to evoke inflammation and result in very insecure knots.[76] Ethibond, coated with polybutilate, is said to evoke less reaction.[45]

Polybutester. A new type of polyester, called polybutester (Novafil), has recently been introduced by Davis & Geck. It is a thermoplastic block copolymer composed of polyglycol terephthate (16%) and polybutylene terephthate (84%). Novafil is monofilamentous and can be purchased blue or clear. It combines many of the advantages of polypropylene with those of polyester. Of significance are its plastic qualities, which increase knot security and allow the suture to expand with wound swelling. However, when wound swelling subsides, the suture contracts somewhat. It has slightly better handling characteristics than polypropylene, and being monofilamentous it evokes less tissue reaction than do other available polyesters, which are braided. Since Novafil is relatively new, few studies have reported its use.

Stainless steel. The use of metal sutures goes back to the time of Galen in the second century AD, who mentions the use of gold wire. Silver wire was used in the latter part of the nineteenth century. With the development of stainless steel in the first half of the twentieth century, its use in surgery as a suture was recognized. Babcock was the early champion of stainless steel sutures; he referred to stainless steel as a "new noble metal" because it was so strong and resistant to chemical or thermal change.[15,16]

Type 316 L (*L* for low carbon) is the usual variety of stainless steel used for surgical sutures. Austenitic stainless steel is corrosion resistant but cannot be hardened by heat treatment. Besides iron it contains chromium, nickel, and carbon. Molybdenum is added to increase resistance to corrosion and pitting.[27]

Physical characteristics and configuration. Monofilamentous and multifilamentous stainless steel can be purchased. The latter is twisted or braided. Regardless of configurations, stainless steel suture material provides the greatest tensile strength and knot security (which is particularly high) of all suture types[76]; it is relatively inert. However, it is difficult to handle, and kinks can occur.

The diameter (gauge) of stainless steel sutures is identified by the B & S (Brown and Sharpe) classification, which is different from the *USP* diameter size classifications. The smallest diameter of stainless steel is size 40 B & S, which corresponds approximately to size 6-0 *USP*. Other useful sizes in cutaneous surgery are 36 B & S (5-0), 33 B & S (4-0), and 30 B & S (3-0).

Absorption and tissue reaction. Stainless steel is nonabsorbable and relatively inert. Although clean wounds closed with stainless steel have been reported to be relatively free of infection,[16] Edlich et al.[55] reported a high incidence of infection. The latter investigators ascribed this to the stiff metal not completely conforming to the suture pathway, and thus leading to tissue damage and infection.

Because surgical stainless steel contains some nickel, one might be concerned about allergic reactions in nickel-sensitive individuals. Since the nickel is rather tightly bound, this is more likely for patients in whom the stainless steel is left buried over a long period of time.

Advantages and uses. Stainless steel is relatively inexpensive. In 1934 a mile of stainless steel could be purchased for $1.00.[16] Undoubtedly the price has risen since then.

The high tensile strength and low reactivity of surgical stainless steel make this suture ideal when there is tension on the wound or in potentially infected areas. They are of particular value where a long-dwelling suture is required.

Udupa studied stainless steel–sutured wounds in guinea pigs and found that they had higher tensile strength at both 7 and 14 days, compared with similar wounds sutured with silk or copper wire.[183] He speculated that perhaps the iron in surgical steel acts as a catalyst in the hydroxylation of proline during collagen formation.

There recently has been some advocacy of the use of surgical stainless steel sutures for running intradermal sutures, especially on the face. However, should the suture break on removal, a retained foreign body may result. Early investigators of these sutures found breakage a frequent problem with this type of suturing technique.[16]

Disadvantages. Stainless steel is subject to mechano-chemical cracking caused by relatively insignificant chemical attack.[27] Thus great care and practice must be exercised in turning and tying wire sutures to avoid "cold working" (excess bending, twisting, or kinking). Kinking can render stainless steel sutures useless. Stainless steel must be handled so that knotting occurs only at the desired point. This prevents cracking points, where body fluids will attack the suture. Such weakening of the wire can lead to breaking in vivo.[27] Multifilamentous stainless steel is easier to handle than the monofilamentous variety because it withstands bending more easily.

Stainless steel sutures have high tensile strength and are very stiff; therefore they may pull or tear tissue if tied too tight. Furthermore, stainless steel does not conform well to suture pathways. This may result in additional tissue damage with tissue movement or swelling and possibly lead to infection.[55] Monofilamentous stainless steel has even been found to pick up *Staphylococcus aureus*.[93]

Barbs may also appear on steel wire strands, piercing gloves or tissue and breaking aseptic technique. Small plastic cuticular needles are not available for stainless steel sutures.

NEEDLES

An understanding of modern needles for sutures is essential for producing good cosmetic results. Surgical needles are designed to bring suture material through tissue with minimal trauma. Selection of a needle should be determined by the type of tissue to be sutured, its accessibility, and the size of the suture material. The nomenclature of needles is more confusing than that of sutures (Table 8-3); however, since needles frequently determine the relative cost of suture materials, their names are important to understand. Surgical needles are made of high-quality corrosion-resistant stainless steel. Needles should be rigid enough to prevent easy bending but flexible enough to bend before breaking. The *strength of a needle* is determined by measuring the force required to bend a needle outward to a 90-degree angle. *Ductility,* on the other hand, is the measurement of the ease with which a needle is broken. It is measured by the number of times the needle can be bent outward to a 90-degree angle without breaking. Ductility is also known as malleability.

Probably the first needles used to sew tissue were made of bone during the Paleolithic period 20,000 to 35,000 years ago.[183] The American Indians, particularly the Winnebago, Dakota, and Tuscaroca tribes, used bone with attached tendon. Threaded needles were known at least from the time of Albucasis in AD 1013. According to Trier, the first swaged suture needle was invented by Mrs. Ella N. Gailland in 1874 and named the Eureka needle[182]; however, MacKenzie gives credit to Merson for this invention and its introduction into surgery in the early twentieth century.[116]

Anatomy (Fig. 8-6)

A surgical needle can anatomically be divided into three separate areas: the point, the body, and the shank. The shank may be with a hole (eye), either closed or open (French), or eyeless (Fig. 8-7). This latter type is referred to as *swaged* (swedged) and is currently almost universally used. The suture is placed inside the hollowed end of the needle and is then slightly crimped by compression of the metal. The hollowed end may be either drilled or flanged, the former being thinner. It does not release during normal wound suturing, but an inadvertent jerk may release it when tying. A specially modified swaged needle is the "controlled-release" type, which may be loosened more easily from the suture.[177] This is particularly useful for running sutures.

It should be noted that the diameter of the swaged end (the *shank*) is the largest part of the needle and is much larger than the suture thread (Fig. 8-6). This part of the needle—not the suture size—therefore determines the size of the suture tract. Sutures that must be threaded by hand on open- or closed-eye needles result in an even wider path, since a double strand of suture is pulled through the suture tract. A major advantage of the swaged needle is that it is used with only one suture thread. This means that the needles are always sharp and are unlikely to break in surgery.

The *body* of the needle may be round, triangular, flattened, or flattened with sides also flattened. The triangular

TABLE 8-3

Comparison of needles

Name	Company	Tip	Body	Needle curvature length (mm)	Uses	Curvature	Finish	Comments
CE-4**	Davis & Geck	Reverse cutting	Triangular	19	Thick skin	⅜	Machine sharpened	Less sharp
FS-2*	Ethicon	Reverse cutting	Triangular	19	Thick skin	⅜	Machine sharpened	Less sharp
PC-5†	Ethicon	Cutting	Rectangular	19	Thick skin	⅜	Machine sharpened	Extra sharp, thinner body
PS-2‡	Ethicon	Reverse cutting	Ovoid	19	Thick skin	⅜	Machine sharpened	Extra sharp
CE-3	Davis & Geck	Reverse cutting	Triangular	16	Moderately thick skin	⅜	Machine sharpened	Less sharp
FS-3	Ethicon	Reverse cutting	Triangular	16	Moderately thick skin	⅜	Machine sharpened	Less sharp
PC-3	Ethicon	Cutting	Rectangular	16	Moderately thick skin	⅜	Machine sharpened	Extra sharp, thinner body
PRE-3¶	Davis & Geck	Reverse cutting	Triangular	16	Moderately thick skin	⅜	Hand sharpened	Extra sharp
PS-3	Ethicon	Reverse cutting	Ovoid	16	Moderately thick skin	⅜	Machine sharpened	Extra sharp
SBE-3§	Davis & Geck	Reverse cutting	Triangular	16	Moderately thick skin	⅜	Hand sharpened	Extra sharp, thinner body
P-3‖	Ethicon	Reverse cutting	Ovoid	13	Thin skin	⅜	Machine sharpened	Extra sharp
PC-1	Ethicon	Cutting	Rectangular	13	Thin skin	⅜	Machine sharpened	Extra sharp, thinner body
PRE-2	Davis & Geck	Reverse cutting	Triangular	13	Thin skin	⅜	Hand sharpened	Extra sharp
SBE-2‖	Davis & Geck	Reverse cutting	Triangular	13	Thin skin	⅜	Hand sharpened	Extra sharp, thinner body
P-1	Ethicon	Reverse cutting	Ovoid	11	Thin skin	⅜	Machine sharpened	Extra sharp
PRE-1	Davis & Geck	Reverse cutting	Triangular	11	Thin skin	⅜	Hand sharpened	Extra sharp
SBE-1	Davis & Geck	Reverse cutting	Triangular	11	Thin skin	⅜	Hand sharpened	Extra sharp, thinner body

*FS, For skin.
†PC, Precision cosmetic.
‡PS, Plastic (skin) surgery.
§SBE, Slim blade ($E = ⅜$ circle).
‖P, Plastic.
**CE, Cutting ($E = ⅜$ circle).
¶PRE, Premium ($E = ⅜$ circle).

bodies have cutting edges along three sides and are found with the FS, CE, PRE, and SBE series needles. The P and PS needles are flattened top and bottom, whereas the newer PC needles are also flattened along the sides, producing a body that is square to rectangular in shape. The side-flattened body makes less of a cut on insertion into tissue (back to front). The round bodies taper gradually to a point. The body may also be ribbed longitudinally on the inner curvature to allow solid grasping by the needle holder.

The cross-sectional shape of the needle *point* (tip) determines the general category of the needle. The three types of needle points useful in cutaneous surgery include the cutting, the reserve cutting, and the round with tapered point (Fig. 8-8). Almost all cutaneous suturing is performed with the reverse cutting needle. This needle is made with a triangular tip in cross section, with two opposing cutting edges and a third cutting edge on the outside edge. Thus when a skin wound is sutured the outside cutting edge is directed away from the

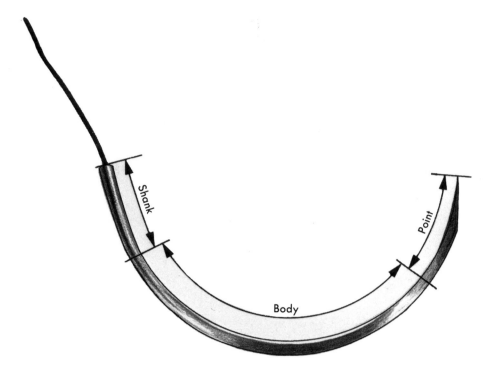

Fig. 8-6. Anatomy of needle.

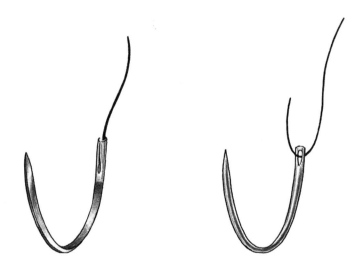

Fig. 8-7. Needle with closed eye, *right;* eyeless (swaged) shank, *left.*

wound edge, and the flat inner surface is directed toward the wound edge (Fig. 8-9). This results in a lesser tendency for sutures to tear through tissue. The CE, FS, P, PS, PRE, and SBE are all reverse cutting needles.

The cutting needle also has a triangular tip but with the third cutting edge directed along the inner surface of the needle and thus toward the wound edge when suturing. This theoretically results in a greater tendency to tear tissue. The newer PC series needles are cutting needles.

The round needle with a tapered point has even less tendency to tear tissue, since it has no cutting edges. It is useful for suturing fascia because it leaves a small hole that does not tear.

Only the edges near the tip of the needle are sharp. Variations in various needles by the same manufacturer are based frequently on the degree of tip sharpness. Some needles are specially sharpened ("hand-honed") and polished and are therefore said to be sharper. This ensures smooth passage through tissue and better placement. Needles may also be coated with very thin plastic surfacing material to allow smooth passage.

The curvature of the needle is an important consideration

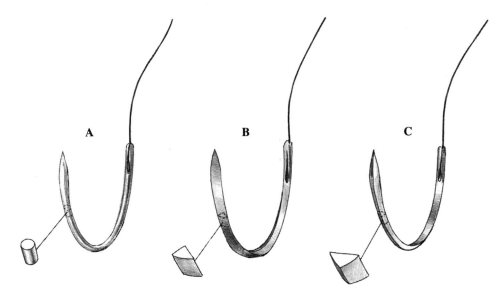

Fig. 8-8. Comparison of three types of needle tips (points). **A,** Round. **B,** Cutting. **C,** Reverse cutting.

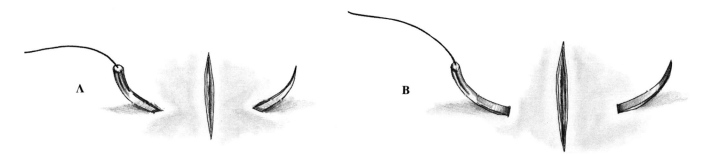

Fig. 8-9. Comparison of puncture wounds made by cutting needle (**A**) and reverse cutting needle (**B**).

(Fig. 8-10). Usually needles for the skin are ⅜ circle rather than ½ circle. The size of the needles can be measured in one of several ways. The *needle curvature length* is the length of the curve from the end of the shank to the tip. The *needle chord length* is the length from the end of the shank to the tip but as seen from the eye to the tip. The *needle radius* is the distance from the center of an imaginary circle in which the needle lies. The caliber of the needle is measured at the swaged end and is related to the gauge of wire used to make the needle.

Uses

For completely buried sutures or for percutaneous sutures where the final cosmetic result is relatively unimportant, an FS-2 (*FS* signifies "for skin") needle (Ethicon) or CE-4 needle (Davis & Geck) is adequate. These are large reverse cutting needles useful in thick skin, where small needles are easily bent. They are relatively inexpensive.

The more expensive P (plastic) and PRE series needles are useful when the skin is thin and the cosmetic results are of utmost importance, such as on the face. These needles are smaller (P-1 or PRE-1 are the smallest) and sharper than in the FS or CE series. The P-2 needle is ½ circle and smaller in chord and curvature length than the P-1 or P-3.

Ethicon also makes a PS (plastic skin) and a newer PC (precision cosmetic) needle, which are sharper than the regular P series needles. The PC-1 is smaller in cross-sectional diameter than the P-3 and has a side-flattened body. Thus a smaller hole is made with it than with the P-3. However, as mentioned earlier, the PC needles are cutting needles.

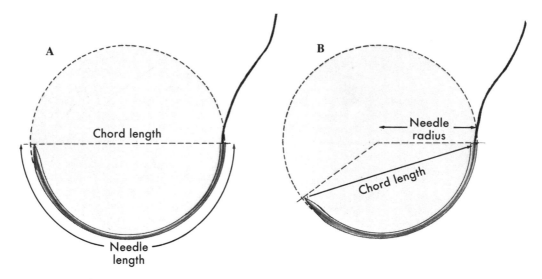

Fig. 8-10. Differences between arcs of needles; relationships of needle curvature length, chord length, and needle radius are shown. **A,** One-half circle needle. **B,** Three-eighths circle needle.

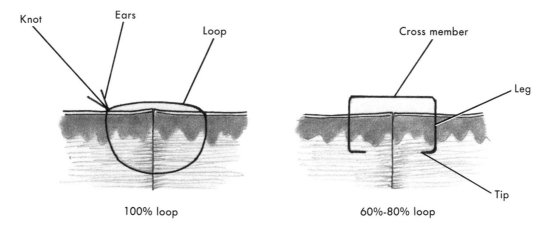

Fig. 8-11. Comparison between complete suture loop, *left,* and incomplete loop formed by staple, *right.*

STAPLES

Since 1980 skin staplers have come into use for cutaneous surgery. The history of their development has been summarized.[160] Staplers are compared in Table 8-4. Important considerations in selecting a stapler are the size of the staples and the ease of visibility for placement of staples.

All surgical staplers produce an incomplete rectangular staple with three components: (1) a top "cross member," or exposed portion, which lies parallel to the skin surface; (2) two legs, representing the height of the staple and extending from the top cross member through the skin; and (3) pointed tips that are bent in and lie beneath the skin parallel to the cross member (Fig. 8-11). The staple is advanced against an anvil and bent into the incomplete rectangular shape just described.[37] The amount of tissue gathered is determined by the size of the cross member (regular or

wide), the leg length, and the angle of insertion (discussed later). Because a staple does not form a complete tract through the wound cavity from the skin surface one wound edge to the other, as suture does, the amount of tissue enclosed by the staple is only 60% to 80% that enclosed by a suture loop.

Note that on Table 8-4 some staplers have a precock mechanism. This allows the staple to protrude partially from the stapler before being bent for insertion, which the manufacturers claim is useful for grabbing one edge of the wound with one tip of the staple and pulling the wound closed before actually inserting the other tip of the staple. I have not found this feature to be very useful.

The angle of insertion of the staple to the plane of the skin may be important, particularly if wound swelling occurs. Rectangular staples tend to rotate or "float" to a 90-degree angle to the skin surface after insertion. The smaller

TABLE 8-4

Comparison of skin staplers

Trade name	Company	Number of staples	Closed width × height (mm)	Wire diameter (mm)	Rotation of head	Angle of insertion (degrees)	Precock mechanism
Appose	Davis & Geck	25, 35	5.7 × 3.8 (Regular)	0.51	No	90	Yes
			6.9 × 3.9 (Wide)	0.56			
Precise II	3M	15, 35	5.0 × 3.5 (Regular)	0.51	No	45	Yes
			6.7 × 3.9 (Wide)	0.55			
Precise disposable skin stapler	3M		5.5 × 4.2 (Regular)	0.55	No	Variable	No
			6.5 × 4.6 (Wide)	0.55			
(5 Shot)		5, 10					
(10 Shot)		5, 15, 25					
Premium (auto suture)	U.S. Surgical	12, 25, 35	4.8 × 3.4 (Regular)	0.51	Yes	60	Yes
			6.5 × 4.7 (Wide)	0.56			
Proximate	Ethicon	15, 25, 35, 55	5.7 × 3.9 (Regular)	0.53	No	90	No
			6.9 × 3.9 (Wide)	0.58			

the angle and the less the purchase of tissue (since the depth of leg penetration is less), the greater the rotation (float) of the staple after insertion (see Fig. 11-4). If the angle of insertion is only 45 degrees, as with the Precise II staplers, when this rotation reaches 90 degrees after insertion, there is more space between the cross member on top and the skin surface below than with a staple inserted 90 degrees to the wound. If wound swelling occurs, having more space results in less chance of cross-hatching.

Special staple removers are purchased separate from the staples and ensure relatively painless staple removal. The greater the distance from the cross member to the skin, the easier it is to remove the staple.

Advantages and uses

Using staples instead of suturing saves time and effort in surgery. One can staple a wound in 25% to 35% the time it takes with conventional suturing techniques.[57,104,126]

When properly placed, staples should ride high so as not to strangulate or compress tissue if swelling occurs. If properly placed, there is no cutting out in tissue, and cross-hatching is thus prevented.[181]

Unlike sutures staples do not form a complete tract from one wound edge to the other. This means there is no foreign body material in the wound and no direct channels of communication from the outside skin surface into the wound itself.

Wounds that are stapled are therefore less likely to become infected, as has been shown with potentially contaminated wounds.[176] In other studies there appear to be no differences in the overall infection rate between stapled wounds and sutured wounds.[57,104]

When there is tremendous tension on wounds—for instance, on the scalp or trunk—staples are very useful to take tension off wound edges. Staples aid in wound edge eversion. This helps to eliminate bolster sutures or buried subcutaneous sutures, ultimately aiding in wound healing. The published cosmetic results from staples are encouraging[173] but warrant further controlled trials and long-term follow-up examinations. It should be pointed out that the wire diameter of skin staples (0.51 to 0.58 mm) is approximately five times the size of 5-0 nylon (0.10 to 0.149 mm).

Disadvantages

Staples on certain areas, such as the back and inguinal or axillary creases, may be uncomfortable for patients. Staples are at least as expensive as sutures and in some instances may be more expensive. Although some physicians recommend sterilizing the unused staples with the staple gun, in my experience this has frequently led to jamming of the mechanism.

Placement of staples may sometimes be difficult, resulting in overlapping skin edges or bunching of the skin if the skin on either side of the wound is of different thickness. Sometimes these problems are surmounted only by placing interrupted sutures between staples.

Skin staples can be removed earlier than sutures because staples remove greater tension from the wound than sutures. However, in some studies, stapled wounds actually were weaker at 2 weeks than sutured wounds were.[73,195] It was hypothesized that this paradox is caused by the lack of tension in the tissue from staples, precluding collagen orientation in the wound for maximal gain in wound strength.

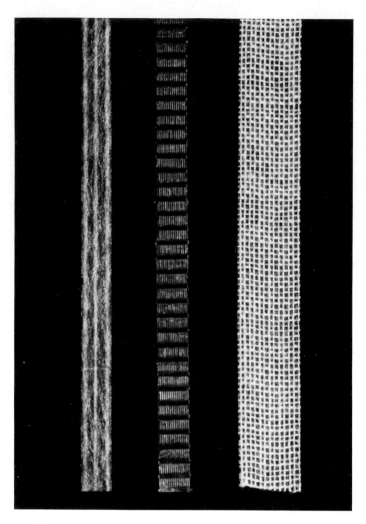

Fig. 8-12. Three types of commercially available skin tapes: *Right,* Steri-Strip. *Middle,* Clearon. *Left,* Cover-Strip.

SUTURELESS SKIN CLOSURES

The use of wound-closing techniques that avoid puncturing the skin is as old as the first medical records. The Egyptians used linen plaster stuck by honey to reinforce wounds.[28] The eminent nineteenth-century surgeon John Hunter advised using plaster across wounds.[114] Paré in the sixteenth century developed a technique to close wounds by suturing together cloth taped on each side of the wound[52] (see Fig. 1-5).

The butterfly bandage was used early in the twentieth century to reinforce wounds or lacerations. However, it was not very useful because the gummy adhesive backing tended to slip.

The evolution of the current use of closing wounds with tapes began in England with the work of Gillman et al., who had seen histologically how much scarring occurred as a result of percutaneous suturing.[68] This led to the development of porous tape and special glues to gain better cosmetic results.[69,70]

Although one usually thinks of skin tapes as the only method of sutureless skin closure, other devices are occasionally investigated that are based on Paré's principle of anchoring a device on each side of the wound and then joining them together.[52] One such device was reported in 1976.[75] However, such devices are used and tested only in areas such as the trunk, where wounds are large and there is enough flat skin surface on both sides for placement of the device. These are of limited use in cutaneous surgery.

Skin tapes

The most satisfactory closure tapes are based on the principle of being nonocclusive. Nonocclusive tape has been shown to reduce the growth of *Staphylococcus aureus* by reducing moisture on the epidermis.[120]

Microporous tape provides the nonocclusive properties desired to tape surgical wounds. This tape is manufactured by coating the backing with a very fine film of adhesive (acrylic polymer) in such a manner that none of the adhesive mass coalesces. This results in a profusion of unobstructed honeycombed fenestrations, which allow air movement. The adhesive does not transfer to the skin and permit creep. It is said to adhere partially by conformation to the surface rather than by actual stickiness; therefore it is more easily removed perpendicular rather than parallel to the skin surface. The adhesive has a high coefficient of adhesion but adheres best to a dry surface. Consequently, it is useful to defat the skin and apply a compound (for example, tincture of benzoin) to promote tackiness of the surface.

There are several types of skin tapes made for taping surgical wounds. They are compared in Table 8-5; a few are shown in Fig. 8-12. All differ in the composition of the backing and, except for Opsite, all are porous. Steri-Strips have a backing that consists of a nonwoven mesh of rayon fibers reinforced by longitudinal rayon fibers running along the long axis. Except for the reinforcing fibers, this is the same material as Micropore surgical tape, which comes in rolls. Steri-Strips are available in various sizes (⅛-, ¼-, ½-inch strips) and mounted on cardboard, which is siliconized for easy removal. The strips are available in sterile polyethylene packets and sterilized by ethylene oxide.

Clearon skin tapes on the other hand, are made from a plastic polymer and are ribbed. This ribbing tends to prevent these tapes from sticking flat like Steri-Strips. Cover-Strips are woven. All these skin tapes are pervious to sweat but not to blood or purulent material.

A study of adherence comparing Steri-Strips with Clearon closures showed that Steri-Strips adhered longer on the average (8.5 days) than did Clearon (3.4 days).[98] The type of skin preparation or presence of a tacky substance (such as tincture of benzoin) did not appear to make a substantive difference in the length of time the skin tapes stuck.

Another recently utilized type of skin closure material used for reinforcing surgical incisions is Opsite.[53] Westaby

TABLE 8-5

Comparison of adhesive skin closures

Trade name	Company	Backing	Adhesive	Sizes (inches)	Comments
Appose Skin Strips	Davis & Geck	Spun-bonded nylon	Acrylic	⅛ × 3, ¼ × 1½ ¼ × 3, ¼ × 4 ½ × 4, 1 × 4	
Clearon Skin Closure	Ethicon	Polypropylene	Acrylic	⅛ × 3, ¼ × 2 ¼ × 3, ¼ × 4 ½ × 4	May not need addition-al adhesive
Cover-Strip	Beiersdorf	Cellulose gauze	Acrylate	¼ × 2, ¼ × 3 ¼ × 4, ½ × 4 1 × 4	
Opsite Wound Closure	Smith & Nephew	Polyurethane	Vinyl ether	5½ × 4	Nonporous
Steri-Strip Skin Closure	3M	Rayon with reinforcing polyester filaments	Acrylic	⅛ × 3, ¼ × 1½ ¼ × 3, ¼ × 4 ½ × 4, 1 × 5	May be purchased with iodophor (Steri-Strip Anti-microbial Skin Closures)

successfully used this material, which is a gas-permeable dressing, for cutaneous incisions on 100 patients who had undergone thoracic or abdominal operations.[190] The only modification was that the Opsite was perforated to allow for better air exchange.

Advantages and uses. Skin tapes are very useful to reinforce incisions after interrupted sutures are removed; they have gained a place in cutaneous surgery almost routinely for this purpose. Their use instead of carefully placed percutaneous interrupted or running intradermal sutures is of questionable value because they do not align wound edges with the same precision as sutures.

There are several distinct advantages of skin tapes. Their use eliminates localized areas of tension and strangulation of tissue as well as the inflammatory response created by suture materials. Therefore in fragile skin (for example, in patients with Cushing's disease) or in ischemic areas, skin tapes are useful even for primarily closing the wound. Suture marks and needle puncture sites are eliminated, lessening the chance for bacteria to gain entrance to the wound. In a 1968 controlled study tape-closed wounds were compared with sutured wounds.[47] There was no difference found between the infection rates for clean wounds, but in potentially contaminated wounds the infection rate was less if the wounds had been taped. This has been shown by other investigators as well.[38,170]

With skin tapes, suture insertion and removal are avoided along with the associated trauma and discomfort; therefore for lacerations on children skin tapes may be desirable. Other advantages include the savings of time and expensive suture materials. Skin tapes may be left on the wound for long periods of time, allowing for wound inspection and for removal by the patient.

Brunius presented experimental evidence in rats to suggest that tape-closed wounds had higher tensile strength than sutured wounds not only initially but up to 12 months later. He speculated that this may have been caused by the lack of early inflammation in taped wounds.[34] Also, the lack of early tension in the sutured wounds leads to weaker wounds compared with wounds closed by tape, which allow more stress on the wound edges.[29] These more stressed tape-closed wounds also seem to have collagen fibers oriented parallel to the wound, whereas in the sutured wounds the collagen was arranged more haphazardly.[33,64] The scars were broader in tape-closed wounds, which may have also contributed to greater measurable tensile strength.[31]

Disadvantages. Despite numerous early reports in the medical literature testifying to the similar or even superior results of skin tapes for primary wound apposition compared with sutures,[47,60,68,70,80] later studies were not so enthusiastic.[47,59] Some of the problems associated with skin-tape closures were pointed out by Ellenberg, who concluded that "Steri-Strips will be valuable to surgeons who have little experience with them."[59] He found that in 3% of patients, skin tape was lifted off by blood or exudate, and secondary wound disruption occurred. In addition, the cosmetic results were only good or fair, since wound edges tended to invert, especially if blood existed in the wound. Eversion of wound edges is difficult to achieve with skin tapes, and wound edge misalignment can occur. Moreover, skin tapes cannot be used easily in hair-bearing areas, in awkward areas (such as nostrils), or on highly mobile parts. They loosen when wet and so should be applied to a dry surface.

The use of skin tapes as the primary method of skin edge apposition frequently requires deep closure first.[47,59,60] Such deep closure brings its own set of problems, which might otherwise be prevented by simple interrupted percutaneous sutures alone.

The use of skin tapes takes experience for when, where, and how to apply them. The difficulties of wound edge alignment should be considered before tape is used as a primary method of wound repair.

Tissue glue

Cyanoacrylate glues have been used on the surface and between wound edges to produce coaptation until initial wound healing is complete. These glues are colorless monomers with a viscosity close to that of water. When applied to any surface, including tissue, they polymerize within 2 to 30 seconds (depending on the moisture).[62] Most glued substances separate in a place other than the joined area.

One may be concerned regarding the safety of applying a foreign substance into the body. An investigation of cyanoacrylate glue (Eastman 910 Adhesive) on dog wounds concluded that it was absorbed within a few weeks.[62] The glue was found to be relatively nontoxic on guinea pigs and is said to be self-sterilizing.

Cyanoacrylates come in different chain lengths. Initially methyl-2-cyanoacrylate (M2C) was used in surgery. This was superceded by isobutyl cyanoacrylate (IBC) and n-butyl cyanoacrylate (NBC), which cause less tissue response.[192] Histoacryl (butyl-2-cyanoacrylate) is another cyanoacrylate commonly used in surgery.[4] These more recent glues have a longer chain length, which increases the speed of polymerization. This results in less contact with the surrounding tissues. The longer chain length, however, results in a longer half-life for biodegradation.

Advantages and uses. The use of cyanoacrylates to close wounds is fast, inexpensive, and convenient. As recently as 1979, Histoacryl was reported to be useful for minor wound apposition, with scars at 1 to 2 weeks no different from those of simply sutured wounds.[171] Other studies confirm these encouraging results[4] and recommend use of these glues for hemostasis, support of wound edges after suture removal, and skin grafts.[192] Tissue glues applied on top of hair transplant plugs are said to reduce plug slippage as well as to minimize plug elevation, which leads to a cobblestone appearance.[193] A further advantage of tissue glue is that it probably seals a wound to bacterial invasion, although no studies have been performed to investigate this.

Of course, cosmesis is of great importance in wound closure. Both animal[11] and human[4] studies attest to better cosmetic results in glued wounds compared with sutured wounds, but these reports are few and unconfirmed. In general, cyanoacrylates are not used at this time in place of sutures for wound apposition.

Disadvantages. Cyanoacrylates polymerize when applied to tissue, producing heat, which may injure surrounding nonepithelial or epithelial tissues.

Cyanoacrylates may also interfere with wound healing. In a careful study of dogs, cyanoacrylate polymer fragments between tissues delayed wound healing by preventing the proliferation of fibroblasts and vessels, which would otherwise have bridged the wounds.[123] Although the early wound strength was greater in this study if the skin edges had been coapted by glue, after 4 days the sutured wounds had greater tensile strength.

FACTORS TO CONSIDER IN SELECTION OF WOUND-CLOSURE MATERIALS

Infection. The presence and degree of infection in a wound are modified if certain types of suture are used.[92] Halsted, although he was an early advocate of silk, recognized that its use was contraindicated in infected tissue and preferred in its stead absorbable catgut suture.[72] Howes also recognized this fact.[89] In general, all sutures should be avoided if possible in contaminated or infected wounds.

The reason that silk tends to prolong wound infection is that it is braided, so its degree of capillarity is increased. This leads to the harboring of organisms in its interstices. Other sutures that tend to harbor bacteria include braided polyester (Dacron or Mersilene), braided nylon (Nurolon), Vicryl,[25] and Dexon.[109]

The ability of sutures to transport bacteria by capillary action was studied in vitro.[24] Mersilene, Ethibond, and silk transported bacteria (immobile *Staphylococcus aureus*), whereas Prolene and catgut did not. In a later experiment buried sutures in rat wounds were inoculated with *S. aureus*. Again, capillary materials—such as Mersilene or Vicryl—resulted in a marked inflammatory infiltrate, whereas there was much less reaction with noncapillary Prolene. It is apparent then that the suture's physical configuration is of great importance in promoting infection. When bacterial counts were performed, a larger number of bacteria were found within the capillary type of suture than in the noncapillary type.[143]

Similar experiments in dogs showed that monofilamentous nylon and steel were best at minimizing the risk of infection in infected wounds, whereas catgut, Dacron (Mersilene), and silk were the worst,[188] and Dexon was intermediate. However, my suture, even monofilamentous nylon, damages the host's ability to resist infection.[162]

Should a wound become inoculated from the surface after suturing, bacteria can be drawn into it. Wounds closed by tape after surface inoculation with the nonmotile *S. aureus* failed to develop infection, but the silk-sutured wounds did.[170] However, with the motile *Escherichia coli*, 7.7% of the taped wounds did develop infection. Interestingly, surface contamination after the third postoperative day did not result in infection of any of the sutured wounds.

In two studies of lacerations sutured in emergency rooms, the incidences of infection after use of different suture types were compared.[1,134] The wounds were considered potentially contaminated. The study by Adams et al.[1] of particular interest because it specified the actual incidence of infection by site. Overall, comparison of polyglycolic acid (Dexon) with silk revealed an incidence of pus on wounds of 1.3% versus 4.4% respectively. On the lower limb there were no problems in 46 wounds sutured with Dexon, but there was pus in 9 of the 71 silk-sutured wounds. The incidence of inflammation was highest on the hand (2.7% for Dexon, 6.8% for silk). On the scalp and face there was no significant difference in infection rate. The authors concluded that silk should definitely be avoided on the hand and lower extremity. In a similar study comparing Dexon, silk, Prolene, and nylon regarding the incidence of infection, Dexon was found to perform as well as nylon or Prolene and better than silk.[134]

In obviously infected or potentially contaminated (traumatized) wounds one should not use braided sutures, particularly silk sutures, since they may form a persistent foreign body. Of the absorbable sutures, catgut is degraded faster and Dexon more slowly in infected wounds.[92,106] The best sutures to use under such circumstances appear to be nylon, polypropylene, or stainless steel. One should not bury sutures in such wounds.

An interesting approach to sutures in infected wounds is to impregnate the sutures with antibiotics or antibacterial substances. Although this idea is not new (catgut used to be iodinized[115]), it is being studied more systematically. Neomycin sulfate in infected wounds works best on monofilamentous nylon, Prolene, and Dexon, but less well on silk, braided nylon, and braided polyester.[163]

Speed. Although physicians should allow suitable time for their surgical procedures, suturing can be tedious. Use of staples or skin tape is much faster and perhaps more desirable under certain circumstances.

Cost. Suture supplies add significant expense to each surgical procedure. In Great Britain, where the National Health Service does not remunerate physicians for their supplies, physicians may be less likely to suture any wound because they lose financially if they do.[21]

In a hospital operating room suture material is the most costly regular supply. It was estimated in 1981 that in an average-sized hospital approximately $2200 worth of suture material is unnecessarily opened and wasted every month.[51]

The cost of modern surgical suturing is determined more by the type of needle used than by the suture material itself. The "plastic" needles that are specially sharpened are very expensive.

Availability. Some types of sutures need to be specially ordered and are not always readily available.

Tissue characteristics. Friable tissue is difficult to close with any type of suture. When vascular supply is low,

or the tissue tears easily, skin tapes may be sufficient.

Location of the wound. As previously mentioned, wounds on the extremities should not be sutured with braided suture material because it tends to enhance infection.

The mucosa, whether oral, vaginal, or nasal, is best sutured with a nonirritating type of suture. Some physicians prefer Mersilene in these locations, but studies indicate that the mucosal tissue reaction to this suture is similar to the reaction to silk.[18] Because Mersilene is more expensive than silk, there is little justification for its use in these locations.

For suturing in very small areas, special needles (for example, the ½-circle ME-2 or P-2 needle) may be useful.

Tension on wound edges. Wounds under great tension need sutures of high tensile strength yet with little tendency to tear through tissue. Staples appear to be ideal for such wounds. Because staples float above the surface of the skin and do not form a complete tract through the wound, there is less likelihood of tissue strangulation than with sutures.

Cosmesis. On the face one desires the best cosmetic result possible. Therefore one should choose the smallest nonreactive suture material that holds the wound together.

Tumor growth. Interestingly, some sutures seem to potentiate the spread of melanoma experimentally.[146] Silk appears to increase early recurrences, whereas chromic catgut and PGA appear to have antineoplastic properties.

Stability. A prime consideration in choosing suture material is its stability.

Sterility. This is not much of a problem in modern times but formerly catgut suture was implicated in cases of tetanus and gas gangrene.[127] Modern sutures are sterilized by ethylene oxide or radiation. The latter is accomplished either by cobalt-60 or electron accelerators. These methods allows sterilization of the final package with little damage to the sutures themselves. The usual dosage is 2.5 megarad. Disadvantages of radiation sterilization include the high cost of the necessary equipment and the fact that some organisms, particularly viruses, may be radioresistant.[81]

Color. Occasionally one may wish to select a blue or green type of suture when suturing in a black-haired area, where black nylon will not be conspicuous when the time comes for suture removal. Clear or undyed sutures are suitable when stitches are buried.

Length. Suture material for cutaneous surgery is usually purchased either in 18-inch or 30-inch lengths. The longer suture is easier to tie by hand and is therefore useful for buried sutures. There appears to be little or no additional cost for the longer sutures.

Uniform diameter. Synthetic sutures are of uniform diameter, whereas nonsynthetic sutures are more variable. In particular, catgut may vary from batch to batch, and some batches may break more easily in tying.

Age of the patient. Children are frequently difficult to suture for obvious reasons. Under some circumstances skin tape works just as well as sutures and should be considered.

In lax, wrinkled skin, surgical scars might not be as apparent as on the young. Consequently, the size and type of needle or suture to use may be less important for older patients.

Medical condition of the patient. Patients who are malnourished are more likely to develop wound dehiscence, infection, and delay in wound healing.[8] Therefore the least reactive sutures should be used; in particular, skin tapes should be strongly considered if possible.

ADVERSE REACTIONS TO SUTURE MATERIALS

Allergy. The possibility of allergic reactions to suture material has been discussed for many years. Catgut, because it is a protein from animals, was thought by some to provoke allergic responses in sensitized individuals, but laboratory studies did not uniformly support this concept[147]; most cases have been anecdotal,[43] although a few clinical studies have been performed.[6] Chromate-sensitive individuals may have an allergic reaction to chromate salts in chromic catgut. Since chromates are the most common cause of industrial allergic contact dermatitis,[63] such reactions are probably more common than formerly recognized. Other suture materials implicated as a cause of allergic reactions are silk[125] and Vicryl.[121]

Hypertrophic scars. Although hypertrophic scars were reported to arise more frequently from wounds sutured with Dexon than with other sutures,[48,165] this observation has been repudiated by several studies.[5,7,95,145] The presence of hypertrophic scars was found to be related to improper placement of incision lines and not to the type of suture used.

Spitting. Buried sutures may occasionally be extruded from wounds through the wound surface in a process known as "spitting." Although this causes the patient some worry, it results in few if any problems with ultimate cosmetic results. Suture spitting has not been well studied. Although it is commonly held to occur if the buried sutures are placed too near the surface of the wound, other factors, such as allergy or granulomatous reactions to the suture material, may be important considerations. Spitting is often an extrusion of walled-off undigested suture, particularly knots.[177] This may occur months or even years after surgery, but in one study of Dexon absorbable sutures, spitting usually occurred between 14 and 34 days (the average was 20 days) after placement.[5] Spitting is common with buried silk, Mersilene, and catgut,[13] as well as with the newer coated Vicryl or Dexon sutures. With experience one tends to use buried sutures less for closures or learns to place the sutures deeper, still achieving good coaptation of wound edges.

Nodules. Buried sutures sometimes result in nodules under the skin surface. Although they usually resolve with time, occasionally they are persistent. The newer coated Vicryl in my experience is more likely to cause such a reaction.

Fire. Catgut suture is routinely packaged in 10% isopropyl alcohol. Fires in operating rooms have been reported when some of this packaging fluid spilled on drapes and was inadvertently ignited by a spark from electrcoagulation apparatus. In one instance second-degree burns were suffered by a patient.[36]

Tissue reactions. Since suture itself is a foreign substance, it is no wonder that tissue reactions occur routinely to even the most nonreactive suture materials. The degree of inflammatory response is proportional to the diameter and quantity of the suture material.[103] The normal reactions to sutures have been discussed under the sections on each suture type.

Excessive tissue reaction to suture may lead to softening of the surrounding tissue with subsequent "cutting out" of the suture—that is, the suture easily comes through mushy tissue so that when one goes to remove it, one finds that it is holding only one side of the wound and that dehiscence may have occurred. Suture materials, such as silk and catgut, that normally produce a marked tissue reaction are most prone to "cut out." Cutting out is also more common with small-caliber sutures, such as 6-0 nylon.

Excessive tissue reaction also delays wound healing. This was shown in the classic experiments of Howes.[89,91,92] Wounds sutured with catgut evoked more inflammatory tissue and delayed the fibroplastic phase of wound healing more than silk-sutured wounds did. As a consequence, wounds sutured with silk gained strength more rapidly.

Sinus formation may occur around any suture, even nylon. Everett feels that when this occurs with nylon, it is because the cut ends are left long and irritate the surrounding tissue.[61] Sinus formation can also occur with persistent infection, which is potentiated by the presence of a foreign body (for instance, suture material). The suture material itself and not the knot is the key element in the development of such sinuses.[71]

Foreign body reaction and granulomas may develop as reactions to suture material or contaminating substances. One such contaminant found on suture is talc from gloves.[96] One may think that talc is no longer used on gloves, but this is untrue. Talc is magnesium silicate, which is insoluble in water and in wounds causes granulomas and faulty wound healing. A practical substitute is cornstarch modified with magnesium oxide, which does not cause these sorts of problems. Sutures contaminated by talc from gloves may cause granulomas in wounds.

Granulomas may also be caused by the suture material itself. Silk has been implicated in granuloma formations,[99,118] sometimes resembling recurrent carcinomas on x-ray films.[173] Shedding of Teflon coating from some suture materials may induce granulomas.

Milia and epithelialization of suture tracts. All suture tracts epidermize to some extent. The degree of epidermization is probably most related to technique and how long sutures are left in place. Aston thought that Dexon and Vicryl were both more likely to result in milia if used as percutaneous instead of subcutaneous sutures but gives no proof.[12]

Infection. Percutaneous suture placement creates an avenue of entrance into a wound for bacteria. Some sutures, such as silk, can suck bacteria into a wound by capillary action better than other "noncapillary" materials can, such as nylon or steel.[24,25]

ORDERING WOUND-CLOSURE MATERIALS

Wound-closure materials are expensive items and it is wise to pay particular attention to how much they cost in an attempt to minimize overhead expense. Local supply houses do not necessarily sell the least expensively, so one should compare costs. Last-minute ordering is expensive; it is much more frugal to stock fairly large quantities of the most frequently used of wound-closure materials.

When ordering suture one needs to specify the type and size of suture, the type and size of needle, the suture color, and the length of the suture. The needle is the most important factor in determining cost, the specially sharpened needles being the most expensive. Be sure to specify the color of the suture material; it is frustrating, when one wants to place interrupted cutaneous sutures, to open a suture pack and discover clear nylon when black or blue sutures are much more visible. Most of the suture materials and needle sizes are listed in Appendix I.

The size of the sutures are between 4-0 and 6-0 for most cutaneous surgery. One should have a few 3-0 sutures, which are larger, for wounds under great tension. Although one may use sutures smaller than 6-0, they probably do not add much to the cosmetic result in the skin.

All nylon sutures with P or PRE series needles come in 18-inch lengths. For hand-tying buried sutures one may wish to order longer lengths.

Quantity is an important consideration. Surgical sutures are packaged in boxes containing either one dozen or three dozen suture packs. Four boxes of 3 dozen form a gross, that is, 144 suture packs. Buying by the gross is definitely less expensive.

A nurse or other appropriate office person should keep track of how much and what kinds of suture material are used each month in the clinic or office. This helps to ensure that suture orders are placed well in advance to prevent the need for last-minute shopping.

Some physicians resterilize unused suture material in an attempt to keep their overhead costs down. Although one may heat-sterilize most nonabsorbable synthetic suture material, it tends to dull the needles. Considering the time and effort of the office personnel in resterilizing suture, this saves little, if any, on costs.

Most suture manufacturers have product representatives who are most willing to come to the office or clinic to demonstrate their product lines. It is a wise idea to contact these sales representatives so that one knows the exact nomenclature for the sutures, needles, and other wound-closure materials that best fulfill one's needs.

REFERENCES

1. Adams, I.W., et al.: A comparative trial of polyglycolic acid and silk as suture materials for accidental wounds, Lancet **2:**1216, 1977.
2. Adamsons, R.J.: The comparative effects of silk and catgut on collagen lysis during the lag phase of primary healing, Surg. Gynecol. Obstet. **121:**1028, 1965.
3. Alexander, J.W., Kaplan, J.Z., and Altemeier, W.A.: Role of suture material in the development of wound infection, Ann. Surg. **165:**192, 1967.
4. Alhopuro, S., et al.: Tissue adhesive vs sutures in closure of incision wounds: a comparative study in human skin, Ann. Chir. Gynaecol. **65**(5):308, 1976.
5. Anscombe, A.R., Hira, N., and Hunt, B.: The use of a new absorbable suture material (polyglycolic acid) in general surgery, Br. J. Surg. **57:**917, 1970.
6. Apt, L., et al.: Catgut allergy in eye muscle surgery. I. Correlation of eye reaction and skin test using plain catgut, Arch. Ophthalmol. **63:**30, 1960.
7. Arabi, Y., and Alexander-Williams, J.: Hypertropic scarring after subcuticular polyglycolic acid sutures [letter], Lancet **1:**724, 1978.
8. Archie, J.P., Jr., et al.: Primary abdominal wound closure with permanent continuous running monofilament sutures, Surg. Gynecol. Obstet. **153**(5):721, 1981.
9. Aries, L.J.: Experimental studies with synthetic fibers (nylon) as a buried suture, Surgery **9:**51, 1941.
10. Artandi, C.: A revolution in sutures [editorial], Surg. Gynecol. Obstet. **150**(2):235, 1980.
11. Ashley, F.L., et al.: Further studies involving wound closure with a rapidly polymerizing adhesive, Plast. Reconstr. Surg. **31:**333, 1963.
12. Aston, S.J.: The choice of suture material for skin closure, J. Dermatol. Surg. **2**(1):57, 1976.
13. Aston, S.J., and Rees, T.D.: Vicryl sutures, Aesth. Plast. Surg. **1:**289, 1977.
14. Auerbach, R., and Pearlstein, M.: A comparison of polyglycolic acid (Dexon), nylon, and silk sutures in skin surgery, J. Dermatol. Surg. **1**(1):38, 1975.
15. Babcock, W.W.: Ligatures and sutures of alloy steel wire, J.A.M.A. **102:**1756, 1934.
16. Babcock, W.W.: Metallic sutures and ligatures, Surg. Clin. North Am. **27:**1435, 1947.
17. Bates, R.R.: Studies on the absorbability of catgut, Am. J. Surg. **43:**702, 1939.
18. Bergenholtz, A.: Tissue reaction in the oral mucosa to catgut silk and Mersilene sutures, Odont. Rev. **18:**237, 1967.
19. Bergman, F.O.: Synthetic absorbable surgical suture material (PGA): experimental study, Acta Chir. Scand. **137:**193, 1971.
20. Berry, A.R., et al.: Polydioxanone: a new synthetic absorbable suture, J. R. Coll. Surg. Edinb. **26**(3):170, 1981.

21. Binnie, G.A.: Stitches in the proper place, Practitioner **226** (1368):1140, 1982.
22. Birdsell, D.C., et al.: "Staying power"—absorbable vs. nonabsorbable, Plast. Reconstr. Surg. **68**(5):742, 1981.
23. Blomstedt, B., and Osterberg, B.: Fluid absorption and capillarity of suture materials, Acta Chir. Scand. **143**(2):67, 1977.
24. Blomstedt, B., Osterberg, B., and Bergstrand, A.: Suture material and bacterial transport, Acta Chir. Scand. **143**(2): 71, 1977.
25. Blomstedt, B., and Osterberg, B.: Suture materials and wound infection, Acta Chir. Scand. **144**:269, 1978.
26. Boruchoff, S.A., et al.: Degradation of "non-absorbable" sutures, Ophthalm. Surg. **8**(5):42, 1977.
27. Brantigan, C.O., Brown, R.K., and Brantigan, O.C.: The broken wire suture, Am. Surg. **45**:38, 1979.
28. Breasted, J.H.: The Edwin Smith surgical papyrus, vol. 1, Chicago, 1930, University of Chicago Press.
29. Brunius, U.: Wound healing impairment from sutures, Acta Chir. Scand. Suppl. 395, 1968.
30. Brunius, U., and Ahren, C.: Healing impairment in skin incisions closed with silk sutures, Acta Chir. Scand. **135**: 369, 1969.
31. Brunius, U., and Ahren, C.: Healing during the cicatrization phase of skin incisions closed by non-suture technique, Acta Chir. Scand. **135**:289, 1969.
32. Brunius, U., and Zederfeldt, B.: Suture materials in general surgery: a comment, Prog. Surg. **8**:38, 1970.
33. Brunius, U., Zederfeldt, B., and Ahren, C.: Healing of skin incisions closed by non-suture technique, Acta Chir. Scand. **133**:509, 1967.
34. Brunius, U., Zederfeldt, B. and Ahren, C.: Healing of skin incisions with intact subcutaneous muscle closed by non-suture technique, Acta Chir. Scand. **134**:187, 1968.
35. Bucknall, T.E.: Factors influencing wound complications: a clinical and experimental study, Ann. R. Coll. Surg. Engl. **65**:71, 1983.
36. Buyers, R.A.: Fire in the operating room caused by fluid from suture packet [letter], J.A.M.A. **237**(6):531, 1977.
37. Campbell, J.P., and Swanson, N.: The use of staples in dermatologic surgery, J. Dermatol. Surg. Oncol. **8**(8):680, 1982.
38. Carpendale, M.T.F., and Soreda, W.: The role of percutaneous suture and surgical wound infection, Surgery **58**:672, 1965.
39. Castelli, W.A., et al.: Cheek mucosa response to silk, cotton, and nylon suture materials, Oral Surg. **45**(2):186, 1978.
40. Chu, C.C.: The in-vitro degradation of polyglycolic acid sutures: effect of pH, J. Biomed. Mater. Res. **15**(6):795, 1981.
41. Chu, C.C.: A comparison of the effect of pH on the biodegradation of two synthetic absorbable sutures, Ann. Surg. **195**(1):55, 1982.
42. Chu, C.C., and Williams, D.F.: Effects of physical configuration and chemical structure of suture materials on bacterial adhesion: a possible link to wound infection, Am. J. Surg. **147**(2):197, 1984.
43. Cochrane, J.C.: Rejection of suture material, Br. Med. J. **2**:634, 1969.
44. Conn, J., Jr., et al.: Vicryl (polyglactin 910) synthetic absorbable sutures, Am. J. Surg. **128**:19, 1974.
45. Conn, J., Jr., et al.: A study of polybutilate lubricated polyester sutures, Surg. Gynecol. Obstet. **144**(5):707, 1977.
46. Conn, J., Jr., et al.: Coated Vicryl synthetic absorbable sutures, Surg. Gynecol. Obstet. **150**(6):843, 1980.
47. Conolly, W.B., et al.: Clinical comparison of surgical wounds closed by suture and adhesive tapes, Am. J. Surg. **117**:318, 1969.
48. Cox, A.G., et al.: Polyglycolic-acid suture material in skin closure [letter], Lancet **1**(7904):452, 1975.
49. Craig, P.H., et al.: A biologic comparison of polyglactin 910 and polyglycolic acid synthetic absorbable sutures, Surg. Gynecol. Obstet. **141**(1):1, 1975.
50. Dahlke, H., et al.: Thrombogenicity of different suture materials as revealed by scanning electron microscopy, J. Biomed. Mater. Res. **14**(3):251, 1980.
51. Dewey, S.: Suture savings only one way to cut costs, Hospitals **55**(13):12, 1981.
52. Dioguardi, D., et al.: Threaded tapes for the sutureless closure of skin wounds, Br. J. Plast. Surg. **30**(3):202, 1977.
53. Eaton, A.C.: A controlled trial to evaluate and compare a sutureless skin-closure technique (Op-Site skin closure) with conventional skin suturing and clipping in abdominal surgery, Br. J. Surg. **67**(12):857, 1980.
54. Edlich, R.F., et al.: Physical and chemical configuration of sutures in the development of surgical infection, Ann. Surg. **177**:679, 1973.
55. Edlich, R.F., et al.: Surgical sutures and infection: a biomaterial evaluation, J. Biomed. Mater. Res. **8**(3):115, 1974.
56. Eilert, J.B., et al.: Polyglycolic acid synthetic absorbable sutures, Am. J. Surg. **121**:561, 1971.
57. Eldrup, J., et al.: Randomized trial comparing Proximate stapler with conventional skin closure, Acta Chir. Scand. **147**(7):501, 1981.
58. Elek, S.D., and Conen, P.E.: The virulence of *Staphylococcus pyogenes* for man: a study of the problems of wound infection, Br. J. Exp. Pathol. **38**:573, 1957.
59. Ellenberg, A.H.: Surgical tape wound closure: a disenchantment, Plast. Reconstr. Surg. **39**:625, 1967.
60. Emmett, A.J.J., and Barron, J.N.: Adhesive suture strip closure of wounds in plastic surgery, Br. J. Plast. Surg. **17**:175, 1964.
61. Everett, W.G.: Suture materials in general surgery, Progr. Surg. **8**:14, 1970.
62. Fischl, R.A.: An adhesive for primary closure of skin incisions: a preliminary report, Plast. Reconstr. Surg. **30**:607, 1962.
63. Fisher, A.A.: The chromates: prime causes of industrial allergic contact dermatitis, Cutis **32**:24, 1983.
64. Forrester, J.C., et al.: Tape-closed and sutured wounds: a comparison by tensiometry and scanning electron microscopy, Br. J. Surg. **57**:729, 1970.
65. Foster, G.E., and Hardcastle, J.D.: Polyglycolic acid as suture material [letter], Lancet **1**:154, 1978.
66. Frazza, E.J., and Schmidt, E.E.: A new absorbable suture, J. Biomed. Mater. Res. **5**:43, 1971.
67. Freeman, B.S., et al.: An analysis of suture-withdrawal stress, Surg. Gynecol. Obstet. **131**:441, 1970.

68. Gillman, T., et al.: Closure of wounds and incisions with adhesive tape, Lancet **2:**945, 1955.

69. Golden, T.: Non-irritating, multipurpose surgical adhesive tape, Am. J. Surg. **100:**789, 1960.

70. Golden, T., Levy, A.H., and O'Connor, W.T.: Primary healing of skin wounds and incisions with a threadless suture, Am. J. Surg. **104:**603, 1962.

71. Greaney, M.G.: A clinical and an experimental study of suture sinuses in abdominal wounds, Surg. Gynecol. Obstet. **155:**712, 1982.

72. Halsted, W.S.: The employment of fine silk in preference to catgut and the advantages of transfixion of tissues and vessels in controlling hemorrhage, J. Am. Med. Assoc. **60:**1119, 1913.

73. Harrison, I.D., et al.: The effect of suture method on the rate of gain of tensile strength in skin wounds: a comparison of skin clips with interrupted nylon sutures, Br. J. Surg. **61**(11):920, 1974.

74. Harvey, S.C.: Concerning the suture, Surg. Gynecol. Obstet. **58:**791, 1934.

75. Hasson, H., et al.: A new sutureless technique for skin closure, Arch. Surg. **111:**83, 1976.

76. Herrmann, J.B.: Tensile strength and knot security of surgical suture materials, Am. Surg. **37:**209, 1971.

77. Herrmann, J.B.: Changes in tensile strength and knot security of surgical sutures in vivo, Arch. Surg. **106:**707, 1973.

78. Herrmann, J.B., Kelly, R.J. and Higgins, G.A.: Polyglycolic acid sutures, Arch. Surg. **100:**486, 1970.

79. Hines, D., and Nichols, W.: Effect of suture materials on healing skin wounds, Surg. Gynecol. Obstet. **140:**7, 1975.

80. Holm, H.H., and Egeblad, K.: Adhesive tape (Steri-Strip) versus suture closure of skin wounds, Nord. Med. **79:**311, 1968.

81. Holm, N., and Christensen, E.A.: Radiation sterilization: background and prospects, Acta Pharm. Suec. **12:**26, 1975.

82. Holmlund, D.E.: Physical properties of surgical suture materials: stress-strain relationship, stress-relaxation, and irreversible elongation, Ann. Surg. **184**(2):189, 1976.

83. Holmlund, D.E.: Knot properties of surgical silk: model study, Br. J. Surg. **64**(9):677, 1977.

84. Holt, G.R., and Holt, J.E.: Suture materials and techniques, Ear Nose Throat J. **60**(1):12, 1981.

85. Homsey, C.A.: Surgical suture—canine tissue interaction for six common suture types, J. Biomed. Res. **2:**215, 1968.

86. Homsy, C.A., et al.: Surgical suture–porcine subcuticular tissue interaction, J. Biomed. Mater. Res. **3:**383, 1969.

87. Hopps, H.C.: Role of allergy in delayed healing and in disruption of wounds. I. Antigenicity of catgut, Arch. Surg. **48:**438, 1944.

88. Hopps, H.C.: Role of allergy in delayed healing and in disruption of wounds. II. Effect of specific sensitivity to catgut on reaction of tissues to catgut sutures and on healing of wounds in the presence of catgut sutures, Arch. Surg. **48:**445, 1944.

89. Howes, E.L.: The strength of wounds sutured with catgut and silk, Surg. Gynecol. Obstet. **57:**309, 1933.

90. Howes, E.L.: Strength studies of polyglycolic acid versus catgut sutures of the same size, Surg. Gynecol. Obstet. **137:**15, 1973.

91. Howes, E.L., and Harvey, S.C.: The strength of the healing wound in relation to the holding strength of the catgut suture, N. Engl. J. Med. **200:**1285, 1929.

92. Howes, E.L., Sooy, J.W. and Harvey, S.C.: The healing of wounds as determined by their tensile strength, J.A.M.A. **92:**42, 1929.

93. James, R.C., and MacLeod, C.J.: Induction of staphylococcal infections in mice with small inocula introduced on sutures, Br. J. Exp. Pathol. **42:**266, 1961.

94. Jenkins, H.P., et al.: Absorption of surgical catgut. III. Duration in the tissues after loss of tensile strength, Arch. Surg. **45:**74, 1942.

95. Jones, S.M., et al.: Polyglycolic-acid suture and scar hypertrophy [letter], Lancet **2:**775, 1975.

96. Khan, M.A., et al.: Suture contamination by surface powders on surgical gloves, Arch. Surg. **118:**738, 1983.

97. Kobayashi, H., et al.: Coated polyglactin 910: a new synthetic absorbable suture, Jpn. J. Surg. **11:**467, 1981.

98. Koehn, G.G.: A comparison of the duration of adhesion of Steri-Strips and Clearon, Cutis **26:**620, (1980).

99. Kronborg, O.: Polyglycolic acid (Dexon) versus silk for fascial closure of abdominal incisions, Acta Chir. Scand. **142**(1):9, 1976.

100. Laufman, H.: Is catgut obsolete? [editorial], Surg. Gynecol. Obstet. **145**(4):587, 1977.

101. Laufman, H., and Rubel, T.: Synthetic absorbable sutures. Surg. Gynecol. Obstet. **145**(4):597, 1977.

102. Lawrie, P., Angus, G.E., and Reese, A.J.M.: The absorption of surgical catgut, Br. J. Surg. **46:**638, 1959.

103. Lawrie, P., Angus, G.E., and Reese, A.J.M.: The absorption of surgical catgut. II. The influence of size, Br. J. Surg. **47:**551, 1960.

104. Lennihan, R., et al.: A comparison of staples and nylon closure in varicose vein surgery, Vasc. Surg. **9**(4):200, 1975.

105. Lerwick, E.: Studies on the efficacy and safety of polydioxanone monofilament absorbable suture, Surg. Gynecol. Obstet. **156:**51, 1983.

106. Liber, A.F.: Splendore-Hoeppli phenomenon about silk sutures in tissue, Arch. Pathol. **95:**217, 1973.

107. Lilly, G.E.: Reaction of oral tissues to suture materials, Oral Surg. **28:**432, 1969.

108. Lilly, G.E.: Reaction of oral tissues to suture materials, Oral Surg. **33:**152, 1972.

109. Lilly, G.E.: Clinical and bacteriologic aspects of PGA, J. Oral Surg. **31:**103, 1973.

110. Lipovan, V.G., et al.: Sensitizing and antigenic action of catgut, Khirurgiia (Mosk.) **6:**68, 1981.

111. Lister, J.: Note on the preparation of cat-gut for surgical purposes, Br. Med. J. **1:**125, 1908.

112. Localio, S.A.: Wound healing: experimental and statistical study. IV. Results, Surg. Gynecol. Obstet. **77:**376, 1943.

113. Localio, S.A., Casale, W., and Hinton, J.W.: Wound healing experimental and statistical study. V. Bacteriology and pathology in relation to suture material, Surg. Gynecol. Obstet. **77:**481, 1943.

114. Longman. In Palmer, J.F., editor: The works of John Hunter, vol. 3, London, 1837.

115. Ludewig, R.M.: Reduction of experimental wound infection

with iodized gut sutures, Surg. Gynecol. Obstet. **133:**946, 1971.

116. Mackenzie, D.: The history of sutures, Med. Hist. **17:**158, 1973.

117. Madsen, E.T.: An experimental and clinical evaluation of surgical suture materials—I and II. Surg. Gynecol. Obstet. **97:**73, 1953.

118. Manor, A., et al.: Unusual foreign body reaction to a braided silk suture: a case report, J. Periodontol. **53:**86, 1982.

119. Marcy, H.O.: The aseptic animal suture: its place in surgery, J.A.M.A. **31:**381, 1898.

120. Marples, R.R., and Kligman, A.M.: Growth of bacteria under adhesive tapes, Arch. Dermatol. **99:**107, 1969.

121. Martin-Casals, A., et al.: Reaction to polyglactin 910 (Vicryl): a case report, J. Pediatr. Ophthalmol. **14**(3):178, 1977.

122. Martyn, J.W.: Clinical experience with a synthetic absorbable surgical suture, Surg. Gynecol. Obstet. **140:**747, 1975.

123. Matsumoto, T., et al.: Tissue adhesive and wound healing: observation of wound healing (tissue adhesive vs. sutures) by microscopy and microangiography, Arch. Surg. **98:**266, 1969.

124. Meade, W.H., and Ochsner, A.: The relative value of catgut, silk, linen, and cotton as suture materials, Surgery **7:**485, 1940.

125. Medicine and the law: Black silk suture allergy prompts malpractice suit, Tex. Med. **71**(4):120, 1975.

126. Meiring, L., et al.: A comparison of a disposable skin stapler and nylon sutures for wound closure, S. Afr. Med. J. **62:**371, 1982.

127. Meleney, F.L., and Chatfield, M.: The sterility of catgut in relation to hospital infections, with an effective test for the sterility of catgut, Surg. Gynecol. Obstet. **52:**430, 1931.

128. Melle, G.J.: The early history of the ligature, S. Afr. Med. J. **8:**290, 1934.

129. Miller, J.M.: A new era of non-absorbable sutures, Exp. Med. Surg. **28:**274, 1970.

130. Miller, J.M. and Kimmel, L.E., Jr.: Clinical evaluation of monofilament polypropylene suture, Am. Surg. **33:**666, 1967.

131. Miller, J.M., Zoll, D.R., and Brown, E.O.: Clinical observations on use of an extruded collagen suture, Arch. Surg. **88:**167, 1964.

132. Moloney, G.E.: The effect of human tissues on the tensile strength of implanted nylon sutures, Br. J. Surg. **48:**528, 1961.

133. Morrill, W.P.: Surgical catgut, Hospitals **10**(2):39, 1936.

134. Mouzas, G.L., et al.: Does the choice of suture material affect the incidence of wound infection?: a comparison of Dexon (polyglycolic acid) sutures with other commonly used sutures in an accident and emergency department, Br. J. Surg. **62:**952, 1975.

135. Narat, J.K., Cangelosi, J.P., and Belmonte, J.V.: Electron sterilization of catgut, Surgery **41:**324, 1957.

136. Nilsson, T.: Mechanical properties of Prolene, Ethilon, and surgical steel loops, Scand. J. Plast. Reconstr. Surg. **15**(2):111, 1981.

137. Nilsson, T.: The relative importance of Vicryl and Prolene sutures to the strength of healing abdominal wounds, Acta Chir. Scand. **147**(7):503, 1981.

138. Nilsson, T.: Mechanical properties of Prolene and Ethilon sutures after three weeks in vivo, Scand. J. Plast. Reconstr. Surg. **16:**11, 1982.

139. Noe, J.M., et al.: Suture material and static electricity, Ann. Plast. Surg. **8:**179, 1982.

140. Ordman, L.J., and Gillman, T.: Studies in healing of cutaneous wounds, Arch. Surg. **93:**857, 1966.

141. Osterberg, B.: Enclosure of bacteria within capillary multifilament sutures as protection against leukocytes, Acta Chir. Scand. **149:**663, 1983.

142. Osterberg, B.: Influence of capillary multifilament sutures on the antibacterial action of inflammatory cells in infected wounds, Acta Chir. Scand. **149:**751, 1983.

143. Osterberg, B., and Blomstedt, B.: Effect of suture materials on bacterial survival in infected wounds: an experimental study, Acta Chir. Scand. **145:**431, 1979.

144. Osterberg, B.O.: Microbiological evaluation of suture items before radiation sterilization, Appl. Microbiol. **26:**354, 1973.

145. Pease, R.: The incidence of hypertrophic scar formation in wounds closed with subcuticular nylon or polyglycolic acid (Dexon), Br. J. Plast. Surg. **29**(4):284, 1976.

146. Pendergrast, W.J., Jr., Futrell, J.W., and Mardiney, M.R.: Differences in potentiation of melanoma growth by absorbable and nonabsorbable suture, J. Surg. Oncol. **8:**223, 1976.

147. Pickrell, K.L.: Studies on hypersensitivity to catgut as a factor in wound disruption, Bull. Johns Hopkins Hosp. **64:**195, 1939.

148. Postlethwait, R.W.: Wound healing. I. Comparison of heat and irradiation, sterilized surgical sutures, Arch. Surg. **78:**958, 1959.

149. Postlethwait, R.W.: Long-term comparative study of non-absorbable sutures, Ann. Surg. **171:**892, 1970.

150. Postlethwait, R.W.: Polyglycolic acid surgical suture, Arch. Surg. **101:**489, 1970.

151. Postlethwait, R.W.: Further study of polyglycolic acid suture, Am. J. Surg. **127:**617, 1974.

152. Postlethwait, R.W.: Five-year study of tissue reaction to synthetic sutures, Ann. Surg. **190:**54, 1979.

153. Postlethwait, R.W., Willigan, D.A., and Ulin, A.W.: Human tissue reaction to sutures, Ann. Surg. **181:**144, 1975.

154. Postlethwait, R.W., et al.: Wound healing. II. An evaluation of surgical suture material, Surg. Gynecol. Obstet. **108:**555, 1959.

155. Preston, D.J.: The effects of sutures on the strength of healing wounds, Am. J. Surg. **49:**56, 1940.

156. Price, P.B.: Stress, strain, and sutures, Ann. Surg. **128:**408, 1948.

157. Racey, G.L., et al.: Comparison of a polyglycolic-polylactic acid suture to black silk and plain catgut in human oral tissues, J. Oral Surg. **36:**766, 1978.

158. Ray, J.A., et al.: Polydioxanone (PDS), a novel monofilament synthetic absorbable suture, Surg. Gynecol. Obstet. **153:**497, 1981.

159. Reti, L.L., et al.: Does subcuticular green polyglycolic acid suture tattoo? Aust. N.Z. Obstet. Gynecol. **22:**153, 1982.

160. Robicsek, F.: The birth of the surgical stapler, Surg. Gynecol. Obstet. **150:**579, 1980.

161. Rodeheaver, G.T., Thacker, J.G., and Edlich, R.F.: Me-

chanical performance of polyglycolic acid and polyglactin 910 synthetic absorbable sutures, Surg. Gynecol. Obstet. **153**:835, 1981.

162. Rodeheaver, G., et al.: Antimicrobial prophylaxis of contaminated tissues containing suture implants, Am. J. Surg. **133**(5):609, 1977.

163. Rodeheaver, G.T., et al.: Biocidal braided suture, Arch. Surg. **118**:322, 1983.

164. Rodeheaver, G.T., et al.: Knotting and handling characteristics of coated synthetic absorbable sutures, J. Surg. Res. **35**:525, 1983.

165. Rose, T.F.: Letter: skin closure with subcuticular polyglycolic acid sutures, Med. J. Aust. **1**(5):140, 1975.

166. Rutledge, G.L., Jr.: Plain catgut for skin closures, Clin. Orthop. **103**:97, 1974.

167. Salthouse, T.N., and Matlaga, B.: Significance of cellular enzyme activity at nonabsorbable suture implant sites: silk, polyester, and polypropylene, J. Surg. Res. **19**:127, 1975.

168. Salthouse, T.N., et al.: Polyglactin 910 suture absorption and the role of cellular enzymes, Surg. Gynecol. Obstet. **142**:544, 1976.

169. Sashchikova, V.G., et al.: Stimulating effect of catgut in treatment of trophic leg ulcers, Vestn. Khir. **116**:116, 1976.

170. Schauerhamer, R.A., et al.: Studies in the management of the contaminated wound. II. Susceptibility of surgical wounds to postoperative surface contamination, Am. J. Surg. **122**:74, 1971.

171. Schultz, A., et al.: Tissue glue in minor skin lesions: a prospective controlled comparison between tissue glue and the suturing of skin minor lesions, Ugeskr. Laeger **141**:3106, 1979.

172. Sharp, W.V., et al.: Suture resistance to infection, Surgery **91**:61, 1982.

173. Shauffer, I.A., et al.: Suture granuloma simulating recurrent carcinoma, Am. J. Roentgenol. **128**:856, 1977.

174. Snyder, C.C.: On the history of the suture, Plast. Reconstr. Surg. **58**:401, 1976.

175. Stegmaier, O.C.: Use of skin stapler in dermatologic surgery. J. Am. Acad. Dermatol. **6**:305, 1982.

176. Stillman, R.M., et al.: Skin staples in potentially contaminated wounds, Arch. Surg. **119**(7):821, 1984.

177. Suture use manual: use and handling of sutures and needles, Somerville, N.J., 1978, Ethicon, Inc.

178. Tera, H., and Aberg, C.: Tensile strengths of twelve types of knot employed in surgery, using different suture materials, Acta Chir. Scand. **142**:1, 1976.

179. Tera, H., and Aberg, C.: Strength of knots in surgery in relation to type of knot, type of suture material, and dimension of suture thread, Acta Chir. Scand. **143**:75, 1977.

180. Tera, H., et al.: The strength of suture knots after one week in vivo, Acta Chir. Scand. **142**:301, 1976.

181. Thompson, D.P., and Ashley, F.L.: Use of stapler in skin closure, Am. J. Surg. **132**:136, 1976.

182. Trier, W.C.: Considerations in the choice of surgical needles, Surg. Gynecol. Obstet. **149**:84, 1979.

183. Udupa, K.N.: Studies on wound healing. II. Role of suture materials in the healing of skin wounds, Indian J. Med. Res. **57**:442, 1969.

184. Ulin, A.W.: The ideal suture material, Surg. Gynecol. Obstet. **135**:113, 1972.

185. United States Pharmacopeia, ed. 15, Rockville, Md., 1980, United States Pharmacopeial Convention, Inc.

186. Van Winkle, W., Jr., Sewell, W., and Wiland, J.: Mechanism of absorption and antigenicity of absorbable collagen suture, J. Am. Geriatr. Soc. **3**:572, 1955.

187. Van Winkle, W., Jr., et al.: Effect of suture materials on healing skin wounds, Surg. Gynecol. Obstet. **140**:7, 1975.

188. Varma, S., et al.: Further studies with polyglycolic acid (Dexon) and other sutures in infected experimental wounds, Am. J. Vet. Res. **42**(4):571, 1981.

189. Webster, R.C., Davidson, T.M., and Smith, R.C.: Broken line scar revision. Clin. Plast. Surg. **4**:263, 1977.

190. Westaby, S.: Evaluation of a new product for sutureless skin closure, Ann. R. Coll. Surg. Engl. **62**:129, 1980.

191. White, J.H., et al.: 6-0 sutures for eyelid skin, Ophthalm. Surg. **12**:195, 1981.

192. Wilkinson, T.S.: Tissue adhesives in cutaneous surgery, Arch. Dermatol. **106**:834, 1972.

193. Wilkinson, T.S.: Tissue adhesive as an adjunct in hair transplantation, South. Med. J. **67**:1408, 1974.

194. Williams, D.F.: The effect of bacteria on absorbable sutures, J. Biomed. Mater. Res. **14**:329, 1980.

195. Williams, D.F., and Harrison, I.D.: The variation of mechanical properties in different areas of a healing wound, J. Biomech. **10**:633, 1977.

196. Williams, D.F., and Mort, E.: Enzyme accelerated hydrolysis of polyglycolic acid, J. Bioeng. **1**:231, 1977.

197. Willie, C.R., et al.: Evaluation of 8-0 chromic collagen suture material, South. Med. J. **67**:54, 1974.

198. Wolff, H.H., et al.: Unusual localized argyrosis, Hautarzt **28**:668, 1977.

Dressings and Miscellaneous Surgical Materials

From the beginning of recorded history and probably earlier, humans have been naturally inclined to cover any wound. Perhaps such inclination resulted from social rather than surgical factors associated with wounds. Nevertheless, this practice has continued to the present day. The orthodoxy of wound coverage is steeped in folklore and surgical lore but is occasionally questioned. Indeed, every generation of physicians has had its proponents of allowing wounds to be exposed to air rather than applying dressings.

This chapter explores the purpose and types of dressing materials with special emphasis on the principles of dressings. The materials and techniques employed may profoundly influence wound healing and the speed and comfort with which it occurs.

HISTORY OF DRESSINGS

The earliest recorded medical treatise, the Edwin Smith Surgical Papyrus, discusses the use of linen strips and adhesive plaster to dress wounds.[22] Sometimes the linen strips were coated with honey, providing a semiocclusive, adherent dressing with antibacterial properties that rivals modern dressings such as Op-Site, which is said to possess the same attributes.

The use of linen fabrics on wounds continued for at least four millenia until the introduction of woven, absorbent cotton gauze in 1871.[59] Gamgee[50] in 1880 realized the importance of gauze dressings and was responsible for their popularization. He first suggested that pads of absorbent cotton be placed behind fine woven gauze to soak up wound drainage and provide a cushion for the wound. This composite dressing became known as the Gamgee dressing. (Gamgee also suggested that diapers for babies be fashioned on the principle of his two-layer dressing. This idea was slow in its

acceptance but is the basis for modern disposable diapers.)

A main problem with plain gauze is that it tends to stick to wounds. This problem was partially solved by impregnating gauze with such substances as paraffin with oil (tulle gras) or petrolatum (Vaseline Gauze, Chesebrough-Ponds, Greenwich, Conn.). Later, antibacterial substances were also included in gauze.

Modern polymer science, which began in the 1930s, resulted in an array of synthetic dressing materials that have been fashioned in conformity with the principles of wound healing. In 1913, three decades before the development of synthetic polymers, Halsted[66] recommended gutta percha, a naturally occurring waterproof polymer. This material is discussed later in the chapter.

PURPOSE OF DRESSINGS

Dressings function in four general ways to assist wounds in healing: absorbing wound drainage, protecting the wound, providing pressure on the wound, and speeding the rate of epidermization of the wound. In addition, dressings help to separate the patient emotionally from the wound and therefore may have psychologic benefits. Dressings allow patients to proceed in life's routines without interference. Pain in open wounds may be relieved by the coverage provided by certain dressings.

Some wounds ooze considerable amounts of exudate, whereas other wounds, such as simple sutured excisions, drain very little. Wounds that drain continuously need a dressing with great absorbency.

Dressings protect wounds from the outside environment, thus preventing direct trauma, as well as contamination by foreign material or bacteria. In a sense a wound dressing assumes the function of normal skin lost by injury. However, dressings may shed and become incorporated into a wound and thus themselves add foreign material to it.

The external pressure that dressings provide has several important benefits to wound healing. Pressure dressings provide hemostasis. (However, pressure dressings should not be used as a substitute for good surgical technique.) Pressure also helps to eliminate dead space within sutured wounds and minimizes wound seepage. Thus moist breeding grounds for bacteria are eliminated. In addition, venous and lymph return is enhanced, which further limits the amount of exudate that seeps into a wound and thus helps to reduce swelling. Pressure helps to splint a wound and immobilize the skin edges and thus eliminates shearing forces between opposed tissue. Splinting and pressure may also help to minimize wound contraction and excess scar tissue. Blair[19] pointed out that maintenance of definite external pressure is essential to the life of the body and the function of many organs. A properly applied pressure dressing helps to recreate this external pressure.

Several studies have established that the rate of epidermization of wounds is faster in wounds with relatively occlusive dressings than in those allowed to be exposed to the atmosphere. This is discussed in more detail later in the chapter.

It seems reasonable, given the advantages of dressings, that their use would be unquestioned. However, this is not the case for all wounds. Several studies have shown that sutured wounds in patients heal with few problems when dressings are not used.

Mengert and Hermes[115] studied abdominal wounds in patients after gynecologic surgery. They compared dressed wounds with undressed wounds and with wounds in which half the wound was dressed and the other half undressed. These investigators noted no difference in the rates of infection or dehiscence, and they concluded that using any type of dressing on a clean abdominal wound was unnecessary, except for the sake of adherence to tradition. Their work was confirmed by subsequent researchers.[65,71,80,127]

These studies do not, however, assess the ultimate cosmetic appearance of the scars produced, nor do they compare wounds in different areas of the body (for example, the face compared with the trunk or extremities). Such variables are undoubtedly important.

Why do undressed sutured wounds not become infected? It is believed that a coagulum of blood and fibrin rapidly forms a seal impermeable to bacteria after closure of a wound. If the wound is protected from microorganisms until this coagulum forms, an artificial covering is unnecessary.

Heifetz, Lawrence, and Richards[70] compared covered wounds with uncovered wounds in rabbits. *Staphylococcus aureus* was rubbed on the wounds at various times after closure. Of the wounds inoculated 30 minutes after closure, only one subsequently developed an infection; of those in-

oculated 60 minutes after closure, none developed infection. These authors concluded that 1 hour after creation of a wound, pathogenic bacteria could come into contact with it without producing infection. Their study contrasts sharply with that of DuMortier,[37] who found that dressed, sutured wounds in guinea pigs could be externally infected up to 5 days after closure if they were inoculated with *Staphylococcus aureus*.

Despite the foregoing studies, dressings continue to be used routinely on both sutured and unsutured surgical wounds. As discussed later in the chapter, evidence suggests that covered wounds heal faster because a scab is prevented or minimized. As a result, less noticeable scarring occurs.

IDEAL SURGICAL DRESSING

There is no single surgical dressing that is beneficial to all types of wounds—wet or dry, clean or contaminated, primarily closed, or allowed to granulate. One needs to approach the surgical wound with an appreciation of its healing requirements and the benefits of various dressings. The number of new dressing materials is rapidly proliferating and undoubtedly will continue to do so.

Scales, Towers, and Goodman[145] and Lawrence[94] listed the properties of an "ideal dressing," which included the following:

1. Is highly porous to water vapor ("breathable") yet keeps wound surface (microenvironment) moist
2. Permits good gas exchange, especially of oxygen
3. Adheres closely but not tightly to wound surface
4. Adequately absorbs wound exudate
5. Provides barrier to passage of microbes or other contaminants
6. Is easy to apply
7. Contours to wound in movement (conformable)
8. Is reasonably strong but not abrasive (does not shear); has low coefficient of friction and provides mechanical support
9. Does not shrink
10. Is free of particulate material that might shed into wound (particle free) and is not likely to shed material from which it is made (fiber fast)
11. Is nontoxic and inert; does not produce tissue reaction, allergy, or hypersensitivity
12. Is compatible with therapeutic agents
13. Is noninflammable
14. Is capable of being sealed to the surrounding normal skin
15. Is easily sterilizable
16. Is available at a low cost
17. Is readily obtainable
18. Is acceptable to patients and nursing staff
19. Has a reasonably long shelf life

MACROSTRUCTURE OF DRESSINGS

To appreciate fully how a dressing functions, one must understand its structural organization. A fully constituted dressing usually has three layers: the contact layer, the absorbent layer, and the outer wrap, or outer covering (see Fig. 10-52). Sometimes the first two layers are spoken of as the primary dressing, whereas the outer covering is the secondary dressing. Each layer has important functions that contribute to the performance of the dressing as a whole.

The contact layer is the portion closest to the wound. It is usually nonsticky so it will not disrupt the wound on removal. Either the dressing material itself is inherently nonsticky (for example, the polyester film in Telfa, Kendall Co., Boston, Mass.) or substances such as petrolatum are incorporated into the dressing material (for example, Vaseline Petrolatum Gauze, Chesebrough-Ponds, Greenwich, Conn.). The following are types of contact dressings:

1. Wet nonadherent gauze-type (for example, Vaseline Petrolatum Gauze, Adaptic, Aquaphor Gauze)
2. Wet nonadherent non-gauze-type (for example, Gelliperm, Vigilon, Mediskin)
3. Dry nonadherent (single layer) (for example, N-Terface, Owens Surgical Dressing, Blister Film)
4. Dry nonadherent (multilayer) (for example, Release, Telfa)
5. Dry with adhesive (for example, Op-Site, Tegaderm)

The absorbent layer is the intermediate layer of the dressing. This portion primarily stores wound secretions and may secondarily cushion the wound.[160] In addition, when wounds occur in concavities or convexities the absorbent layer further functions to contour the contact layer so that the latter remains on the wound surface. The absorbent layer should be capable of absorbing both vertically and horizontally. Frequently an absorbent layer and a contact layer are combined in one conveniently packaged dressing, such as Telfa, which is composed of two sheets of polyester film that serve as nonadherent layers on either side of absorbent cellulose. The following are types of absorbent dressings:

1. Cotton
2. Gauze pads
3. Multiple different layers (different contact and absorbent layers)
   a. Sheets (for example, Telfa, Release)
   b. Slight bulk (for example, Cover-Pad)
   c. Very bulky (for example, eye pads, Surgipad)

The outer wrap, also called the outer covering or binder, holds the underlying components in their proper position (see the following outline). It also provides firm, comfortable pressure on the underlying wound and renders support to the area of surgery. Usually the outer wrap is composed of stretchable dressing material and tape or merely tape. It gives the dressing a neater, more finished appearance. The structure and composition of these dressings are fully described later. The following are outer wrap (secondary dressings:

I. Nonadhesive gauze-type (woven)
   A. Low stretch
      1. Conforming Gauze (Professional Medical Products, Inc.)—6 ply, medium bulk
      2. Intersorb Roll Gauze (Chesebrough-Ponds)—6 ply, medium bulk
      3. Kling (Johnson & Johnson)—2 ply
      4. Sof-Band Bulky Bandage (Johnson & Johnson)—6 ply, high bulk
      5. Sta-Tite (Chesebrough-Ponds)—2 ply
      6. Stretch Gauze (Prof. Med.)—2 ply
   B. Medium stretch
      1. Kerlix (Kendall Co.)—6 ply, high bulk
   C. High stretch
      1. Elastomull (Beiersdorf)—1 ply
      2. Sof-Band High Stretch Bandage (Johnson & Johnson)—1 ply
II. Nonadhesive knitted
   A. Tubular Gauze (Burlington Industries)
   B. Tubegauze (Scholl)
III. Nonadhesive elastic
   A. Roll wrap
      1. Ace Wrap (Becton-Dickinson)
      2. Dynaflex (Johnson & Johnson)
      3. Readi-Flex (Prof. Med.)
      4. Tensor (Kendall)
   B. Tubular net
      1. JetNet (Hyginet Co.)
      2. Scholl Tubegauze Net (Scholl)
      3. Spandage (MediTech International)
      4. Surgitube (Carlton Corp.)
      5. Surgiflex (Hyginet Co.)
      6. X-Span (concept)
IV. Self-adherent (adheres to itself but not to patient)
   A. Coban (3M)—crepe construction
   B. PEG (Becton-Dickinson)
IV. Adhesive (adheres to itself and to patient)
   A. Conform (Kendall Co.)
   B. Cover-Roll Stretch (Beiersdorf)—acrylic adhesive
   C. Elastoplast (Beiersdorf)—rubber-based adhesive
   D. Elastikon (Johnson & Johnson)—rubber-based adhesive
V. Elastic tape
   A. MicroFoam (3M)

FUNCTIONAL ASPECTS OF DRESSINGS

The performance of a dressing is intimately related to its basic structure and composition. This interrelationship of

TABLE 9-1

Structure-function relationships of dressings

Dressing	Adherence	Absorbability	H_2O permeable	H_2O vapor permeable	O_2 permeable	Bacteria permeable
Plain gauze	Yes	Yes	Yes	Yes	Yes	Yes
Ointment-impregnated gauze	No	No	Yes	No/yes*	No/yes*	Yes
Perforated polyester sheets (e.g., Telfa)	No	Yes	Yes	Yes	Yes	Yes
Polyurethane film	No/yes*	No	No	Yes	Yes	No
Colloid dressing	No/yes*	Yes	No	Yes	No/yes*	No
Rubber	No	No	No	No	No	No
Cellophane	No	No	No	Yes	Yes	No
Saran Wrap	No	No	No	No	No	No
Amnion	Tight	No	No	Yes	Yes	No
Skin graft	Tight	No	No	Yes	Yes	No

*Certain dressings in category may perform differently during wound healing.

structure, composition, and function is the key to understanding why some dressings work well for some wounds but not others. Appreciation of both the macrostructure (just discussed) and the microstructure of dressings (to be discussed later) will assist the physician in choosing the proper dressing for the task at hand. Table 9-1 compares several types of dressing and the important functional aspects to be discussed below.

Absorbability

Since many wounds drain continuously, some dressings need to be fashioned to absorb the transudate or exudate. A dressing performs this function through capillarity,[122] defined as the process by which the surface of a liquid where it is in contact with a solid (here dressing fibers) is elevated (soaked up) or depressed depending on the relative attractiveness of the liquid molecules for each other and for those of the solid. If the attractive force between the molecules of the liquid and solid is greater than the force of attraction between the same molecules of the liquid, adhesive capillarity occurs as evidenced by liquid rising within a solid structure.

Plain gauze is constructed so that it wicks away wound secretions or blood by capillary action (Fig. 9-1, *A*). This is due to the multiple twisted fibers in the gauze threads. Absorption occurs between these fibers. This may cause swelling of the threads and thus prevent further absorption. The soaked-up secretions dry and may form a barrier over the wound, preventing further capillary action. In addition, drying of the secretions makes it difficult to remove the dressing at the time of the dressing change.

When an absorbent layer is placed above the gauze layer, some wound exudate is wicked through the gauze into the upper layer. This minimizes the formation of dried secretions and helps preserve the capillarity of the gauze.

A dressing's ability to absorb exudate is related to the rate at which the exudate soaks into the dressing and the maximal quantity of exudate the dressing is capable of absorbing. The speed with which a liquid soaks into a dressing is known as absorbency. The maximal quantity of fluid that can be absorbed by a dressing is termed the water retention coefficient or absorbing capacity. The water retention coefficient is related to the fiber arrangement of the dressing. The most regular structures, such as finely woven gauze, have the lowest water retention coefficients, whereas the most irregular, such as cotton wool, have the highest. Sphagnum moss, used by the American Indians for dressings, has a very irregular structure and thus a high water retention coefficient.[101,144]

For good wicking action of a dressing, close contact must exist between the dressing and the wound, as well as between the various layers of the dressing. Therefore close adhesion between the dressing layers is important to ensure.

The contact layer of dressing next to the wound, as mentioned previously, is frequently impregnated with ointment to keep the dressing from sticking to the wound. Three different types of ointment are used to cover gauze:

1. *Ointment that is both water insoluble and water nonabsorbent (hydrophobic).* Petrolatum, such as Vaseline, is such an ointment. When ointment of this type is used, the wound exudate is trapped beneath the dressing and cannot pass through it easily (Fig. 9-1, *B*). Antibiotic ointments containing petrolatum placed beneath gauze produce a similar situation.

2. *Ointment that is water insoluble but water absorbent (hydrophilic).* Hydrophilic petrolatum is an example

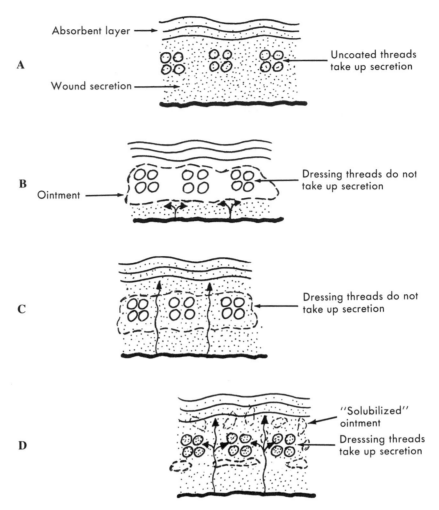

Fig. 9-1. Capillarity of dressings. **A,** Uncoated contact dressing threads. **B,** Hydrophobic non-water-soluble ointment coating contact dressing threads. **C,** Hydrophilic non–water soluble ointment coating contact dressing threads. **D,** Hydrophilic water-soluble ointment coating contact dressing threads. (Modified from Noe, J.M., and Kalish, S.: Surg. Gynecol. Obstet. **143:**454, 1976.)

of this type of ointment. The wound exudate, which is water soluble, is absorbed by the hydrophilic petrolatum and usually is passed into the absorbent layer above (Fig. 9-1, *C*). Since the hydrophilic petrolatum is not water soluble it remains on the threads and keeps them from soaking up secretions and swelling. An example of this type of ointment-gauze combination is Aquaphor Gauze (Beiersdorf, Norwalk, Conn.). The term "gauze" here does not mean cotton gauze but rather gauze-type construction (woven or otherwise constructed with interstices). Aquaphor Gauze is composed of woven cellulose acetate, a semisynthetic material.

3. *Ointment that is water soluble and water absorbent (hydrophilic).* An example of this type of ointment is hydrophilic ointment. In this situation the wound exudate is drawn into the ointment. Because the

ointment is also soluble in the exudate, both ointment and exudate pass into the absorbent layer above (Fig. 9-1, *D*). Xero-Flo Gauze* (Chesebrough-Ponds, Greenwich, Conn.) is impregnated with a hydrophilic ointment base containing 3% bismuth tribromophenate. Several other antibacterial creams and ointments in similar bases are available and may be combined with gauze *at the same time* the dressing is applied. For instance, Silvadene Cream (Marion Laboratories, Kansas City, Mo.) is a hydrophilic ointment that is commonly applied to gauze over burns. A substance that functions in a manner similar

---

*Do not confuse with XeroForm Gauze Dressing (Chesebrough-Ponds, Greenwich, Conn.), which is impregnated with a more occlusive petrolatum blend but also contains 3% bismuth tribromophenate.

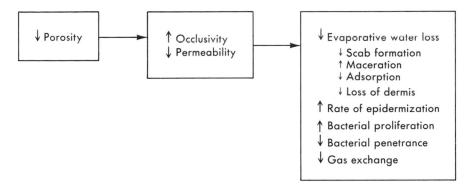

Fig. 9-2.. Relationship of dressing porosity to wound healing.

to hydrophilic ointment is polyethylene glycol, which is used as a base for other antibacterial agents such as Furacin Water Soluble Dressing (Norwich Eaton, Norwich, N.Y.).

In dressings for sutured excisional wounds the contact layer serves mainly to protect the wound from outside contaminants and allow painless removal of the dressing; sorptive capacity for secretions is usually a lesser priority. Therefore petrolatum impregnated gauze may be preferred. Since petrolatum is hydrophobic, it protects the wound from within and minimizes soaking of the absorbent portion of the dressing, which only serves to draw organisms into the wound.

Adherence

The phenomenon of a dressing sticking (adsorbing) to a wound is seen frequently but is rarely discussed. If a dressing adheres unduly to a wound, it can disrupt partially healed tissue and pull off new epidermis at the time of removal, delaying wound healing. Therefore knowledge of this seemingly simple phenomenon and its causes are essential when dressing wounds.

Adhesion of a dressing may occur through three mechanisms[123,146]: the exudate of the wound may act as a glue, the interstitial size of the contact layer may be large enough to permit penetration by granulation tissue, or the fibrous exudate of the wound may physically entrap the dressing. Thus the absorbency of a dressing is related to its adherence. The more absorbent the dressing material, the more it is likely to stick. Conversely, the less absorbent, the less it will stick. A compromise dressing should be selected based on the characteristics of the wound.

The exudate acts as a glue because of its protein content.[146] As the exudate dries by evaporation, the protein content steadily increases. If there is little evaporation loss through drying, the dressing is unlikely to stick.

A single-layer dressing applied alone directly to a weeping wound will stick to some degree whether it is impregnated with an ointment or not. Without a secondary absorbent layer, which draws secretions away from the contact layer by capillary action, the secretions dry by exposure to air, forming a crust that entraps the dressing. Dry gauze is the dressing most likely to become entrapped; gauze impregnated with hydrophobic ointment sticks less because the fibers are filled with the ointment and thus cannot be penetrated by the exudate (Fig. 9-7).

If the contact layer of a dressing has an absorbent layer above it, the secretions are to some degree drawn into this layer and the contact layer sticks less. If the absorbent layer or even the outer wrap is occlusive, this prevents drying of secretions and minimizes adherence to the wound even more.

The intersticial size of gauze varies with the number of threads running in either direction per square inch. The smaller the interstice, the less likely granulation tissue will penetrate. Fine-mesh gauze has very small interstices. Conversely, the larger the interstice, the greater the likelihood that the gauze will be penetrated and entrapped by granulation tissue. If penetration of the dressing by granulation tissue is desired for debridement, wide-mesh fabric should be used. Such material provides absorption without occlusion. If entrapment would impede wound healing, fine-mesh fabrics or, preferably, nonperforated dressings are suggested. A more complete description of gauze construction is given later in the chapter.

Occlusivity

One of the most important factors affecting the events of wound healing is the occlusivity of a dressing. The occlusivity is inversely related to the permeability to water vapor and is a function of the pore size of the dressing material (Fig. 9-2). The smaller the pore size, the greater the occlusivity and the less the permeability. Conversely, the larger the pore size, the less the occlusivity and the greater the permeability. Dressings may be ranked with respect to relative occlusivity as shown in Fig. 9-3. Pore size of a dressing also affects whether bacteria will be able to penetrate it.

Intact human skin could be considered an ideal dressing with which synthetic or nonsynthetic dressings should be compared. Human epidermis allows gas exchange and in-

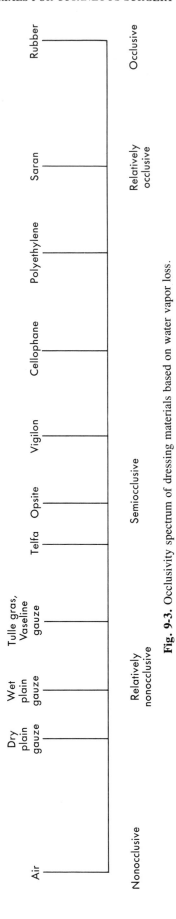

Fig. 9-3. Occlusivity spectrum of dressing materials based on water vapor loss.

sensible water loss. When applied to wounds, it is tightly adherent and may have antibacterial properties by virtue of this tight seal.

In nature, the epidermis forming the roof of an intact blister acts as a dressing. Gimbel et al.[58] studied the rate of epidermization of blister burns in humans. These investigators found that the wound bed epithelialized 40% faster when the roof of the blister was left intact than when it was unroofed. If the blister fluid was aspirated, the rate of epithelialization was slowed down, but not as much as when the blister roof was removed. Therefore a blister roof helps to maintain a moist microenvironment that favors the rapid reepithelialization of superficial wounds.

Evaporative water loss

How does the blister roof help provide an ideal environment for wound healing? One answer is that the blister roof allows the diffusion of oxygen and limits the insensible water loss. Winsor and Burch[167] found that the water diffusion loss through a blister roof that was left intact was about the same as through normal skin. However, if the stratum corneum was removed, the diffusion rate markedly increased. Therefore, within the epidermis itself, it is the stratum corneum that provides the greatest barrier to water loss. These investigators calculated that the tissue fluid loss was 10 times greater from the floor of an uncovered blister or superficial wound than from a blister covered by epidermis.

When the blister roof limits evaporative water loss, a wet environment is maintained that bathes the wound bed and the regenerating epidermis. Such a moist environment decreases desiccation of the wound bed, which increases both collagen synthesis and the rate of epithelialization. A moist environment recreates the original milieu in which wound healing must have first occurred, the primordial ocean.

Forage[45] investigated identical burns on the legs of patients. He noted that where the blister top was left intact, the patient's wound healed more rapidly with a better cosmetic result at 1 year. Also, the healing wound was less painful. The water loss following epidermis removal was almost 20 times greater than if the epidermis was left intact.

Obviously, different dressings and even different ointments applied to wounds result in different rates of water loss. For instance, Dempski, DeMarco, and Marcus[34] found that petrolatum was the most effective barrier to water loss and was five or six times more effective than Saran Wrap. Therefore topical wound preparations must be considered important in influencing wound healing.

Occlusive dressings that are impervious to both water and water vapor can produce maceration and sodden-appearing wounds. Materials that cause such effects include rubber compounds[25] and nonperforated polyethylene film.[151]

Rate of epidermization

Several studies have demonstrated that the actual rate of epidermization of superficial type I wounds is faster with relatively occlusive dressings both in animals[38,99,168,169,172] and humans.[77,98,140,149] It should be stressed that the wounds investigated in these studies extended only into the superficial dermis and therefore did not involve extensive fibroplasia or granulation tissue formation. Furthermore, although the pig has been the favored animal model for such studies because its skin is superficially similar to human skin, there are several important differences, such as the lack of eccrine glands and almost universal presence of apocrine glands in the pig's skin.[119] Since reepithelialization occurs from adnexal structures as well as from the sides of wounds, these differences may be significant.

In contrast to the speed of healing in superficial wounds, the speed of healing in full-thickness wounds may not be significantly faster with occlusion than if air exposed.[131,151] Knudsen and Snitker[89] compared punch biopsy sites (full thickness of dermis) that were occluded by Telfa with those left uncovered. They found no significant difference in the rate of wound healing. This study, however, was not substantiated by a later investigation, which found that occlusion increased healing of punch biopsy wounds.

How do dressings affect superficial wound epidermization? One effect is on the migration rate of the epidermis. Krawczyk[90] studied the epidermal cell migration when agents such as colchicine or vinblastine were administered. Although these drugs interrupted the mitotic activity, no difference was seen in the epidermal migration rates in blisters on mice. Therefore it is the migration rate and not the mitotic rate that is affected by wound coverage. Fisher and Maibach[43] actually found a decrease in mitotic rate for human skin stripped of stratum corneum and then covered with a dressing.

Although the weight of the evidence just cited seems to minimize the importance of mitotic rate in occluded wounds, the less occlusive the dressing, the higher the mitotic rate that may occur. Rovee et al.[140] found that air-exposed skin stripped of stratum corneum had a greater mitotic peak than similarly stripped occluded skin. This could be interpreted to mean that, with occlusion, migration occurs so fast that mitosis makes little contribution to resurfacing the wound. However, with no occlusive dressing and subsequent dehydration, epidermal mitosis plays a greater role because of the longer or more tortuous route that the epidermis must travel in such a desiccated environment.

In contrast to the foregoing studies, Salomon, Diegelmann, and Cohen[143] found that dressings increased epidermal cell mitoses in split-thickness skin graft donor sites. Their study, however, did not employ highly occlusive dressings, but mainly highly porous medicated dressings. Therefore these wounds were relatively nonoccluded and air exposed. In addition, the drugs incorporated into such

dressings need to be taken into account when studying their effects on wound healing and epidermal cell mitotic rates.

Whether migration or mitosis or a combination of both influences epidermal cell migration, the rate of regeneration is about 0.25 to 0.5 mm per day. This is approximately one cell diameter per hour, the same rate as the growth of hair, which is about 0.3 to 0.5 mm per day.[172]

Effects on dermis and scab formation

The effect of occlusive dressings on the dermis, although little discussed, is also important. Such dressings help to keep the base of a wound from drying out. If wounds are allowed to dry and form a scab, a portion of the superficial dermis will also dry out and be incorporated into the scab.[82,140] Therefore recognizable collagen fibers can be seen in scabs, especially at their edges.[178]

Winter and Scales[169] performed a classic study of wound healing in large white pigs. Superficial wounds were created and then either occluded with a dressing or left undressed with a stream of air blown over their surface. These investigators found that the air-blown wounds developed a much thicker scab and epithelialized more slowly than the occluded wounds. This led to the concept that a scab represented an impediment to wound reepidermization. The slower rate of epidermal regeneration was related to the fact that the epidermis must migrate down, below dehydrated fibrous tissue where the environment is sufficiently moist for cells to live.[170] The greater the desiccation of the dermis, the thicker and deeper the scab, and the farther the epidermal cells must travel to bridge the gap in a wound (see Fig. 2-24).

An additional reason why a thick scab may also cause slower epidermization in superficial wounds is that the contribution from the adnexal structures will be less. As pointed out in Chapter 2, superficial (type I) wounds extending only to the superficial dermis heal not only from the skin edges but from the adnexal structures as well. This is the case with dermabrasion wounds or most wounds resulting from curettage and electrodesiccation. Scabs may also become infected, further slowing epidermization.

Lawrence[93] performed an interesting experiment on guinea pigs with piebald skin (Fig. 9-4). He grafted black skin onto white areas of prospective burn sites. This was done in such a way as to produce squares of white skin surrounded on all sides by black skin (Fig. 9-4, *C*). The white squares were then burned and covered with either a relatively nonocclusive or a semiocclusive (Op-Site) dressing (Fig. 9-4, *D*). If covered by the nonocclusive dressing, the resultant healed wounds were black, indicating that the new epidermis had come from only the pigmented edges of the wound. However, if the wounds were covered by a semiocclusive dressing, the wound was covered by white skin. This white skin could have come only from the nonpigmented adnexal structures deep in the dermis.

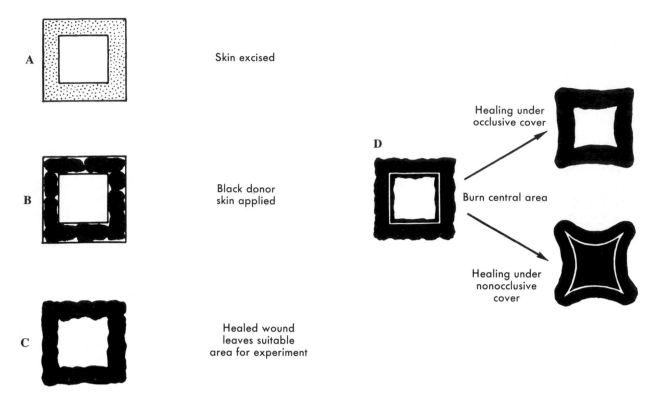

Fig. 9-4. Experiments with piebald guinea pigs. See text for details. (From Lawrence, J.C.: Injury **13:**500, 1982.)

Lawrence's study is important because it points out the greater loss of the dermis that can occur with nonocclusive dressings. This loss of collagen can lead to unsightly scars, since they cast a great shadow because of their depth.[140] Skin flaps in rats have also been shown to lose less tissue if covered with a semiocclusive cream rather than being allowed to air dry.[113]

Other effects of occlusive dressings on the dermis include an early decrease in the inflammatory response[99,140] and a less intense fibroblastic response at 7 days in comparison with air-exposed wounds.[99] The lack of inflammation helps to increase the rate of wound healing by providing less debris for the cells, whether dermal or epidermal, to remove. The decreased fibroblastic response[99] may result from the lessened early inflammation as well as the earlier, more efficient collagen synthesis. Alvarez, Mertz, and Eaglstein[6] found that collagen synthesis was increased with occlusion of superficial wounds by Op-Site (Smith & Nephew, Massillon, Ohio) or Duoderm (ConvaTec, Princeton, N.J.).

The relationship between occlusion of deep (type II) wounds and wound contraction has also been noted. Zahir[177] believes that the loss of moisture in wounds aids the contraction process. Perhaps this can be explained by the heightened prolonged fibroplasia induced by air exposure and scab formation.

Bacterial entrance and proliferation

Since the time of Lister, over a century ago, dressings have been viewed both as barriers to infection and as a means to combat the presence of bacteria. The latter function is why dressings may be impregnated with various antibacterial agents.

Moisture within a dressing appears to be the key factor in whether organisms are drawn into a wound. If wet, a dressing acts as a wick, bringing microbes into or out of the wound. This phenomenon of bacterial penetration is sometimes referred to as *bacterial strike-through.* Owens[125] in 1943 showed that it was possible to draw organisms into a wound model from the outside through 64 layers of moist gauze. This was prevented, however, by interposing cellophane within the gauze. Cellophane is waterproof but permeable to water vapor. It apparently also prohibits the passage of bacteria.

Colebrook and Hood[28] performed in vitro experiments with a cotton gauze and wool dressing soaked with plasma. Like Owens, they found that bacteria traversed the full thickness of the dressing within 4 to 48 hours. *Pseudomonas* were the fastest bacteria, appearing in as little time as 4 hours. Hemolytic *Streptococcus* took from 24 to 48 hours to appear, and *Staphylococcus aureus* was the slowest in initial appearance at 42 hours. The motility of *Pseudomonas* probably affected its ability to pass through dressings relatively quickly. Cellophane also prevented the passage of bacteria in this dressing model.

These experiments point out the general misconceptions that the outside of dressing may be handled with impunity and that dressings are an effective barrier to microbial passage. Once a dressing becomes wet, bacteria that come in contact with it can be easily drawn to the wound surface. Therefore dressings should be changed when wet. In addition, hand washing before and after handling a dressing should be encouraged, if not required.

Based on the previously described experiments, modern dressings are frequently designed to prevent bacterial or moisture strike-through. For instance, the Curity Wet-Pruf ABD Pad (Kendall Co., Boston, Mass.) is constructed with two kinds of cotton in the absorbent inner pad. The outer cotton has not been treated (bleached) to remove natural oils and therefore is water repellent. The inner cotton closest to the wound is treated (bleached) and water absorbent. This dressing absorbs some wound exudate but prevents it from reaching the surface of the dressing, which would draw bacteria into the wound. Moisture from the environment is also prevented from entering the wound.

Some dressing materials commonly used on wounds may not be sterile as packaged, especially the outer covering. Pearson, Valenti, and Steigbigel[128] reported five cases of clostridial wound infections associated with the use of elastic outer wraps. All five patients had adult-onset diabetes and wounds on the lower extremities. The elastic bandages used as the outer wraps were nonsterile and found to contain *Clostridium perfringens*. These investigators concluded that the bacterium had gained access to the wound from the outer elastic wrap through the inner gauze barrier.

Rhizopus has also been reported to have caused wound infections from contamination of Elastoplast wound dressings.[51] This fungus has been cultured from unopened nonsterile packages.[87] The manufacturer now makes this elastic outer wrap available in a sterile package.

The best methods of sterilizing various products, especially dressing materials, have not been determined. Although many dressings are sterilized by gamma radiation from cobalt-60, at the current recommended radiation dosage (2.5 megarad) some bacteria and fungi have been found to be radioresistant when placed in fabrics.[91] Infection from these "sterilized" products, especially in immunocompromised hosts, is a conceivable although remote possibility.

The bacterial flora present on the skin and probably in all wounds is influenced by dressing occlusivity. A more porous dressing is more likely to be invaded by bacteria but also produces a drier wound, which is unfavorable for bacterial growth. Conversely, a more occlusive dressing is a greater barrier to environmental bacteria but provides a moist environment conducive to survival of any bacteria present under the dressing.[13] Dressings that are semipermeable and semiocclusive, that is, that resist passage of water but not water vapor, usually form an effective barrier to environmental bacteria and keep the underlying skin or wound moist, yet minimize the survival of indigenous bacteria.[25]

In general, organisms applied to wet skin live longer than those applied to dry skin.[133] When the skin is covered with occlusive dressings, the resident flora increases by a factor of about 10^4.[8,16] This increase is thought to be due to greater hydration that occurs with occlusive dressings, since they allow less insensible water loss. Although the increase in organisms is usually in the lipophilic diphtheroids and micrococci, pathogenic organisms may also thrive in a moist environment if they happen to be present. These organisms may then become dominant.

Both gram-positive and gram-negative pathogenic organisms can survive and grow under occlusive dressings. Bibel and LeBrun[16] found that Enterobacteriaceae (especially *Enterobacter aerogenes*) were the most successful pathogenic colonizers. Other investigators have noted these same gram-negative bacteria in wounds occluded with Saran Wrap.[109]

Staphylococcus aureus is a common pathogen that survives and multiplies rapidly in a moist environment.[145] Marples and Kligman[109] found that *S. aureus* was the most frequent invader and became the dominant organism in 20% of individuals with stripped skin occluded with Saran Wrap and was present in moderate numbers in another 20%.

Although occlusive dressings may result in an apparent qualitative and quantitative increase in pathogenic organisms, delayed wound healing or other signs of true infection may be absent.[116] This seeming paradox may be explained by several factors. The number of bacteria per square centimeter or per gram of tissue is more significant than the mere presence of an organism. Signs of infection or delay in wound healing may not occur until the population reaches a critical number.[98,102] This concept is discussed more fully in Chapter 4.

Another possible explanation for the lack of true clinical infection with the presence of an increased bacterial population may be the moist microenvironment created on the wound surface. With a moist environment, viable leukocytes and phagocytes are likely to be present at the wound surface and to dispose of bacteria. Nonviable tissue, which serves as a haven for bacterial growth, is also minimized under occlusive dressings.[140] In addition, it has been suggested that occlusive dressings may enhance the vascular supply to the wound and thus increase the local concentration of systemic antibiotics, if given.[94]

Gas exchange

Winter[172] and Silver[150] noted that the speed of superficial wound epidermization is correlated with the oxygen permeability of dressings. The positive effects of oxygen on

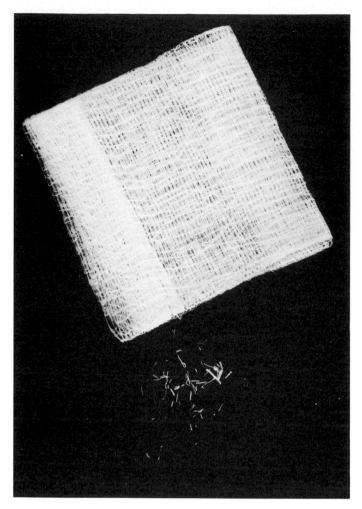

Fig. 9-5. Lint shed from gauze that has rubbed against itself.

wound healing may be due to its direct action on energy production by glycolysis in cells or the known necessity for oxygen by phagocytic leukocytes in killing of bacteria.[78]

Oxygen may have other effects on deep, full-thickness wounds. Knighton, Silver, and Hunt[88] showed that oxygen inhibited rather than stimulated granulation tissue in the rabbit ear model. Hypoxia thus appears to be necessary for wound healing angiogenesis. This may explain the good results on full-thickness wounds seen with dressings, such as Telfa, that have a relatively low oxygen concentration between the dressing and the wound.

Of the dressings tested by Silver,[150] cellophane had a relatively high permeability to oxygen, whereas polyester (Telfa) had a relatively low permeability. Interestingly, wet gauze was less permeable than dry gauze, pointing up the fact that exudate-soaked dressings can be a barrier to oxygen diffusion from the air.

Incorporation of dressing materials into wounds

Dressings may fray, and the detached materials may become incorporated into the wound. Such ravelings occur

during wear or use of fabrics, especially cotton, and are known as lint. Lint from plain gauze may be seen if this material is rubbed upon itself (Fig. 9-5). Cellulose wadding appears to fray the most.[94] Although foreign body reactions in the skin from such free fibers are rare, they have been reported and may impair wound healing and the cosmetic result.[9,153]

The microscopic appearance of the tissue reaction to lint is characteristic. One sees small granulomas or scattered multinucleated giant cells containing minute, unstained, refractile inclusions that are slightly curved or bent sharply on themselves in a hairpin configuration. In one study lint was 3 to 7 μm in diameter and refractile.[9]

New sponges made from nonwoven cellulose fibers that produce one-sixth the lint of regular cotton gauze are under investigation.[161]

Toxicity

Although direct toxic effects of dressings would seem to be a remote possibility, various plastics carry traces of potentially toxic substances. Substances in some dressings (perforated terylene and cellulose acetate) have been shown to impede skin respiration.[94]

WOUND DRESSING MATERIALS

The term "wound dressing" is applied to many products, from Band-Aids to skin grafts. Dressings may be classified in a number of ways. Dressings may be categorized by usage relative to the wound surface as contact layer, absorbent layer, or outer wrap. Dressings may also be categorized according to composition, as is done here. For the purposes of this discussion, dressings are divided into three general categories: natural fabrics, synthetic dressings, and biologic membranes. All three groups of dressings may be modified by impregnation with substances such as glues, ointments, antibiotics, or other materials to modify the behavior of the dressing. In addition, synthetic materials may be combined with natural materials or even biologic materials to produce dressings of complex composition. Therefore some overlap occurs among these three categories.

Natural (nonsynthetic) dressings

Natural dressings are those composed of materials occurring in nature. They include the following:
I. Nonimpregnated
  A. Linen
  B. Silk
  C. Cotton
    1. Threads (bleached)
      a. Cotton balls (Johnson & Johnson)
      b. Cotton roll
    2. Woven gauze (bleached) sponges
      a. Curity Gauze Sponges (Kendall Co.)—
        U.S.P. type VII
      b. Gauze Sponges (Johnson & Johnson)—

U.S.P. type VII
- c. Melrose Gauze Sponges (Professional Medical)
- d. Steri-Pad Gauze Pads (Johnson & Johnson)
3. Woven gauze (bleached) outer wrap roll (see also p. 312)
    - a. Kling (Johnson & Johnson)—2 ply
    - b. Sta-Tite (Chesebrough-Ponds)—2 ply
    - c. Kerlix (Kendall Co.)—6 ply
    - d. Sof-Band (Johnson & Johnson)—6 ply
4. Gauze packing strips
    - a. Nu Gauze Packing Strip (Johnson & Johnson)
5. Knitted tubular gauze (see also p. 312)
    - a. Tubegauze (Scholl)
6. Felted gauze
    - a. Band-Aid Brand Moleskin (Johnson & Johnson)

II. Impregnated
   A. Woven gauze (bleached)
   1. Soft paraffin and vegetable oil
       - a. Tulle gras
   2. Hydrophilic ointment (oil emulsion)
       - a. Xero-Flo (Chesebrough-Ponds)
   3. Hydrophilic petrolatum
   4. Petrolatum
       - a. Vaseline Petrolatum Gauze (Chesebrough-Ponds)
   5. Zinc oxide, calamine, and gelatin (Unna boot)
       - a. Gelocast (Beiersdorf)
       - b. Dome-Paste (Miles, West Haven, Conn.)
       - c. Medico Paste (Graham-Field, New Hyde Park, N.Y.)
   6. Antibacterials
       - a. Betadine Gauze (Purdue-Frederick)
       - b. Iodoform Gauze
       - c. Xeroform Gauze (Chesebrough-Ponds)
       - d. Xeroflo Gauze (Chesebrough-Ponds)
       - e. Nu-Gauze Packing Strips with Iodoform (Johnson & Johnson)
       - f. Sofra-Tulle (Roussel)
       - g. Bacti-gras (Smith & Nephew)
   7. Epithelial stimulants
       - a. Scarlet Red Gauze (Chesebrough-Ponds)

Cotton gauze. The most common wound dressing material used today is cotton. Raw cotton (cotton wool) is relatively nonabsorbent. It must be bleached to remove oils before it becomes absorbent. The bleached cotton is then carded, spun, and woven into gauze. Other natural materials formerly used for dressings include linen and wool.

As pointed out by Baron,[13] textile dressings should be viewed in both two and three dimensions. The two-dimensional view takes into account the cut size of the woven material, the size of the threads themselves, and the sizes of the interstices in the fabric. The three-dimensional view considers in addition the thickness of the material (related to the size of the threads) making up the fabric, as well as the number of layers (ply).

Dressings may be woven, knitted, carded, or felted. Woven fabric has spun threads running in two directions perpendicular to one another. The threads are composed of twisted fibers originating in the basic material. Threads running lengthwise are the warp, whereas those running crosswise are the woof. Such woven fabrics are classified by the number of warp and woof threads per square inch. The U.S. Pharmacopeia[2] divides woven cotton gauze into the following eight types defined by the warp versus woof: I (41-47 × 33-39), II (30-34 × 26-30), III (26-30 × 22-26), IV (22-26 × 18-22), V (20-24 × 16-20), VI (18-22 × 14-18), VII (18-22 × 10-14), and VIII (12-16 × 8-12). The interstices are smallest in type I gauze and largest in type VIII (Fig. 9-6). Gauze is also defined by the final folded cut size (for example, 2 × 2, 3 × 3, 4 × 4 inches) and the ply. The ply is the number of layers resulting after the gauze is folded; commonly this is 8, 12, or 16 ply. The greater the ply, the thicker each piece of gauze and the greater its rate of absorption (absorbency) as well as absorptive capacity.

Dressing fabrics may also be knitted, usually by looping of a single thread (in contradistinction to weaving of two threads). Knitted fabrics generally have more stretch than woven fabrics. Carded fabrics are composed of unwoven, unknitted wool or cotton or both to provide bulk. The carding process gives uniform direction to the threads. If glue is used to glue the cotton or wool threads together, the carded fabric becomes compressed into felt (felted).

Tightly woven fabrics allow little ventilation to the wound and have minimal absorptive capacity. With absorption the threads may swell, closing the interstices and rendering the dressing impermeable. This inhibits further evaporative loss from the wound.

Impregnated gauze. Cotton gauze may be used uncoated or impregnated with various substances. Antibacterials, such as povidone-iodine (Betadine Gauze, Purdue Frederick, Norwalk, Conn.) or bismuth tribromophenate (Xeroform Petrolatum Dressing, Chesebrough Ponds, Greenwich, Conn.), are added to provide an antibacterial effect in wounds. Gauze impregnated with petrolatum or other ointments to render it less likely to stick on the wound surface is also available. Dry gauze uncoated with ointment readily soaks up secretions and holds them in contact with the wound. Another advantage of ointment-impregnated gauze is that in deep wounds it is easily moldable and able to fill defects of any size, thus functioning as a tampon.

Petrolatum is a good impregnant because it is relatively inert, nontoxic, nonsensitizing, and nonirritating. Petrolatum is hydrophobic and is not water soluble. Therefore it provides good occlusion to the wound and good protection

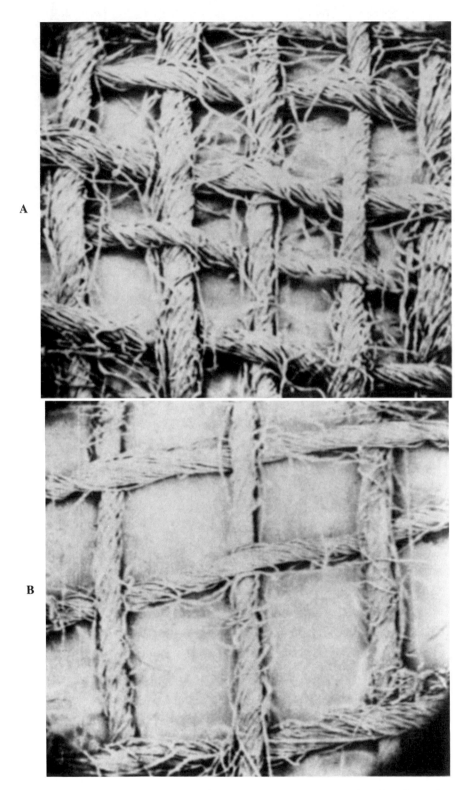

Fig. 9-6. A, U.S.P. type I gauze. (×25.) **B,** U.S.P. type VII gauze. (×25.) Note larger interstices for type VII gauze. (From Noe, J.M., and Kalish, S.: Surg. Gynecol. Obstet. **147:**185, 1978.)

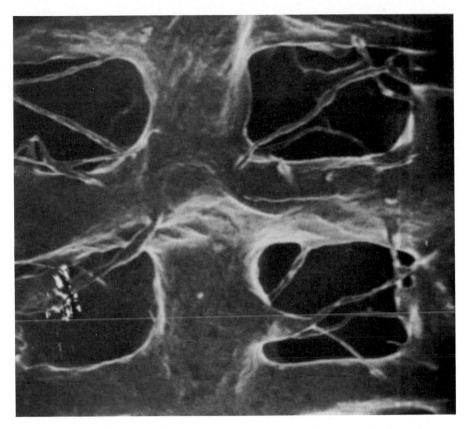

Fig. 9-7. Petrolatum-impregnated gauze (U.S.P. type I). (×53.) Note strands of petrolatum spanning the interstices. (From Noe, J.M., and Kalish, S.: Surg. Gynecol. Obstet. **147:**185, 1978.)

from outside contaminants. Gauze that is impregnated with hydrophobic petrolatum (Vaseline Petrolatum Gauze) is a fine mesh (USP type I gauze) that is easy to remove from the wound. It is flexible and does not tend to slip on the wound surface. Because the petrolatum blocks the interstices to some extent (Fig. 9-7), secretions are deterred from penetrating the interstices and ventilation of the wound surface is impaired. As a result, maceration may occur if this dressing is left in place for long periods of time. Interestingly, the "inert" materials with which gauze may be impregnated or combined may affect wound reepithelialization. In one study Vaseline Petrolatum Gauze and Xeroform Petrolatum Dressing seemed to help epidermization, whereas Furacin Cream was not helpful.[152] Geronemus, Mertz, and Eaglstein[53] found that Furacin actually decreased the rate of epithelialization. In a study by Gemberling et al.[52] on split-thickness skin graft donor sites in humans, gauze impregnated with Vaseline, Xeroform, or other impregnants had no more effect on the healing rate of wounds than plain gauze. Therefore these authors concluded that plain gauze was as good for this purpose as any other commercially available gauze whether or not it was impregnated by an antibacterial substance or ointment. However, plain gauze probably causes more pain than other dressings when used on split-thickness skin graft donor sites because this fabric

constantly shears as the threads of the fabric move and because it shrinks when wet.

Although most of the substances contained in dressings are nontoxic, they may have harmful effects if applied to wide areas and absorbed. For instance, polyethylene glycol in Furacin-soluble dressing has been reported to be absorbed when this dressing was used on burn patients and resulted in renal failure, particularly in patients with renal impairment.[158] Allergic sensitization may occur with prolonged use of antibiotic-impregnated dressings.

Tulle gras. In Western Europe, especially France and England, a specially prepared gauze called tulle gras is used. This is a fine-mesh gauze (cotton or silk) impregnated with soft paraffin wax, balsam of Peru, and vegetable oil. It allows some air to reach the wound and at the same time permits drainage.[111] The paraffin helps keep the dressing from sticking to draining wounds. However, the oxygen tension is low under such dressings.[150] Tulle gras may be impregnated with various antibiotics, such as silver sulfadiazine, framycetin (Sofra-Tulle), or chlorhexidine (Bactigras). It is currently used for dressing burns and split-thickness graft donor sites. Gillman and Hathorn[55] found that it promoted granulation and contraction of rabbit wounds.

Extensible outer wrap cotton gauze. Modified cotton bandages with coarse weaves and wide meshes are extensible but have minimal elastic qualities (see outline on p. 312). These products are used as the final contouring outer wraps to provide cushioning, compression, and support to wounds, as well as to keep the other dressings in place. They are particularly useful on the scalp and extremities. Because they are extensible, they expand somewhat to accommodate any significant swelling. Kling (Johnson & Johnson, New Brunswick, N.J.) is all woven cotton, chemically treated to give it elasticity. It tends to cling to itself and other dressings, which prevents telescoping and slipping. In other products elastic or nylon threads have been added to impart elasticity.

Kerlix (Kendall Co., Boston, Mass.) is another useful extensible bandage. It is especially woven and dried to give it bulk and elasticity. Its open weave pattern provides good wicking and excellent aeration of the underlying wound. It has slightly more elasticity than Kling. In addition, it is a six-ply product and thus more absorbent than Kling, which is two-ply.

Synthetic and semisynthetic dressings

The drawbacks of cloth dressings have been known for centuries. When soaked with exudate, such materials are painful to remove and damage the underlying wound. Halsted[66] in 1913 proposed that gutta percha be used as a surgical dressing. This material is a nonelastic, naturally occurring polymer that resembles rubber and is used today in dentistry, as well as to cover golf balls and underwater cables. Its use as a surgical dressing was based on its ability to help seal a wound and to be removed without disturbing the wound bed. However, its almost totally occlusive property makes it less than ideal. Gutta percha was, nevertheless, a forerunner of modern polymer dressings.

With the development of polymer chemistry in the 1930s, synthetic dressings made their appearance. These are usually constructed to be semipermeable. Perhaps the first use of a synthetic or semisynthetic dressing was reported by Bloom[20] in 1945. The material used was cellophane, which was obtained from the wrapping of blood transfusion equipment and was first used while Bloom was a prisoner of war during World War II. He noted that the pain from wounds disappeared after application of cellophane. Cellophane (regenerated cellulose) is waterproof but allows water vapor to escape from the wound surface. Therefore it is semipermeable rather than totally occlusive. Since it is made from a regenerated, naturally-occurring substance (cellulose), it is considered semisynthetic.

Bull[25] in 1948 tested nylon fabric as a dressing and thought that it performed well. Schilling, Roberts, and Goodman[149] showed that nylon dressings significantly shortened healing time for abrasions and lacerations compared with totally occlusive dressings. This was probably the first well-controlled trial of dressing materials. However, this dressing material never caught on. Polyvinyl-

chloride film that was made microporous was the next material to be investigated. Scales, Towers, and Goodman[145] showed that on the fingers this microporous film significantly shortened the healing time for minor cuts and abrasions compared with more occlusive dressings. In addition, it was associated with a lower infection rate with *Staphylococcus aureus* than more occlusive dressings. These studies represent the beginning of the manufacture of dressing materials based on the physiology of wound healing and wound problems. The microporous polyvinylchloride dressing was subsequently marketed as Airstrip (Smith & Nephew, Massillon, Ohio).

The following are synthetic and semisynthetic dressings:

I. Regenerated Cellulose
   A. Sheets (from cellulose xanthate)
      1. Cellophane
   B. Threads (from cellulose xanthate)
      1. Rayon
      2. Curity Rayon Ball (Kendall Co.)
   C. Woven (from cellulose acetate)
      1. Aquaphor Gauze (Beiersdorf)—with Aquaphor
      2. Adaptic Gauze (Johnson & Johnson)—with hydrophilic petrolatum
   D. Plastic film (from cellulose nitrate)
      1. Collodion (pyroxylin)
      2. New-Skin (MedTech)
   E. Multilayer (distinct contact and absorbent layers)—rayon facing and cellulose/cotton interior
      1. Adherent to wound, nonbulky
         a. Topper (Johnson & Johnson)
      2. Adherent to wound, bulky
         a. Combine Pad (Chasten Medical)
         b. Composite Padding (Prof. Med.)
         c. Curity Wet-Pruf ABD Pad (Kendall Co.)
         d. Curity Oval Eye Pads (Kendall Co.)
         e. Eyepad (Johnson & Johnson)
         f. Surgi-Pad (Johnson & Johnson)
         g. Triple (Prof. Med.)
II. Polyamide (for example, nylon)
   A. Woven
      1. Owens Surgical Dressing (Davis & Geck)—"parachute silk"
   B. Gauze-type (open mesh, nonwoven)
      1. Cover-Roll Stretch (Beiersdorf)
III. Polyester (for example, Dacron)
   A. Film (see also polyurethane film below [VII]) for comparison)
      1. Blister Film (Chesebrough-Ponds)—without adhesive over wound
      2. Co-Film (Chesebrough-Ponds)—with adhesive over wound
IV. Polymer blend (nonwoven)

A. N-Terface (Winfield Laboratories)
V. Polyester-cellulose (rayon) combination
  A. Gauze-type blend (nonwoven)
    1. Excilon (Kendall Co.)—6 ply
    2. Nu Gauze (Johnson & Johnson)
    3. Soft-Wick (Johnson & Johnson)
    4. Sorb-It (Prof. Med.)
    5. Tendersorb (Kendall Co.)—6 ply
    6. Versalon (Kendall Co.)—4 ply
VI. Polymer film—cellulose-polyester combination (distinct contact and absorbent layers)
  A. Nonadherent to wound, nonbulk
    1. Airstrip (Smith & Nephew)—with adhesive on edges
    2. Microdon Non-Adherent Sheeting (3M)
    3. Microdon Surgical Dressing (3M)—with Micropore tape on edges
    4. Release (Johnson & Johnson)
    5. Telfa (Kendall Co.)
    6. Telfa "Ouchless" Sterile Adhesive Pad (Kendall Co.)—with adhesive on edges
  B. Slight adherence to wound, slight bulk
    1. Band-Aid Brand Surgical Adhesive Dressing (Johnson & Johnson)—with Dermicel tape
    2. Coverlet (Beiersdorf) with paper tape
    3. Cover-Pad (Beiersdorf)
    4. Steri-Pad Sterile Pads (Johnson & Johnson)
    5. Yield Non-Adherent Dressing (Prof. Med.)
VII. Polyurethane film (see also polyester film above [III])
  A. With adhesive
    1. Bioclusive (Johnson & Johnson)
    2. Ensure (Deseret Med.)
    3. OpraFlex (distributed by Professional Medical)
    4. Op-Site (Smith & Nephew)
    5. Polyskin (Kendall Co.)
    6. Tegaderm (3M)
    7. Uniflex (United Division, Pfizer)
  B. Without adhesive
VIII. Polyurethane foam
  A. With adhesive
    1. Reston Self-Adhering Foam Pad (3M)
  B. Without adhesive
    1. Epi-Lock (Derma-Lock Medical Corp.)
    2. Synthaderm (Derma-Lock Medical Corp.)
IX. Silastic foam
X. Colloid dressings
  A. Bard Absorptive Dressing (Bard Home Health Care, Inc.)
  B. Comfeel (Colloplast)
  C. Debrisan (Johnson & Johnson)
  D. Duoderm (ConvaTec)
  E. Gelliperm (Geistlich Pharmaceuticals)
  F. Johnson & Johnson Ulcer Dressing (Johnson & Johnson)
  G. Vigilon Primary Wound Dressing (Bard Home Health Care, Inc.)
XI. Plastic film (from acrylate)
  A. Hydron (Hydron Laboratories)

Cellulose-derived dressings. Cellulose is the main structural component of wood and plant fibers. Cotton, for instance, is almost pure cellulose. Starch, on the other hand, is also derived from plants but makes up the reserve food supply.

Various acids or alkalis may act on cellulose, yielding semisynthetic materials. Cellulose nitrate results from the action of nitric acid on cellulose. Pyroxylin is a common cellulose nitrate that is the main component of collodion. Cellulose acetate results from the reaction of acetic acid, acetic anhydride, and sulfuric acid on cellulose. Cellulose acetate may be formed into filaments, which are known as acetate rayon. Finally, cellulose may react with carbon disulfide and aqueous sodium hydroxide to form cellulose xanthate. When this is dissolved in alkalis, a viscous colloidal dispersion called viscose is produced. If the viscose is forced through holes, fine filaments known as rayon are produced. On the other hand, if viscose is forced through narrow slits, thin sheets known as cellophane are made.

Many of the cellulose products just mentioned are important components of dressings (see preceding outline). For instance, Aquaphor Gauze is gauze made from cellulose acetate and impregnated with Aquaphor.

Several bulk-type dressings are mainly derived from cellulose. Usually these have a nonwoven rayon facing (covering) and an interior (inner) composed of rayon or cotton fibers, or both. For example, Surgi-Pad (Johnson & Johnson, New Brunswick, N.J.) is composed of a rayon facing and a cotton/cellulose inner. The inner provides bulk and cushioning for the wound. Although this type of dressing is more absorbent than regular gauze, it is also more likely to get wet and thus more susceptible to bacterial or moisture strike-through. To avoid this problem, some composite cellulose dressings are constructed so the outer portion of the bulk inner layer is waterproof, preventing penetration of water from inside or outside.

Cellulose products may also be combined into dressings that have little bulk and good wicking action. Topper (Johnson & Johnson, New Brunswick, N.J.) is an example of this concept. These pads have a gauze-type rayon covering and a cellulose filler for better wicking action. However, if the pads are used during surgery, the filler material may fray and shed.

The multilayer regenerated cellulose dressings just mentioned are not coated with materials that prevent adhesion of the dressing to the wound. Therefore, if applied to heavily draining wounds, such dressings tend to stick at the time of dressing changes.

Semi-synthetic gauze. Modern materials such as regenerated cellulose and polyester may be fashioned into fabrics that resemble cotton gauze (see outline on p. 324). Nu Gauze (Johnson & Johnson, New Brunswick, N.J.), made from rayon and polyester fiber, is an example. These semisynthetic gauzes are more absorbent than a comparable layer of cotton gauze.

Nonadherent dry dressings. Telfa was one of the first widely used dressings that was nonadherent and dry. Telfa dressings are thin pads composed of two uniformly perforated polyester films between which is an inner composed of absorbent cellulose. The film is ¼ mil (0.00025 inch) thick and has about 200 perforations per square inch. Each perforation is 0.2 to 1 mm in diameter. The inner is about 2 mm thick.[134]

Telfa pads have been in wide use since they were first introduced in the mid-1950s. Early studies showed that these dressings did not stick to wounds.[62,134] They have continued to enjoy popularity because of this property and because they have been used for many years without ill effects.

Telfa pads are not totally occlusive, especially underneath the small holes in the polyester film. Significant water loss occurs from the dermis opposite these perforations. When the wound is highly exudative, the absorbent inner becomes soaked, which renders the dressing occlusive. In addition, with excessive exudate the dressing tends to stick to the wound surface at the location of the small holes if left in place for long periods.

Winter[171] performed biopsies in pigs of split-thickness wounds that were dressed with Telfa pads. The areas underneath the holes showed evidence of superficial necrosis, and the wounds in general took longer to epithelialize than if covered by a more occlusive, nonperforated, inert film. If Telfa pads are left in place until healing is complete over split-thickness skin graft donor sites, a uniform pattern of these dried-out areas of tissues may be seen localized underneath the small uniform perforation patterns.[117]

The ability of Telfa to promote wound healing has been questioned. As mentioned, Winter showed that epidermization was slowed by Telfa.[171] Early studies in rabbits showed that Telfa inhibited granulation tissue formation and wound contraction.[55,56] The oxygen tension underneath Telfa is about the same as under dry gauze.[150] Punch biopsy wounds in humans either allowed to heal by exposure to air or covered with Telfa pads showed no difference in the rate of healing.[89] On the other hand, Stark[152] in a study on rabbit ear wounds noted that Telfa helped epidermization.

Despite conflicting data, Telfa pads have survived the test of time. I routinely use these dressings on almost all excisional wounds and wounds allowed to heal by granulation and epithelialization. The pads may be easily cut to conform to the wound shape or depth. There is minimal fraying of the cut edges. If the pads are changed daily, the drying-out effect underneath the perforations is minimized. In addition, an antibiotic may be used with this dressing, which further minimizes drying and any sticking that might otherwise occur.

The drawback of dressings such as Telfa is the low absorbency of the dressing pad. For wounds that drain continuously, this dressing must be changed frequently (twice a day) or a more absorbent dressing may be used.

Other nonadherent dry dressings that are similar to Telfa include Release (Johnson & Johnson, New Brunswick, N.J.), and Airstrip. Telfa Ouchless Sterile Adhesive Pads are also available; these have adhesive on the edges so they may be applied as a large adhesive bandage.

Owens Surgical Dressing (Davis & Geck) is a woven nylon similar in texture to parachute silk. This fine-mesh material is another nonadherent dry dressing because nylon does not absorb water. Therefore this dressing does not stick to draining wounds. A new product composed of a nonwoven polymer blend is N-Terface (Winfield Laboratories, Richardson, Tex.), which like pure nylon is nonadherent.

Vapor-permeable films. Within the past decade a new class of surgical dressings usually composed of polyurethane has appeared. These dressings are permeable to water vapor but not to water. Op-Site is the prototypic dressing in this class of dressings, since it was the first to be developed and has been the most widely investigated. Polyurethane film was initially used as a surgical drape, but with the development in understanding of moist wound healing, it came to be used as a postoperative wound cover.

Op-Site is a thin, transparent, polyurethane membrane coated on one side with a polyvinyl ethyl ether adhesive that sticks only to dry surfaces. It is gas permeable, allowing the passage of oxygen, carbon dioxide, and water vapor but preventing the efflux of larger molecules, such as protein and water. Because it is permeable to water vapor, Op-Site allows the escape of insensible water and vaporization of sweat from the skin. This helps to preclude maceration of the wound. Op-Site is nonirritant and prevents the passage of bacteria, thus protecting the wound from outside contamination. Because this dressing is transparent, the wound may be covered and yet directly inspected. Op-Site is slightly elastic, conforming well to superficial wounds in nonhairy areas.

Although theoretically Op-Site may be useful in any wound that is not unduly contaminated, it is ideally suited for split-thickness skin graft donor sites.[14] The dressing is applied after bleeding has stopped and is left in place until healing is complete, usually in 7 to 10 days depending on the wound depth. The Op-Site is allowed to separate spontaneously. Usually a compression dressing is used on top of the Op-Site for the first few days to minimize wound exudate and absorb leakage that may occur around the dressing edge.

When used as a wound cover for split-thickness skin graft donor sites, Op-Site has been shown to result in a faster rate of epithelialization than gauze (Fig. 9-8).[12,15,17] Wound collagen synthesis is also increased.[6] Moreover, patients are more comfortable and have less pain than those with more traditional gauze dressings, which tend to rub the wound surface as the patients move about.[36,83]

Op-Site has been reported to be useful for ulcers on the lower extremities or elsewhere that have resisted conventional methods to promote wound healing. In Alper's study[5] of patients who had more than one leg ulcer, one of which was treated with Op-Site, the Op-Site-treated wound healed 2.6 times faster than the control wound. Another advantage of Op-Site therapy for leg ulcer patients is that they may be treated as outpatients, since they require less frequent dressing changes.

Op-Site has been used in Britain both as a wound cover for sutured incisional wounds and as sutureless skin closures in place of percutaneous sutures.[26,157] It allows direct inspection of the wound, and as a sutureless skin closure it is said to be adequate for bringing the wound edges together. The advantages and disadvantages of sutureless skin closures are discussed in Chapter 8.

Another interesting use for Op-Site is on skin grafts at the recipient site. Its use over pinch grafts has been recommended.[57] Op-Site may also be used as a "backbone" for thin split-thickness skin grafts to keep them from folding or crinkling at the time of harvesting. When used in this manner, Op-Site is applied on the skin donor area before the time of harvesting a split-thickness skin graft. As the skin graft is cut with a dermatome, the Op-Site keeps the skin graft stiff. The harvested skin graft with the Op-Site attached is then sutured into place at the recipient site.[155] Another sheet of Op-Site may be used instead of sutures over the skin graft with the Op-Site attached.

Op-Site has been reported to be associated with some wound problems. If the dressing, which adheres to dry surfaces, is removed too soon after the new epidermis forms underneath, it may dislodge this epidermis.[6,179] This is because the newly formed epidermis is not tightly adherent to the underlying dermis and thus adheres preferentially to the adhesive on the dressing material. Therefore Op-Site should be allowed to separate spontaneously.[83]

An exudate, usually serosanguineous but sometimes purulent, is present under Op-Site in 50% to 70% of wounds.[36,114] Aside from its appearance, the exudate does not present any problems. Occasionally the serum works its way to a free edge of the dressing where it drains. Therefore an absorbent dressing over the Op-Site for the first few days is recommended to catch this leakage.[83] A No. 21 butterfly needle may be used to provide drainage from underneath the Op-Site. Its attached tubing (with holes cut in the side first to provide drainage) is placed under the Op-Site and the needle is inserted into a Vacutainer tube.[132] An alternative

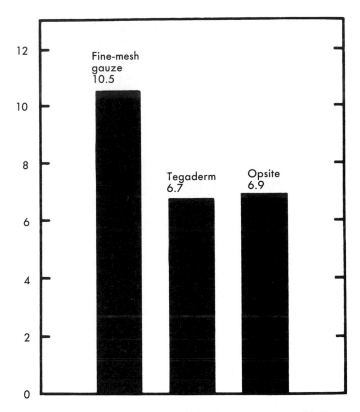

Fig. 9-8. Days (expressed on vertical axis) to complete epithelization of split-thickness skin graft donor sites covered by fine-mesh gauze, Tegaderm, or Op-Site. (From Barnett, A., et al.: Am. J. Surg. **145**:379, 1983.)

method of removing the exudate is by aspiration through the membrane with a small-gauge needle. If the needle hole does not reseal itself, it may be patched with another piece of Op-Site.[159] Excessive fluid accumulation may necessitate changing the dressing.

The problem of infection underneath Op-Site dressings was reported in the early clinical evaluations of this material.[14,36,83,100] but was not emphasized. As clinical experience was gained, it became a more widely recognized phenomenon.[42,106] It would seem reasonable that the semiocclusivity of Op-Site would promote the proliferation of bacteria, particularly in the moist wound environment provided by this dressing. However, with Op-Site the wound infection rates range from 2% to 12% depending on the reasons for its use.*

Mertz and Eaglstein[116] studied the bacterial proliferation underneath Op-Site placed on superficial wounds on pigs. They found a significant increase in the bacterial population (to the level of 10^7) after 48 hours. The composition of the bacterial population shifted toward the gram-negative types. Although these authors did not believe that the mere pres-

---

*References 14, 36, 83, 100, 114, and 147.

ence of such bacterial populations necessarily interferes with wound healing or leads to infection, they cautioned that physicians and nurses should be alert to possible clinical wound infection.

The premise that the presence of bacteria underneath Op-Site dressings does not necessarily presage infection and delayed wound healing is supported by the poor association of bacterial presence with clinical wound infection. Alper[5] noted that 15 of 16 wounds treated with this dressing healed despite gross bacterial contamination. Schein and Dunn[147] cultured underneath Op-Site dressings and had positive cultures in 38% of the cases, but only one third of these developed clinical infection.

Infection underneath Op-Site may also occur even though no exudate is present. McLean and MacKinlay[114] studied 103 patients in whom Op-Site was used as a postoperative wound dressing. Infection occurred in eight patients, only five of whom had an exudate.

Part of the explanation for the low infection rate despite large numbers of bacteria appears to be that the exudate that collects underneath Op-Site is bactericidal. This exudate may be either purulent or serosanguineous. When the exudate is examined under the microscope, large numbers of polymorphonuclear leukocytes, some of which have intracellular bacteria, are seen.[100]

Buchan[24] studied the exudate under Op-Site and found that it had significant bactericidal activity. He found that the cell type and number of cells were typical of an inflammatory exudate and that the protein content appeared to be indistinguishable from that of plasma. The neutrophils in the exudate killed *Staphylococcus aureus* at the same rate as in whole blood. Lysozyme levels were increased in the exudate, probably because of death of or leakage from neutrophils. This enzyme is particularly active against gram-negative bacteria such as *Pseudomonas*. Op-Site has also been shown to activate the third component of complement (C3), which aids in microbial killing by facilitating opsonization and phagocytosis.[79]

Other polyurethane membranes similar to Op-Site include Tegaderm (3M, Minneapolis, Minn.), Ensure (Deseret Med., Inc., Sandy, Utah), Bioclusive (Johnson & Johnson, New Brunswick, N.J.), and Polyskin (Kendall Co., Boston, Mass.). These products may not all be equivalent, however. In one study,[79] Op-Site was found to be superior to Tegaderm in both bacterial killing and ability to activate C3. Apparently Tegaderm does not activate complement.

Two new vapor-permeable films composed of polyester but similar in function to the polyurethane films just discussed are Blister Film and Co-Film (Chesebrough-Ponds, Greenwich, Conn.). Co-Film is made with an adhesive that covers the wound surface, whereas Blister Film has the adhesive just along the edges of the film and not in contact with the wound. Thus when Blister Film is removed from newly formed epidermis, it theoretically will not pull the epidermis with it as sometimes happens with adhesive-backed polyurethane films.

Polyurethane foam. Two newly available dressings, Epi-Lock and Synthaderm (Derma-Lock Medical Corp., Englewood, Colo.), are dry dressings composed of modified polyurethane. Epi-Lock is smaller (5 × 5 cm) than Synthaderm (10 × 10 cm). These dressings have hydrophilic properties on one side of the dressing and hydrophobic properties on the other. Thus they absorb wound exudate yet are waterproof to the outside environment. Because they are gas and water vapor permeable, they promote epidermal proliferation under ideal conditions.

Wayne[165] compared Epi-Lock with Xeroform as dressings on burns, abrasions, and lacerations seen in an emergency room. He found that "quality of healing," speed of healing, and ease of use, were statistically better in all three groups with Epi-Lock. In addition, use of Epi-Lock was less expensive for the patients. Therefore Epi-Lock was shown to be superior to the other dressing tested.

Two cases of contact dermatitis associated with Synthaderm have been reported.[72] However, the exact allergen was not established.

The Reston Self-Adhering Foam Pad (3M, Minneapolis, Minn.) is a thick polyurethane foam pad adhesive on one side. This product is useful for placing pressure on skin grafts or other wounds.

Silastic foam. Silicone may be made into a rubber foam (Silicone Foam Elastomer, Dow Corning, Midland, Mich.) by means of a catalyst. This rubber foam can be used as a packing, especially for deep ulcers such as pilonidal sinuses. It contours to the wound, is nonadherent, and yet is absorptive. Although experience with this material is limited in the United States, it has reportedly been used successfully in Britain[166,174] and Canada.[60] Its main advantages over other types of packing for deep wounds are that it is less expensive, requires little skilled nursing care for dressing changes, and is comfortable for patients.

Colloid dressings. Colloid dressings are based on principles of colloid chemistry, which must be understood to appreciate the mechanism of action of these materials. All colloid systems are composed of two phases of matter, the dispersed or internal phase and the dispersion medium or external phase. The dispersed phase is composed of colloid particles that are suspended in the dispersion medium. These particles generally range in size from 1 to 100 μm. When water is the dispersion medium, the colloid is known as a hydrosol. Colloids exist because of the mutually unattractive charges between the colloid particles.

The term "colloid sol" or simply "sol" is synonomous with "colloidal solution," but it is important to realize that a colloid sol is not a true solution. A solution is composed of a single phase, with the molecules dissolved rather than suspended.

A gel is a special type of colloid in which the colloid particles are particularly attracted to the dispersion medium. Cooling a colloid solution usually produces a substance that is jellylike. Jellies are a special subclass of gels characterized by the presence of large amounts of water.

Gels have a property called imbibition, which is a tendency to take up liquid and swell. This is based partially on the fact that the gel acts as a semipermeable membrane to diffusible electrolytes in the solution surrounding the gel. Because the colloid particles in the gel cannot diffuse through its surface into solution, a Donnan equilibrium is set up between the gel and the surrounding solution. Since the concentration of particles is usually higher in the gel than in the surrounding solution, water diffuses from the solution into the gel, and the gel swells.

Gels as wound dressings have several advantages besides absorption (imbibition) of wound exudate. Gels cool the wound area and are air permeable. They conform to the wound surface and adhere to the wound by gel tension. Gels may also be safely applied over antibacterial agents.

Colloid membranes are ubiquitous in the cells and tissues of the body. Therefore it is not surprising that colloid dressings promote wound healing by providing an environment similar to that seen on the surface of cells. In addition, colloid membranes provide a surface charge that may have stimulatory effects on wound healing.

Debrisan (Johnson & Johnson, New Brunswick, N.J.) is a powder of dry, porous, spherical hydrophilic beads (0.1 to 0.3 mm in diameter) composed of Dextranomer. Dextranomer is composed of macromolecular chains of cross-linked dextran. When placed into oozing wounds the beads swell, acting as a hydrogel, and form a gelatinous mass. Small molecules are absorbed into the beads themselves, and large molecules (greater than 5000 molecular weight) are sucked into the spaces between the beads. Plasma proteins and fibrinogen in particular are found between the swollen beads. Thus the principles of colloid swelling and capillarity underlie Debrisan's ability to function. A suction force is generated that removes wound exudate and possibly bacteria from the wound surface.

Debrisan is directly applied to a wound by pouring the beads into it. However, if left until dry, Debrisan is difficult to wash off and delays healing. Therefore it should not be left in a wound for more than 24 hours. Although initial clinical studies with Debrisan were encouraging,[120,121] it has not been widely accepted because it is expensive and requires a high level of nursing care. There have been relatively few adequately designed studies establishing the advantages of Debrisan over other types of dressings, especially outside the hospital environment.[120] However, it may be worth considering as an alternative dressing for removal of pus or necrotic debris when other methods are difficult or unsuccessful because of the wound's depth.

Duoderm (ConvaTec, Princeton, N.J.) is an adhesive colloid dressing. It is composed of gelatin, pectin, sodium carboxymethylcellulose and polyisobutylene. Duoderm is applied as a dry dressing with a polyurethane backing. When it interacts with the wound exudate, it swells, forming a soft, moist hydrocolloid gel. Duoderm molds easily to the contours of the body surface and is adherent to it because it is coated with an adhesive (modified Stomadhesive). Although it is relatively occlusive and impermeable to oxygen, these characteristics do not appear to adversely affect the rate of wound repair. In pigs, Duoderm was shown to increase the rates of reepithelialization of wounds and collagen synthesis.[5]

Friedman and Su[49] compared Duoderm with conventional treatment of leg ulcers in seven patients with 20 ulcers. Although the healing time was the same in both groups, Duoderm was more convenient because it was changed much less frequently (every few days). In addition, patients said that they had much less pain. One disadvantage of Duoderm is that it sticks to the underlying dry tissue, so newly formed epidermis may come off with the dressing and thus actual healing time may be prolonged.[179]

Vigilon Primary Wound Dressing (Bard Home Health Care, Inc., Berkeley Heights, N.J.) is a new, moist, hydrogel sheet composed of a colloidal suspension of 4% polyethylene oxide and 96% water. The inert cross-linked polyethylene oxide is the dispersed phase, and the water is the dispersion medium. Vigilon is oxygen permeable and transparent. On both surfaces is a thin polyethylene film. The occlusivity of (and thus water vapor loss through) the membrane may be altered by removing only one or both films. The film on one side is usually removed so the gel is in direct contact with the wound. This results in some water vapor transmission, yet provides a moist wound cover on a moist wound surface with little danger of maceration. The outer film is usually left in place. If it is removed, water vapor transmission is increased and the wound exudate may seep through the hydrogel sheet, necessitating the use of outer absorbent dressings. Like other gels Vigilon absorbs considerable wound exudate by imbibition. It is so absorptive that it can soak up its own weight in wound exudate within 24 hours.

Like other gels, Vigilon has a cooling effect because it induces a high rate of evaporative water loss. Therefore it is mildly anesthetic and feels soothing on burns or abrasions. It contains no glues but is slightly adherent (gel adherence); some type of tape or overlying bandage must be used to keep it in place. It is also flexible, conforms well to body contours, and provides some cushioning that protects the wound. Therefore it does not disrupt the epidermis when dressing changes are performed. Like other colloids it is compatible with topical medications.

Clinical experience with Vigilon has been mixed. Mandy[106] reported that two patients with dermabrasion wounds had less pain and more rapid healing with Vigilon

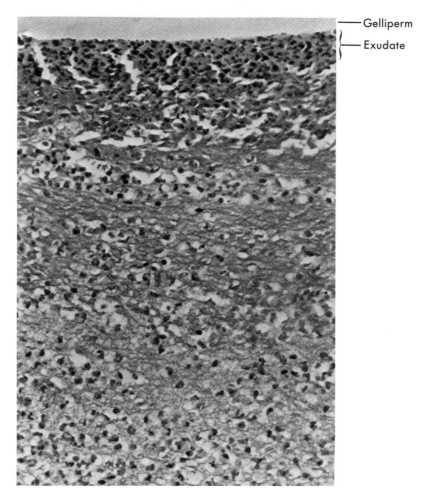

Fig. 9-9. Gelliperm on wound surface. Note exudate between the dressing and wound surface. (From Wokalek, H., et al.: Aktuel. Dermatol. **5:**255, 1979.)

than with Adaptic dressings (Johnson & Johnson, New Brunswick, N.J.). Geronemus and Robins[54] showed that in pigs superficial wounds treated with Vigilon had a 44% faster rate of epithelialization than untreated wounds. However, when Yates et al.[176] evaluated Vigilon for emergency room abrasions, four wounds became infected and five patients had a minor hypersensitivity reaction, the exact cause of which was not determined. These authors concluded that Vigilon was no better than standard dressings for suppurative wounds. The same material as Vigilon may be purchased less expensively in nonsterile form in athletic stores under the name Cool Skin (Spenco Medical Corp., Waco, Tex.).

Gelliperm (Geislich Pharmaceuticals, Inc., Washington, D.C.) is a hydrogel similar to Vigilon. Gelliperm is composed of true agar copolymerized with acrylamide and dispersed in water. This gel is thicker than Vigilon and therefore gives more support to wounds. In addition, it has the ability to absorb pigment particles and therefore may be useful after dermabrasions for tattoos. Wokalek et al.[173] evaluated Gelliperm in 100 patients. These authors pointed out that a wall of fibrinous exudate appears to form between the gel dressing and the wound surface (Fig.9-9). Within this exudate are a considerable number of leukocytes. Gelliperm may be purchased either as a sheet or as a minced gel that may be packed into wounds.

An additional hydrogel product that may be useful on exudative ulcers is Bard Absorptive Dressing (Bard Home Health Care, Inc., Berkeley Heights, N.J.). This is a copolymer of cornstarch packaged as a dry powder. When hydrated it forms a moldable hydrogel that may be placed in the wound. It absorbs approximately 14 times more blood than a piece of gauze. In pigs it was found to increase the superficial wound epithelialization rate by 24%.[54]

Plastic film dressings. Plastic spray dressings that form a thin film over wounds were formerly used but are no longer available. A plastic is a high–molecular weight, synthetic organic compound to which plasticizers may be added to change the compound's character. Although plastics in liquid form were initially used as wound dressings,[135,163] spray dressings forming films were later used.[164] These plastic films were transparent and were said to be permeable to oxygen as well as water vapor. Plastic spray dressings were popular for use on sutured wounds, especially in hair-bearing areas such as the scalp, where they remained in position until the sutures were removed. These dressings were not found to accelerate wound healing but did appear to protect wounds from bacteria.[131,163] Some products were actually shown to be antibacterial.[164]

Although plastic dressings were convenient and theoretically protected wounds, a number of problems associated with them led to their decreased usage. First, plastic compounds may contain products theoretically toxic to wounds. Second, some researchers found that plastic film dressings formed a mechanical barrier to epithelialization and thus impeded wound healing.[59] Third, the thickness of the film over a sutured wound was difficult to adjust accurately. If the film was too thick, it was more occlusive than necessary and resulted in an increased bacterial flora. Finally, although these films provided a measure of protection from bacteria, some bacteria still penetrated.[164]

A recently developed polyacrylate dressing is the Hydron Burn Dressing (Hydron Laboratories, Inc., New Brunswick, N.J.).[130] This dressing is a polyhydroxyethylmethacrylate that forms a thin, transparent, unilaminate membrane in situ on wounds. Although it does not appear to interfere with wound healing, it does allow infection if colonization of the wound surface occurs. Usually this happens when small cracks develop in the dressing membrane.

Another use of plastic films is on skin irritated by wound secretions, urine, or feces. Products such as Bard Protective Barrier Film (Bard Home Health Care, Inc., Berkeley Heights, N.J.) are available as liquids or aerosols. Although these products are designed for use around stomas or for incontinent patients, they may also be used on tape-irritated skin when further use of skin tapes will be necessary for dressing changes.

Collodion may be used in the same manner as plastic spray dressings without the problem of toxic side effects. It forms a tenacious, sticky film that adheres to the skin on drying. Collodion has been used as a paint-on dressing for wounds for at least a century. It is a viscous solution of cellulose nitrate (nitrocellulose) in ether and alcohol. Although it is a semi-synthetic dressing, it is mentioned here for comparison. Collodion may also be painted on either side of a wound as a glue for gauze, which is then splinted over the wound.[69]

Elastic bandages. Elastic bandages are bandages with considerable stretch and elasticity. They are used as outer cover (secondary) dressings (see p. 312) and when it is essential to place pressure on a wound. Usually elastic bandages are composed of synthetic fibers and rubbers, although rubber may also be combined with more traditional cotton. It is important to distinguish between elastic bandages and stretchable gauze. Stretchable gauze is specially treated or woven gauze that has some stretch, but less than an elastic bandage.

Elastic bandages can be divided into those that are nonadhesive, those that adhere to the skin, and those that are mostly self-adherent (that is, sticking mostly to the substance of which they are made). Ace Wrap (Becton-Dickinson, Rochelle Park, N.J.) is a typical elastic nonadhesive bandage. Self-adherent elastic bandages are frequently crepe designed. The elastic adhesive bandages include Elastoplast (Beiersdorf, Norwalk, Conn.). Microfoam tape (3M, Minneapolis, Minn.) has been added to this dressing category, since this tape stretches and thus provides a good pressure dressing.

Another way in which dressings may be made elastic and stretchable is by knitting rather than weaving. For example, tubular gauze is knitted and therefore more stretchable than woven gauze. Some of the knitted fabrics have rubber or Spandex added for elasticity. X-Span Tubular Dressing (Concept, Clearwater, Fla.) is an example of this type of construction. These dressing materials are excellent for placing pressure on the digits or extremities.

Adhesive bandages. Adhesive bandages are bandages with a nonadhesive contact layer, a thin absorbent layer, and tape, all packaged as a single unit in individually wrapped packages (see following outline).

The following are adhesive bandages:
  I. Spots
   A. Band-Aid Brand Sheerspot (Johnson & Johnson)
   B. Coverlet Spot (Beiersdorf)*
   C. Curad Spot (Kendall Co.)
   D. Ready Bandage Spot (Prof. Med.)
   E. Salvesept Plastic Spot (Cedarroth)
   F. Salvesept Woven Cloth Spot (Cedarroth)*
 II. Strips
   A. Band-Aid Brand (Johnson & Johnson)
    1. Flexband*
    2. Medicated (benzalkonium chloride)
    3. Plastic
    4. Sheer Strip
    5. Tricot Mesh
   B. Coverlet (Beiersdorf)*
   C. Curad (Kendall Co.)
   D. Curad Flexible (Kendall Co.)*
   E. Nichi-Aid (Nichiban)
   F. Ready Bandage Strip (Prof. Med.)
   G. Salvesept Plastic Strip (Cedarroth)
   H. Salvesept Woven Cloth Strip (Cedarroth)*
   I. Stik-Tite Adhesive Bandage (American White Cross)

---

*Significant stretch.

J. Super-Band (American White Cross)*
III. Special cut adhesive bandages (for knuckles, fingers, and so on)
 A. Band-Aid Brand Flexible Fabric (Johnson & Johnson)*
 B. Coverlet (Beiersdorf)*
 C. Salvesept Plastic (Cedarroth)
 D. Salvesept Woven Cloth (Cedarroth)*
 E. Super-Band (American White Cross)*
IV. Patches
 A. Airstrip (Smith & Nephew)
 B. Band-Aid Brand Sheer Patch (Johnson & Johnson)
 C. Coverlet Patches (Beiersdorf)*
 D. Ready Bandage Patch (Prof. Med.)
 E. Salvesept Plastic Patch (Cedarroth)
 F. Salvesept Woven Cloth Patch (Cedarroth)*
 G. Super-Band Patch (American White Cross)*
V. Surgical dressing-type adhesive bandages
 A. Airstrip (Smith & Nephew)
 B. Band-Aid Surgical Dressing (Johnson & Johnson)—with Dermicel tape
 C. Coverlet O.R. (Beiersdorf)
 D. Microdon Surgical Dressing (3M)—with Microspore tape
 E. Telfa "Ouchless" Sterile Adhesive Pad (Kendall Co.)
 F. Yield Non-Adherent Dressing (Prof. Med.)

The prototypic adhesive bandage is the plastic Band-Aid Strip (Johnson & Johnson, New Brunswick, N.J.). Adhesive bandages are available as small "spots," which are excellent after small skin biopsies, as plastic strips, or as patches or pads. Some adhesive bandages (such as Coverlet, Beiersdorf, Norwalk, Conn.) are knitted and thus stretchable to provide some pressure on wounds. A large, nonadherent bandage that is convenient for use over wounds is the Telfa "Ouchless" Sterile Adhesive Pad (Kendall Co., Boston, Mass.), which is a flesh-tone Telfa pad with adhesive on two edges.

Biologic dressings

Biologic dressings are dressings composed wholly or partially of tissue derived from human or animal sources. They include the following:
 I. Homograft
 A. Autograft
 1. Skin graft
 2. Cultural skin
 B. Isograft
 II. Heterograft
 A. Allograft

1. Human amniochorionic membrane
 2. Skin graft
 B. Xenograft
 1. Porcine
 a. Mediskin (Genetic Lab, Inc.)
 b. Mediskin with Silver (Genetic Lab, Inc.)
 c. E-Z Derm (Genetic Lab, Inc.)
III. Synthetic-biological dressing
 A. Silicone-porcine
 1. Biobrane (Woodroof Laboratories)

The best biologic dressing is the cutaneous autograft, to which other dressings should be compared to determine their relative effectiveness. The autograft is a graft from one part of the body to another in the same individual. An isograft is a graft between genetically identical twins. An allograft is a graft from another person who is genetically different, usually a relative or cadaver. A xenograft is a graft from an animal to a human or vice versa. Human amnion is a special type of allograft from the fetal membranes. Other biologic dressings include combinations of synthetic materials and animal tissues.

The major benefit of biologic dressings is that, if they adhere tightly to the wound bed, the microbial population density falls dramatically. This concept, which is basic to understanding how a biologic membrane (or any dressing) functions, was appreciated as early as 1924 by Dr. V.P. Blair.[19] Even if biologic membranes do not adhere tightly, they may hasten debridement of wounds because of the submembrane suppuration that occurs; presumably both bacterial and white blood cell enzymes assist in debridement of nonviable tissue. In addition, biologic membranes function in the same way as other dressings to decrease desiccation of the wound bed, reduce contamination, protect the wound, and lessen the patient's pain.

One benefit of a cutaneous graft is its antibacterial effects. It is sometimes stated that skin coverage of a contaminated wound results in its sterilization. Burleson and Eiseman[27] tested the effect of both homografts and xenografts (porcine skin) on wound bacteria in rats as well as in vitro. These investigators found that bacterial counts were decreased within granulation tissue, but not on the wound surface itself. On petri dishes with bacteria, skin grafts did not inhibit bacterial proliferation. Therefore it appears that the antibacterial effect of skin grafts has more to do with tight adherence to the wound bed than with intrinsic antibacterial effect. Interestingly, viability of the skin was not essential for the antibacterial effect.

Amniochorionic membrane. Human amniochorionic membrane has been used as a wound covering since 1910.[33] Although the initial reported experiences with this tissue were not successful, Sabella[141] recorded its successful use in five wounds in 1913. Amniochorionic membrane is composed of two layers, the amnion and the chorion. Amnion is histologically similar to fetal skin. It is formed from the

---

*Significant stretch.

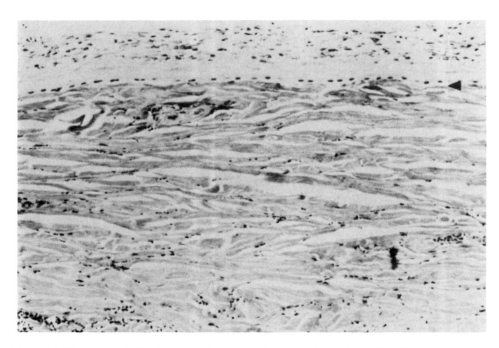

Fig. 9-10. Human amniochorionic membrane dressing on wound with amnion side in contact with wound. The chorion is above the amnion. Note lack of wound exudate at dressing-wound interface *(arrowhead)* compared with that in Fig. 9-9. (From Kucan, O., Robson, M.C., and Parsons, R.W.: Ann. Plast. Surg. **8:**523, 1982.)

ectoderm as is the cutaneous surface of a fetus. Amnion is a thin membrane consisting of an epithelial layer that rests on thin connective tissue. The epithelial layer is directed toward the fetus and is composed of cuboidal or flattened epithelial cells. The connective tissue has delicate processes that pass to the chorion. The chorion is the membranous portion of the fetal membrane and has villous attachments to the endometrium. It is composed of loosely spaced mesenchymal tissue. The amnion and chorion may be used together on wounds, or the amniotic membrane may be used alone. Robson et al.[139] suggest that for partial-thickness wounds amnion should be used alone, whereas for full-thickness wounds amniochorionic membrane should be used with the chorion side down. This allows some vascularization of the chorion, which helps to reduce bacteria. Since vascularization does not occur with amnion alone, amnion is a more temporary biologic cover.

Amniotic membranes have been used successfully for human wounds[40,112,139] and are particularly successful for dermabraded surfaces. Kucan, Robson, and Parsons[92] described a series of 33 patients who had amniochorionic membrane used as a dressing after dermabrasion. They reported excellent results and stressed that the whole amniochorionic membrane could be used but that the amnion side should be placed directly *down* on the wound surface. Their method for preparation of this membrane is as follows. The membranes are aseptically removed from the placenta, with no attempt to separate the amnion from the chorion. The membrane is then passed through four separate rinses of sterile saline, one rinse of 0.025% sodium hypochlorite solution, and four more rinses with sterile saline. Each rinsing solution is agitated to clean any clots or other extraneous matter from the membranes. The membranes are then refrigerated at 4° C in sterile containers, cultured at weekly intervals, and discarded after 6 weeks of storage.

Amniotic membrane is pliable and adheres tightly to wound surfaces. Use of amniotic membrane has resulted in the rapid appearance of clean, healthy granulation tissue in wounds, faster healing, and decreased bacterial growth on wounds. It has thus been suggested that amnion may have both angiogenic and antibacterial effects.[112] Human amniotic membranes are not immediately rejected when placed on wounds, perhaps because this tissue contains glycoproteins that block the rejection phenomenon or because amniotic epithelial cells do not express HLA antigens.[3]

Amnion appears to be superior to other biologic membrane grafts for lowering bacterial counts in wounds.[138,139] This may be because this tissue adheres to wound surfaces and does not allow the formation of a significant wound exudate (Fig. 9-10). Another possible explanation is that allantoin, a purine breakdown product associated with amniotic fluid and thus the amnion, may be bacteriostatic.[40]

Pig skin. Pig skin (porcine xenograft) has also been reported to be useful as a temporary biologic dressing.[23] The use of pig skin for this purpose was partially predicated on the close structural similarity of pig skin to human skin.

However, pig skin has several limitations and is inferior to most other types of biologic membranes.[64] Porcine xenografts are short lived and bond only weakly to human wounds. This results in poorer bacteriostatic properties than those of human allografts or amniotic membranes.[138] When pig skin for dressing split-thickness skin graft donor sites was used and compared with gauze or air exposure, no differences in the rate of wound healing were noted.[142] An additional potential problem with this biologic dressing is that pig skin breakdown products can be absorbed, giving rise to increased human antiporcine cytotoxic antibodies.[64] Therefore pig skin is probably not as useful as other types of biologic dressings.

Biobrane. Biobrane (Woodroof Laboratories, Inc., Santa Ana, Calif.) is considered here as a biologic membrane dressing although it is mostly synthetic. It is a bilaminate structure, with an inner knitted nylon fabric bonded to a thin, semipermeable silicone rubber membrane on the outside. The inner nylon fabric is coated with type I porcine collagen, which allows the Biobrane to adhere to tissue without inflammation. This dressing is semipermeable, allowing passage of water vapor but not bacteria. It is elastic and easily draped on wounds. However, it may directly affect the contraction of wounds. In a study of rats, contraction took three times longer to occur in wounds dressed with Biobrane than it did to occur in open wounds.[46]

Although for the present the ultimate wound dressing is the skin autograft, tissue culture–derived skin grafts are being investigated.[130] Since the time needed to form a significant amount of tissue in culture for grafting can be several weeks, skin autografts are much faster. However, with improved technology, skin grafting as it is now known may become a thing of the past.

MISCELLANEOUS SUBSTANCES COMBINED WITH DRESSINGS

As mentioned previously, dressing materials may be used with various substances to modify wound healing. Some of these substances also modify the dressing itself and thus require separate discussion.

The art of surgical dressings changes in much the same way as clothing fashions—on a yearly or even seasonal basis. Whether new dressing materials or old dressings impregnated or combined with various substances (such as antibiotics) make any difference in facilitating wound healing is open to question. Andersen[10] studied 32 infected wounds and calculated the rate of wound healing using various types of antiseptics, as well as packing. He tried dry gauze, saline, alcohol, iodoform, Merthiolate, Dakin's solution, and zinc peroxide cream. None of these substances seemed to make a difference with respect to the healing of the wounds studied, provided that drainage and debridement of devitalized tissue were adequate.

Saline

Saline is used with gauze to keep wounds moist and relatively clean before reparative surgery (wet-to-wet dressings) or to debride wounds (wet-to-dry dressings). Saline-soaked gauze left in an open, draining wound eventually dries and adheres to the wound bed. Thus for wet-to-wet dressings the gauze must be changed every hour or a plastic sheet must be used to reduce evaporative loss. For wet-to-dry dressings the gauze is allowed to air dry, but not necessarily completely. The gauze adheres to the wound, and thus the act of removal debrides the wound. Secretions from the wound potentiate this debridement by being absorbed between the cotton gauze fibers and within the interstices of the fabric.

Saline is innocuous and does not damage tissue or interfere with wound healing.[175] Brånemark[21] studied the microcirculatory effects of various disinfectants and saline on the hamster cheek pouch. Saline induced no recognizable changes in the microcirculation, whereas the other agents tested (tap water, distilled water, soap, and iodophor) did.

Astringents

Astringents (see Chapter 4) placed in contact with wounds have a drying effect and a mild antibacterial action. Useful astringents include hypertonic saline, 5% aluminum acetate solution (Burrow's solution), zinc sulfate (0.5% to 1%) acetic acid, potassium permanganate (0.025% to 0.1%), and silver nitrate (0.25% to 0.5%). Potassium permanganate and silver nitrate may stain the skin.

The drying effect of astringents combined with gauze is due to their hypertonicity, which draws wound secretions into the gauze and then permits evaporative water loss. Usually gauze with astringents is used as a wet-to-semidry compress to absorb exudate from a weeping wound and thus prevent the buildup of debris and keep a crust from forming. Saturated gauze is changed every 10 to 15 minutes for 30 minutes to 1 hour depending on the amount of drainage. This process is repeated three or four times a day. Between the wet-to-dry compresses the wound is dressed.

Some astringents, such as Burow's solution or potassium permanganate, may be used as a bath or soaking solution for particularly eczematous, oozing skin or leg ulcers. Usually the patient bathes once or twice a day in such a solution.

Petrolatum

Petrolatum combined with gauze (Vaseline Gauze) is readily available. Sterile petrolatum is also available in individually packaged containers for one time use (U.S.P. White Petrolatum, E. Fougera, Melville, N.Y.).

Petrolatum is generally considered inert and, aside from its moisture-retaining properties, is not considered to influence the wound healing process, but this may not be the case. Eaglstein and Mertz[38,39] showed that petrolatum (Vaseline) decreases the epithelialization rate of with superficial wounds in pigs. Less occlusive creams or lotions applied to similar wounds increased the rate of epithelialization. The reasons for these differences in the epithelialization rates are unclear but may be related to the highly occlusive properties of Vaseline. Petrolatum has been shown to be a much more effective barrier to water loss than even Saran Wrap.[34] It should be remembered that Vaseline Petrolatum Gauze is not totally occlusive and indeed is probably less occlusive than plain Vaseline applied to a wound. This helps to explain the fact that Vaseline Petrolatum Gauze, rather than pure Vaseline, increased the epithelialization rates in other animal experiments.[152]

Benzoyl peroxide

Benzoyl peroxide dressings have been recommended to facilitate wound healing, especially on wounds that are slow to heal.[103] Benzoyl peroxide is a powerful oxidizing agent. It releases molecular oxygen, which helps provide energy to cells involved in wound healing. It may also have an indirect bacteriostatic effect by providing phagocytes with the oxygen necessary for bacterial destruction. In addition, benzoyl peroxide helps to stimulate granulation tissue. To release oxygen effectively, the benzoyl peroxide must be kept moist and at 37° C.[126] This is done by covering it with plastic film and a thick pad. Benzoyl peroxide is known to be a potent contact sensitizer, and it would be reasonable to assume that with the high concentration recommended for use in wounds (10% to 20%), a high degree of sensitization would result.

Pace[126] reported on the use of benzoyl peroxide (20% and 50%) in 133 nonhealing ulcers with only 13 failures. In 5% of his patients either an irritant or a contact allergic reaction occurred. The benzoyl peroxide did not have a bactericidal effect on any organisms in the wounds in which it was tested. Later studies using 20% benzoyl peroxide in both animals[7,29] and humans[103] seemed to substantiate the benefit of this substance on wounds. However, Lookingbill, Miller, and Knowles[102] did not demonstrate any benefit from using 10% benzoyl peroxide on chronic leg ulcers. Whether this was because of the lower concentration used or the different types of wounds is open to speculation.

Alvarez et al.[7] in an interesting experiment in piglets showed that 20% benzoyl peroxide lotion increased the rate of superficial wound epithelialization by 33% over a 7-day period, compared with untreated wounds. The benzoyl peroxide that had the highest zinc level had the greatest effect on wound healing. Meleney, an early worker in surgical microbiology, recommended zinc peroxide to stimulate wound healing, so perhaps there is some basis for this recommendation.[126]

Hydrogen peroxide

When hydrogen peroxide is instilled into wounds, it comes into contact with catalase, an enzyme found in blood and most tissues. This enzyme rapidly decomposes the hydrogen peroxide to oxygen and water. The released oxygen probably has little antibacterial effect. However, the effervescent effect of the peroxide helps to loosen the dried exudate or debris on the wound surface.

Although some physicians believe that hydrogen peroxide is more injurious to wounds than normal saline, I have found it to be innocuous in open wounds. Hydrogen peroxide should not be placed under pressure into closed wounds because of the possibility that gas could be released to the vascular system and result in embolism.

Antibacterial agents

The use of topical antibiotics and antiseptics in wounds is discussed in Chapters 2 and 3. The ointments commonly used on cutaneous wounds are Bacitracin Ointment (Eli Lilly & Co., Indianapolis, Ind.); Neomycin Ointment (Upjohn Co., Kalamazoo, Mich.); Ilotycin Ointment (Dista Products Co., Indianapolis, Ind.), containing erythromycin; Polysporin Ointment (Burroughs Wellcome Co., Research Triangle Park, N.C.), containing bacitracin and polymyxin B; and Neosporin Ointment (Burroughs Wellcome), containing bacitracin, neomycin, and polymyxin B. These ointments are compounded in a petrolatum base that, as previously discussed, is both water insoluble and water nonabsorbent (hydrophobic).

Besides having an obvious effect on the flora of a wound, antibiotics may enhance or depress events in wound healing such as epithelialization. For instance, Neosporin Ointment and Silvadene Cream (silver sulfadiazine) were found to increase the rate of epithelialization, whereas nitrofurazone (Furacin) decreased it.[53,152] Possibly nitrofurzone inhibits the induction of ornithine decarboxylase, an enzyme normally increased in healing wounds.[97]

Nitrofurazone (Furacin) is available for topical use on wounds as either a cream or a water-soluble base. The latter contains mainly polyethylene glycol. When the water-soluble base dressing is combined with gauze, the wound secretions are drawn into the gauze. If an absorbent layer is placed over the gauze, which is usually the case, the nitrofurazone is drawn with the secretions into the absorbent layer. As just mentioned, nitrofurazone may impede epithelialization. In addition, if applied to large areas, as in burn patients, polyethylene glycol is absorbed and can result in renal failure, especially in patients with renal impairment.[158]

Silver sulfadiazine (Silvadene) is available as a 1% cream that is water soluble and water absorbent. When combined with gauze, it performs like Furacin Soluble Dressing with respect to absorption of wound drainage. The base in Silvadene is particularly good for keeping wounds from drying out and provides an ideal microenvironment for wound healing. McGrath[113] showed that this base increased tissue survival of skin flaps under experimenal conditions in rats.

Mafenide acetate (Sulfamylon, Winthrop-Breon Laboratories, New York, N.Y.) is available as a water-soluble cream with the same antibacterial spectrum as silver sulfadiazine. The antibacterial action is not inhibited by pus or other secretions. However, the cream may cause pain on application, and allergic skin reactions can occur (see Fig. 13-4). When used in widespread areas, it has been reported to cause acid-base disturbances.

Topical antibiotics in open or closed wounds may induce sensitization to either the antibiotics or components of the vehicle used (see color plate 2). Although this is uncommon, it usually presents little difficulty once the problem is recognized. If a local allergic reaction to an antibiotic ointment occurs, discontinuation of the offending antibiotic ointment is adequate. Use of a topical steroid for a few days hastens resolution of the allergic reaction. Rare cases have been reported of anaphylaxis occurring when ointments containing antibiotics (neomycin or bacitracin) were applied to leg ulcers.[39,129]

Scarlet red

Scarlet red is an aniline dye with a brilliant scarlet color that has been used since the beginning of the twentieth century to facilitate wound healing. Davis[32] in 1909 reported 60 cases in which this substance was applied to wounds and enthusiastically endorsed its use. Since that time there have been many other proponents. It is currently available in ointment form (5% Scarlet Red, with lanolin oil and petrolatum, Cheseborough-Ponds, Greenwich, Conn.), either alone or as an impregnant of fine-mesh gauze.

Data concerning the effect of scarlet red in wound epithelialization are conflicting. Salomon, Diegelmann, and Cohen[143] evaluated the effect of various dressings on healing of split-thickness skin graft donor sites as measured by incorporation of tritiated thymidine. These investigators found that scarlet red gauze dressing and Xeroform gauze were superior to plain gauze. However, other investigators have not found scarlet red in ointment form to be especially helpful with respect to epithelialization.[52]

Scarlet red has been shown to induce epithelial proliferation. Vasiliev and Cheung[162] injected scarlet red into the ears of rabbits. These investigators found epithelial proliferation with invasive ingrowth, as well as proliferation of young undifferentiated fibroblasts in the underlying dermis. These events have been interpreted by some investigators as evidence for carcinogenesis, but by others as evidence for enhancement of wound healing.

Scarlet red apparently has no antibacterial effect.[44] Sensitivity (allergic or irritant) is rare but can occur.[32,44]

Gold leaf, silver foil, and aluminum foil

Gold and silver foils have been reported to aid wound healing.[66] However, these materials are seldom used today. When subjected to more modern clinical evaluation with suitable control wounds, gold leaf and aluminum foil were found to be only as effective as the controls.[68,151]

Zinc oxide–calamine–gelatin

The Unna boot is a roll of gauze impregnated with zinc oxide, calamine and gelatin. Its use to wrap leg ulcers was described by Unna in 1883.[67] The use of gelatin was a forerunner of modern gelatin dressings, which as discussed previously can be helpful in healing wounds. The Unna boot is discussed in more detail later in this chapter.

MISCELLANEOUS MATERIALS USED IN WOUNDS
Cotton-tipped applicators

Six-inch wooden sticks with cotton wrapped at one end are useful for sponging blood during surgery (see Fig. 10-25). Cotton-tipped applicators may also be purchased with plastic rather than wooden handles, but the plastic ones are much less useful in cutaneous surgery because they do not allow the surgeon to place as much pressure on the wound.

Cotton fibers tend to fray. Therefore some surgeons prefer the cellulose sponge Weck-Cell (Edward Weck Co., Research Triangle Park, N.C.). However, cellulose sponges are much more expensive than cotton-tipped applicators. I have never encountered a problem from cotton fibers that may have been inadvertently trapped in wounds.

Hemostatic agents

Dermatologists have traditionally used Monsel's solution (ferric subsulfate) or aluminum chloride (hydrous) 35% in isopropyl alcohol 50% as hemostatic agents on wounds. However, Monsel's solution may destroy a significant amount of connective tissue[69] (making it a caustic) and may cause pigmentation of the skin (see Fig. 13-9). The overzealous use of Monsel's solution for deep wounds (full thickness of the skin) is therefore discouraged. Other, more rarely used caustics include silver nitrate (75%) on applicator sticks, phenol, and dichloroacetic acid. Frequently pressure alone, which does not adversely affect wounds, stops bleeding if applied for 10 to 20 minutes with no peeking underneath the dressing material to see if the bleeding has abated.

Occasionally the need arises for a material to facilitate hemostasis when simple electrocoagulation, pressure, caustics, or styptics are inadequate or when vessels cannot be visualized and clamped. Hemostatic materials are rarely needed in cutaneous surgery, since bleeding sites are normally easily seen. However, if the surgeon wishes to injure as little tissue as possible, materials are available to help stop bleeding. These include oxidized cellulose (Oxycel, Deseret Med, Inc., Sandy, Utah; Surgicel, Surgikos Div., Johnson & Johnson, New Brunswick, N.J.); gelatin sponge (Gelfoam, Upjohn Co., Kalamazoo, Mich.); microfibrillar collagen (Avitene, Alcon, Inc., Fort Worth, Tex.); and topical thrombin (Parke-Davis, Morris Plains, N.J.). It should be emphasized that these agents are not a substitute for meticulous surgery. Also, these hemostatic materials can potentiate infection and should be used with caution where significant bacterial contamination exists.

Oxidized cellulose was developed in the early 1940s as an absorbable gauze.[47] The oxidation process, which shrinks the fabric and makes it smoother, is carefully controlled on cellulose (or regenerated cellulose). Although there is tissue reaction on implantation, the material disappears in time. Oxidized cellulose swells when saturated with blood and fills the wound cavity. The hemostatic action depends more on swelling of material, which provides internal pressure, than on clotting.[47] If oxidized cellulose is placed in locations where expansion may compromise surrounding structures, care should be exercised.

Oxidized cellulose has been shown to possess antibacterial properties, an attribute not shared by gelatin sponge or topical thrombin.[35,148,154] Therefore in infected wounds it does not appear to potentiate infection to the same degree as Gelfoam or Avitene. Oxidized cellulose is available as a gauze-type knitted fabric (Surgicel) or as cotton-type carded cellulose (Oxycel).

Gelatin sponge (Gelfoam) is a water-insoluble foamed gelatin preparation made from a select grade of animal skin gelatin. It is pliable and said to be a nonspecific, nonantigenic protein rich in proline and glycine.[73] The foam has a uniform porosity and is soft yet springy when dry. When placed into a wound cavity, the gelatin rapidly absorbs fluid and becomes mushy. This sponge is capable of absorbing and holding in its meshes many times its weight in whole blood. It adheres to bleeding surfaces and facilitates blood clotting through the release of thromboplastin within the sponge to produce a clot. Gelfoam is usually completely digested by proteolytic enzymes and absorbed by phagocytosis in 4 to 6 weeks if left in the wound.[18,124] However, prolonged lymphocytic reactions,[124] fibrous tissue reactions,[73] infection,[35] and abscesses[76] have been reported to occur with this material. Gelfoam potentiates infection in wound colonized by bacteria.[35] Therefore it should be viewed as a foreign body even though it is absorbable and usually nonreactive. Gelfoam is available as both a sponge and a powder. The sponge may be ordered in sheets or as smaller dental packs. The dental packs are more convenient for cutaneous surgery.

When Gelfoam is used in punch biopsy sites or other small spaces to stop bleeding, an exposed portion must be left above the skin surface as a wick (see Fig. 14-7). Gelfoam action in stopping bleeding apparently involves its functioning as a physical plug, which it does best when a portion is exposed and dry. If Gelfoam completely covers the wound, it becomes soggy and loses its physical strength.

Gelfoam may be used as a packing in open wounds, such as nail bed excisions, in which it helps counteract the bleeding that frequently continues after nail surgery. Since the wound is allowed to heal by granulation and epidermization, the Gelfoam absorbs without much likelihood of infection. In closed wounds, however, Gelfoam should not be used as a packing, especially if infection is likely; as mentioned previously, this material may become a nidus for infection.

Microfibrillar collagen (Avitene) is a new hemostatic agent made from edible bovine collagen as a water-soluble partial acid salt of natural collagen.[4] It is a fluffy, white, fibrous material that adheres firmly to bleeding surfaces. Microfibrillar collagen is superior to both Gelfoam and Surgicel in stopping bleeding.[4] The mechanism underlying its hemostatic action is based on the interaction of platelets with collagen, resulting in platelet aggregation and platelet plug formation. Avitene is thus less active when the patient has a platelet deficiency than when the patient is receiving heparin.[1] This material is absorbed, usually without a foreign body reaction, although a low-grade inflammatory reaction may occur.[4] Avitene has been reported to potentiate infection in contaminated wounds.[148] Compared with other hemostatic materials, Avitene is expensive.

Topical thrombin is another hemostatic agent to consider for oozing wounds. It is available as a powder in 1000, 5000, and 10,000 unit containers. Usually the 1000 unit dosage is used in cutaneous surgery, dusted on wounds as a powder. It is of bovine origin and is prepared from prothrombin, which is converted to thrombin in the presence of tissue thromboplastin and calcium chloride.[35] The thrombin clots fibrinogen of the blood directly. It does not adversely affect wound healing[69] and may be useful after such procedures as dermabrasion.[106]

SURGICAL ADHESIVE TAPES
History

Adhesive tapes have been used in one form or another since the first recorded surgery.[22] Currently these materials are readily available in pharmacies and even grocery stores. Prepackaged adhesive bandages such as Band-Aids have been produced in the United States in essentially their current form since 1899.[85]

In the nineteenth century the term "adhesive tape" was not used, but rather "adhesive plaster" or "emplastrum adhaesivum."[85] There were originally two main types of adhesive plasters: emplastrum resinae and emplastrum plumbi. Emplastrum plumbi, also known as lead plaster, was a mixture of lead oxide, olive oil, and water. If resin was added to the mixture, it was known as emplastrum resinae, or sticking plaster. The resin used was the residue remaining after the volatile oil of turpentine from pine trees had been distilled. It was also known as rosin (colophony). Resin made lead plaster more adhesive.[75]

The use of lead plaster can be traced to Celsus (30 BC to 25 AD), who termed it Coacon plaster, from the Greek word

Κῷος (of or belonging to Cos, the birthplace of Hippocrates). These sticky mixtures were applied to cloth strips that in turn were used to splint wounds or hold dressings in place. Some interesting variations used in the last century include application of emplastra to elastic webbing to provide elastic tension[136] (the forerunner of elastic tapes) and the incorporation of antibacterials such as zinc chloride into the cloth tapes[110] (the forerunner of antibacterial tapes).

Definitions

Adhesive tape has two components: the adhesive mass and the backing, that is, the carrier of the adhesive. The modern adhesive mass is usually a non–rubber based acrylic polymer that has a great ability to stick (high coefficient of adhesion). The older, more traditional cloth adhesive tapes, which were used almost exclusively until the 1950s and are still available, contain a rubber-based adhesive mass composed of zinc oxide, natural rubber, resins, and turpentine. The exact composition of the adhesive mass may thus be somewhat complex. The backing may be any of several materials such as cloth, paper, plastic, or foam.

Surgical adhesive tapes are described as pressure sensitive; that is, the tape can be applied with hand pressure without the use of adjunctive substances such as solvents or heat.

Types of tape

The types of surgical tape differ mainly in the type of backing. Cloth and some plastic backings commonly use a rubber-based adhesive, whereas rayon backings use more modern, hypoallergenic acrylates.

The development of microporous paper (nonwoven rayon) tape was an important contribution to surgery. During manufacture of this type of tape the adhesive mass is applied without coalescing, producing a tape that is quite porous. Such a highly porous tape results in few irritant reactions.[61]

The following are common types of surgical tape:
- I. Cloth (cotton)
  - A. Nonporous
  - B. Porous (areas without adhesive)
    1. Curity Cloth Tape (Kendall Co.)
    2. Zonas Porous Tape (Johnson & Johnson)
    3. Regular Surgical Tape (American White Cross)
    4. Orthaletic Tape (Prof. Med.)
  - C. Waterproof (vinyl coated)
    1. Wet Pruf (Kendall Co.)
    2. Waterproof Surgical Tape (American White Cross)
    3. Johnson's Waterproof Tape (Johnson & Johnson)
    4. Orthaletic Waterproof Tape (Prof. Med.)
- II. Polyester gauze-type (open mesh, woven)
    1. Cover-Roll Adhesive Gauze (Beiersdorf)
- III. Plastic
  - A. Without holes
    1. Benderm (3M)
    2. Leukoflex (Beiersdorf)
  - B. With holes
    1. Transpore (3M)
    2. Leukofix (Beiersdorf)
    3. Demaclear (Johnson & Johnson)—nonhypoallergenic
    4. Curity Clear Tape (Kendall Co.)
- IV. Paper
  - A. Nonwoven rayon
    1. Micropore (3M)
    2. Ultrapore (3M)
    3. Tender Skin (Kendall Co.)
    4. Dermalite II (Johnson & Johnson)
    5. Scanpore (Hollister Stier)
    6. Leukopor (Beiersdorf)
  - B. Woven rayon
    1. Dermicel (Johnson & Johnson)
    2. Curasilk (Kendall Co.)
    3. Durapore (3M)
    4. Dermiform (Johnson & Johnson)
    5. Hypoallergenic Tape (American Cross)
    6. Leukosilk (Beiersdorf)
- V. Foam
  - A. Microfoam (3M)

Occlusivity of tapes

Tapes may be occlusive, permeable, or semiocclusive (semipermeable). Occlusivity means that water loss from the surface of the skin or wound is prevented. The degree of occlusivity is determined by both the adhesive and the backing. Plastic backings are occlusive but may be perforated to give some degree of exposure to the underlying skin and wound. Paper, cloth, or other fabric backings are usually permeable to some degree. Of the adhesives used, rubber-based adhesives are occlusive, whereas acrylate adhesives are permeable.

Occlusivity of tapes is important in determining the hydration of the underlying skin and wound, as well as proclivity for bacterial proliferation. In a study of second-degree burns, Miller[118] found that occlusive tapes that have a low porosity result in minimal evaporative water loss and may lead to infected wounds that are moist and purulent. On the other hand, tapes with high porosity and high evaporative water loss result in smooth, dry wounds that have a low incidence of infection.

Marples and Kligman[108] studied the growth of bacteria on the skin under various types of adhesive tapes. These investigators found an increased bacterial growth under all plastic-backed tapes whether perforations were present or not. Micropore tape, an acrylate adhesive on a paper back-

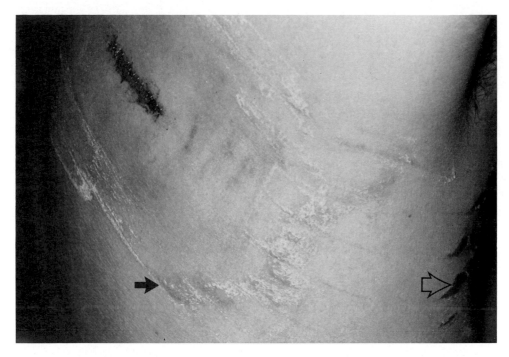

Fig. 9-11. Blisters *(closed arrow)* and wound from stripped epidermis *(open arrow)* due to shearing forces of rubber-based elastic bandage used for wound dressing.

ing, did not increase bacterial growth. Interestingly rubber-based adhesive tape with a fabric backing also did not show an increased bacterial growth.

Untoward reactions

Tape may produce several different types of untoward reactions (Fig. 9-11). Traumatic reactions include dermographism or actual stripping of the skin. Dermographism, which is seen in suspectible individuals, is transient erythema at the site of the tape after its removal. Shearing forces between the tape and the skin may be followed by stripping of the skin or blister formation. Occlusion, as previously pointed out, can result in bacterial proliferation; increased hydration of the skin and swelling shut of the sweat pores, leading to miliaria or follicular occlusion; and maceration.

If wounds require frequent dressing changes with reapplication of tape, the skin may become irritated because of the stripping of the stratum corneum that occurs with each dressing change. Montgomery straps are a special type of outer binder with a tape and a nontape portion. The nontape portion is laced over the top of the absorbent portion of the dressing. With each dressing change the tape portion is left in place and only the nontape portion is disturbed. It is unlaced, a fresh dressing is applied to the underlying wound, and it is then relaced over the new dressing. Thus the irritation from the frequent dressing changes is avoided. Modern Montgomery straps are available with relatively porous tape, such as Dermicel Montgomery Straps (Johnson & Johnson, New Brunswick, N.J.). These may be easily modified to fit wounds of any size and are especially useful for trunk wounds that require frequent dressing changes.

True allergic reactions to tapes are uncommon but can occur. Allergic contact dermatitis is a cell-mediated immunologic reaction whose cause can be determined by patch testing to the appropriate materials. It should be differentiated from irritant dermatitis, which is not based on an allergic reaction. Older rubber-based tapes were associated with a fairly high incidence of reactions, many of which were erroneously thought to be allergic. True allergic reactions were stated to be due to resins, turpentine, or the rubber itself. More commonly, however, the presumed "allergic" reactions were actually irritant dermatitis.[63] For instance, Humphries[81] lowered the incidence of tape irritation from 30% to 4% by the addition of antimicrobial substances into the adhesive plaster. Therefore irritant tape dermatitis probably is multifactorial but is at least partially due to overgrowth of microbes. In a recent study[107] of 100 surgical patients, 12 patients developed an irritant dermatitis to adhesive tape. In all 12 patients the tape used was a rubber-mass adhesive tape. Patch test results were negative, so it was believed that the dermatitis was nonallergic.

Other substances associated with allergic reactions to rubber mass adhesive tapes include abietic acid, dihydroabietic acid, and dihydroabietic alcohol.[31,48] These components are found in colophony (rosin), which is apparently still a component of some adhesives.

Newer adhesive tapes with acrylic polymer adhesives and porous paper backing cause fewer reactions, at least of a irritant nature. Allergic reactions are also uncommon because the amount of monomer present in the tape glue is negligible. New methods of production (dispersion polymerization) have further decreased the amount of these prepolymers, making allergic reactions even more unlikely.[105] Nevertheless, allergic reactions to both the adhesive mass[11,74,86] and the tape backing[48] have been reported. Such reactions may be due to 2-ethylhexylacrylate, methyl methacrylate, or maleamic acid. Tapes such as Scanpor Tape (Hollister Stier, Spokane, Wash.), which is itself used routinely in patch testing, may contain traces of formaldehyde, which can be a cause of allergic contact dermatitis.[11]

Skin degreasers and tape removers

Substances are manufactured specifically for removal of adhesive tape, especially rubber-based adhesive, which may remain on the skin after the tape is removed. Usually these are organic solvents. They may also be used to degrease the skin before application of tape in order to make the tape stick more firmly.

Tape remover may be purchased in individually wrapped towelettes (such as Clinipad, Clinipad Corp., Guilford, Conn.) or as a liquid (such as Detachol, Ferndale Laboratories, Inc., Ferndale, Mich.). Acetone, isopropyl alcohol, or ether can also be used to degrease the skin or remove tape adhesive, but these substances are inflammable. Some compounds are specifically made for degreasing the skin (such as T/Prep, Ferndale Laboratories, Inc., Ferndale, Mich.).

Liquid tactifiers

Certain substances may be used to make the skin tacky and increase adhesive tape adhesion. One such substance, compound tincture of benzoin, is widely available and has been used for at least 100 years.[85] It contains benzoin, styrax, balsam of tolu, and aloe. Allergic contact dermatitis to one or all of these components may occur.[84,107]

An alternative tactifier, Mastisol (Ferndale, Laboratories, Inc., Ferndale, Mich.), contains gum mastic and styrax. Once sensitization to tincture of benzoin has occurred, cross-reaction to Mastisol is likely.[84] Unlike compound tincture of benzoin, Mastisol is colorless.

Skin-Prep (United Division, Pfizer, New York City) is a tactifier that contains citric acid polymer in alcohol. The alcohol helps to degrease the skin, and the polymer leaves a coating that helps tape to stick. With subsequent dressing changes, the latter material helps to protect the skin from tape irritation.

CONTENTS OF A DRESSING TABLE

I have found it convenient to designate a space in the treatment or surgical room as the dressing table and cabinet (see Fig. 5-2). This table should contain the materials and substances most commonly used to make dressings. The contents of this table should include the following:

1. Bandage scissors
   a. Lister or Universal bandage scissors
2. Hemostatic agents
   a. Monsel's solution
   b. Aluminum chloride (hydrous) 35% in isopropyl alcohol (50%)
   c. Silver nitrate (75%) sticks
   d. Oxidized cellulose (Surgicel [Johnson & Johnson] or Oxycel [Deseret Med])
   e. Gelatin sponge (Gelfoam [Upjohn Co.])
3. Irrigation solutions
   a. Hydrogen peroxide 3%
   b. Sterile normal saline
   c. Ophthalmic irrigation solutions such as Blinx (Barnes-Hind/Hydrocurve, Inc.) or Dacriose (Coopervision Pharmaceuticals)
4. Ointments
   a. Sterile and nonsterile petrolatum such as Vaseline (Johnson & Johnson) or White Petrolatum, U.S.P. (Fougera & Co., Melville, N.Y.)
   b. General antibiotic ointments such as Polysporin Ointment (Burroughs Wellcome Co.)
   c. Ophthalmic antibiotic ointments such as Polysporin Ophthalmic Ointment (Burroughs Wellcome Co.)
5. Skin cleaners or degreasers
   a. Isopropyl alcohol (wipes or in container with cotton balls)
   b. Solvent tape remover or degreaser such as Detachol (Ferndale Laboratories, Inc.)
   c. Prepackaged antibacterial solutions such as Pharmadine Solution Microbicidal Swabstick (Sherwood Pharmaceuticals Co., Mahwah, N.J.)
6. Nonadherent dressings
   a. Perforated polyesters such as Telfa (Kendall Co.) or Release (Johnson & Johnson)
   b. Petrolatum-impregnated gauze such as Vaseline Gauze (Chesebrough-Ponds) or Adaptic (Johnson & Johnson)
7. Absorbent dressing materials
   a. Gauze (3 × 3), sterile in metal containers (dressing jars)
   b. Cotton balls
   c. Cotton dental packs
   d. Eye pads
   e. Gauze packing strips (plain and iodoform)
8. Sponge forceps (Forester, serrated 7- to 9 inch) and forceps holder (jar) (Alcohol is placed in the jar. Sponge forceps may be used to place the gauze from the sterile metal gauze container on the dressing table.)

9. Applicators
   a. Cotton-tipped applicators (wooden), 6-inch
   b. Tongue depressors
10. Outer cover dressing materials (see p. 312)
    a. Stretchable gauze on rolls such as Kerlix (Kendall Co.)
    b. Elastic wraps such as Ace Bandages (Becton-Dickinson)
11. Surgical tapes (see p. 338), paper backed, such as Micropore flesh-colored tapes, ¼, ½, and 1 inch (3M)
12. Skin tactifiers such as compound tincture of Benzoin or Mastisol (Ferndale Laboratories, Inc.)
13. Sutureless skin closures (see Table 8-5), paper backed, such as Steri-Strips (3M)
14. Bandages combined with adhesive (see p. 331)
    a. Spot bandages such as Coverlet (Beiersdorf)
    b. Strip bandages such as Coverlet (Beiersdorf)
    c. Pad bandages such as Telfa Adhesive Pads (Kendall Co.)
15. Special dressing materials
    a. Polyurethane such as Op-Site (Smith & Nephew)
    b. Colloid such as Duoderm (ConvaTec) or Vigilon (Bard Home Health Care, Inc.)
16. Gloves (sterile and nonsterile)

DRESSING TECHNIQUES

Dressing methods vary with the anatomic site and the type of injury or surgery. Physicians should be actively involved in constructing and applying dressings and not simply delegate the task to a nurse or assistant. How a dressing is made and applied can greatly influence the surgical result. The wrong dressing properly applied or the right dressing improperly constructed and applied can delay wound healing. Unfortunately, little instruction in dressing technique is given during a physician's training. Indeed, this is nearly a lost art and one that requires common sense, improvisation, and ingenuity.

Dressings for closed wounds

Most postsurgical dressings fall into one of two categories: pressure or nonpressure. Pressure dressings are used when continued bleeding into the wound site is possible or edema is likely. They are also used over skin grafts to minimize slippage between the graft and wound bed. Nonpressure dressings are simple dressings that may exert minimal pressure on the wound.

The dressing, whether pressure or nonpressure is usually composed of a number of layers. Each layer must be in close contact with the adjacent layers, without gaps or dead spaces. This ensures that maximal wound drainage will occur. The lowest layer in direct contact with the wound bed should be adherent to the underlying tissue for the same reason.

The nonpressure, composite, dressing is shown in Fig. 10-52. Basically this is constructed of a contact layer, an absorbent layer, and an outer wrap (outer covering or binder). The contact layer is usually a nonadherent material such as Telfa or Vaseline Gauze. Beneath the contact layer one may use an ointment, such as sterile Vaseline or an antibiotic ointment, to help to keep the contact layer from sticking to the wound. The absorbent layer is an eye pad, cotton balls, the bulk in the Telfa, or even gauze (folded or fluffed). This layer not only absorbs wound drainage but also helps the dressing to conform to the wound cavity and cushions the wound. The outer wrap is usually folded gauze and paper tape such as Micropore tape. This outermost layer retains (with or without pressure) the underlying dressing components in their proper positions. As the dressing is constructed, the bottom layers are the smallest, barely overlapping the wound. Subsequent layers are larger, overlapping the lower layers. The final layer overlaps the wound on all sides for some distance. The simple composite dressing for sutured wounds is changed after 24 hours. The wound is cleaned with sterile saline or hydrogen peroxide, and another similar dressing is applied. Usually dressing changes once a day suffice for sutured wounds.

The pressure dressing is similar to the nonpressure dressing but provides more pressure on the wound, usually by a bulkier absorbent layer and a stretchable outer layer. Bulk within the absorbent layer can be built up with fluffed gauze, cotton, sponge (the sponges in suture boxes may be used), or eyepads. The Reston Self Adhesive Foam Pad (3M, Minneapolis, Minn.) may also be useful to put pressure on large areas such as dermabrasion sites on the face.

It should be pointed out that the outermost layer of a pressure dressing is either a stretchable overlayer or a stretchable wrap. The choice depends on the size and location of the wound, as well as on the amount of pressure needed. Elastic tape is useful as a stretchable overlayer where the wound cannot easily be included in a wraparound dressing. Special, composite pressure dressings are also available as adhesive bandages that provide both bulk absorbency and tape (for example, Coverlet operating room bandages). If a wraparound dressing is essential, stretchable gauze (such as Kerlix) or elastic wraps (such as Ace Wraps) are useful. Elastic wraps produce greater pressure on the wound.

Pressure dressings are usually applied immediately postoperatively and may be exchanged for a lighter covering in 24 hours. The first 24 hours is important, since swelling will be the greatest during that time.

Pressure dressings are commonly used on digits, extremities, and the scalp. Such bandages have several important functions: they limit bleeding into the wound, support injured tissue, splint the wound, minimize edema, and hold other dressings in place. As long as the pressure exerted does not exceed the intravascular hydrostatic pressure, the

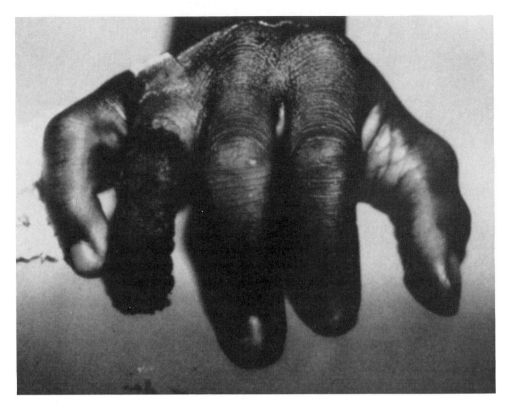

Fig. 9-12. Necrosis of finger caused by tight elastic tubular dressing. (From Ersek, R.A.: Tex. Med. **78**:47, 1982.)

bandage successfully limits edema without impeding blood flow. However, it is possible to cut off the circulation with a dressing and perhaps cause tissue necrosis, particularly on the extremities.[41] In addition, the hydrostatic pressure changes with the patient's posture and the position of the extremity relative to the heart. Elevating a dressed hand may actually decrease the blood supply.

The pressure resulting from a wraparound pressure dressing depends on the tension applied on the bandage at the time of application, the number of layers, the degree of overlap between successive turns, and the radius of curvature of the limb.[156] The smaller the radius, the larger the resultant pressure is likely to be. Therefore, when bandaging an arm or leg, one should be careful when moving from a larger area in radius to a smaller one. Since the relatively small radius of the extremities or digits in children is likely to result in great pressure within bandages, one needs to be careful under such circumstances. Pressure also increases if one twists the bandage 180 degrees when wrapping it around an anatomic structure.[104]

Tube dressings for the fingers are a popular method for providing a neat pressure dressing. However, such dressings may be highly constrictive if not applied properly. Fig. 9-12 shows necrosis that occurred on a finger with use of an elastic net bandage as reported by Ersek.[41] In this case a 16-year-old boy had his finger dressed in an elastic net

bandage applied in many layers. The elastic net dressing increased the pressure on the finger with each successive layer. Cotton tube gauze can also be used as a finger dressing. Because it is thicker than elastic net, few layers are usually applied. Ersek showed that cotton tube gauze produces less pressure on fingers than the elastic net dressing.

Dressings for open wounds

Dressings for small, superficial or deep wounds (such as punch biopsy wounds) can be fashioned from ointment, nonadhesive dry dressing (such as Telfa), and tape. Alternatively, several types of adhesive dressings are made for this purpose, including Band-Aids and Coverlet dressings.

Dressings for wide, deep, open wounds must be constructed to provide drainage and be absorbent. The contact layer should not stick to the wet wound unless debridement is desired. Usually Telfa covered with an antibiotic ointment, if changed once or twice a day, suffices for such wounds. Fluffed gauze or eye pads are used for bulk, and tape secures the bandage in position. Deep wounds that are allowed to heal by secondary intention because of bacterial contamination may be packed with gauze strips, such as Iodoform Gauze. When this is done, the packing may be gradually removed by the patient or physician over 2 or 3 days. The gauze srip provides an avenue for egress of bacteria as well as exudate.

Wide, superficial, open wounds heal faster if covered by a semiocclusive dressing. The transparent semipermeable polyurethane membranes are excellent for this purpose. When dressings must be changed frequently, colloid dressings are a good alternative because they do not stick tightly to underlying new epidermis.

Cutaneous thermal burns produce a unique type of wound that requires special dressings. The area of the burn can be divided into three separate zones seen visually and histologically: coagulation, stasis, and hyperemia. Necrotic tissue exists in the zone of coagulation and may extend into the zone of stasis with time. If an occlusive or semiocclusive dressing is applied, the extent of subsequent tissue loss will be minimized.[93] Since necrotic tissue provides a nidus for infection and there may be considerable fluid loss and wound drainage, a broad-spectrum topical antibiotic cream, such as 1% silver sulfadiazine (Silvadene) cream, is recommended, followed by fine-mesh gauze, an absorbent layer, and nonocclusive microporous tape.

The Unna boot is a special dressing used to wrap a leg that has a nonhealing ulcer. This dressing, which is gauze impregnated with zinc oxide, calamine, and gelatin, is wrapped circumferentially around the extremity. The Unna boot dressing is a semiocclusive dressing that reduces edema of the extremity and keeps the wound moist. It is purposely left in place for a prolonged period, usually a week, to discourage the patient or others from meddling with the wound. Harnar et al.[67] demonstrated that the Unna boot is an excellent dressing for skin graft recipient sites on the lower extremity. It permits early ambulation, usually the day following the skin graft. The incidence of graft takes with the Unna Boot is as high as with conventional therapy and bed rest.

Dressings for specific anatomic areas

Each different anatomic area has a unique surface anatomy and blood supply that influence how dressings should be constructed. This section explores the ways in which dressings are modified and tailored to areas difficult to fit with dressings or prone to problems. Many additional examples are provided in subsequent chapters.

Scalp. The presence of hair on the scalp makes taping of dressings impractical. Therefore dressings in this location are usually fashioned by wrapping successive layers of Kerlix or Kling around the head as an outer wrap. This provides some pressure and, more important, helps to keep the underlying dressings in place. If additional pressure is needed, an elastic wrap such as an Ace Wrap may be used on top of the underlying cotton wrap dressing. Such wraparound dressings should be secured by tape, both at the edges to the skin on the forehead and between successive wrapped layers. Tape between the overlapped layers keeps them from slipping on each other.

Applying the head wrap dressing is a matter of practice.

Usually, wrapping the whole scalp (the turban dressing) is unnecessary except for aesthetic reasons. Bringing the wrap under the jaw is also unnecessary in most cases but is recommended by some physicians.[95]

Scalp dressings may also be held in place by means of elastic net or stockinette dressings. Robinson[137] recommends using panty hose on the scalp with the elastic waistline tightened by means of a coin.

Ear. The ear has many curved surfaces and is therefore more difficult to bandage than a flat surface. A successful dressing is the result of providing bulk; an easy way to do this is to open a 3 × 3 or 4 × 4 piece of gauze and fluff it (Fig. 9-13). This fits easily into crevices and particularly into the postauricular sulcus. Tape may then be applied directly to the gauze and surrounding skin. If additional pressure is required, an outer wrap Kerlix or Kling dressing may then be applied around the scalp to include the ear.

Nose. Because the side of the nose is concave, some bulk may be needed to fill out the dressing. Bulking may be accomplished by means of fluffed gauze as on the ear or alternatively by means of a small dental pack (Fig. 9-14). Dental packs are the cylindrical rolls of cotton used by dentists to absorb secretions and blood in the mouth.

Sometimes the nose must be packed to provide adherence between a skin flap on the cutaneous surface of the nose and the underlying mucosa. Such counterpressure is best accomplished by means of a finger cut from a rubber glove and filled with gauze. The outside of the cut rubber glove finger is lubricated with ointment so it slips smoothly inside the nostril and may be easily extracted at the appropriate time. Vaseline Gauze packing may also be used, but it sometimes sticks to wounds inside the nose if there is much drainage.

Hand. Instead of tube dressings on the digits, I usually employ gauze cut and folded as shown in Fig. 9-15. The gauze is then taped, with the tape applied snugly in an *oblique* fashion. Theoretically, the vascular supply may be impeded by wrapping tape circumferentially around digits. This bandlike constricting effect can be avoided by wrapping the tape around the digit diagononally or cutting it so one piece does not totally encircle the digit. Such a dressing provides adequate pressure to preclude bleeding, a frequent occurrence in nail surgery.

Finger dressings may also be wound lightly round the finger and then secured back around the wrist.[96] This allows as much function as possible for the fingers. In general, however, movement of the wound should be avoided to speed healing.

A sling may be advisable after surgery on the upper extremity. This reduces pain, especially if the wound is on the fingers. However, the hand should not be elevated more than horizontally to avoid diminishing the blood supply.

Occasionally the physician may wish to splint the fingers to minimize tension on the wound. Flexible aluminum

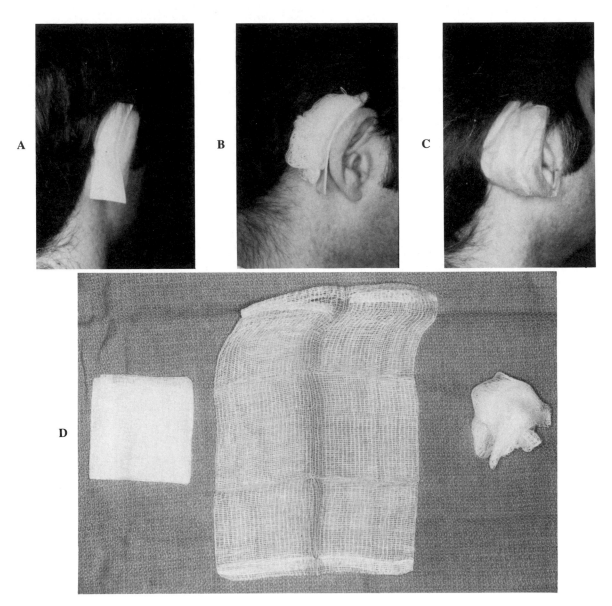

Fig. 9-13. Dressing behind ear. **A,** Nonadherent dressing cut to size and applied directly to wound. **B,** Fluffed gauze to provide bulk and contour. **C,** Cut tape applied to ear going from anterosuperior to posterior and around to anteroinferior ear. Alternatively, bulk wrap-around dressing (such as Kerlix or Kling) on head including ear can be used. **D,** To fluff gauze, unfold *(middle)* and ball up lightly *(right)*.

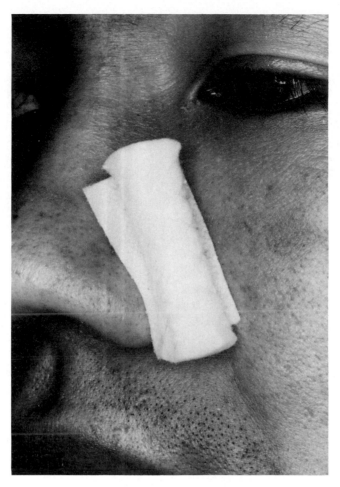

Fig. 9-14. Dressing beside nose. Dental roll used to provide bulk and contour.

splints padded with foam arc excellent for this purpose. Splinted fingers should be flexed in the direction of motion.

Foot. The main problem with dressings on a foot is that the patient cannot get the foot into a shoe. Special shoes are available that allow the patient to walk after surgery. The Reese boot and Zimmer boot are wood-soled shoes with canvas uppers that can be laced up the front so the toes are open. This allows the patient to walk while at the same time immobilizing the foot and toes.

Occasionally the physician desires to avoid movement of the foot so tension on the wound is minimized. This may be accomplished by means of a support cast made of plaster of Paris or other orthopedic material. Usually such support casts are posterior splints that wrap about halfway around the limb and under the heel. Such splints are secured on the extremity by wraparound dressings and are easily removed at the time of dressing changes.

As with wounds on the upper extremities, elevation of the limb should be stressed to the patient. This will minimize pain, decrease edema, and promote healing.

Principles of wound care

Based on knowledge of wound healing and the manner in which dressings function, certain principles of dressing care are clear and need to be stressed to patients. The main principle of wound care is to *keep the wound covered and moist*. This has several advantages, not the least of which is that it minimizes scarring. A wound should not be exposed to air and allowed to form a scab. A second principle of wound care is to *keep the wound clean*. Cleaning the wound with sterile saline or hydrogen peroxide helps to rid it of exudate. After the first 24 hours patients may get their wounds wet when bathing. However, if the dressing becomes wet with blood, exudate, or fluid from an external source, it should be changed, since a wet dressing allows bacteria to penetrate the wound.

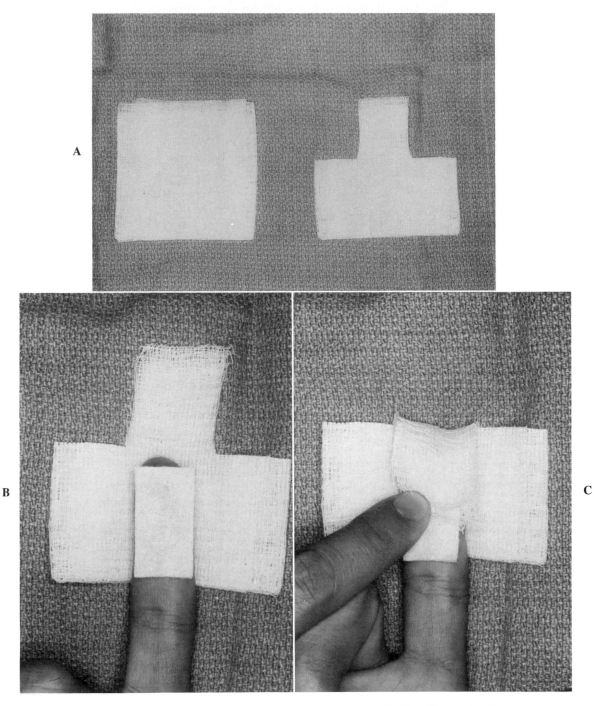

Fig. 9-15. Dressing for finger. **A,** Gauze *(left)* cut to pattern *(right)*. **B,** Nonadherent dressing cut to size and applied to wound. Cut gauze under finger; then fold over top of finger **(C)** and sides **(D** and **E)**. Paper tape is applied **(F** and **G)**. Note oblique direction of tape **(G)**.

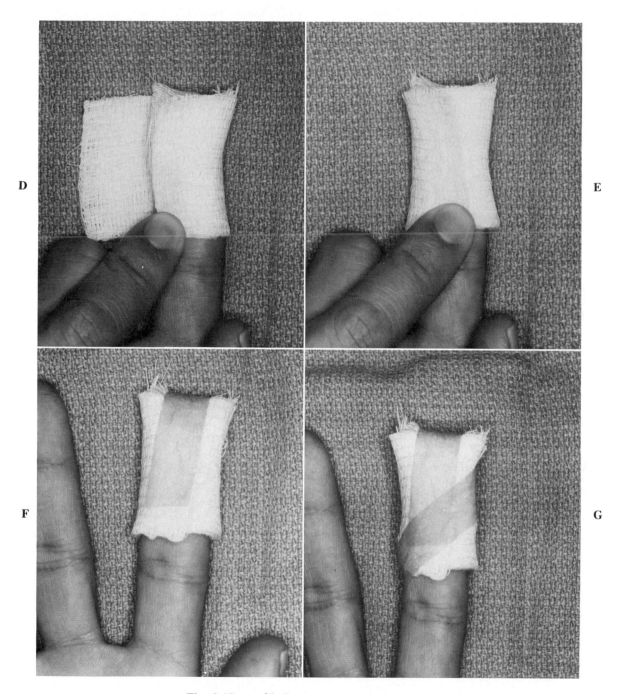

Fig. 9-15, cont'd. For legend see opposite page.

REFERENCES

1. Abbott, W.M., and Austen, W.G.: Effectiveness and mechanism of collagen induced topical hemostasis, Surgery **78:**723, 1975.
2. Absorbent gauze. In United States pharmacopeia, ed. 21 Rockville, Md., 1985, United States Pharmacopeial Convention, Inc.
3. Akle, C.A., et al.: Immunogenicity of human amniotic epithelial cells after transplantation into volunteers, Lancet **2:**1003, 1981.
4. Alexander, J.M., and Rabinowitz, J.L.: Microfibrillar collagen (Avitene) as a hemostatic agent in experimental oral wounds, J. Oral Surg. **36:**202, 1978.
5. Alper, J.C., et al.: Moist wound healing under vapor permeable membrane, J. Am. Acad. Dermatol. **8:**347, 1983.
6. Alvarez, O.M., Mertz, P.M., and Eaglstein, W.H.: The effect of occlusive dressings on collagen synthesis and re-epithelization in superficial wounds, J. Surg. Res. **35:**142, 1983.
7. Alvarez, O.M., et al.: Benzoyl peroxide and epidermal wound healing, Arch. Dermatol. **119:**222, 1983.
8. Aly, R., et al.: Effect of prolonged occlusion on the microbial flora, pH, carbon dioxide, and transepidermal water loss on human skin, J. Invest. Dermatol. **71:**378, 1978.
9. Amromin, G., Saphir, O., and Goldberger, I.: Lint granuloma, Arch. Pathol. **60:**467, 1958.
10. Andersen, D.P., Jr.: The problem of wound healing: the effect of local antiseptic agents on infected wounds, Ann. Surg. **108:**918, 1938.
11. Andersen, K.E., et al.: Formaldehyde in a hypoallergenic non-woven textile acrylate tape, Contact Dermatitis **9:**228, 1983.
12. Barnett, A., et al.: Comparison of synthetic adhesive moisture vapor permeable and fine mesh gauze dressings for split-thickness skin graft donor sites, Am. J. Surg. **145:**379, 1983.
13. Baron, H.: Standardization of wound textiles, Nature **175:** 760, 1955.
14. Bergman, R.B.: A new treatment of split-skin graft donor sites, Arch. Chir. Neerl. **29:**69, 1977.
15. Bergman, R.B., and Tolhurst, D.E.: A comparative trial of skin donor site dressings, Chir. Plastica (Berl.) **4:**137, 1978.
16. Bibel, D.J., and LeBrun, J.R.: Changes in cutaneous flora after wet occlusion, Can. J. Microbiol. **21:**496, 1975.
17. Birdsell, D., Hein, K., and Lindsay, R.: The theoretically ideal donor site dressing, Ann. Plast. Surg. **2:**535, 1979.
18. Blaine, G.: Absorbable gelatin sponge in experimental surgery, Lancet **2:**427, 1951.
19. Blair, V.P.: The influence of mechanical pressure on wound healing, Ill. Med. J. **46:**249, 1924.
20. Bloom, H.: "Cellophane" dressing for second-degree burns, Lancet **2:**559, 1945.
21. Brånemark, P.I.: Local tissue effects of wound disinfectants, Acta Chir. Scand. **357**(suppl):166, 1966.
22. Breasted, J.H.: The Edwin Smith surgical papyrus, Vol. 1, Chicago, 1930, University of Chicago Press.
23. Bromberg, B.E., Song, I.C., and Mohn, M.P.: The use of pig skin as a temporary biologic dressing, Plast. Reconstr. Surg. **36:**80, 1965.
24. Buchan, I.A., Andrews, J.K., and Lang, S.M.: Clinical and laboratory investigation of the composition and properties of human skin wound exudate under semipermeable dressings, Burns **7:**326, 1981.
25. Bull, J.P., Squire, J.R., and Topley, E.: Experiments with occlusive dressings of a new plastic, Lancet **2:**213, 1948.
26. Bunker, T.D.: Problems with the use of Op-Site sutureless skin closures in orthopaedic procedures, Ann. R. Coll. Surg. Eng. **65:**260, 1983.
27. Burleson, R., and Eiseman, B.: Mechanisms of antibacterial effects of biologic dressings, Ann. Surg. **177:**181, 1973.
28. Colebrook, L., and Hood, A.M.: Infection through soaked dressings, Lancet **2:**682, 1948.
29. Coleman, G.J., and Roenigk, H.R.: The healing of wounds in the skin of piglets treated with benzoyl peroxide, J. Dermatol. Surg. Oncol. **4:**705, 1978.
30. Comaish, J.S., and Cunliffe, W.J.: Absorption of drugs from varicose ulcers: a cause of anaphylaxis, Br. J. Clin. Pract. **21:**97, 1967.
31. Cronin, E., and Calnan, C.D.: Allergy to hydroabietic alcohol in adhesive tape, Contact Dermatitis **4:**57, 1978.
32. Davis, J.S.: The effect of scarlet red in various combinations upon the epithelization of granulating surfaces, Bull. Johns Hopkins Hosp. **20:**176, 1909.
33. Davis, J.S.: Skin transplantation with a reveiw of 550 cases at the Johns Hopkins Hospital, Johns Hopkins Hosp. Rep. **15:**307, 1910.
34. Dempski, R.E., DeMarco, J.D., and Marcus, A.D.: An in vitro study of the relative moisture occlusive properties of several topical vehicles and Saran Wrap, J. Invest. Dermatol. **44:**361, 1965.
35. Dineen, P.: Antibacterial activity of oxidized regenerated cellulose, Surg. Gynecol. Obstet. **142:**481, 1976.
36. Dinner, M.I., Peters, C.R., and Sherer, J.: Use of semipermeable polyurethane membrane as a dressing for split-skin graft donor site, Plast. Reconstr. Surg. **64:**112, 1979.
37. DuMortier, J.J.: The resistance of healing wounds to infection, Surg. Gynecol. Obstet. **56:**762, 1933.
38. Eaglstein, W.H., and Mertz, P.M.: New method for assessing epidermal wound healing, J. Invest. Dermatol. **71:**382, 1978.
39. Eaglstein, W.H., and Mertz, P.M.: "Inert" vehicles do affect wound healing, J. Invest. Dermatol. **74:**90, 1980.
40. Egan, T.J., O'Driscoll, J., and Thakar, D.R.: Human amnion in the management of chronic ulceration of the lower limb: a clinico-pathologic study, Angiology **34:**197, 1983.
41. Ersek, R.A.: Ischemic necrosis and elastic net bandages, Tex. Med. **78:**47, 1982.
42. Field, L.M.: Over-sight on Op-Site (letter to the editor), J. Dermatol. Surg. Oncol. **7:**597, 1981.
43. Fisher, L.B., and Maibach, H.I.: The effect of occlusive and semipermeable dressings on the cell kinetics of normal and wounded human epidermis. In Maibach, H.I., and Rovee, D.T. (eds.): Epidermal wound healing, Chicago, 1972, Year Book Medical Publishers, Inc.
44. Fodor, P.B.: Scarlet red, Ann. Plast. Surg. **4:**45, 1980.
45. Forage, A.V.: The effects of removing the epidermis from burnt skin, Lancet **2:**690, 1962.
46. Frank, D.H., et al.: Decrease in rate of wound contraction

with the temporary skin substitute Biobrane, Ann. Plast. Surg. **12**:519, 1984.

47. Frantz, V.K., Clarke, H.T., and Lattes, R.: Hemostasis with absorbable gauze, Ann. Surg. **120**:181, 1944.

48. Fregert, S., et al.: Contact allergic reactions to diphenylthiourea and phenylisothiocyanate in PVC adhesive tape, Contact Dermatitis **8**:38, 1982.

49. Friedman, S.J., and Su, W.P.D.: Management of leg ulcers with hydrocolloid occlusive dressing, Arch. Dermatol. **120**:1329, 1984.

50. Gamgee, J.S.: Absorbent and medicated surgical dressings, Lancet **1**:127, 1880.

51. Gartenberg, G., et al.: Hospital-acquired mucormycosis (Rhizopus rhizopodiformis) of skin and subcutaneous tissue, N. Engl. J. Med. **299**:1115, 1978.

52. Gemberling, R.M., et al.: Dressing comparison in the healing of donor sites, J. Trauma **16**:812, 1976.

53. Geronemus, R.G., Mertz, P.M., and Eaglstein, W.H.: The effects of topical antimicrobial agents, Arch. Dermatol. **115**:1311, 1979.

54. Geronemus, R.G., and Robins, P.: The effect of two new dressings on epidermal wound healing, J. Dermatol. Surg. Oncol. **8**:850, 1982.

55. Gillman, T., and Hathorn, M.: Profound modification by dressings of wound healing and of site behavior of donor and recipient sites (preliminary report), Transplantation **4**:64, 1957.

56. Gillman, T., Hathorn, M., and Penn, J.: Is skin homografting necessary? Plast. Reconstr. Surg. **18**:260, 1956.

57. Gilmore, W.A., and Wheeland, R.G.: Treatment of ulcers on legs by pinch grafts and a supportive dressing of polyurethane, J. Dermatol. Surg. Oncol. **8**:177, 1982.

58. Gimbel, N.S., et al.: A study of epithelization in blistered burns, A.M.A. Arch. Surg. **74**:800, 1957.

59. Gissane, W., Bull, J. and Jackson, D.: Current therapeutics CXXXI: wound dressings, Practitioner **181**:640, 1958.

60. Gledhill, T., and Waterfall, W.E.: Silastic foam: a new material for dressing wounds, Can. Med. Assoc. J. **128**:685, 1983.

61. Golden, T.: Non-irritating, multipurpose surgical adhesive tape, Am. J. Surg. **100**:789, 1960.

62. Gray, G.H., and Jones, H.W., Jr.: A satisfactory non-adherent intranasal pack, Plast. Reconstr. Surg. **17**:471, 1956.

63. Grolnick, M.: Factors involved in the production of adhesive plaster irritation, Am. J. Surg. **50**:63, 1940.

64. Habal, M.B.: Pig skin over open wounds (editorial), Surg. Gynecol. Obstet. **149**:395, 1979.

65. Haeger, K., and Liedberg, C.F.: Are postoperative dressings necessary? Nord. Med. **66**:960, 1961.

66. Halsted, W.S.: Ligature and suture material: the employment of fine silk in preference to catgut and the advantage of transfixion of tissues and vessels in controlling hemorrhage, J.A.M.A. **60**:1119, 1913.

67. Harnar, T., et al.: Dr. Paul Unna's boot and early ambulation after skin grafting the leg: a survey of burn centers and a report of 20 cases, Plast. Reconstr. Surg. **69**:359, 1982.

68. Harris, D.R., and Keefe, R.L.: A histologic study of gold leaf treated experimental wounds, J. Invest. Dermatol. **52**:487, 1969.

69. Harris, D.R., and Youkey, J.R.: Evaluating the effects of hemostatic agents on the healing of superficial wounds. In Maibach, H.I., and Rovee, D.T. (eds.): Epidermal wound healing, Chicago, 1972, Year Book Medical Publishers, Inc.

70. Heifetz, C.J., Lawrence, M.S., and Richards, F.O.: Comparison of wound healing with and without dressings, Arch. Surg. **65**:746, 1952.

71. Heifetz, C.J., Richards, F.O., and Lawrence, M.S.: Wound healing without dressings, Arch. Surg. **67**:661, 1953.

72. Helland, S., Nyfors, A., and Utne, L.: Contact dermatitis to Synthaderm, Contact Dermatitis **9**:504, 1983.

73. Hellström, S., Salén, B., and Stenfors, L.-E.: Absorbable gelatin sponge (Gelfoam) in otosurgery: one cause of undesirable postoperative results—an experimental study in the rat, Acta Otolaryngol. (Stockh.) **96**:269, 1983.

74. Heskel, N.S., Samour, C.M., and Storrs, F.J.: Allergic contact dermatitis from dodecyl maleamic acid in Curad adhesive plastic bandages, J. Am. Acad. Dermatol. **7**:747, 1982.

75. Hewsen, A.: On substitutes for adhesive plaster, Boston Med. Surg. J. **103**:339, 1880.

76. Hinman, F., Jr., and Babcock, K.O.: Local reaction to oxidized cellulose and gelatin hemostatic agents in experimentally contaminated renal wounds, Surgery **26**:633, 1949.

77. Hinman, C.D., and Maibach, H.: Effect of air exposure and occlusion on experimental human skin wounds, Nature **200**:377, 1963.

78. Hohn, D.C.: Host resistance to infection: established and emerging concepts. In Hunt, T.K. (ed.): Wound healing and wound infection: theory and surgical practice, New York, 1980, Appleton-Century-Crofts.

79. Holland, K.T., et al.: A comparison of the in-vitro antibacterial and complement activating effect of Opsite and Tegaderm, J. Hosp. Infect. **5**:323, 1984.

80. Howells, C.H.L., and Young, H.B.: A study of completely undressed surgical wounds, Br. J. Surg. **53**:436, 1966.

81. Humphries, R.E.: New factors in adhesive formulas which lessen irritation, J. Invest. Dermatol. **9**:219, 1947.

82. James, D.W.: A connective tissue constituent in the scab formed over cutaneous wounds, J. Pathol. Bacteriol **69**:33, 1955.

83. James, J.H., and Watson, A.C.H.: The use of Opsite, a vapour permeable dressing, on skin graft donor sites, Br. J. Plast. Surg. **28**:107, 1975.

84. James, W.D., White, S.W., and Yanklowitz, B.: Allergic contact dermatitis to compound tincture of benzoin, J. Am. Acad. Dermatol. **11**:847, 1984.

85. Jelenko, C., III, et al.: The evolution of adhesive tape, Surg. Gynecol. Obstet. **126**:1083, 1968.

86. Jordan, W.P.: Cross sensitization patterns in acrylate allergies, Contact Dermatitis **1**:13, 1975.

87. Keys, T.F., et al.: Nosocomial outbreak of rhizopus infections associated with elastoplast wound dressings, M.M.W.R. **27**:33, 1978.

88. Knighton, D.R., Silver, I.A., and Hunt, T.K.: Regulation of wound-healing angiogenesis-effect of oxygen gradients and inspired oxygen concentration, Surgery **90**:262, 1981.

89. Knudsen, E.A., and Snitker, G.: Wound healing under plastic-coated pads, Acta Dermatovenerol. **49**:438, 1969.

90. Krawczyk, W.S.: Some ultrastructural aspects of epidermal repair in two model wound healing systems. In Maibach,

H.I., and Rovee, D.T. (eds.): Epidermal wound healing, Chicago, 1972, Year Book Medical Publishers, Inc.

91. Kristensen, H., and Christensen, E.A.: Radiation-resistant micro-organisms isolated from textiles, Acta Pathol. Microbiol. Scand. **89:**303, 1981.

92. Kucan, J.O., Robson, M.C., and Parsons, R.W.: Amniotic membranes as dressings following facial dermabrasion, Ann. Plast. Surg. **8:**523, 1982.

93. Lawrence, J.C.: The perinecrotic zone in burns and its influence on healing, Burns **1:**197, 1975.

94. Lawrence, J.C.: What materials for dressings? Injury **13:**500, 1982.

95. Lebovits, P.E., and Dzubow, L.: Surgical gems: a pressure dressing on the scalp by a modified Russian technique, J. Dermatol. Surg. Oncol. **6:**259, 1980.

96. Lebovits, P.E., Dzubow, L., and Leider, M.: The art of bandaging: fingers and hands, toes and feet, the gauntlet (or glove) and the sock, J. Dermatol. Surg. Oncol. **7:**611, 1981.

97. Lesiewicz, J., and Goldsmith, L.: Inhibiter of rat skin ornithine decarboxylase by nitrofurazone (letter), Arch. Dermatol. **116:**1225, 1980.

98. Leyden, J.J.: Effects of bacteria on healing superficial wounds, Clin. Dermatol. **2:**81, 1984.

99. Linsky, C.B., Rovee, D.T., and Dow, T.: Effects of dressings on wound inflammation and scar tissue. In Dineen, P., and Hildick-Smith, G. (eds.): The surgical wound, Philadelphia, 1981, Lea & Febiger.

100. Lobe, T.E., et al.: An improved method of wound management for pediatric patients, J. Pediatr. Surg. **15:**886, 1980.

101. London, P.S.: Current therapeutics CCXXVIII: wound dressings, Practitioner **197:**824, 1966.

102. Lookingbill, D.P., Miller, S.H., and Knowles, R.C.: Bacteriology of chronic leg ulcers, Arch. Dermatol. **114:**1765, 1978.

103. Lynch, W.S., and Bailin, P.: The promotion of wound healing following chemosurgery (Mohs' technique) by dressings with a lotion of benzoyl peroxide, J. Dermatol. Surg. Oncol. **4:**91, 1978.

104. Malimson, P.D.: On twisting bandages: an experimental study, Br. J. Plast. Surg. **37:**626, 1984.

105. Malten, K.E.: Dermatological problems with synthetic resins and plastics in glues. II., Derm. Beruf Umwelt **32:**118, 1984.

106. Mandy, S.H.: A new primary wound dressing made of polyethylene oxide gel, J. Dermatol. Surg. Oncol. **9:**153, 1983.

107. Marks, J.G., Jr., et al.: Cutaneous reactions to surgical preparations and dressings, Contact Dermatitis **10:**1, 1984.

108. Marples, R.R., and Kligman, A.M.: Growth of bacteria under adhesive tapes, Arch. Dermatol. **99:**107, 1969.

109. Marples, R.R., and Kligman, A.M.: Bacterial infection of superficial wounds: a human model for *Staphylococcus aureus*. In Maibach, H.I., and Rovee, D.T. (eds.): Epidermal wound healing, Chicago, 1972, Year Book Medical Publishers, Inc.

110. Martin, H.A.: A new adhesive plaster especially adapted to the requirements of modern surgery, Boston Med. Surg. J. **97:**407, 1877.

111. Matthews, D.N.: Dressing of open wounds and burns with tulle gras, Lancet **1:**43, 1941.

112. Matthews, R.N., Bennett, J.P., and Faulk, W.P.: Wound healing using amniotic membranes, Br. J. Plast. Surg. **34:**76, 1981.

113. McGrath, M.H.: How topical dressings salvage "questionable" flaps: experimental study, Plast. Reconstr. Surg. **67:**653, 1981.

114. McLean, N.R., and MacKinlay, J.: 'Op-Site' as a postoperative dressing in general surgery, Br. J. Clin. Pract. **35:**356, 1981.

115. Mengert, W.F., and Hermes, R.L.: Simplified gynecologic care, Am. J. Obstet. Gynecol. **58:**1109, 1949.

116. Mertz, P.M., and Eaglstein, W.H.: The effect of a semiocclusive dressing on the microbial population in superficial wounds, Arch. Surg. **119:**287, 1984.

117. Mikhail, G.R., Farris, W., and Gimbel, N.S.: The pattern of superficial blood vessels in healing skin donor site, J. Invest. Dermatol. **44:**75, 1965.

118. Miller, T.A.: The healing of partial-thickness skin injuries. In Hunt, T.K. (ed.): Wound healing and wound infection: theory and surgical practice, New York, 1980, Appleton-Century-Crofts.

119. Montagna, W.: Cutaneous comparative biology, Arch. Dermatol. **104:**577, 1971.

120. More on Debrisan for ulcers and infected wounds, Drug. Ther. Bull. **22:**15, 1984.

121. Mummery, R.V., and Richardson, W.W.: Clinical trial of Debrisan in superficial ulceration, J. Int. Med. Res. **7:**263, 1979.

122. Noe, J.M., and Kalish, S.: The mechanism of capillarity in surgical dressings, Surg. Gynecol. Obstet. **143:**454, 1976.

123. Noe, J.M., and Kalish, S.: The problem of adherence in dressed wounds, Surg. Gynecol. Obstet. **147:**185, 1978.

124. Olson, R.A., Roberts, D.L., and Osbon, D.B.: A comparative study of polylactic acid, Gelfoam, and Surgicel in healing extraction sites, Oral Surg. **53:**441, 1982.

125. Owens, N.: Use of pressure dressings in the treatment of burns and other wounds, Surg. Clin. North Am. **23:**1354, 1943.

126. Pace, W.E.: Treatment of cutaneous ulcers with benzoyl peroxide, Can. Med. Assoc. J. **115:**1101, 1976.

127. Palumbo, L.T., Monnig, P.J., and Wilkinson, D.E.: Healing of clean surgical wounds of thorax and abdomen with or without dressings, J.A.M.A. **160:**553, 1956.

128. Pearson, R.D., Valenti, W.M., and Steigbigel, R.T.: *Clostridium perfringens* wound infection associated with elastic bandages, J.A.M.A. **244:**1128, 1980.

129. Pippen, R.: Anaphylactoid reaction after chymacort ointment (letter), Br. Med. J. **1:**1172, 1966.

130. Pruitt, B.A., Jr., and Levine, W.S.: Characteristics and uses of biologic dressings and skin substitutes, Arch. Surg. **119:**312, 1984.

131. Raekallio, J., Möttönen, M., and Nieminen, L.: Evaluation of three synthetic films as wound covers, Acta Chir. Scand. **139:**1, 1973.

132. Ramirez, O.M., et al.: Optimal wound healing under Op-Site dressing, Plast. Reconstr. Surg. **73:**474, 1984.

133. Rebell, G., et al.: Factors affecting the rapid disappearance of bacteria placed on the normal skin, J. Invest. Dermatol. **14:**247, 1950.

134. Rice, R.H., and Vogt, P.R.: New material for surgical dressings, Northwest Med. **54:**162, 1955.

135. Rob, C.G., and Eastcott, H.H.G.: A plastic surgical dressing, Br. Med. J. **2:**17, 1954.

136. Roberts, M.J.: Elastic tension therapeutically utilized in adhesive and medicated plasters, Med. Record **21:**348, 1882.

137. Robinson, J.K.: An effective pressure dressing on the scalp that is easily made and is cosmetically acceptable, J. Dermatol. Surg. Oncol. **7:**607, 1981.

138. Robson, M.C., Samburg, J.L., and Krizek, T.J.: Quantitative comparison of biologic dressings, J. Surg. Res. **14:**431, 1973.

139. Robson, M.C., et al.: Amniotic membranes as a temporary wound dressing, Surg. Gynecol. Obstet. **136:**904, 1973.

140. Rovee, D.T., et al.: Effect of local wound environment on epidermal healing. In Maibach, H.I., and Rovee, D.T. (eds.): Epidermal wound healing, Chicago, 1972, Year Book Medical Publishers, Inc.

141. Sabella, N.: Use of the fetal membranes in skin grafting, Med. Record **83:**478, 1913.

142. Salisbury, R.E., et al.: Biologic dressings for skin graft donor sites, Arch. Surg. **106:**705, 1973.

143. Salomon, J.C., Diegelmann, R.F., and Cohen, I.K.: Effect of dressings on donor site epithelization, Surg. Forum **25:**516, 1974.

144. Savage, R.M., Bryce, D.M., and Elliot, J.R.: The water retention coefficient of surgical dressings, J. Pharm. Pharmacol. **4:**944, 1952.

145. Scales, J.T., Towers, A.G., and Goodman, N.: Development and evaluation of a porous surgical dressing, Br. Med. J. **2:**962, 1956.

146. Scales, J.T., and Winter, G.D.: The adhesion of wound dressings: an experimental study. In Slome, D. (ed.): Wound healing, Oxford, 1961, Pergamon Press.

147. Schein, M., and Dunn, S.: What grows beneath Op-Site surgical wound dressing? S. Afr. Med. J. **66:**752, 1984.

148. Scher, K.S., and Coil, J.A., Jr.: Effects of oxidized cellulose and microfibrillar collagen on infection, Surgery **91:**301, 1982.

149. Schilling, R.S.F., Roberts, M., and Goodman, N.: Clinical trial of occlusive plastic dressings, Lancet **1:**293, 1950.

150. Silver, I.A.: Oxygen tension and epithelization. In Maibach, H.I., and Rovee, D.T. (eds.): Epidermal wound healing, Chicago, 1972, Year Book Medical Publishers, Inc.

151. Smith, K.W., Oden, P.W., and Blaylock, W.K.: A comparison of gold leaf and other occlusive therapy, Arch. Dermatol. **96:**703, 1963.

152. Stark, R.B.: The rabbit ear as an experimental tool, Plast. Reconstr. Surg. **19:**28, 1957.

153. Sturdy, J.H., Baird, R.M., and Gerein, A.N.: Surgical sponges: a cause of granuloma and adhesion formation, Ann. Surg. **165:**128, 1967.

154. Sugar, O.: Oxidized cellulose hemostat (Surgicel) (editorial), Surg. Neurol. **21:**521, 1984.

155. Swanson, N., et al.: Skin grafting: the split thickness skin graft in 1980, J. Dermatol. Surg. Oncol. **6:**524, 1980.

156. Thomas, S., Dawes, C., and Hay, P.: A critical evaluation of some extensible bandages in current use, Nurs. Times **76:**1123, 1980.

157. Tinckler, L.: Surgical wound management with adhesive polyurethane membrane: a preferred method for routine usage, Ann. R. Coll. Surg. Engl. **65:**257, 1983.

158. Topical PEG in burn ointments, FDA Drug Bull. **12:**25, 1982.

159. Transparent wound dressings, Med. Lett. Drugs Ther. **25:**103, 1983.

160. Turner, T.D.: Hospital usage of absorbent dressings, Pharm. J. **222:**421, 1979.

161. Van Way, C.W., III, et al.: Clinical evaluation of a low lint surgical sponge, Surg. Gynecol. Obstet. **155:**529, 1982.

162. Vasiliev, J.M., and Cheung, A.B.: Evolution of epithelial proliferation induced by scarlet red in the skin of normal and carcinogen-treated rabbits, Br. J. Cancer **16:**238, 1962.

163. Wallgren, G.R.: Plastics as surgical dressings: one year's experience with Nobecutane, Ann. Chir. Gynaecol. **43:**279, 1954.

164. Wallgren, G.R.: Bacteriological experiments with surgical plastic dressings, Acta Chir. Scand. **112:**161, 1957.

165. Wayne, M.A.: Clinical evaluation of Epi-Lock: a semiocclusive dressing, Ann. Emerg. Med. **14:**20, 1985.

166. Williams, R.H.P., et al.: Multicentre prospective trial of Silastic foam dressing in management of open granulating wounds, Br. Med. J. **282:**21, 1981.

167. Winsor, T., and Burch, G.E.: Differential roles of layers of human epigastric skin on diffusion rate of water, Arch. Intern. Med. **74:**428, 1944.

168. Winter, G.D.: Formation of scab and the rate of epithelization of superficial wounds in the skin of the young domestic pig, Nature **193:**293, 1962.

169. Winter, G.D., and Scales, J.: Effect of air drying and dressings on the surface of the wound, Nature **197:**91, 1963.

170. Winter, G.D.: Comment to Hinman, C.D., and Maibach, H.: Effect of air exposure and occlusion on experimental skin wounds, Nature **200:**377, 1963.

171. Winter, G.D.: A note on wound healing under dressings with special reference to perforated film dressings, J. Invest. Dermatol. **45:**299, 1965.

172. Winter, G.D.: Epidermal regeneration studied in the domestic pig. In Maibach, H.I., and Rovee, D.T. (eds.): Epidermal wound healing, 1972, Year Book Medical Publishers, Inc.

173. Wokalek, H., et al.: First experiences with a transplant liquid gel in the treatment of fresh operation wounds and chronic epithelial defects on the skin, Aktuel. Dermatol. **5:**255, 1979.

174. Wood, R.A.B., Williams, R.H.P., and Hughes, L.E.: Foam elastomer dressing in the management of open granulating wounds: experience with 250 patients, Br. J. Surg. **64:**554, 1977.

175. Wright, A.E., Fleming, A., and Colebrook, L.: The sterilisation of wounds by physiological agency, Lancet **1:**831, 1918.

176. Yates, D.W., et al.: Clinical experience with a new hydrogel wound dressing, Injury **16:**23, 1984.

177. Zahir, M.: Contraction of wounds, Br. J. Surg. **51:**456, 1964.

178. Zahir, M.: Formation of scabs in skin wounds, Br. J. Surg. **52:**376, 1965.

179. Zitelli, J.A.: Delayed wound healing with adhesive wound dressings, J. Dermatol. Surg. Oncol. **10:**709, 1984.

FUNDAMENTALS OF EXCISIONAL SURGERY

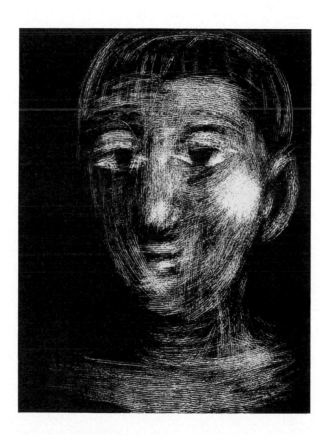

La Tête de Garçon, lithocut by Picasso. Note artist's accentuation of many maximal skin tension lines. (From the author's collection.)

CHAPTER

10

Basic Excisional Surgery

The skilled excision of cutaneous lesions and repair of the resulting surgical defects require the development of tissue-handling techniques. Such techniques are based on a thorough understanding of the principles of wound healing and a knowledge of microbiology, anatomy, instruments, and other surgical materials at one's disposal. These topics have been discussed previously.

The appearance of the closed surgical wound and the inevitable scar that results is perhaps the best index of the quality of work performed throughout the operation. Surgical scars reflect the surgeon's skills and are an important visible means by which the patient judges the surgeon. The method of wound closure is performed by each surgeon in a highly individual manner. Excellent results usually are obtained, but some techniques are better than others.

An important realization for any physician operating on the skin is that every incision produces a permanent scar. The goal in excisional surgery is the production of ''good'' scars. A good scar is a scar that can be seen only close up and which does not cast a shadow; it is a fine line that is level with the surrounding tissue. The color of a good scar should approach that of the nearby skin, and there should be no contractures visible to the eye. Good scars are not a matter of chance but instead are the result of well-planned and well-executed surgery. This includes correct design of the wound and incision of tissue with appropriate tension and no injury to the surrounding tissues.

No one textbook in cutaneous surgery can be all inclusive. Every author has developed personal surgical tricks from which everyone can benefit. Textbooks that I have found useful and to which I frequently refer include Borges,[11] Converse,[25] Grabb and Smith,[55] Petres and Hundeiker,[110] and Stegman, Tromovitch, and Glogau.[133]

ARTISAN PHYSICIAN-SURGEON

Excisional surgery is not merely a technique, but an art form. The surgeon, like an artist, can previsualize the end result and achieve it, whereas a technician can only repetitiously and mechanically perform tasks.

Some physician-surgeons perform this art better than others, in that the resultant scars are hardly perceptible. Such physicians have a keen awareness of the end result and of how a scar will ultimately appear.

Although it is difficult if not impossible to measure one's ability at excisional surgery, we all recognize these artisan physician-surgeons by the types of wounds and scars they leave: wounds with minimal problems and scars that are inconspicuous in placement and appearance. Although several methods are available to remove a lesion adequately, they do not always produce the same end result. The artisan physician-surgeons appear to choose the ideal method of wound creation, the ideal method of closure, and proper postoperative management.

What are the qualities of the artisan physician-surgeon? These physicians first and foremost have developed their senses, particularly the ability to see rather than look and to feel rather than touch. Not only can they perceive the end result, but they have trained themselves to see or feel their way to a diagnosis before surgery. They detect subtle changes in the texture or tension of the skin that will influence the end cosmetic result.

Artisan physician-surgeons constantly search for excellence. They are critical of themselves and others. They continually seek to improve surgical techniques in search of the ideal. They realize that success depends on the mastery of many details. When a wound dehisces or other problems arise within a surgical site, these physicians question what happened and ponder methods of preventing such problems in the future. They are in constant movement from the patient to the medical literature to teachers or colleagues and back to the patient again. They turn current surgical failures into future victories.

The ability to learn from one's mistakes is the foundation of excellent surgical judgment. Only from both bad and good experiences can one gain surgical judgment. These are not lessons learned from textbooks alone but from the continual evaluation of one's experience with many patients.

Artisan physician-surgeons develop the ability to handle tissue carefully with a minimum of motion. Their movements appear effortless, well-controlled, and smooth—much like those of a concert pianist. Their techniques are not learned in a short time; on the contrary, they are the result of years of practice, refinement of technique, and development of concentration.

Some authorities[23,124] propose that a surgical technique such as suturing can be readily taught by means of pig skin,[129] turkey skin,[83] chicken skin, or even electronic devices[124]—but I disagree. One can easily be taught to sew but not to suture. Good suturing is a matter of the many factors already mentioned. It is learned by those with a sense of perfection and an attention to detail. These qualities are rarely found even among physicians.

ATRAUMATIC TECHNIQUE

The one principle underlying every type of surgery is that gentle, minimal handling of tissues results in the best possible surgical wound and the least apparent scar.[20,40,59,60] The surgeon should know how to handle the skin carefully. The skin is a delicate fabric that shows reaction to gross handling.[143] Atraumatic technique minimizes the two major obstacles to successful surgery—fibrous tissue proliferation and infection—which are related to the amount of injured, devitalized tissue in a wound.[67,91,126]

The rough handling of tissue frequently results in fluid accumulation and edema. Edema interferes with wound healing by separating tissues that need to unite, by impairing venous return, and by interfering with tissue metabolism. Devitalized tissue in a wound is as detrimental as bacteria.[118] The presence of tissue debris diverts the energies of the cells, which normally should be concerned with repair, to the elimination of dead material. Therefore every physician performing surgery should strive to handle tissue gently to minimize dead tissue.

Minimal tissue injury is achieved in various ways. Sharp instruments should be selected; dull knives or scissors tend to compress tissue on cutting and do more damage than sharp ones. Skin hooks rather than pickups should be chosen to reduce compression of wound edges.[114,115] Tissue destruction at the time of hemostasis (with hemostats, suture, or electrosurgery) should be minimized. Operating lights that produce little heat should be used; otherwise tissue tends to desiccate. Conservation of movement, concentration, and deliberate effort all help to reduce the duration and trauma of surgery. A physician performing surgery needs to develop the use of all fingers and a gracefulness of motion. Every effort to steady his or her movements should be made.

In 1921 Bunnell best described the techniques of physicians who do not understand gentle tissue-handling techniques.[20] "Tissue is torn, pinched, crushed, twisted, pulled, rubbed, scraped and picked to shreds with gross disregard for not only its microscopic structure, but even for its macrostructure . . . " The magnitude of damage to tissues with only minor trauma is emphasized by Schilling.[125] He points out that one hemostat may be responsible for the death of $10,000,000$ (10^7) cells. Also, a cubic centimeter of blood contains about 5 billion (10^9) cells. Therefore one should reduce the trauma to tissue as much as feasible and keep blood in a wound to a minimum.

PREOPERATIVE EVALUATION

Every patient for whom surgery is contemplated should be evaluated for the appropriateness of the surgery and the risks involved. This involves a preoperative history and physical examination, assessment of the problem, discussion about the proposed procedure, obtaining of informed consent, and preoperative instructions. A record should be made of all these different parts of the preoperative evaluation. Every effort should be made to establish a diagnosis before treating the patient.

Preoperative history

The preoperative history is a subjective record of the patient's recollections of the lesion or condition under consideration. This should incude the length of time the lesion or condition has been present, any associated symptoms (such as pruritus or bleeding), and previous forms of therapy (and their results). Any other attendant factors, such as preceding injury or infections in the areas of concern, should also be noted.

For complex surgical procedures (such as large excisions, grafts, or skin flaps) a complete review of systems and detailed medical history should be obtained. I have found it useful to use a preoperative checklist so that important conditions are not overlooked (see Appendix A).

The review of systems should include a history of problems with wound healing or scarring, bleeding problems, heart problems (including pacemaker), high blood pressure, glaucoma, diabetes, mental problems, liver disease, kidney disease, allergies (to anesthetics, antibiotics, and pain medications), and prior episodes of jaundice or hepatitis (Table 10-1). Certain dermatologic conditions, such as lichen planus or psoriasis, tend to localize in cutaneous scars, a reaction known as the Koebner phenomenon (Fig. 10-1). One should inquire about the medical history, including current medications, previous surgery, and prior hospitalizations.

Two common forms of medical therapy that need thoughtful evaluation before surgery are anticoagulation and pacemakers. If the patient is on warfarin (Coumadin) and an extensive procedure is planned, the physician who has prescribed the anticoagulant should be consulted. An anticoagulant given for minor reasons is frequently discontinued

TABLE 10-1

Review of systems in cutaneous surgery

System	Problem	Perioperative problem
Endocrine	Thyrotoxicosis	↑ Cardiac sensitivity to epinephrine
	Myxedema	↑ Sensitivity to depressant drugs
	Cushing's disease	↓ Liver synthesis of pseudocholinesterase
	Addison's disease	Hyperpigmentation
	Pregnancy	Effects of local anesthetics on fetus
	Diabetes	↑ Time of wound healing (if poorly controlled)
Pulmonary	Asthma	↑ Histamine release with morphine
	Emphysema	↑ Toxicity of local anesthetics (caused by respiratory acidosis)
Renal	Renal failure	↑ Toxicity of local anesthetics
	Hypokalemia	↑ Cardiac arrhythmia with epinephrine
Cardiac	Heart failure	↑ Toxicity of local anesthetics
	Arrhythmia	↑ Toxicity of epinephrine
	Pacemakers	Interference by electromagnetic radiation
Gastrointestinal	Cirrhosis	↑ Toxicity to anesthetics
		↑ Bleeding
	Hepatitis	Possible inoculation
Hematopoietic	Bleeding disorder	↑ Bleeding or hematoma
	Anticoagulation	↑ Bleeding
Cutaneous	Ehlers-Danlos syndrome	Widening of scars
	Discoid lupus erythematosus, lichen planus, psoriasis	Koebner phenomenon
	Infection other than operative site	↑ Wound infection
	Keloids	↑ Scar formation
Central nervous system	Neurosis	Noncooperative patient
	Psychosis	
	Depression	
Immunologic	Allergy	Allergy to medication
	Cryoglobulinemia	Cold (for example, from liquid N_2) could cause precipitation of cryoglobulins
Miscellaneous	Pseudocholintesterase deficiency	↓ Plasma clearance of ester anesthetics
	Porphyria	Barbiturates can cause attack
	Herpes simplex (recurrent)	Herpes simplex reactivation
	AIDS	Possible inoculation

3 to 4 days before surgery and begun again immediately after surgery without undue risk of bleeding. However, if continuous anticoagulation is necessary, one should arrange for heparinization during the surgery. In this situation I usually discontinue the warfarin 3 or 4 days before surgery and then on the day of surgery begin heparin, 5000 units every 12 hours until the day after the surgery. This requires hospitalization and monitoring of the blood coagulation profiles.

Pacemakers also are of concern during surgery if the surgeon is using an electrosurgical apparatus. In general, pacemakers are not interfered with during minor surgery on the cutaneous surfaces. Modern pacemakers are coated with materials that shield them from extraneous electromagnetic interference; therefore such interference is unusual but of theoretical interest.[155] However, it should be appreciated

that every patient with a permanent pacemaker has significant underlying cardiovascular disease. Simon recommends that all patients with pacemakers should be monitored during surgery to detect any arrhythmias and verify proper pacemaker function.[127] The current on the electrosurgical apparatus should be set as low as possible and the ground plate be placed as remotely as possible from the pacemaker generator and leads. The use of the active electrocoagulation electrode over or near a pacemaker is potentially a dangerous situation; in these instances patients should be carefully evaluated during surgery. More on pacemakers is discussed in Chapter 16.

A family history may be important information to obtain as well, particularly in regard to the current problem. For instance, I have occasionally seen patients with skin cancers

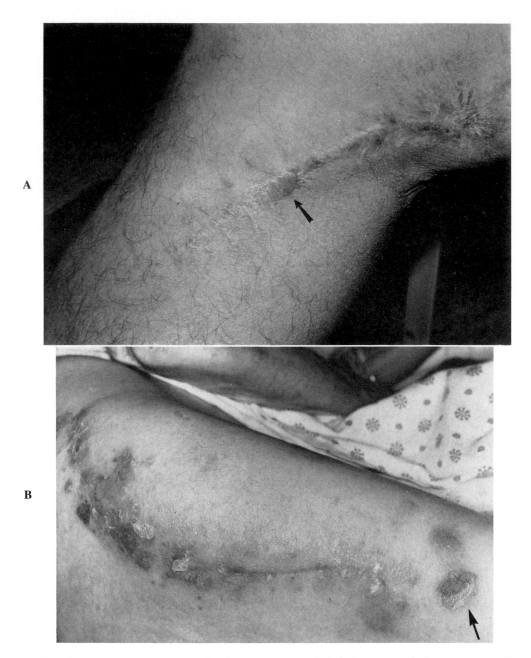

Fig. 10-1. Koebner phenomenon. **A,** Biopsy-proven psoriatic lesion *(arrow)* in linear scar on calf. **B,** Pemphigus foliaceus localizing to scar from hip replacement. Note crusted bullous lesion *(arrow)* on right.

who were anxious because of previous bad experiences with the same condition in their mother or father.

A social history helps to put the patient in perspective and may impinge on the current problem. For instance, knowledge of excessive sun exposure in certain occupations may be important for patients with skin cancer so that one can properly advise them with respect to future sun exposure.

Physical examination

Careful examination of the lesion or condition forms the basis of objective data, with which a diagnosis can be considered. Observation is the basis of surgical diagnosis.[44] A complete description of the lesion to be excised should include its location (and distribution, if relevant), color, texture (smooth, scaly, ulcerated, and so on) and form (macule, papule, and so on). The two largest diameters of the

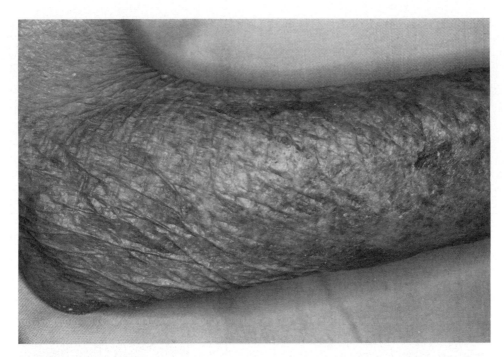

Fig. 10-2. Thinned skin on arm of elderly patient, which is readily torn by sutures and bruises easily.

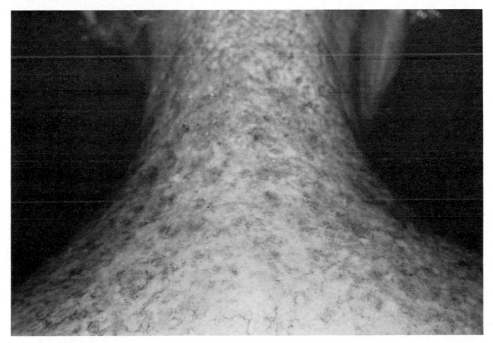

Fig. 10-3. Radiodermatitic skin of posterior neck.

lesion should be precisely measured perpendicular to each other. A diagram of the lesion's anatomic location is an excellent and more accurate record than mere description and is thus highly recommended. The lesion should be palpated, and its softness, hardness, or mobility should be noted.

The physical examination should consider the texture (porous or smooth) of the skin near the surgical site and the patient's complex type. Some elderly patients or those chronically on corticosteroids have very fragile skin (Fig. 10-2), which tears easily when sutured with materials of high tensile strength. Such thin skin is also more susceptible to bruising. Radiodermatitic skin is poorly vascular (Fig. 10-3) and may demonstrate impaired wound healing. The patient should be inspected for other surgical scars to see if

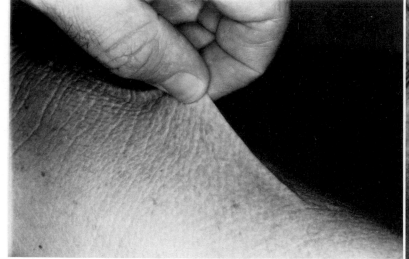
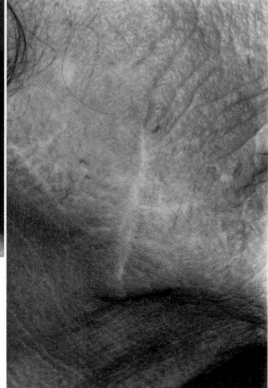

Fig. 10-4. A, Very stretchable skin in "double-jointed" patient. **B,** Spread scars on cheek of same patient.

they are spread, hypertrophic, or depressed. Patients with very stretchable skin and those who are double jointed tend to get spread scars (Fig. 10-4). Patients who are known keloid formers are more likely to form keloids with any surgical procedure.

It is important to note preoperatively any neurologic deficits around the contemplated surgical site. Occasionally nerves are severed at the time of surgery, but neurologic damage may also have existed preoperatively. Unless this is specifically looked for before surgery, it is most likely to be overlooked.

For patients with cutaneous malignancies it is important to feel for enlarged nodes in the lesion's possible drainage areas. If nodes are found, their character (hardness, softness), mobility, location, and size should be recorded; if they are not found, their absence should be recorded.

If surgery is performed around the eyes, visual acuity should be measured. This is a simple procedure that requires only an eye chart.

A general physical examination is usually unnecessary before cutaneous surgery unless a large amount of local anesthetic or general anesthesia is contemplated. It is nonetheless wise to note the overall nutritional status since poorly nourished patients may have healing difficulties.

Laboratory examination

Before surgical therapy it may be useful to obtain a biopsy of the tissue to be removed so that the precise type of lesion and its depth of penetration can be determined. This allows a thoughtful approach to treatment, which may be planned and discussed with the patient. Preoperative biopsies are particularly essential for malignancies of the skin, for which a more aggressive approach to treatment may be necessary. Specimens removed at the time of surgery should be sent for pathologic examination. If patients are admitted to the hospital, prior biopsy specimens should be made available to the hospital pathologist for examination and issuance of an official report for the hospital record.

Assessment of the problem and informed consent

Based on the subjective and objective data gathered, the physician should discuss with the patient the evaluation of the problem, the proposed surgical procedure, alternative methods of therapy, and any consequences that are likely to occur as a result of either the surgery or of the problem being left untreated. It is important for patients to understand that all surgical procedures leave a scar.

A consent form for both the surgical procedure and any photographs taken is highly recommended. Although verbal consent to a surgical procedure is always obtained before surgery, a written consent is proof that the procedure was discussed in detail with the patient. A form that I have found convenient is in Appendix B. It is important that consent forms be readable at about the eighth-grade level of education.[57]

TABLE 10-2

Historical considerations of skin tension lines

Investigators	Date of pertinent publication(s)	Name for lines	Method	Remarks
Dupuytren[38]	1831	—	Stiletto in cadavers	Noted that circular wounds became elliptic in chest
Malgaigne[88]	1838	—	Circular instrument in cadavers	Noted that pattern of elliptic wounds was transverse on chest and like rays around eyes
Langer[79]	1861	Langer's lines	Awl in cadavers	Noted longitudinal lines on extremities
Kocher[76]	1902	Kocher's lines	Incisions in patients	Noted longitudinal lines on extremities
Cox[29]	1941	Cleavage lines	Marlinspike in cadavers	Noted longitudinal lines on extremities
Rubin[122]	1948	Skin lines	Ink (special) in volunteers	Noted horizontal and vertical wrinkle lines on upper lips
Kraissl and Conway[78]	1949	Excision lines	Clinical observation	First to notice favorable lines for excision on extremities run circularly (not longitudinally)
Hutchinson and Koop (infant studies)[70]	1956	Skin-cleavage lines	Awl in infant cadavers	Noted that some areas had triangular wounds
Borges and Alexander[12]	1962	Relaxed skin-tension lines (RSTLs)	Clinical observation	Emphasized placing skin in relaxed position for determination of lines
Stegman[132]	1980	Skin-tension lines	Cutaneous punches into face and trunk of patients	Noted that round punch holes do not become elliptic in certain areas of face

Preoperative instructions

It is a good idea to give patients a written preoperative instruction sheet for the most commonly performed operations. It would state that they should arrive at the office with no makeup (for surgery on the face), freshly bathed, and having eaten a light meal. If surgery is performed on the scalp, preoperative washing with pHisoHex is recommended. Patients should be advised against taking aspirin for approximately 1 week before surgery, if the surgery is extensive.

Preoperative sedation may be requested by the patients but in my experience is unnecessary. Sometimes preoperative sedation may be achieved by having the patient take diazepam (Valium) orally (5 to 10 mg) 30 to 45 minutes before the procedure. If such sedation is used, one must have the patient arrange for transportation before and after surgery, which may be a good idea in any case.

PLANNING LINES FOR EXCISION

Before the injection of a local anesthetic one should plan the direction, shape, and length of a cutaneous excision. The most appropriate lines for an excision are those that produce the least amount of scarring when the wound is completely healed. The direction of an excision is important, since tension on its wound edges are usually greatest in one direction.

Historical background (Table 10-2)

In 1831 Dupuytren made the observation that a virtually round instrument piercing the skin of the chest produced an elliptically shaped wound.[38] This physician was called to the Hôtel-Dieu in Paris to treat a merchant who had attempted suicide. The attempt had been made with a stiletto, a cylindrically bladed knife, but the wounds were nevertheless practically linear. Dupuytren found this difficult to believe, so he performed experiments on a cadaver and confirmed that a round instrument piercing the skin produces a slitlike (not circular) defect. He mapped these slits into lines on certain areas of the body.

In 1838 Malgaigne demonstrated that the long axes of elliptic wounds produced in a cadaver with a round instrument lay along a pattern of lines.[88] He reviewed the pattern of these lines on the entire body, and his patterns differed somewhat from those of Dupuytren. Thus even at this early time tension lines differed from one investigator to another.

In the early 1860s Langer performed a series of experiments in cadavers of all ages.[79,80,81] He pierced the skin with a spike, symmetrically ground to a conical point, and produced linear-shaped wounds. Piercing the skin just ahead of the point of the linear defect produced another linear-shaped wound. Producing a number of such stab wounds resulted in lines that varied somewhat in different bodies but were in general rather uniform. These lines became known as Langer's lines.

Although Langer performed his experiments in cadavers that were in rigor mortis, he nevertheless stressed the relationship of the direction of the slitlike clefts to the position of the underlying joints and muscles. It is interesting to note that Langer himself realized the phenomenon he was describing was caused by the cleavage of the dermis between adjacent groups of collagen fibers. He proposed that these fibers had definite orientation in the skin. Histologically Langer saw collagen bundles running longitudinally and parallel to the slitlike wounds but obliquely if viewed perpendicular to the slits. Based on both microscopic and functional considerations, Langer thought that the collagen fiber in the skin functioned as though in a rhomboidal, or honeycomb, pattern.

In 1902 Kocher suggested that excision lines should be based on a pattern determined by the direction an incision in a patient spreads the least.[76] Thus Kocher devised charts showing the favorable lines of incision, based on the direction that incisions spread the least at the time of incision. These lines became known as Kocher's lines. Although many of these lines were similar to Langer's lines, there were some differences.

General acceptance of Langer's lines as the best guide to cutaneous excisions persisted in the early part of the twentieth century in dermatology and surgery textbooks.[36,111] Even recent surgical textbooks still recommend basing excision lines on Langer's lines.[100] However, it was suggested in 1935 by Webster that wrinkle lines, especially on the face, should be followed in making incisions rather than Langer's lines.[143] Many of Langer's lines ran across natural creases and flexion lines such as on the forehead or over joints. Straatsma[136] also suggested the use of tension lines or natural folds as guides to incision making.

The first modern reevaluation of Langer's work was performed by Cox in 1941.[29] This investigator worked on 28 unclaimed bodies, confirming the earlier studies by Langer. Like Langer, Cox used a marlinspike to produce slitlike holes in succession, and called the resultant lines cleavage lines. Cox pointed out, however, that the line pattern varied according to the body build; also, in certain areas the punctures formed triangular wounds (not round) and came to lie in nonpatterned groups. (Interestingly, Langer had also found such nonpatterned groups of lines and triangular defects.[79]) In these areas the skin tension is the same in all directions rather than being greater in one direction. On the face these triangular wounds occurred between the aesthetic zones on the lateral malar prominence; on the trunk they occurred on the upper chest and back, corresponding to areas of prominent scar formation.

In 1948 Rubin became the first investigator to suggest that the most favorable lines for excision on the face paralleled the wrinkle lines and were perpendicular to the underlying muscle groups.[122] He studied the face by mapping out the wrinkle lines with a colorless chemical used by police in a technique similar to fingerprinting. Cox found a fairly consistent relationship between the wrinkle lines and the orientation of the underlying muscle bundles. In general they ran perpendicular to each other. He concluded that the most favorable lines for excision were generally perpendicular to the underlying muscle group. Rubin pointed out that around the mouth, particularly on the upper lip, the wrinkle patterns of different individuals may vary by as much as 90 degrees. This point is discussed later.

In 1949 Kraissl and Conway[78] and Kraissl alone in 1951[77] suggested, as did Rubin,[122] that the wrinkle lines are the most favorable lines for excision on the face and that these lines are at right angles to the pull of the underlying muscle groups. They demonstrated histologically connections (insertions) of muscles to the overlying skin and emphasized the importance of dynamic forces producing skin tension lines, concluding that these insertions pulled skin into folds and wrinkles. Kraissl extended Rubin's findings on the face to the whole body, comparing his lines, drawn perpendicular to the underlying muscles, with Langer's lines. In several places, such as the back and neck, and over joints, these new favorable lines of excision were quite different from those of Langer and Cox. The forehead's wrinkle lines frequently run at angles to Langer's lines.

In 1956 Hutchinson and Koop investigated the lines of cleavage on 50 stillborn infants.[70] In general they were the same as those found by Langer; however, on the scalp there seemed to be no pattern. Also, as Langer and Cox had reported, in a few areas triangular rather than slitlike wounds occurred; in those areas no consistent line occurred.

Borges and Alexander published their concept of relaxed skin-tension lines (RSTLs) in 1962.[12] These lines correspond to the directional pull that exists on skin when the individual is in a state of repose and are influenced by the draping effect of skin over bone and cartilage. Thus the relaxed skin-tension lines are formed by the tenting of skin over the framework of the body. These lines are usually but not necessarily the same as the wrinkle lines, creases, or folds of the body that are related to the underlying muscles. The authors suggest that fusiform excisions should parallel these RSTLs if possible.

In 1980 Stegman published an extremely important and interesting study.[132] He recorded the direction and shape of facial wounds created with a cutaneous punch followed by undermining. His findings showed that although many of the circular holes become elliptic in the direction of the wrinkle lines, in many cases either an ellipse did not form and the round hole remained a round hole, or the direction of the ellipse was contrary to the proposed favorable excision lines of other studies.[29,77] For instance, on the forehead

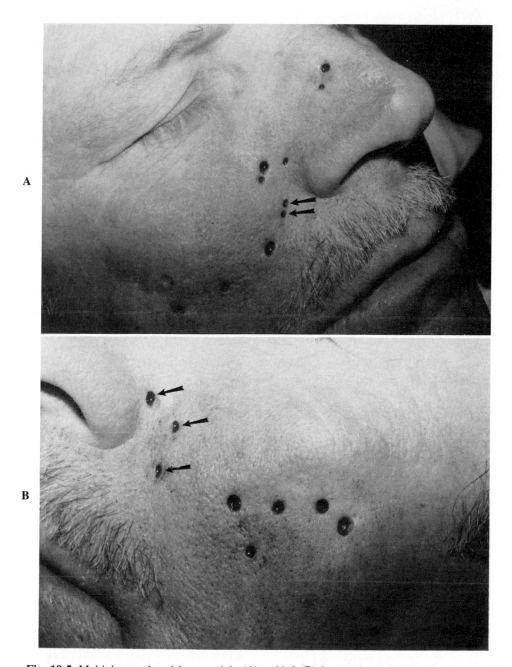

Fig. 10-5. Multiple round excisions on right **(A)** and left **(B)** face performed with cutaneous punch. Note that some of round excisions have oriented themselves into elliptic configurations *(arrows)* being pulled by MaxSTLs.

several ellipses were directed vertically rather than horizontally along wrinkle lines. On the nose, round holes remained round holes, indicating perhaps that the skin tension was the same in all directions.

The findings of Stegman are further supported by Bulacio-Nuñez,[19] who also observed the presence or absence of elliptic configurations subsequent to round excisions on the skin. Unlike Stegman, however, Bulacio-Nuñez did not undermine in all directions; nevertheless, he found that on the scalp, nose, malar eminences, and anterior

chest that the force of tension seemed to be as great in one direction as another. This is similar to Stegman's findings and my own clinical observations.

In the patient shown in Fig. 10-5, numerous round incisions were made in the skin of the face with 3 and 4 mm punches, planned as recipient sites for punch grafts. As can be seen *(arrows),* some of the round holes became elliptic with their axis in the direction of the maximal skin tension lines (MaxSTLs), discussed later; however, some of the circular defects remained as circular defects. Undermining

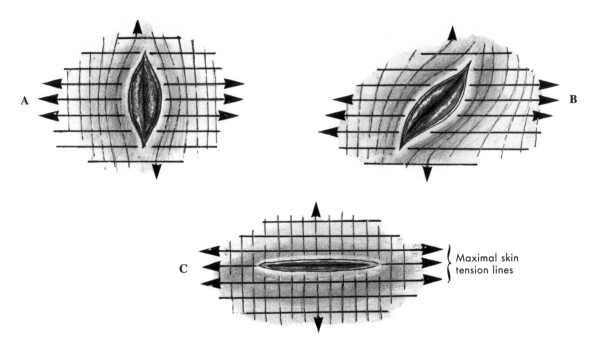

Fig. 10-6. Incisions in the skin that are, **A,** perpendicular, **B,** oblique, and **C,** parallel to MaxSTLs. Note that incision spreads most in **A** and least in **C**. Therefore least tension is on wound edges in **C**.

was not performed around any of the circular holes, but if it had been, some of the circular defects might have been converted to elliptic configurations and some would have remained circular. These findings are similar to those found by Stegman.[132]

In summary, a number of investigators have by various means attempted to determine the most favorable lines for cutaneous excisions. Although there is agreement in most areas of the body, differences of opinion still exist. Probably wrinkle lines (both with muscle contraction and in relaxation), crease lines, contours, and the direction of underlying muscle groups all contribute to the most favorable lines for excision.

Significance of lines of tension

The MaxSTLs are imaginary lines along which maximal forces are generated by the skin in conjunction with the underlying muscle groups. Practical experience has shown that excisions made parallel to the MaxSTLs heal with minimal problems and produce scars with little spreading. Additionally, such scars are stronger, as reflected in tensile strength measurements.[13] Such scars lie along lines of higher tension than those placed perpendicular to the MaxSTLs. Excisions placed in other directions will probably result in more noticeable scars, regardless of the amount of suturing performed to bring the wound edges together. Therefore the relationship that an excision line bears to the MaxSTLs is more important than any other single factor in the production of a fine linear scar.

In all areas of the body these skin tension lines exist like a network in every direction, but the strength of this network is almost always greatest in one direction (the MaxSTL) (Fig. 10-6). Tension lines in the skin are probably the result of functional adaptation during development, since the skin is continually stretched and pulled in one direction more than another by the underlying muscles. The collagen and elastic fibers come to be aligned in the direction of the stretch. This is not surprising: Weiss demonstrated that connective tissue cells grown on culture orient themselves along lines of tension.[145]

There are probably three main factors that generate the MaxSTLs: the orientation of the collagen fibers; the orientation of the underlying muscle groups; and the orientation of the fibrous bands between the muscle groups and the overlying skin.[28] Moreover, joint mobility, presence or absence of elastic fibers, and gravity also probably contribute to the tension forces.

Collagen fibers and their orientation are important determinants of maximal and minimal skin-tension lines. Cox[29] and Langer[79] excised skin and found that it maintained its cleavage line pattern; they therefore concluded that the maintenance of the skin lines was largely intrinsic. Perhaps even more suggestive of the large influence of collagen fibers is the fact that microscopic sections cut parallel to the cleavage lines show a parallel arrangement of collagen fibers, whereas those cut perpendicular to the cleavage lines show collagen bundles cut transversely. Thus the cleavage lines are really a reflection of the layout of collagen fibers. This pattern of collagen fiber orientation was also demonstrated by x-ray diffraction, which showed that the orientation of the majority of collagen fibers was parallel to the crease lines and thus perpendicular to the underlying muscles.[64] Since the collagen fibers are more randomly oriented perpendicular to the MaxSTLs, pulling on the skin in that direction allows for greater stretch, whereas the collagen fibers are already stretched to some degree along the MaxSTLs. Pulling in that direction is not as easy because the collagen fibers are already stretched.[16]

Investigators have also studied the pattern of collagen fibers by light and scanning electron microscopy.[50] In deference to the previous studies, these investigators found that in relaxed skin the dermal fibers were randomly oriented and aligned themselves in parallel array only when the skin was stretched. Perhaps these differences between investigators can be explained by the differences in the anatomic locations examined.

The underlying muscles and their insertions into the skin are also important determinants of skin-tension lines. Kraissl demonstrated microscopically the anatomic connections (fibrous bands) between the skin and the underlying muscles[77] (see Fig. 2-2). Thus the MaxSTLs were related to the pull of the underlying muscles and could not be considered to exist in isolation in the skin. In general these bands to the skin run in lines perpendicular to the underlying muscles. When the muscles contract, the skin is thrown into accordion like folds or wrinkles.

When skin is incised, it separates (Fig. 10-6). If the incision is parallel to the MaxSTLs, the gap in the wound is minimal (Fig. 10-6, *C*). If the incision is perpendicular to these lines of tension, the gap is maximal[29,80] (Fig. 10-6, *A*). Incisions cut obliquely to the MaxSTLs retract an amount in between (Fig. 10-6, *B*). Thus incisions are easier to bring together if parallel to the MaxSTLs.

If wounds are produced and then allowed to contract, the maximal contraction occurs in the direction of minimal resistance, parallel to the lines of minimal skin tension (MinSTLs).[142] The MinSTLs are perpendicular to the MaxSTLs. In an experiment by Catty[22] 1 cm × 1 cm wounds were produced on the arms of young men. Contraction occurred with healing, producing linear wounds running transversely on the arm, and perpendicular to the underlying muscles. This seems to support the work of Kraissl,[77] in contrast to Langer,[79] who thought the greatest forces of tension on the arm to be longitudinal. Thus maximal wound contraction occurred perpendicular to the MaxSTLs. We have also seen similar examples of such contraction in Chapter 2, which produced scars with the long axis oriented along the MaxSTLs (see Fig. 2-15 and 2-16).

The forces of tension have been measured parallel and perpendicular to Langer's lines on the trunk.[117] Excised human skin was found to be one third weaker at right angles to Langer's lines than along them. It should be emphasized that these values were calculated only for skin on the trunk and probably would show a much greater difference in certain areas of the face. Langer himself performed similar studies on excised skin from the trunk and extremities and obtained similar results.[81]

A study on the extensibility of human skin on the chest in vivo found that it was most extensible perpendicular to Langer's lines (MaxSTLs).[51] Orienting excisions along MaxSTLs results in being able to close the resultant wounds more easily, because the wound edges (not the apices) are perpendicular to the MinSTLs.

As an interesting observation, striae on the abdomen of a pregnant woman or patients with Cushing's disease (see Fig. 2-5) run *perpendicular* to Langer's lines. This may be explained by the fact that the collagen fibers rupture first at certain points along the MaxSTLs (Langer's lines), producing a line of their own perpendicular to Langer's lines.

Collagen fibers in scars orient themselves along the long axis of the scar, regardless of the orientation of the scar to the MaxSTLs.[64,96] Therefore scars that are oriented along the MaxSTLs have their collagen fibers oriented in the same direction as most of the surrounding collagen and thus conform to the normal architecture of the skin. This results in scars that have great tensile strengths[151] and show little tendency to spread.[153] Furthermore, there is little tendency for such scars to contract because of the great forces at each end. On the other hand, scars oriented perpendicular to the MaxSTLs show maximal contraction, since they have less resistance to contraction. Hypetrophic scars may then result.

Clinical experience has shown that wounds heal better with more inconspicuous scars when incisions are made parallel to the MaxSTLs.[70] For several years general surgeons have observed that incisions parallel to MaxSTLs on the chest or abdomen were flat and spread minimally, whereas incisions perpendicular to MaxSTLs were frequently hypertrophic or spread maximally.[26] Moreover, in children wounds at right angles to the lines of cleavage tend to ''grow'' in length out of proportion to the growth of the body.[70]

An important study measured the skin tension forces required to approximate the skin edges of human cutaneous wounds on the chest.[153] These forces were correlated with the direction of the wounds with respect to the MaxSTLs. In general the more the wound differed in direction from the local MaxSTLs, the greater was the force required for approximation, and the greater was the width of the scar at 1 year.

Determining the maximal skin tension lines

In planning an excision one must carefully consider and choose the orientation of the incision lines. Composite drawings of MaxSTLs may serve as a useful guide or reference (Fig. 10-7); however, no composite drawing can uni-

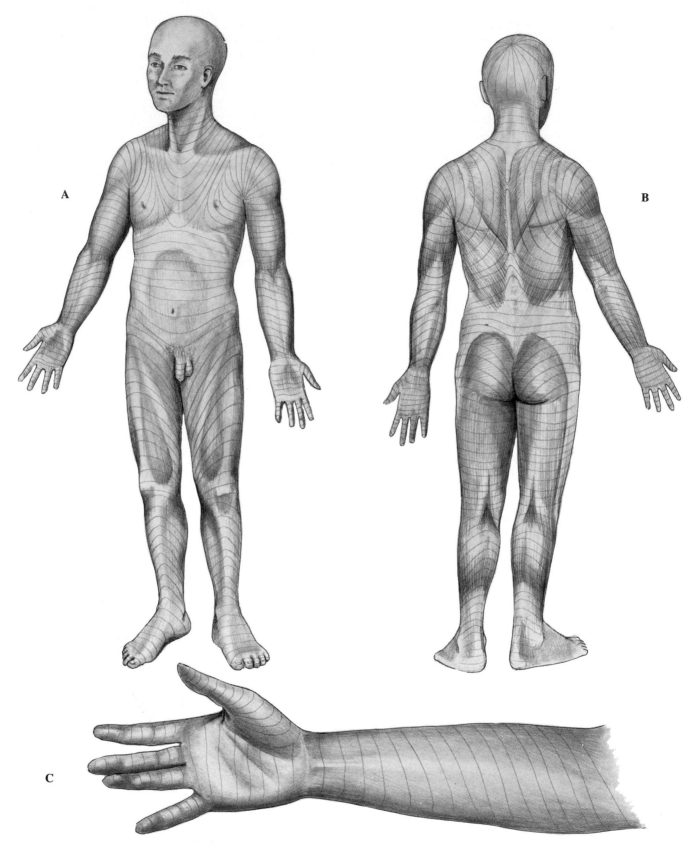

Fig. 10-7. MaxSTLs for trunk and extremities. **A,** Anterior view. **B,** Posterior view. **C,** Ventral forearm and palm. Note generally perpendicular alignment to underlying muscles.

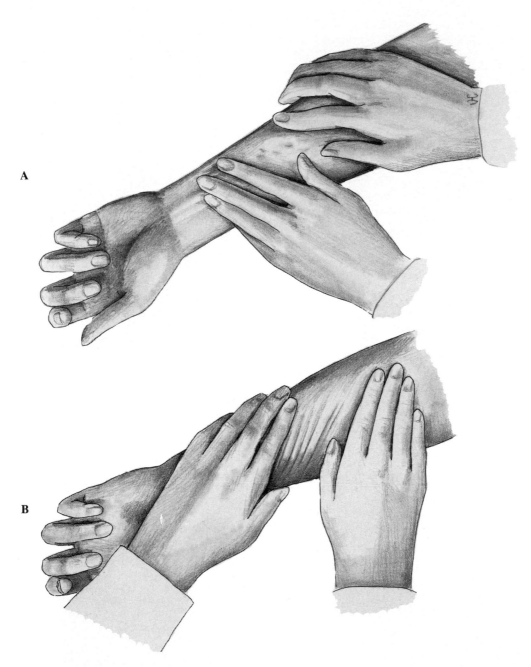

Fig. 10-8. Compression of skin on forearm, **A,** along MaxSTLs, which produces minimal wrinkling, and **B,** along MinSTLs, which produces maximal wrinkling.

versally predict the skin-tension lines in all individuals.

On the trunk and extremities, since wrinkles do not usually exist, it is best to determine the skin-tension lines by compressing the skin (Fig. 10-8). Compressing the skin in the direction of the force of minimal tension results in ready wrinkling (Fig. 10-8, *B*), whereas if one compresses the skin in the direction of the maximal forces of tension, few wrinkles appear (Fig. 10-8, *A*). On the extremities the maximal lines of tension are in general circumferential. On the trunk, particularly the upper back above the scapula, the maximal lines of tension are very difficult to determine,

since the forces of tension may be almost equal in all areas in this location.

The face and neck are different from other areas of the body in that their wrinkles and skin folds appear and deepen with age. These wrinkle lines are generally the visible expression of the MaxSTLs. Incisions on the face in general should follow the wrinkle or crease lines that run perpendicular to the underlying muscles; they may be readily apparent, especially in the elderly. Having the patient grimace, smile, whistle, or make other facial expressions exaggerates wrinkle lines, making them more apparent[26] (Fig. 10-9).

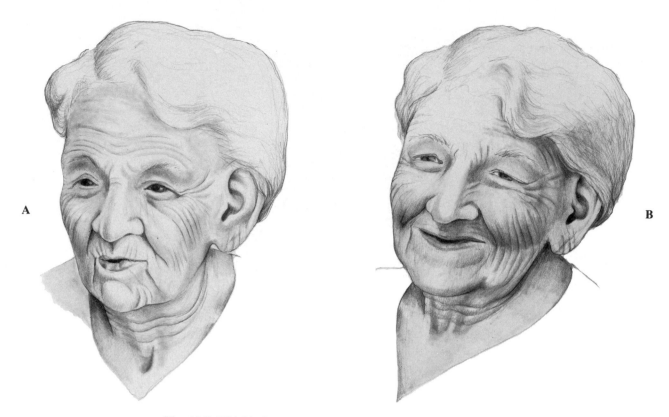

Fig. 10-9. Wrinkle lines of face with **A,** whistling, and, **B,** smiling.

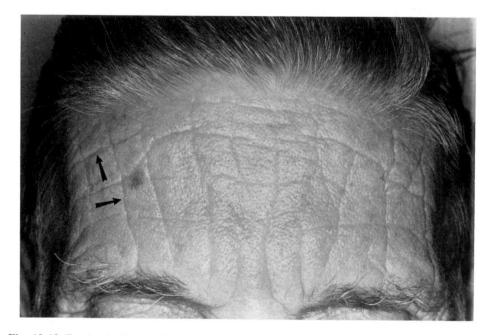

Fig. 10-10. Forehead of man with extremely sun-damaged skin. Note primary crease lines *(vertical arrow)* and secondary crease lines *(horizontal arrow)*.

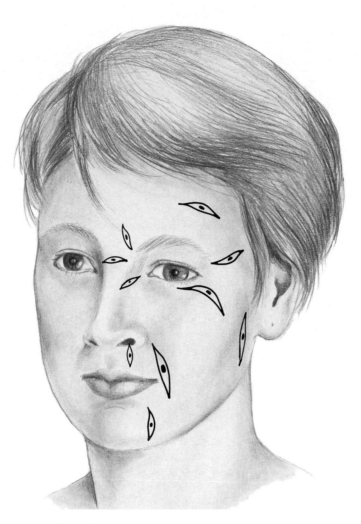

Fig. 10-11. Suggested lines for excisions on face.

This maneuver is quite important in the young, where wrinkle and creases are not seen on relaxation but become apparent on contraction of the muscles.

Excisions made parallel to or in wrinkle lines result in scars with several advantages. The scars may be mistaken for crease lines. In addition, since they are also parallel to the MaxSTLs, such scars are thinner, heal more quickly and result in higher tensile strength.

On the forehead the transverse wrinkle lines are caused by the contraction of the frontalis muscle. The melolabial fold is caused by the pull from the zygomaticus and quadratus labii superioris muscles. Several of the more important skin creases and lines of the face are shown in Fig. 3-2.

Although it is frequently taught that the wrinkle line invariably lies perpendicular to the underlying muscles,[7] this is not always the case. For instance, the wrinkle lines of the eyelids are parallel to the underlying muscles, and on the upper lip the underlying muscles run in two directions perpendicular to each other (see Fig. 3-15).

Sometimes in extremely sun-damaged individuals, secondary crease lines appear, running at right angles to the primary crease lines (Fig. 10-10). They usually appear on the forehead or on the malar prominence of the cheeks. They should not be used in planning excisions, since they are perpendicular rather than parallel to the maximal skin-tension lines.

An illustration of several suggested lines for excisions on the face is shown in Fig. 10-11. The axes of these excisions in general parallel the wrinkle lines previously shown (Fig. 10-9) in a more aged individual. Note that some of the excisions are gently curved so as to fit in with the natural curves of the face. This ultimately helps to make the resultant scars less noticeable.

It has been suggested that if unsure of the most favorable line of excision, one may excise the lesion using a circular incision and then after undermining in all directions, the long axis of the excision becomes apparent as the circle is pulled into an ellipse by the surrounding MaxSTLs.[33,130] If there is no ellipse, one may also use skin hooks to pull the edges of the wound together to determine the direction of minimal or maximal tension. Proponents of this technique feel that less tissue is sacrificed when the dog ears are

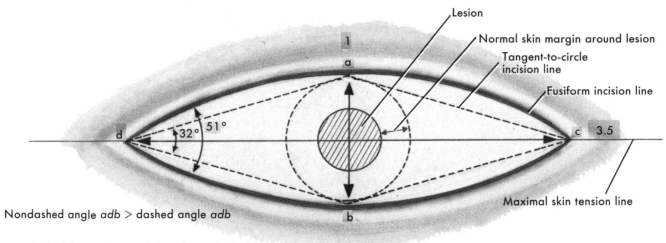

Nondashed angle *adb* > dashed angle *adb*

Nondashed (curved incision) line *dac* > dashed line *dac*

Fig. 10-12. Proper method of determining incision lines for excision.

subsequently removed than if a larger excision is done. Moreover, the orientation of the excision is more favorable than if determined by guesswork or an idealized illustration.

It should be appreciated, however, that there are certain areas where a circular excision cannot be easily pulled into an ellipse. In these areas the lines of tension radiate equally in all directions rather than course in a straight line. Langer,[79] Cox,[29] and Hutchinson and Koop[70] describe these areas as triangular and stated that the skin tension lines there were nonpatterned. As previously mentioned, the main regions for the location of these triangular areas are over the scapula, the anterior chest, and the lateral malar prominence of the face.

Size and shape of excision

Having selected the direction of an excision, one should draw the pattern of excision on the patient. The most favorable pattern (tangent-to-circle) is constructed in the following steps:

1. Draw the outer border of the margin on all sides of the lesion. A benign lesion's normal skin margin is not much larger than the lesion itself. A malignant lesion's normal skin margin may be 0.5 cm or more beyond the perimeter of the clinical lesion. This is shown as the outer circle in Fig. 10-12.
2. One then draws straight-line *(ac, bc, ad, bd)* tangents from the borders of the circular excision defect to intersect (points *d* and *c*) on the MaxSTL *(cd)*, which bisects the lesion itself. The points of intersection of the tangents are at a distance so that the length-to-width ratio of excision is 3:1 or 4:1. The ratio shown is 3.5:1. The angle between two tangents at the apex should be about 30 degrees.

Planning excisions in this manner reduces the likelihood of tissue distortion and dog ear formation.

Fig. 10-12 compares the tangent-to-circle incision lines *(dashed lines)* with those of a more standard fusiform excision *(nondashed lines)* between points *a, c, b,* and *d.* If one looks carefully, one can see there are two important differences between these two configurations. First, the straight-line tangents are shorter than the curved lines of the elliptic excision. Since the shorter arms of the tangents more closely approximate the length of the final incision line *(dc),* there is less lateral tissue distortion on closure.

The second major difference between the tangent-to-circle configuration and the elliptic excision is the angle formed at the apex. In the example shown, the angle at which the two tangents meet is smaller (32 degrees) than the angle formed by the nondashed lines of the elliptic excision (51 degrees). The smaller the angle formed between the sides of an excision, the less rotation of tissue occurs, and thus less tissue distortion takes place.[119]

A comparison between an ellipsoidal, a lenticular or fusiform, and a tangent-to-circle excision is shown in Fig. 10-13, *A.* The ellipse has rounded ends and is mathematically based on the parabola. Obviously this is not useful in excisional surgery. Circular skin punches in the skin may assume this shape. The lenticular shape has slightly curved sides and comes to a point at each end. Lenticular (from the Latin *lenticula,* meaning lentil) refers to the cross-sectional shape of a biconvex lens; it is also described as spindle shaped, or fusiform (from the Latin *fusus,* meaning spindle).[11,72] As seen in Fig. 10-13, *B,* the longer the length of a fusiform excision, the straighter are its sides, and the more it approximates the tangent-to-circle excision shape. Therefore fusiform excisions with almost straight sides are fairly good approximations to the tangent-to-circle shape.

The tangent-to-circle excision most closely resembles a parallelogram with all sides equal. A parallelogram is a plane geometric figure in which the opposite sides are parallel and equal. In Fig. 10-13, *A,* all sides of the tangent-to-circle excision are of equal length. However, since the midpoints of the sides of the excision (points *a* and *b* in Fig. 10-12) may not form angles but rather rounded edges, technically the configuration is not a parallelogram.

One may also construct a closure in which the tangents on one side intersect the axis at a farther point than the tangents on the opposite side do (Fig. 10-14). In this situation two tangents on one side are equal in length but differ in length from the tangents on the opposite side *(ad = bd ≠ ac = cb).* Since the angle between the two tangents farther from the midpoint of the excision (angle *acb*) is smaller, the possibility of dog-ears is less on that side. Alternatively, the two tangents on the opposite side meet with a greater angle (angle *adb*). This makes dog-ears more likely at this location, other factors being equal. The triangle *(abd)* closing the right side of the excision in Fig. 10-14 is sometimes called Ammon's triangle. This triangle is almost equilateral; its value is that it may be used to modify for closure one end of a triangular wound such as *acb* or either end of a rectangular wound.[11]

Constructions such as Fig. 10-14 are made when one knows that dog-ears are less likely on one side than another because of a different tissue tension. By making the tangents smaller on one side, less tissue is sacrificed. Such constructions can be made retrospectively where circular defects are pulled together and the dog-ears repaired at each end. The amount of tissue removed is frequently unequal because the tissue tension differs on both sides (Fig. 10-70, *B*).

The recommended proportion between length and width of a standard fusiform excision is 3:1 or 4:1. This is based on clinical experience but has been substantiated mathematically in two dimensions by both tension-field theory[32] and finite element analysis.[34] When one grasps the skin on

A

Tangent-to-circle

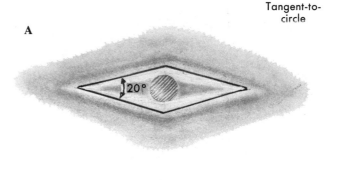

Fusiform

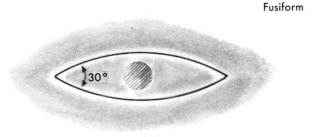

Elliptic

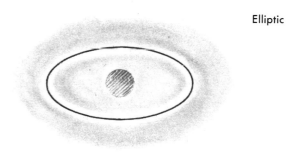

B

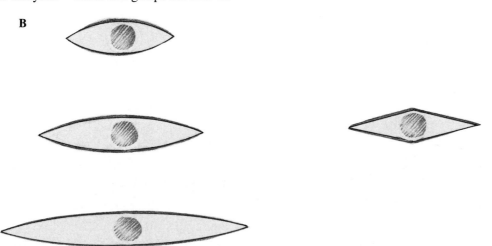

Fig. 10-13. A, Comparison between elliptic, fusiform (or lenticular), and tangent-to-circle excision. **B,** Increase in length of sides of fusiform excision *(left)* effectively results in straighter sides and smaller angles at apices, the approximating a tangent-to-circle excision *(right).*

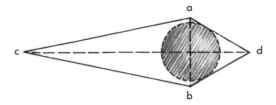

Fig. 10-14. Tangent-to-circle excision with unequal opposite tangents.

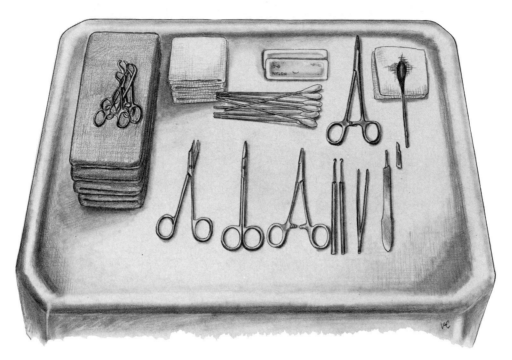

Fig. 10-15. Sterile tray. On bottom row from right to left are No. 15 blade, scalpel handle, Adson serrated forceps, two skin hooks, hemostat, iris scissors, and Stevens tenotomy scissors. On top row are prepackaged antibacterial skin swab, needle holder, suture material, numerous cotton-tipped applicators, gauze, and muslin towels for draping with towel clips. Local anesthetics may also be included in sterile tray but are frequently given before skin preparation and draping.

the back of the hand, rays of tension may be seen radiating from the pinched skin. The summation of forces from these rays may be shown to approach a minimal value when the length-to-width ratio of an excision is 3:1 to 4:1.

Other factors to consider in planning excisions

Structures of cosmetic or functional importance need to be considered in planning excisions. Eyebrows, eyelids, lips, nose, ears, and hairlines are all important boundaries to attempt to preserve. Excisions involving these structures may represent special situations; these are dealt with separately later.

On occasion, to perform an adequate excision, the surgeon may need to create an excision with a long axis that does not parallel the MaxSTLs. In this circumstance it may be wisest simply to suture the defect rather than to create a more complicated closure. Under other circumstances, it may be preferable to redirect the lines of the excision. If the excision is small, usually redirection of the lines is easily accomplished.

The fusiform and tangent-to-circle excisions are the simplest and most basic methods of surgically excising skin lesions. As a general rule it is wisest to make the simplest possible excision; therefore all skin lesions should be excised with these patterns if possible.

STERILE TRAY

A sterile tray with the instruments commonly used for excisonal surgery is shown in Fig. 10-15. A Mayo stand on which the sterile tray may be placed is standard equipment. As an alternative to the Mayo stand, holding drapes are available; they can be draped on the patient, and instruments adhere to them without falling to the floor (Insta-Hold Nonmagnetic Reusable Surgical Instrument Holding Drape,

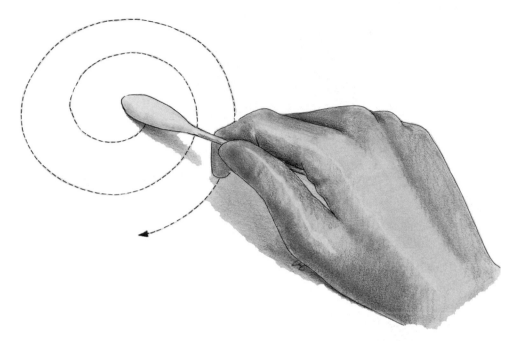

Fig. 10-16. Proper method for preoperative preparation of surgical site.

distributed by McGhan Medical, Santa Barbara, CA, 93111). Instruments should not be left to lie free on the patient's body. Local anesthetics (not shown) may also be included on the standing sterile tray; however, they are frequently administered separately.

The sterile tray should be covered with a sterile towel until ready to be used, to keep the instruments as sterile as possible. Exposed instruments may also be a bit unnerving to anxious patients; inconspicuous equipment helps to make them feel less apprehensive.

PATIENT AND PHYSICIAN PREPARATION

The physician should wash his or her hands and wear sterile gloves. Masks are not required for cutaneous surgery. Special gowns for physicians or patients are also optional.

The operative site should be cleansed first with a detergent to rid the area of dirt and then with an antiseptic solution such as chlorhexidine gluconate (Hibiclens) or povidone-iodine (Betadine). Alcoholic solutions should not be used when use of electrocoagulation is contemplated. The sparks may ignite such solutions to cause a fire that may burn a patient.[42]

There are no data relating the length of time of scrubbing the cutaneous surfaces to subsequent wound infection for removal of superficial cutaneous lesions. Probably scrubbing from 1 to 3 minutes is adequate. Much of the information available on skin preparation is presented in Chapter 4. One basically desires to reduce the skin flora to a minimum so that postsurgical infections are less likely.

The proper method to prepare an area surgically is shown in Fig. 10-16. The suggested motion is centrifugal from the center of the wound toward the periphery. This prevents dragging organisms from the dirty area to the clean area. Avoid back-and-forth motions while cleaning the area. A firm rubbing action is essential because the physical abrasion by itself helps to reduce bacteria. One should extend the cleansing well beyond the operative site. With contaminated wounds draining pus, one should cleanse in the opposite direction—from the surrounding skin into the wound; otherwise one theoretically will contaminate the surrounding skin.

Convenient prepackaged applicators or pads with either detergent or antibacterial solutions are available. They are better to use than stock solutions of antibacterials, which may become contaminated with pathogenic microorganisms.

If hair may interfere with the surgery, shaving is optional. If there is an immediate cosmetic benefit to not shaving, the patient can safely be left unshaved. Shaving induces small knicks in the skin, which may become havens for bacterial proliferation, and wound infection may result. If the patient is shaved, it should be done just before scrubbing the skin with an antibacterial agent. If the hair is not shaved, it may still be necessary to get the hair out of the way during surgery. This can be done in a number of ways. My usual method is simply to use paper adhesive tape; other methods to consider are bobby pins or hair clips, rubber bands, hair nets, or an ointment. The latter has the marked disadvantage of being messy. Eyebrow hair should not be shaved or clipped because this hair takes 6 to 12 months to regrow, and the cosmetic deficit is readily apparent.

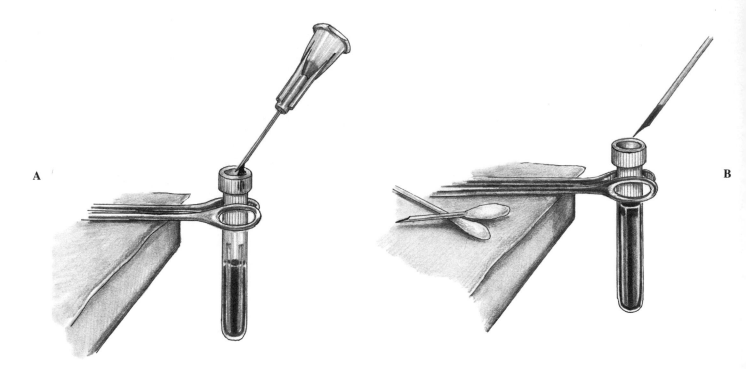

Fig. 10-17. "Ink well" for sterile tray. **A,** Use of syringe to place marking solution into plastic needle-cover. **B,** Use of broken cotton-tipped applicator as stylus.

MARKING INCISIONS

It is frequently advantageous to mark the planned excision on the skin after scrubbing but directly before infiltration of an anesthetic, since the anesthetic may distort the tissue. Also, marking is best performed before draping so the appropriate landmarks and skin-tension lines can be visualized and appreciated. For marking the skin one should use a marker that is readily washable: either gentian violet or Bonney's blue may be used. (The latter is a mixture of gentian violet and malachite green mixed in water and alcohol.[73]) Another possible marker is Berwick marker, also a mixture of malachite green and gentian violet but in alcohol only.[133] On a sterile tray one may create an "ink well" by use of a syringe plastic needle-cover and sponge forceps, as shown in Fig. 10-17. The marking solution is introduced into the plastic needle-cover *(A)*. Cotton-tipped applicators with wooden handles are broken to form sharp points *(B)*. To break an applicator one must hold it *at each end*. Another alternative for marking the skin is disposable skin marking pens, which are packaged sterile and contain gentian violet. Although they are convenient, the cost is somewhat high.

Some physicians suggest marking not only the lines of incision but perpendicular lines across the wound to orient the surgeon to the points of apposition later. I have not in general found this to be helpful; this practice may even become a problem if the perpendicular lines are not drawn precisely.

ANESTHESIA

The injection and use of various anesthetic agents is covered in Chapter 6, so it is not covered here. For particularly anxious patients the radios with stereo headphones are relaxing and are highly recommended. The most important person present at the operation is the patient, and every possible step should be taken to make the experience as pleasant as possible.[97]

DRAPING

Once cleansed and anesthetized, the operative site may be draped. Draping serves to protect the operative site from bacteria and keep the field of surgery as aseptic as possible. The draping also helps to keep the suture and instruments from becoming contaminated. Moreover, draping helps to make the patient feel detached from the wound, which may be important for anxious individuals.

Two types of drapes are available for cutaneous surgery: disposable and nondisposable. There are many disposable drapes on the market; some of them are compared in Table 10-3. Some drapes have apertures in the center, some adhesive backing, and some are translucent. Disposable drapes have replaced cloth drapes in cutaneous surgery to a large extent for several reasons. Disposable drapes are convenient, are less expensive, present fewer problems with lint, and are more impermeable to blood, fluid, and bacteria than cloth drapes are.

TABLE 10-3

Disposable drapes for cutaneous surgery

Name	Manufacturer	Size (inches)	Fenestration (diameter in inches)	Translucent	Self-adhesive	Material
American Aperture Drape	American Hospital Supply	16 × 16	2	Yes	Yes	Polyethylene
Barrier	Johnson and Johnson	17 × 27	3	No	No	Cellulose/polyethylene/cellulose*
Converters Fenestrated Towel	American Converters	18 × 26	2½	No	No	Two layers 100% cellulose thermally laminated with low-density polyplastic
Steri-Drape (aperture drape)	3M	15⅝ × 15⅝	2¼	Yes	Yes	Polyethylene
Steri-Drape (minor procedure)	3M	22⅜ × 25⅞	2⅜	No	Yes	Rayon/polyethylene/rayon*

*Three layers.

Disposable drapes do have a few drawbacks. Drapes with small round apertures cause one to lose perspective on the relationship of the wound to surrounding structures and the MaxSTL. Some plastic drapes tend to get hot under lighting that produces heat. Plastic drapes also tend to allow blood to flow over the drape instead of absorbing the blood.

Some disposable drapes are still a fire hazard despite manufacturing standards regarding impregnation with fire-retardant materials.[106] Fires can occur when nonevaporated alcohol or other inflammable materials are on the wound or drape at the same time that the electrosurgical apparatus is sparking.

When disposable drapes are used over the nose or mouth, patients may feel claustrophobic or suffocated. Some ingenious devices have been invented to lift the drape off the patient's face,[139] but they are probably unnecessary. An adjustment of the draping is usually sufficient to alleviate any feelings of suffocation.

Nondisposable drapes are usually cloth muslin drapes, which are also acceptable and offer a number of advantages. They may be folded and placed to provide the necessary size of the aperture for surgery. The absorbency of muslin is greater than that of prepackaged drapes. Also, muslin drapes can be situated in such a way as to prevent the patient from feeling uncomfortable or suffocated. The disadvantage of muslin drapes is that they are a less effective barrier to bacteria than paper or plastic drapes.[5,48] When wet, cloth drapes tend to act like a wick, drawing bacteria toward the wound. Towel clips must be used to hold cloth drapes in place.

INCISION

The method of making incisions is shown in Fig. 10-18. For most skin incisions a No. 15 scalpel blade is preferred. The scalpel is held like a pencil, and the skin is slightly stretched by the opposite hand as one incises. Only gentle tension should be placed on the skin by the non–scalpel bearing hand, lest undue distortion occur. The hand with the scalpel is stabilized and braced by placing the fifth finger on the patient. Therefore 2- or 3-point traction is produced by use of both hands.[148] This tension and countertension immobilize the skin as the incision is made and help the surgeon to control more accurately the direction and depth of the scalpel blade. Tissue must be placed under some tension to be incised with precision. This produces clean, sharp, straight edges and prevents production of beveled edges.

As the blade is gently placed on stretched skin, the tissues can be divided a millimeter at a time. In contrast to this, when one cuts lax tissue with a scalpel, the scalpel itself creates tension, pushing rather than cutting through the tissues. This does not allow for fine dissection.[75]

The incision begins at one end of the proposed excision and is curled toward the physician. One should not cut tissue by pushing the scalpel blade away from one's center of gravity; this results in less control over the direction of the blade and may cause inadvertent cuts in the tissue. To begin the incision, one need cut only lightly at first; then as one continues the incision, the blade is pressed harder into the skin. The depth of penetration should be appropriate for the type of lesion being excised. It should also be uniform along the incision's length. Thus a certain touch needs to be

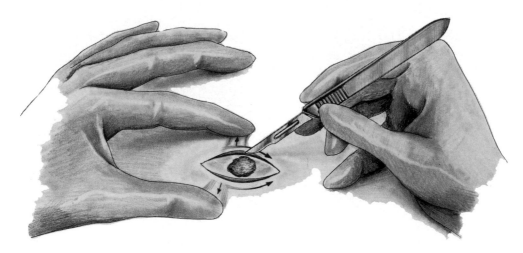

Fig. 10-18. Making incisions with three-point traction.

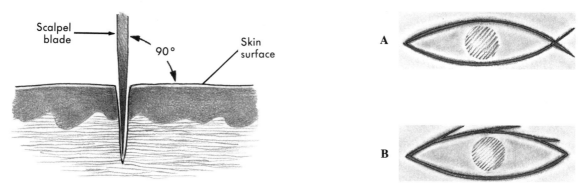

Fig. 10-19. Scalpel blade is oriented perpendicular (90 degrees) to plane of skin surface.

Fig. 10-20. Unnecessary incisions at time of excision. **A,** "Fishtailing." **B,** Nicked edges.

developed to gauge the depth of the blade's penetration. This incision-making method is emphasized by Zoltan.[156]

Borges recommends that for fusiform excisions the middle segments of the lateral sides should be incised first and the apices last.[11] Although I have not personally used this technique, it does emphasize the concentrated, gentle motions that should be employed for incision.

Some physicians feel that one should begin the incision with the tip of the scalpel blade at the apex.[133] I do not think this is necessary. The scalpel blade tip is not as sharp as the scalpel blade belly, so one gets a cleaner, less traumatic cut without using the tip.

One should hold the blade belly at a 90-degree angle to the skin surface (Fig. 10-19). This ensures the shortest incision through tissue and wound edges, which are approximated with minimal surface distortion. The natural tendency is to slant or bevel the blade toward the center of the lesion rather than hold it perpendicular to the skin; neophytes in surgery frequently make this mistake.

One exception to the advisability of holding the blade perpendicular to the skin is in a hair-bearing area, where the blade may be angled obliquely to avoid cutting the hair follicles, which are oriented obliquely to the skin surface. Thus one cuts parallel to the hair shafts. If one cuts perpendicular to the skin in hair-bearing areas, one transects hair follicles and causes a loss of hair for a variable distance around the scar that is ultimately produced. This alopecia is apt to be cosmetically unacceptable. Cutting parallel to the obliquely angled hair shafts is particularly important in locations such as the eyebrow, where the loss of hair cannot be covered over by surrounding hair, as is possible in the scalp.

When beginning or ending the incision, avoid carelessly extending the incisions, or "fish-tailing" (Fig. 10-20, *A*). Also avoid nicking the lateral skin edges (Fig. 10-20, *B*). A clinical example of such a nick is shown in Fig. 10-81, *B*. These needless incisions are best prevented by *concentration* during surgery.

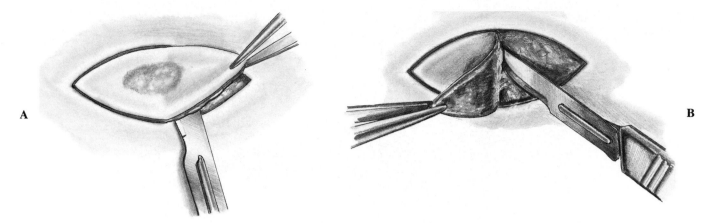

Fig. 10-21. Undercutting tissue. If tissue is pulled over scalpel blade **(A)**, tissue is cut in less depth than if tissue is pulled away from scalpel blade **(B).**

EXCISION

Once the proper incisions are made, one grasps the tissue at one end, usually with pickups but a skin hook may also be used if one wishes not to damage the tissue. The scalpel blade is then used to undercut the tissue in a back-and-forth motion. A scissors may also be used to cut tissue. It is best to use either the Stevens tenotomy scissors or the Gradle scissors for this purpose. Iris scissors tend not to have enough fulcrum power for tissue cutting and thus may cause tissue damage.

If the tissue is brought *over* the scalpel blade as one undercuts (Figs. 10-21, *A,* and 10-78, *B*), the blade does not cut as deeply as if the tissue is pulled away from the blade (Fig. 10-21, *B*). As the blade sweeps from side to side, one should keep from nicking the edges of the tissue and producing slashes (Fig. 10-20, *B*).

After removal of a fusiform piece of tissue, as in Fig. 10-21, *A,* there is frequently more fat or dermis left at either end, so that the base of the wound is not uniformly deep. As much tissue should be removed at the ends as at the center. Fleury emphasizes removal of this excessive tissue so as to make the wound the same depth in all directions.[45]

UNDERMINING
Purposes

On completion of an adequate excision, it is usually a good idea to undermine the surrounding area. The main reason for undermining is to take tension off the wound edges, both laterally and vertically, when the subsequent closure is complete. In areas at which the tension is not great or the wound is small, undermining might not be necessary.

Returning to basic anatomy, one remembers that there are numerous fibrous bands running between the underlying muscles and the overlying skin (see Fig. 2-2). Removal of the majority of these bands surrounding excision sites frequently helps to release the vertical and lateral tension forces on the wound edges and underlying tissue. That these tension forces are related to the subdermal fibrous bands of tissue can be seen experimentally.[33,132] If one produces a round surgical defect and then undermines in all directions, the round defect may be converted into an elliptic defect, since one has removed the tissue bands maintaining the circular shape.

Undermining also helps to restore the skin surface contour on wound closure. If the excision is particularly deep, mobilization of the surrounding tissue helps to fill out what would otherwise be a gap in the tissue under a sutured overlying epidermis. With tension taken off the surrounding subepidermal tissues, careful coaptation of the wound edges with layer-by-layer approximation can be obtained. This results in a stronger wound and less tendency for inversion of wound edges.

Undermining also adds strength to the wound by another mechanism. The general concept that all scars contract is used to advantage in undermining wounds. Scar tissue forms during wound healing in the plane of undermining. It contracts, tending to hold the wound together (see Fig. 10-34) and minimizing subsequent scar spreading.

The disadvantage of undermining is that tissue relationships are changed in the plane of dissection. Usually this has no significant consequence; however, when a cutaneous malignancy has been removed, the change in tissue planes may be significant if the neoplasm has not been totally removed, because it may be difficult to locate residual tumor extensions. Another disadvantage of undermining is that a new space is created for potential fluid or blood accumulation. When undermining, one must weigh the advantages against the disadvantages.

Method

One method of holding the tissue when undermining is shown in Fig. 10-22. Elevation of the skin by use of a skin hook is an ideal way to hold tissue because traumatic dam-

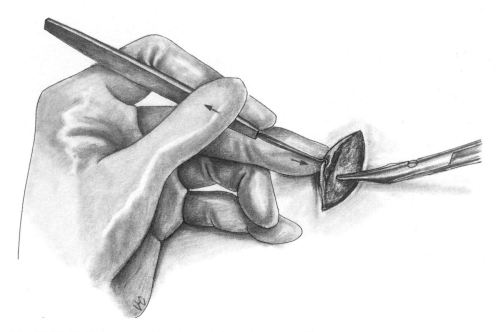

Fig. 10-22. Holding tissue with skin hook for undermining. Note that tissue is draped over middle finger, which in turn is used to push skin forward.

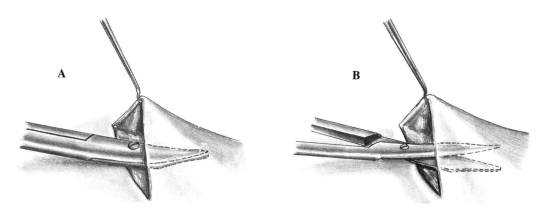

Fig. 10-23. Undermining skin. Scissors should be inserted closed underneath skin (**A**) before they are opened (**B**).

age to cells is minimized.[114,115] The middle finger on the hand holding the skin hook pushes forward underneath the skin that is folded up on the finger, while the skin hook is drawn the opposite way. This tends to stretch the underlying tissues forward (provide countertraction) as they are undermined. Although pickups, such as the Adson forceps, can be used to pick up the wound edges, they tend to cause more tissue damage.

In undermining it is important to use blunt-tipped scissors, such as a tenotomy scissors for small lesions or a Lahey scissors for larger lesions. The use of sharply pointed scissors or scalpel blades is discouraged. Undermining is mainly a technique for pushing underlying attachments free rather than cutting all the attachments completely. It is

necessary on rare occasions to cut some of the attachments, but this is exceptional; one tries to injure as few vascular or neural structures as possible. Severed nerves often do not regenerate,[14] and vascular structures may provide important nutrition to cut wound edges.

As one introduces the scissors under the skin edge, the scissors should be closed (Fig. 10-23, *A*). Only when they are under the tissue to the distance required or when they can go no further should the scissors be opened (Fig. 10-23, *B*). In this manner important structures are not actually cut but rather pushed to the side. In undermining, the overlying skin is pulled over the scissors as the scissors are pushed gently under the skin. This produces traction and countertraction that help to keep the plane of undermining from

```
┌─────────────────────────────────────────────┐
│                                               │
│        SUGGESTED LEVELS OF UNDERMINING        │
│                                               │
│   Scalp          Below hair follicles or below galea
│   Forehead       Low subcutaneous tissue      │
│   Temple         High subcutaneous tissue     │
│   Cheeks, chin   High subcutaneous tissue     │
│   Lips (mucosa)  Beneath mucosa               │
│   Nose           Mid or low subcutaneous tissue
│   Neck           Mid or high subcutaneous tissue
│   Trunk          Any level above muscle fascia│
│   Extremities    Any level above muscle fascia│
│   Hands, feet    Below dermis                 │
│                                               │
└─────────────────────────────────────────────┘
```

going deeper and deeper. This is the same principle shown previously regarding excision of tissue, with which one pulls the tissues over the blade (Fig. 10-21, *A*).

When one begins to undermine, one searches for the plane of separation of tissue. Usually this becomes apparent on the first or second foray with the scissors. This plane is where the tissues above and below easily separate from each other. One tries to keep this same plane of separation on all sides of the excision, so that the depth of undermining is uniform.

Extent of undermining

The question as to how deeply to undermine is not easily answered, since it depends on the depth of the lesion excised, the anatomic site, the ease with which the tissue planes separate, and the potential injury to surrounding structures (see box above). As a general rule, try to undermine in the most superficial layer possible. Most of the time this is somewhere in the superficial fat layer slightly above the deepest part of the excision. Where the skin and subcutaneous tissues are thin, as on the eyelids or dorsum of the hands, one undermines superficially; the subcutaneous tissue is scant, and the dermis lies practically juxtaposed on top of the muscle. In these locations one essentially separates the dermis from the underlying tissue as one undermines. In contrast, where the skin and subcutaneous tissues are thick (such as on the back), one undermines at a deep level in the deepest part of the subcutaneous tissue.

In some locations anatomic peculiarities must be taken into account. On the scalp, where the fibrous bands in the subcutaneous tissue are well developed, it may be very difficult to undermine in this layer. In addition, undermining superficially in the scalp inevitably results in considerable bleeding, since blood vessels are profuse and easily torn. Therefore one may have to go all the way into the subgaleal space to loosen the tissue and may even need to cut the galea from below.

On the face and neck, try to undermine in the superficial subcutaneous tissue for less injury to nerves and blood vessels that tend to run in the deeper subcutaneous tissue in most areas. On the temple one needs to be particularly careful to undermine very superficially (just beneath the dermis), because the temporal branch of the facial nerve runs superficially (above the muscle fascia) in this area (see Fig. 3-18).

On the trunk and extremities undermining can be done in the superficial or deep subcutaneous tissue as required without fear of injuring nerves or blood vessels. Frequently undermining in these areas is done just above muscle fascia.

The lateral extent of undermining is a matter of clinical judgment. Some authorities suggest undermining an area in all directions, equivalent to the size of the defect created.[130] This may or may not be necessary, depending on the tension upon the wound edges. The tension may be checked periodically during undermining by using two skin hooks to draw the wound edges together. Since there is rarely tension on the apices of fusiform or tangent-to-circle excisions, it may be unnecessary to undermine in these areas. The main undermining is under the lateral wound edges. However, it has been suggested that undermining at the apices of the excision helps to reduce the dog-ear phenomenon immediately or helps dog-ears to flatten out with time. This has not been systematically studied, but on the basis of my experience I do not think that undermining has much influence on dog ears. Dog-ears are more often the result of excess tissue.

Sometimes one may wish to undermine only under one lateral wound edge of a fusiform or tangent-to-circle excision rather than under both wound edges. This helps to place the sutured incision line slightly off center, since the tissue is mobilized more in one direction than another. By doing this, one may more easily camouflage the sutured incision line in wrinkle lines, skin creases, or furrows. This technique is of some value in the area between the lateral nose and cheek (the nasofacial angle).

HEMOSTASIS

Blood vessels are inevitably transected or nicked during surgery. Many of these vessels stop bleeding almost immediately as the vessels go into spasm. Continuous bleeding from vessels should be stopped; otherwise blood accumulates in wounds. This results in hematomas that produce tension on wound edges and unnecessary debris.

One method to stop bleeders is to spot coagulate by use of pickups and an electrosurgical apparatus (Fig. 10-24). One should be careful to grasp with the pickups only as much tissue as necessary. A jeweler's forceps or other fine pickup is preferred. The active electrode of the high-frequency electrosurgical apparatus is then touched to the pickups, usually on the lower one-third, which transmits the electrical energy to the tips. It should be emphasized that the area at the tips of the forceps and the immediately adjacent area

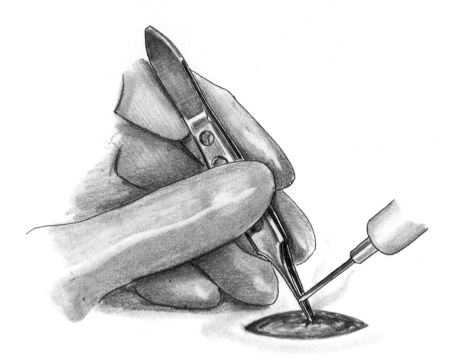

Fig. 10-24. Spot coagulation with forceps and high-frequency electrosurgical apparatus.

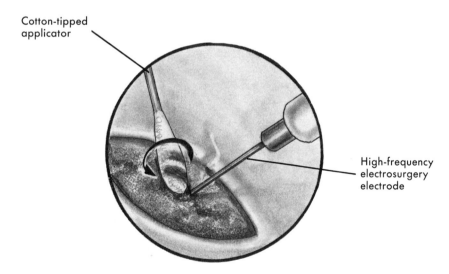

Cotton-tipped
applicator

High-frequency
electrosurgery
electrode

Fig. 10-25. Use of cotton-tipped applicator to soak up blood so as to facilitate use of electrosurgical apparatus.

need to be dry of blood for efficient and adequate coagulation by the electrosurgical apparatus to occur. When the tissue at the tips of the pickup becomes visibly coagulated, it can be released. Specialized ''bipolar'' forceps for coagulation may be purchased, which are attached directly to an electrosurgical apparatus. In my experience they are unnecessary for most cutaneous surgery. They are discussed more fully in Chapter 16.

Another method to stop bleeding is to touch any bleeding areas directly with the active electrode of the high-frequency electrosurgical apparatus. Although fast, this method tends to destroy more tissue than accurate use of pickups with electrocoagulation does. However, by use of cotton-tipped applicators, the bleeding points can be accurately located, and thus the amount of tissue destruction can be minimized (Fig. 10-25). One simply rolls the applicator in the wound until the bleeding point is exposed. The cotton-tipped applicator is ideal for this purpose because it helps soak up the blood near the electrode tip of the electrosurgical apparatus, making coagulation more effective. In addition, the cotton-tipped applicators place gentle focal pressure on a wound and thus stop bleeding with little trauma.

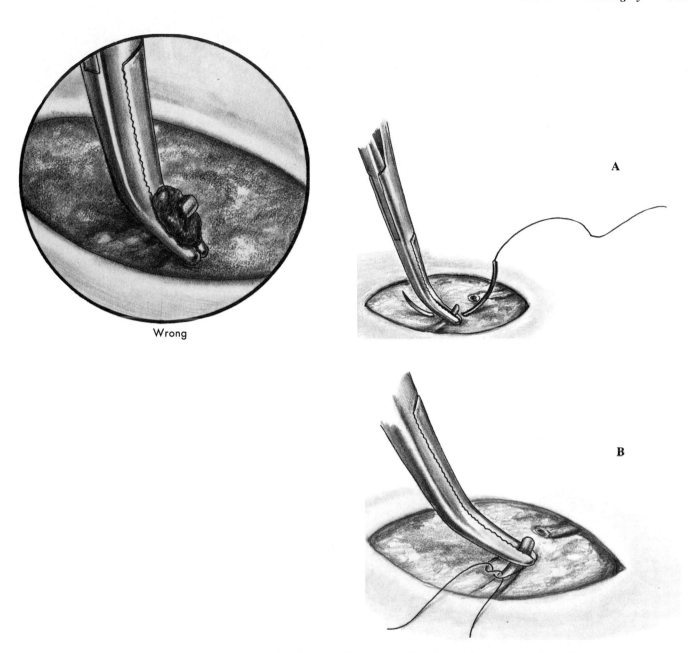

Wrong

A

B

Fig. 10-26. Method of securing bleeding vessel to surrounding tissue. **A,** Insertion of needle in tissue. **B,** Tying vessel to tissue.

Novices tend to abuse the electrosurgical apparatus by destroying much more tissue than necessary to stop bleeding. Excessive tissue destruction can lead to higher infection rates.[87] This is partially caused by the fact that living cells can combat bacteria, whereas dead tissues, such as those produced by electrosurgery, are powerless against them. One also needs to be careful not to electrocoagulate adjacent tissue edges inadvertently when using an electrosurgical apparatus deep in a wound.

When a large vessel is cut it may be preferable to tie it off, so that bleeding does not occur hours after the wound is closed (Fig. 10-26). The vessel should be visualized first and then grasped with a fine-tipped hemostat. One should not concomitantly crush the surrounding tissue with the hemostat (*insert,* Fig. 10-26, *A*). I prefer to tie the vessel by grasping a small amount of supporting tissue to anchor the tied vessel. Some authorities think that it is best not to tie the vessel to adjacent tissue, in an attempt to minimize devitalized tissue in a wound.[67,91] If the pressure in the vessel is high, however, a suture may slip off the vessel. I therefore prefer the extra reassurance of anchoring the vessel.

The amount of suture buried in a wound should be minimized, so vessels should not be tied off unless they are bleeding profusely. Although it seems that burying foreign bodies such as a suture in a wound predisposes to infection more than electrocoagulation does, this is not supported in the literature.[113]

Sometimes brisk bleeding that is difficult to localize occurs underneath skin edges, which have been undermined or exists in deep crevices within tissue. The scalp may present a particular problem with such bleeding, because blood vessels tend to be held open by the rich fibrous stroma, sometimes retracting into the recesses of the subcutaneous tissue. The secret to finding these vessels so that they can be compressed with a hemostat is exposure. This requires a good light and a suction machine. Blind pinching of tissue with large-tipped hemostats is discouraged in the skin or subcutaneous tissue, since it leads to tissue necrosis. Fine-tipped Halsted or Hartmann hemostats are excellent for grasping small arterial vessels in the skin. Use of a suction machine helps to eliminate the needless sponging of tissue, which itself causes trauma.[40]

When attempting to clamp a vessel, one sometimes cannot completely see the cut end. If the hemostat tips are near but not exactly on the vessel itself, bleeding may continue but at a slower rate. Twisting the clamp a fourth to half a turn may completely stop the bleeding. If this is the case, a suture can then be placed at the tip of the hemostat on the side from which the bleeding occurs. Figure-eight sutures are rarely necessary in cutaneous surgery; they are used when bleeding points cannot be accurately determined.

It is important to stress that bleeding in a wound need not be completely stopped but only be mostly controlled.[118] As previously emphasized, one should avoid excessive electrocoagulation and burying sutures to tie off vessels. A caustic such as ferric subsulfate (Monsel's solution), should not be used in wounds to be closed, since those substances probably destroy otherwise viable cells.

A wound should not be sutured until all brisk bleeding is stopped. Although wound closure provides some hemostasis, it is unwise to rely on sutures at the time of closure for this purpose. Placing a drain in a cutaneous wound because of continuous blood flow is also usually unwise. A drain is a two-way street, providing a conduit for bacteria into the wound, and should not replace careful, painstaking control of hemostasis. The one legitimate indication for a drain in cutaneous surgery is to drain an infected abscess. Only rarely does the situation arise in which a wound is so large and deep that bleeding is inevitable after the local anesthesia wears off. A drain may be considered for this, but it is better to rely on a good pressure dressing.

HEMOSTATIC PACKING SUBSTANCE

Agents to stop bleeding in cutaneous surgery are available but are unnecessary in simple excisional surgery except under unusual circumstances, which are specifically cited later. These substances include oxidized cellulose (Oxycel, Surgicel), microcrystalline collagen (Avitene), absorbable gelatin sponges (Gelfoam), and tissue thromboplastin.

DEBRIDEMENT

Before closure the surgical wound should be inspected for any free devitalized tissue or extraneous foreign material, such as hair or lint from gauze. This material—and any free devitalized tissue—should be meticulously removed. Left in a wound, foreign matter may evoke a foreign body reaction.

TECHNIQUE OF WOUND CLOSURE

The usual method of apposing wound edges is with sutures. Sutures function to restore the proper anatomic relationships so that healing occurs at an optimal rate. Still, every suture tract is a covert intradermal incision.[104] As long as the suture remains in situ, surface epidermis and epidermis from transected appendages grow perisuturally.[54] Some types of sutures may evoke inflammation of the same degree or even greater than that evoked by a scalpel incision. Suture tracts are also avenues for bacterial spread.[21]

Every suture produces injury to tissue that is proportional to the tension it places on the skin. When sutures are removed, the suture tracts inevitably fibrose, causing suture marks. Therefore a surgeon should take great pains to use a minimal number of sutures and to place them with the least tension possible. Furthermore, needle punctures themselves can be a source of inflammation,[41] so careful atraumatic technique should be used, with as few misplaced sutures as possible.

Method of holding needle

The suture needle is placed in the needle holder midway between the tip and the swage (*inset* in Fig. 10-27), much as one would hold a spear (Fig. 10-28). Although some authorities recommend the needle be held three-fourths of the way back from the tip,[65] I feel that with the fine suture needles used in cutaneous surgery it is preferable to hold the needle only halfway back.[150] This results in less tendency for bending a delicate needle in tissue. Also, when insertion of the needle into the skin occurs, one needs to pronate the wrist less to achieve a 90-degree angle.

Method of holding needle holder

The method I prefer for grasping the needle holder is shown in Fig. 10-27. Note that the index finger is placed on the jaws near and posterior to the needle; the thumb is almost on the spring, and the handle rests gently in the palm encircled by the middle, ring, and little fingers. The thenar and hypothenar eminences are in a position of slight adduction. With this technique the thumb and index finger control

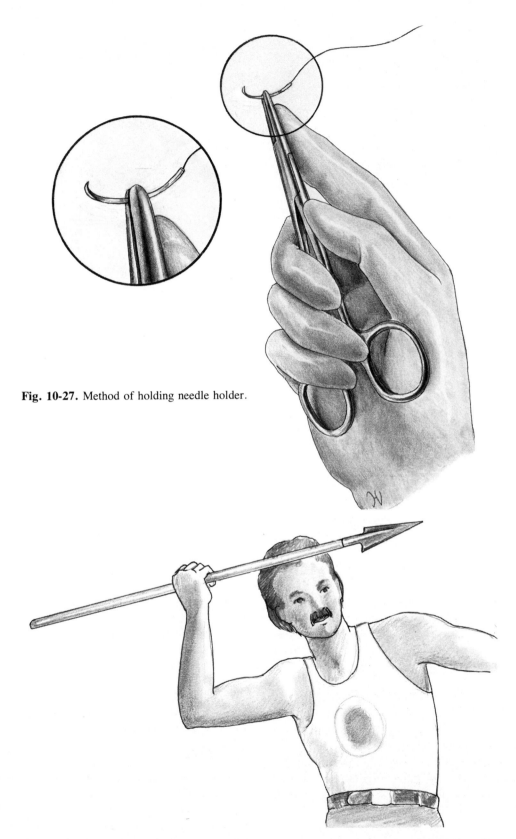

Fig. 10-27. Method of holding needle holder.

Fig. 10-28. One holds fine needle in needle holder like one holds a spear—in middle. (Modified from Troutman, R.: Microsurgery of the anterior segment of the eye. Vol. 1: Introduction and basic techniques, St. Louis, 1974, The C.V. Mosby Co.)

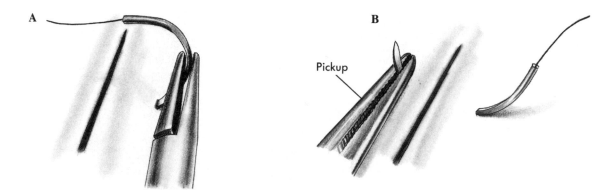

Fig. 10-29. A, Inserting needle 90 degrees to skin surface. **B,** Using pickups to grasp needle coming through opposite skin edge.

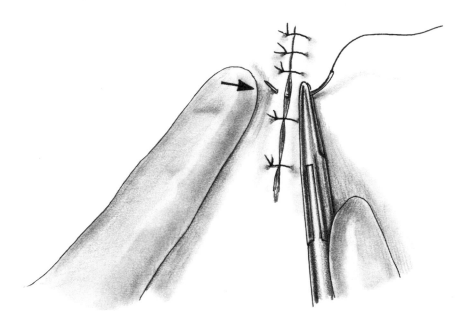

Fig. 10-30. Using finger on opposite hand to produce eversion of wound edge.

the needle's passage. Placing the finger on the jaws almost behind the needle is essential, since it gives the physician greater control over placement of the needle. It is unnecessary to place one's fingers through the rings of the needle holder's handle while placing sutures in the skin.[146]

SIMPLE INTERRUPTED PERCUTANEOUS SUTURES

Simple interrupted sutures are used in all branches of surgery. If the wound is not deep—extending only to the dermal-subdermal junction, or where there is little tension on the wound edges and no significant tissue loss, or dead space has occurred—simple interrupted sutures may be used alone.

Placement

The needle is inserted approximately 90 degrees to the skin surface. This requires slight hyperpronation of the hand

at the wrist. The needle is then brought through the opposite side, where it is grasped with pickups (Fig. 10-29).

When bringing the needle through the opposite wound edge, it occasionally gets hung up, especially if the skin is thick. In such a situation the tips of the pickup should be held horizontally on the skin to provide tension, and the needle can then be pushed between these tips. Instead of pickups one may use the needle holder to grasp the needle as it comes through the skin, but one needs to be careful not to injure the needle itself. As the needle exists from the wound on the opposite side, its path should also be 90 degrees to the skin surface. This is usually ensured by everting the opposite skin edge with a finger[25] (Fig. 10-30).

Sometimes to ensure that the needle will enter the skin perpendicularly, it is necessary to pick up the skin edge for proper placement of the suture, especially where the skin is thin and the edge tends to curl under. A skin hook is ideal for this purpose (Fig. 10-31, *A*), whereas toothed forceps

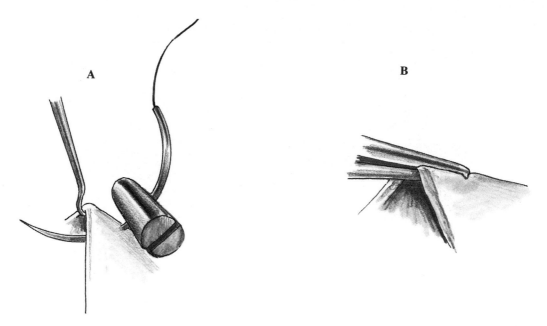

Fig. 10-31. A, Using skin hook to elevate edge of tissue. **B,** Crimping of tissue with toothed forceps.

tend to crimp and tear tissue (Fig. 10-31, *B*). Such compression of wound edges has been shown to enhance infection[126] and should be avoided.

A suture that produces some slight eversion of the wound edges counteracts the natural tendency of all wound edges to invert. The proper path of a simple interrupted suture is illustrated on the right in Fig. 10-32; an improper path is shown on the left. As can be seen, the suture enters the skin at an angle 90 degrees to the skin surface, as already described. It then travels perpendicularly or obliquely and laterally as it descends in depth. The needle is brought out of the wound in the center and reenters the wound on the opposite side, where it reenters the skin. It is then angled perpendicularly or obliquely and medially to the wound so that on exiting from the skin the needle is 90 degrees to the skin surface. This method of exiting the wound in the center is good technique for making a suture loop broader at the base than at the points of entrance and exit from the skin. Albom recommends this method and to avoid going through both skin edges with one turn of the needle.[3] It is essential that when tied, the suture loop should be slightly larger at the bottom than the top[39] and wider than it is deep.[52] This configuration has been likened to the outline of a flask; it ensures that the skin edges are everted. Knots are best placed to the side of the wound so the tails do not rest in the wound itself, thereby interfering with wound healing (Fig. 10-38).

The improper method of suturing, shown on the left in Fig. 10-32, results in overlapping skin edges. This occurs because of the uneven and nonsymmetric pathway the needle has taken on each side of the wound. Note that the needle did not exit the middle of the wound before entering the opposite side. Eversion of the wound edge with a single finger (Fig. 10-30) was not performed. Such unevenness of skin edges results in slower epidermization of the wound.[104]

The consequences to the final scar of orienting the needle 90 degrees to the skin surface with a resultant suture path that produces in slight eversion of the epidermal skin edges is illustrated in Fig. 10-33. All wound scars contract with time. The contraction becomes an additional tension force within the skin, but occurring after the wound is made and modified with time. An incisional scar contracts in all directions along its length—vertically, horizontally, and side-to-side. The vertical contraction flattens the slightly everted skin edges with time (Fig. 10-33, *A*). If the wound edges are sutured flat initially, there may ultimately appear a slightly depressed scar (Fig. 10-33, *B*). Such depressed scars cast a shadow. If the wound is sutured with obvious depression, this depression only gets worse with time (Fig. 10-33, *C*). A wound cut tangentially tends to buckle with time at one epidermal surface, as the oblique wound contracts (Fig. 10-33, *D*). This scar contraction contributes to the so-called trapdoor phenomenon.

Rarely it is desirable to cause purposeful inversion in a scar—for instance, at a location where one wishes to recreate a skin fold such as the melolabial or upper eyelid fold. This is performed by changing the normal pathway of the needle, so as to form a loop that is wider at the top than at the bottom, (Fig. 10-33, *C*). Inversion also tends to occur if the sutures are placed very superficially.

Exemplifying the same principle of scar contraction over

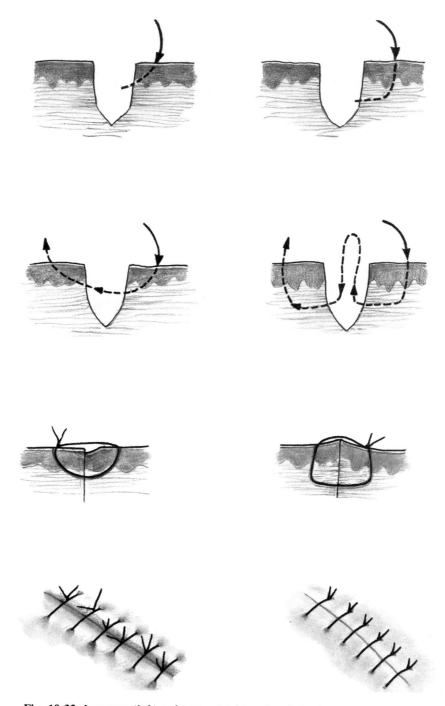

Fig. 10-32. Improper *(left)* and proper *(right)* paths of simple percutaneous suture.

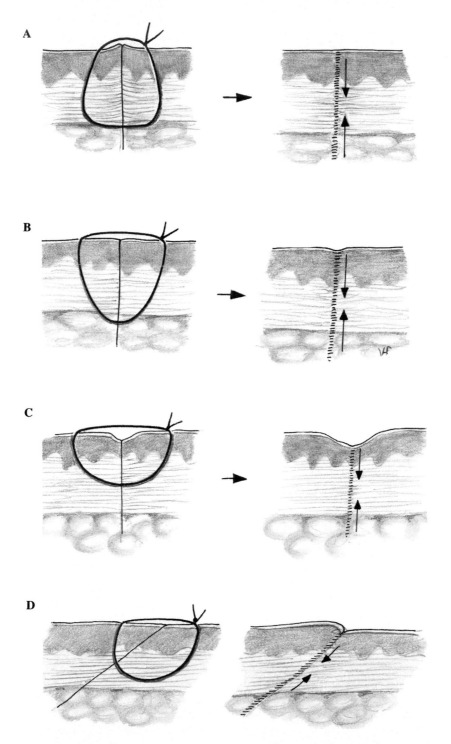

Fig. 10-33. Relationship of suture path and wound edges *(left)* to ultimate scar formation *(right)*. **A,** Sight eversion; **B,** flat; **C,** inversion; **D,** beveled edge. Arrows indicate lines of contraction.

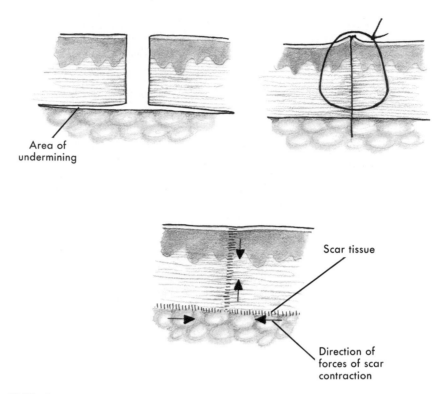

Fig. 10-34. Scar contraction in undermined wounds helps to hold wounds together. *Top left,* Undermined wound. *Top right,* sutured wound. *Bottom,* Healed wound with scar tissue. Note direction of scar contractions *(arrows).*

time, is the contraction that occurs in wounds that have been laterally undermined. The scar that occurs at the interface of the undermined planes contracts, helping to hold the wound together and thereby preventing spread of the scar (Fig. 10-34).

Suture tying

For interrupted cutaneous sutures, tying with a needle holder is preferred (Fig. 10-35). Note that the first loop is teased down to coapt the wound edges (Fig. 10-35, Step C). At the same time the first throw is snugged down, the suture is slightly lifted to align and evert the skin edges. The second loop sets the knot (shown square); by this I mean the knot still slips enough to tease the wounds together just enough without undue tension. When suturing with nylon or polypropylene, additional loops in opposite directions are necessary to prevent knot slippage.

Tying sutures is a very important part of excisional surgery. Sutures should be tied just tight enough to bring the wound edges together without tension, pressure, or cutting into the tissue. *Approximate, do not strangulate.* Remember, edema may occur after closure and make sutures too tight. Sutures tied too tight strangulate tissue, cause tissue necrosis,[98] and may lead to subsequent wound infection.[41] In addition, overlapping or inversion of the skin edges may occur. Attempting to remove totally the lateral tension on the wound edges by numerous tightly tied sutures can induce

fibrous tissue hyperplasia,[109] delay wound healing,[17] and produce a weaker wound.[82,102] On the other hand, if there is too much lateral tension on a wound, spreading of a scar or scar hypertrophy may result.[49] One attempts by suturing to balance the extrinsic tension acting to separate a wound by intrinsic tension generated from sutures.[31]

The basic types of surgical knots are shown in Fig. 10-36. A tied suture has three components: a loop, a knot, and ears (tails). The loop is a fixed perimeter whose geometry is secured by a knot. When the ear and loop of a two-throw knot are on the same side of the knot and are parallel with each other, the knot is square. The knot is a granny if the ear and loop cross on different sides of the knot. The granny knot is thus built with two half-knots in the same direction. Since it slips easily, if used, additional throws in the opposite direction are necessary to secure proper tension on the wound and to keep the knot from slipping. However, it should be pointed out that the square knot can be transformed into a half hitch if both throws are not pulled with approximately equal tension.[46,137,149]

A square knot (also known as a reef knot) has a flat plane.[85] To be tied properly it requires either opposite motions of the same hand (bimotility) or identical movements of opposite hands (ambidexterity). These must be conscious motions, since the natural tendency is for one to tie a knot by movements in the same direction with the same hand.

The square (reef) knot is the workhorse of cutaneous

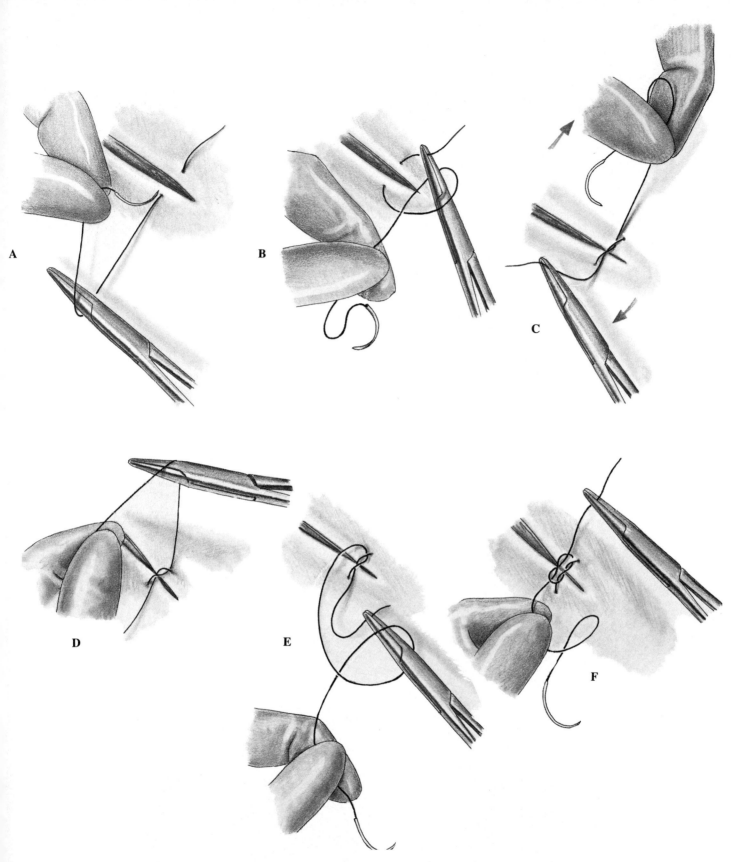

Fig. 10-35. Steps in instrument tie. **A,** Suture looped over needle holder. **B,** Free end of suture is grasped with needle holder and then pulled through loop created in step **A** to produce first throw of knot (**C**). **C,** Knot is eased down so skin edges are teased together. **D,** Suture on opposite side of wound is looped over needle holder. **E,** Free end of suture is again grasped with needle holder and pulled through loop created in step **D**. This creates second throw of square knot (**F**).

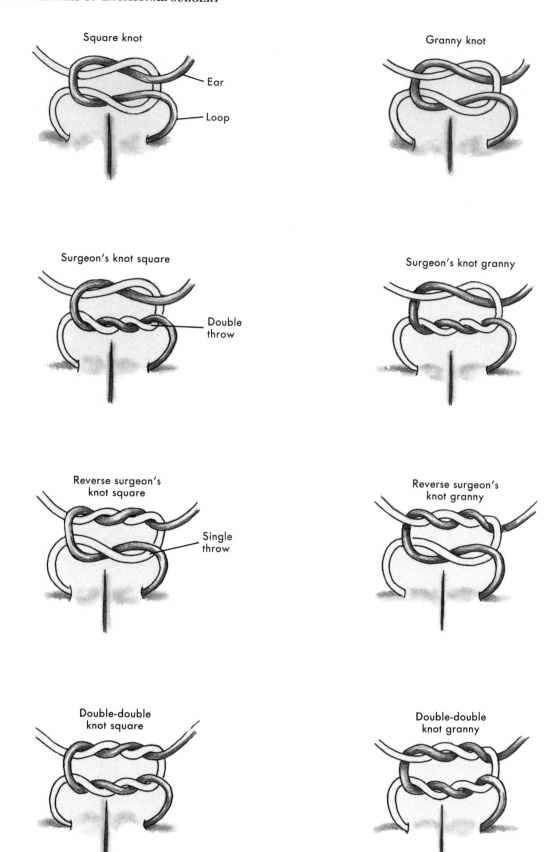

Fig. 10-36. Types of knots used in cutaneous surgery.

surgery. Some surgeons prefer the surgeon's knot square because it is more secure and the first double-throw temporarily holds the wound edges together while the surgeon throws and sets the second loop. However, the surgeon's knot tied square does not easily allow the physician to set the knot after the second throw and in my experience requires extra effort to tie. Returning to Fig. 10-35, Step C, when the first throw of the simple square knot is set, if the wound edges do not hold together, one may help keep the knot from slippage by rotating the hand and needle holder counterclockwise for 90 degrees. This helps to lock the loop in place so that the second throw may be made without the first throw coming loose.

Sutures may become loose because of knot slippage or tearing into tissues as swelling occurs in the wound. All knots probably slip to some degree, but swelling may actually help the knot to become more secure.[46] Knots themselves do not break but may become untied. If a break occurs, it is usually adjacent to the knot and caused by a weak point where the fibers have been fractured in tying.[138]

Knot security increases with the number of throws but the percentage of increase is reduced with each one[138]; however, a third and fourth throw still add considerably to knot strength. For modern silk, three throws versus two throws improve the holding capacity of a suture fivefold.[63] For suture materials that slip easily (have a low coefficient of friction), such as nylon or polypropylene, four throws are recommended. The type of suture material influences knot slippage, being worse with nylon or polypropylene but much better with silk or polyester (uncoated).[6]

Suture and needle selection

The principles of suture and needle selection are discussed at length in Chapter 8. Some additional discussion at this point reemphasizes some of that discussion.

Since no ideal suture exists, selection of suture involves a series of compromises. The strength and size of the suture material and needle should be chosen with the strength of the tissue to be sutured in mind. Suturing cheesecloth with rope does not increase the strength of the sutured line any more than suturing with 4-0 silk.

Other factors to consider in the selection of suture include the tension to which the wound edges must be subjected and the state of the tissue being sutured. Inflamed tissue does not hold sutures well, for instance. The holding power of any tissue is a function of the amount and density of the fibrous tissue it contains.[68] Where the dermis is thick, such as on the back, the holding power is greater than where the skin is thin, such as on the eyelid. If the dermis is thinned by administration of corticosteroids, the holding power is also diminished. The strength of a wound cannot be greater than the holding power of the tissue for the sutures. *A wound is held together by the surrounding tissue and not by the sutures*. It is unnecessary to employ a suture

that is stronger than the tissue through which it passes. Therefore one should select the smallest suture that can appose the wound edges without cutting through the tissues. Larger sutures than necessary do not add to the strength of a healing wound.[101] Also, larger suture material places a greater amount of foreign material in a wound and thus may provoke a greater inflammatory response than is normal.[41] Using the smallest suture possible was taught by Halsted as part of good surgical technique.[60]

The tendency of sutures to cut through tissue depends on the tensile strength of the suture, the strength of the tissue, and the suture size; therefore, given two tissues of equal strength and the same suture material, a smaller suture is more likely to cut through the tissues.[69,150] This is caused by greater force per unit area of tissue exerted by the thinner suture than that exerted by a thicker suture tied with the same tension.

Some sutures are more likely than others to promote wound infection. In general, braided materials are more prone to harbor or draw organisms into wounds, so nonbraided nylon or polypropylene are best in this regard. Vicryl and Dexon should not be used percutaneously because they are said to enhance not only bacterial infection but also epidermization of suture tracts (see Fig. 4-16).[4]

Synthetic materials appear to be less reactive in tissues than naturally occurring material, such as silk.[1] Enthusiasts of mild chromic catgut for cutaneous placement do not emphasize that chromic sutures left in tissue provoke a pronounced inflammatory reaction.[144]

The size of the needle should be chosen on the basis of the size of the suture. In general, one should use the thinnest, smallest needle possible. Do not use wide, large needles with thin suture material, since this results in a larger suture tract than necessary and promotes epidermal ingrowth and bacterial contamination.

Size of the loop

The smallest bite that can comfortably appose the wound edges both superficially and in depth without crimping or cutting through the tissue should be used. This keeps the amount of tissue under tension to a minimum and minimizes any subsequent scarring from sutures. Usually this means placing the suture within 1 to 3 mm of the wound edges. If the tissue is thin, one may need to come closer to the wound edges to prevent inversion and obtain slight eversion. Thicker skin under tension may require a larger bite; however, with larger bites one tends to tie sutures tighter, which may lead to strangulation of tissue and necrosis. Because the fibrous component of tissue is the determining factor holding a wound together, an increase in the size of the bite does not necessarily increase the holding power of a suture. In general, the more tension on the wound edges the farther the sutures should be placed from the wound edges.

When a suture is placed in tissue, various forces act on

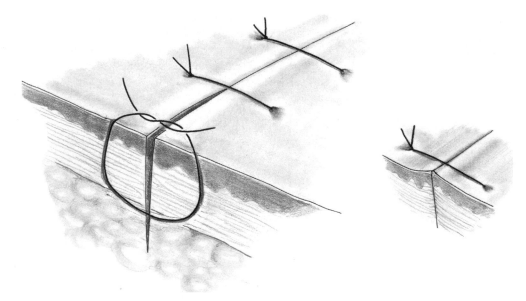

Fig. 10-37. Simple percutaneous suture. Knots should be tied and then pulled gently to side of wound.

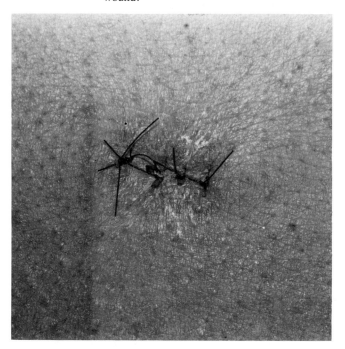

Fig. 10-38. Excision site 1 week after operation. Tails of sutures are inadvertently caught in incision line. This will delay wound healing.

the suture loop.[116] These include the lateral pull of the musculature and tissue tension outside the loop (extrinsic tension). Inside the loop edema and inflammation create pressure (intrinsic tension). The tension in the suture loop is proportional to the area enclosed by the suture. The larger the loop, the more tension is placed on the suture. Therefore smaller bites place less tension on sutures.

The depth of the loop is determined by the thickness of the dermis and how deep the incision is. In general, the suture loop is slightly larger in the horizontal direction than in depth[39] (Figs. 10-32 and 10-37).

Spacing and number of sutures

Wound strength is partially determined by the number of sutures but, more important, by the holding power of the tissue. Sutures should be placed along an incision line so that the tension is minimized but not eliminated on the wound edges. The number of sutures required is the minimum needed to hold the wound edges exactly apposed without crimping. Generally speaking, the more tension on a wound, the closer the sutures should be placed; however, very closely spaced sutures result in wounds of decreased strength and destruction of tissue.[68] Increasing the number of sutures in a wound increases the holding power, but less than one might think. The holding power of two stitches is less than double that of one.[69] The holding power also reaches a maximum.[68] The sutured wound is only about 70% as strong as intact tissue.[84] In contrast, a scarcity of sutures leaves gaps in the wound.

The spacing between sutures is thus commensurate with the tension on the wound edges. In a fusiform excision, this tension is usually not uniformly distributed along the whole length of the skin edges but is greatest in the center and less at the ends. Therefore even spacing of sutures along the length of an incision (Figs. 10-32, *right,* and 10-39, *A*) is not necessarily proper technique. When a fusiform wound is sutured, the spacing between the sutures may not be equal but is less in the center where the wound tension is greatest and more at the apices where the tension is less (Fig. 10-39, *B*).

When sutures are uniformly spaced in an incision line,

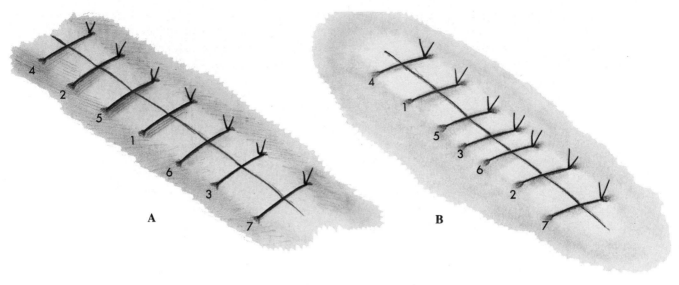

Fig. 10-39. Suggested sequence for placement of sutures in simple excision. **A,** Excision wound with minimal tension in center. First suture may be placed in center. **B,** Excision wound with great tension on wound edges. Initial sutures (*1* and *2*) are lateral to center. Also, note that more sutures are placed more closely together in center of wound than in **A**. This helps take tension off wound edges when it is too great.

the total tension is distributed equally among the sutures. If the number of sutures in a wound is increased, the tension on the wound is divided into smaller portions, and the stress borne by each suture becomes less with each additional suture. Thus the functional strength of each suture is increased. If the tension of the wound is increased, the sutures can be placed closer together. In contrast, if one uses fewer sutures more widely spaced, each suture is subject to more tension. If in an incision line one of the sutures subsequently breaks or becomes undone, the tension it bore is transferred to the surrounding sutures. If these sutures break or tear through the tissue because of increased tension, more strain is thrown on the remaining sutures; thus a chain reaction may disrupt an entire row of sutures.

PLACEMENT OF KNOTS

Knots should be placed on the side of the suture line

Away from
Vital structures (such as eye)
Sources of contamination (such as mouth)
Structures they will irritate (such as nostril)

Toward
A better blood supply
Where it is easier to tie
Where a mark is least noticeable (e.g., on hairline)

Modified from Noe, J.M.: Ann. Plast. Surg. **5**(2):145, 1980.

Placement of the knot (see box below)

For cutaneous sutures the knot should be placed to the side of the incision line after it is tied (Fig. 10-37). This keeps the cut ends (tails) from getting caught in the wound and thus interfering with healing (Figs. 10-32, *bottom left,* and 10-38). Also, if placed in the wound's center, the knot's increased pressure sometimes makes the skin edges invert.

Knots and suture tails can also irritate structures such as the eye, nose, and mouth and should be placed away from these structures. Since knots tend to harbor bacteria, they are best placed away from any source of wound contamination (for example, the mouth and nose).[103]

Sequence of tying sutures

Although much of the time it makes little difference as to the sequence of individual suture placement in a straight-line closure, sometimes it may be best to begin in the center to even out the pressure and properly align the wound edges (Fig. 10-39, *A*). Starting at one end and suturing to the other end can occasionally increase one's chances of getting a dog-ear. Therefore alternating the sutures between those previously placed more evenly distributes any discrepancy, however small, in wound edge length on either side. Note also in Fig. 10-39 that the knots on the sutures are placed neatly to the side.

Some authors recommend beginning to suture a wound from the end rather than in the middle.[39] This is acceptable as long as one keeps any discrepancy in the length of the cut edges from forming. When the tension on the wound edges in the center of the wound is particularly high, one may be forced to begin suturing at either end, since beginning in the center may break the suture or tear the skin. One should go one step at a time and "feel one's way," taking the tension on the tissue as a guide. As previously emphasized, sutures in the center of a wound may need to be placed closer together to take tension off the wound edges where it is highest.

When placing sutures it is also essential to keep in mind the surrounding vital structures, such as the mouth, eye, ear, and so forth. The first sutures placed should properly align the skin so as to cause as little distortion of such structures as possible and to restore the proper anatomic relationships. One may begin suturing anywhere along the incision line to accomplish this.

BURIED INTERRUPTED SUTURES

If excisions are deep into subcutaneous tissues and significant tissue loss has occurred, buried sutures should be considered. A buried suture is a suture whose loop is tied so that it does not pass through the epidermal surface. Buried sutures may be placed at many different levels and in several different tissues. Buried sutures may unite not only skin but nerve, muscle, fascia, and even bone.

Types

Cutaneous surgery is concerned with two basic buried interrupted sutures—the dermal and the subcutaneous—which differ in the depth at which they are placed. The dermal suture is confined mainly in the dermis with the knot beneath the dermal-subdermal junction. The subcutaneous suture is placed within the subcutaneous tissue exclusively. A third suture, actually a variant of the buried dermal suture, is the dermal-subdermal suture, which has a variable amount of its loop in the dermis and subcutaneous tissue but always contains a portion of the dermal-subdermal tissue plane.[2] It differs from the buried dermal suture by containing a greater amount of the subcutaneous tissue in its loop.

Purpose

The strength of scars resides in the fibrous tissue below the epidermis at every level. How this tissue is handled and realigned greatly affects the ultimate functional strength and cosmetic appearance of the scar.[53] Buried sutures helps to realign deep tissues into their normal position relative to each other.

Not infrequently the tension on the wound edges is greater than can be easily handled by simple interrupted percutaneous sutures. This tension occurs because of the location, the size, or the depth of a surgical defect. When significant tissue is removed at a level below the superficial dermis, closure of a wound puts considerable lateral and vertical tension on the wound edges. Thus one of the main functions of buried sutures is to take tension off the wound edges at all levels.

If placed properly, intradermally buried sutures help to coapt the overlying epidermis and even up the wound edges. Ideally, this leads to the use of fewer percutaneous sutures and the production ultimately of finer, more inconspicuous scars. Fewer percutaneous sutures mean less visible scarring from sutures and less likelihood of infection.[112] If there is a considerable amount of dead space in a wound, buried sutures also function to close the dead space and thus help to prevent hematoma formation.

History and background

The earliest description of buried interrupted sutures came from Halsted in 1889.[58] Halsted devised these sutures for experiments on dogs. He found that stitch abscesses around percutaneous sutures were such a problem with these animals that some other means had to be devised to close the wounds. By burying sutures Halsted avoided puncturing the skin surface, which had previously led to abscesses. Later he employed this same suturing in humans.

Fig. 10-40 is a photograph of a herniorrhaphy scar that resulted from Halsted's use of buried sutures in 1891.[59] This photograph is remarkable for the almost imperceptible linear scar (between the two crosses) achieved by a general surgeon who was very respectful of all tissues he encountered, particularly the skin.

The idea that buried sutures reduce wound infection was confirmed experimentally[21,112] and is certainly true in wounds with little contamination. Also, if buried sutures are placed so that percutaneous sutures are not used, less inflammatory response may occur.[15] Buried sutures themselves may, however, potentiate infection if significant contamination in the wound has occurred. Thus these sutures are a double-edged sword. In most clean cutaneous wounds contamination is negligible, so the chance of subsequent infection is minimal. In grossly contaminated wounds this is not the case. Two studies on lacerations sutured in emergency rooms showed that the use of buried sutures in such wounds was associated with a higher rate of infection.[10,140] Experimentally in rats, crushing contaminated tissue with ligatures has been shown to lead to an increased incidence of infection.[91] Therefore when wounds are contaminated, buried sutures should not be used, if possible.

Closure of dead space

Buried sutures are said to help eliminate dead space and thereby the subsequent wound drainage or bleeding that occurs into such dead spaces. Although it seems logical that one should try to obliterate dead space if possible,[89] its value has not been demonstrated. In fact, Halsted, the first to advocate buried sutures, was also a great advocate of not trying to obliterate all dead space. He realized early on that too many sutures, when used for this purpose, "enfeeble the circulation and impair the vitality of tissues."[59] It is doubtful if dead space is ever completely eliminated in a wound. Halsted advised surgeons of his generation to let

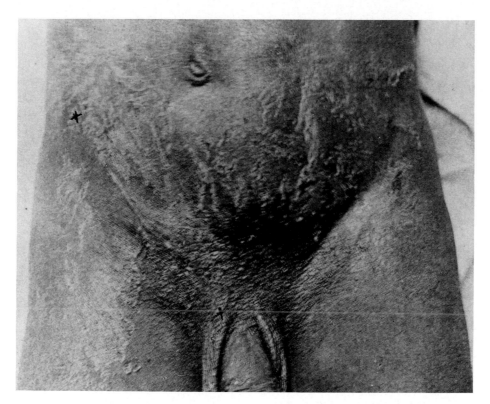

Fig. 10-40. Herniorrhaphy scar (between 2 crosses) produced in 1891 by Halsted, who used buried sutures. The wound dressing has not been totally wiped free. From Halsted, W.S.: Johns Hopkins Hosp. Rep. **2:**255, 1891.

dead space take care of itself. Based on my experience, I agree. Extra effort in attempting to eliminate dead space is of questionable benefit. The small amounts of tissue held in multiple-layered closures are likely to cause tissue necrosis and cutting out.

A recent study tested the use of sutures placed in subcutaneous fat to obliterate the dead space and to reduce hematoma formation in 208 patients.[94] The investigators found no difference in wound infection or hematoma formation rates in comparable groups. Because fat is mostly water and has little tensile strength, sutures in this layer probably have little overall benefit. They concluded that the disadvantages of subcutaneous sutures (tissue strangulation, promotion of infection, and foreign material) outweighed the advantages (closure of a portion of the dead space).

The idea that blood in a wound is necessarily harmful appears to be ingrained in the minds of many surgeons. Although one should try to eliminate blood if possible, since it is material that a wound must absorb and therefore does perhaps slow up wound healing, some bleeding is inevitable. A point of diminishing returns is quickly reached if one attempts to eliminate all blood from a wound. Excessive use of buried sutures for this purpose is counterproductive. Equally harmful are drains routinely placed in wounds because of minor continuous blood flow. Such drains are to

be avoided, since they may provide a direct avenue for the entrance of bacteria into the wound.

Welch in 1891 reported experiments in dogs in which wounds were allowed to fill with blood and then were inoculated with *Staphylococcus aureus*.[147] The wounds did not suppurate. Therefore the presence of blood does not necessarily make a wound more susceptible to infection.

Two important studies should be discussed at this point. One 1961 study showed in dogs that a seven-layered abdominal wall closure of contaminated wounds resulted in less wound infection that a four-layered closure.[24] The investigators concluded that the more meticulous the closure of the dead space, the less the chance of infection. Thus the idea arose and seemed to be substantiated in animals that careful closure of the dead space alone was a deterrent to wound infection.[40] An interesting footnote to the 1961 study is that silk and Dacron were found to have equal power to potentiate infection and much more such power than nylon has.

In a 1974 study, dead space closure was examined in rabbits.[35] The authors studied the presence of dead space versus no dead space in contaminated wounds and found that the presence of dead space alone potentiated infection. But sutured closure of the dead space—compared to not closing the dead space—did not lower the infection rate and even made it worse. This supports the work cited earlier regarding the higher wound infection rates in emergency room wounds with buried sutures.[10,140] Ferguson came to similar conclusions regarding closure of dead space in general surgical wounds[43] and refuted the clinical application of his earlier work.[24]

Based on the foregoing and my own clinical experience, it is best to prevent *production* of dead space during surgery. Excessive undermining and unnecessary cutting lead to larger amounts of dead space and bleeding and thus theoretically help to potentiate infection in contaminated areas. Therefore, one should do only what is necessary. The main use of buried sutures should be to take tension off the wound edges, with closure of dead space being of only secondary importance.

Buried "permanent" sutures

Burying sutures, particularly intradermally, is said to take tension off the wound edges, which helps to prevent subsequent spreading of scars. Some authorities recommend the use of completely buried clear nylon or polyester sutures for this purpose, since those materials remain in tissue long enough for the wound to gain substantial tensile strength.[61] Use of such "permanent" buried sutures for this purpose is not universally supported in the literature and remains controversial.[130]

A study of rectus sheath plication on patients with either Vicryl or nylon revealed that there was no difference in the width of the scars at 6 months.[9] The authors concluded that the strength of the bond holding tissue together is in the scar tissue produced, and is not related to the suture type that may be buried. A study of 70 wounds (mammoplasty or facelifts) in 23 patients compared buried Dexon to buried coated polyester sutures.[154] There was no difference in either the ultimate cosmetic appearance or the width of the scars produced.

A similar study compared cutaneous scars in laminectomy patients; the wounds were partially closed with either subcutaneous clear nylon or subcutaneous Dexon and the scars were compared with each other and with the remaining portions of the scar that had undergone no subcutaneous closure.[152] The type or presence of subcutaneous sutures had no effect on the subsequent scar width. The authors concluded that the most important determinant of scar width is the individual patient.

Buried sutures versus no buried sutures

My own experience is that where the surrounding forces of tension are great, for example on the trunk, it makes little difference whether buried sutures are used or which buried sutures are used with respect to the ultimate cosmetic result. This seems to be supported in the references previously cited.[9,152,154] In areas where the tension is much less in one direction than another, for instance the face, burying sutures helps in producing finer scars. Part of the reason for this

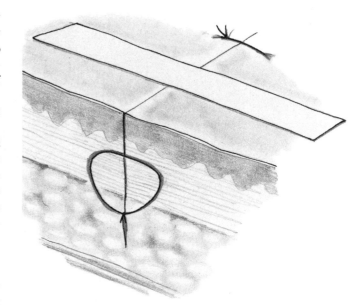

Fig. 10-41. Buried interrupted dermal suture.

may be that healing is faster on the face than the trunk, so that sufficient wound tensile strength is formed faster and before adequate tensile strength of the buried sutures is lost.

Buried interrupted dermal or dermal-subdermal sutures

Tension on the epidermal wound edges may be greatly alleviated by the use of buried dermal or dermal-subdermal sutures. Since these buried sutures are left in the underlying tissue for an indefinite period of time until absorbed, the tension on the skin is alleviated for a time beyond when the cutaneous sutures are normally removed. In addition, properly placed buried dermal sutures help to evert the wound edges, which is difficult to do with interrupted percutaneous sutures, even with careful placement.

Buried sutures may be placed at different levels. One may place a buried suture so that much or most of the loop is in dermis (Fig. 10-41); this is the buried interrupted dermal suture. Alternatively, most of the loop may be placed in the subcutaneous fat with only a small superficial portion in the dermis (Fig. 10-42). Such sutures are known as dermal-subdermal sutures.[2] The reason for the slight amount of dermis in the suture loop is to provide a greater amount of fibrous tissue for a more stable closure than can be provided by the subcutaneous tissue alone. By placing the suture deeper than a normal buried dermal suture, more space is left above for interrupted or running intradermal sutures. The buried dermal-subdermal suture may not appose the wound edges as well as the buried dermal suture does.

The proper method of placing a buried dermal-subdermal suture is shown in Fig. 10-43. Note that one begins the stitch deep in the wound (on the left side if the surgeon is right handed) beneath the dermis, first passing vertically

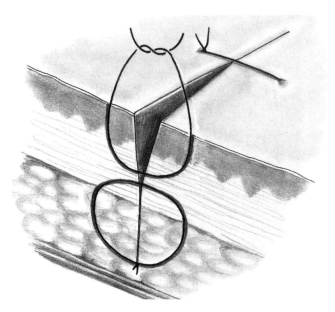

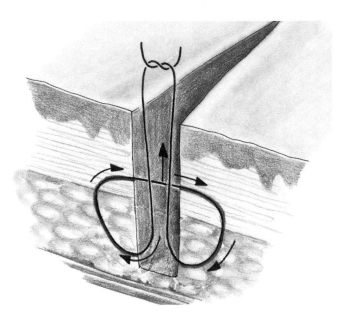

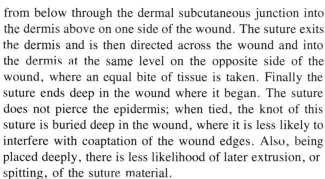

Fig. 10-42. Buried interrupted dermal-subdermal suture with interrupted cutaneous suture. Note deeper position of suture with more subcutaneous tissue than in Fig. 10-41. Overlying epidermal wound edges are not apposed but only approximated.

Fig. 10-43. Method of placing buried interrupted dermal-subdermal suture.

from below through the dermal subcutaneous junction into the dermis above on one side of the wound. The suture exits the dermis and is then directed across the wound and into the dermis at the same level on the opposite side of the wound, where an equal bite of tissue is taken. Finally the suture ends deep in the wound where it began. The suture does not pierce the epidermis; when tied, the knot of this suture is buried deep in the wound, where it is less likely to interfere with coaptation of the wound edges. Also, being placed deeply, there is less likelihood of later extrusion, or spitting, of the suture material.

Properly tied, the buried dermal or dermal-subdermal suture should approximate the cutaneous surfaces so that they may subsequently be reinforced easily by skin tapes (Fig. 10-41), interrupted sutures (Fig. 10-41), or a running intradermal suture (see Fig. 11-25). The distance between the skin edges before the final layer of percutaneous sutures or tapes is placed gives a good indication of the potential width of the final scar, because the forces acting on the skin edges at that time are still present when the percutaneous sutures or tapes are removed.

Variations on the vertically placed buried dermal suture include oblique or even horizontal placement in the dermis. These techniques may be useful when there is little space for the needle in the wound. The knot with horizontally buried dermal sutures is closer to the skin surface than that with vertically placed buried sutures; the higher position of the knot may interfere with dermal coaptation.

Tying intradermal or dermal-subdermal buried sutures can sometimes be difficult. I use a one-handed tie, so that

tension can be maintained on the first throw while the second throw is made and the knot is set. If an instrument tie is used with this suture, one usually needs to use a surgeon's knot square, since the first loop will otherwise slip undone. When this happens, the second loop sets the knot with difficulty. Also, when tying buried knots one should pull the suture ends parallel to the closed incision line and not perpendicular to it. Occasionally there is significant tension on the wound edges, and it may be easier to have an assistant hold the wound together while tying down and setting the knots in these buried sutures. One may even first place a few cutaneous sutures to take the tension off the buried sutures.

The commonly used suture materials for buried sutures—Vicryl or Dexon—are of high tensile strength and tend to cut through tissues, so a back-and-forth sawing motion should be minimized. The number of throws used for knotting these materials is less than for nylon, either two or three. More than three throws should not be used because to do so adds greatly to the amount of buried foreign suture material.[121] The tails (ears) on the knot should be short, almost on the knot itself.

Aligning wounds properly in the horizontal direction for not only buried dermal sutures but also simple interrupted sutures can sometimes be troublesome. The use of two skin hooks, one on each apex of a fusiform excision, helps to line up the skin edges at the time of suture placement.[114,115]

The most common mistake made by novices in placing the buried dermal or dermal-subdermal suture is that not enough tissue *laterally* is included in the suture path. The greater the amount of lateral dermal tissue included, the

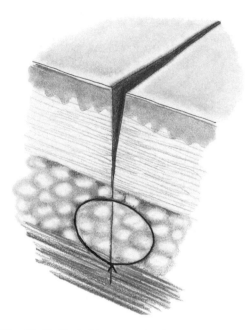

Fig. 10-44. Buried interrupted subcutaneous suture.

closer the epidermal wound edges come. It should be noted, however, that if too much tissue is grabbed laterally, a skin surface dimples on either side of the wound.

Another problem with this stitch is that if it is placed too near to the epidermal surface, suture extrusion may occur within the first month after closure. Extrusion of sutures has not been well studied but is probably caused by a combination of events. First, there is a tissue reaction to the suture itself, which is inevitable. Second, if this tissue reaction is high in the dermis, it interferes with normal epidermal healing. Third, the suture itself may represent a physical barrier to epidermization of the wound. Not until extrusion takes place can normal epidermal healing occur.

Buried interrupted subcutaneous sutures

Sometimes cutaneous wounds are deep enough to warrant sutures placed more deeply than the dermis. Such sutures are placed entirely within the subcutaneous tissue, where they help to obliterate the dead space and remove tension from the final cutaneous closure. The pros and cons of deeply placed sutures for these purposes have already been discussed.

Buried subcutaneous sutures, unlike buried dermal sutures, do not result in complete coaptation of the cutaneous wound edges but only approximation. Therefore higher buried dermal sutures may be required.

Like the buried dermal or dermal-subdermal suture, the buried subcutaneous suture is begun deep so that the knot is buried deeply (Fig. 10-44). It is tied like the buried dermal suture, and the ends are cut short. Frequently after placement of the subcutaneous sutures, buried dermal sutures are placed, and finally cutaneous sutures. Thus the wound may be closed with three ''layers'' of sutures.

CUTTING SUTURES

The cutting of sutures should not be approached in a cavalier manner but with a certain precision, like other techniques in wound closure. The proper method for cutting is shown in Fig. 10-45. One places the index finger on the fulcrum screw of the scissors and the thumb and fourth fingers through the rings of the handle. The placement of the index finger over the fulcrum is critical, since it allows the operator full control over the elevation or descent of the scissors' points. Any assistants who cut sutures should be instructed in this technique.

The preferable scissors for cutting sutures is the iris scissors. One should make it a habit to use this type of scissors for cutting sutures because the cutting of sutures dulls scissors. Other types of scissors, for instance, the tenotomy scissors, should be reserved for cutting tissue rather than sutures to keep them from dulling quickly.

The ideal length of the tails of sutures varies with the type of sutures being used and whether they are buried or not. For nonburied sutures, usually tails that are 2 to 3 mm long are sufficient. One may use shorter tails of 1 to 2 mm for silk, which does not tend to slip or untie. For more slippery sutures, longer tails are required: 3 to 4 mm. Around the eyes one may be forced to cut the tails short to keep them from irritating the conjunctiva.

For buried sutures one should bury as little suture material as possible. One should cut the suture just slightly (about 1 mm or less) away from the knot, using the suture to guide the tips of the iris scissors to the knot and then turning the hand 45 to 90 degrees clockwise (if right handed) before cutting. This allows a slight safety area of suture length to prevent one from cutting the knot directly.

PROBLEMS WITH SUTURING

Very minor but common problems may occur during placement of the sutures previously described, which should be addressed.

Misplaced sutures

Sometimes after a suture has been tied it becomes obvious that the suture is not ideally situated. Misplacement may involve the suture being too shallow, too deep, too close to one edge, different distances from the edges, tied too tightly, or tied so that the wound edges are not properly aligned. Do not hesitate to remove such sutures and replace them with properly placed or tied sutures. However, needle holes themselves can be sources of inflammation[41] and tracts for bacteria, so the number of unnecessary perforations of the skin should be minimized.

Uneven skin edges

This common problem is particularly vexing to the novice cutaneous surgeon. As pointed out previously, uneven edges should be evened up by vertical adjustment because they result in a prolonged period of epidermization and

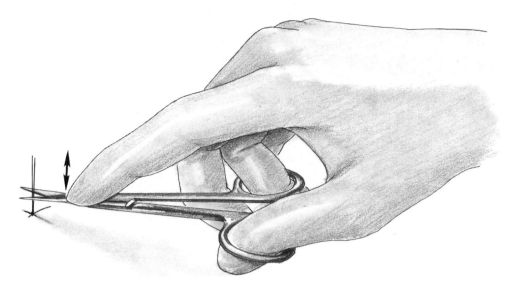

Fig. 10-45. Proper method of holding scissors to cut suture. Index finger overlies screw on scissors, allowing placement control of scissors tips.

greater tissue loss.[104] The latter may lead to a broader, more unsightly scar.

There are four ways to even up uneven skin edges. The easiest method is to shift the knot from one side of the wound to the other (Fig. 10-46). This helps to redistribute the tension slightly on the wound. One may need to play around with the knot and the wound edges to determine the side of the wound edge on which the knot seems to be better placed, so as to even up the wound edges. There are no hard-and-fast rules regarding knot placement with respect to such "fine-tuning" of the skin edges; however, a knot set on the low side tends to lower the opposite elevated side. Dushoff recommends setting the first loop of the square knot to the low side to adjust the wound edges when tying.[39] If one uses the surgeon's knot square (with a double throw), one cannot fine-tune the skin edges as easily.

In a second method of evening up uneven skin edges, one must place the needle the same distance from the skin surface on both sides of the wound (Fig. 10-47). Because the low side is more difficult to reach with the needle and may be slightly more bound down, one may need to go seemingly a little deeper on the low side. In reality one cannot easily measure distances in tissue depth; therefore one should try to go high (superficially) on the high side and low (in greater depth) on the low side, and will probably end up as shown in Fig. 10-47.

A third method, shown in Fig. 10-48, is to use a half-buried horizontal mattress suture. This method is particularly useful when one side is much more bound down than the other. When tied, this suture may actually pull the high side down rather than the low side up—but the wound edges nevertheless end up at the same level.

A fourth method, shown in Fig. 10-49, does not require tying the suture and takes advantage of the stiffness of

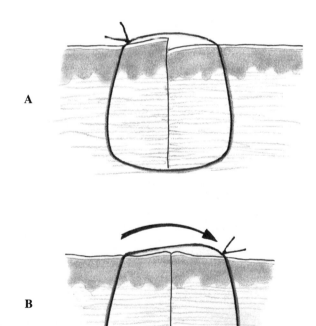

Fig. 10-46. Shifting knot of suture to even up epidermal wound edges.

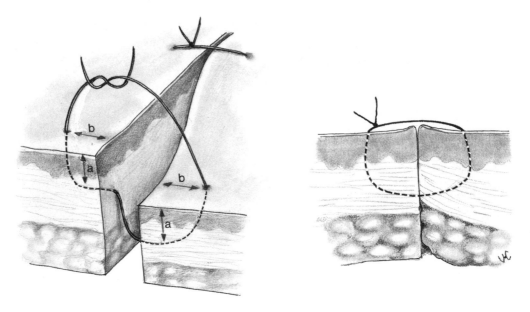

Fig. 10-47. High-on-high side–low-on-low side method of evening up epidermal wound edges.

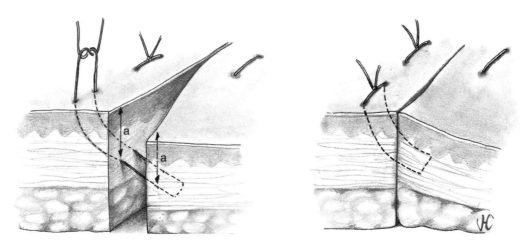

Fig. 10-48. Half-buried horizontal mattress suture used to even up epidermal wound edges.

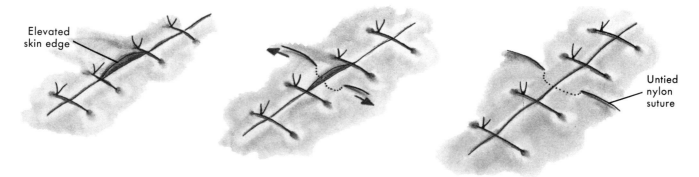

Fig. 10-49. Untied nylon suture used to even up epidermal wound edges.

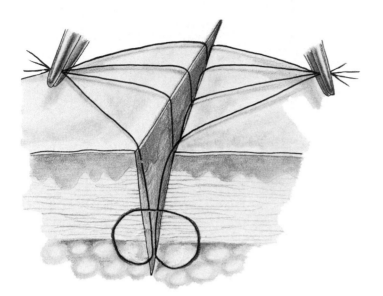

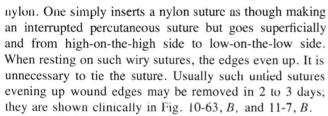

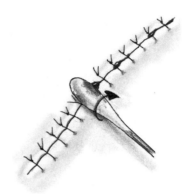

Fig. 10-50. Placement but delayed tying of dermal-subdermal sutures. Sutures are held together at sides of wound by hemostatic forceps.

Fig. 10-51. Expressing blood from wound by means of cotton-tipped applicator. This should be performed before application of dressing.

nylon. One simply inserts a nylon suture as though making an interrupted percutaneous suture but goes superficially and from high-on-the-high side to low-on-the-low side. When resting on such wiry sutures, the edges even up. It is unnecessary to tie the suture. Usually such untied sutures evening up wound edges may be removed in 2 to 3 days; they are shown clinically in Fig. 10-63, *B,* and 11-7, *B.*

Some authors advise taking unequal bites to even up wound edges[108,120]; however, this method is not geometrically sound. It is important to understand that the surface of the wound on each side must be the same distance from the point at which the suture crosses the incision (Fig. 10-47). When the suture is pulled tight, the edges even up.

Which of the four methods to use for evening up epidermal wound edges is determined by the degree of vertical malalignment of the epidermal edges and the forces from below holding one edge lower than the other. If the epidermal edges are apposed but slightly malaligned vertically, a simple method like an untied suture may be all that is necessary. If one epidermal edge is bound down firmly and far below the other, then a more secure method is used, such as the half-buried horizontal mattress suture.

Insufficient space to place buried sutures

Sometimes when burying sutures, especially dermal or dermal-subdermal sutures in a long wound, one closes the deep wound a suture at a time and gets to a point where one cannot place any further sutures because the space remaining is too small—even though more sutures may be required to coapt the wound edges fully. This problem can be circumvented by putting the suture loops in place but not tying them until all the sutures are ready[2] (Fig. 10-50). The

strands from the individual sutures may be placed to the side in a hemostat to keep them from getting tangled. When all the sutures are in place, they can be tied one at a time.

Buried dermal sutures do not appose wound edges

This again is a common problem for the novice. Dermal sutures do not appose wound edges because the lateral portion of the dermal loop is not wide enough. Placing it wider usually results in coaptation of the wound edges. However, placing the dermal buried sutures too far laterally may cause a dimpling in the skin, so one must find a compromise distance from the wound edges.

AFTERCARE OF THE WOUND

The aftercare of the sutured wound is just as important as the planning and closure.[44] Aftercare includes preparing the wound for the dressing, application of the dressing, and instructions to the patient regarding care of the wound.

Preparation of the wound for dressing

The wound and surrounding skin are cleansed of blood and other debris. For this purpose I use hydrogen peroxide, although saline can also be used. One should be careful to remove any clots or hair caught in the sutures or wound. A cotton-tipped applicator is rolled with pressure over the incision to express any blood that may have settled in the wound (Fig. 10-51). Should a continuous blood flow be noticed coming between the sutures, steady pressure should be applied for 5 to 10 minutes. If the bleeding continues after the pressure, the wound should be opened and explored for the source of bleeding, and the bleeding stopped appropriately.

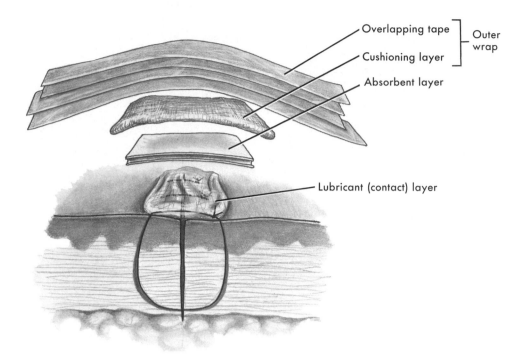

Fig. 10-52. Anatomy of dressing. For purposes of illustration, overlying tape is placed perpendicular rather than parallel to length of wound.

If the dressing is to be left in place for more than a day, a tacky substance may be placed on the skin to help the dressing adhere more securely. Either compound tincture of benzoin or Mastisol (Ferndale Laboratories, Inc., 780 West Eight Mile Road, Ferndale, Michigan 48220) may be used. The skin is first degreased with an organic solvent (ether or adhesive tape remover). It is important that the tacky substance be kept out of the wound, since it may be harmful to wound healing and potentiate infection.[107]

There have been occasional reports of contact dermatitis from compound tincture of benzoin used to secure dressings.[134] This compound contains many chemicals of plant origin including benzoin, storax, tolu balsam, and aloes in alcohol. Steiner and Leifer showed that once a patient was sensitized to the benzoin portion of this compound, sensitization occurred to storax as well.[134] Mastisol contains storax and gum mastic. Therefore one probably cannot use Mastisol on those sensitized to compound tincture of benzoin because cross reactions will occur.[71] Whether Mastisol is less sensitizing than compound tincture of benzoin is unknown; however, it does contain fewer sensitizing agents. For patients sensitized to tincture of benzoin, Coskey recommends the use of a tape adherent composed of abietic anhydride, para-chloro-metaxylenol, and chlorinated solvents.[27]

Dressings

The purposes of a wound dressing are many. Dressings serves to protect the wound from contaminants and the outside environment. Properly applied, dressings main-

tain some pressure on the wound, helping to minimize bleeding, edema, and potential dead space. Dressings assist in taking tension off the wound edges; they also cusion the wound from extraneous trauma and help to restrict motion in the area of the wound. The last function serves to place the wound at rest, which promotes better wound healing without problems.[118]

The anatomy of a typical dressing is shown in Fig. 10-52, and a clinical example is in Fig. 10-53. As can be seen there are a number of layers, each with a specific function. A thin layer of sterile petrolatum (usually an antibiotic ointment) is first applied to the wound so that moisture is maintained and the overlying layers are less likely to stick. A porous contact layer of nonadherent material is used, followed by an absorbent layer. Vaseline gauze may be used for the porous layer and plain gauze or eye pads for the absorbent layer. Eye pads are particularly useful because they serve the dual purpose of being absorbent and cushioning the wound. Nonadherent Telfa or Release pads may also be used in place of Vaseline gauze and the absorbent layer. One problem with these nonadherent pads is that they are thin, should there be considerable oozing from a wound, they become quickly saturated. In addition, as the blood or exudate dries, these nonadherent pads may stick slightly to the wound. A cushioning layer is added, either an eye pad or more gauze (fluffed or unfluffed); finally tape a layer is added. I almost exclusively use paper tape because it is less irritating and has been shown to help minimize the growth of bacteria by its relatively nonocclusive properties.[90] It is important always to cut neatly the ends of the tape, since the

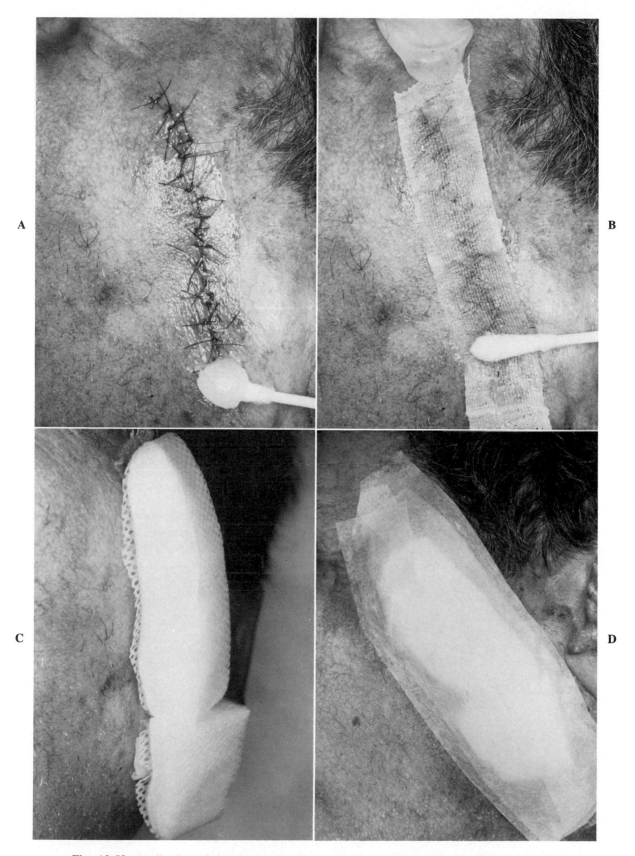

Fig. 10-53. Application of dressing to wound. **A,** Antibiotic ointment. **B,** Vaseline gauze. **C,** Eyepad cut to cover wound. **D,** Overlapping tape.

Continued.

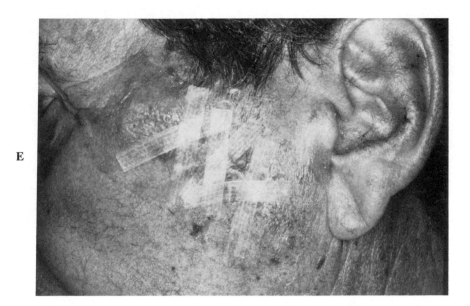

E

Fig. 10-53, cont'd. E, Reinforcement of wound with skin closure tapes subsequent to suture removal 5 days later.

tape is what the patient sees. How neatly the tape is cut and applied is perceived as a reflection of the neatness of the job underneath the tape. The tape is overlapped and is usually placed parallel to the underlying wound.

Some materials used in dressings perform more than one function, and therefore the actual number of layers that comprise a dressing may change with the material used. Thus a dressing is comprised of a number of layers that provide the functions shown in Fig. 10-52, yet not necessarily in the same number of layers. For instance, an eye pad within a dressing functions as both an absorbent and a cushioning layer to the wound (Fig. 10-53, *C*). Because this one material provides both of these dressing functions, an additional cushioning layer might not be necessary. A more complete discussion of dressings is found in Chapter 9.

It should be noted in passing that at the turn of the century, collodion was used as a hermetic seal for wounds.[89] It helped to keep bacteria out and may have speeded up epidermization. In an interesting study the use of collodion painted on wounds in mice resulted in a lower incidence of infection than that in wounds where it was not used.[135] Other substances, such as gutta-percha and foils, were also used with success to seal wounds.[60] Such substances should probably be reexamined in light of our current knowledge about wound healing.

Prophylactic antibiotics

The use of prophylactic antibiotics for simple excisional surgery is discouraged. This subject is discussed at some length in Chapter 4. Antibiotics should not be used to cover up poor surgical technique; nevertheless under certain circumstances use of prophylactic antibiotics may be justifi-

able. Such circumstances include obviously contaminated wounds, poor host defenses, or remote preexisting infection. Because of the poor vascular supply on the lower extremities, wounds in this location are more likely to become infected, and therefore prophylactic antibiotics may be useful.

I usually start prophylactic antibiotics while the patient is still in the office or clinic, within at least a few minutes of the completion of surgery. If possible, beginning the antibiotic administration before surgery is even better. I have found it convenient to keep in the office a supply of erythromycin, Keflex, and tetracycline to give to the patient orally; if one gives the patient a prescription, it may be hours before it is filled. It has been determined that for prophylactic antibiotics to work, they must be instituted within a few hours of the surgery.

Immediate postoperative instructions

Written postoperative instructions should be given to all patients, which include the supplies necessary for the patient to buy, the time for dressing changes, and a telephone number by which a physician can be contacted. Patients frequently do not or cannot concentrate well enough after surgery to understand completely how to make dressing changes. Having *simple* written instructions minimizes telephone calls and increases the chances of an uneventful postoperative course. A sample postoperative dressing instruction sheet is found in Appendix D.

Postoperative medications are usually unnecessary but may be useful when surgery has been extensive. Usually Tylenol or Tylenol 3 (containing ½ grain of codeine) is sufficient. Aspirin or aspirin-containing products should be avoided because they interfere with platelet adherence and thus increase the probability of extensive postoperative bleeding. The newer nonsteroidal antiinflammatory medications may cause a prolonged bleeding time. When surgery has been performed on an extremity, elevation of it helps to decrease pain.

Usually I have patients or their families remove the dressing 24 hours after surgery and cleanse the wound gently with hydrogen peroxide on cotton-tipped applicator sticks. The wound is then dried with gauze, and a fresh dressing is applied. The dressing to be placed by the patient is simpler than that applied in the office, usually consisting of an antibiotic ointment, Telfa, gauze, and paper tape. It is normally necessary for the patient to change the dressing only once a day, assuming that no unusual drainage is occurring.

Patients should be instructed to contact the physician or the physician's staff if excessive bleeding, redness, swelling, or fever occurs. With wounds of the head or neck, patients may usually get their wounds wet and may shampoo or shower the day after surgery.

The length of time a dressing should be left in place after surgery until the first dressing change is a matter of surgical experience. In 1933 the sutured wounds of guinea pigs were inoculated with bacteria at various time intervals following closure. Within the first 6 to 12 hours the wounds were most susceptible to infection.[37] After that period of time there was a steady decrease in the incidence of wound infection over 5 days. After 5 days sutured wounds could not be infected by bacterial inoculation of their surface. These experiments led to the practice of keeping all wounds covered for 5 to 7 days after surgery. In another study similar experiments to these were performed, but in rabbits.[62] Those investigators, however, found that sutured wounds exposed to bacteria 1 hour after closure do not become infected and concluded that dressings are unnecessary after that time to protect wounds from microbes.

Practical experience has shown that beginning dressing changes after 24 hours does not seem to affect the incidence of wound infection or other problems. Philosophically it is advantageous to enlist the patient in the care of his or her wound. Problems with wounds usually occur when the patient is noncompliant. Patients should be told to protect the wound by keeping a dressing on and not traumatizing the area. Strenuous physical activity affecting the wound area should be avoided for 2 weeks after surgery

An exception to beginning dressing changes after the first 24 hours is for wounds on the extremities, particularly the digits. In these locations I prefer to allow the dressing to remain for 2 to 3 days and then to perform the initial dressing change myself during the first week, because the incidence of infection is higher in these areas than it is in other areas.

The proper method for removing dressings is shown in Fig. 10-54. Note that the final layer is removed along the

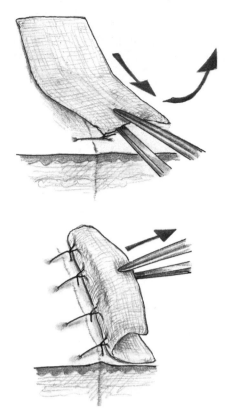

Fig. 10-54. Proper *(top)* and improper *(bottom)* method of dressing removal.

length and not across the wound. Should the sutures adhere to the dressing, pulling it across the wound tends to reopen the wound.

SUTURE REMOVAL

In his classic paper on wound healing, Reid remarks that a frequent question asked by students is, "When should skin sutures be removed?"[118] Those with much experience in the healing of wounds know that there is no set formula for suture removal; it depends on the progress of wound healing. The physicians with little experience are frustrated by having no clearly established routine. Reid goes on to stress that routines of wound care and thoughtlessness or ignorance of wound healing go hand in hand.

Time for removal

The proper time to remove percutaneous sutures is as soon as the wound has healed to a point at which removal would not result in dehiscence. This depends on the anatomic location, amount of wound tension, and presence of buried sutures. In places where the dermis is thin and supplied by a good vasculature, such as on the eyelids, sutures can be removed safely as early as 2 to 3 days. Where the dermis is thick and under considerable tension, such as on the back, sutures should be left longer, from 8 to 12 days

TIMETABLE FOR INTERRUPTED PERCUTANEOUS SUTURE REMOVAL

Scalp	5 to 6 days
Eyelid	2 to 3 days
Face	3 to 6 days
Neck	5 to 7 days
Trunk (anterior)	7 to 10 days
Trunk (posterior)	7 to 12 days
Extremities	7 to 14 days

(see box above). Other variables concerning wound healing that should be taken into consideration include the patient's age, medical condition, infection, and type of wound.

Usually I see the patient back for suture removal in from 5 to 7 days, depending on where the wound is and other variables, such as the patient's schedule. Although I may want to see the wound to remove sutures in 5 days, this may fall on a Sunday and it becomes necessary to wait until Monday. Usually waiting an extra day or two makes little difference, unless this extends beyond a week—all patients should be seen within a week.

When removing sutures early, within 2 to 5 days, I begin by removing every other or every third suture. If the wound appears slightly unstable, I stop and have the patient return in a few days, when the wound is more completely healed. If the wound appears well healed, I remove all the sutures. If the wound is well healed but under considerable tension, I may remove most of the sutures but leave one or two sutures for removal within a few days.

As a general rule one should remove skin sutures as early as possible. Most of the literature agrees that 7 days seems to be the critical time. Sutures removed before 7 days are less painful to remove, result in less obvious suture marks,[30] and are less likely to interfere with wound healing. In fact, sutures removed in less than 4 days result in wounds with greater tensile strength than wounds over which sutures remained longer.[18,99] Sutures remaining for more than 7 days delay wound healing,[17] result in higher infection rates,[10] and are more likely to cause suture tracks.[30]

Based on histologic examination of sutured guinea pig wounds the authors of one study recommended suture removal at no earlier than 6 days but no later than 10 days.[105] That study showed *complete* epidermization of suture tracts in 8 to 12 days.[104] However, from the time the suture is initially placed the surface epidermis and the epidermis from transected appendages grow perisuturally along the suture tract. Extrapolation of these data to man should be made cautiously.

In an interesting 1959 study an investigator removed cutaneous sutures the day after surgery in 200 general surgical cases.[123] The wounds were then reinforced with butterfly bandages. A comparable number of similar cases was also studied, and the sutures were left in place for the recommended time (about 1 week). When the sutures were removed the day after surgery, there were no dehiscences and no infections; the cosmetic results were also better. In contrast, when the sutures were left in place longer, 10% of the patients developed stitch abscesses, and 2% of patients had deep wound infections.

Technique for removal of sutures

Before the removal of sutures, the wound should be cleansed gently with hydrogen peroxide or sterile saline to remove dried blood or exudate. One method for cutting sutures before removal is shown in Fig. 10-55. The suture is lifted slightly with forceps by one of the tails, and a No. 11 scalpel blade is placed under the knot. A quick but gentle flick of the blade toward the operator is sufficient to cut the suture (Fig. 10-56, *left*). Note that the hand holding the scalpel blade is steadied on the skin, giving the operator more control over the position of the blade tip. After the suture is cut, it is then pulled *across* the wound (Fig. 10-56, *right*). Pulling the suture in the opposite direction to that shown puts tension on the wound edges and could result in dehiscence.

Other instruments can be used to cut the sutures. Stitch-removal scissors are specifically designed for this purpose. My experience is that these scissors are slightly large at their tips for small percutaneous sutures. Fine, extra-delicate iris scissors are ideal. Their tips are so small that they can easily get under even the smallest suture loop.

It should be noted that a percutaneous suture loop has most of the loop buried under the skin surface, but a small portion is exposed to the environment. This latter part of the loop is subject to contamination; therefore one should try to keep from pulling this portion of the suture through the suture tract where it may contaminate the wound. When one lifts gently on the tail to cut under the knot (Fig. 10-55 and 10-56), one exposes a small area of the suture that is "clean" because it had been sitting beneath the skin surface.[3] Cutting this clean end and dragging it through the wound minimizes any chance of contamination.

As an alternative, one may cut the suture at the side of the wound opposite the knot, where it exits from the skin. Pulling the suture through the wound from that point also pulls clean suture through. Personally, I prefer to cut underneath the knot because it is easier to get an instrument under the loop by pulling the tail to lift the knot.

An exception to the foregoing guidelines on suture removal occurs when a small suture abscess exists at one of the two points of suture exit from the skin. When this happens, cut the suture at the skin edge opposite the abscess and pull the clean suture toward the abscess. Pulling the suture in the opposite direction serves only to contaminate the wound.

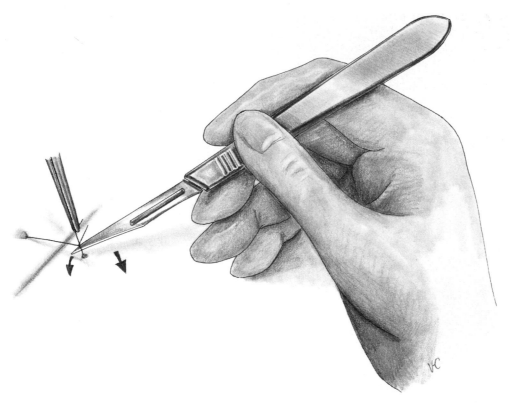

Fig. 10-55. Technique for cutting sutures to be removed with use of No. 11 scalpel blade.

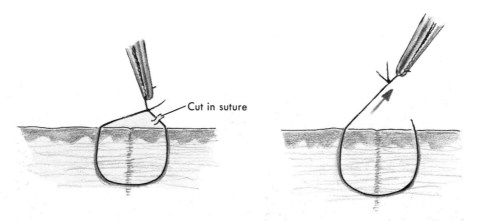

Fig. 10-56. Location for cutting suture *(left)* and direction to pull suture for removal *(right)*. Pull *across* wound, not away from wound.

Resistance to suture removal

The longer the sutures have been in place, the more difficult they are to remove—that is, the more force it takes to pull the suture through the suture tract. This resistance to withdrawal is caused by the interaction taking place between sutures and the surrounding tissues. An epithelial sleeve grows down the suture tract, surrounding the suture and sometimes adhering to it. On withdrawal of a suture, a perisutured sleeve may be present and grossly seen.

At the points of perforation through the skin a crust is formed, which adheres to the suture extending from the epidermis. Approximately 70% to 85% of the work of withdrawal is caused by the tissue interactions at the points of perforation of the skin.[66] Therefore there are at least two reasons for existence of a measurable force resisting the withdrawal of sutures.

In a calculation of the withdrawal work for various sutures at 1 week, silk had the highest amount, Prolene had the lowest, and nylon was intermediate.[47] Because it is multifilamentous, silk invites tissue encrustation. The concerns

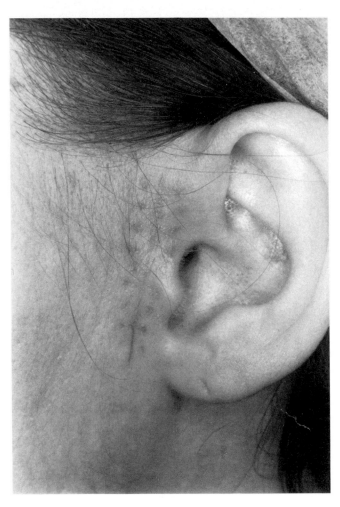

Fig. 10-57. Suture marks on preauricular area.

that patients have about the pain of suture removal are usually based on memories of the resistance encountered when silk sutures were used routinely.

The newer monofilamentous sutures are less likely to cause such tissue interactions and therefore are much less painful to remove. Rarely is there any noticeable resistance to removal of nylon or polypropylene sutures. One interesting idea is that sutures should be cut one day and removed the next.[8] This gives time for the tissues to relax and accommodate. Removing sutures in this manner supposedly causes less pain for very apprehensive patients.

Origin of suture marks

Although there are several reasons for the presence of cutaneous suture marks and "tracks" (Figs. 10-57 and 10-58), the most common cause is leaving the sutures in the skin for a long time. In a study of 6 patients who were sutured on the trunk, no suture marks appeared if the sutures were removed at or before 7 days.[30] On the other hand, if the sutures were removed at 14 days, suture marks were invariably present. This was found to be true regardless of suture size. Apparently, greater epidermization of the suture tracts occurs with time, leading to more pronounced scarring at the site of sutures.[86]

As a corollary to the ever-present epidermization of suture tracts, in places where the skin contains an abundance of well-developed adnexal structures (such as in markedly porous skin), suture marks are more likely because of the ready epidermization of suture tracts from the inevitably transected follicular structures in this type of skin.

A suture tract is a covert cutaneous incision.[104] All such incisions end in scars. Therefore whatever enlarges scars

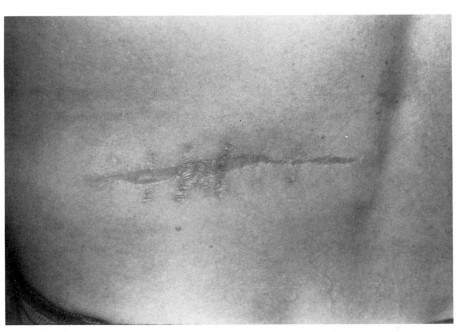

Fig. 10-58. Suture "track" on lower back.

also makes suture marks more visible. On removal of the sutures these tracts fibrose like any other incisional wound.

An important factor in the production of suture marks is tension. This may result from extrinsic factors, such as inherent tension in surrounding tissues, and/or intrinsic fac-

tors, such as sutures being tied too tightly.[30,31] Figs. 10-59 and 10-60 show examples of poor suture technique caused by unnecessary tension. Sutures that are pulled too tightly tend to tear through tissues. The skin intervening between tightly tied sutures tends to evert and pucker, producing

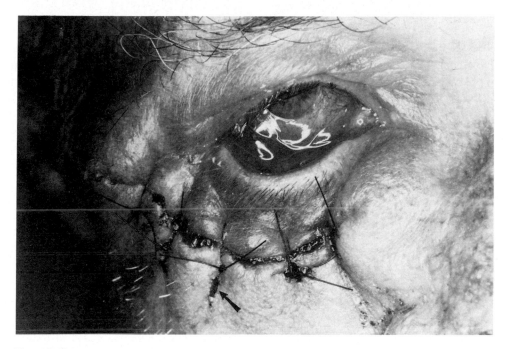

Fig. 10-59. Extreme example of tension on wound sutured closed because referring physician erroneously believed patient was better off with wound closed even if only temporarily. Note tearing of tissue *(arrow)* by suture and ectropion with chemosis of conjunctiva.

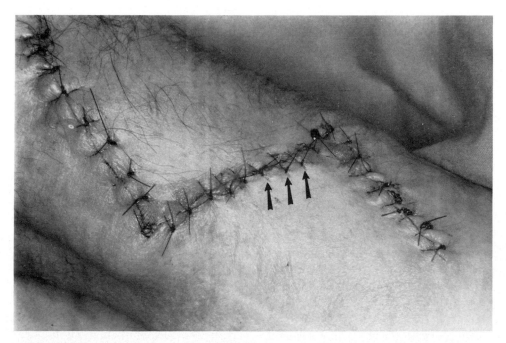

Fig. 10-60. Poor suturing technique on arm. Tension on wound edges produces bunching of skin, or "fish-mouthing," of wound edges between sutures and some tearing of tissue by sutures *(arrows)*.

''fish-mouthing.'' Sometimes edema in a wound forces a suture through the tissue, producing small tears. Such tears go on to produce scars, seen as suture tracks. Even if perceptible tears do not occur in the tissue, too much tension can produce inapparent necrosis.[98] As the devitalized tissue is sloughed, it is replaced by scar tissue.

Some types of suture are more prone to produce suture marks. Silk, which has little elasticity and only rare knot slippage, tends to strangulate swelling tissue. Nylon, because of its high tensile strength, tends to cut through swollen tissue. Polypropylene, on the other hand, stretches with tissue swelling and stays stretched when the swelling subsides, leading to less chance of suture marks; however, the wound edges may not stay tightly coapted.

Other factors associated with the production of suture marks include improper placement of sutures (producing inversion on wound edges) and factors within the patient, such as a predisposition to keloids.

Infected wounds and sutures

Sutures in wounds that subsequently become infected are a special problem. Such sutures should be immediately removed, since they act as a nidus for persistence of the infection. If the sutures are far enough away from the point of wound infection and they appear to be holding the tissues together, one may consider leaving them and reassessing the wound again within a short period of time (1 to 2 days). Usually, however, leaving such sutures adds very little to the already lowered tensile strength of the wound.

REINFORCEMENT OF THE WOUND

After removal of sutures the wound and surrounding tissue are again gently cleared of all crusts and debris. The wound is then reinforced with cutaneous wound-closure skin tapes (Fig. 10-53, *E*). The surrounding skin is degreased first with an organic solvent (such as tape remover), followed by application of a tacky substance (such as compound tincture of benzoin), followed by application of skin tapes. Patients are instructed to leave the tapes in place and let them fall off by themselves, which usually occurs in 1 week. This requires keeping the wound area dry, since water loosens skin tapes. Continuous reinforcement of wounds for 1 to 2 weeks after suture removal is essential. Young wounds only a few days to a week in age do not have enough strength to withstand minor trauma or the forces that normally occur in the area from regular activity.

Some physicians recommend the use of regular paper tape for immediate reinforcement of the wound because of the much decreased cost of this material compared to products specially made for taping wounds (such as Steri-Strips). My own preference is to use the specially made products because of their sterility and superior design for this purpose (skin-closure tapes are reinforced).

Some physicians recommend that wounds be continu-

ously reinforced for many months with tape.[56,130] This is said to result in less conspicuous scars. I have no experience with this, and the medical literature does not address it specifically.

FUTURE CARE AND EVOLUTION OF THE WOUND

A healed surgical wound is a scar that goes through an evolution of healing in several phases that take months to years. Patients need to be told what to expect. Scars are the most unsightly within the first month or two after the sutures are removed because of increased vascularity and collagen deposition. Initially scars are erythematous but with time (6 months to a year) become less red as the neovascularization becomes less. Sometimes scars become pruritic and hypertrophic. These events also usually become better in time. Scar maturation takes about 1 or even 2 years. Patients need to be reassured that the appearance of scars will probably improve with time. Occasionally scars spread. Many of these problems are discussed in Chapter 13. Patients with large scars should be seen at intervals to evaluate the progress of healing and to offer reassurance if necessary. Time is almost always the best treatment of scars.

EXAMPLES OF EXCISIONS AND CLOSURES

Although most carefully planned excisions are straightforward and simple, each area of the body has certain peculiarities that I have personally found to need careful consideration. The following summarizes my own experience in these areas.

Scalp

The scalp is very vascular, and for that reason excisions in this area tend to be bloody. Excisions should follow the course of nerves and blood vessels, which in general run vertically in the scalp. The MaxSTLs in the scalp are of little consequence, since the forces of tension are almost as great in one direction as in another. Even with extensive undermining, the skin has little stretch because of the extensive fibrous network in the subcutaneous tissue. Therefore linear excisions in the scalp are limited in size. If undermining is done, it should be beneath the hair follicles or, if necessary, below the galea. One may need to incise the galea from below to get more mobility,[93,133] but in my experience this is of limited value, because the basic problem is that the fibrous tissue component of the scalp above the galea just does not allow the skin to stretch like it does elsewhere.

Forehead

The forehead is one of the easiest areas on which to perform a fusiform or tangent-to-circle excision. Usually such excisions are oriented parallel to the primary crease lines so that the ultimate scar is well camouflaged.

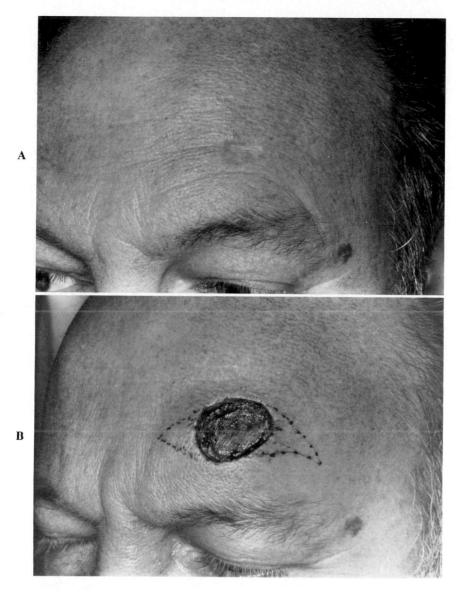

Fig. 10-61. Excision and closure of basal cell carcinoma of forehead. **A,** Preoperative. **B,** Wound immediately after excision of tumor with planned repair.

Continued.

The biggest mistake made in repairing lesions on the forehead is failing to make a fusiform or tangent-to-circle excision. A fairly large amount of tissue may be removed in this area, and the wound closed in a linear manner. Fig. 10-61 shows the results of a modified fusiform excision performed after extirpation of a basal cell carcinoma. Note that the fusiform excision is modified slightly (Fig. 10-61, *B*), so that the final scar fits nicely into the crease lines. The resultant surgical scar (Fig. 10-61, *C*) is hardly apparent 1 year later. On a full-face view (Fig. 10-61, *D*) one can see that there is no elevation of the eyebrow; one can also see that the scar is not noticeably spread, even after many months.

There is an alternative procedure that can be chosen to close defects on the forehead like that in Fig. 10-61, *B:* skin flaps, which would entail other incisions (whose resultant scars with time might become very apparent). Therefore one should do the simplest possible closure that will result in the fewest possible incisions.

If the eyebrow is elevated after suturing above it, it almost always comes down in time (from 2 to 6 months) without significant spreading of the scar. This is because the muscles depressing the eyebrow are relatively strong and produce a good counter force.

Occasionally the long axis of a lesion in the forehead is perpendicular to the crease lines. If this occurs in the central forehead, the wound can be sutured directly. Perpendicular excisions in the central forehead hardly spread at all

C

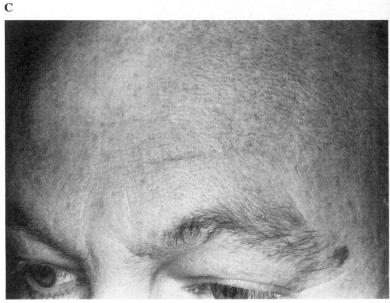

D

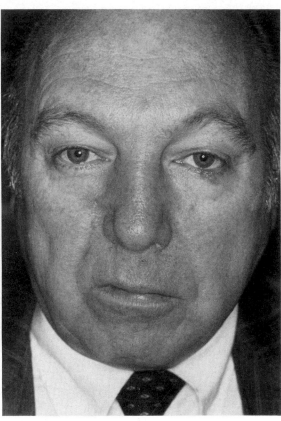

Fig. 10-61, cont'd. C, Scar 1 year later. **D,** Full-face view 1 year later.

because the two frontalis muscle bellies are not completely joined together underneath, leaving a virtual void of underlying musculature in this area.

A potential problem with excisions on the forehead is anesthesia from transection of the underlying nerves. If excisions are carried down to the muscle fascia, there is a good chance that the supratrochlear or supraorbital nerves will be severed. The patient would then experience a loss of sensation superior to this area. Usually this loss of sensation recedes at least partially within 2 years. Keeping the number of incisions to a minimum lowers the probability of such sensory nerve damage.

Temple

Excisions in the temple should follow the wrinkle lines radiating out around the eyes as seen when the patient squints. Examples of closures in this area are shown in Figs. 11-5, 11-6, and 11-7.

A danger zone is discussed in Chapter 3 (see Fig. 3-17). It extends about 2 cm above the lateral eyebrow and laterally to the anterior temporal hairline. There the temporal branch of the facial nerve courses in the subcutaneous tissue above the muscle. Excisions in this area should be superficial, and undermining, if done, should be performed gently and carefully to prevent nerve damage.

Periorbital area

Excisions on the upper eyelid follow the pretarsal crease. In this area fairly large amounts of tissue may be removed without compromising the patient's ability to close the eye.

The problem area in the periorbital region is the lower eyelid, where—regardless of the direction in which the lesion lies—the direction of closure should be parallel to the lower eyelid (Fig. 10-62). The surgical defect shown in Fig. 10-62, *A,* can be closed either with a full-thickness skin graft or directly. The arrow indicates the proper direction of closure. To accomplish this, the first sutures pull the skin medially and parallel to the lower eyelid. Dog-ears are removed superiorly and inferiorly. Note that with full wound closure (Fig. 10-62, *B*), there appears to be a slight ectropion, but this was caused by swelling of tissue from infiltration of local anesthesia. The final healed result (Fig. 10-62, *C*) shows an imperceptible scar and an excellent cosmetic result.

Surgical defects that occur partially over the medial orbital rim or slightly into the inner canthal region should be closed with the same principle of going parallel to the lower eyelid. Fig. 10-63 shows closure of such a defect. Note the direction of closure, as indicated by the arrow. This closure was made with the first few sutures (in this case, buried absorbable sutures) being placed in a horizontal position.

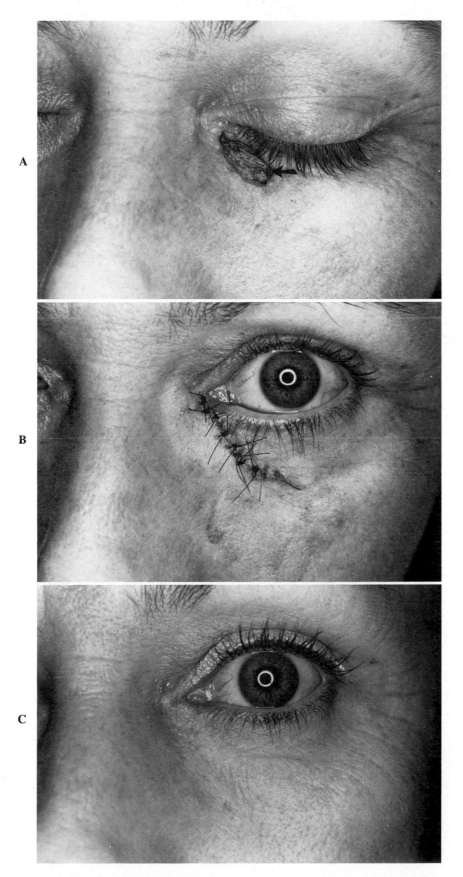

Fig. 10-62. Closure of surgical defect on lower eyelid. **A,** Surgical defect. Arrow indicates direction of closure, horizontal and parallel to lower eyelid. **B,** Sutured wound with slight ectropion caused by anesthesia. **C,** Healed result.

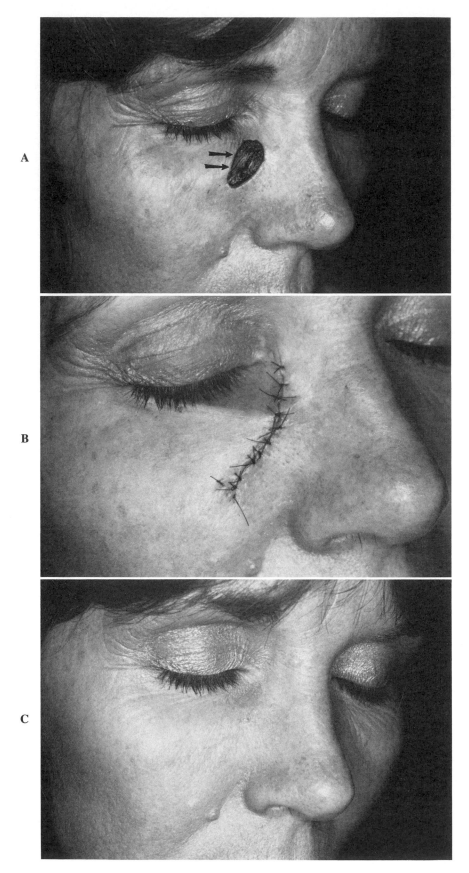

Fig. 10-63. For legend see opposite page.

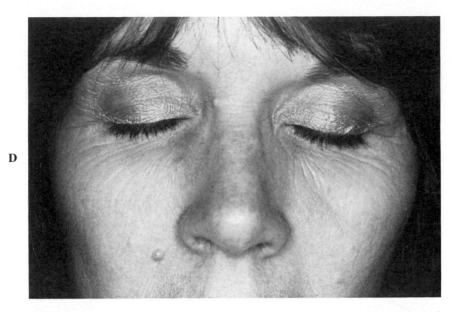

Fig. 10-63, cont'd. Closure of surgical defect on side of nose toward inner canthal area. **A,** Surgical defect. Arrows indicate direction of closure. **B,** Closure in horizontal direction. **C,** Final healed result. **D,** Full-face view 2 years postoperatively.

Dog-ears were then removed superiorly and inferiorly. Note that on Fig. 10-63, *B,* the last inferior suture is not tied. This suture is placed simply to even up the skin edges and is unnecessary to tie. Note also the extreme medial horizontal tension shown by the medially directed folds of skin from the lower eyelid toward the wound. With time, the scar is almost imperceptible (Fig. 10-63, *C*), and the tension on the eyelid settles out. On frontal view (Fig. 10-63, *D*) there is no tenting in the medial canthal area.

The horizontal closure in Fig. 10-63 has a very important consequence, which is not readily apparent. If an oblique wound is sutured horizontally, dog-ears are maximized at each end (see Fig. 12-15). They are repaired in the standard manner. The production of dog-ears at the ends of excisions and their repair, however, effectally lengthens scars. This lengthening is critical in areas where a shortened band of tissue is noticeable on scar contraction; it tents the skin over concave surfaces such as the inner canthus, or constricts over convex surfaces such as the malar eminence or arm. This is discussed in greater detail in Chapter 12.

If wounds such as that shown in Fig. 10-63, *A,* are closed in a simple, direct side-to-side manner rather than horizontally, an extracanthal fold results from shortening of the medial canthal tissue with scar contracture. In Fig. 10-64, *A* and *B,* the directional forces of wound closure were in a simple side-to-side manner *(upper closed arrows)* rather than horizontally directed *(lower open arrows).* The resultant scar contracted, leaving an extracanthal fold (Fig. 10-64, *C* and *D*). Therefore around the lower eyelids, the directonal forces of closure are critical.

To correct the extracanthal fold in Fig. 10-64, *C* and *D,* a

V-to-Y incision was made (Fig. 10-64, *E*). The flap of skin created by making incisions on each side of the band of tissue was advanced superiorly, in effect, lengthening the scar. The resultant surgical defect at the lower end of the incision was then closed horizontally (Fig. 10-64, *F*), and not side to side (which would have been oblique to the lower eyelid). This in effect also lengthened the incision, but at the lower end. The healed surgical result 2 months later is shown in Fig. 1-64, *G* and *H.*

Nose

It is difficult to achieve a good cosmetic result on the nose with fusiform excisions unless the closures are very small. It has been suggested that large defects on the nose can be closed directly in a side-to-side manner.[95] Fig. 10-65 shows that this does not result in a fine-line scar. To close the wound shown in 10-65, *A,* it was converted into a tangent-to-circle defect and sutured directly (Fig. 10-65, *B*). Even though initially the wound held together, spreading of the scar eventually occurred, resulting in a broad scar (Fig. 10-65, *C*). The broad spread scar that results on the nose is shiny and smooth, and stands out in contrast to the surrounding porous skin; therefore it is not considered an acceptable cosmetic result. The best alternative for repair of the defect in Fig. 10-65, *A,* is performance of a flap procedure.

Cheek

The cheek should be considered as three separate areas that differ in their degree of tension. The medial cheek is relatively loose, and large defects can be closed without a
Text continued on p. 420.

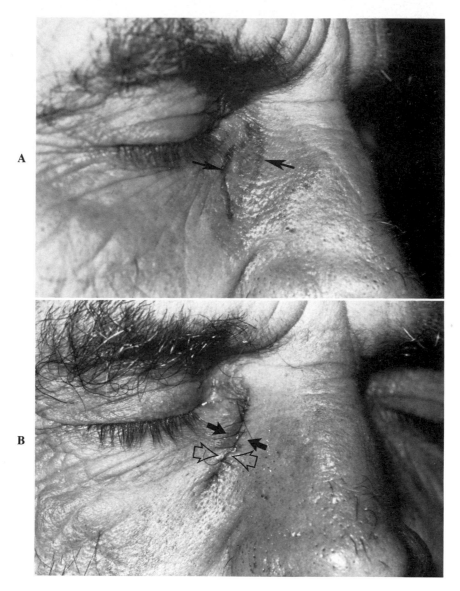

Fig. 10-64. Closure of a wound on side of nose toward inner canthal area. **A,** Surgical lesion to be excised with planned excision size. **B,** Slightly oblique direction of closure *(upper closed arrows).* Proper direction of closure in this area (but not performed) is horizontal *(lower open arrows).* Compare this with the horizontal direction shown in Fig. 10-63, *A.* **C,** and **D,** Healed incision line scar. Note that this has produced extracanthal fold. **E,** V incision at base of canthal band with redirection of incision scar horizontally, as shown by lower open arrow in **B.** This extends incision line inferiorly.

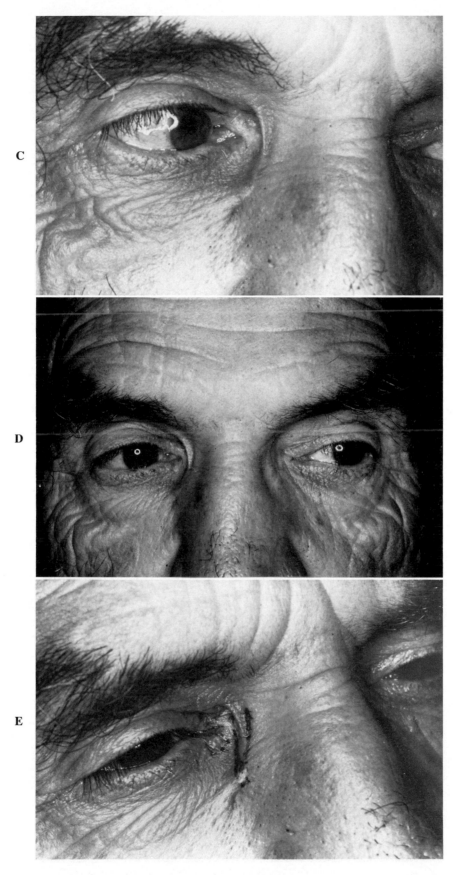

Fig. 10-64. For legend, see opposite page.

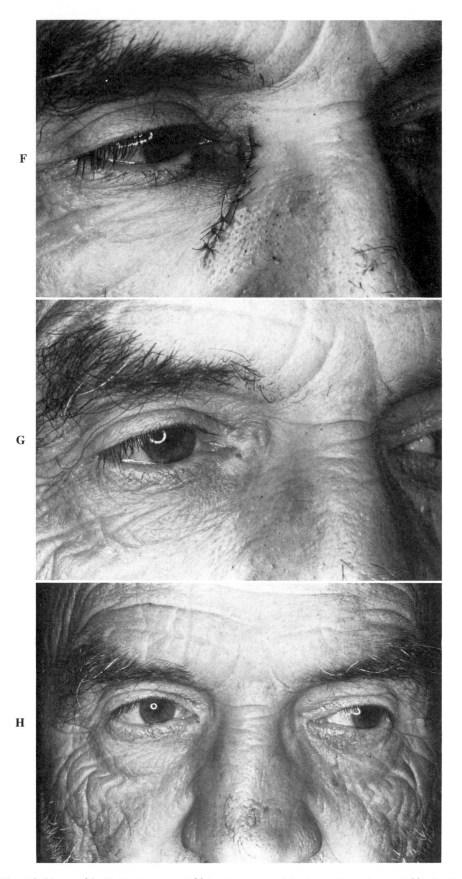

Fig. 10-64, cont'd. F, Production of Y incision sutured horizontally at base of Y. **G,** Healed surgical result at 2 months. **H,** Full-face view at 2 months.

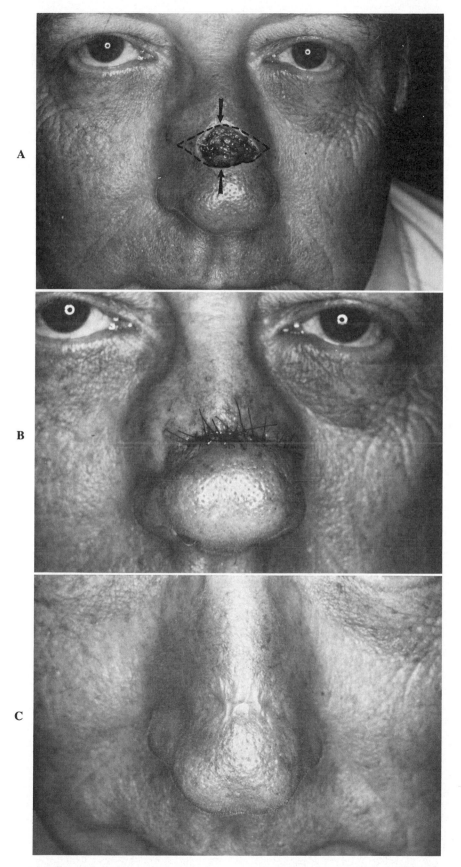

Fig. 10-65. Closure of surgical defect on nose. **A,** Surgical defect subsequent to excision of basal cell carcinoma. Arrows indicate direction of closure. **B,** Defect sutured closed subsequent to excision of lateral tissue converting wound into tangent-to-circle defect. **C,** Healed result 1 year later. Note smooth spread scar.

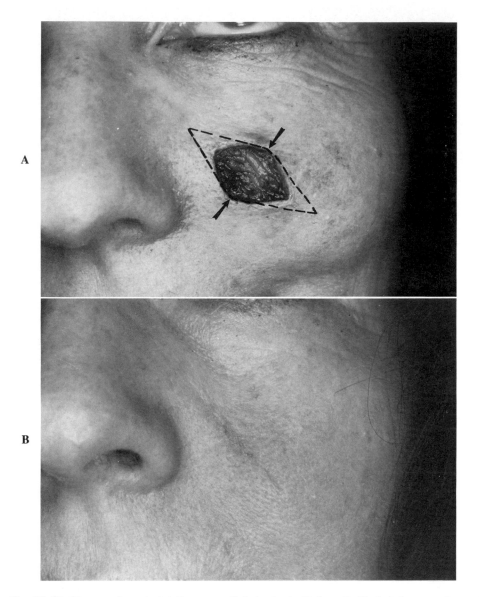

Fig. 10-66. Closure of surgical defect on medial cheek. **A,** Defect. **B,** Healed closure at 1 month. Apparent hyperpigmentation is caused by purple Vicryl.

problem. The buccal cheek also can usually accommodate closure of large lesions, particularly in the elderly. The malar cheek, however, especially over the lateral zygomatic process on some individuals, may be quite tense and result in spreading of scars. This is one area where Langer found triangular rather than slitlike defects produced by his round piercing instrument; in other words, the tension forces in this area are not greater in one direction than another.

A typical closure in the medial cheek is shown in Fig. 10-66. The surrounding tissue was undermined and closed with absorbable suture material. Interestingly, the absorbable suture material in the case shown was purple Vicryl, which at first showed through the wound (Fig. 10-66, *B*). With time, this was absorbed (Fig. 10-66, *C* and *D*). The

cosmetic result is excellent. Because the patient's skin is "nonporous" the smooth scar does not offer any contrast to the smooth skin.

A fusiform wound on the lateral cheek can usually be easily closed where there is abundant loose tissue, especially in the elderly. The sizeable defect shown in Fig. 10-67, *A*, was closed in a linear fashion after undermining and the use of buried dermal sutures (Fig. 10-67, *B*). The cosmetic result is excellent (Fig. 10-67, *C*), with the scar blending in nicely with the other wrinkle lines on the face. One could have considered a more complex type of closure on this wound, such as a flap; however, skin flaps require more incisions, which ultimately become scars. The pattern of such scars is usually not hidden by wrinkle lines.

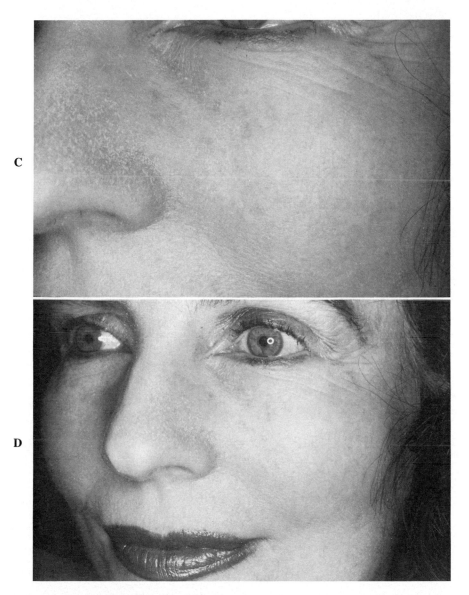

Fig. 10-66, cont'd. C and **D,** Final result 2 years later.

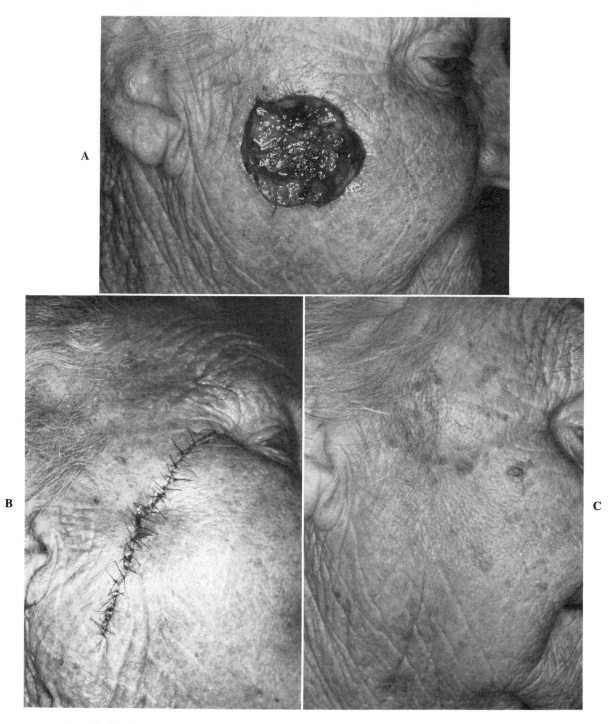

Fig. 10-67. Closure of large surgical defect on lateral cheek in elderly woman. **A,** Defect. **B,** Closure in linear fashion. **C,** Healed result at 1 year.

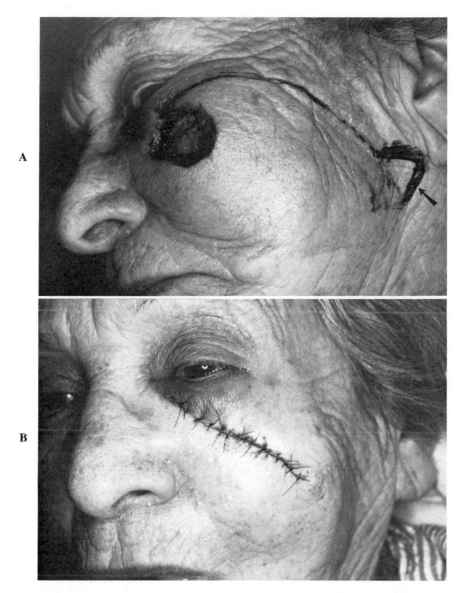

Fig. 10-68. Closure of surgical defect on anterior cheek in elderly woman. **A,** Defect with contemplated rotation cutaneous flap and Burow's triangle marked on patient's skin *(arrow)*. **B,** Closure in linear fashion instead of skin flap.

Continued.

If this patient had been younger, without an abundance of loose tissue, a skin flap would have been strongly considered.

Another variable to be considered on cheek closures is the thickness of the dermis. If the epidermis is porous, the underlying dermis is usually thicker and less stretchable. If the epidermis is smooth, the dermis is thinner, and is usually the case in elderly women (Fig. 10-67, *A*), the skin can be more easily stretched. In the patients with thicker dermis, skin flaps may be preferable.

The concept that one should do the simplest possible closure is highlighted in Fig. 10-68. The surgical defect in Fig. 10-68, *A,* was situated on the mid anterior cheek. A

contemplated flap was designed in anticipation of closure; however, it was decided to rethink the closure in terms of the simplest method, which was a linear closure. Thus the wound was closed side to side with elimination of dog-ears (Fig. 10-68, *B*). The resultant scar fits in well with the patient's wrinkles (Fig. 10-68, *C* and *D*). Closure of the wound in this manner prevented longer incisions in the patient's face and mobilization of large amounts of tissue. Note, however, that there is a slight bandlike constriction over this convex surface of the face with such a closure.

The malar prominence can be a problem area for large fusiform excisions. An example of a relatively small wound that when closed had a good cosmetic result is shown in

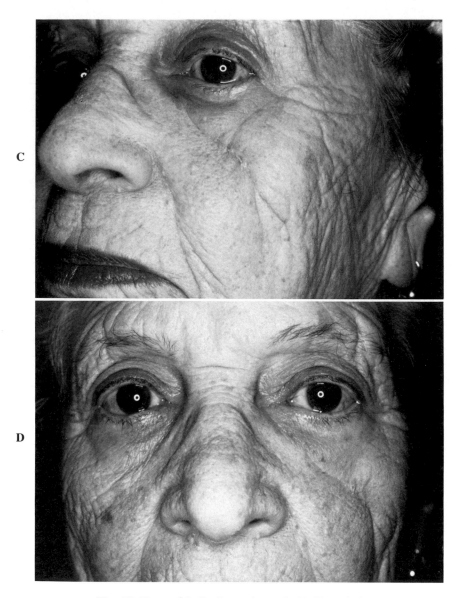

Fig. 10-68, cont'd. C, Cosmetic result. **D,** Frontal view.

Fig. 10-69. A recurrent basal cell carcinoma is present in Fig. 10-69, *A*. The wound following Mohs surgery (fresh tissue technique) is shown in Fig. 10-69, *B*. Note the extension of the ends of the fusiform excision drawn as tangents to the circular defect. After undermining of the surrounding tissue and burying of absorbable dermal sutures, the closure was completed (Fig. 10-69, *C*). The cosmetic result (Fig. 10-69, *D*) is excellent.

A case that did not turn out nearly so well is shown in Fig. 10-70. This was a recurrent basal cell carcinoma in a 25-year-old man. The darker area is the site of a recent biopsy (Fig. 10-70, *A*). After extirpation of the tumor, it was decided to close the wound as shown in Fig. 10-70, *B*. The lower triangle can be considered an example of Ammon's triangle, which is a triangle of tissue at the end of a rectangular or large triangular defect made to close the defect in a linear fashion. The defect was closed uneventfully, as shown in Fig. 10-70, *C*. At 1 week the wound has little apparent tension on the sutures. The patient did develop a slight hematoma in the upper and lower eyelids—not uncommon when surgery is performed around the eyes. Seen 1 year after the operation, the scar had spread because of the relentless tension on the wound in this area (Fig. 10-70, *D*).

The patient shown in Fig. 10-70 was younger, was a man, and had a larger wound; the skin itself was under greater tension. The patient in Fig. 10-69, on the other hand, was a middle-aged woman who had a smaller wound and whose skin was looser. All these factors affect the success of closures over the malar eminences.

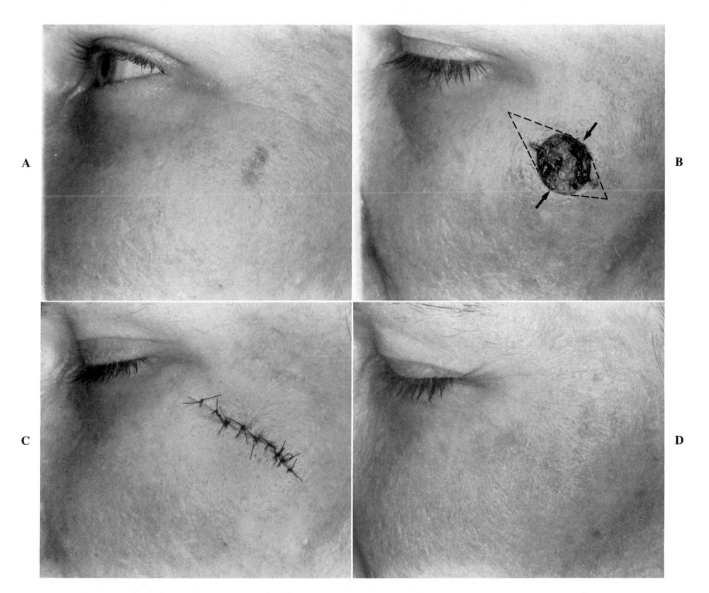

Fig. 10-69. Repair of surgical defect on anterior malar prominence. **A,** Preoperative view of recurrent basal cell carcinoma. **B,** Surgical defect following extirpation of tumor. **C,** Sutured wound. **D,** Cosmetic result at 1 year.

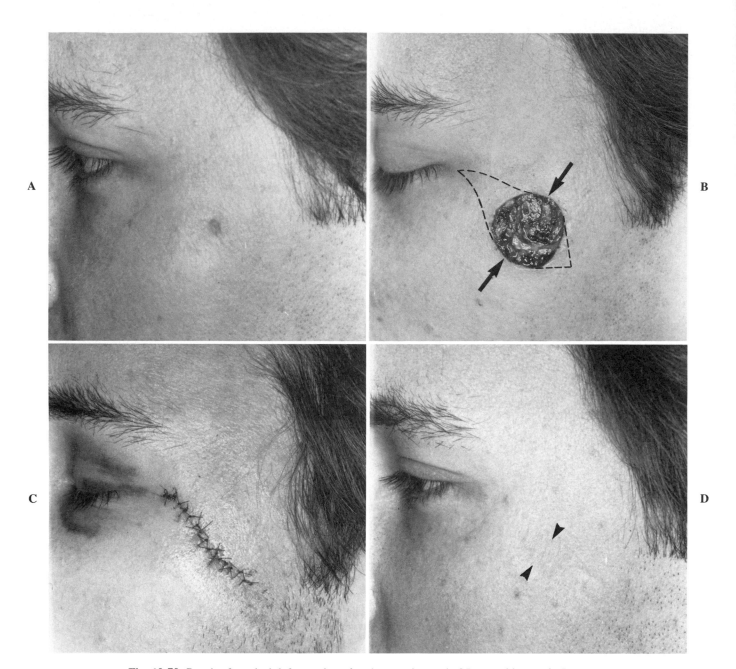

Fig. 10-70. Repair of surgical defect on lateral malar prominence in 25-year-old man. **A,** Preoperative view of recurrent basal cell carcinoma. **B,** Surgical defect following extirpation of tumor with lines of excision used to close defect. Lower triangle could be considered an example of Ammon's triangle. **C,** Closure at 1 week just before suture removal. **D,** Scar at 1 year postoperatively. Note spreading of scar *(arrows)*.

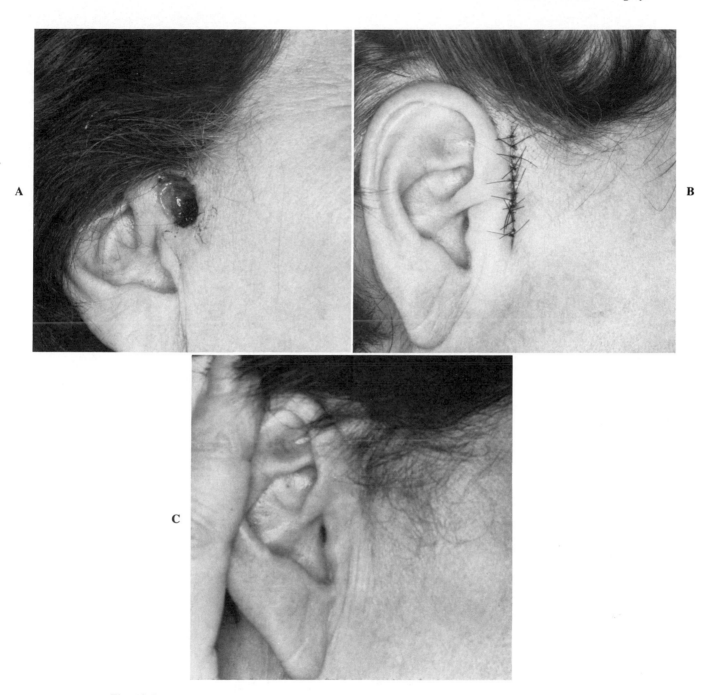

Fig. 10-71. Repair of preauricular surgical defect. **A,** Defect. **B,** Closure. **C,** Postoperative view at 1 year.

Preauricular area

The area immediately in front of the ear is usually easily closed vertically, as shown in Fig. 10-71.

Ear

Like the nose, the ear is a specialized area where closures may be complicated as to require specialized closure techniques of skin flaps.

The areas of the posterior ear and sulcus are easier to reconstruct than the anterior ear is. The sulcus in particular

is an easy area in which to do excisional surgery; one directs the axis of the excision longitudinally down the sulcus. However, malignant tumors in this area may go very deeply and therefore frequently require specialized techniques for total removal.

Lips

The recommended axis of a fusiform excision in the external lip is vertical and parallels the usual wrinkle lines in this area (Fig. 10-11). However, wrinkle lines on the exter-

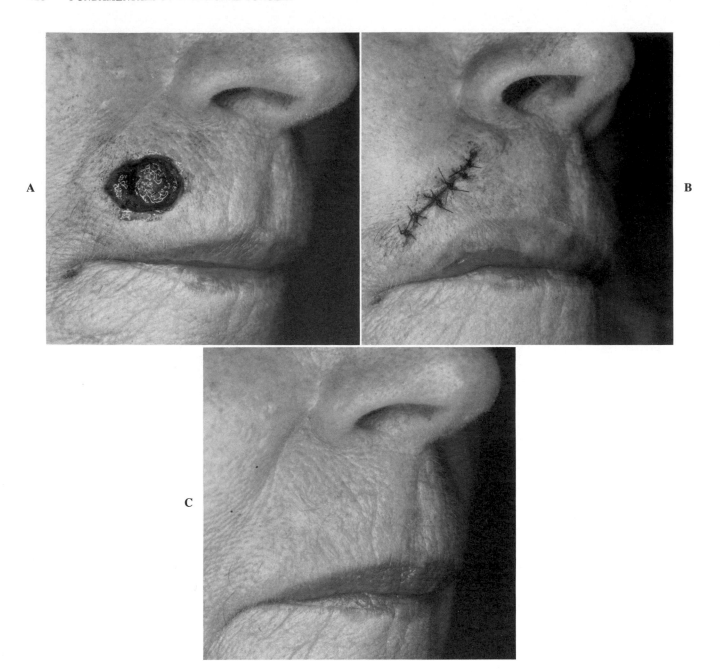

Fig. 10-72. Repair of surgical defect of upper lip. **A,** Defect. **B,** Closure, obliquely rather than vertically placed. **C,** Healed scar 3 months later.

nal upper lip may be either vertical or horizontal and vary between individuals,[122] since the underlying muscles of the lip run in more than one direction and in some patients are more dominant in one direction than another.

The patient in Fig. 10-72 was left with an elliptic defect oriented parallel to the upper lip. Rather than suturing this defect vertically, I chose to orient the closure somewhat obliquely (Fig. 10-72, *B*). This resulted in an immediate upturning of the upper lip; however, within 3 months this distortion corrected itself, and the patient's scar was ultimately cosmetically good (Fig. 10-72, *C*). The same self-

correction phenomenon of distorted structures was discussed with reference to eyebrows. Although there is some slight spreading of the scar, this is minimal and hardly noticeable. A vertically placed closure would have been under more tension in this patient; moreover, such a closure would have required small lateral advancement flaps—but the cosmetic result would have been excellent.

The vermilion portion of the lip is quite vascular and heals readily with imperceptible scars regardless of the direction of closure. Tension forces in this area are less of a factor in producing a good cosmetic result if the tissue ex-

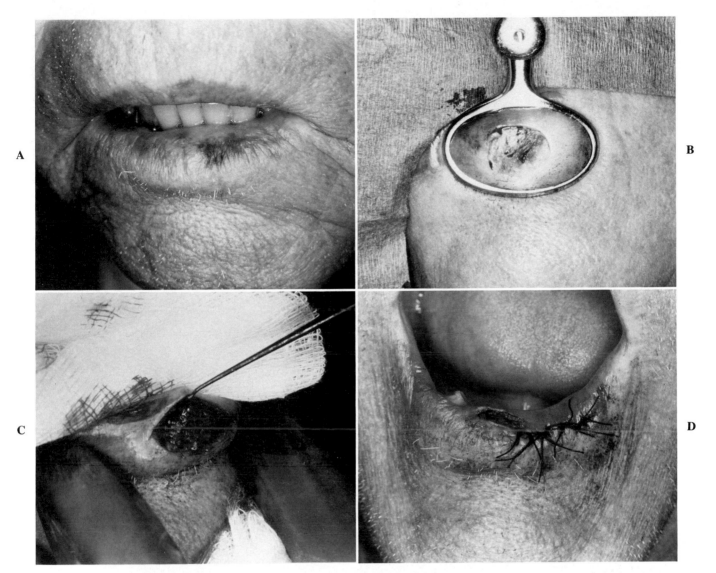

Fig. 10-73. Excision of lentigo maligna and repair of surgical defect. **A,** Preoperative view. **B,** Excision using chalazion clamp to help control bleeding and grasp lip. **C,** Advancing mucosa forward with skin hook after undermining. Note second wound superior to initial wound shown in **B.** This second wound resulted from removal of small superficial squamous cell carcinoma. **D,** Sutured wound. Note small wound in central lip (second wound in **C**), allowed to heal by secondary intention.

Continued.

cised is superficial. Deeper excisions extending into muscle require reapposition of the muscle and other structures to maintain full function.

Fig. 10-73 shows a patient with a superficial lentigo maligna of the lower lip. To help control the bleeding at the time of surgery, a chalazion clamp was used (Fig. 10-73, *B*). After undermining posteriorly to free the mucosa, it was advanced forward with a skin hook (Fig. 10-73, *C*). The mucosa was then sutured with silk so as to cause the patient less irritation than from the bristly tails of monofilamentous nylon sutures (Fig. 10-73, *D*). Note the small wound located centrally that was not sutured—the result of

removal of a small superficial squamous cell carcinoma. The cosmetic result is excellent (Fig. 10-73, *E*). Note also that the area allowed to heal by granulation has a scar broader than the area sutured. Although this is acceptable, suturing would have probably resulted in a thinner scar.

The tongue, like the vermilion, is quite vascular. Removing lesions from this area can be tricky. Fig. 10-74 is a fibroma of the tongue. Excision was performed with the long axis running parallel with the side of the tongue (Fig. 10-74, *B*). By using gauze an assistant can hold the tongue and maintain pressure at the sides of the excision. This allows one to work in a virtually bloodless field. The wound

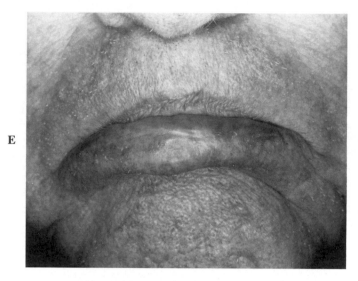

Fig. 10-73, cont'd. E, Healed result. Sutured wound has less noticeable scar tissue than central wound allowed to heal by granulation and epidermization.

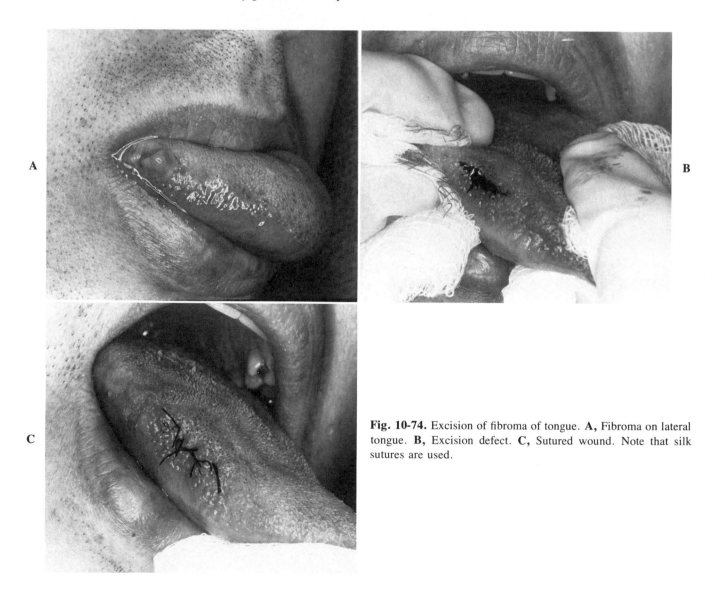

Fig. 10-74. Excision of fibroma of tongue. **A,** Fibroma on lateral tongue. **B,** Excision defect. **C,** Sutured wound. Note that silk sutures are used.

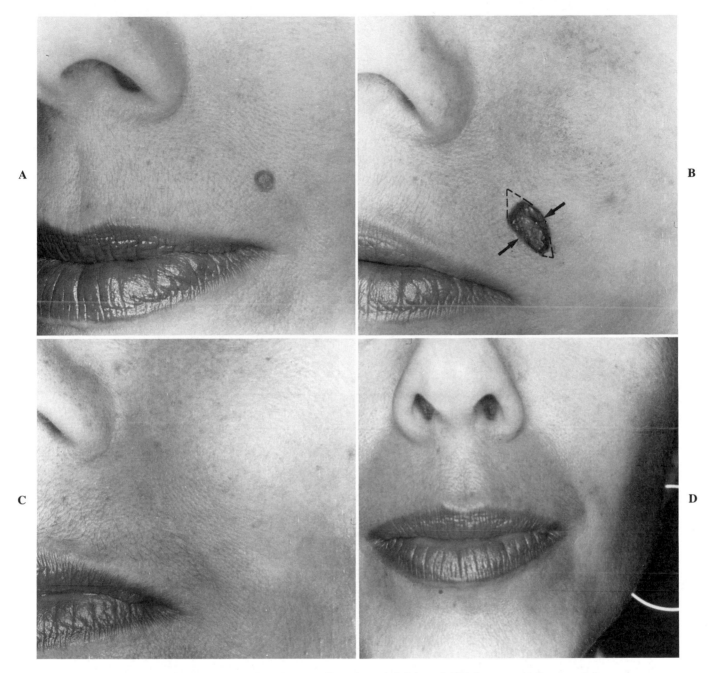

Fig. 10-75. Excision and repair of basal cell carcinoma of right melolabial crease. **A,** Preoperative view. **B,** Surgical defect with planned excision. **C,** Healed surgical scar at 1 year. **D,** Frontal view.

was sutured, as the vermilion was, with silk (Fig. 10-74, C). The sutures should be tied tight enough to stop the bleeding in this area. Buried sutures are usually unnecessary.

Other techniques can be used to excise lesions on the tongue. Sponge forceps or chalazion clamps can be used to steady the tongue and stop bleeding. (Patients find it impossible to hold their tongues in one position by themselves.) One may also use a temporary 4-0 silk suture through the tongue and pull it forward to gain exposure to

the area where the surgery is to be performed. In this vascular area sutures may be placed under a lesion to be excised before the actual excision so that they can be tied immediately after the extirpation.

Melolabial crease

The crease between the lips and cheek offers a good camouflage for excision lines. Like those in the forehead, excisions in these creases are eventually hardly perceptible. Fig. 10-75 demonstrates closure of a defect resulting

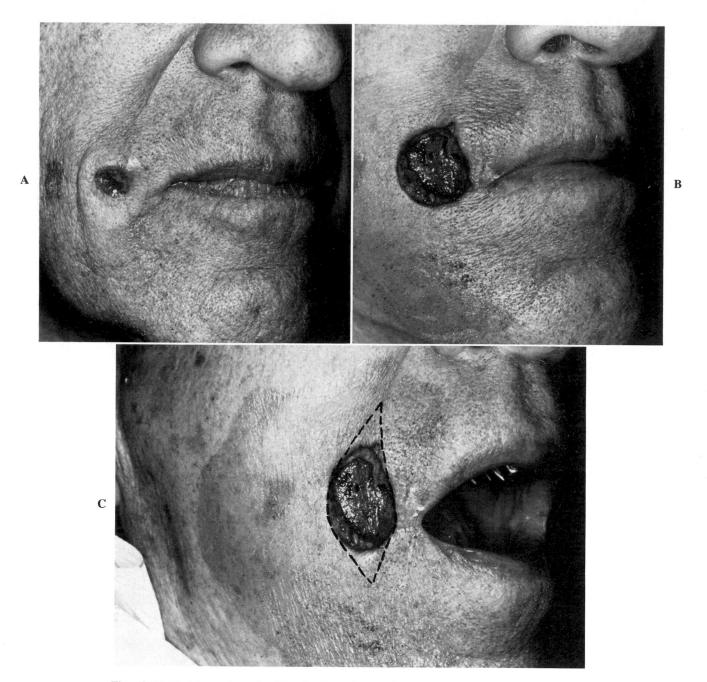

Fig. 10-76. Excision and repair of basal cell carcinoma. **A,** Preoperative view. **B,** Surgical defect after extirpation. **C,** Elongation of defect with opening mouth and planned repair.

from removal of a basal cell carcinoma. Fig. 10-75, *A,* shows the basal cell carcinoma slightly medial to the melolabial crease. Fig. 10-75, *B,* shows the resultant surgical defect after total removal of the neoplasm as well as how the defect was converted into a tangent-to-circle configuration with the long axis directed along the melolabial crease. Closure was made in the normal manner with undermining and buried dermal sutures. The resultant cosmetic appearance of the scar is excellent (Fig. 10-75, *C* and *D*).

The patient shown in Fig. 10-76 has a larger tumor in the same area, the melolabial crease; it proved to be a nodular basal cell carcinoma (Fig. 10-76, *A*). After total extirpation the resultant wound was circular (Fig. 10-76, *B*). By asking the patient to open his mouth (Fig. 10-76, *C*), one can see that the directional forces on the wound are greater superiorly and inferiorly as the wound is pulled in these directions. Therefore the proper closure to take advantage of these directional forces is perpendicular to them (Fig. 10-

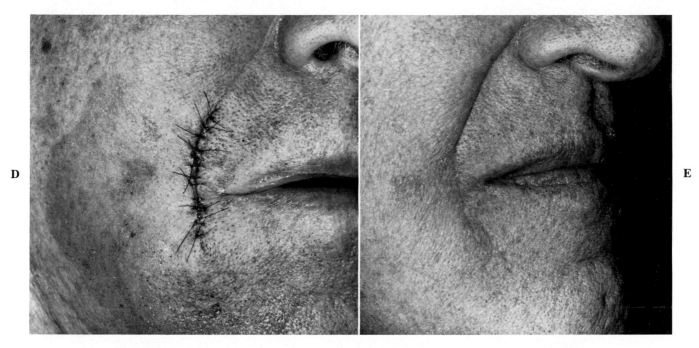

Fig. 10-76, cont'd. D, Closure along long axis of defect determined in **C. E,** Healed surgical scar at 6 months.

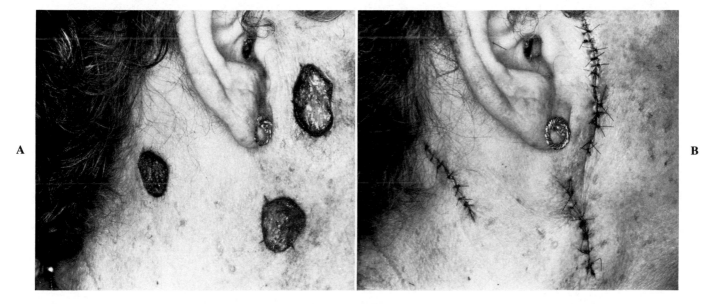

Fig. 10-77. Repair of three postoperative wounds after removal of basal cell carcinomas of cheek and neck. **A,** Immediate postoperative wounds. **B,** Sutured wounds.

Continued.

76, *D*). This eventuated in a well-hidden scar (Fig. 10-76, *E*). Note that the mouth was slightly distorted laterally at the time of closure (Fig. 10-76, *D*). Like distortions of the upper lip and eyebrow, this eventually settles out.

Neck, trunk, extremities

Excisions on the neck (Fig. 10-77), trunk, and extremities are fairly straightforward and should follow the Max-

STLs, which have been outlined. In some areas of the trunk, especially the areas overlying the scapula and anterior chest, the lines of maximal tension are not much greater in one direction than another. This results in spread scars no matter how well planned the excisions may be. Patients should be warned about this eventuality.

On the convex surfaces of the back of the hand, arms, and legs it is preferable to plan tangent-to-circle rather than

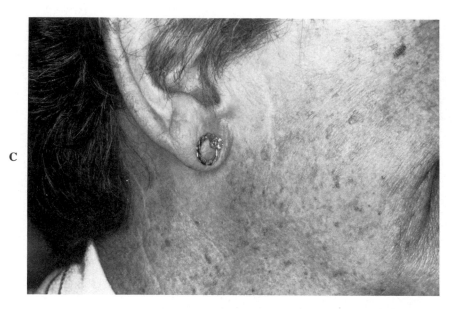

Fig. 10-77, cont'd. C, Healed scars at 1 year.

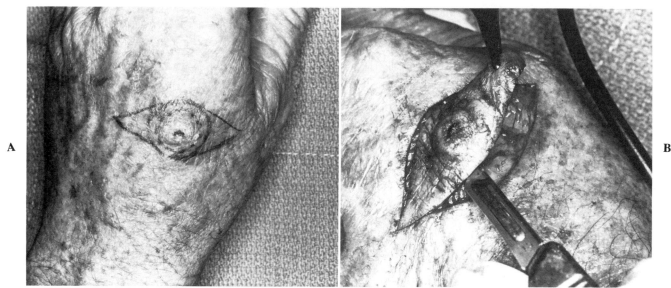

Fig. 10-78. Excision and repair of squamous cell carcinoma of dorsum of hand. **A,** Preoperative appearance. Note straight-line tangents drawn from central circle. **B,** Excising tissue. Note tissue is pulled over blade.

fusiform excisions (Fig. 10-78). Dog-ears are more readily formed over these curved surfaces but can be minimized by tangent-to-circle excisions planned.

VARIATIONS OF FUSIFORM EXCISIONS
Crescent excisions

Under some circumstances, especially on the face, one may wish to modify a standard fusiform excision by making one of the sides slightly concave rather than convex. This is done so that the long axis of the excision is curved and

conforms to a curved MaxSTL (Fig. 10-79). A good example of where this technique is useful is near the melolabial crease (Fig. 10-80). By making the medial side of the excision slightly concave or even straight, one produces an excision line that when sutured will be slightly curved and fit into this crease. If the sides of an excision are drawn, as on Fig. 10-80, one side will be longer than the other. This should be sutured using the "rule of halves" to ensure that the tension on closure is evenly distributed and that dog-ears do not form at the ends. The rule of halves proposes that

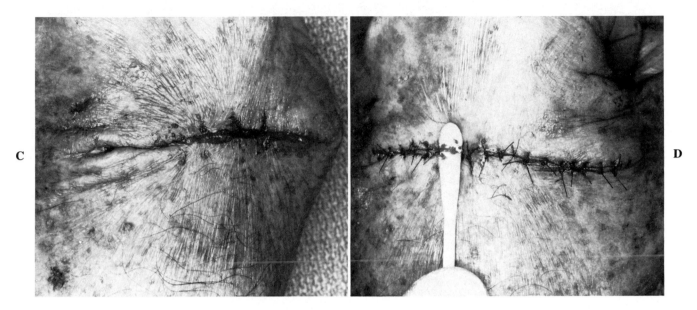

C   D

Fig. 10-78, cont'd. C, Wound initially closed with buried sutures. **D,** Completely sutured wound.

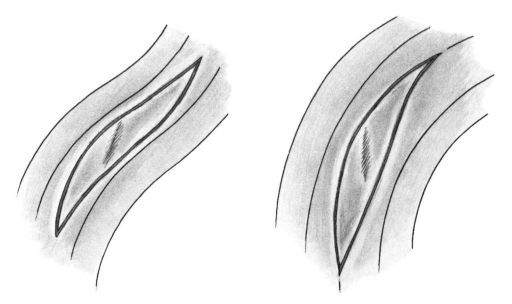

Fig. 10-79. Modifications of fusiform excisions to conform to curved MaxSTLs.

A   B

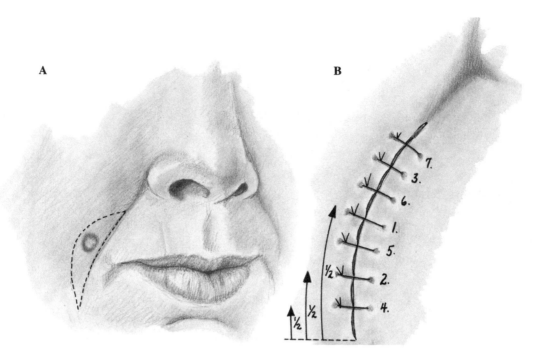

Fig. 10-80. Modified fusiform excision near melolabial crease **(A).** Closure is best accomplished by rule of halves **(B).**

sutures be placed half way between the excision ends, a suture and an excision end, or two sutures. The first suture (No. 1) is placed halfway between the two ends of the excision. The next sutures (Nos. 2 and 3) are placed halfway between the first suture and one of the ends. Additional sutures (Nos. 4, 5, 6, and 7) are then placed halfway between the previously placed sutures or between the previously placed sutures and one of the ends of the excision.

A patient with a basal cell carcinoma over the anterior malar eminence is shown in Fig. 10-81, *A.* The excision is planned so that the lower edge will be slightly concave and the suture line will fit into the curved MaxSTL in this area. Fig. 10-81, *B,* shows the surgical defect. Note the small nick in the tissue medially *(arrowhead),* which should be avoided during excisions. The sutured surgical defect is shown in Fig. 10-81, *C,* after being sutured by the rule of halves. The curve to the excision line at this point is not dramatic but still enough to make a small difference. The final healed surgical scar fits in nicely with the patient's cheek curve (Fig. 10-81, *D* and *E*).

The use of modified fusiform incisions are just described is somewhat controversial. Kraissl recommended such incisions, as can be seen in his illustrations,[77,78] and Fleury likewise recommended crescent excisions.[45] In contrast, other authorities think that a modified fusiform excision producing a curved scar will result in a trap-door deformity.[12,74] In other words, because of scar contraction with time, a curved scar contracts and inevitably bunches the skin on the inner side. Borges thinks that such curved excision scars

frequently do not follow his skin-tension lines anyway and therefore are nonphysiologic.[12] For small excisions this is probably so, but for larger excisions the scars can follow the skin-tension lines nicely. However, the arguments against curved scars do have some basis in fact. If one looks critically at Fig. 10-81, *E,* there is a slight bowing of the left cheek. However, the alternative would have been a straight-line closure, which would not lie in the skin folds of the face. Therefore this controversy is basically aesthetic and a matter of personal preference. A slightly curved but bowed excision scar line among skin creases may look better than a straight, nonbowed excision line running oblique to the natural creases of the face.

Stages excisions

Occasionally when the skin tension is too great or the lesion to be excised too large for comfortable closure with a single excision, a staged excision may be considered. This is based on the principle that the skin stretches with time. The first excision only partially removes the lesion. The surrounding skin is stretched, which results in less tension when the next excision is performed.[50] By sequentially staging excisions over a period of time a large lesion can be completely excised; however, there is a limit on how much the skin can be stretched before a permanent deformity, such as striae, develops or the scar spreads markedly. Thus the "law of diminishing returns" comes into effect.[131] After a year there is only about a 70% relaxation in the increased tension that occurs after an elliptic excision.[50]

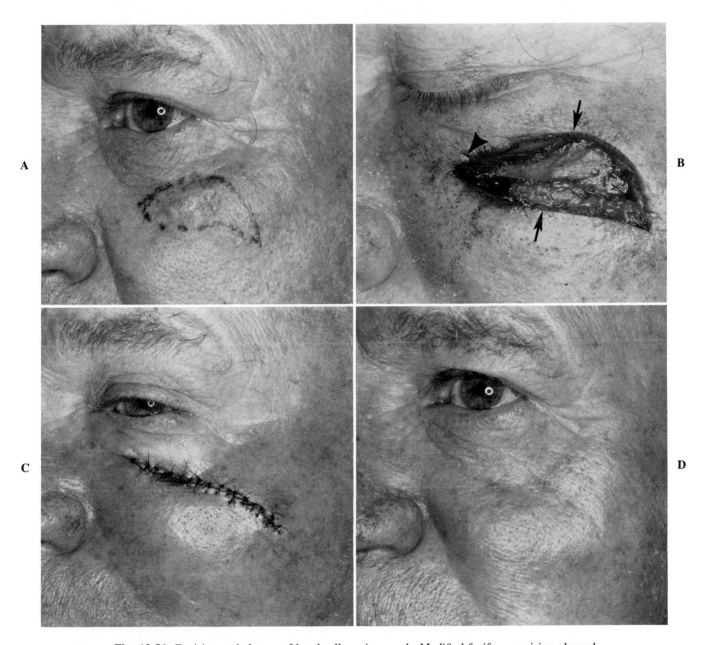

Fig. 10-81. Excision and closure of basal cell carcinoma. **A,** Modified fusiform excision planned with concave and convex surfaces. **B,** Surgical defect. Arrows show direction of closure. Note small nick on wound edge medially *(arrowhead)*. **C,** Closure using rule of halves. **D,** Healed scar at 3 years.

Continued.

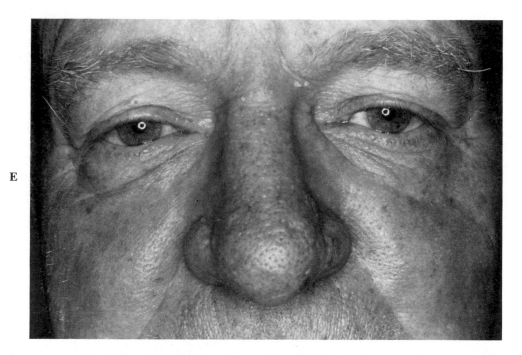

Fig. 10-81, cont'd. E, Frontal view. Note slightly curved, depressed scar.

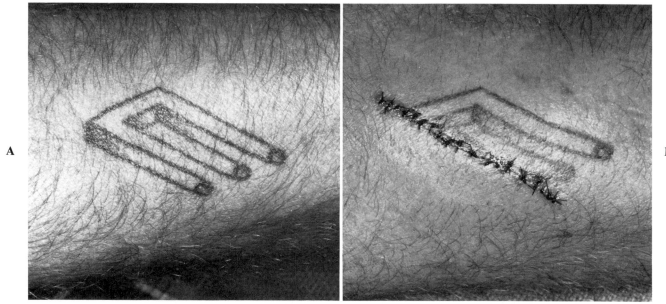

Fig. 10-82. Staged excision of tattoo from forearm. **A,** Preoperative. **B,** First excision.

Fig. 10-82 demonstrates a staged excision of a tatoo on the lower forearm. The lesion was too large for a single excision, so three separate excisions were made, all parallel with one another at 2- to 3-month intervals (Fig. 10-82, *B, C,* and *E*). Regardless of the stretch that occurs in the surrounding skin, the scars inevitably stretched (Fig. 10-82, *D*). It has been my experience that all staged excisions result in spread scars. Nevertheless, the ultimate scar is probably less extensive than would otherwise occur with a simple large excision.

Staged excisions are particularly useful on congenital nevi (see Fig. 21-6).

TRAUMATIC INCISIONS

Cutaneous incisions caused by trauma are relatively frequent, and all physicians at some point in their training are

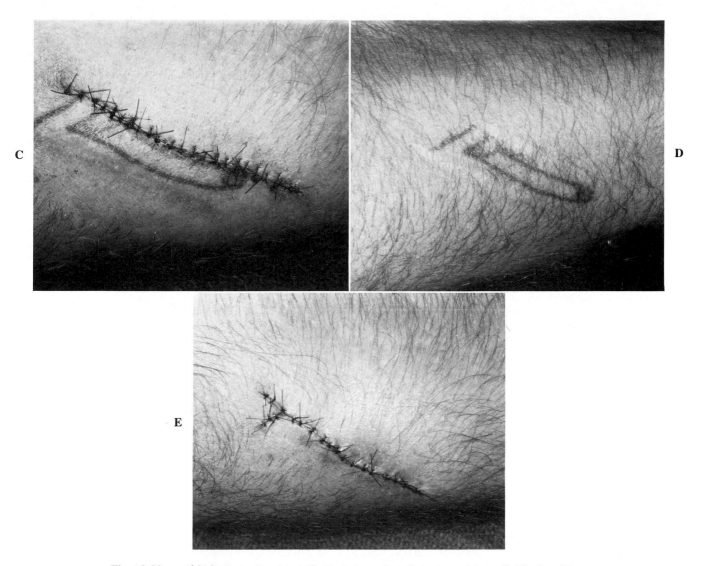

Fig. 10-82, cont'd. C, Second excision. **D,** Healed scar from first two excisions. **E,** Final excision.

called on to manage such wounds. It is essential to realize that all such wounds are potentially contaminated and therefore differ from elective incisions. The first thing one does after anesthetizing the area of the laceration is to clean the wound. Usually normal saline is excellent for this purpose. Flushing the wound with normal saline hung as an IV and using the pressure from the IV line works very well. As a general rule it is best to keep detergents and other antibacterials out of fresh wounds. Foreign substances such as dirt, gunpowder, or other materials that can tattoo the skin, should be picked out of the wound with forceps. A toothbrush may also be gently used to clean such wounds.

Frequently lacerations may be tangential to the skin surface—rather than perpendicular, as occurs with a scalpel excision. Such tangential wounds should be converted to more perpendicular ones because, if sutured tangentially, such a wound produces a trapdoor deformity (also called a

toilet-seat deformity) (Fig. 10-33, *D*). One exception to squaring off such tangential lacerations is if they are very superficial, in which case they can be simply approximated with skin-closure tape.

Traumatic lacerations may produce devitalized tissue; it is important, however, not to be too vigorous in removing this tissue. Debridement alone cannot "sterilize" a heavily contaminated wound. It may be best to suture as well as one can or even allow the wound to heal by secondary intention and then later perform a scar revision. Conservation of normal tissue where possible is preferable. Extravagant treatment of routine lacerations is unsafe and unnecessary.[92]

For contaminated wounds older than 4 hours, one should consider freshening the edges; this helps to reduce the possibility of wound infection.[128] Traumatic wounds older than 12 hours should not be closed immediately. One can delay closure of such wounds for 2 to 6 days without an increased incidence of infection. Allowing such wounds to heal by secondary intention should also be strongly considered.

Lacerations can be sutured or taped, depending on the depth, anatomic location, and extent of the injury. If sutured, it is preferable not to bury dermal or subcutaneous sutures, since buried sutures under such circumstances tend to increase the incidence of infection.[10,140] One should begin suturing traumatic lacerations by using the anatomic landmarks as a guide for the first key sutures. Also, prophylactic antibiotics used in patients with simple lacerations do not appear to decrease the incidence of wound infection, except possibly if the wound closed is older than 4 hours.[140]

OPERATIVE REPORTS

All surgical procedures should have an operative report typed as a record. A sample operative report I currently use can be found in Appendix C. Basically the following facts should be mentioned in the operative report:

1. *Name of patient* and any in-office or hospital identification number.
2. *Status of patient* at the time of surgery (whether inpatient or outpatient).
3. *Place of surgery,* which could be an outpatient operating facility, office, clinic, or operating room.
4. *Date of surgery.*
5. *Time of surgery* should include time the anesthetic was begun and time the surgery was finished.
6. *Preoperative diagnosis,* which is usually based on a prior pathology report or clinical judgment.
7. *Postoperative diagnosis,* which is usually based on events that happen at the time of surgery. If a lesion is found to extend beyond the area mentioned in the preoperative diagnosis or if unusual findings make themselves known, these should be mentioned here.
8. *Name of operation or procedure performed.*
9. *Surgeon's name.* If surgical assistant physicians are present, they should be mentioned too.
10. *Nurse's name.* If other types of assistants are used, they should be mentioned specifically, by name with educational degree.
11. *Anesthesia used.* The type, the concentration, and the amount should be specified.
12. *Preoperative medications.*
13. *Anesthetist,* who is usually the same person as the surgeon if a local anesthetic is given.
14. *Preparation of patient,* which should include the position in which the patient is placed on table and how the operative site is prepared and draped.
15. *Procedure.* The manner of local anesthetic injection, if used, is mentioned, as is a full description of the surgical procedure from incision to dressing. This includes undermining, hemostasis, type of sutures used, and their depth of placement.

16. *Size of sutured wound.*
17. *Estimated blood loss.*
18. *Complications.* Include unusual bleeding problems or reactions to medications.
19. *Condition of patient after surgery.*
20. *Postoperative medications.*
21. *Postoperative dressing instructions.* State either the specific directions given for dressing changes or whether a dressing instruction sheet was given.
22. *Disposition of patient.* State where the patient was sent to recuperate (home, friend's home, hospital, and so forth) and when the patient was instructed to return to physician's office for a wound check or suture removal. One may also state how the patient can get in touch with the physician in case of emergency.
23. *Physician's signature.*

BILLING AND FEES

Physicians during their training are not taught how to deal with either patients or insurance companies regarding fees and payments. Most patients have questions about the costs of surgical procedures, which are best handled honestly and in a straightforward manner. Usually a well-trained office staff is essential in handling these questions.

Billing is best done in accordance with the CPT (*Current Procedure Terminology,* ed. 4, Chicago, 1987, American Medical Association; edited by Fanta, C.M., et al.) Every surgical or medical procedure has a corresponding CPT-4 code, which is recognized by most insurance carriers. Along with each procedure code on a bill one must list a diagnosis. This is simplified by the ICD codes for diagnoses, found in the ICD-9-CM code book (International Classification of Diseases, revision 9 of ed. 2, U.S. Department of Health and Human Services, DHHS Publication No. (PHS) 80-1260, U.S. Government Printing Office, Washington, D.C. 20402).

Fees are best determined by assessing what the physicians in one's surrounding geographic area normally charge for a procedure. One should develop a flow sheet of the procedures one commonly performs and get a price range that is charged by a number of different physicians. Some insurance companies, including Medicare carriers, also give a range of payments they make for certain procedures listed by CPT-4 codes; these payment schedules are available on request. In some states the insurance companies deny any requests for payment schedules. Inquiry should be made anyway.

Another source of information on physicians' charges is found in *Physician's Fee Reference.* This contains a computerized average of physicians' fees from all stages given by CPT code numbers. It is available by writing to Physician's Fee Reference, 2703 West Wisconsin Avenue, Milwaukee, Wis. 53208.

Physicians should be reasonable and fair regarding the assignment of CPT-4 codes to the procedures performed. Simple lacerations or complex repairs should not be billed as skin flaps, and skin flaps should not be used when simpler procedures suffice. Such extravagant treatment and billing unfortunately and undoubtedly exist.[92]

REFERENCES

1. Adams, I.W., et al.: A comparative trial of polyglycolic acid and silk as suture materials for accidental wounds, Lancet **2:**1216, 1977.
2. Albom, M.J.: Dermo-subdermal sutures for long, deep surgical wounds, J. Dermatol. Surg. Oncol. **3:**504, 1977.
3. Albom, M.J.: Scalpel and scissors surgery. In Epstein, E., and Epstein E., Jr., editors: Techniques in skin surgery, Philadelphia, 1979, Lea & Febiger.
4. Aston, S.J.: The choice of suture material for skin closure, J. Dermatol. Surg. **2:**57, 1976.
5. Beck, W.C.: Aseptic barriers in surgery: their present status, Arch. Surg. **116:**240, 1981.
6. Becker, H., and Davidoff, M.R.: The physical properties of suture materials are related to knot holding, S. Afr. J. Surg. **15:**105, 1977.
7. Bernstein, L.: Incisions and excisions in elective facial surgery, Arch. Otolaryngol. **97:**238, 1973.
8. Bialostozky, L.: Painless removal of sutures [letter], Surgery **76:**356, 1974.
9. Birdsell, D.C., et al.: ''Staying power'': absorbable vs. nonabsorbable, Plast. Reconstr. Surg. **68:**742, 1981.
10. Bodiwala, G.G., and George, T.K.: Surgical gloves during wound repair in the accident-and-emergency department, Lancet **2:**91, 1982.
11. Borges, A.F.: Elective incisions and scar revision, Boston, 1973, Little, Brown & Co.
12. Borges, A.F., and Alexander, J.E.: Relaxed skin tension lines, Z- plasties on scars, and fusiform excision of lesions, Br. J. Plast. Surg. **15:**242, 1962.
13. Borgström, S., and Sandblom, P.: Suture technic and wound healing: an investigation based on animal experiments, Ann. Surg. **144:**982, 1956.
14. Bradley, W.G.: Disorders of peripheral nerves, Oxford, U.K., 1975, Blackwell.
15. Bridgens, N.K.: A comparative study of surgical suture materials and closure techniques, J. Am. Osteopath. Assoc. **82**(9 Suppl.):715, 1983.
16. Brown, I.A.: A scanning electron microscopic study of the effects of uniaxial tension on human skin, Br. J. Dermatol. **89:**383, 1973.
17. Brunius, U.: Wound healing impairment from sutures, Acta Chir. Scand. (Suppl.)**395:**1, 1968.
18. Brunius, U., and Åhrén, C.: Healing impairment in skin incisions closed with silk sutures, Acta Chir. Scand. **135:**369, 1969.
19. Bulacio-Nuñez, A.W.: A new theory regarding the lines of skin tension, Plast. Reconstr. Surg. **53:**663, 1974.
20. Bunnell, S.: An essential in reconstructive surgery: ''atraumatic'' technique, Calif. State J. Med. **19:**204, 1921.
21. Carpendale, M.T.F., and Sereda, W.: The role of the percutaneous suture in surgical wound infection, Surgery **58:**672, 1965.
22. Catty, R.H.C.: Healing and contraction of experimental full-thickness wounds in the human, Br. J. Surg. **52:**542, 1965.
23. Clarke, J.S., et al.: Suture technicians for emergency services in a Children's Hospital, Ohio State Med. J. **73:**371, 1977.
24. Condie, J.D., and Ferguson, D.J.: Experimental wound infections: contamination versus surgical technique, Surgery **50:**367, 1961.
25. Converse, J.M.: Reconstructive plastic surgery: general principles, ed. 2, vol. 1, Philadelphia, 1977, W.B. Saunders Co.
26. Conway, J.H.: Notes on cutaneous healing in wounds, Surg. Gynecol. Obstet. **66:**140, 1938.
27. Coskey, R.J.: Contact dermatitis owing to tincture of benzoin, Arch. Dermatol. **114:**128, 1978.
28. Courtiss, E.H., et al.: The placement of elective skin incisions, Plast. Reconstr. Surg. **31:**31, 1963.
29. Cox, H.T.: The cleavage lines of the skin, Br. J. Surg. **29:**234, 1941.
30. Crikelair, G.F.: Skin suture marks, Am. J. Surg. **96:**631, 1958.
31. Crikelair, G.F.: Surgical approach to facial scarring, J.A.M.A. **172:**160, 1960.
32. Danielson, D.A., and Natarajan, S.: Tension field theory and the stress in stretched skin, J. Biomechan. **8:**135, 1975.
33. Davis, T.S., Graham, W.P., III, and Miller, S.H.: The circular excision, Ann. Plast. Surg. **4:**21, 1980.
34. De Hoff, P.H., and Key, J.E.: Application of the finite element analysis to determine forces and stresses in wound closing, J. Biomechan. **14:**549, 1981.
35. De Holl, D., et al.: Potentiation of infection by suture closure of dead space, Am. J. Surg. **127:**716, 1974.
36. Duhring, L.A.: Cutaneous medicine, Philadelphia, 1905, J.B. Lippincott Co.
37. DuMortier, J.J.: The resistance of healing wounds to infection, Surg. Gynecol. Obstet. **56:**762, 1933.
38. Dupuytren, G.: Traite theorique et pratique des blessure par armes de guerre, vol. 1, Paris, 1834, J.B. Bailliere.
39. Dushoff, J.M.: A stitch in time, Emerg. Med. **5:**21, 1973.
40. Dykes, E.R., and Anderson, R.: Atraumatic technique: the sine qua non of operative wound infection prophylaxis, Cleveland Clin. Q. **28:**157, 1961.
41. Edlich, R.F., et al.: Studies in management of the contaminated wound. I. Technique of closure of such wounds together with a note on a reproducible experimental model, J. Surg. Res. **8:**585, 1968.
42. FDA Drug Bulletin: Burns with hibitane tincture, **15**(1):9, 1985.
43. Ferguson, D.J.: Clinical application of experimental relations between technique and wound infection, Surgery **63:**377, 1968.
44. FitzGibbon, G.M.: The commandments of Gillies, Br. J. Plast. Surg. **21:**226, 1968.
45. Fleury, A.F.: Minor surgery in the office of the primary care physician, Med. Times **109:**31, 1981.
46. Flinn, R.M.: Knotting in medicine and surgery, Practitioner **183:**322, 1959.

47. Freeman, B.S., et al.: An analysis of suture withdrawal stress, Surg. Gynecol. Obstet. **131:**441, 1970.

48. French, M.L.V., Eitzen, H.E., Ritter, M.A.: The plastic surgical adhesive drape, Ann. Surg. **184:**46, 1976.

49. Gibson, T.: Biomechanics in plastic surgery. In Kenedi, R.M., editor: Biomechanics and related bio-engineering topics, Oxford, U.K., 1965, Pergamon Press.

50. Gibson, T., and Kenedi, R.M.: Biomechanical properties of the skin, Surg. Clin. N. Am. **47:**279, 1967.

51. Gibson, T., Stark, H., and Evans, J.H.: Directional variation in extensibility of human skin in vivo, J. Biomechan. **2:**201, 1969.

52. Gilles, H.: Techique of good suturing, St. Bartholomew's Hosp. J. **47:**170, 1943.

53. Gillman, T.: Some aspects of the healing and treatment of wounds, Triangle **4:**68, 1959.

54. Gillman, T., et al.: A reexamination of certain aspects of the histogenesis of healing cutaneous wounds, Br. J. Surg. **43:**141, 1955.

55. Grabb, W.C., and Smith, J.W.: Plastic surgery, ed. 3, Boston, 1979, Little, Brown & Co.

56. Gross, D.: Personal communication, 1985.

57. Grundner, T.M.: The readability of surgical consent forms, N. Engl. J. Med. **302:**900, 1980.

58. Halsted, W.S.: The radical cure of hernia, Bull. Johns Hopkins Hosp. **1:**13, 1889.

59. Halsted, W.S.: The treatment of wounds with especial reference to the value of blood clot in the management of dead space, Johns Hopkins Hosp. Rep. **2:**255, 1891.

60. Halsted, W.S.: Ligature and suture material: the employment of fine silk in preference to catgut and the advantage of transfixing tissues and vessels in controlling hemorrhage, J.A.M.A. **60:**1119, 1913.

61. Hartman, L.A.: Intradermal sutures in facial lacerations: comparative study of clear monofilament nylon and polyglycolic acid, Arch. Otolaryngol. **103:**542, 1977.

62. Heifetz, C.J., Richards, F.O., and Lawrence, M.S.: Comparison of wound healing with and without dressings, Arch. Surg. **65:**746, 1952.

63. Holmlund, D.E.: Suture technic and suture-holding capacity: a model study and a theoretical analysis, Am. J. Surg. **134:**616, 1977.

64. Holmstrand, K., Longacre, J.J., and de Stefano, G.A.: The ultrastructure of collagen in skin, scars, and keloids, Plast. Reconstr. Surg. **27:**597, 1961.

65. Holt, G, R., and Holt, J.E.: Suture materials and techniques, Ear Nose Throat J. **60:**12, 1981.

66. Homsy, C.A., et al.: Surgical suture-porcine subcuticular tissue interaction, J. Biomed. Mater. Res. **3:**383, 1969.

67. Howe, C.W.: Experimental studies on determinants of wound infection, Surg. Gynecol. Obstet. **123:**507, 1966.

68. Howes, E.L.: The immediate strength of the sutured wound, Surgery **7:**24, 1940.

69. Howes, E.L., and Harvery, S.C.: The strength of the healing wound in relation to the holding strength of the catgut suture, N. Engl. J. Med. **200:**1285, 1929.

70. Hutchinson, C., and Koop, C.E.: Lines of cleavage in the skin of the newborn infant, Anat. Rec. **126:**299, 1956.

71. James W.D., White, S.W. and Yanklowitz, B.: Allergic contact dermatitis to compound tincture of benzoin, J. Am. Acad. Dermatol. **11:**847, 1984.

72. Jobe, R.: When an "ellipse" is not an ellipse, Plast. Reconstr. Surg. **46:**295, 1970.

73. Johnson, H.A.: Bonney's blue marking ink, Plast. Reconstr. Surg. **56:**155, 1975.

74. Ju, D.M.: The physical basis of scar contraction, Plast. Reconstr. Surg. **7:**343, 1951.

75. Karakousis, P.: Principles of surgical dissection, J. Surg. Oncol. **21:**205, 1982.

76. Kocher, T.: Chirurgische-Operationslehre, Jena, Germany, 1902, Fisher-Verlag.

77. Kraissl, C.J.: The selection of appropriate lines for elective surgical incisions, Plast. Reconstr. Surg. **8:**1, 1951.

78. Kraissl, C.J., and Conway, H.: Excision of small tumors of the skin of the face with special reference to the wrinkle lines, Surgery **25:**592, 1949.

79. Langer, K.: Zur Anatomie und Physiologie der Haut. I. Über die Spaltbarkeit der Cutis, S. B. Akad. Wiss. [Wien] **44:**19, 1861.

80. Langer, K.: Zur Anatomie und Physiologie der Haut. II. Die Spannung der Cutis, S. B. Akad. Wiss. [Wien] **45:**133, 1862.

81. Langer, K.: Zur Anatomie und Physiologie der Haut. III. Über die Elasticität der Cutis, S. B. Akad. Wiss. [Wien] **45:**156, 1862.

82. Lascelles, A.K.: The effect of suture materials and suture techniques on the healing of wounds in the skin of sheep, Aust. J. Exp. Biol. Med. Sci. **38:**111, 1960.

83. Lawrence, T.L., and Wiviott, W.: Use of turkey skins for surgical teaching, J. Fam. Pract. **6:**169, 1978.

84. Lichtenstein, I.L., et al.: The dynamics of wound healing, Surg. Gynecol. Obstet. **130:**685, 1970.

85. Livingston, E.M.: Study of the square knot, Am. J. Surg. **6:**121, 1929.

86. Macht, S.D., and Krizek, T.J.: Sutures and suturing: current concepts, J. Oral Surg. **36:**710, 1978.

87. Madden, J.E., et al.: Studies in the management of the contaminated wound. IV. Resistance to infection of surgical wounds made by knife, electrosurgery, and laser, Am. J. Surg. **119:**222, 1970.

88. Malgaigne, J.F.: Traité d'anatomie chirurgicale et de chirurgie expérimentale, vol. 1, Paris, 1838, J.B. Baillére.

89. Marcy, H.O.: The aseptic animal suture: its place in surgery, J.A.M.A. **31:**381, 1898.

90. Marples, R.R., and Kligman, A.M.: Growth of bacteria under adhesive tapes, Arch. Dermatol. **99:**107, 1969.

91. McDowell, A.J.: Wound infections resulting from the use of hot wet sponges, Plast. Reconstr. Surg. **23:**168, 1959.

92. McDowell, A.J.: Extravagant treatment of garden variety lacerations, Plast. Reconstr. Surg. **63:**111, 1979.

93. McGregor, I.A. Fundamental Techniques in Plastic Surgery, and their Surgical Applications, ed. 6, New York, 1975, Churchill Livingstone.

94. Milewski, P.J., et al.: Is a fat stitch necessary? Br. J. Surg. **67:**393, 1980.

95. Mohs, F.: Personal communication, 1977.

96. Motegi, K., Nakano, Y., and Namikawa, A.: Relation between cleavage lines and scar tissues, J. Maxillofac. Surg. **12:**21, 1984.

97. Moynihan, R.G.A.: The ritual of a surgical operation, Br. J. Surg. **8:**27, 1920.
98. Myers, M.B., and Cherry, G.: Functional and angiographic vasculature in healing wounds, Am. Surg. **36:**750, 1970.
99. Myers, M.B., Cherry, G., and Heimburger, S.: Augmentation of wound tensile strength by early removal of sutures, Am. J. Surg. **117:**338, 1969.
100. Nealon, T.F., Jr.: Fundamental skills in surgery, ed. 3, Philadelphia, 1979, W.B. Saunders Co.
101. Nelson, C.A., and Dennis, C.: Wound healing, Surg. Gynecol. Obstet. **93:**461, 1951.
102. Nilsson, T.: Effect of increased and reduced tension on the mechanical properties of healing wound in the abdominal wall, Scand. J. Plast. Reconstr. Surg. **16:**101, 1982.
103. Noe, J.M.: Where should the knot be placed? Ann. Plast. Surg. **5:**145, 1980.
104. Ordman, L.J., and Gillman, T.: Studies in the healing of cutaneous wounds. II. The healing of epidermal, appendageal, and dermal injuries inflicted by suture needles and by the suture material on the skin of pigs, Arch. Surg. **93:**883, 1966.
105. Ordman, L.J., and Gillman, T.: Studies in the healing of cutaneous wounds. III. A critical comparison in the pig of the healing of surgical incisions closed with sutures or adhesive tape based on tensile strength and clinical and histological criteria, Arch. Surg. **93:**911, 1966.
106. Ott, A.E.: Disposable surgical drapes: a potential fire hazard, Obstet. Gynecol. **61:**667, 1983.
107. Panek, P.H., et al.: Potentiation of wound infection by adhesive adjuncts, Am. Surg. **38:**343, 1972.
108. Perry, A.W., and McShane, R.H.: Fine tuning of the skin edges in the closure of surgical wounds: controlling inversion and eversion with the path of the needle—the right stitch at the right time, J. Dermatol. Surg. Oncol. **7:**471, 1981.
109. Pers, M.: Some general surgical principles as applied to aesthetic surgery, Scand. J. Plast. Reconstr. Surg. **17:**187, 1983.
110. Petres, J., and Hundeiker, M.: Korrektive Dermatologie, Operationen an der Haut, New York, 1975, Springer-Verlag.
111. Pincus, F.: Die normale Anatomie der Haut. In Jadassohn, J., editor: Handbuch der Haut und Geschlechtskrankheiten, Berlin, 1927, Springer.
112. Polglase, A., et al.: A comparison of the incidence of wound infection following the use of percutaneous and subcuticular sutures: an experimental study, Aust. N. Z. J. Surg. **47:**423, 1977.
113. Pollock, A.V.: Surgical wound sepsis, Lancet **1:**1283, 1979.
114. Popkin, G.L., and Brodie, S.J.: The versatile skin hook, Arch. Dermatol. **86:**343, 1962.
115. Popkin, G.L., and Gibbs, R.C.: Another look at the skin hook [surgical gems], J. Dermatol. Surg. Oncol. **4:**366, 1978.
116. Price, P.G.: Stress, strain, and sutures, Ann. Surg. **128:**408, 1948.
117. Ragnell, A.: The tensibility of the skin: an experimental investigation, Plast. Reconstr. Surg. **14:**317, 1954.
118. Reid, M.R.: Some considerations of the problems of wound healing, N. Engl. J. Med. **215:**753, 1936.
119. Robbins, T.H.: Elliptical excision and closure, J.R. Coll. Surg. Edinb. **25:**59, 1980.
120. Robinson, J.K.: Even coaptation of wound edges of unequal thicknesses or unequal heights, J. Dermatol. Surg. Oncol. **5:**844, 1979.
121. Rodeheaver, G.T., Thacker, J.G., and Edlich, R.F.: Mechanical performance of polyglycolic acid and polyglactin 910 synthetic absorbable sutures, Surg. Gynecol. Obstet. **153:**835, 1981.
122. Rubin, L.R.: Langer's lines and facial scars, Plast. Reconstr. Surg. **3:**147, 1948.
123. Sakson, J.A.: First-day removal of skin sutures, Arch. Surg. **78:**304, 1959.
124. Salvendy, G., et al.: The development and validation of an analytical training program for medical suturing, Hum. Factors **22:**153, 1980.
125. Schilling, J.A.: Wound healing, Surg. Clin. North Am. **56:**859, 1976.
126. Silvola, H., et al.: Tissue trauma in surgical wound infection, Ann. Chir. Gynec. Fenniae **57:**548, 1968.
127. Simon, A.B.: Perioperative management of the pacemaker patient, Anesthesiology **46:**127, 1977.
128. Singleton, A.O., Jr., and Julian, J.: An experimental evaluation of methods used to prevent infection in wounds which have been contaminated with feces, Ann. Surg. **151:**912, 1960.
129. Snell, G.F.: A method for teaching techniques of office surgery, J. Fam. Pract. **7**(5):987, 1978.
130. Spicer, T.E.: Techniques of facial lesion excision and closure, J. Dermatol. Surg. Oncol. **8:**551, 1982.
131. Steffensen, W.H., and Worthen, E.F.: Limitations of multiple excision, Am. J. Surg. **95:**237, 1958.
132. Stegman, S.J.: Excisions on the face, Dermatology **3**(4):43, 1980.
133. Stegman, S.J., Tromovitch, T.A., and Glogau, R.G.: Basics of dermatologic surgery, Chicago, 1982, Year Book Medical Publishers, Inc.
134. Steiner, K., and Leifer, W.: Investigation of contact-type dermatitis due to compound tincture of benzoin, J. Inves. Dermatol. **13:**351, 1949.
135. Stillman, R.M., Bella, F.J., and Seligman, S.J.: Skin wound closure: the effect of various wound closure methods on susceptibility to infection, Arch. Surg. **115:**674, 1980.
136. Straatsma, C.R.: Surgical technique helpful in obtaining fine scars, Plast. Reconstr. Surg. **2:**21, 1947.
137. Strickler, J., and Gannon, P.G.: The "square knot" that slips, Minn. Med. **62:**643, 1979.
138. Taylor, F.W.: Surgical knots, Ann. Surg. **107:**458, 1938.
139. Taylor, G.A.: A new drape support for ophthalmic surgery, Am. J. Ophthalmol. **97:**391, 1984.
140. Thirlby, R.C., et al.: The value of prophylactic antibiotics for simple lacerations, Surg. Gynecol. Obstet. **156:**212, 1983.
141. Troutman, R.: Microsurgery of the anterior segment of the eye. Vol. 1; Introduction and basic techniques, St. Louis, 1974, The C.V. Mosby Co.
142. Watts, G.T.: Wound shape and tissue tension in healing, Br. J. Surg. **47:**555, 1960.
143. Webster, J.: Deforming scars, their causes, prevention, and treatment, Penn. Med. J. **38:**929, 1935.

144. Webster, R.C., Davidson, T.M., and Smith, R.C.: Broken-line scar revision. In Borges, A.F., editor: Clinics in plastic surgery, vol. 4, Philadelphia, 1977, W.B. Saunders Co.

145. Weiss, P.: In vitro experiments on the factors determining the course of the outgrowing nerve fiber, J. Exp. Zool. **68:** 393, 1934.

146. Weiss, Y.: Simplified method of needle-holder handling, Arch. Surg. **106:**735, 1973.

147. Welch, W.H.: Conditions underlying the infection of wounds, Trans. Cong. Am. Phys. Surg. **2:**1, 1891.

148. Werth, J.L.: Basic skin closure, Ear Nose Throat J. **60:**25, 1981.

149. Westreich, M., and Kapetansky, D.I.: Avoiding the slippery knot syndrome [letter], J.A.M.A. **236:**2487, 1976.

150. White, J.H., and Stern, R.U.: A theoretical consideration of suturing technique, Ann. Ophthalmol. **3:**509, 1971.

151. Wianko, K.B.: Wound healing: incisions and suturing, Can. Med. Assoc. J. **84:**254, 1961.

152. Winn, H.R., et al.: Influence of subcuticular sutures on scar formation, Am. J. Surg. **133:**257, 1977.

153. Wray, R.C.: Force required for wound closure and scar appearance, Plast. Reconstr. Surg. **72:**380, 1983.

154. Wray, R.C., Jr., Holtmann, B., and Weeks, P.: Factors in the production of inconspicuous scars, Plast. Reconstr. Surg. **56:**86, 1975.

155. Zaidan, J.R.: Pacemakers, Anesthesiology **60:**319, 1984.

156. Zoltan, J.: Cicatrix optima; Baltimore, 1978, University Park Press.

11

Alternative Suture Techniques

There are endless variations of suture techniques for skin closure, many of which seem to work better for some surgeons than for others. All of these techniques have certain indications, advantages, and disadvantages. Mastery of these different methods and understanding of the geometry of tissue movements affected by these techniques can give the surgeon more versatility and better cosmetic results.

In comparing various suturing methods, the following factors are important to keep in mind:

1. Likelihood of complications (such as infection)
2. Cosmetic results, especially the long-term rather than just the short-term results
3. Patient comfort and acceptability
4. Ease of placement
5. Ease of postoperative management

As shown in the following outline, cutaneous closure techniques may be divided into interrupted (noncontinuous) and continuous. Interrupted closures require separate sutures or other materials to close a wound; continuous closures are closed by one continuous thread or other material.

Closure techniques can be further subcategorized into nonburied, partially buried, and totally buried. It is important to appreciate the existence of these three possible locations of wound closure material because depth of placement affects wound healing and the possibility of subsequent wound infection. Sutures with a portion of the suture material on the surface and a portion below the surface are only partially buried. Even sutures with only a minor component exiting the skin—for instance, running intradermal sutures—are considered partially buried.

I. Interrupted (noncontinuous)
  A. Nonburied
    1. Skin tapes
  B. Partially buried
    1. Staples
    2. Interrupted (simple) suture

    3. Vertical mattress suture
    4. Half-buried vertical mattress suture
    5. Horizontal mattress suture
    6. Half-buried horizontal mattress suture
    7. Near-far–far-near suture
    8. Figure-eight suture
  C. Totally buried (dermal, dermal-subdermal, subdermal)
    1. Simple vertical interrupted
    2. Simple horizontal interrupted
II. Continuous
  A. Nonburied
    1. Skin tapes
    2. Tissue glue
  B. Partially buried
    1. Running continuous suture
    2. Running vertical mattress suture
    3. Running locked suture
    4. Running horizontal mattress suture
    5. Running intradermal suture
  C. Totally buried
    1. Dermal running suture
    2. Subcutaneous running suture

INTERRUPTED CLOSURES
Skin tapes

Skin tape designed for closure of wounds is probably the most underutilized wound-closure material in cutaneous surgery. Skin tape closure materials, their advantages and disadvantages, and their effects on wound healing are all discussed in Chapter 8; however, a few highlights are mentioned here for emphasis.

Investigators working on guinea pigs realized that skin tapes cause no trauma and that their use to close wounds therefore makes more sense than percutaneous sutures from a histologic point of view.[22,38] Sutures create additional

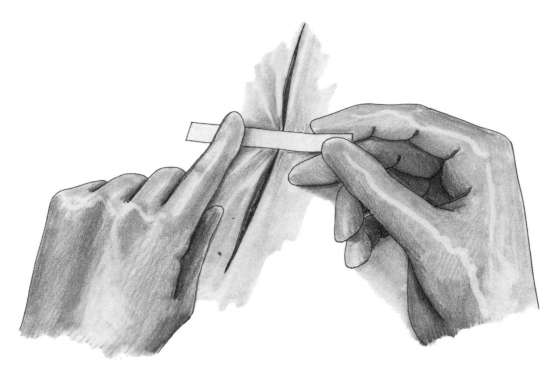

Fig. 11-1. Application of skin tapes.

wounds within suture tracts that are subject to infections and scarring. Since taped wounds do not develop suture tracts, routine use of tape was recommended. Naturally this suggestion was met with much resistance.

The use of skin tapes to close wounds has been shown in several studies to be biologically sound and useful for a number of reasons. Skin tapes provide relatively strong mechanical support for wound edges and can be used for long periods of time. Because suture tracts are not formed, the cosmetic results may be better than if percutaneous sutures are used.[26,40] Wounds closed with skin tapes are also less likely to get infected.[45] The lack of additional trauma beneath the skin surface results in less inflammation and aids wound healing. Taped wounds show greater early gains in tensile strength, than sutured wounds.[16,17]

One common indication for skin tape is primary closure of wounds where the skin edges are under little tension— for instance, where buried sutures have been placed that coapt the wound edges. Skin tapes may also be used in conjunction with interrupted percutaneous sutures (see Fig. 10-41). Perhaps the most common use of skin tapes is to reinforce wounds after percutaneous sutures have been removed[21] (see Fig. 10-53, *E*). Skin tapes are also recommended to close wounds when sutures are otherwise undesirable (for example, in uncooperative adults or children).

Skin tapes are not without problems, however.[9] Alignment of the wound edges is not as precise as with percutaneous sutures. Sometimes skin tapes do not adhere or slip. This may particularly be a problem if the wound oozes blood or serum. Skin tapes do not stick in hair-bearing areas or where there is maceration. Wounds have also been known to dehisce with skin tapes. Buried dermal sutures will help to prevent this.

The method for application of skin tapes is shown in Fig. 11-1. Note that one finger holds the skin tape in place and at the same time pushes one wound edge toward the other while the opposite end of the tape is fixed. Before application of skin tapes, the skin should be cleansed of dried blood and debris and degreased with an organic solvent (such as tape remover), and a tackefier should be applied (such as compound tincture of benzoin). The tackefier is allowed to dry, since moisture prevents sticking of the skin tapes. One should be careful not to inadvertently let the tackefier get into the wound itself because it may potentiate wound infection.[39] The patient should be instructed to keep the wound dry, since water weakens the tape's bond to the skin.

The pattern of skin tape application depends on the clinical situation. Normally, to reinforce wounds when sutures are removed in a week, singly placing the tapes straight across (and perpendicular to length of) the wound is sufficient (Fig. 11-2, *A*). If the wound is under more tension, alternative methods may be useful to hold the wound together better (Fig. 11-2, *B* and *C*). Note that the methods shown are interrupted skin tape closures.

One may also apply a skin tape running along and over the length of the wound in a continuous nonburied skin-closure technique. Some skin tapes (Clearon Skin Closures) are reinforced perpendicular to the long axis of the strip for

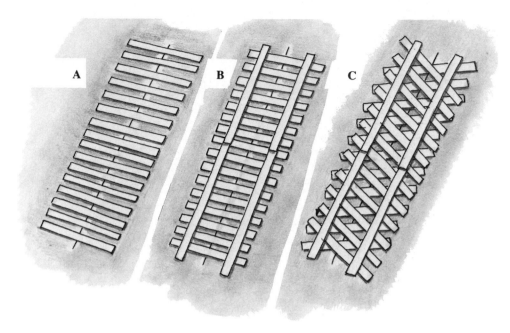

Fig. 11-2. Different patterns of skin tape application. **A,** Perpendicular to length of wound. **B,** Perpendicular to wound and reinforced. **C,** Criss-cross and reinforced. (Modified from Converse, J.M.: Reconstructive plastic surgery, Philadelphia, 1977, W.B. Saunders Co.)

this purpose. Op-Site may also be used for this purpose.[59] This material is of some value during the first week after closure, when occlusion enhances epidermization.

Staples

Staples are discussed in some detail in Chapter 8. The advantages of staples are their ease and speed of placement and the good wound edge eversion achieved.[11,31,51] Also, because a staple does not form a complete 360-degree loop like a suture, tracts leading from the cutaneous surface into the wound are unlikely (see Fig. 8-11). Theoretically this results in less likelihood of wound infection. For the same reason, staples lead to less tissue strangulation than percutaneous sutures do. Staples are very strong and nonreactive and are therefore of use in areas under great tension.

The main problem with staples is that it is sometimes difficult to get good wound edge alignment, and therefore the cosmetic results cannot be expected to be as good as with fine percutaneous sutures. However, I have found the cosmetic results surprisingly good.

For the proper placement of skin staples, the wound edges should first be completely apposed. If subcutaneous or dermal buried sutures have been used, this may have already been accomplished; however, frequently one finds that the skin edges have not been apposed. Sometimes during staple placement the skin edges can be temporarily apposed by hand, with or without an assistant. Other techniques to appose the skin edges temporarily include using a Backhaus towel clip or using a silk suture. The latter technique is shown in Fig. 11-3, on the next page. Once the

staples have been placed, the temporary suture is removed.

Skin hooks, either at the ends of an excision or at the sides, may also be used to bring the wound edges together. This has the advantage of not perforating the cutaneous surface.

A staple after placement should ride high, so that subsequent wound swelling does not cause crimping of the tissue and cross hatching to occur.[31] If a staple is inserted at an angle to the surface of the skin (Fig. 11-4), it will naturally rotate so that its cross member is higher (*b* in Fig. 11-4) than if the staple is inserted straight down into the tissue (*c* in Fig. 11-4). Some staple manufacturers currently make staple guns specially designed so that the staple is inserted at an angle of 45 to 60 degrees to the skin surface.

The excellent cosmetic results from staples is shown in Fig. 11-5. A surgical defect is shown on the temple, which resulted from removal of a cutaneous neoplasm (Fig. 11-5, *A*). The wound was closed with staples and a few interrupted nylon sutures (Fig. 11-5, *B*). The latter were necessary to provide good wound apposition and eversion where malaligned edges had occurred. This is not uncommon with staples, particularly on the skin. The wound, before the insertion of staples, was brought together by buried dermal absorbable sutures, and dog-ears at each end were repaired. The cosmetic result at 1 year (Fig. 11-5, *C*) is excellent. There are no cross-hatch suture marks even though the staples were removed 1 week later.

For the sake of comparison one should turn to two other cases with similar surgical defects: Figs. 11-6 and 11-7. Fig. 11-6, *A,* is a wound in a similar location and of similar

Text continued on p. 453.

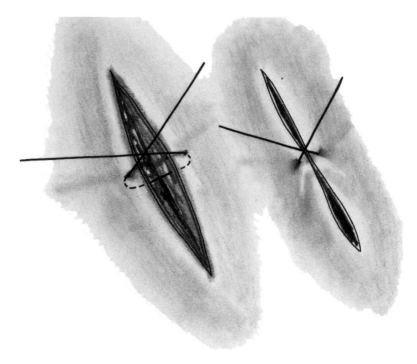

Fig. 11-3. Use of temporary silk suture to appose wound edges for staple placement.

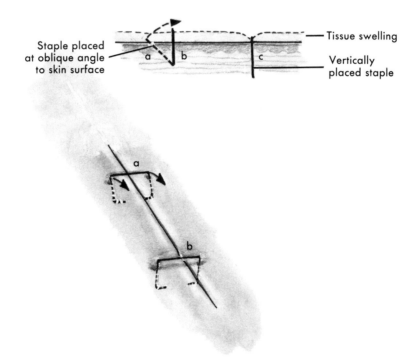

Fig. 11-4. Relationship of initial staple-placement angle to final height of cross member above skin surface. Staple placed *(a)* obliquely to skin surface rotates to new vertical position *(b)* naturally. Vertically placed staple *(c)* cannot rotate. With tissue swelling, vertically placed staple *(c)* tends to constrict tissue, whereas obliquely placed staple does not constrict tissue because its cross member is higher.

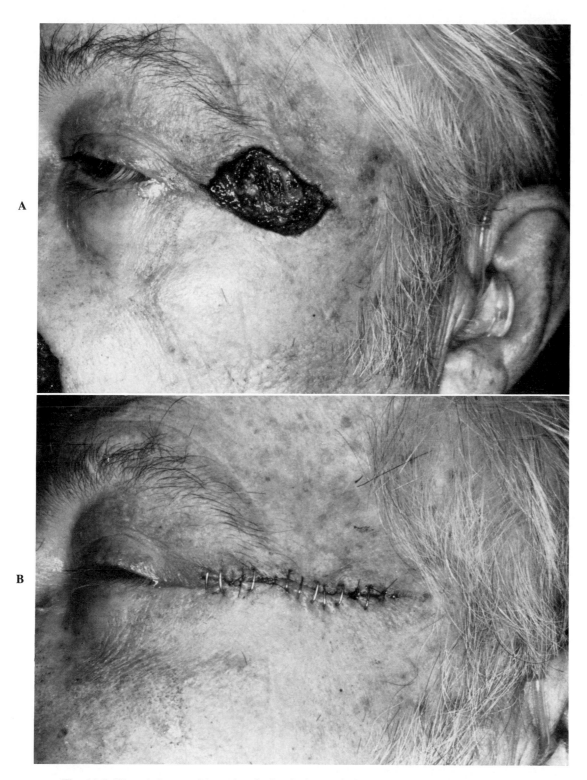

Fig. 11-5. Wound closure with staples. **A,** Surgical wound after removal of basal cell carcinoma. **B,** Wound closed with staples and a few interrupted nylon sutures. Straight dog-ear repairs made at each end of wound. *Continued.*

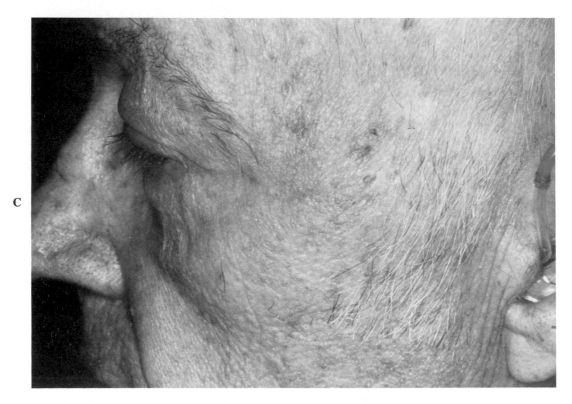

Fig. 11-5, cont'd. C, Healed surgical wound 1 year after surgery. Note excellent cosmetic result.

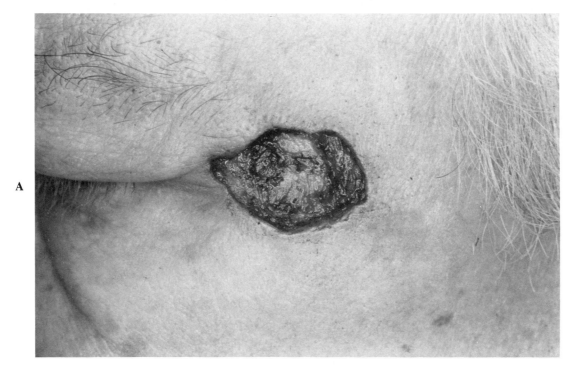

Fig. 11-6. Wound closure with interrupted sutures. **A,** Surgical wound after removal of basal cell carcinoma.

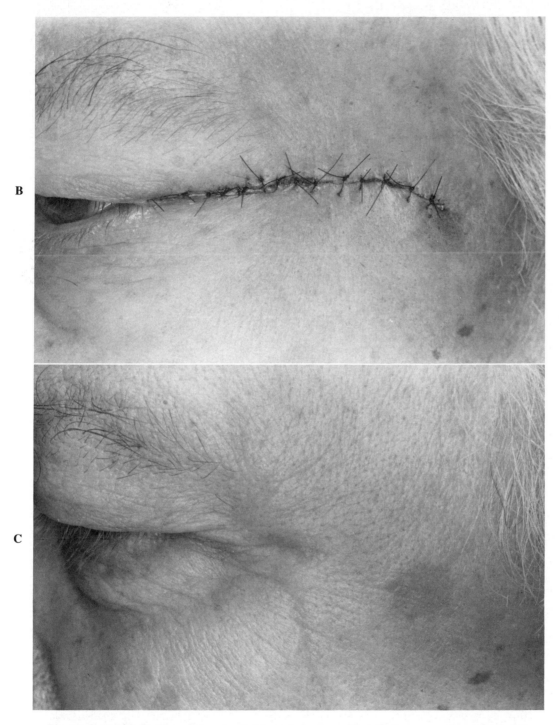

B

C

Fig. 11-6, cont'd. B, Wound closed with interrupted sutures. Straight dog-ear repair anteriorly but slightly curved dog-ear repair posteriorly. **C,** Healed surgical wound 1 year after operation; note excellent cosmetic result. Compare with Fig. 11-5, *C.*

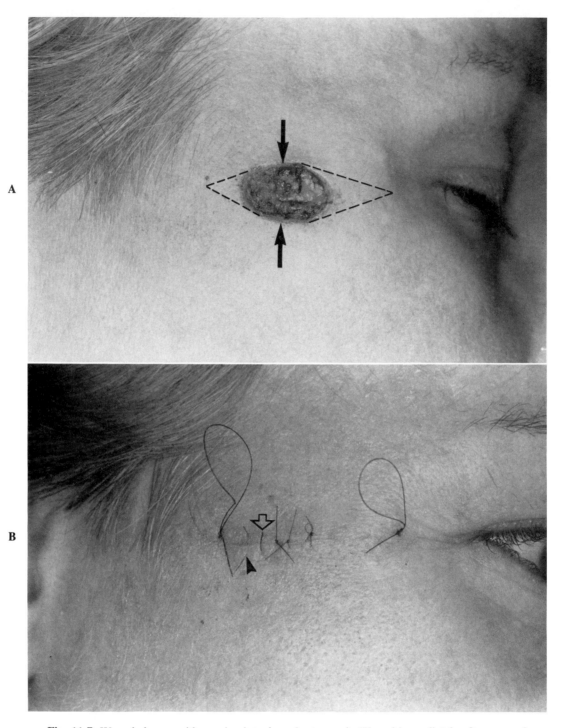

Fig. 11-7. Wound closure with running intradermal sutures. **A,** Wound immediately after removal of basal cell carcinoma. Wound closed initially with buried absorbable sutures in direction of arrows. Dog-ears were removed anteriorly and posteriorly. Dashed lines represent the tissue removed in dog-ear repairs. Alternatively, one could have excised tissue along dashed lines before initial closure. **B,** Wound sutured with running intradermal suture, knotted on skin surface at each end of incision line. Note that running intradermal suture is looped above the skin surface *(open arrow),* where lateral wound tension is high. Also, a few interrupted sutures are placed to even up wound edges precisely. One suture *(arrowhead)* is left untied purposely to even up wound edges without bunching tissue.

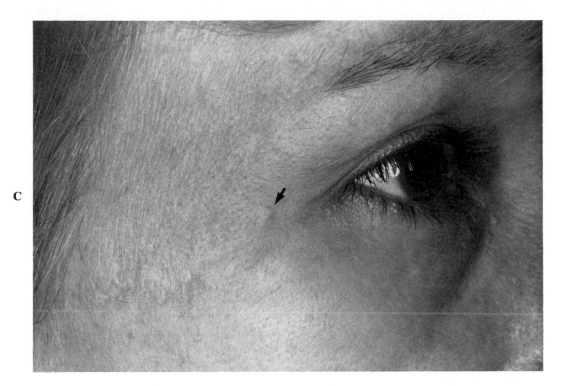

C

Fig. 11-7, cont'd. C, Healed surgical wound 1 year after operation. Compare with Figs. 11-5 and 11-6. Note slight protuberance *(arrow)* where running intradermal suture is knotted. This sometimes occurs because knot works its way into tissue. Therefore I prefer to tape ends of running intradermal sutures, as shown in Fig. 11-26.

size to that of the patient in Fig. 11-5, A; however, the cutaneous edges of the wound were sutured totally with interrupted nylon sutures (Fig. 11-6, *B*). As in the previous case the wound was first brought together by buried dermal absorbable sutures and then the dog-ears were repaired. The healed surgical scar 11-6, *C*, is barely apparent and comparable to that in Fig. 11-5, *C*.

A third approach to suturing a wound in this area is shown in Fig. 11-7: the wound was closed as before with buried dermal absorbable sutures, and the dog ears at both ends were repaired, requiring tissue to be removed as shown on the dashed line (Fig. 11-7, *A*). However, a running intradermal suture was placed (Fig. 11-7, *B*); one point of exit of the suture from the wound (where the tension was highest) is shown by the open arrow. The arrowhead points to a purposely untied nylon suture placed to even up the wound edges. The cosmetic result is, as in the previous cases, excellent (Fig. 11-7, *C*). Nevertheless, if one looks closely *(arrow),* one can see a small protuberance, the point of entrance of the running intradermal suture. This is why I do not recommend knotting the ends to secure this suture, as is shown here (Fig. 11-7, *B*). More about this is discussed later.

To summarize, staples can lead to excellent cosmetic results when one would not normally expect this to be the case. In addition, different types of surgical closures may lead to essentially comparable cosmetic results. Perhaps more important than which technique is used is *how* it is used. Gentle handling of tissue cannot be overemphasized.

Modifications of simple interrupted sutures

Certain modifications of simple interrupted sutures have been described. Webster, Davidson, and Smith described using 6-0 mild chromic suture (made by Davis & Geck) as interrupted simple percutaneous sutures.[60] They thought that this suture is absorbed so fast that skin suture marks are unlikely. Because this chromic suture is "mild," only a minimal inflammatory reaction usually occurs; still, some individuals may have a greater reaction to chromic sutures than others. In addition, buried portions of this suture remain in the tissue and must be absorbed. Another disadvantage of this technique is the unpredictability of the absorption time. A more recently described catgut suture used for the same purpose that mild chromic catgut is used is a nonchromatized catgut—"fast-absorbing gut" (made by Ethicon). This new suture, however, probably has disadvantages similar to those of mild chromic catgut.

Interrupted sutures tied in locations where considerable tension exists crimp the tissue, cutting into it and ultimately leaving suture marks. Some rarely used techniques have been devised to prevent this. Special clamps have been described to grasp the suture when it exists from the skin so

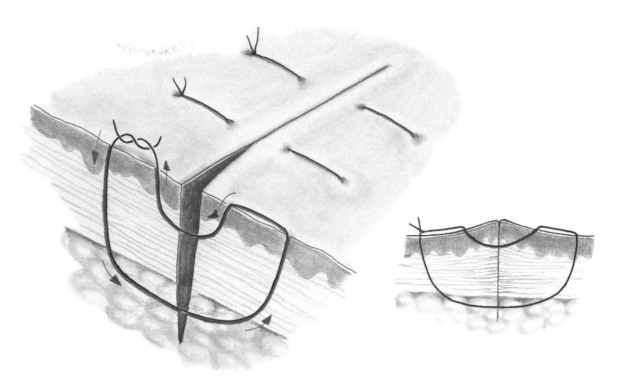

Fig. 11-8. Vertical mattress suture. Note eversion of epidermal wound edges *(right)*.

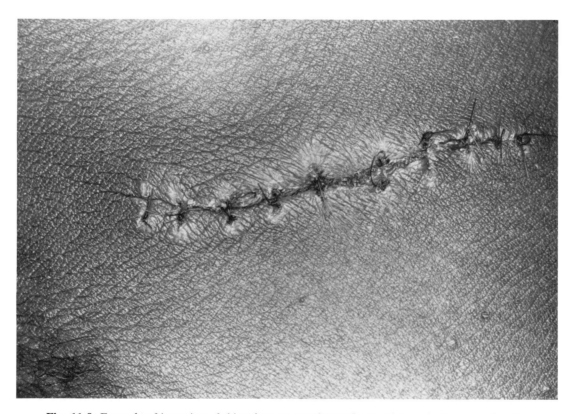

Fig. 11-9. Example of inversion of skin edges on anterior neck wound 1 week after operation. In this case small-caliber interrupted sutures were used in very thin skin. Vertical mattress sutures would have prevented inversion and produced more exactly apposed wound edges.

it is unnecessary to tie suture over the top of a wound.[44] Another described technique is to use plastic tubing, much thicker than normal sutures, as suture material.[12] This prevents the tearing of tissue seen with thinner, more conventional sutures.

Vertical mattress suture

The vertical mattress suture (Fig. 11-8) has three basic functions. First, it helps to evert epidermal wound edges when they tend to invert. Second, it helps to close the deeper areas of the wound. Third, it adds strength to a wound closure.

Infolding of the epidermal wound edges is particularly a problem where the skin is thin, such as on the eyelids or anterior neck (Fig. 11-9). Problems with the entire wound edge alignment also occur when a thin wound edge abuts a thick one. Vertical mattress sutures are ideal in these situations because they help to even up the epidermal and dermal layers of a sutured cutaneous wound.

As can be seen in Fig. 11-8 the vertical mattress suture is composed of two loops whose ends are symmetrically placed and equidistant from the wound cavity. One begins this stitch farther from the wound edge than one would a simple interrupted suture. Usually one enters the skin about 2 to 3 mm from the wound edge, goes through the dermis or fat to the other wound edge, and exits through the epidermis at a point opposite to the point of entrance on the other side. These initial points of exit and entrance are equidistant from the wound edges. One then reenters the wound edge close (within 1 mm) to the wound cavity, exits through the dermis, crosses the wound, and exits through the opposite wound edge, where the knot is tied. When the knot is tied the epidermal wound edges are forced up into a position of eversion (Fig. 11-8, *right*).

Mattress sutures, because they have a greater amount of dermal tissue within their loops, have greater holding power than simple interrupted sutures have.[30] This holding power is increased as the amount of tissue within the suture increases.[28] Therefore, this suture is occasionally useful to take tension off a sutured wound. Vertical mattress sutures do, however, tend to constrict the blood supply, more so than interrupted sutures,[35] so when they are used, they should be tied very carefully and very gently.

Vertical mattress sutures tend to constrict and crimp the epidermal tissue between the loops of the sutures on each epidermal surface. This sometimes leads to noticeable suture scars, so in areas of great cosmetic concern this suture should be used sparingly. If it is necessary to evert the wound edges, sometimes only a few vertical mattress sutures do the job, and in between them simple interrupted sutures may be used.

As already discussed, vertical mattress sutures help to align and appose more completely the dermal and epidermal wound edges. This can result in faster wound healing with greater tensile strength earlier than if simple interrupted sutures are placed (Fig. 13-5, *C*). Locations such as the anterior neck, inguinal areas, and eyelids seem to heal with better scars if vertical mattress sutures are used (for at least part of the wound). Fig. 11-9 shows inversion of the skin edges at 1 week, where simple interrupted sutures were used on the skin of the anterior neck. This probably would have been prevented by use of a few vertical mattress sutures.

A modification of the vertical mattress suture that is sometimes useful is shown in Fig. 11-10. The suture deviates in depth from its usual horizontal course by diving to pick up some deep fibrous tissue. Thus it encloses more tissue within its loop and eliminates additional dead space. This suture may also be used when one wishes to orient the incision line more to one side of a surgical defect than another. If the tissue at the base of the surgical defect is fairly fibrous, placing the deep loop to one side helps to anchor the wound there. This is occasionally of benefit to help place incision lines more precisely into the contours of the face. The same deep anchoring deviation pathway can be used with simple interrupted buried sutures as well.

When suturing mucosa from the nonmucosal side—as, for example, with a lip wedge—a vertical mattress suture is used so that the mucosa is everted toward the inside of the mouth.[32] This is similar to the Gambee suture used on the mucosa of the gastrointestinal tract.[46]

Condon reported a modification of the vertical mattress suture: on exiting the wound just before being tied, the suture is looped under the loop on the opposite side and then brought over the wound and tied.[7] He claimed that this "locked vertical mattress suture" takes tension off the deeper part of the wound. However, this modification probably tends to invert the wound edges and contributes to a certain asymmetry on the wound surface.

Another variation of the vertical mattress suture has been described, in which the vertical mattress suture is placed by two passes of the needle in the same direction.[36] The first pass goes through the skin edges on both sides near the wound. One can then use the suture to tent up the skin edges and pass a second suture loop—again, through both skin edges and in the same direction as the first but further back from the wound. When tied, this vertical mattress suture is a cross stitch, going from the near skin edge to the opposite far side. The problem with this variation is that it tends to invert the skin edges, although it is more quickly placed than the classic vertical mattress suture.

Half-buried vertical mattress suture

The half-buried vertical mattress suture (Fig. 11-11) is used to align wound edges when cosmesis is important and vascular impairment must be minimized. Since this stitch has only one loop rather than two above the skin surface (as in the vertical mattress suture), there is less crimping of

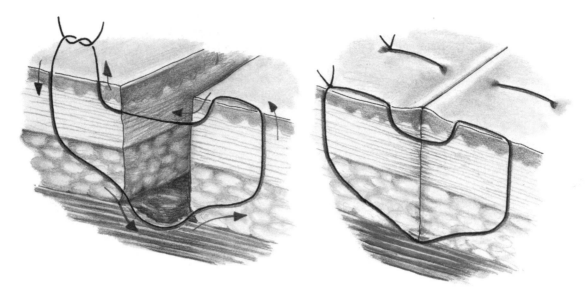

Fig. 11-10. Modified vertical mattress suture. Deep loop catches underlying deep subcutaneous tissue and fascia, thereby facilitating elimination of dead space.

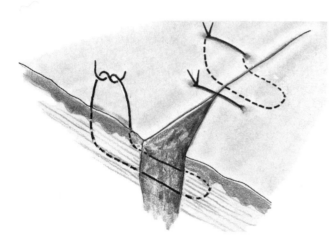

Fig. 11-11. Half-buried vertical mattress suture.

epidermal tissue. This suture may occasionally be useful for suturing flaps. Note in Fig. 11-11 the closer distance from the wound edge of the simple interrupted suture, compared to where the half-buried vertical mattress suture enters the skin.

Horizontal mattress suture

The horizontal mattress suture (Fig. 11-12) is used to take tension off wound edges. Because it includes a copious amount of tissue, it is useful to stop bleeding from wound edges in vascular areas, such as the scalp. The larger the amount of deep tissue contained in this suture, the larger the amount of dead space eliminated.

The horizontal mattress suture begins on one side of the wound about 2 to 3 mm from the skin edge, which is farther from the edge than where a simple interrupted suture is usually placed (about 1 to 1.5 mm). It enters the skin, passing through the dermis or subcutaneous tissue to the opposite side of the wound, where it passes up through the dermis and exits the skin. At this point the suture courses parallel to the wound for 2 to 3 mm and reenters the skin, passing through the dermis. After crossing the wound cavity, the suture passes through the dermis and exits through the epidermis, where it is tied. Therefore this suture is composed of two loops, as the vertical mattress suture is; however, the planes of the two loops face one another, and the strands crossing the wound cavity do so parallel to one another but in a horizontal plane. (In a vertical mattress suture the strands cross the wound cavity parallel to each other but in a vertical plane.)

The loops of the horizontal mattress suture enclose epidermis, which is inevitably crimped. This is particularly true when significant tension occurs in the wound. Strangulation of tissue, necrosis, infection, and obvious suture marks may all result. These problems may be minimized somewhat by the placement of bolsters (Fig. 11-12). A bolster is a material placed under the suture to distribute the tension of the sutures on the underlying skin more evenly. Bolsters thus help prevent sutures from cutting into the tissue. Many substances can be used as bolsters, including cotton, plastic tubing, flat buttons,[41] or the cardboard paper in which the suture material is packaged.

Horizontal mattress sutures may be used to take some tension off wound edges, especially when large amounts of dead space exist. When used in this manner, they are placed both wide (5 to 10 mm) of the wound edges and deep into the subcutaneous tissue. Wide horizontal mattress sutures act as holding sutures. They cinch and ease the

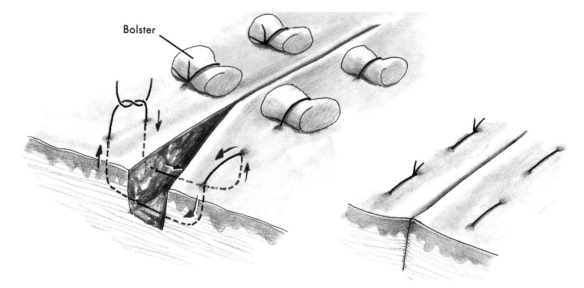

Bolster

Fig. 11-12. Horizontal mattress sutures, tied with bolsters *(left)* and without bolsters *(right).*

wound edges together when simple subcutaneous or dermal-subdermal sutures are not quite strong enough by themselves. Usually simple interrupted sutures are then placed more proximal to the wound than these wide horizontal mattress sutures. The wide horizontal mattress sutures may be only temporary, being removed when the deep and other percutaneous sutures are all placed. They are removed before the dressing is applied. If likelihood of dehiscence of the wound exists on removal of the horizontal mattress sutures, they are left in place and removed at a later time.

Significant tension occurs on wide horizontal sutures placed to hold wound edges together, so large-caliber suture material, such as 3-0 silk or nylon, must be used. Significant pressure on the enclosed epidermis also occurs with wide horizontal mattress suture, so bolsters must be used to minimize the cutting into tissue by the suture material itself.

Simmonds has written about the use of horizontal mattress sutures with bolsters to prevent dehiscence.[47,48] He states that the bolstered sutures may be left in place until healing is adequate to prevent dehiscence. He recommends removal of these sutures from 1 to 2 days on the face to 2 to 3weeks on the back or extremities.

My own experience with bolstered horizontal mattress sutures used to hold a wound together because of tension on the wound edges is not good. Unfortunately, if these sutures are removed in only a few days, the wound is likely to dehisce. If left until after the other cutaneous sutures are removed and the wound has gained significant wound strength, the risk of necrosis and scarring is high. Fig. 11-13 shows areas of necrosis that occurred under cotton bolsters. Compared with horizontal mattress sutures, staples hold wounds together with less tissue constriction when the wound edges

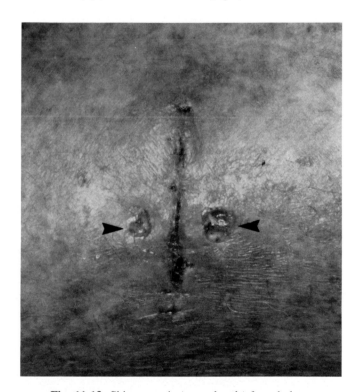

Fig. 11-13. Skin necrosis *(arrowheads)* from bolster.

are under great tension and thus with less likelihood of necrosis. Since the introduction of staples, horizontal mattress sutures have become less commonly used as holding sutures.

Like the vertical mattress stitch, horizontal mattress stitches undoubtedly are stronger than interrupted stitches. Also, because of the amount of tissue enclosed within their loops, these sutures are more likely to create avascular areas and necrosis.

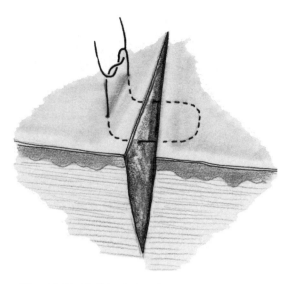

Fig. 11-14. Half-buried horizontal mattress suture.

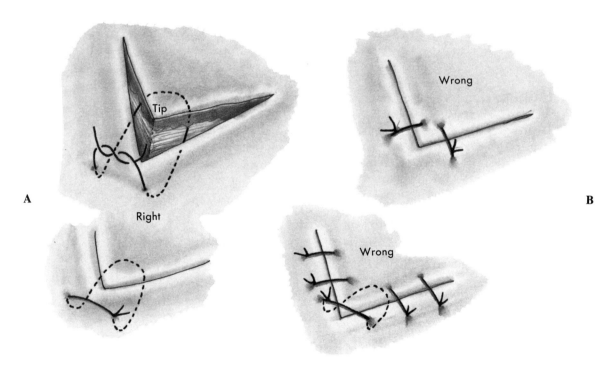

Fig. 11-15. Proper (**A**) and improper (**B**) methods of placing three-point suture.

In one study a horizontal mattress suture was buried except at the four corners in an attempt to prevent necrosis of tissue and suture marks.[10] This method does not prevent suture marks, however, and in fact is likely to cause tissue necrosis because of the tissue entrapped at the corners.

Half-buried horizontal mattress suture

The half-buried horizontal mattress suture is similar to the horizontal mattress suture except that one of the loops

is totally buried (Figs. 10-48 and 11-14). Like a half-buried vertical mattress suture, a half-buried horizontal mattress suture results in only 2 punctures through the skin instead of four.

The main use for a half-buried horizontal mattress suture is in securing the edges of flaps, when a more secure suture than a simple interrupted suture is required. However, theoretically the half-buried horizontal mattress suture impedes the blood supply to the epidermis on the buried side more than a simple interrupted suture does.

Another important use of the half-buried horizontal mattress suture is to even up even wound edges, particularly when one edge is bound down and rather immobile. This is discussed and illustrated in Chapter 10 (Fig. 10-48).

Three- and four-point suture

The three- and four-point sutures can be considered half-buried horizontal mattress sutures. They are used to secure tips of tissue into corners without strangulating the tips. Such tips of tissue are found in skin flaps, Z-plasties, and multiple W-plasties. Star-shaped traumatic lacerations also include triangular tips of tissue. The three-point suture is also referred to as the corner stitch, or Gillies' corner stitch.[34] The latter term is a misnomer, since Gillies really described closure of triangular defects and not a corner suture.

The three-point suture is shown in Fig. 11-15. In placing this suture there are four important considerations with respect to the suture's location relative to the skin surface, skin edges and tip. These include the following:
1. Location of the points of entrance and exit
2. Vertical level of the suture in the surrounding tissue immediately after the exit and before the entrance
3. Vertical depth of the suture loop in the tip
4. Horizontal distance the loop is placed proximally in the tip

If all four of these considerations are kept in mind, the three-point suture will be well placed.

The suture is begun in the skin behind and slightly to the side of the apex of the recipient corner for the tip of tissue. It is initially carried to about the mid dermis, then crosses the wound to loop through the tip of the triangular piece of tissue. It is essential that this loop be horizontal to the skin surface and placed at the same level in the dermis of the tip as the point at which the suture exits the skin to cross the wound. After the loop is made in the tip, the suture enters the other side of the wound, also at the same level of the dermis, and exits the skin near its entrance point. The final exit point and the initial entry point are equidistant from the wound edge. When the suture is tied, there should be minimal tension on the tip of tissue. Also, the tip should be level with the surrounding tissue.

The portion of the suture on the skin surface outside the wound should not cross the tip of tissue. If this does happen, as shown in Fig. 11-15 *(lower right),* it tends to promote strangulation of tissue.

It should be pointed out that suturing a tissue tip in this way does not obliterate the dead space underlying the tip. Dead space is exacerbated under a tip of tissue because a tip is frequently cut obliquely on the undersurface, or the undersurface of the tip on stretching pulls the tissue into a more oblique position relative to the surface epidermis. Although this dead space usually is not a source of problems, one needs to keep it in mind.

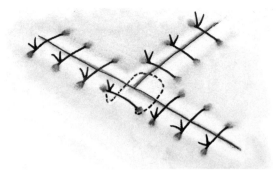

Fig. 11-16. Four-point suture.

Vertical suture placed directly through the tip or two vertical sutures (one on either side of the tip), are to be avoided[32] (Fig. 11-15, *upper right*). It is felt that a three-point suture allows more blood flow to the tip, especially in the epidermis, which may necrose if its vascular supply is impeded. However, this concept is not based on scientific evidence but on clinical impression. In pigs there was virtually no difference in tip survival whether vertical sutures through the tip or three-point sutures were used.[34] Nevertheless, I prefer a three-point suture.

A four-point suture is shown in Fig. 11-16. This suture is similar to a three-point suture, except that two tips of tissue are sutured instead of one. Therefore there are four points of tension on the suture instead of three.

Sometimes 3- or 4-point sutures do not result in tips perfectly aligned with surrounding tissues. Usually this means that the loop of suture in the tip is not level with the entrance and exit points in the surrounding tissue. If the tip is riding high, the suture loop is relatively too deep from the skin surface in the tip; alternatively, if the tip is too low, the suture loop is too high in the dermis of the tip. If the tip's surface does not lie flat and at the same level as the adjacent tissue surface, the suture should be removed and replaced so that the loop's depth of placement on the tip is level with the entrance and exit points in the lateral dermis of the corner.

The distance the suture loop is placed from the end of the tip is variable. As already mentioned tips of tissue are frequently cut obliquely so that it is difficult to get an adequate amount of tissue close to the cut edge in the loop. Ideally the loop should be placed just far enough back in the tip to obtain good security of tissue but not far enough back that the tip would ride high when tied. The proper distance is a matter of judgment, practice, and finesse. Usually 1 mm or less is enough distance in the tip to get an adequate amount of tissue.

Six-point suture

The six-point suture is a horizontal mattress suture with three loops instead of two, and six points of tension (Fig. 11-17). This suture is useful in closing triangular defects of

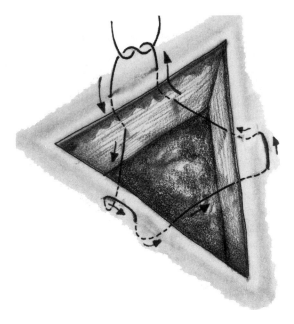

Fig. 11-17. Six-point suture.

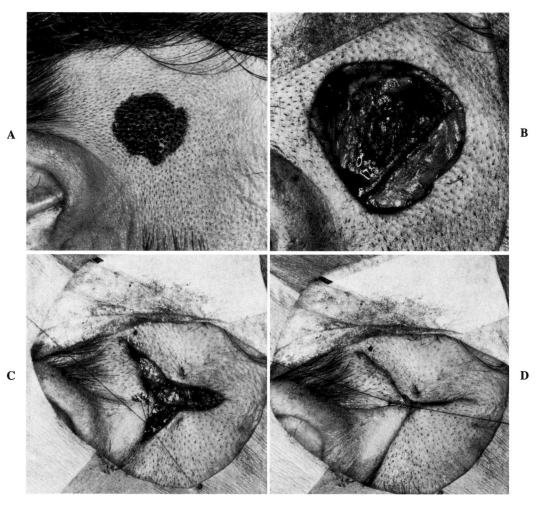

Fig. 11-18, For legend, see opposite page.

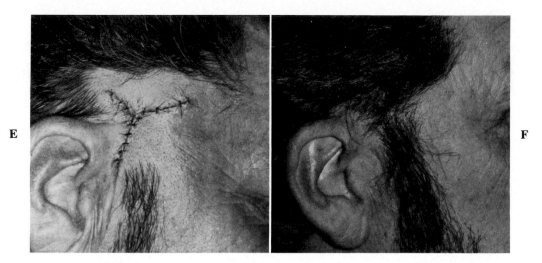

Fig. 11-18, cont'd. Six-point suture used to close a surgical defect. **A,** Preoperative photograph of melanoma (Clark's level II) in congenital nevus on parietal scalp. **B,** Excision with adequate margins on sides and bottom. **C,** Conversion of rounded defect to Y with six-point suture. **D,** Total apposition of skin edges with six-point suture. **E,** Sutured wound after repair of dog-ears and placement of interrupted sutures. **F,** Healed wound at 3 months. Note that tension on anterior helix (seen in **D** and **E**) has resolved.

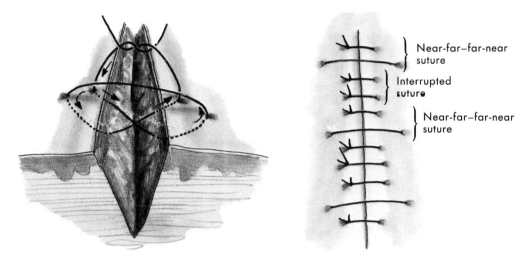

Fig. 11-19. Near-far–far-near suture.

equal sides, so that when tied the edges are drawn together with equal tension and are everted. The triangular defect is thus converted into a Y-shaped closure. This suture is particularly useful in closing defects that are under considerable tension and can be used as the initial key suture (Fig. 11-18, *C* and *D*).

The suture is placed in the mid to lower dermis or even below the dermis; however, below the surface of the skin the suture should be at the same depth where it crosses the wound cavity. Bolsters are rarely necessary. Once the wound is drawn together by the six-point suture, interrupted sutures are placed at the three sides. These help take the tension off the skin held by the six-point suture.

Gillies described a modification of the six-point suture in which two of the three horizontal loops were completely buried, leaving only one loop above the skin between the entrance and exit points.[34] My experience is that this usually does not work nearly as well as when all three loops of the six-point suture are above the surface of the skin.

Near-far–far-near suture

When the skin is thin but under some tension, the near-far–far-near suture is a good alternative (Fig. 11-19). This suture combines the strength of a vertical mattress suture with the careful tissue approximation of an interrupted suture. Compared with the horizontal and vertical mattress

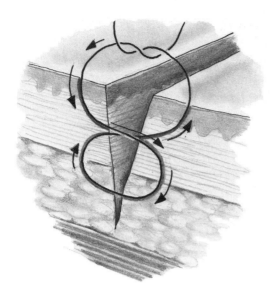

Fig. 11-20. Figure-eight suture (superficial).

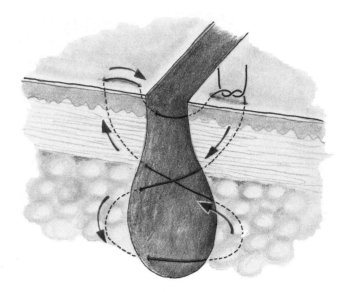

Fig. 11-21. Figure-eight suture (deep). Note that superficial loop is placed with vertical mattress suture pathway.

sutures, the near-far–far-near suture has less of a tendency to strangulate tissue. It is composed of two loops, one closer to the skin edges than the other. The near-far–far-near suture was popularized for suturing on the eyelids, where the skin is thin.[49]

The suture is begun near the wound edge at the usual distance (1.0 to 1.5 mm) at which one would enter the skin to place a simple interrupted suture. It then crosses the wound at an angle and enters the opposite wound edge at the same level; but it exits further from the wound edge (usually 2 or 3 mm) than the initial point of entrance. Therefore one has gone from near the wound edge to far from the wound edge. The suture is then brought over the wound surface directly across to the opposite side, where it enters the skin—again, far from the wound edge and equidistant to the opposite side. Finally the suture again crosses the wound, enters the skin on the opposite side, and exits from the skin near the wound edge. The second portion of the suture thus goes far from the wound edge to near the wound edge. The suture is then tied. It results in two portions crossing the wound above the surface of the skin, one with and one without the knot.

Figure-eight suture

The dead space in wounds may be lessened without the use of buried sutures by use of figure-eight sutures (Figs. 11-20 and 11-21). Basically this suture is composed of two loops, deep and superficial. When the wound is superficial and the dead space is minimal (Fig. 11-20), the deeper loop is a dermal-subdermal loop, and the superficial loop is placed like a simple interrupted suture. However, if the wound is deep and contains a larger amount of dead space (Fig. 11-21), the deep loop is entirely subdermal, and the

superficial loop is placed with a vertical mattress suture pathway. This latter modification is necessary because with larger, deeper wounds, the skin edges tend to invert, caused by the downward tension from the deep suture loop. The vertical mattress type of pathway on the superficial loop counteracts this tension.

Figure-eight sutures have been used for many years. In 1892 Fowler described their use to close many layers of skin, subcutaneous tissue, and muscle at one time.[19] Various modifications have been proposed.[3,53] Stephens described what he called a "safety pin suture" for suturing scalp, in which the deep loop of the figure-eight is inverted and enclosed within the larger superficial loop.[53]

One of the advantages of using a figure-eight suture or one of its modifications is that one can lessen dead space without a completely buried suture. These sutures can more quickly close a wound, since they close with one suture an area that would normally take two. When the sutures are removed, the deep loop is removed along with the superficial loop. Thus no suture remains in the wound. More permanently buried sutures are a foreign body that serves as a source of inflammation and possible infection.

The major disadvantage of the figure-eight suture is that the deeper part of the wound may not be adequately healed when the suture is removed. This suture is therefore best used in areas where wound healing is relatively fast, for instance, on the head and neck.

Modification of totally buried sutures

The usual technique for placement of vertical buried sutures is discussed in Chapter 10. An interrupted buried suture (either dermal or subdermal) can be modified by being placed horizontally, either as a single loop[52] or a double

TABLE 11-1

Comparison between interrupted and continuous sutures

	Continuous	Interrupted
Speed	Fast	Slow
Distribution of tension	Even	Uneven
Approximation	Less even	Even
Crimping of tissue	Yes	Controllable
Suture mass buried in wound	Same or greater	Same or less
Strength of sutured wound	Same	Same
Breakage of suture	Results in total dehiscence	Results in small dehiscence
Early removal of alternate sutures	Impossible	Possible
Spread of infection	Tends to travel length of wound	May be confined to area around one suture

loop (figure-eight suture).[24] However, in each case tissue is enclosed and compressed in the horizontal direction, which is more likely to interrupt blood supply to the overlying skin. Sometimes a horizontal buried suture is easier to place because of the constraints of either too little space within the wound or too large needle being used.

Another modification proposed for totally buried sutures is in the material used. Usually buried sutures are readily absorbable, so that their effective period of actually holding tissue together extends for only a week or two. This is discussed in greater depth in Chapter 8. Some authorities recommend using nylon or polyester as completely buried suture materials thinking that these materials hold tissue together indefinitely. Although this idea at first glance seems logical, in reality there is no published scientific or clinical data that support it. Polyester may remain intact indefinitely, but nylon is degraded over time. Studies that compare buried nylon to the more quickly absorbed sutures or to no subcutaneous sutures at all do not demonstrate significant differences in spreading of scars.[61,63] Scar widths are affected more by tension on wound edges than by the type of materials used to close the wound.[62]

CONTINUOUS CLOSURES

Compared with interrupted closures, continuous closures close a large portion, if not the whole, of a surgical defect by means of a single suture (Table 11-1) or other material. Continuous sutures are fast and distribute the tension evenly on surgical wound edges, although accurate approximation of the tissue edges may be less than with interrupted sutures. Continuous sutures crimp tissue, whereas with interrupted sutures crimping is easily controlled. One cannot easily make final adjustments with continuous sutures. Continuous sutures are therefore useful on areas where the type of suturing technique has less influence on the ultimate cos-

metic result and the vascularity is excellent. Decreased blood supply to tissue occurs with crimping of tissue, especially if the suture is interlocked for hemostasis.

The strength of a wound at the time of closure appears to be the same whether it is closed by interrupted sutures or one continuous suture.[29] The likelihood of dehiscence also appears to be the same clinically.[43] However, breakage of a continuous suture results in total wound disruption, whereas a broken interrupted suture rarely leads to anything but a small and limited dehiscence.

Infection is no more likely with a continuous suture than with interrupted sutures.[33] Nevertheless, should infection occur, it is more likely to spread through the length of a wound sutured with a continuous suture, because such a suture forms a continuous pathway for bacteria. Such an infection may require removal of the entire continuous suture, and the whole wound may open up. It is possible to remove only a portion of the continuous suture by cutting it at the point of maximal inflammation and unwinding it through the wound until reaching a point of no redness. Then the new ends are secured with tape.[33] Infections with interrupted sutures are frequently confined around only one suture. This suture may be removed without disrupting the whole wound.

A major advantage of interrupted sutures over a continuous suture is that the patient may have alternate sutures removed at different times. With a continuous suture the whole suture is usually removed at once.

In 1979 the effect of continuous versus interrupted sutures on healed wound strength and microcirculation in pigs was studied.[50] The investigator found that wounds closed by interrupted sutures had 30% to 50% greater bursting strength, less edema and induration, and less impaired microcirculation. He concluded that interrupted sutures are preferable for wounds with impaired circulation or with significant tension on the wound edges. Another investigator also found weaker rounds resulted when continuous sutures were used.[42] A 1956 study, however, concluded that there was no difference in the tensile strength of rabbit healed wounds closed by either interrupted or continuous sutures.[5]

Skin tape

A skin tape, as previously mentioned, may be applied as a continuous strip running lengthwise over a wound surface. It thus forms a continuous wound closure in contrast to an interrupted closure formed by skin tapes that are laid perpendicular to the wound surface at intervals (Fig. 10-2).

Tissue glue

Acrylic compounds are made to glue the skin together. These are discussed in Chapter 8. I have no experience with these substances.

Running continuous suture

The running continuous suture (Fig. 11-22) is the simplest continuous suture. It is also known as the over-and-over suture or the whipstitch. After a simple, interrupted suture is tied at one end of a wound, the end with the needle attached is not cut. This suture is then looped continuously over and through the wound until the entire wound edge is closed. When one arrives either at the end of the suture thread or at the end of the wound, a knot is tied between the end of the suture and the last loop.

The method of tying the running continuous suture is shown in Fig. 11-22. One uses an instrument tie, looping the free end of the suture over the instrument and grabbing the last loop. After this throw is placed, one again loops the free end around the instrument and places a second throw,

setting the knot. A square knot tied in this way at the end of a running continuous suture is not strong, since it is strained from three directions instead of two; a bowline knot is recommended.[14] Noe recommends not tying the initial knot at the very beginning of a continuous suture until the suture is completed, so that bunching of the skin may be prevented and the tension on the wound adjusted.[37]

The running continuous suture is useful when the skin is under minimal tension and the exact adjustment of skin edges has little to do with the ultimate cosmetic result. A skin graft can quickly be sutured into place by these means.

An interesting variation of the running continuous suture to help alleviate the problem of epidermal inversion is a vertical mattress suture bite of tissue, taken on one side after exiting through the epidermis but before crossing the wound.[57] One can place this bite anywhere along the length of the wound where inversion is a problem, or one may simply incorporate it into every other loop or even every loop (continuous vertical mattress suture).

Another variation of the running continuous suture is the "baseball" or cross-stitch.[4] After the wound is sutured with the running continuous suture, the suture is not tied—but the wound is then sutured from the opposite direction, with the suture overlapping the previously placed sutures. This results in a cross-stitch pattern over the wound and a more even distribution of tension along the wound edges.

Running locked suture

The running locked suture is shown in Fig. 11-23. This stitch is also known as the blanket stitch. One begins this suture by placing an interrupted stitch, with one long end of the thread attached to the needle and the knot to one side of the wound. The suture is brought down the incision line without crossing it and enters the skin. After exiting the skin

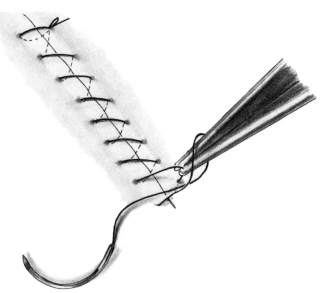

Fig. 11-22. Running continuous suture.

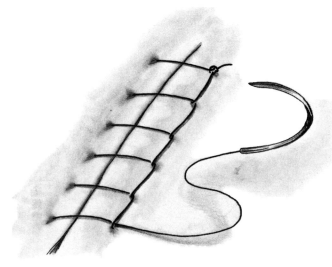

Fig. 11-23. Running locked suture.

on the opposite side of the wound, the suture is brought straight across the wound and looped under the suture where it last entered the skin. It is then continued down the wound.

The running locked suture is useful for wounds under moderate tension when the end cosmetic result is of no consequence. The degree of inversion of the edges and overall tension along the suture is difficult to adjust. One might consider using this stitch on areas such as the scalp or behind the ear, especially for full-thickness skin graft donor sites. However, running locked sutures may decrease the blood supply to tissue slightly more than a simple continuous suture does, so this suture should be used cautiously when the blood supply is impaired. There appears to be no difference in the tensile strength of wounds (at 5 days) sutured with either the running continuous suture or the running locked suture.[5]

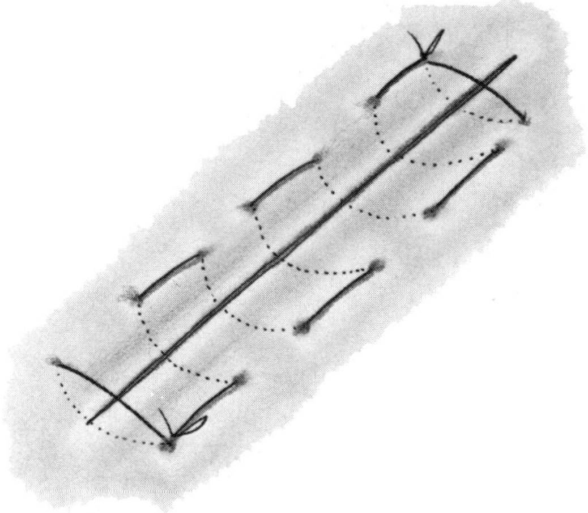

Running horizontal mattress suture

The running horizontal mattress suture (Fig. 11-24) is also known as the quilted suture. It was described as early as 1863 in the American surgical literature.[30] This suture is useful for fast closure of wounds with moderate tension and in which slight eversion of the skin edges is necessary; therefore it can be used for lesions of the face, but it still has the other disadvantages of running sutures.

Running intradermal suture

The running intradermal suture (Fig. 11-25) is also known as the running subcuticular suture, which is a poor

Fig. 11-24. Running horizontal mattress suture.

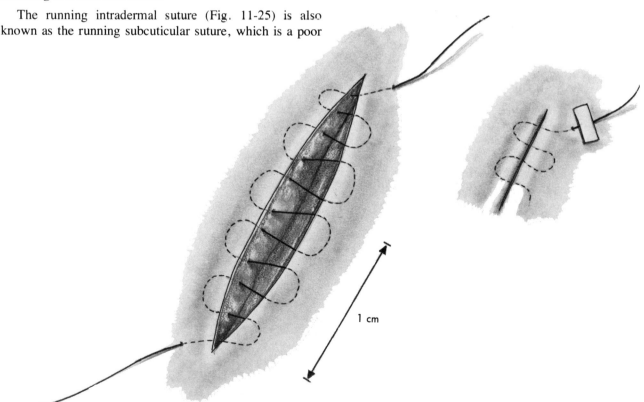

1 cm

Fig. 11-25. Running intradermal suture. Note taped end *(upper right);* also note that multiple loops are placed per centimeter of wound.

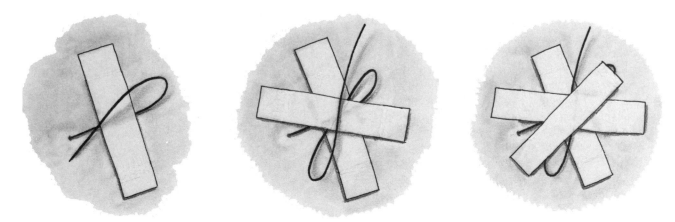

Fig. 11-26. Securing end of running intradermal suture thread with tape.

term because of its nonspecificity. The running intradermal suture is the most important running suture to master, since it is clearly superior to interrupted percutaneous sutures under some circumstances.[58]

The concept of the running intradermal suture was initially described by Halsted in 1913.[23] In 1919 Davis reported that this suture helps to minimize scarring.[13] It was later popularized by Straith in a key article that appeared in 1961.[56] The running intradermal suture is the most difficult suture to master, but once mastered it becomes indispensible for cutaneous surgery.

The running intradermal suture begins at one end of an incision, entering percutaneously into the wound through the dermis. It traverses the wound, where dermal tissue is grabbed in a horizontal loop. It then crosses the wound to the opposite side, grabbing additional tissue in another horizontal loop. This continues for the length of the incision. At the end, the suture is brought out of the wound through the dermis and epidermis. It is helpful to hold the needle holder like a pencil when placing the intradermal loops (see Frontispiece). The needle holder is then perpendicular to the wound during placement of the suture.

Several key features of this suture exist that I have personally found make the difference between a good closure and an almost perfect one. First, before placement of the running intradermal suture, almost all tension should be removed from the dermal wound edges by buried dermal or dermal-subdermal sutures. Therefore the epidermal wound edges should be apposed or almost so at the time this suture is used. Second, the initial entrance and final exit points of the suture are *to the sides* of the wound ends and not beyond the ends and on the long axis of the incision line. The forces on the free ends of the suture are thus directed straight in line with the suture loops rather than at a right angle to them. This ensures that when tension is placed on the suture, there is no bunching of tissue at the apices of the wound.

The third point is that the loops must be on the same level within the dermis. Note also that this suture lies en-

tirely within the dermis (usually mid to upper dermis) except at the entrance and exit points and thus, as pointed out earlier, is most properly referred to as running intradermal suture.

Fourth, when placing the loops in the dermis one should backtrack slightly, because when the suture is tied and the forces of tension are exerted on the loops, the arms of the loops straighten out. Backtracking too much, however, can be just as much of a problem as not backtracking at all. Forrest feels that backtracking should be avoided completely[15]; however, I am sure he refers to excessive backtracking, which tends to put uneven tension on the wound edges. Only slight backtracking is required.

Fifth, multiple loops are required to close a surgical defect. Most illustrations usually do not indicate the multitude of loops required. Six loops per centimeter is not unusual.[65] My experience is that the more loops placed, the better the closure.

Sixth, do not place knots in the ends of the suture thread. It should be taped at each end (Fig. 11-26). One degreases the skin, applies a tacky substance, and then place a skin tape over the suture. The suture is then looped over the tape and a second piece of tape is placed. Finally, the suture is looped over the second piece of tape and a third piece of tape is placed. Taping both ends as shown more than adequately holds the ends and does not result in wound dehiscence. Other methods to secure the ends of a running intradermal suture have been suggested, such as tying slip knots, tying lead shots, and even tying the suture over the wound. All these methods place unnecessary tension on the wound edges. Tied ends in particular are notorious for working their way into the wound at the ends and may leave small scars or puckerings (*arrow* in Fig. 11-7, *C*).

Seventh, the best suture to use for this stitch is polypropylene (Prolene).[2] Polypropylene has the lowest coefficient of friction of any suture, so it slips easily through tissue when pulled out.[20] Other sutures, such as nylon, tend to drag through tissue or to get hung up in the wound. Multi-

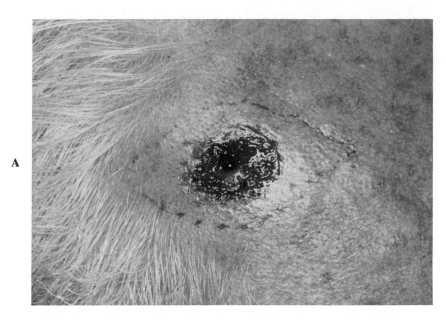

A

Fig. 11-27. Wound closure with running intradermal and interrupted sutures. **A,** Lesion in center of planned tangent-to-circle excision.   *Continued.*

filamentous sutures especially silk, should not be used as running intradermal sutures. Recently there has been a resurgence of interest in the use of multifilamentous steel wire sutures for running intradermal suturing.[1,8] This material is difficult to use, however, and should it break at the time of suture removal, it may be a source of irritation for the patient.

Eighth, if the wound being sutured is fairly long (greater than 4 to 5 cm), one may wish to bring the suture through the epidermis in the middle of the wound or at other intervals. This suture is then looped directly over the wound, and it reenters the epidermis on the opposite side (Fig. 11-7, *B, open arrow*). Such percutaneous suture loops along the course of running intradermal sutures help to hold the wound edges together in a stronger manner and during suture removal may be cut, making it easier to remove the suture. A shorter suture is easier to pull through the wound than a longer one is.

Ninth, the wound edges should be reinforced with skin tapes after placement and after removal of the running intradermal suture. This helps to take additional tension off the wound edges and leads to faster healing.[58]

The time for removal of the running intradermal suture is variable. Usually the minimum is 1 week, although it may be left 3 weeks or longer.[54] The longer the suture is left, the more difficult it is to remove and the more likely it is to leave small suture scars at the points of exit and entrance, caused by epidermization of the suture tracts. These factors must be balanced against the progress in wound healing and tension on the incision line.

Occasionally a running intradermal suture strongly resists removal. Usually this occurs when nylon has been used

rather than polypropylene. Should this occur, one may cut the suture at the point of exit or entrance as it is pulled on tension so as to "permanently" bury it.[8] Since nylon and polypropylene are relatively nonreactive, they may be buried safely. A clever method for removing a hung-up running intradermal suture was described by Hockly.[25] One tapes a rubber band on the skin beyond but in line with the suture. One then puts the rubber band on stretch and attaches it to the running intradermal suture by means of a small hemostat. Thus over time gentle elastic traction pulls the suture out of the wound.

A way to prevent sutures from getting hung up has been mentioned previously: exit from the wound to form loops crossing the wound on the surface of the skin.

Even in the best of hands, the running intradermal suture might not totally approximate the skin edges. When a small gap occurs, it may be closed with small interrupted sutures, which may be removed in a day or two (Fig. 11-7, *B, arrowhead*).

An alternative to the suture just described is a running intradermal suture that is completely buried. The suture is tied as a buried interrupted suture at the level of the dermis, is run the length of the wound as a running epidermal suture, and is tied at the opposite end with the knot buried. If one uses this technique, either nonreactive "nonabsorbable" materials such as nylon or polypropylene or, alternatively, absorbable sutures such as Dexon, Vicryl, or PDS should be buried. Completely buried running intradermal sutures may be useful, especially in children, to obviate the need for suture removal.[64]

A clinical example of a running intradermal suture is shown in Fig. 11-27. The lines of excision of a basal cell

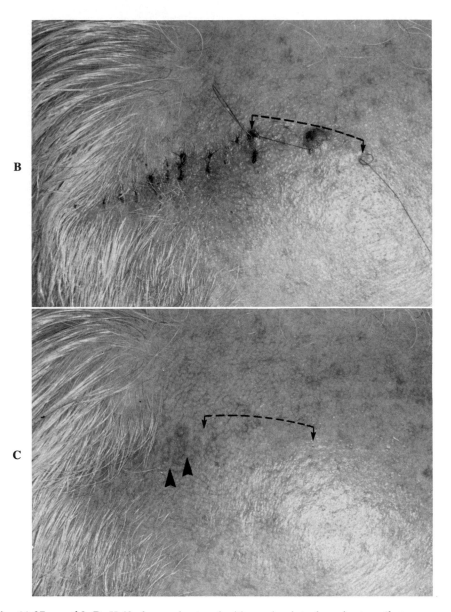

Fig. 11-27, cont'd. B, Half of wound sutured with running intradermal suture *(between arrows);* remaining wound closed with interrupted sutures. **C,** Cosmetic result 6 months later. Note that wound scar between small arrows, where running intradermal suture was placed, is imperceptible, but suture tracks are visible as white linear scars *(arrowheads)* where interrupted sutures were placed.

carcinoma of the forehead are shown in Fig. 11-27, *A*. A portion of the wound (between the arrows and under the dashed line on Fig. 11-27, *B*) was sutured by a running intradermal suture. The remainder of the wound was sutured with simple interrupted sutures. One finds it hard to locate the scar from the running intradermal suture 6 months later (Fig. 11-27, *C, dashed line* and *arrows*); however, suture tracks that appears as small hypopigmented linear scars *(arrowheads)* are visible where the wound was closed by interrupted sutures. It has been my my experience that such small scars become more apparent in time, particularly

in individuals with a ruddy complexion. The stark white scar becomes more apparent against a red background. Therefore areas that are ruddy, such as the forehead, are excellent regions for use of the running intradermal suture.

Another example of a running intradermal suture is found in Fig. 11-7, *B*. Note that in this earlier example the suture was knotted at the ends rather than taped. As I mentioned earlier, knotting is not preferable, and I have abandoned its use in favor of taping the ends. Also note that small gaps in the wound were closed by fine interrupted sutures. The open arrow points to the location at which the

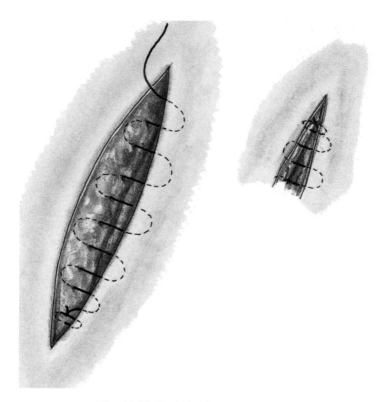

Fig. 11-28. Buried subcutaneous suture.

running intradermal suture was brought out of the wound through the skin and looped over the incision line. A suture thread *(arrowhead)* is placed to even up the wound edges but is untied because tying is not necessary. The stiffness of the untied nylon maintains even wound edges.

A wound closed by one running epidermal suture contains many fewer percutaneous routes into the wound edges than a wound closed by several interrupted sutures. Fewer tracts are therefore present where ingrowth of epidermis[28] or ingress of bacteria can occur.[55] The result is less scarring. Percutaneous suture tracts, not the incision itself, are the main routes of infection.[6] However, if a wound closed by a running intradermal suture is contaminated, the well-coapted wound edges may seal off infection.[18]

Running intradermal sutures close a wound more tightly and completely than simple interrupted sutures do, which have gaps between them. Such total apposition helps to eliminate superficial dead space in wounds.

Running subcutaneous closure

The running subcutaneous suture (Fig. 11-28) is placed with loops, as is the running intradermal suture; however, it is usually completely buried and entirely confined to the fat layer. Therefore one should use nonreactive material, such as nylon, or absorbable sutures for burying.

The running subcutaneous suture is useful where the fat is thick and fibrous. It is faster to place but may not coapt

the tissue as securely as interrupted sutures. Running subcutaneous sutures do not by themselves close wound edges and cannot be depended on to provide the main force holding a wound closed. They are therefore used with more superficial intradermal or percutaneous sutures. In one study wounds sutured with running subcutaneous sutures tended to dehisce in cachetic malnourished patients.[2]

Zoltan describes wound closure using a running subcutaneous suture brought through the skin in the same manner as a running intradermal suture.[65] It is layered below a running intradermal suture, also brought out through the skin. On adequate wound healing, both sutures are removed. I have no experience with this technique.

REFERENCES

1. Alt, T.: Personal communication, 1982.
2. Archie, J.P., Jr., and Feldtman, R.W.: Primary abdominal wound closure with permanent, continuous running monofilament sutures, Surg. Gynecol. Obstet. **153:**721, 1981.
3. Bentley, P.G., et al.: Wound closure with Dexon (polyglycolic acid) mass suture, Ann. R. Coll. Surg. Engl. **60:**125, 1978.
4. Borges, A.F.: Elective incisions and scar revision, Boston, 1973, Little, Brown & Co.
5. Borgström, S., and Sandblom, P.: Suture technique and wound healing: an investigation based on animal experiments, Ann. Surg. **144:**982, 1956.
6. Carpendale, M.T.F., and Sereda, W.: The role of the percu-

taneous suture in surgical wound infection, Surgery **58**:672, 1965.

7. Condon, R.E.: Locked vertical mattress stitch for skin closure, Surg. Gynecol. Obstet. **127**:839, 1968.

8. Converse, J.M.: Introduction to plastic surgery. In Converse, J.M., McCarthy, J.G., and Littler, J.W., editors, Reconstructive plastic surgery, Philadelphia, 1977, W.B. Saunders Co.

9. Ellenberg, A.H.: Surgical tape wound closure: a disenchantment, Plast. Reconstr. Surg. **39**:625, 1967.

10. Epstein, E.: The buried horizontal mattress suture, Cutis **24**:104, 1979.

11. Farringer, J.L., Jr.: An auto-suture instrument: preliminary report, Am. J. Surg. **125**:382, 1973.

12. Faxén, A., et al.: A new kind of ''deep retention suture,'' Acta Chir. Scand. **142**:13, 1976.

13. Fisher, G.T., et al.: Origin of the use of subcuticular sutures, Ann. Plast. Surg. **4**:144, 1980.

14. Flinn, R.M.: Knotting in medicine and surgery, Practitioner **183**:322, 1959.

15. Forrest, J.F.: An improved technique for delayed primary closure of potentially infected incisions, Surg. Gynecol. Obstet. **149**:401, 1979.

16. Forrester, J.C., et al.: Tape-closed and sutured wounds: a comparison by tensiometry and scanning electron microscopy, Br. J. Surg. **57**:729, 1970.

17. Forrester, J.C., et al.: Wolff's law in relation to the healing skin wound, J. Trauma **10**:770, 1970.

18. Foster, G.E., et al.: Subcuticular suturing after appendectomy, Lancet **1**:1128, 1977.

19. Fowler, G.R.: The crossed suture, Ann. Surg. **15**:351, 1892.

20. Freeman, B.S., et al.: An analysis of suture withdrawal stress, Surg. Gynecol. Obstet. **131**:441, 1970.

21. Gibson, E.W., and Poate, W.J.: The use of adhesive surgical tape in plastic surgery, Br. J. Plast. Surg. **17**:265, 1964.

22. Gillman, T., et al.: Closure of wounds and incisions with adhesive tape, Lancet **2**:945, 1955.

23. Halsted, W.S.: Ligature and suture material: the employment of fine silk in preference to catgut and the advantages of transfixion of tissues and vessels in control of hemorrhage; also an account of the introduction of gloves, gutta-percha tissue and silver foil, J.A.M.A. **60**:1119, 1913.

24. Hill, T.G.: More surgical gems: simplified closure of fusiform defects by one or more continuous spiral sutures of two turns, J. Dermatol. Surg. Oncol. **6**:986, 1980.

25. Hockly, G.: Easy removal of the obstinate subcuticular suture, Plast. Reconstr. Surg. **63**:275, 1979.

26. Holm, H.H., and Egeblad, K.: Adhesive tape (Steri-Strip) versus suture closure of skin wounds, Nord. Med. **79**:311, 1968.

27. Holmlund, D.E.W.: Suture technic and suture-holding capacity: a model study and a theoretical analysis, Am. J. Surg. **134**:616, 1977.

28. Homsy, C.A., et al.: Surgical suture–porcine subcuticular tissue interaction, J. Biomed. Mater. Res. **3**:383, 1969.

29. Howes, E.L.: The immediate strength of the sutured wound, Surgery **7**:24, 1940.

30. Howes, E.L., and Harvey, S.C.: The strength of the healing wound in relation to the holding strength of the catgut suture, N. Engl. J. Med. **200**:1285, 1929.

31. Lennihan, R., Jr., and Mackereth, M.: A comparison of staples and nylon closure in varicose vein surgery, Vasc. Surg. **9**:200, 1975.

32. McGregor, I.A.: Fundamental techniques of plastic surgery and their surgical applications, Edinburgh, 1975, Churchill Livingstone.

33. McClean, N.R., et al.: Comparison of skin closures using continuous and interrupted nylon sutures, Br. J. Surg. **67**:633, 1980.

34. McQuown, S.A., et al.: Gillies' corner stitch revisited, Arch. Otolaryngol. **110**:450, 1984.

35. Myers, M.B., and Cherry, G.: Functional and angiographic vasculature in healing wounds, Am. Surgeon **36**:750, 1970.

36. Nghiem, D.D.: New technic for skin closure, South. Med. J. **73**:1290, 1980.

37. Noe, J.M., and Gloth, D.A.: A technique for the placement of a continuous suture, Surg. Gynecol. Obstet. **150**:404, 1980.

38. Ordman, L.J., and Gillman, T.: Studies in the healing of cutaneous wounds. III. A critical comparison in the pig of the healing of surgical incisions closed with sutures or adhesive tape based on tensile strength and clinical and histological criteria, Arch. Surg. **93**:911, 1966.

39. Panek, P.H., et al.: Potentiation of wound infection by adhesive adjuncts, Am. Surg. **38**:343, 1972.

40. Pedersen, V.M., et al.: Skin closure in abdominal incisions: continuous nylon suture versus Steri-Strip tape suture—a controlled trial, Acta Chir. Scand. **147**:619, 1981.

41. Pinto, S.S.: A button for holding tension sutures, Am. J. Surg. **48**:477, 1940.

42. Preston, D.J.: The effects of sutures on the strength of healing wounds, Am. J. Surg. **49**:56, 1940.

43. Richards, P.C., et al.: Abdominal wound closure: a randomized prospective study of 571 patients comparing continuous vs. interrupted suture techniques, Ann. Surg. **197**:238, 1983.

44. Samuels, P.B., et al.: Mechanized skin suturing, Arch. Surg. **109**:838, 1974.

45. Schauerhamer, R.A., et al.: Studies in the management of the contaminated wound. II. Susceptibility of surgical wounds to postoperative surface contamination, Am. J. Surg. **122**:74, 1971.

46. Shureih, S.F., et al.: Modified Gambee stitch: safe, easy, and fast modification, Am. J. Surg. **141**:304, 1981.

47. Simmonds, W.L.: Excision surgery as an office procedure, Cutis **6**:1221, 1970.

48. Simmonds, W.L.: Uses of bolsters in dermatologic surgery, J. Dermatol. Surg. Oncol. **3**:281, 1977.

49. Smith, B.C., and Nesi, F.A.: Practical techniques in ophthalmic plastic surgery, St. Louis, 1981, The C.V. Mosby Co.

50. Speer, D.P.: The influence of suture technique on early wound healing, J. Surg. Res. **27**:385, 1979.

51. Stegmaier, O.C.: Use of skin stapler in dermatologic surgery, J. Am. Acad. Dermatol. **6**:305, 1982.

52. Stegman, S.J.: Suturing techniques for dermatologic surgery, J. Dermatol. Surg. Oncol. **4**:63, 1978.

53. Stephens, H.W. Jr.: An alternative for scalp wounds, Med. Times **104**:81, 1976.

54. Stephenson, K.L.: Suturing, Surg. Clin. North Am. **57**:863, 1977.

55. Stillman, R.M., Bella, F.J., and Seligman, S.J.: Skin wound closure: the effect of various wound closure methods on susceptibility to infection, Arch. Surg. **115:**674, 1980.

56. Straith, R.E., Lawson, J.M., and Hipps, J.C.: The subcuticular suture, Postgrad. Med. **29:**164, 1961.

57. Talamas, I.: A fast and good way of suturing the skin, Aesthetic Plast. Surg. **6:**59, 1982.

58. Taube, M., Porter, R.J., and Lord, P.H.: A combination of subcuticular suture and sterile micropore tape compared with conventional interrupted sutures for skin closure: a controlled trial, Ann. R. Coll. Surg. Engl. **65:**164, 1983.

59. Watson, G.M., Anders, C.J., and Glover, J.R.: Op-Site skin closure: a comparison with subcuticular and interrupted sutures, Ann. R. Coll. Surg. Engl. **65:**83, 1983.

60. Webster, R.C., Davidson, T.M., Smith, R.C.: Broken line scar revision. In Borges, A.F., editor: Clinics in plastic surgery, vol. 4, Philadelphia, 1977, W.B. Saunders Co.

61. Winn, H.R., et al.: Influence of subcuticular sutures on scar formation, Am. J. Surg. **133:**257, 1977.

62. Wray, R.C., Jr.: Force required for wound closure and scar appearance, Plast. Reconstr. Surg. **72:**380, 1983.

63. Wray, R.C., Jr., Holtmann, B., and Weeks, P., Jr.: Factors in the production of inconspicuous scars, Plast. Reconstr. Surg. **56:**86, 1975.

64. Wright, J.E.: Absorbable subcuticular sutures: how to avoid the childhood ordeal of suture removal, Med. J. Aust. **2:**874, 1975.

65. Zoltan, J.: Cicatrix optima, Baltimore, 1977, University Park Press.

12

Complex Closures

Complex closures require adjustments of surrounding tissues to effect a flat inconspicuous scar. These adjustments include undermining, placement of multiple layers of sutures, and usually removal of excessive skin at the ends of the excision. Undermining and multiple-layered closures are discussed in Chapters 10 and 11. This chapter focuses primarily on an approach to elimination of excess tissues at the sides or apices of excisions.

DOG-EARS

Although the name *dog-ear* leaves something to be desired, this term is deeply embedded in surgical parlance. A dog-ear refers to the fold of tissue seen, usually protruding above the surface of the skin, at the ends or sides of excisions. Other terms used to refer to dog-ears are "pig's ears" or simply "puckering." When discussing this excess skin in front of patients, it is probably best to refrain from the use of the term "dog-ear," and to use *pucker* instead.

The cause

Dog-ears are caused by an excess amount of tissue at the ends or sides of an excision.[15] This excess tissue comes about in four ways.

Discrepancy of length. As a fusiform excision is closed (Fig. 12-1) the cut edges fall together in the central axis. Since the cut edges (*acb* and *adb*) are always longer than this long axis (*ab*), pressure is extended at the ends of the excision, pushing the tissue away from the wound. This causes some bunching of the tissue at the ends and less tension on the skin surrounding the ends. Quite the opposite occurs at the midpoints of the cut edges (*c* and *d*), at which points, on closing the excision, the tension is the greatest. If the bunching of tissue at the ends is minimal, a dog-ear is not formed.

When the discrepancy between the cut edges and the long axis is great (Fig. 12-1, *right*), the bunching at the corners of the excision is great, and obvious dog-ears are produced. As an extreme example, a circular excision on closure results in even more apparent dog-ears.

Angle of rotation. The second reason for dog-ears is the size of the angle of closure at the end of an excision. When a fusiform excision is closed, the tissue on either side of the angle at each end is rotated around a pivotal point toward the center. Rotation around this pivotal forces tissue into the corners of the fusiform excision. This tissue is unnecessary and redundant. If the angle is small (usually less than 15 degrees), a small rotation is ensured (Fig. 12-1, *left*). If the angle is large (much greater than 30 degrees), the rotation of tissue is greater (Fig. 12-1, *right*). When this occurs, excessive tissue is brought into the corner of an excision, and a pucker occurs.

Elasticity of skin. The formation of dog-ears depends partially on the inherent elasticity of the skin in a given area and on how tightly the dermis is bound down to the underlying muscle fascia. Remember that the subdermal tissue has fibrous attachments from the dermis to the underlying muscle fascia. When these attachments are well developed, the excess tissue caused by rotation and axis–cut edge length discrepancy will be partially counterbalanced by tension in a third plane; that is, that caused by the fibrous attachments to the tissue below. Sometimes these attachments are very tight, causing an infolding of skin (an inverted dog-ear) rather than a puckering above the surface. Alternatively, when the skin is very loosely attached to the underlying tissue and is less elastic (for example, on the back of the hand, or on the eyelids), everted dog-ears are more prominent.

Nonflat tissue planes. Dog-ears form regularly at the ends of an excision over convex surfaces such as the arm or lip (Fig. 12-2, *left*). A tissue at the ends of an excision in these locations is more easily elevated since this tissue is below the midpoint of the excision's long axis.

Gormley[10] has likened cutaneous tissue being sutured to a "sheaf of fibers" (Fig. 12-2, *right*). This is partially a valid concept because of the fibrous nature of cutaneous collagen and orientation of many of its fibers, particularly along the maximal skin tension lines (MaxSTLs). The sheaf of fibers has substantial bulk, which helps to explain the

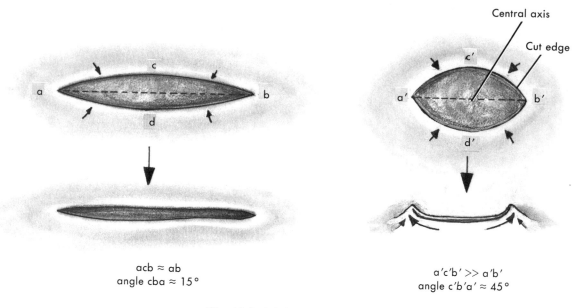

acb ≈ ab
angle cba ≈ 15°

a′c′b′ >> a′b′
angle c′b′a′ ≈ 45°

Fig. 12-1. Origin of dog-ears.

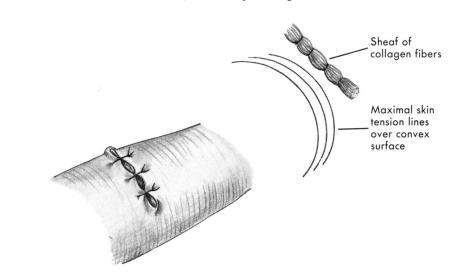

Fig. 12-2. Accentuation of dog-ears over curved surfaces. (Modified from Gormley, D.E.: J. Dermatol. Surg. Oncol. **3:**194. Copyright 1977, The Journal of Dermatologic Surgery and Oncology, Inc.)

slight gaping of sutured wound edges. As an excision crosses a convex surface such as the convex surface over the radius of the forearm, the fibers in the tissue beyond the corners of the excision come to lie almost at right angles to the fibers within the sutured excision itself. This divergence of fibers further accentuates the dog-ears formed.

Dog-ears as cones

Dog-ears can be visualized as cones of tissue that either stand or lie at the sides or ends of excisions. A cone is a solid figure bounded by a circular base, the sides of which slope evenly from the base's perimeter to one point (the apex or vertex). The sides are formed by line segments joining every point of the boundary of the circular base to the common vertex or apex. Limberg was one of the first physicians[12] to visualize geometrically the resemblance of dog-ears to conical deformations of tissue; he divided cones into two types: standing and lying. A typical dog-ear formed at the end of a wide fusiform excision resembles a standing cone. With the standing cone the axis is perpendicular, and the base is parallel to the skin surface. A lying cone, on the other hand, is a cone with its central axis parallel to and its base perpendicular to the cutaneous surface. A dog-ear that resembles a lying cone is formed when one side of an excision is longer than the other. This discrepancy commonly occurs at the end of a rotation or advancement flap (see Fig. 12-8).

Distinguishing between these two types of dog-ears (ly-

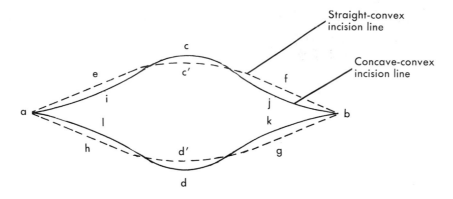

$$\text{straight-convex incision line} < \text{concave-convex incision line}$$

$$aec'fb < aicjb$$

$$ahd'gb < aldkb$$

Fig. 12-3. Comparison of length of concave-convex *(nondashed line)* to straight-convex *(dashed line)* incision lines.

ing or standing cones) is important because their repairs are different. The standing cone requires almost complete removal of the cone. However, the lying cones require excision of only the half of the cone that protrudes above the surface of the skin for correction. The lying cone might have tissue distortion below the surface of the skin similar to that seen above. Therefore its correction must frequently include undermining to minimize the underlying subdermal fibrous connections that are a partial cause of dog-ear distortions.

Avoidance of dog-ears

Physicians performing surgery on the cutaneous surfaces should not be afraid of the formation of dog-ears; dog-ears are a natural and frequently unpredictable result of suturing excisional wounds and should be considered a challenge. Rather than trying to prevent dog-ears, one should work on improving and expanding one's repertoire of ways to remove them.

Some physicians[7,18] recommend the purposeful formation of dog-ears by making every excision circular. The surrounding skin is then undermined so that the most favorable lines of closure can be determined. Subsequent closure of such a circular excision inevitably results in dog-ears. However, these physicians argue that removal of purposely formed dog-ears in this way results in more favorable excision lines and sacrifice of less tissue than would have occurred with standard fusiform or tangent-to-circle excisions that are planned to prevent dog-ears. In my experience this is true.

Dzubow[8] recommends avoiding dog-ears by formation of concave-convex incision lines rather than the straight-convex incision lines of a typical fusiform or tangent-to-circle excision (see Fig. 12-3). This maneuver cannot be recommended in general for a variety of reasons. First, concave-convex incision lines produce longer lines for excision (than straight or slightly convex lines) and thus help bring about dog-ears, despite the fact that they decrease the angle of closure. Second, concave-convex lines help to place more tension on the midpoint of the excisions, whereas at the ends there is less pressure. Third, even with the best of planning, dog-ears cannot be avoided, because, as already discussed, the geometry of the situation is not the only factor influencing dog-ear formations. Tissue tension and elasticity also are important and at times difficult to gauge.

Leaving dog-ears

Occasionally, dog-ears form at the ends of excisions and, instead of being repaired immediately, are left to take care of themselves (''fall out''). Because of swelling from infiltration of anesthetic, particularly in loose tissue, it is sometimes difficult to know how much puckering at the end of an excision is a true dog-ear and how much is just artifactual. Much of the time it is a combination of both.

Sometimes a dog-ear appears because of excess fat that underlies the apex of an excision and that was inadvertently left at the time of excision. This has been referred to as a ''pseudo-dog-ear.''[19] Usually, if excessive fat is the problem, this can be excised easily, or the pseudo-dog-ear will probably flatten out by itself in time.

Over time some true dog-ears resolve on their own. This commonly happens over firm surfaces such as the forehead and is probably caused by contracture of the linear excision scar both longitudinally and vertically. But if the skin is loose, contracture has less of an effect on dog-ears. One cannot always depend on scar contracture and time to correct dog-ears; in fact, dog-ears can interfere with wound healing by working to evert skin edges in their proximity.[4] Final-

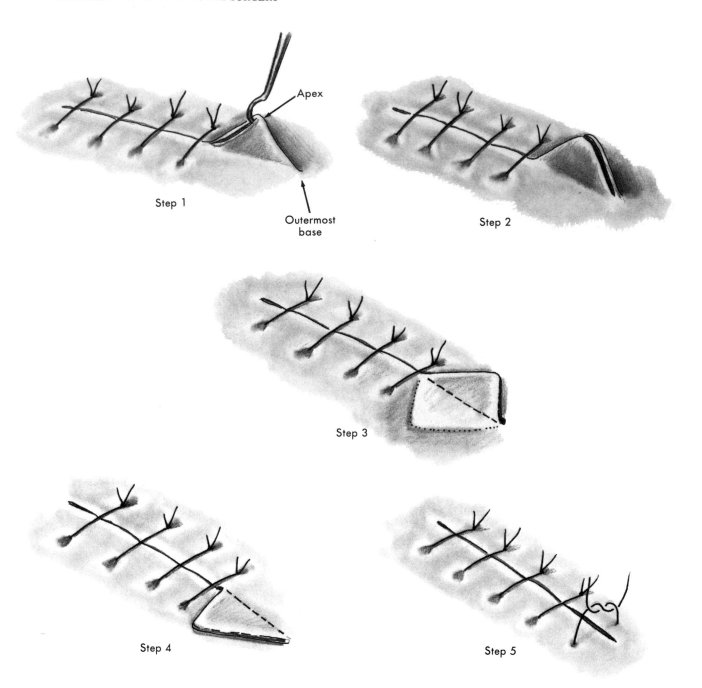

Fig. 12-4. Straight dog-ear repair.

ly, most patients become annoyed at the appearance of dog-ears and prefer that they would have been taken care of at the time the wound was originally closed. If dog-ears do persist, they mar an otherwise excellent cosmetic result. Therefore I believe it is preferable to remove them at the time of surgery.

A large angle of rotation (up to 90 degrees) sometimes occurs at the base of a rotation flap. Because of this relatively large angle, a dog-ear is inevitable at one side of the base of the flap. Frequently it is the best course of action to leave this dog-ear until the flap is well vascularized (1 to 2 weeks), at which time it can be removed. If the removal is done on the same day that the flap is created, it might impede precious blood supply to flap tissue and thereby jeopardize the ultimate success of the flap.

If a dog-ear is left after surgery and it does not resolve on its own, a standard fusiform excision usually corrects the problem. Alternatively, local injection of a steroid (for example, Kenalog 10 mg/ml) into the dog-ear may bring about its resolution.

Repair of dog-ears

There are several different ways to excise dog-ears that differ in the direction of the resultant excision line.* On the face in particular, it is essential for the physician to position the dog-ear correction properly so it fits neatly into wrinkle lines or crease lines. Borges thinks that it is particularly important to position dog-ear excision lines so that they fall into the MaxSTLs.[4]

Dog-ears are very common, and the methods of their repair need to be mastered to operate successfully on the cutaneous surfaces. Dog-ear repairs are based on the concept of increasing the length-to-width ratio of excisions by delineation and excision of excess tissue. Every physician operating on the cutaneous surfaces needs to know the first two types of dog-ear repair shown, the straight and the curved. Other types of dog-ear repairs are useful under unusual circumstances. Knowledge of all these types of repairs gives the physician more options with which to operate and more flexibility in repairing wounds.

Before repair of a dog-car, the physician should suture the wound until the elevation becomes pronounced. This procedure, together with the relationship of the dog-ear to the MaxSTLs, more clearly defines the amount of excess tissue that needs to be excised and gives a more accurate visualization of the best direction for the dog-ear repair.

Straight dog-ear repair (Fig. 12-4). This method is useful when it is desirable to extend the excision as a straight line. The excess tissue is picked up by a skin hook *(Step 1)* so that the geometry of excess tissue (dog-ear) is better defined as the shape of a cone. The apex and base of the cone are thus visualized. It is essential to define the outermost base, since this delineates the necessary amount of tissue that must be excised to eliminate the dog-ear and thus the stopping point of the dog-ear excision. An incision is made from the top of the excess tissue (the apex of the cone) to the outermost base *(Step 2)*. This forms two equal triangles of tissue. One triangle is folded under one side of the wound and the other triangle is folded over the opposite side *(Step 3)*. These folded triangles underlapping and overlapping normal skin represent the amount of excess tissue that needs to excised. The overlapping triangle is excised first *(dashed line, Step 3)*. The underlapping triangle is then flipped up on top of the skin *(Step 4)*. Again, this excess triangular piece of tissue is excised. Finally, the wound is sutured closed as a straight line *(Step 5)*.

The bases of the triangles to be incised (dashed lines in steps 3 and 4) are determined by an imaginary extension of the main excision line. The triangles should not be pulled laterally when they are incised, since this leads to more tissue removal than necessary. It is a good idea to conserve as much normal tissue as possible.

An alternative straight line dog-ear repair is simply to excise a fusiform piece of tissue containing the dog-ear. This method is not as precise as the one shown and in my opinion should not be used.

Curved dog-ear repair (Figs. 12-5 and 12-6). The curved dog-ear repair is useful when one wishes to extend an excision line to fit into a curved wrinkle or crease. Since a wrinkle or crease beyond an excision might curve in one of several directions, it is necessary to know how to tailor a dog-ear excision to fit into the curve.

Fig. 12-5 demonstrates curving a dog-ear to fit a wrinkle line lateral to the eye, if the excision line comes from below. The dog-ear is lifted up with a skin hook at the apex *(Step 1)*. The excess tissue is gently pulled down so that a curved incision can be made at its base from the cut edge to the outermost base of the excess tissue *(Step 2)*. This curved incision is important, since it represents the direction of the final line of extension from the excision itself. The newly cut edge is then freed up and unfolded over the opposite side of the wound *(Step 3)*. Underlying this new triangular piece of skin is the new cut edge extension of the excision line formed in *Step 2*. This underlying cut edge is used as the underlying pattern for excision of the new triangular piece of tissue as it is cut along at its base *(dashed line, Step 3)*. The wound is finally sutured as a curved excision *(Step 4)*.

Fig. 12-6 shows an excision line with the dog-ear removal so that the curve goes in the opposite direction. One can direct the curve of a dog-ear repair in either direction. In this case, the choice of direction is determined by the wrinkle lines in the vicinity of the excision.

Hockey stick dog-ear repair (Fig. 12-7). A more acute angle might be required to fit a dog-ear excision line into a wrinkle line or MaxSTL. The hockey stick dog-ear repair can then be used. The excess tissue is pulled up, and an incision *(dashed line)* is made tangential to the base of this tissue (the dog-ear) as well as oblique to the main incision line *(Step 1)*. Note how this incision differs from those in Figs. 12-5 and 12-6. The angle to the main incision line in the hockey stick dog-ear repair can be adjusted to fit surrounding wrinkles. The new triangular piece of tissue is then unfolded on top of the skin *(Step 2)*. The underlying new cut edge *(dotted line)* is used as a template for the incision *(dashed line)* at the base of the overlying triangle of excess tissue. The triangle is cut off, and the wound sutured *(Step 3)*. The repair results in an excision line that forms roughly a 120-degree angle to the main excision line and resembles a hockey stick.

L-shaped dog-ear repair (Fig. 12-8). When a flap is rotated or advanced, one side of tissue moves a greater distance than the other. This creates an excessive amount of tissue on one side of the wound. When the excess tissue is picked up with a skin hook, it is seen to be a lying half-cone with the other half represented by tissue deep to the surface of the skin. The dog-ear is incised from the far cut edge of the excision (really the outermost base of the cone) to the apex

---

*References 1, 3, 4, 6, 11, 13, 19, 23.

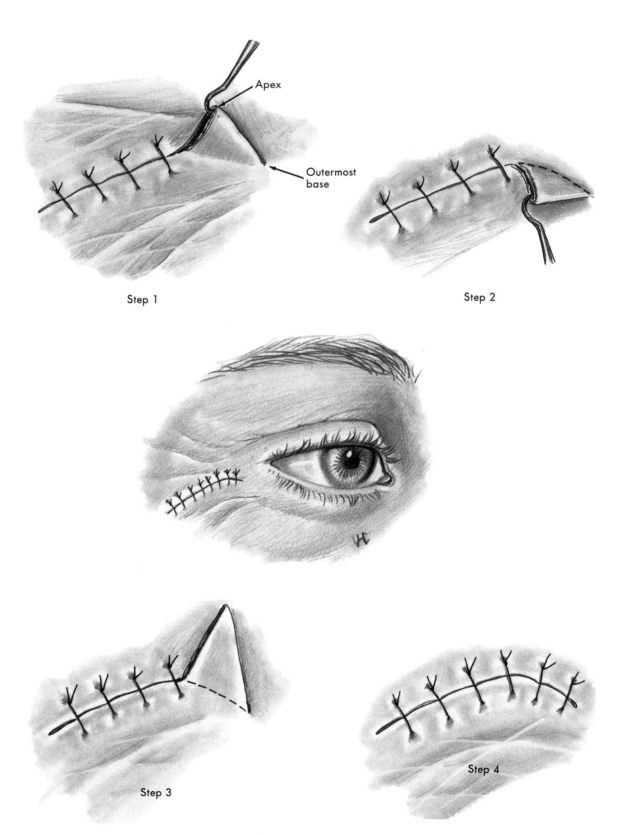

Fig. 12-5. Curved dog-ear repair.

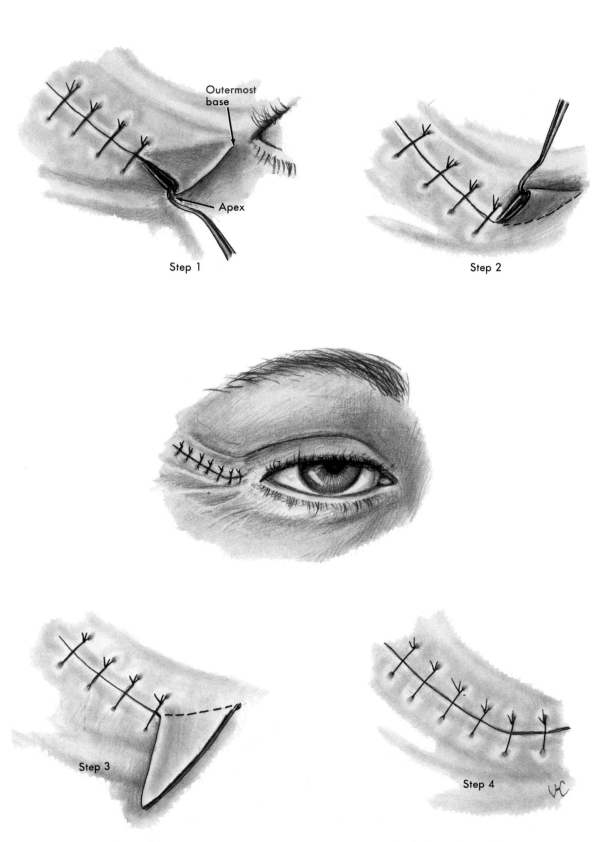

Fig. 12-6. Curved dog-ear repair (curve opposite to that in Fig. 12-5).

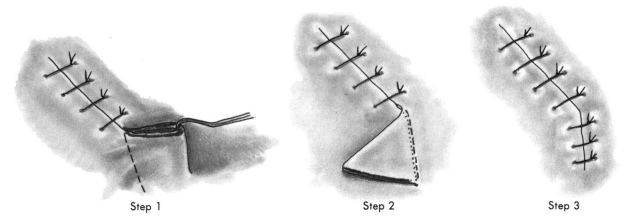

Fig. 12-7. Hockey stick dog-ear repair.

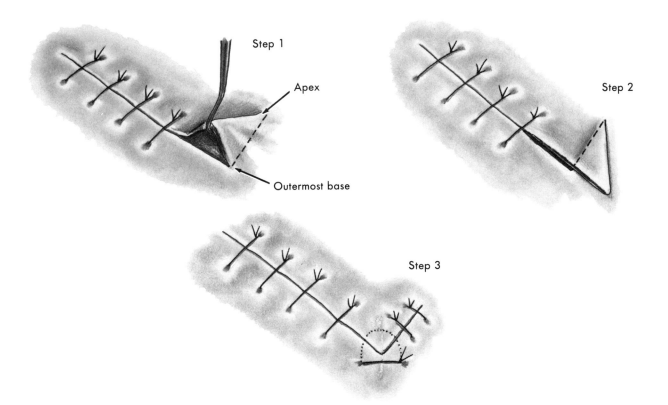

Fig. 12-8. L-shaped dog-ear repair.

of the excess tissue (the apex of the lying half-cone). The new triangle of excess tissue is unfolded over the surrounding tissue *(Step 2)*. It is trimmed at its base overlying the cut tissue below. The new cut edges are then sutured into place with interrupted sutures and a three-point suture *(Step 3)*. It should be noted that the angle of the new incision relative to the main incision line might be slightly less than the 90-degree angle shown in Fig. 12-8.

This dog-ear in a rotation or advancement flap could have been anticipated and prevented by excision of a Burow's triangle.[5] This is a triangular piece of skin excised at the end of the cut edge that is longer than its corresponding cut edge on the opposite site. Such excess tissue on one skin edge is common in rotation or advancement flaps. This is drawn on the proposed rotation flap depicted in Fig. 10-68, *A*.

T-shaped dog-ear repair (Fig. 12-9). When tissue is bunched up at both sides of the end of an excision, it can be excised in a fusiform pattern *(Step 1)*. It is then closed with

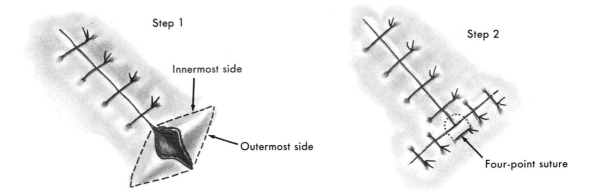

Fig. 12-9. T-shaped dog-ear repair.

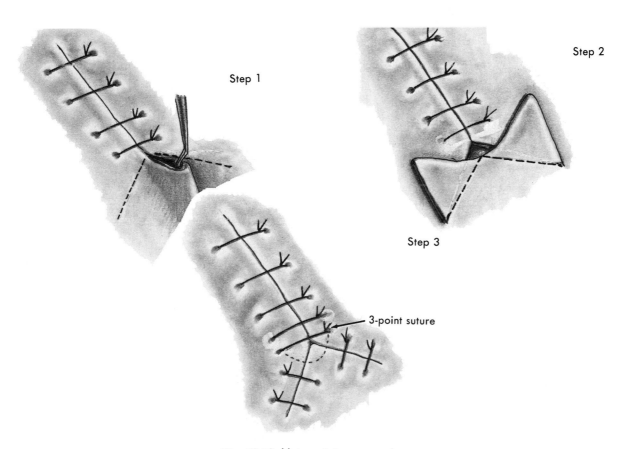

Fig. 12-10. V-shaped dog-ear repair.

interrupted sutures and a four-point suture in the center *(Step 2)*. It should be noted that the dog-ears shown in Fig. 12-9 are geometrically two half-cones on their sides.

An alternative way to deal with the above excess tissue pattern is to incise the dog-ears only along their outermost (or the innermost) sides to their apices. As the tissue is advanced, the excess is trimmed off. This alternative method probably sacrifices less tissue overall, but results in either a T with bent cross arms (↑) like an arrow (if the outermost sides are incised first) or a T with cross arms bent in the opposite direction, almost like a Y (if the outermost sides are incised first).

V-shaped dog-ear repair (Fig. 12-10). Occasionally, an excision extends to a vital area such as the eye, nose, or mouth, where it would be best for the excision line (if it must be extended because of a dog-ear) to diverge into two paths rather than continue straight. Such a dog-ear repair is called the V-shaped dog-ear repair, but it is based on the

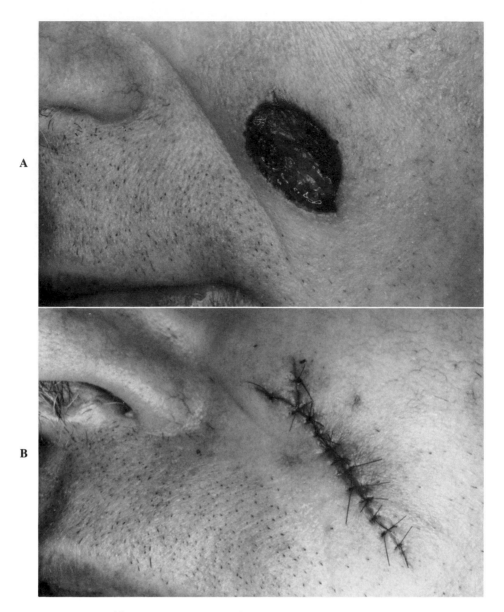

Fig. 12-11. Use of V-shaped dog-ear repair. **A,** Surgical wound of cheek immediately after extirpation of basal cell carcinoma. **B,** Sutured wound with straight dog-ear repair inferiorly and V-shaped dog-ear repair superiorly.

M-plasty repair that is described later in this chapter. It was described by Straith, Lawson, and Hipps in 1961[20] and again in 1979 by Grabb[11] but only recently popularized by Salasche and Roberts.[17]

The excess tissue forming the dog-ear is elevated with a skin hook, and an incision is made on either side tangential to the base of the dog-ear *(Step 1)* at about the same angle to the excision line as in the hockey stick dog-ear repair (Fig. 12-7). The excess tissue is unfolded and fanned out, forming two new triangles that overlie the lateral tissues *(Step 2)*. The bases of these triangles are cut along a line overlying the cut edge of the tissue below. The V-shaped tissue thus formed is then sutured into place with a three-point suture *(Step 3)*.

A clinical example of the V-shaped dog-ear repair is shown in Fig. 12-11, *A* through *D*. A surgical wound following excision of a basal cell carcinoma occurred on the cheek. The wound was sutured side-to-side. The lower dog-ear repair resulted in a straight line, whereas the upper dog-ear repair resulted in divergent lines forming a V-shape (Fig. 12-11, *B*). Note that a side view of the scar on the healed photo looks excellent (Fig. 12-11, *C*). However, a frontal view (Fig. 12-11, *D*) reveals that there is a slight fullness on the cheek at the site of the V-shaped dog-ear repair *(arrows)*. This is caused by slight scar contraction along both arms of the V. Such slight puckering is not uncommon with this type of dog-ear repair and is considered less than ideal. Thus it is the best course of action to

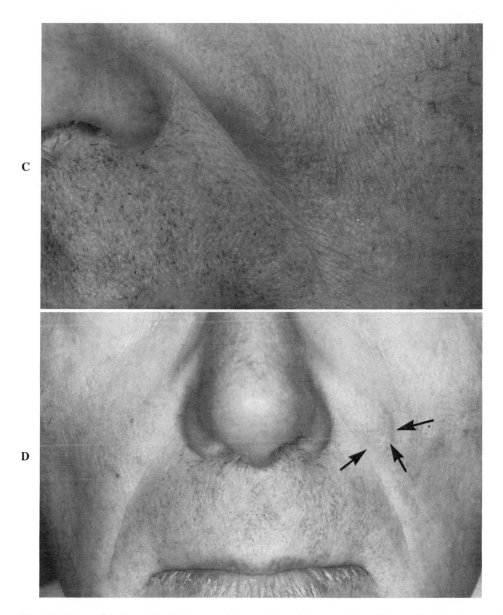

Fig. 12-11, cont'd. C and **D,** Healed result 1 year later. Note small but distinct elevation *(arrows)* at site V-shaped dog-ear repair.

use the V-shaped dog-ear repair only when necessary.

Another clinical example of the V-shaped dog-ear repair is shown in Fig. 12-12. Two separate basal cell carcinomas were removed from the cheek. Also present is a superficial wound at which site an actinic keratosis was curetted superior to the lower surgical defect. After excision of the piece of normal tissue between the two full-thickness wounds, the resultant wound was brought together primarily. Dog-ears were corrected with a straight dog-ear repair superiorly and a V-shaped dog-ear repair inferiorly (Fig. 12-12, *B*). One can observe the fact that 3 months later the patient has an excellent cosmetic result (Fig. 12-12, *C*). The reason why the V-shaped dog ear repair was chosen inferiorly was that the skin folds beyond that end of the partially closed wound appeared to diverge in two different directions. Thus the two arms of the V followed these radiating lines.

WOUND EDGES OF UNEQUAL LENGTH

Occasionally excision wounds are made so that the two lateral edges are of unequal length. This situation occurs when it is desirable to end up with a curved excision line rather than a straight one (see Fig. 10-80 and 10-81). It can also occur by chance with excisions and especially with skin flaps.

There are three basic methods used to even out wounds with unequal sides (Fig. 12-13). A small triangular portion of tissue can be removed from the longer side either in the

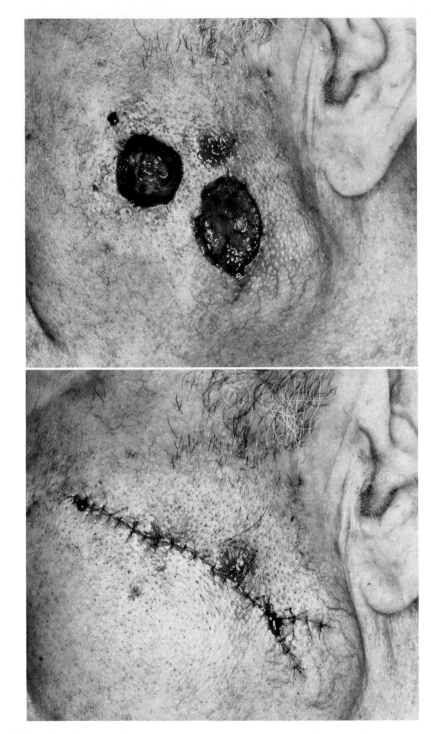

Fig. 12-12. Use of V-shaped dog-ear repair. **A,** Two surgical wounds on cheek after extirpation of two unconnected basal cell carcinomas. The smaller superficial wound (superior to the most posterior of larger wounds) is result of curettage of small actinic keratosis. **B,** Sutured wound. Portion of normal uninvolved tissue between the two large wounds in **A** was excised, wound was brought together initially by buried sutures, and dog-ears were superomedially and inferolaterally repaired. Superomedially a straight dog-ear repair was used, whereas inferolaterally a V-shaped dog-ear repair was chosen.

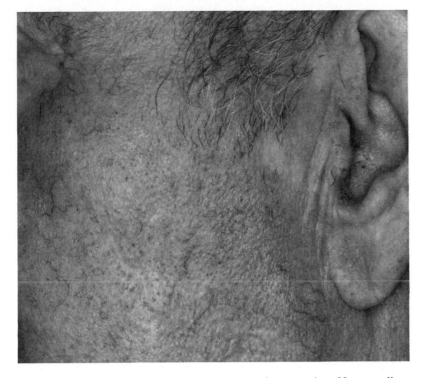

Fig. 12-12, cont'd. C, Healed surgical wound 6 months after operation. Note excellent cosmetic result.

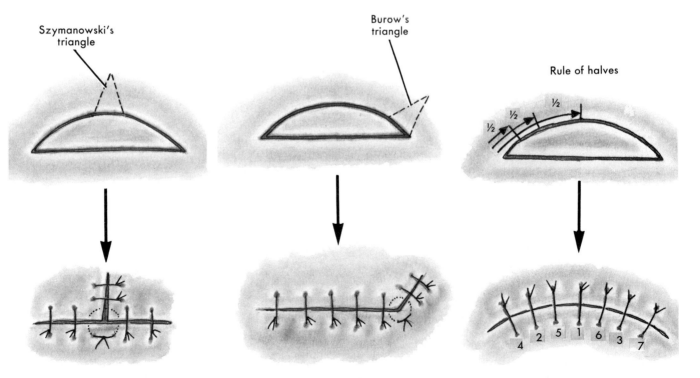

Szymanowski's triangle

Burow's triangle

Rule of halves

½ ½ ½ ½

4 2 5 1 6 3 7

Fig. 12-13. Wounds of unequal length.

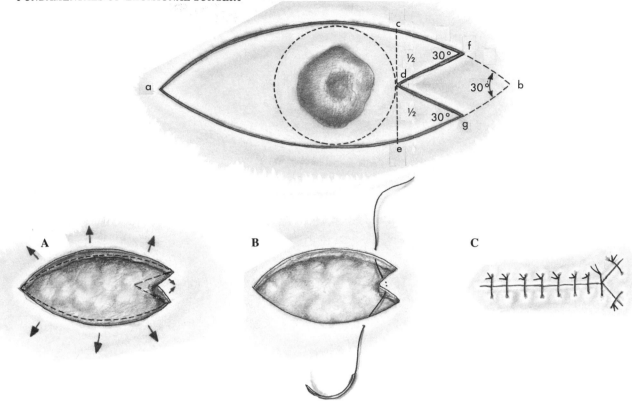

Fig. 12-14. *Top,* M-plasty repair design. **A,** Tissue expansion after excision. Normal position of wound edges is shown by dashed line. **B,** Suturing slightly ahead of tip. **C,** Sutured M-plasty.

center (Szymanowski's triangle)[21] (Fig. 12-13, *left*) or at the end (Burow's triangle) (Fig. 12-13, *middle*). The result is that the longer side is shortened and the lengths of the two sides of an excision are evened up. The third and perhaps most common method of dealing with this situation is by using the rule of halves to suture the surgical defect (Fig. 12-13, *right*). The rule of halves uses the principle of even distribution of tension by placing the sutures halfway between two points where wound edges come together, either excision ends or suture closure points. The numbered sequence of placement is shown (Fig. 12-13, *right bottom*). The first suture (suture *1*) is halfway between the two ends of the excision. The next two sutures (sutures *2* and *3*) are halfway between the first suture (placed in the middle) and each end of the excision. The remaining sutures (*4* through *7*) are placed between the ends of the incision and previously places sutures or between two previously placed sutures.

Other less common methods of repairing wounds with unequal sides include excision of triangles at both ends of the longer side or excision of tissue forming multiple W-plasties at one end or both.[4]

It should be noted that any of the methods used to correct the side length inequity just described can either be planned and executed in advance or dictated by one's closure technique. If the unequal-sided defect in Fig. 12-13 is closed by suturing from both ends toward the center, it is necessary to remove a Szymanowski's triangle to even up the sides. If

suturing begins on one end and proceeds to the far end, the excess tissue is at the far end, and it is necessary to excise a Burow's triangle to even up the wound edges. If one begins in the center and sutures toward the ends, it is necessary to remove two small Burow's triangles, one on each end. It should be noted that each of these two Burow's triangles will be one half the size of the triangles previously mentioned for removal in the center or at either end. Finally, suturing can be performed with the rule of halves and excision of any extra tissue can probably be avoided.

M-PLASTY

A variation of a fusiform excision that modifies one or both ends is the M-plasty. This technique helps to reduce the length of the excision line and the amount of tissue removed.[1,22] Therefore it is useful when the excision line abuts structures or when tissue conservation is essential. In addition, the divergent line that results from the M-plasty is less discernible to the eye than the straight line of a fusiform or tangent-to-circle excision.

The proper method for designing an M-plasty is shown in Fig. 12-14, *top*. The border of normal tissue around the lesion to be excised is marked *(dashed circle)*. Then a fusiform (or tangent-to-circle) pattern for excision is drawn in the standard manner between points *a* and *b*. A straight line tangent (line *ce*) to the border of normal tissue *(dashed circle)* is drawn within the fusiform pattern and running

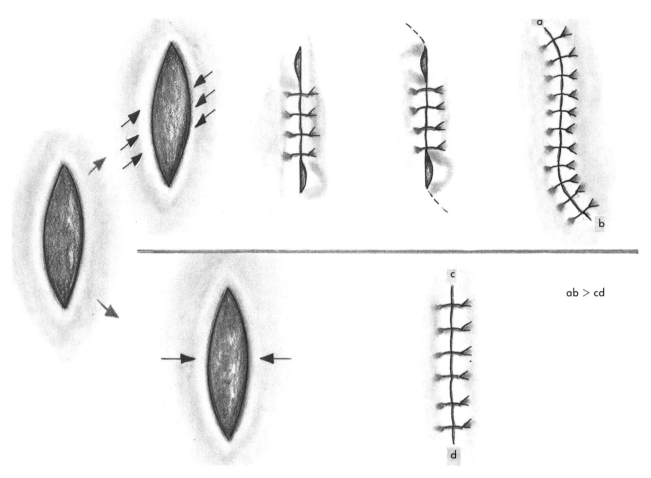

ab > cd

Fig. 12-15. Oblique closure *(top)* and simple side-to-side closure *(bottom)* of fusiform excision.

parallel to its short axis. At the midpoint of this tangent (point *d*) two additional lines are drawn that bisect on each side the distance from the ends of the tangent (points *c* and *e*) to the apex of the ellipse (point *b*). Thus two new points are created, points *f* and *g*. Therefore, *cf* = *fb* = *eg* = *gb*. The lesion and surrounding border of tissue are then excised after incising from point *a* to *f* and *a* to *g* and then from *g* to *d* and *f* to *d*. The area of tissue bounded by points *d, f, b, g* is not excised. This represents the area of tissue that would otherwise have been excised in a fusiform excision and is thus salvaged.

The resulting surgical defect (drawn on a different scale) is shown in Fig. 12-14. Note that all the margins of the wound normally expand with excision. Consequently, the tip *(fdg)* retracts back as well. Therefore, when this V-shaped tip is sutured, it is brought forward by placement of the suture at the lateral wound edges slightly ahead of the tip (Fig. 12-14, *B*), so that when the three-point suture is tied, the tip is advanced into its normal position (Fig. 12-14, *C*).

An M-plasty can be formed at one end or both ends of a fusiform or tangent-to-circle excision. It is essential that, for good results, the lines of excision must be carefully planned on the basis of the geometry shown in Fig. 12-14.

The M-plasty is useful in areas where the skin is loose and wrinkles diverge in two directions or more (for example, around the eyelids). At the point of divergence the two arms of the resultant V from the M-plasty can be directed to fit into the radiating wrinkles.

There are some disadvantages to the M-plasty. Returning to our concept that all scars contract longitudinally over time, it is possible for the area bounded by points *fdg* to develop a trap-door phenomenon (Fig. 12-11, *C*). This bunching of skin is also accentuated if the design of the M-plasty is not carefully measured.

Another disadvantage of the M-plasty is that the broken lines at the end may look somewhat unnatural compared to a straight line. Therefore this technique is not useful on the middle back or forehead. Remember that with time scars become hypopigmented and sometimes more noticeble than immediately following surgery.

S-PLASTY

The S-plasty is a special type of excision that is shaped like an S but with both ends slightly curved. This has thus also been called the "lazy S" (Fig. 12-15). Such a configuration can occur by accident from suturing a fusiform excision obliquely and repairing the dog-ears at each end in opposite directions (Fig. 12-15, top) or by purposeful design. Milford[14] recommends S-shaped excisions for hand surgery, because they give more wound space for a better view of underlying structures and conform better to natural lines. The gently curving scars that result from such excisions are then less noticeable in that area.

The S-plasty, besides giving a unique-appearing scar, differs from a standard fusiform closure in two ways. First, it lengthens the scar (Fig. 12-15). This becomes important in areas where one wishes to minimize bandlike constriction of scars that may occur over the convex or concave body surfaces. Convex surfaces include the extremities and digits. Here bandlike constrictions result in tethered depressed scars. Concave body surfaces include the inner canthus or between digits. Contraction of scars in the inner canthus can lead to an extracanthal fold (Fig. 10-64, *C* and *D*) that may be lengthened at the time of surgery by use of the S-plasty.

The second thing accomplished by an S-plasty is to alter slightly the direction of the long axis of the excision (not shown on Fig. 12-15). This slight alteration in direction might minimize the tethering depressions or the bandlike elevations just discussed.

The S-plasty can be simply created by obliquely suturing a fusiform excision (Fig. 12-15). This results in effectively lengthening a portion of each side of the excision relative to the opposite side. Thus dog-ears are produced at each end of the excision that can be repaired as shown. Note that this dog-ear repair is slightly different from the other types shown previously. The excision line is simply extended to conform to the shape of the lazy S. The excess tissue is then pulled over the extended incision and trimmed. Thus a crescent- or half moon–shaped piece of skin is excised.[16]

One ideal place to use the S-plasty is on a forearm excision over the radial bone. Because of the prominence of the radial bone, which produces a convex cutaneous surface, excisions can ultimately form constricting bands. By oblique suturing of the excision, dog-ears are produced at each end. On the dorsal side of the arm, the end of the S is directed toward the hand. On the ventral side, it is directed toward the elbow.

Although recommended by some,[14] the creation of S-plasty without dog-ear formation and repair is fraught with problems. By proceeding one step at a time, one makes fewer mistakes with respect to proper adjustment of the direction of the long excision axis and the curved ends.

PARTIAL CLOSURE

It is better to allow some surgical defects to granulate and epidermize rather than to cause the patient to undergo a major rearrangement of tissue planes or a skin graft. However, allowing wounds to contract occasionally results in noticeable distortion of surrounding structures. To minimize such distortion, a surgical defect can be partially closed and partially allowed to heal by secondary intention. Fig. 12-16, *A* through *D*, demonstrates a partial closure.

Fig. 12-16, *A,* is a large surgical defect from excision of a squamous cell carcinoma. Because I thought that allowing this wound to heal completely by granulation would result in some distortion of the lateral canthus, I partially closed the wound in the direction of minimal tension with a large (no. 3-0) silk suture and repaired the dog-ears that occurred on two sides of the wound (Fig. 12-16, *B*). Because of the great tension on the wound, these dog-ear corrections were closed with staples. At 1 month, the wound was healing nicely, although the one dog-ear repair had broken down, probably as a result of the great tension on that area (Fig. 12-16, *C*). At 1 year postoperatively (Fig. 12-16, *D*) the patient has a good cosmetic result without any distortion of the lateral canthus. There is a small extra fold of skin on the lateral lower eyelid (the result of not repairing the dog-ear in that area at the time of surgery), but the patient refused further surgery to correct this.

Although partial closure has been used for many years, the time and place for its use depend greatly on experience. Epstein[9] described the use of partial closure to prevent dog-ears and other distortions of tissue. Although I agree that partial closure may be used to prevent distortion, it should not be used to prevent dog-ears, because the dog-ear repairs usually look better than the scars resulting from the partial closure. Furthermore, as just seen, partial closure can lead to dog-ears.

Albright[2] referred to the use of "guiding sutures" to direct the skin tension so that open wounds would heal in the most favorable position possible. In Fig. 12-16, *B*, the silk suture acted as the guiding suture to give direction to the wound. I have found silk to be the best for this purpose, since it does not cut through tissue as easily as other sutures. Since the guiding sutures are frequently under considerable tension, this is important. Also if possible, I try to keep the guiding sutures from coming through the skin to minimize necrosis of the cutaneous surfaces. If it is necessary to come through the skin, it is best to use bolsters under the sutures. Guiding sutures are left in place from 1 or 2 weeks up to 1 month, depending on the progress of wound healing. The partially buried and partially exposed silk suture in Fig. 11-16, *B* was left in place 4 weeks without any problems. Usually by that time the wound is well on its way to being healed and the silk suture has loosened up considerably; it is found to be functioning as a foreign body rather than holding tissue together.

Repairs of all cutaneous wounds involve a series of compromises. With partial closures, these compromises are particularly apparent. Knowing the probable end result of a partial closure compared to a full closure, the physician can choose the closure that is in the patient's best interest. A full closure of the wound in Fig. 12-16, *A,* might have looked as good cosmetically but would have subjected the patient to a much more complicated and involved surgical procedure. The end functional results, however, are the same. There-

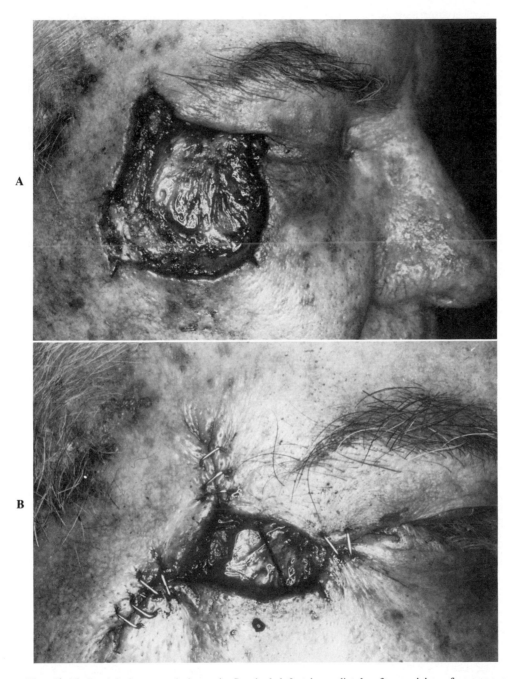

Fig. 12-16. Partial closure technique. **A,** Surgical defect immediately after excision of squamous cell carcinoma. **B,** Partial closure of surgical defect with staples. Note that silk suture in right center of wound was first placed along lines of minimal tension to guide wound partially closed. Also note that dog-ear from outer canthus along lower lid is not repaired. *Continued.*

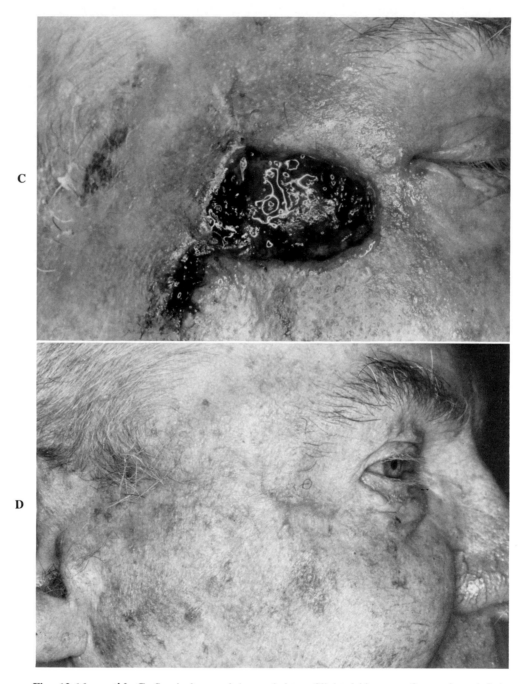

Fig. 12-16, cont'd. C, Surgical wound 1 month later. Slight dehiscence of most lateroinferior dog-ear is present. **D,** Healed surgical wound at 1 year after operation; note excellent cosmetic result. Note also that dog-ear from outer canthus along lower eyelid still persists. Patient refused correction.

fore a partial closure was chosen. It should be emphasized that a partial closure is not selected because a full closure cannot be done. Rather, it is performed with the patient's best interest in mind.

REFERENCES

1. Albom, M.: Scalpel and scissors surgery. In Epstein, E., and Epstein, E., Jr.: editors: Techniques in skin surgery, Philadelphia, 1979, Lea and Febiger.
2. Albright, S.D., III: Placement of "guiding sutures" to counteract undesirable retraction of tissues in and around functionally and cosmetically important structures, J. Dermatol. Surg. Oncol. 7(6):446, 1981.
3. Borges, A.F.: Elective incisions and scar revision, Boston, 1973, Little, Brown & Co.
4. Borges, A.F.: Dog-ear repair, Plast. Reconstr. Surg. **69:**707, 1982.
5. Burow, C.A.: Beschreibung einer neuen Transplantations: Methode zum Wiederersatz verlorengegangener Theile des Gesichts, Berlin, 1855, A. Nauck.
6. Converse, J.M.: Introduction to plastic surgery. In Converse, J.M., editor: Reconstructive plastic surgery, Philadelphia, 1977, W.B. Saunders Co.
7. Davis, T.S., Graham, W.P., III, and Miller, S.H.: The circular excision, Ann. Plast. Surg. **4**(1):21, 1980.
8. Dzubow, L.M.: The dynamics of dog-ear formation and correction, J. Dermatol. Surg. Oncol. **11**(7):722, 1985.
9. Epstein, E.: Surgery of skin tumors: excision with partial suture closure, Cutis **18**(3).384, 1976.
10. Gormley, D.E.: The dog-ear: causes, prevention and correction, J. Dermatol. Surg. Oncol. **3:**194, 1977.
11. Grabb, W.C.: Basic techniques of plastic surgery. In Grabb, W.C., and Smith, J.W., editors: Plastic surgery, ed. 3, Boston, 1979, Little, Brown & Co.
12. Limberg, A.A.: Design of local flaps. In Gibson, T., editor: Modern trends in plastic surgery, vol. 2, London, 1966, Butterworths.
13. McGregor, I.A.: Fundamental techniques of plastic surgery and their surgical applications, Edinburgh, 1975, Churchill Livingstone.
14. Milford, L.: The hand. Edmonson, A.S., and Crenshaw, A.H., editors: Campbell's operative orthopaedics, ed. 6, St. Louis, 1980, The C.V. Mosby Co.
15. Robbins, T.H.: Elliptical excision and closure, J.R. Coll Surg. (Edinb) **25**(1):59, 1980.
16. Robinson, D.W.: Simple revision of scars, Clin. Plast. Surg. **4:**217, 1977.
17. Salasche, S.J., and Roberts, L.C.: Dog-ear correction by M-plasty, J. Dermatol. Surg. Oncol. **10:**478, 1984.
18. Spicer, T.E.: Techniques of facial lesion excision and closure, J. Dermatol. Surg. Oncol, **8**(7):551, 1982.
19. Stegman, S.J., Tromovitch, T.A., and Glogau, R.G.: Basics of dermatologic surgery, Chicago, 1982, Year Book Medical Publishers, Inc.
20. Straith, R.E., Lawson, J.M., and Hipps, C.J.: The subcuticular suture, Postgrad. Med. **29:**164, 1961.
21. von Szymanowski, J.: Handbuch der Operativen Chirurgie, Braunschweig, 1870, Druck und verhag von Friedrick Vieweg und Sohn.
22. Webster, R.C., et al.: M-plasty techniques, J. Dermatol. Surg. **2:**393, 1976.
23. Zoltan, J.: Cicatrix optima, Baltimore, 1978, University Park Press.

13

Problems Associated with Cutaneous Surgery

Any surgical or medical procedure has associated with it a certain risk of producing problems for the patient. Although usually these problems are of a minor nature and rarely result in permanent injury, their recognition and proper management result in faster healing and frequently lead to improved cosmetic results. This chapter explores several problems seen either during or subsequent to surgery on the cutaneous surfaces. Many of these problems are discussed in greater detail elsewhere in this text.

SURGICAL PROBLEMS VERSUS SURGICAL COMPLICATIONS
Definitions

The term "complication" is loosely used by patients and physicians alike to refer to any event that occurs unexpectedly. However, many wound conditions predictably occur at the time of or soon after surgery and therefore should not be considered complications but rather expected problems.

The French philosopher Pascal remarked that everything depends on the point of view. Patients in general have limited first-hand knowledge of what to expect in terms of healing. Therefore physicians need to appreciate this fact and be as informative as possible. A problem that the surgeon views as normal or expected might be totally unexpected to the patient, who would thus consider it a complication.

Problems associated with surgery are either expected or unexpected. An expected problem is one that occurs in the majority of individuals undergoing a procedure. It is the natural result of surgery or wound healing. An unexpected problem, or complication, on the other hand, is more unusual and happens in only a small proportion of patients. (This concept is graphically depicted in Fig. 13-1.) Problems that are expected are inevitable and not generally under the control of the physician or patient—but unex-

pected problems are, to some extent. These distinctions are important, because physicians need to consider what unexpected problems they can minimize as well as what expected problems they must accept. Perhaps the term "complication" should be abandoned as applied to medical or surgical procedures, since it does not accurately reflect the likelihood of a specific event occurring.

Before surgery, physicians need to explain to patients what problems to expect. This helps to make patients more informed and accepting of any problems, whether expected or unexpected. Although most wounds heal uneventfully, it is impossible to guarantee to every patient an excellent result without problems. Therefore patients need to be informed that all wounds heal slightly differently and all people heal slightly differently.

Prevention of problems

Frequently, there are several causes for surgical problems, whether expected or unexpected. However, it should be recognized that both the patient and the physician have certain responsibilities to ensure that the chances of any untoward events are minimized. Too often blame is laid on the physician for problems or for a poor result, when in fact the patient has been guilty of noncompliance. The best surgical results come about because of teamwork between the patient, the patient's family, the physician, and the physician's staff.

It is the physician's responsibility to ensure that the patient is totally informed both preoperatively and postoperatively as well as intraoperatively about what problems are definitely going to occur and what problems are reasonably likely to occur. The physician must also explain what is required in terms of wound care and follow-up visits.

Patients should be as informed as possible and assume the responsibility for and help participate in the care of their wounds. The patient should carefully follow any preopera-

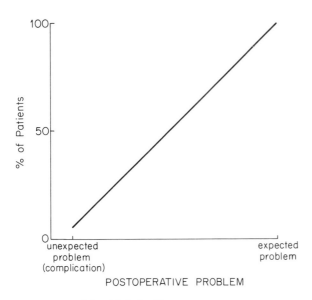

Fig. 13-1. Problem spectrum.

tive, intraoperative, or postoperative instructions given by the physician or by other members of the medical team. The patient has the responsibility to report any problems associated with wound healing to the physician.

Causes of problems

Either the patient or the physician may make surgical problems more likely in several ways. The patient may be a poor historian and not give valuable information to the physician. Medical problems may exist that effect untoward reactions to surgery (see Table 10-1, p. 357). The patient might not inform the physician of various medications he or she is taking unless specifically asked. Sometimes this is not the fault of the patient, but rather of the physician who does not specifically ask questions such as "Have you ever had any drug reactions?" The patient may also cause problems by improperly carrying out preoperative or postoperative instructions.

Physicians may increase the risk of surgical problems or complications because of one or more of the following: (1) poor history and physical examination, (2) poor technique during the time of surgery, or (3) poor instructions given the patient following surgery. Before surgery, the physician should inquire about any allergies, previous surgery, and medical problems.

Questions should be specific. A poor medical history and physical examination may fail to uncover medical problems that might influence the surgery. Patients frequently do not offer information unless asked specifically. For example "Do you have any allergies to drugs, medications, or creams?" is specific and more likely to uncover the important information one needs than "Do you have any allergies?" If the question is too general, patients may be

more likely to tell you about their pollen allergies than about their drug allergies.

The physician should specifically ask about pacemakers or anticoagulants. The physical examination should include examination of other scars the patient may have, and these should be documented. In addition, any problems with hyperpigmentation should be noted. If surgery is contemplated on the face, the physician should carefully examine the operative site for any nerve damage that may already be present. A sample routine preoperative history and physical examination form is included in Appendix A.

Physicians can cause complicatons with poor surgical technique. Good surgical technique is stressed elsewhere in this book. A sound knowledge of surgical principles and materials is the backbone of good technique.

Physicians may contribute to poor results by giving poor instructions to patients either preoperatively or postoperatively. Patients are frequently very nervous both before and after the surgery and may easily forget what is said to them. This problem can be avoided by carefully writing out preoperative and postoperative instructions for patients. The written instructions should be simple and easy to read. They should also contain information on how to contact the physician should any problems arise. Appendix D contains a typical postoperative instruction sheet.

DISSATISFIED PATIENT

The patient is usually satisfied with the surgical result. However, occasionally one encounters a patient who feels disappointed with it or the manner in which the surgery was performed. This may occur for a variety of reasons. The patient may (1) have had unrealistic expectations of the surgery, (2) be dissatisfied with the bill or the manner in which it was handled by the office staff, or (3) be very demanding and never be satisfied with any surgical result at the hands of any physician. Whatever the reason, the physician should be reassuring and demonstrate a caring attitude toward such dissatisfied patients. Even though this may be difficult to do at times, it certainly does no harm and may possibly mean the difference between a happy outcome and one that is a bother to the physician in the future.

It is usually obvious before surgery which patients will be dissatisfied with the surgical result. These are the patients who are demanding to the office staff before they even enter the office, who complain about minor bills, and who shop around from physician to physician. One should be wary of operating on such individuals unless absolutely necessary. It has been said that one makes a reputation not by the cases one does but rather by the cases one does not take on.

DISSATISFIED PHYSICIAN

The physician needs to aim for excellence to provide his or her patients with the best surgical results. This requires continuous self-criticism. It means recognizing poor results and trying to discover the reasons for complications (unexpected problems) of surgery so that they can be avoided in the future. Dissatisfaction with less than optimal results provides motivation to improve one's skills.

A physician should be wary of criticizing the surgical results of others, particularly in front of patients. Such commentary is usually self-serving and provides only an ''ego trip'' for the expositor; it is doubtful if it serves any useful function; it can make the patient more anxious; and, such criticism, no matter how inadvertent or unintentional, might come back later to haunt the criticizing physician.

PROBLEMS AT THE TIME OF SURGERY
Bleeding

Perhaps the most common problem encountered during surgery is bleeding that is not easily controlled. It is always reassuring to remember a remark made by an otolaryngology colleague that ''all bleeding can be stopped.'' One should place continuous pressure on the bleeding area until the necessary equipment is available to control the bleeding. The key to stopping the bleeding is visualization. This requires a good light and possibly a suction machine. This is covered in Chapter 10.

All arterial bleeding that is visibly ''pumping'' the blood vessel should be stopped before excisional wounds are repaired. The pressures of time are no excuse for providing good hemostasis. A good precaution to take is to roll a sterile cotton-tipped applicator over the wound bed before closing to make certain there are no oozing areas that need to be stopped (see Fig. 10-51).

Fainting

Another problem occasionally seen with surgery is fainting. This can be minimized by operating on patients in the prone or supine position rather than in a sitting position. The surgical table should be capable of being tilted easily into the Trendelenburg position so that the patient's head is positioned below his heart and feet. Rarely are smelling salts necessary, but they should be readily available.

The most frequent cause of fainting during surgery is vasovagal syncope, in which anxiety provokes vasodilation of the arteries with a subsequent fall in blood pressure. However, other reasons for fainting must also be considered and include reactions to medications or cardiac problems such as pacemaker malfunction. If these latter causes are probable, an intravenous line should be established, and the correct resuscitation equipment should be made available.

Allergic reactions

Allergic reactions to the medications given at the time of cutaneous surgery are rare, but they are a theoretic possibility. Minor reactions, such as urticaria, can be treated by intravenous or intramuscular steroids or antihistamines.

Life-threatening laryngeal edema and bronchospasm caused by anaphylaxis require resuscitative equipment and medical support. These should be readily available (see Appendix F).

Seizures

Although unusual, seizures may occur during cutaneous surgery. Three of my patients have had a seizure in the past 10 years. One case was related to vasovagal syncope, another to syncope caused by cardiac malfunction, and a third to a grand mal seizure unrelated to the surgery. All three patients had gone through similar episodes previously. Therefore it is probably a good idea to include an inquiry about previous seizures or fainting episodes in the preoperative evaluation form. Lack of adequate blood to the brain for whatever reason can result in seizures. The patient should be protected during the seizure and should not be allowed to drive a car during the postictal period.

Cardiac arrhythmia and arrest

The problem most feared during surgery is ventricular fibrillation or cardiac arrest. If patients have a strong history of prior episodes, careful monitoring during the surgery may be required. This involves use of a cardiac monitor, measuring heart rate and rhythm, and a blood pressure monitor. In addition, appropriate resuscitative equipment (including oxygen) should be readily available. This is listed in Appendix F.

It cannot be too strongly emphasized that as many as possible of the office or clinic personnel, including the physicians should receive certification in cardiopulmonary resuscitation (CPR). There should also be a well-organized plan worked out in advance to provide the necessary care for the patient if an arrest does occur.

PROBLEMS FOLLOWING SURGERY

The problems that occur after surgery can be divided into those that occur (1) after surgery until the wound is healed, and (2) after the wound is healed. Although such a classification is somewhat arbitrary and some overlap may occur, it is useful to consider problems in these two general time frames since the causes are frequently different. Problems occurring soon after the surgery are usually related to the surgery itself, whereas problems occurring after the wound is healed are frequently related to the healing ability of the patient.

Bleeding or hematoma

Some bleeding after closure of a wound will occur and may threaten the speed of healing and the cosmetic result. This is particularly likely when a local anesthetic with epinephrine has been used. As the epinephrine diffuses out of the wound locality, vasoconstriction becomes less, and bleeding ensues. Therefore it is helpful if most wounds are supported by a dressing that provides some pressure for the first day after surgery.

Hemorrhage may unexpectedly occur directly into a wound and into the surrounding skin as well. The latter results in bruising (Fig. 13-2). However, in some cutaneous areas, bruising is expected after any procedure. For example, around the eyes, bruising of the skin surrounding a wound occurs in many if not most patients. This is because of the shearing trauma to the blood vessels with poor dermal support in this area. Patients need to be informed about this so they know what to expect and thus do not become unnecessarily alarmed.

Occasionally the patient inadvertently causes trauma to the wound after leaving the office. This can possibly induce bleeding into the wound, which may interfere with wound healing. If this occurs, the patient should call the physician.

Some patients are more prone to bleeding than others. Those who have been on anticoagulants and those who are heavy imbibers of alcohol are at high risk for excessive bleeding. Some patients whose nutritional status is poor tend to be bleeders as well. Wounds in these patients should be watched carefully. These patients should be instructed to return more frequently than other patients for follow-up visits and to be more careful with their wounds.

All patients leaving the office should be told specifically how to stop bleeding. They should be reminded that if bleeding occurs they should lie down and put steady pressure on the wound for at least 15 to 20 minutes without peeking. Pressure should be placed as directly over the bleeding area as possible with a small piece of gauze. A large towel should not be used, since it diffuses the pressure over a large area and is thus ineffective.

Fig. 13-3, *A* shows a patient in whom bleeding occurred into the wound and continued for 2 days after surgery. The patient was an aspirin abuser but did not tell the treating physicans. Such wounds need to be opened (Fig. 13-3, *B*), the bleeding controlled (Fig. 13-3, *C*), and the wound immediately resutured (Fig. 13-3, *D*). Alternatively, the wound may be allowed to heal by granulation and epidermization. If resutured, the wound heals normally and usually without infection (Fig. 13-3, *E*). It should be remembered that, if the wound is opened and resutured (without freshening the edges) within 3 to 4 days after the surgery, the sutures may still be removed on the same day suture removal was originally scheduled (assuming this is 7 days after the original surgery). Usually little interruption of the wound-healing process occurs by opening a wound before collagen and vascular tissue has bridged the wound (within the first 4 days or so).

Infection

Wound infection subsequent to cutaneous surgery is infrequent, since this is clean surgery and therefore not subject to heavy contamination as is other types of surgery (for

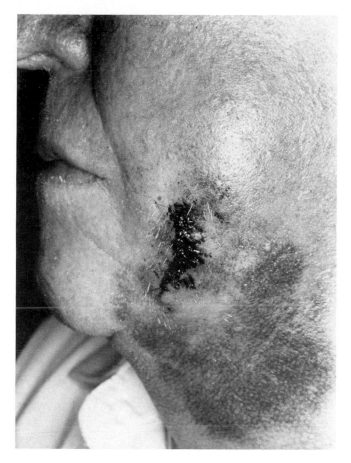

Fig. 13-2. Bruising of skin surrounding wound and bleeding from wound itself 3 days after surgical excision of basal cell carcinoma.

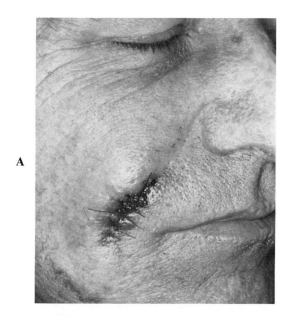

A

Fig. 13-3. For legend, see next page.

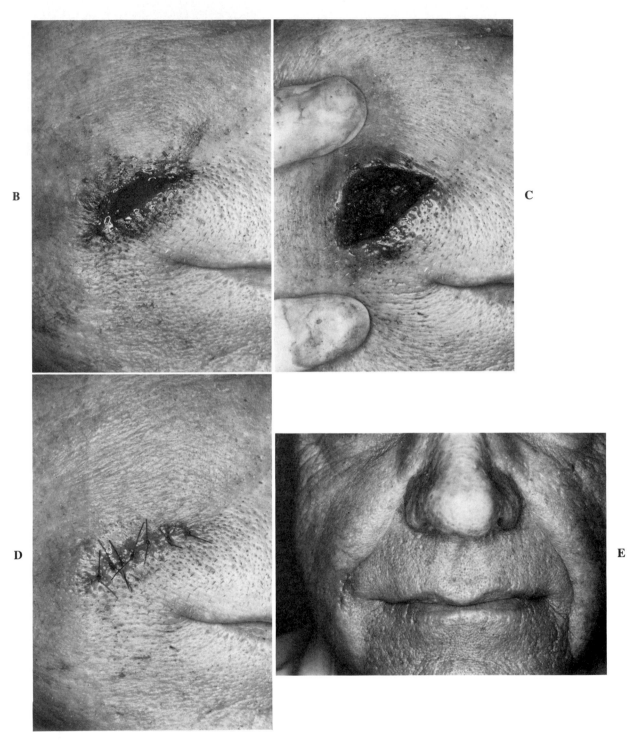

Fig. 13-3, cont'd. A, Bleeding into and from a wound 3 days after surgery for extirpation of keratinous cyst. Note tension of skin around sutures is increased from blood in wound. Such increased tension is forcing sutures to strangulate tissue. **B,** Fresh blood in wound seen after removal of sutures. **C,** Bleeding localized and stopped by means of electrocoagulation. **D,** Wound was immediately resutured without freshening edges. **E,** Wound at time of suture removal 4 days later.

example, bowel surgery). The causes and treatments of infections have been extensively reviewed in Chapter 4. Wounds that are heavily colonized (more than 10^5 bacteria per gram of tissue) with pathogens at the time of closure are likely to become infected.[6]

If a sutured wound becomes infected, it is best to remove all the sutures as soon as possible. Sutures become a nidus for infection and have little holding power in highly inflamed tissue. A bacteriologic culture should be obtained, the patient should be started on the most appropriate antibiotic (subject to change depending on the culture report), and the wound should be reinforced by means of wound-closure tapes.

One poorly recognized type of infection seen occasionally in cutaneous surgery is that which results from *Candida albicans* (Plate 1-A). Usually the dermatitis that results from heavy colonization by this organism is fairly well localized and demarcated compared to contact dermatitis, which is more diffuse and ill defined (Plate 1-B). For reasons unknown, *C. albicans* can infect wounds in patients who are not immunosuppressed. These infections may be related to topical antibiotic ointments (which are frequently used on both sutured or granulating wounds) selecting out yeast or to the moisture and maceration of the dressing that provide a haven where microbes tend to thrive. Treatment with a topical antifungal agent, such as Nystatin, is usually sufficient to clear such yeast infections.

Acute tissue reactions

Surgery naturally traumatizes tissue, and tissue responds initially with an inflammatory reaction, the earliest response in wound healing (see Chapter 2). Placement of sutures with needles similarly causes inflammation and fibroplasia.[25] An increase in this reaction is seen with tissue compression from a tightly tied suture.[18] Wounds may thus normally have a slight degree of erythema around them and no pus. If erythema persists or purulence appears, an infection should be suspected.

One specific form of inflammation appears to be chondritis of the pinna, which frequently occurs if cartilage is left exposed subsequent to surgery. This situation may arise after even a simple procedure such as a punch biopsy. Chondritis is characterized by exquisite pain in the cartilage, especially with the application of pressure, and erythema in the skin surrounding and underlying the exposed cartilage. Should chondritis occur, tetracycline by mouth and warm vinegar (acetic acid) soaks four times a day have been found to be very useful. The recommended vinegar is white vinegar mixed 1:2 with water. In my experience tetracycline, begun immediately after surgery that has exposed ear cartilage, appears to prevent chondritis much of the time. Postoperative analgesics such as codeine may be necessary because of the pain.

The cause of ear chondritis is not well studied and there-

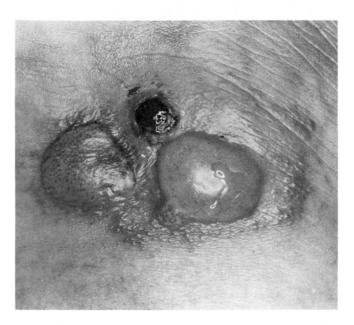

Fig. 13-4. Bullous contact dermatitis caused by topical sulfur-contaning antibiotic cream. Hypergranulation tissue superiorly was found to be caused by wood splinter.

fore is speculative. Some theories are that it is caused by exposure of the cartilage, destruction of the cartilage with heat generated near the electrode tip of an electrocoagulation device, or infection. If a bacterial infection is involved, it is often caused by gram-negative rods. Stegman, Tromovitch, and Glogau[33] believe that ear cartilage chrondritis is usually caused by *Pseudomonas aeruginosa*. However, as just mentioned, this has not been well studied.

Contact dermatitis

Contact dermatitis is an allergic reaction of the delayed hypersensitivity type. It may be reproduced by appropriate patch testing with the offending allergen. Allergic reactions to any of the antibacterial ointments frequently placed on wounds can be seen. Such ointments are used for their bacteriostatic and occlusive properties as well as to keep overlying dressings from sticking. These ointments usually contain not only antibacterial substances but also other chemicals such as preservatives. When an allergic reaction to one of these ointments occurs, the patient usually complains of pruritus around the wound. There is intense redness that is poorly demarcated and tends to blend into the adjacent, normal skin (Plate 1-B) surrounding the wound. Rarely one may see a bullous reaction as an extreme form of contact dermatitis (Fig. 13-4). Treatment consists of use of a topical fluorinated steroid for a few days and discontinuance of the offending substance. Short-term use of topical steroids on wounds does not appear to have any deleterious effects of a practical nature on wound healing. Plain petrolatum may be substituted for an antibacterial ointment if an ointment is needed on the wound for several weeks in the allergic patient. Sterile white petrolatum is available in individually packed, single-use containers. (*USP* White Petrolatum, E. Fougera, Melville, N.Y.)

Contact dermatitis may occur to other surgical supplies besides antibacterial ointments. Such reactions to adhesive tape, compound tincture of benzoin, or even surgical scrub solutions used to prepare the operative site have all been reported.[19,20,26] Allergic tape reactions usually occur just under the adhesive tape and are *sharply demarcated.*

Dehiscence

Wound edge separation can occur for a variety of reasons. Pressure on sutures can cause tearing of the tissue. Pressure can result from external trauma, bleeding into the wound, or edema. Infection softens tissue and allows sutures to pull through it more easily. Poor tissue handling at the time of surgery results in necrotic tissue and malalignment of wound edges that will delay wound healing.

Removal of sutures before adequate union of two sides of a wound occurs may also result in dehiscence. Delayed union can occur in areas slow to heal such as the lower extremities. On rare occasions nutritional problems such as vitamin C deficiency may also cause a delay in healing.

The use of buried sutures at the time of wound closure may help to prevent dehiscence at the time of suture removal. However, if extreme tension exists in wound edges, buried sutures do not by themselves stop a wound from opening up.

If a wound does dehisce during the first few days after closure, assuming there is no infection, it may be resutured without trimming the epidermal-dermal edges. Trimming the epidermal-dermal edges may make a slightly neater appearance at first, but the final result is frequently about the same. If the epidermal-dermal edges are trimmed, the sutures used for resuturing must be left in a longer time for adequate healing than if the edges are not trimmed (see Chapter 2).

If obvious infection is present at the time of dehiscence, it is best to get a culture, place the patient on appropriate antibiotics, and allow the wound to heal by granulation and epidermization. The cosmetic result is usually acceptable. If not, a scar revision may be safely performed at a later time.

It is interesting to note that certain suture techniques may result in faster, more firm healing than others. Vertical mattress sutures, for instance, result in a stronger wound earlier with less likelihood to dehisce than simple interrupted sutures. This is nicely shown in Fig. 13-5. Here a wound in the pubic area was sutured with simple interrupted sutures superiorly and vertical mattress sutures inferiorly (Fig. 13-5, *B*). At 1 week all sutures were removed and the wound dehisced, but only superiorly, where the simple interrupted sutures had been placed (Fig. 13-5, *C*). The dehisced portion of the wound was resutured without freshening the wound edges (Fig. 13-5, *D*), and the sutures were

removed 5 days later without any signs of dehiscence.

To help minimize dehiscence, all wounds are usually supported for 1 week after suture removal with wound-closure tapes.

Delayed wound healing

Delayed wound healing can be caused by many factors, which are discussed in depth in Chapter 2. In open wounds, infection is the main reason for delayed wound healing, and careful quantitative bacterial cultures should be obtained if a wound does not heal within a reasonable time.[6,16] Other reasons for delayed wound healing such as nutritional or metabolic problems are rare but can occur. Poor vascular supply in the lower extremities in patients with arteriosclerosis also delays wound healing.

Tissue necrosis

Death of tissue occurs because of poor blood supply. Whether this is the result of tension on vessels, vessels being transected at surgery, poor tissue handling, or inadequate blood supply, the result is the same. Tissue necrosis first appears as superficial blistering of the epidermis and a dusky appearance of the underlying dermis (Fig. 13-6). Within a few days the zone of tissue death becomes well demarcated and can usually be debrided with scissors to facilitate wound healing. The patient experiences no pain, since the dead tissue has no feeling.

Hypergranulation

Exuberant granulation tissue can occasionally form in a wound allowed to heal by secondary intention. This appears as bright red spongy tissue that covers the wound bed and extends above the surface of the surrounding skin (Plate 1-C). This is commonly referred to as "proud flesh." In my experience, hypergranulation tissue appears to be more common in wounds of the scalp and upper back.

The cause of hypergranulation tissue is unknown. Where cultures have been done, *C. albicans* has frequently grown; whether it is the cause or is a secondary invader is unknown. Histopathologically, numerous newly formed blood vessels can be seen.

If left to persist, hypergranulation tissue delays or even impedes wound healing by providing a mechanical barrier to migrating epidermis; therefore it is best and often necessary to remove it. The easiest way to do this is simply to curette hypergranulation tissue away with a dermal curette. This may be done without local anesthesia. The subsequent bleeding can be easily controlled with pressure or a nonstaining styptic, such as 35% aluminum chloride (hydrous) in 50% isopropyl alcohol. The patient should be seen again at 3- to 4-week intervals to see if the exuberant granulation tissue has reformed. If it has, it is again removed with the curette and the bleeding stopped. Occasionally it is necessary to remove the hypergranulation tis-

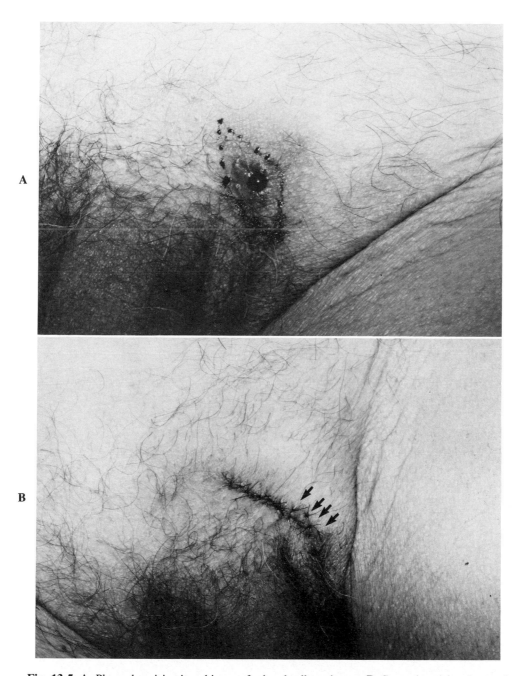

Fig. 13-5. A, Planned excision in pubic area for basal cell carcinoma. **B,** Sutured excisional wound in pubic area. Superior portion of wound sutured with simple interrupted sutures. Inferior portion of wound sutured with vertical mattress sutures *(arrows)*. *Continued.*

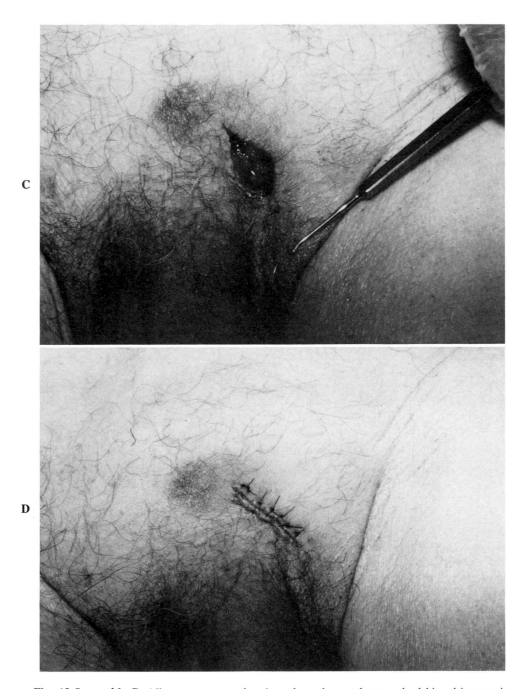

Fig. 13-5, cont'd. C, All sutures removed at 1 week, and wound promptly dehisced in superior portion, where simple interrupted sutures had been placed. Inferior portion of wound sutured by vertical mattress sutures did not dehisce. Inferior extent of wound is demonstrated by skin hook. **D,** Upper dehisced portion of wound was immediately resutured (without freshening the wound edges) with vertical mattress sutures, and second group of sutures was removed 1 week later. Healing was then uneventful. (Photographs courtesy Dr. Stuart Kaplan, Los Angeles.)

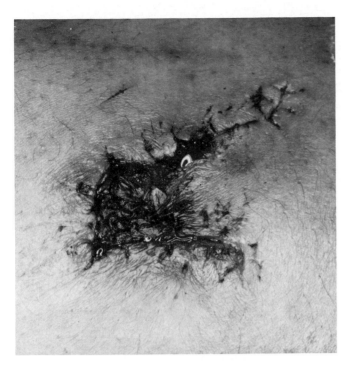

Fig. 13-6. Tissue necrosis in distal portion of skin flap on arm.

suc several times before complete epidermization occurs.

An alternative method used to remove exuberant granulation tissue is to touch the excessive tissue with silver nitrate (75%) on sticks until the tissue turns white. However, this method has one drawback; that is, silver nitrate tends to stain, especially if it is applied to a large area.

Pain

Pain can follow any surgical procedure. Fortunately, after most cutaneous operations, severe pain is not present. Patients are frequently surprised to find how little pain occurs compared to their expectations. However, perception of pain is a highly individual phenomenon. Some patients appear to be more sensitive to it than others. For minimal pain, two tablets of acetaminophen (Tylenol) every 4 hours is sufficient. For more intense pain one or two tablets of acetaminophen with one-half grain of codeine (Tylenol No. 3) every 4 hours may be given if necessary. Patients should be advised not to take aspirin for 1 week after surgery.

Pain may be a sign of other problems such as infection or pressure subsequent to bleeding. Therefore if pain becomes severe or becomes continually worse, patients should be instructed to consult their physician.

Immediate nerve damage

When one performs surgery on the skin and subcutaneous tissue, damage to either the motor or sensory nerves may occur. Usually this occurs in the face or scalp and is

evident soon after surgery is complete. All patients should be examined preoperatively to assess whether nerve damage is present in the area of the surgery. The patient may not have noticed subtle changes in nerve function that would pass unnoticed unless specifically looked for. If present, these should be well documented in the patient's chart.

The best means of avoiding damage to nerves at the time of surgery is by having a thorough knowledge of the anatomic structures through which one is cutting. The major superficial nerves of the head and neck have been discussed in Chapter 3. Careful *blunt* dissection and *gentle* technique help to prevent damage to nerves. Minimizing the number and size of incisions necessary by doing the simplest possible surgery for a given problem also helps to lessen the chance of nerve damage. If a skin flap is necessary for closure of a surgical defect, part of the reason for choosing a particular design for the flap should be based on the likelihood of damage to nearby nerves.

Sometimes skin tumors may invade the perineural nerve sheath (see Fig. 20-27) as well as deeper structures such as muscle or bone. However, one should not excise deeply without histologic or obvious visual confirmation that the tumor has encroached on such structures.

Edema

Swelling within and around wounds is common following any surgery, since injury to tissue has occurred. Use of a pressure dressing helps to minimize this. Fortunately edema in cutaneous surgical wounds is usually minimal and of little consequence. However, if edema does occur to a significant extent, considerable pressure is placed on sutures as well as on tissue, and necrosis may result.

Edema may also occur following surgery in areas where the surgery has interrupted the lymphatic drainage. One place this commonly occurs is in the periorbital area after surgery on the malar eminence. The patient may experience swelling of the eyelids caused by interruption of the lymphatic flow that courses down over the zygomatic arch. Usually such swelling is temporary and disappears in weeks to months, depending on the extent of the lymphatic blockage.

PROBLEMS AFTER WOUND HEALING
Scar nodules

Nodules may occur in surgical scars for the following reasons*:

I. **Related to Surgical Procedure**
   A. Hypertrophic scar
   B. Keloid
   C. Foreign body
      1. Suture
      2. Starch, Talc

---

*Modified from Batres, E., and McGavran, M.: Cutis **23:**609, 1979.

D. Bone formation
E. Irritation (mechanical, caused by implanted suture)
F. Traumatic nodule
G. Epidermal inclusion cyst

II. **Related to Underlying Disease**
  A. Metastatic neoplasm
  B. Locally recurrent neoplasm

III. **Disease with a Predilection for Scars**
  A. Psoriasis
  B. Sarcoidosis
  C. Discoid lupus erythematosus
  D. Lichen planus

IV. **Miscellaneous**
  A. Desmoid tumor
  B. Endometriosis
  C. Prurigo nodularis

Various foreign bodies such as suture material,[29] lint,[2] or talc[7] may provoke nodules to form in scars. Usually such nodules are associated with chronic granulomatous reactions to these materials. Talc is still used on most surgical gloves during their manufacture.[34] This talc may be transferred from the surface of gloves to suture material[14]; thus the talc is implanted in tissue by means of the sutures. It has been suggested that many tissue reactions to suture materials may in fact be tissue reactions to talc.[28]

On rare occasions bone formation in surgical scars can occur and form nodules.[23] This is thought to occur because fibroblasts are pleuripotential and may differentiate in a number of ways to produce various connective tissues.[3] The extracellular conditions in which the fibroblast finds itself may help determine its secretory pattern so that it produces different extracellular matrices in different environments. Orda, Baratz, and Wiznitzer[23] reported two cases of bone formation in abdominal wound scars. The bone formation occurred months after the original surgery and was asymptomatic. It was thought that bone formation was not related in these cases to suture material, keloid formation, or postoperative wound infection.

Mechanical irritation caused by steel wire suture implanted below the skin can cause nodules.[4] Irritation from without such as that seen in prurigo nodularis, can also cause nodules to appear.

Milia (small epidermal inclusion cysts) may form in a scar and appear as small white papules.[24] These are discussed later in this chapter and in Chapter 26.

Rarely, metastatic malignancy or endometriosis may localize to a surgical scar.[32] Probably this occurs during the vasodilatory phase of scar maturation. Desmoid tumors may also appear in scars, especially on the abdominal wall.[1]

Following removal of a malignancy, one should be suspicious of nodular growths in or around the scar. Such nodules may represent persistent malignancy (see Fig. 13-

14). This should be considered particularly when the nodule is unresponsive to local injection of steroids.

Certain skin conditions have a predilection for localization in scars. Psoriasis (see Fig. 10-1, *A*), lichen planus, discoid lupus erythematosus, or sarcoidosis may all result in papules, small nodules, or chronic inflammation in scars.[15,27]

The treatment for nodules in scars is determined by the underlying cause. If underlying suture material is causing irritation, it must be removed. Frequently, injections of triamcinolone acetonide (Kenalog), 10 mg/ml, are given at monthly intervals until flattening is sufficient. If there is no regression of the nodule after a few steroid injections, a skin biopsy should be considered.

Hypertrophic scar

Scars that are hypertrophic may occasionally occur despite carefully planned excisions. Some patients have a predisposition to form such scars. Therefore it is important to examine other scars that the patient may have to see if they evidence such a propensity. If other hypertrophic scars are found, the patient should be advised regarding the likelihood of any such scars after the planned surgery.

The causes of hypertrophic scars and their relationship to keloids are discussed in Chapters 2 and 23. Fig. 13-7, *A* shows a hypertrophic scar that developed in a full-thickness skin graft soon after placement. The scar was injected with triamcinolone acetonide, 10 mg/ml, at monthly intervals until flattening occurred. It was also necessary to perform a slight scar revision at the inferior edge of the graft where the steroid injection seemed to have little effect. The hypertrophic scar faded, and the final cosmetic result was much more acceptable (Fig. 13-7, *B*).

Some anatomic locations are more prone to hypertrophic scar formation. For example, the chest, shoulders, and upper back are notorious for the production of hypertrophic scars. This is probably related to the extreme tension put on almost any wound in these areas.

Spread scar

Spreading of scars may occur with time because of tension on the wound edges. Although various techniques have been proposed to minimize such spreading, none has been shown to be of great value. If significant tension exists on a wound at the time of closure, some scar spreading occurs. The same areas prone to hypertrophic scar formation are also prone to spread scars; that is, the chest, shoulders, and upper back. Wound infection may also lead to spread scars.

Depressed scar

Depressed scars are unusual with excisional surgery but may occur with scar spreading. The shadow cast by the de-

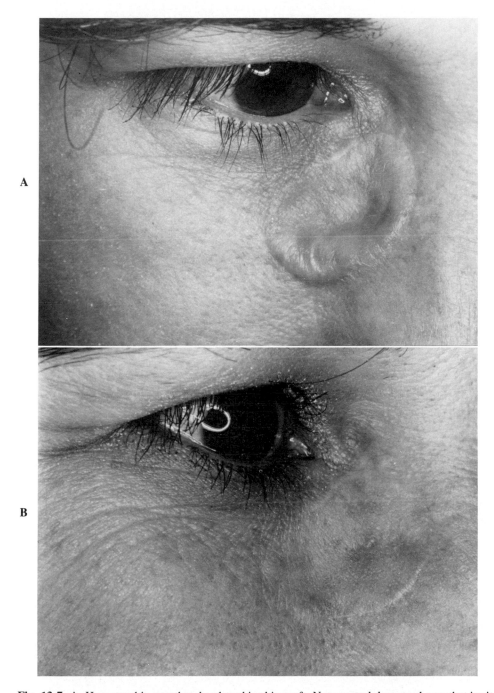

Fig. 13-7. A, Hypertrophic scar that developed in skin graft. Note central depressed area that is site of atrophy from initial steroid injection. **B.** Final result after five additional steroid injections at different times and scar revision of inferior edge of graft.

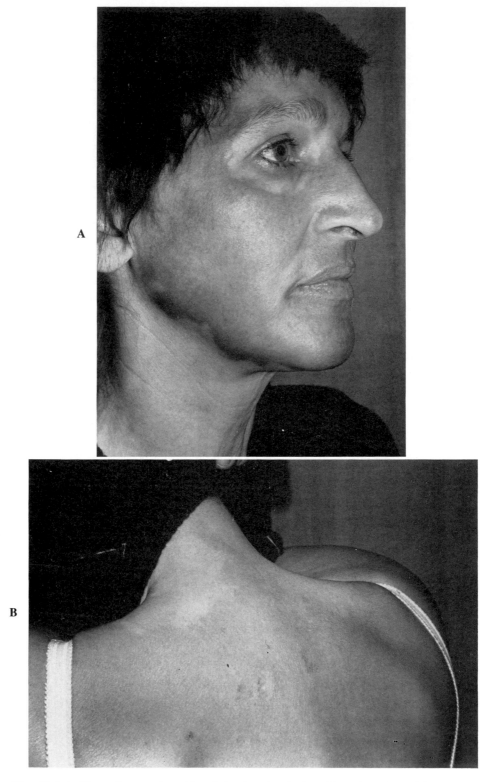

Fig. 13-8. A, Hyperpigmentation of face following chemical peel in patient with Addison's disease. **B,** Hyperpigmentation of back in same patient as in **A.**

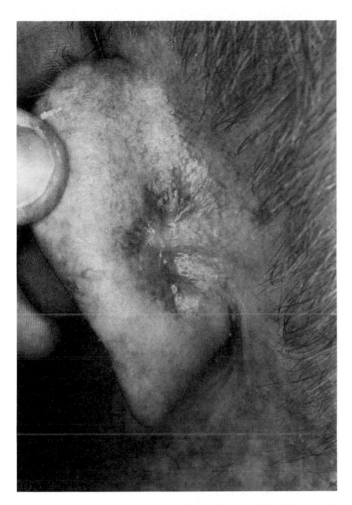

Fig. 13-9. Hyperpigmented scar of posterior ear following wound healing by granulation and epidermization. Excessive Monsel's solution was applied to provide hemostasis at time of surgery.

pressed scar may be somewhat unsightly. Depressed scars frequently result from "shaving" of a lesion such as a nevus when excessive tissue is taken in depth (see Fig. 21-11). Curettage and electrodesiccation may also result in depressed scars, particularly on the nose (see Fig. 15-7).

Where the cutaneous surface is very oily and the pilosebaceous apertures are abundant as well as patulous, it is particularly difficult to obtain a fine-line smooth scar flush with the surrounding skin. Scars in such locations tend to be depressed, slightly spread, and hypopigmented with time. Highly sebaceous skin does not hold sutures firmly, thus predisposing to fine cutaneous sutures tearing through tissue.

Hyperpigmentation and hyperpigmented scar

Fortunately, hyperpigmentation following surgical procedures is unusual. However, if a patient has Addison's disease, caution is advised. Fig. 13-8, *A* depicts a patient with Addison's disease who developed hyperpigmentation following a chemical peel of the face. She was referred for suggestions as to how to bleach the excess pigmentation. Fig. 13-8, *B* shows the diffuse hyperpigmentation over this patient's upper back. This case points out the need for careful preoperative evaluation in all patients.

Hyperpigmentation of surgically treated skin can occur in genetically susceptible patients, especially on sun-exposed areas. Following dermabrasions or chemical peels, this may be seen in dark-complexioned individuals with dark-colored eyes, especially if they expose themselves more than casually to the sun during the first 3 to 6 months after surgery. Patients with melasma are also more susceptible to hyperpigmentation. Therefore these patients should be instructed regarding sunscreens and limited sun exposure. The recommended sunscreen should contain a chemical to limit effectively cutaneous absorption of long-wave ultraviolet light (UVA), which is the spectrum mainly responsible for inducing additional pigmentation in the skin.

Hyperpigmentation can also occur in scars because of *excessive* use of ferric subsulfate solution (Monsel's solution*). It is believed that the iron pigment is deposited in the dermis and thus provides an iatrogenic tattoo. Fig. 13-9 shows a large healed hyperpigmented scar on the posterior aspect of the ear. Excessive ferric subsulfate solution was used in this case, because the patient had a pacemaker and the wound was literally soaked in the solution to stop the bleeding subsequent to excision of a large neoplasm. High-frequency electrosurgery at the site of Monsel's solution application may cause the precipitation of elemental iron and insoluble iron compounds, which results in tattooing.

Hypopigmentation and hypopigmented scar

Hypopigmentation is much more common than hyperpigmentation. In fact, almost all excisional scars become hypopigmented over time if viewed carefully. The portion of the new epidermis that bridges the wound is without melanocytes. Early scars (3 to 6 months) look better than later scars (6 months and later), because in the early stages the scar is slightly red because of hyperemia and vasodilation. With time, however, the redness fades and hypopigmentation becomes obvious.

Plate 1-D shows a hypopigmented scar of the forehead 1 year after surgery. This hypopigmented scar is particularly noticeable because the patient has a ruddy complexion. Also note that the suture marks are seen as white lines perpendicular to the line of the scar. Therefore, on the forehead, particularly in plethoric patients, a running intradermal suture is the suture of choice so that hypopigmented suture marks will not be present in the future.

---

*$Fe_4O\ (SO_4)_5$ formed by the action of hot sulfuric and nitric acids on ferrous sulfate.

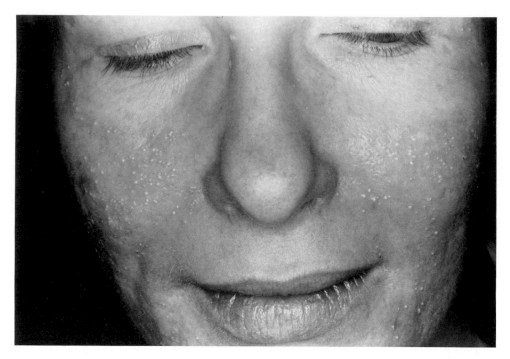

Fig. 13-10. Multiple milia following dermabrasion.

Hypopigmentation is common after certain procedures such as dermabrasion, chemical peels, cryosurgery, or curettage. Both dermabrasion and cryosurgery cause a loss of melanocytes in the skin.

Suture spitting

Suture spitting is a common phenomenon seen in cutaneous surgery. This happens when buried sutures are extruded through the wound, usually without inflammation. Spitting can occur whether the buried suture is absorbable or nonabsorbable. The usual cause is that the suture is placed too high in the dermis. Either the suture loop is too close to the skin surface or the knot is too close because it was tied proximal to the skin surface rather than buried distally. Once the suture material is extruded, the wound heals uneventfully.

Another possible cause of suture spitting is a heightened inflammatory reaction to the suture itself. With modern suture materials this is unusual. However all buried sutures should be viewed as foreign material. The more material buried, the more likely it is that a reaction will occur.

Chronic tissue reactions

Chronic tissue reactions may occur in wounds that never completely heal or heal and then break down at a later time. They may or may not be associated with nodules in scars. Chronic tissue reactions may have several causes. Bits of foreign material may have inadvertently been left in the wound before closure. Such foreign matter could include small bits of hair, lint from gauze, talc from gloves, suture material, or other contaminants. Suture spitting is sometimes associated with a chronic tissue reaction.

One distinct form of chronic tissue reaction, the granulomatous reaction, is possible in a wound. Both lint from cotton gauze[2] and suture materials[8,31] have been associated with such reactions. In addition, systemic sarcoidosis may form sarcoid nodules in scars.[27] Although rarely seen in cutaneous surgery, granulomas caused by talc from gloves are possible. Talc is magnesium silicate, which is insoluble in water, cold acids, or alkalies. It is commonly used on gloves during the manufacturing process. During surgery, talc is transferred from gloves to the suture material. Modified cornstarch, an alternative to talc in the manufacture of gloves, is much less likely to cause problems in wounds. However, use of talc is still widespread in the surgical glove industry.[14] Some surgical gloves (Deseret Surgical Gloves, Deseret, Sandy, Utah) are manufactured with no surface powder on them, but they are very tight and frankly uncomfortable to wear during surgery.

Milia

Small keratinous cysts may be formed where the skin reepidermizes. These may be seen after dermabrasion[21] (Fig. 13-10) and may also be seen along sutured incision lines or at suture tract entrance or exit points. Possible reasons for their formation around or within excision scars include epidermization of the suture tracts or wounds and transection of adnexal structures by either scalpel blade[24] or suture needle (Fig. 26-13).[25] As wounds epidermize, hyperplastic epidermis appears, particularly in the central area of the

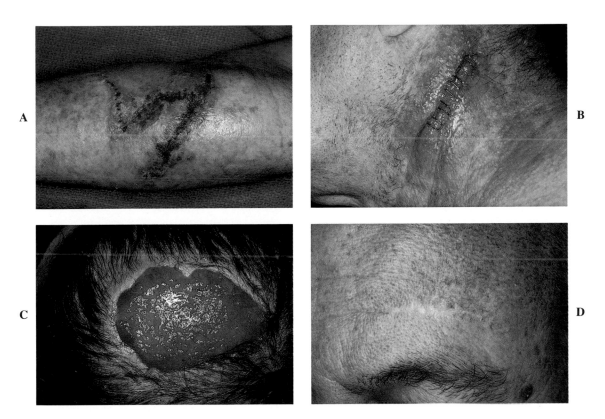

Plate 1. A, Erythematous, eczematous dermatitis surrounding incision line of skin flap. Skin culture was positive for *C. albicans* and infection cleared readily with Nystatin cream. Note relatively sharp demarcation of skin reaction compared to Plate **B** (contact dermatitis). **B,** Allergic contact dermatitis caused by antibiotic ointment used on wound for daily dressings. Note relatively poorly demarcated border of dermatitis, which blends into adjacent normal skin. **C,** Exuberant granulation tissue on scalp 4 weeks following extirpation of basal cell carcinoma. This wound had been allowed to heal by granulation and epidermization. After removing exuberant granulation tissue with curette, wound uneventfully healed. **D,** Hypopigmented scar of forehead particularly prominent 1 year after surgery because of surrounding telangiectasias of skin. Note that a few suture marks are also apparent.

wound. If fragments of this epidermis remain below the skin surface, small cysts may form.[12] Epidermal hyperplasia also occurs along the outer portion of suture tracts.[25] Because adnexal structures such as hair follicles or sweat ducts are invariably transected during surgery, their remains may also be involved in cyst formation. This is similar to cyst formation that ordinarily occurs in the hairless mouse where the hair papillae and strands of hair cells are stranded in the dermis.[22] Experiments in humans with implanted skin has been shown to lead to cyst formation.[10] Epstein and Kligman[9] feel that the development of keratinous cysts is related to the pluripotentiality of epidermal cells that, if trapped in the dermis, may give rise to cystic structures.

Histologically, milia are similar to epidermal cysts but are smaller.[17] They contain laminated, horny, keratinized material (keratin). The treatment depends on the extent of the milia. For a few localized lesions, simply removing the top with a sterile needle and expressing the milium are sufficient (see Fig. 26-14). If there are several lesions, as seen in Fig. 13-7, topical Retin-A and a Buff-puff are usually sufficient to resolve them.

Pruritus

Pruritus in scars after healing usually occurs to some degree, especially in scars that are hypertrophic or keloidal. Although the exact cause of this phenomenon is unknown, it may be related to an increased local histamine level.[35] Increased levels of histamine have been found in keloids[5] and may be a stimulus for the growth of fibroblasts.[11] Kahlson et al.[13] showed that wounds in rats heal with an increased amount of histidine decarboxylase activity and that the rate of healing can be increased by increasing the histamine-forming capacity.

Topol, Lewis, and Benveniste[35] found that fibroblasts from some keloids were more growth-sensitive to stimulation by histamine. These stimulated fibroblasts could be inhibited by the antihistamine diphenhydramine (Benadryl). Diphenhydramine has been reported in an uncontrolled study to be useful for pruritus associated with keloids.[5]

An increased number of mast cells may occasionally be seen in scar tissue, especially in certain areas such as around the eyes. These mast cells may release histamine, which results in pruritus. Steroids, either applied topically or injected into the scar tissue, help to relieve the itching by perhaps interfering with this release of histamine. As the scars flatten out with steroid injections, the pruritus disappears as well. Perhaps cortisone interferes with wound healing by thus interfering with histamine availability.

Mild pruritus may also occur in flat scars, particularly in those that are spread or have been allowed to heal by secondary intention. This may be because of the lack of sebaceous glands in the new epidermis that covers such scars. Usually a bland ointment (for example, Vaseline) is sufficient to relieve this symptom.

It has been noted that skin tumors, especially basal cell carcinomas, during their growth give patients a sensation of pruritus best described as "a worm crawling in the skin." If this sensation in a scar is noted by a patient following removal of a cutaneous neoplasm and is persistent, a biopsy may be indicated to rule out the presence of tumor.

Pain

Pain that exists after wound healing may conceivably have a number of causes. The most serious cause is persistence of a skin tumor within the perineural nerve sheath (see Fig. 20-27). In this situation, the tumor in its growth pushes its way along the path of least resistance. As it grows perineurally along the nerve, it tends to compress the nerve and give rise to pain.

Scar tissue may also entrap a nerve and give rise to shooting pains in the distribution of the nerve. I have seen this happen in the neck, where the great auricular nerve may become entrapped, giving rise to sharp, shooting pains behind the ear. Cut nerves may also heal with the production of traumatic neuromas.

Persistent nerve damage

Nerves may be severed at the time of surgery; this results in loss of sensation or motor function. The loss of sensation gives the patient a feeling of numbness along the distribution of the nerve. Numbness is a nuisance, but the patient will most probably regain full or partial feeling within months to years, normally by 2 years. The mechanism for this return in sensation is not fully understood. Either there is some regrowth of sensory nerves with time; or other nerves, not normally supplying an area of skin, take over some of the function of the injured or severed nerves.

The loss of motor function caused by nerve injury or transection is more likely to be permanent. If the nerve is injured but not completely severed, return of motor function is possible. However, if the nerve is totally transected, motor function is probably permanently lost. When there is return in function, it is difficult to state with certainty whether the nerve was completely severed or only partially.

Fig. 13-11, *B* shows a patient with injury to the temporal branch of the facial nerve that occurred during surgery to remove a large basal cell carcinoma of the right zygomatic and temple areas (Fig. 13-11, *A*). This nerve courses across the temple area and innervates the frontalis muscle, which raises the eyebrow. Note how the patient's right eyebrow is depressed and there is a lack of wrinkles on the right forehead. Since there was no return of function at 2 years, a crescent-shaped excision was performed above the drooping eyebrow to lift it into parallel position with the opposite eyebrow (Fig. 13-11, *C*). Anchoring sutures from the inferior edge of the excision to the periosteum were not placed. Such sutures are frequently unnecessary for this procedure, but initial overcorrection is necessary. The

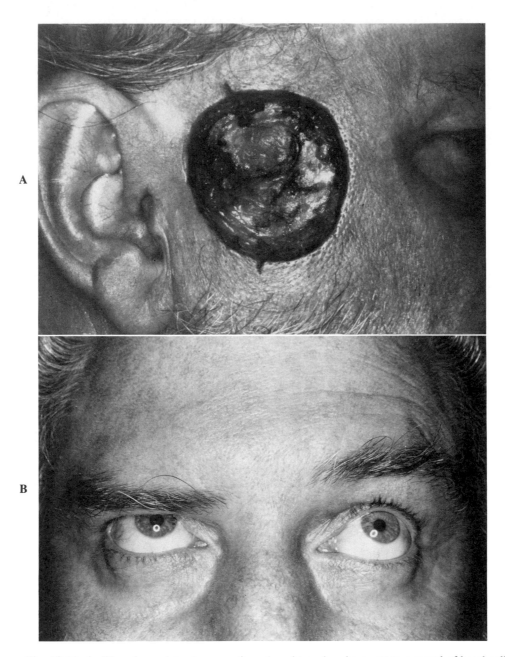

Fig. 13-11. A, Wound over lateral zygomatic arch and temple subsequent to removal of basal cell carcinoma. This surgery transected temporal branch of facial nerve that innervates frontalis muscle. **B,** Depressed right eyebrow caused by lack of innervation of right frontalis muscle. **C,** Crescent excision superior to right eyebrow to even up eyebrow levels. Suturing to periosteum was not performed. **D,** Patient 1 year after crescent type of excision in **C.** Note inconspicuous scar superior to eyebrow and excellent cosmetic result.

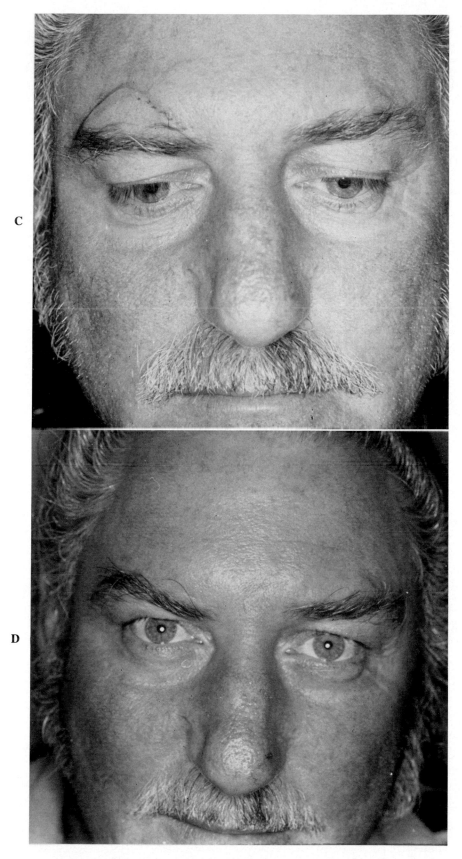

Fig. 13-11, cont'd. For legend, see opposite page.

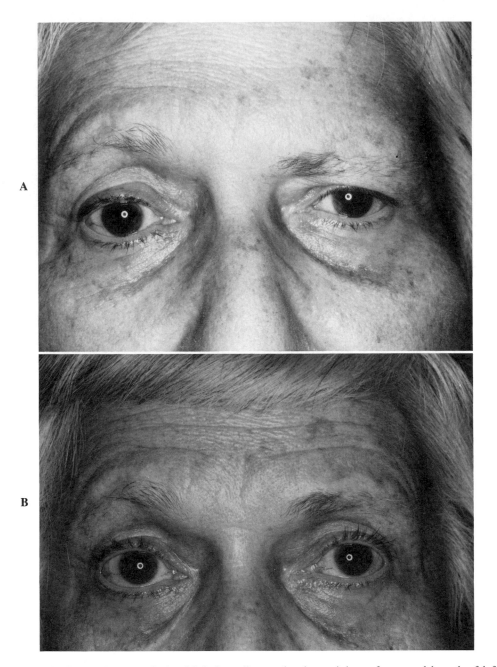

Fig. 13-12. A, Motor paralysis of left frontalis muscle, due to injury of temporal branch of left facial nerve 1 month after removal of squamous cell carcinoma on left temple. Note depressed left eyebrow, depressed left upper eyelid, and lack of wrinkles on left forehead. B, Significant return of function to frontalis muscle 1 year after surgery.

cosmetic result 1 year after surgery is excellent (Fig. 13-11, *D*).

Fig. 13-12, *A* shows a patient who suffered similar motor impairment of the temporal branch of facial nerve 1 month subsequent to removal of a squamous cell carcinoma of the left temple. At 1 year postoperatively (Fig. 13-12, *B*), almost complete recovery of motor function had occurred. In my experience, such return of function is rare.

Within 6 months after surgery for removal of a squamous cell carcinoma on the face, I have seen two patients develop progressive motor nerve weaknesses in the seventh facial nerve (CN VII). In both cases the patients proved to have infiltration of CN VII by squamous cell carcinoma *without* concurrent palpable nodal metastases. Therefore careful evaluation of such patients is warranted.

On the basis of the foregoing, if there is lack of sensation after surgery, the physician can tell the patient that sensation will probably return with time but it will take 1 to 2 years. If there is motor function loss, the physician should tell patients that this function will probably not return.

If major branches of the facial nerve have been severed, nerve grafts or direct nerve repair may be considered. Usually such procedures are either unsuccessful or not totally satisfactory. However, each case should be judged individually.

Contraction

If a wound heals by granulation and epidermization, contraction of the wound edges occurs to some degree. After reepidermization is complete, the patient notes an increased sensation of drawing, pulling, or tightening in the wound. This is because of continuous contraction of fibrous tissue, which persists for approximately 2 months after reepidermization is finished. Patients should be reassured that this is very common and will subside.

Contracture

Contracture is the resultant distortion of nearby structures such as the eyelid, lip, or nose by scar contraction (see Fig. 2-17). Usually this is avoided by proper placement of incisions and proper closure techniques. If wounds are allowed to heal by granulation and epidermization, contracture may be less predictable. If contracture does occur, it will be maximal 2 months after reepidermization of wounds is complete (3 to 4 months after wound creation for wounds healing by secondary intention). With time, contraction relaxes and the contracture may become less. Usually such relaxation lasts from about 3 to 4 months following surgery until 1 year or longer. The process of relaxation may be hastened by the injection of steroids such as Kenalog, 10 mg/ml, into the contracted scar.

Chronic edema

Edema of tissue near surgical wounds may persist chronically. Such edema is frequent on the extremities, particularly on the lower extremities. Long-term swelling of digits is not uncommon. Unlike on the face, where edema frequently corrects itself within a few months, on the extremities edema may take many months to resolve. The cause of edema may also be more complex on the extremities than simple interruption of the lymphatic drainage. Low-grade infection of the lymphatic channels may have occurred with the surgery and become persistent. Therefore, long-term use of antibiotics (for example, erythromycin) may be indicated and useful where edema persists.

Temperature lability

New scars contain blood vessels that are not under the same vasomotor control as normal blood vessels. These newly formed blood vessels are more prone to vasodilation with heat and cannot constrict as easily in cold. Patients may complain of some pain in scars caused by this vasomotor instability. This is most noticeable when the patient goes out in the cold air or during hot showers. Usually with maturation of the scar, these dilated vessels regress or come under neural control, and the patient's symptoms lessen.

Telangiectasia

Occasionally scars contain very dilated vessels coursing just under the epidermal surface. Such vessels may be particularly apparent where considerable tension exists on the wound edges at the time of closure. Although the exact cause is unknown, it has been speculated that the lack of nerve regeneration into new blood vessels leads to persistent dilation.[30] As nerves grow into scars with time, these vessels come under some vasomotor control. If they do not regress, they may be treated by either injections of sclerosing agents or an epilating needle with low epilating current.

Arteriovenous fistula

An arteriovenous (AV) fistula may occur following surgery in the skin, usually on the scalp after a hair transplantation or a punch biopsy but is theoretically possible after any surgery in any location. The reason why an AV fistula is more common in the scalp than other areas is probably because of the high degree of vascularity in this area. A misaligned regrowth of blood vessels results in a direct connection between an artery and vein. If this occurs in the scalp near the ear, the patient complains of a buzzing or a "choo-choo" sound like that of a train in motion. Usually the AV fistula can be palpated. The treatment is surgical visualization and ligation of the involved vessels.

Local recurrence of lesion

Local recurrence of either benign or malignant lesions can occur following their removal (Fig. 13-13). For malignant lesions of the skin, evidence of recurrence usually appears within 1 year but may take much longer (5 to 10 years). Careful follow-up of all patients treated for malignancies is recommended to detect recurrences so that early retreatment may be instituted.

Metastatic spread

Some skin cancers, including squamous cell carcinomas that are small and on sun-exposed areas, are capable of metastases (see Fig. 20-27). Therefore all patients treated for squamous cell carcinomas should have their regional lymph nodes examined before treatment and at intervals after treatment to detect metastases.

Lymph node swelling may occur following surgery because of infection or inflammation in the surgical wound. Usually such swelling is painful and resolves within a few

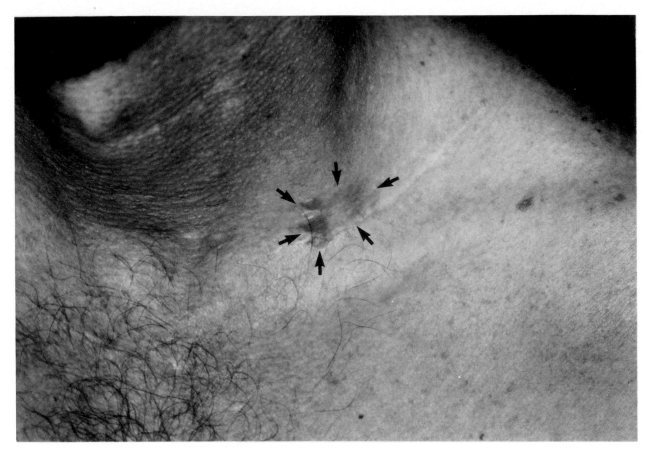

Fig. 13-13. Local recurrence *(arrows)* of dermatofibrosarcoma protuberans in supraclavicular area at medial superior edge of excision scar 3 years following local excision.

weeks with antibiotics. Persistent lymph node swelling that lasts more than a few weeks following removal of a cutaneous malignancy should be looked upon suspiciously, and a biopsy should be performed to rule out the possibility of metastatic spread.

REFERENCES

1. Ackerman, L.V.: Desmoid of the abdominal wall. In Warren, S.: Tumor seminar. J. Mo. M. A. **45:**354, 1948.
2. Amromin, G., Saphir, O., and Goldberger, I.: Lint granuloma, Arch. Pathol. **60:**467, 1958.
3. Bassett, C.A.L., and Herrmann, I.: Influence of oxygen concentration and mechanical factors on differentiation of connective tissues in vitro, Nature **190:**460, 1961.
4. Batres, E., and McGavran, M.: Traumatic nodule in surgical scar, Cutis **23:**609, 1979.
5. Cohen, I.K., et al.: Histamine and collagen synthesis in keloid and hypertrophic scar, Surg. Forum **23:**509, 1972.
6. Duke, W.F., Robson, M.C., and Krizek, T.J.: Civilian wounds, their bacterial flora and rate of infection, Surg. Forum **23:**518, 1972.
7. Eiseman, B., Seelieg, M.G., and Womack, N.A.: Talcum powder granuloma: a frequent and serious postoperative complication, Ann. Surg. **126:**820, 1947.
8. Epstein, A.J., et al.: Suture granuloma: an unusual cause of an enhancing ring lesion in the postoperative brain, J. Comput. Assist. Tomogr. **6:**815, 1982.
9. Epstein, W.L., Kligman, A.M.: The pathogenesis of milia and benign tumors of the skin, J. Invest. Dermatol. **26:**1, 1956.
10. Epstein, W.L., and Kligman, A.M.: Epithelial cysts in buried human skin, Arch. Dermatol. **76:**437, 1957.
11. Fitzpatrick, D.W., and Fisher, H.: Histamine synthesis, imidazole dipeptides, and wound healing, Surgery **91:**430, 1982.
12. Gillman, T., et al.: Reactions of healing wounds and granulation tissue in man to auto-Thiersch, autodermal, and homodermal grafts, Br. J. Plast. Surg. **6:**153, 1953.
13. Kahlson, G., et al.: Wound healing as dependent on rate of histamine formation, Lancet **2:**230, 1960.
14. Khan, M.A., et al.: Suture contamination by surface powders on surgical gloves, Arch. Surg. **118:**738, 1983.
15. Löfgren, S., Snellman, B., and Nordenstam, H.: Foreign body granulomas and sarcoidosis: a clinical and histolopathological study, Acta Chir. Scand. **108:**405, 1955.
16. Lookingbill, D.P., Miller, S.H., and Knowles, R.C.: Bacteriology of chronic leg ulcers, Arch. Dermatol. **114:**1765, 1978.
17. Love, W.R., and Montgomery, H.: Epithelial cysts, Arch. Dermatol. Syph. **47:**185, 1943.

18. Madsen, E.T.: An experimental and clinical evaluation of surgical suture materials, Surg. Gynecol. Obstet. **97:**73, 1953.
19. Marks, J.G., Jr.: Allergic contact dermatitis to povidone-iodine, J. Am. Acad. Dermatol. **6:**473, 1982.
20. Marks, J.G. Jr., and Rainey, M.A.: Cutaneous reactions to surgical preparations and dressings, Contact Dermatitis **10:1,** 1984.
21. Monash, S., and Rivera, R.M.: Formation of milia following abrasive treatment for postacne scarring, Arch. Dermatol. Syph. **68:**589, 1953.
22. Montagna, W., Chase, H.B., and Melaragno, H.P.: The skin of hairless mice. I. The formation of cysts and the distribution of lipids, J. Invest. Dermatol. **19:**83, 1952.
23. Orda, R., Baratz, M., and Wiznitzer, T.: Heterotopic bone formation in abdominal operation scars, Injury **15:**334, 1984.
24. Ordman, L.J., and Gillman, T.: Studies in the healing of cutaneous wounds. I. The healing of incisions through the skin of pigs, Arch. Surg. **93:**857, 1966.
25. Ordman, L.J., and Gillman, T.: Studies in the healing of cutaneous wounds. II. The healing of epidermal, appendageal, and dermal injuries inflicted by suture needles and by the suture material in the skin of pigs, Arch. Surg. **93:**883, 1966.
26. Osmundsen, P.E.: Contact dermatitis to chlorhexidine, Contact Dermatitis, **8:**81, 1982.
27. Paslin, D.A., Heaton, C.L., and Wood, M.G.: Scar biopsy in sarcoidosis, Dermatologica **146:**315, 1973.
28. Perou, M.L.: Iatrogenic foreign body granulomas: a study of selected cases with the polarizing microscope, Int. Surg. **58:**676, 1973.
29. Postlethwait, R.W., Willigan, D.A., and Ulin, A.W.: Human tissue reaction to sutures, Ann. Surg. **181:**144, 1975.
30. Remensnyder, J.P., and Majno, G.: Oxygen gradients in healing wounds, Am. J. Pathol. **52:**301, 1968.
31. Shauffer, I.A., and Sequeira, J.: Suture granuloma stimulating recurrent carcinoma, Am. J. Roentgenol. **128:**856, 1977.
32. Steck, W.D., and Helwig, E.B.: Cutaneous endometriosis, J.A.M.A. **191:**167, 1965.
33. Stegman, S.J., Tromovitch, T.A., and Glogau, R.G.: Basics of Dermatologic Surgery, 1982, Chicago, Year Book Medical Publishers, Inc.
34. Tolbert, T.W., and Brown, J.L.: Surface powders on surgical gloves, Arch. Surg. **115:**729, 1980.
35. Topol, B.M., Lewis, V.L., Jr., and Benveniste, K.: The use of antihistamine to retard the growth of fibroblasts derived from human skin, scar, and keloid, Plast. Reconstr. Surg. **68:**227, 1981.

COMMON PROCEDURES IN CUTANEOUS SURGERY

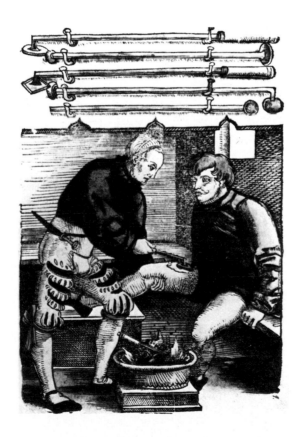

Woodcut by Johannes Wechtlin from Hans von Gersdorff's *Feldt-buch der Wundartzney* (1540), showing variety of cautery irons. Patient is having thigh lesion cauterized. (From Smith, Kline, and French Collection, Philadelphia Museum of Art.)

CHAPTER

14

The Skin Biopsy

The skin biopsy is probably the most common surgical procedure performed by dermatologists. It is very rewarding, because it frequently informs a diagnosis that aids in the management of a patient's medical problem. Although a skin biopsy is generally regarded as a simple procedure,[12] its proper performance requires knowledge of both cutaneous surgical principles and cutaneous pathology. One needs to know why, where, when, and how to remove a piece of tissue.[1] The inappropriate and unnecessary removal of normal cutaneous tissue such as a large wedge resection for an obvious seborrheic keratosis often occurs when the physician is unfamiliar with the subtleties of dermatologic diagnosis and the excellent cosmetic results that can be obtained by surgical procedures other than scalpel excision.

According to at least one authority,[3] too many residents in dermatology finish their training unable to perform a simple adequate biopsy. The submission of tissue that is inadequate in amount, inappropriately selected, or poorly handled at the time of surgical removal is a problem that needs to be addressed to ensure that the most accurate and helpful information is obtained from a biopsy.

This chapter contains a description of (1) the surgical techniques available for performing a skin biopsy and (2) which technique might be useful under a given set of circumstances. It must be stressed, however, that the physician's judgment concerning which lesion to biopsy, the number of lesions to biopsy, and the technique to use are developed only by experience.

PURPOSE OF A SKIN BIOPSY

There are several reasons for obtaining a skin biopsy,[1] the most obvious of which is to provide histopathologic information that leads to the correct diagnosis.[9] A skin biopsy can either establish a diagnosis when there is none or confirm a clinical diagnosis that is in doubt. Rarely a cutaneous biopsy may lead to the discovery of a previously undescribed disease entity. Such histopathologic information may aid or even be required by the clinician before embarking on a method of treatment.

Additional reasons for performing a skin biopsy include the following: to determine the extent of a disease process (both in depth and breadth), to assess the efficacy of therapy, and to provide tissue to clarify a disease process. The cutaneous organ has been metaphorically described as a natural "kymograph" that reflects the changing waves of pathologic processes, both locally in the skin and systemically.[12] The histopathologic assessment of the skin thus provides a glimpse in time of a pathologic process.

Every lesion removed from the surface of the skin deserves pathologic examination. Often, this examination should be performed before definitive therapy (especially destructive treatment) of a lesion. This is particularly important in the case of suspected skin malignancies in which histologic study reveals degree of differentiation and depth of invasion.[4] Because growths in the skin are visible to the naked eye, clinical diagnosis of malignancy is more obvious than in other organs. However, this does not obviate the necessity and importance of pathologic examination. Information gained from such examination is frequently useful if not crucial to the selection of the most appropriate form of therapy.

Careful histologic examination of obvious clinical entities occasionally yields unsuspected results. For example, basal cell carcinomas can occasionally underlie benign seborrheic keratoses (Fig. 14-1). Histologic examination of known clinical conditions also aids in understanding pathologic processes better.

Many disease entities are described years after their occurrence by retrospective review of biopsy specimens. Therefore biopsy specimens should be kept for the lifetime of a physician and passed on so that the next generation may benefit as well.

SELECTION OF LESION TO BIOPSY

If there is only one lesion in question, the problem of which lesion to biopsy does not exist. However, frequently the physician is confronted with a patient who has several lesions. Haphazard selection of lesions to be biopsied may

517

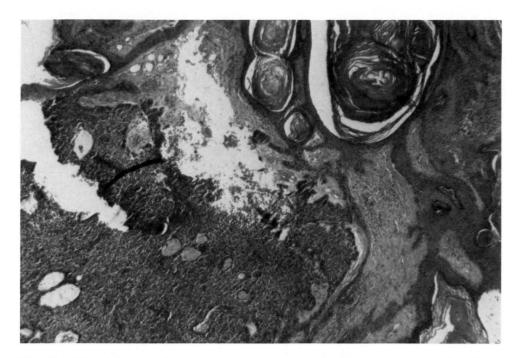

Fig. 14-1. Seborrheic keratosis *(upper right)* overlying a basal cell carcinoma *(lower left)*. (Hematoxylin and eosin ×100.)

lead to no helpful information or, even worse, to erroneous conclusions.

In conducting a clinical examination, the cutaneous surgeon is actually performing a study of gross pathology. Only by first determining the type, size, color, texture, distribution, and extent (laterally and in depth) of the visible lesions present, can a thoughtful approach to selection of the most appropriate lesions to biopsy be made.

Lesions selected for biopsy are best if fully developed and untreated. In general, immature or, alternatively, "burned-out" lesions should be avoided. However, there are some exceptions. For example, the pathologic processes in dermatitis herpetiformis may be best seen in very early lesions. "Secondary" skin lesions, those produced by the patient or physicians, should also be avoided as the underlying pathologic process is invariably obscured.

If multiple lesions are present and heterogeneous, it might be best to obtain multiple biopsy specimens of lesions at different stages of development. This usually gives more information than a single specimen and is thus more likely to help establish a diagnosis.

HANDLING OF A BIOPSY SPECIMEN

The cutaneous biopsy is only one step in a cycle that links the cooperative efforts of the clinician and pathologist. However, the cycle begins and ends with the clinician.[1] The clinician, acting as a gross pathologist, must select with care the lesion and optimally remove and carefully handle the specimen. The pathologist must process the specimen carefully and render a histopathologic diagnosis. The biopsy

report returns to the clinician who then must interpret the report in the context of the patient. It is advisable for the clinician to review the biopsy specimen personally. Just as no written description of a patient's lesion can convey its gross appearance with total accuracy, so too no written description of a pathologic process can convey entirely its histologic appearance. Thus the pathologist and clinician must work together cooperatively on the same team to ensure that the most knowledge possible is obtained from the study of a biopsy specimen. Each person needs to appreciate the other's unique problems and limitations in the handling of tissue and understand the difficulties encountered in reaching a correct diagnosis.

The physician submitting a biopsy specimen has several responsibilities. The tissue should be obtained as atraumatically as possible and handled gently. This is discussed in more detail below. It is also the physician's responsibility to orient the specimen and to ensure that it is placed in the proper fixative, usually 10% formalin, or transport medium. If the specimen is small or curled, it should be placed flat on a small piece of filter paper or white paper towel, properly oriented, before being placed in the fixative. This enables the pathologist to more readily find and more accurately orient the specimen,[9] to gross the tissue properly, and thus to render the most meaningful interpretation.[16] If a border of a lesion that includes normal skin is biopsied, the specimen should be marked so that it is sectioned properly; otherwise, only the normal half of the specimen might be processed. If a tumor specimen is submitted to determine adequacy of excision, it should be marked at one end with a suture or

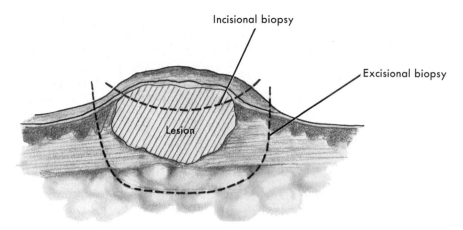

Fig. 14-2. Comparison between incisional and excisional biopsy.

dye so that the pathologist can orient the tissue to assess which margin might be involved with the tumor. Other more complex but complete methods for submitting tissue have been described that involve separate assessment of each side of the specimen as well as the bottom.[28] These techniques are rarely used, however. If multiple specimens are taken, each needs to be placed in a separate bottle that is labeled with the patient's name, the date, and the site from which each specimen was obtained.[6]

Most routine specimens are placed in 10% formalin (4% solution of formaldehyde) buffered to a pH above 6 with either calcium carbonate or magnesium carbonate.[1,9] The amount of formalin should be roughly 20 times that of the specimen by volume.[1] If special stains or other histologic studies need to be performed, the clinician is instrumental in suggesting such studies. If fat is to be investigated, alcohol fixation and processing must be avoided. Special transport media are also available for electron microscopy and immunofluorescence.

A biopsy form is submitted with the biopsy specimen bottle. This form should contain the patient's name, the date, and the site of the biopsy. In addition, the method of biopsy (for example, curette, punch, or incision) should be stated. Biopsy specimens of tumors obtained by the curette cannot be accurately assessed for adequacy of excision. Such assessment with curetted specimens may be unnecessary and unwarranted, but the pathologist must know that the specimen was curetted.

The biopsy form should contain a description of the lesion and a tentative diagnosis. Giving the pathologist as much information as possible is helpful in establishing an accurate diagnosis and ultimately benefits the patient. As Highman once remarked, ''The possession of a microscope does not endow the pathologist with supernatural powers.''[8]

BIOPSY RESULTS

The pathology report should be typed and should contain a description including the measurement of the gross speci-

men and how it was sectioned (for instance, longitudinally), a histologic description of the microscopic sections, and a diagnosis. The pathologist should avoid written recommendations regarding further therapy.

When the biopsy report is received in the office, the physician should personally review it and indicate on it whether further therapy is warranted. The physician will find it helpful to keep a biopsy log to use for cataloging results and for keeping track of biopsy specimens. All patients should be asked to call the physician's office to obtain biopsy results.

TYPES OF CUTANEOUS BIOPSIES

Three categories of biopsies are available for obtaining tissue: needle biopsy, incisional biopsy, and excisional biopsy. All three types have certain limitations and applications that need to be understood.

Needle biopsy

The needle biopsy is performed by aspiration of tissue, followed by smearing the aspirate onto glass slides that are subsequently stained. A pathologist making the diagnosis must have experience in the interpretation of such slides. The needle biopsy is rarely used in the skin, since the tissue to be biopsied is so readily accessible. It may be considered when an incisional or excisional biopsy is inconvenient, and it may rarely be used for aspiration of potentially metastatic lymph nodes; however, implantation of tumor along the needle tracts is a theoretic possibility.[4]

Incisional biopsy

Most cutaneous biopsies are either incisional or excisional (Fig. 14-2). An incisional biopsy removes only part of a lesion, whereas an excisional biopsy removes the total lesion visibly or palpably present. The choice between an incisional or excisional biopsy is based on several factors. Although every effort should be made to obtain adequate tissue for diagnosis, cosmetic considerations should also be

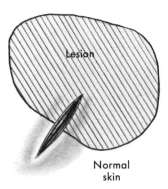

Fig. 14-3. Incisional wedge biopsy including normal tissue at edge of lesion.

taken into account. Both the pathologist and the patient should be told whether a biopsy is excisional or incisional.

Incisional biopsies are frequently performed on large lesions or lesions prone to local recurrence despite "total" excision, for example, on lesions in inflammatory conditions such as psoriasis or lupus erythematosus.

Incisional biopsies must be deep enough for proper histologic assessment of involvement of the dermis or subcutaneous tissue, particularly in cases of verrucous carcinomas or other low-grade malignancies in which knowledge of the extent of invasion is essential. Sometimes it is advantageous for the pathologist to view a piece of tissue that contains both the pathologic process and adjacent normal tissue, so the transition of the abnormal process in the skin can be seen and more readily compared to normal tissue. Such an incisional biopsy is usually performed as a wedge (Fig. 14-3).

A special type of incisional biopsy for keratoacanthomas was described in 1966.[25] Keratoacanthomas are difficult to diagnose histologically unless adequate tissue, properly oriented, is submitted for histologic examination. If only a small portion of the lesion is biopsied, a report of squamous cell carcinoma instead of the benign condition keratoacanthoma may be returned to the clinician. Since the overall histologic morphology of this lesion is equally important to the cellular morphology, this study[25] recommends a fusiform excision extending completely through the center of the lesion from normal skin on one side to normal skin on the other side. Care should be taken to include an adequate amount of subcutaneous tissue in depth beneath the lesion. This recommendation arose from the inadequate specimens frequently submitted as suspected keratoacanthomas.

This study[25] also claims that an added advantage of subtotal fusiform excisions for keratoacanthomas is that their evolution is hastened. However, this statement is not supported by any data in the original paper and is thus purely anecdotal.

Controversy exists regarding the wisdom of obtaining incisional biopsies of obvious invasive melanomas.[21,26]

Such lesions have the potential for being highly metastatic, and thus the theoretic possibility exists for spread of tumor as a result of a simple biopsy. However, comparisons of recurrences and survival rates between patients whose tumors were removed following incisional biopsies and patients whose tumors were removed in toto without previous biopsies have shown no significant differences.[1,4,13]

Based on the concept that a complete biopsy yields the best information possible, most clinicians recommend that if suspected melanomas are small, they be excised completely.[26] However, if a suspected melanoma is large and the total removal cannot be performed with a simple closure or the resultant excision would be cosmetically deforming, an incisional biopsy is warranted and recommended.[16]

Some authorities[21] emphasize that total removal of a pigmented lesion helps the pathologist not only to classify the lesion routinely but in addition to assess the histopathologic picture in terms of the lesion's depth, breadth, symmetry, and circumference.[21] Such a panoramic view is not afforded by a small incisional biopsy. These authors feel that large biopsies lead to few errors on the part of the pathologist and are therefore essential for lesions such as melanomas, the misdiagnosis of which could conceivably lead to extensive and unnecessary lymph node dissection. This is supported by another study,[26] in which differences of opinion regarding the histopathologic diagnosis of melanoma occurred in 9% of the cases.

The inability to assess depth of melanomas biopsied by methods other than excision was also studied.[21] In six of 25 specimens obtained by punch biopsy and 14 of 33 specimens obtained by shave biopsy, not enough tissue was taken in depth. This would seem to support the use of only a scalpel blade to biopsy melanomas, and if possible the excision of the lesion in toto rather than in part.

Excisional biopsy

An excisional biopsy totally removes a skin lesion. Thus it is both diagnostic and therapeutic. Excisional biopsies are preferred for small lesions that can be removed easily and in which the subsequent defects are repaired or allowed to heal by second intention.

If possible, an excisional biopsy specimen should be removed in one piece so that the pathologist can assess if removal is complete. If the surgeon wishes margin assessment, a border of the excised specimen should be tagged with a suture or marked with India ink.

When an excisional biopsy of a melanoma is performed, it should be planned with the excision's long axis along the lines of lymphatic drainage, which do not always follow the MaxSTLs usually recommended for excisions.[16] On the extremities, excisional biopsies for melanomas should be placed longitudinally, and longitudinally on the trunk, toward the nearest axilla or groin. Subsequent surgery (lymph node dissection in continuity with the lesion) may be more

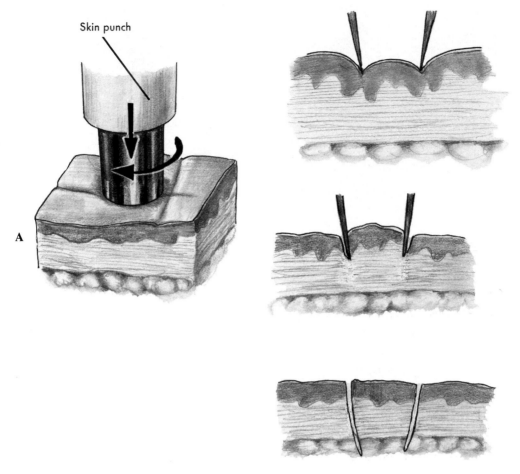

Skin punch

A

Fig. 14-4. Schematic diagram showing technique of punch biopsy. **A,** Vertical and circular motion of the cutaneous punch. Note that inward slant to outer walls of punch result in piece of tissue with base narrower than its top. *Continued*

difficult to perform if initial excisions are not oriented in these directions.

CUTANEOUS BIOPSY TECHNIQUES

There are several methods of performing cutaneous biopsies. In choosing a method, two objectives should be kept in mind: (1) obtaining an adequate amount of tissue for histologic examination, and (2) causing the least possible cosmetic disfigurement for the patient.

Punch biopsy

Early on, dermatologists recognized the need for an instrument that made possible a rapid, convenient, easy removal of small samples of tissue for histologic examination. The "cutisector" of Piffard was an early attempt to meet this need.[24] This instrument had two parallel blades adjusted in width by means of a screw. After incision in the skin, a band of incised tissue was produced that could be picked up, cut at both ends, and sutured closed. This method of performing small skin biopsies is no longer used and has been superseded by the cutaneous punch (see Fig. 7-25),

which has been in use for about 100 years. It was originally described by Watson as the "discotome"[37] in 1878; in 1887 Keyes' more widely recognized description of the cutaneous punch was published.[12,17] Both authors developed this cutaneous trephine to remove gunpowder pigmentation from the face of a patient. Keyes[17] also used it to remove basal cell carcinomas from the lower eyelid and side of the nose. For nevi on the back he recommended going only to the mid dermis with the punch, excising the tissue plug, and then allowing the wound to heal by secondary intention.

The technique for obtaining a punch biopsy is shown in Fig. 14-4. After properly cleansing the skin and anesthetizing the operative site, the physician holds the skin punch vertically to the skin and firmly pushes it into the skin at the same time as it is being turned, usually in a clockwise motion. This vertical pressure and circular motion are maintained until the cutting edge descends into the fat. Turning the punch in only one direction rather than back and forth is preferable, since the latter technique tends to distort tissue. The cutaneous punch is then withdrawn, leaving a cylindrical column (broader at the top than at the bottom) of

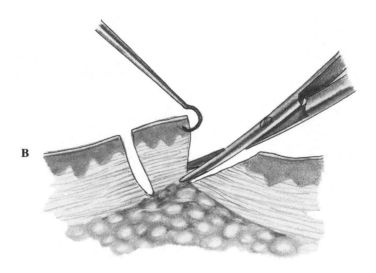

Fig. 14-4, cont'd. B, Use of skin hook to lift out biopsy plug.

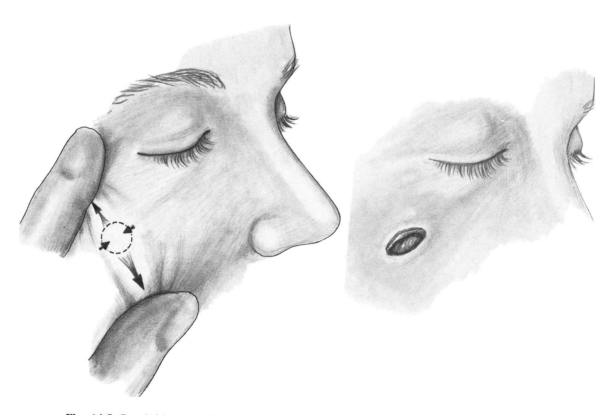

Fig. 14-5. Punch biopsy performed under traction. Note direction of stretch is perpendicular to future excision line. This results in elliptic, rather than round, incision.

epidermis, dermis, and fat attached by a pedicle at the base. After cutting its pedicle, the physician removes the tissue from the cylindrical hole and places it in the fixative. The surgical defect can be closed with a suture or allowed to heal by granulation and epidermization after bleeding is stopped.

In areas of cosmetic concern, such as the face, it might be preferable to close the surgical defect created by a cutaneous punch. Since an elliptic defect closes with less dog-ear formation than a round hole does, creation of an elliptic defect is desirable. This is done by putting lateral traction on the skin *perpendicular* to the maximal skin tension lines at the time the punch biopsy is performed (Fig. 14-5). Thus the tension is also perpendicular to the long axis of the ellipse

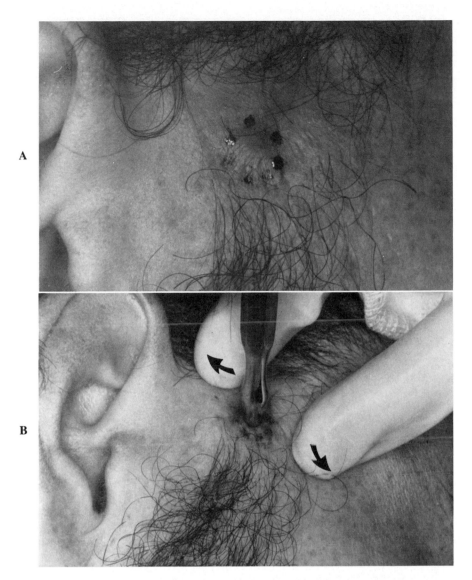

Fig. 14-6. Punch biopsy. **A,** Location of lesion marked with gentian violet before infiltration of anesthetic. **B,** Punch biopsy in use with lateral stretching of skin *(arrows).*   *Continued.*

eventually produced. Tension in this direction narrows the amount of tissue removed in one direction and at the same time lengthens the wound in the opposite direction. The result is an elliptic wound; that is, a wound with rounded ends with one axis longer than the other. This technique is also shown in Fig. 14-6. Note that, in Fig. 14-6, *A,* gentian violet is used to mark the site of the biopsy. Marking the site before injection of a local anesthetic can be useful, when the injected anesthetic is likely to obscure the lesion to be biopsied because of tissue expansion.

The reason a cylindrical piece of tissue from a punch biopsy is wider at the top than the bottom is shown on the right in Fig. 14-4. As vertical pressure is exerted on the tissue, the surface epidermis expands into the punch. This results in slightly more tissue at the top of the punch biopsy

specimen. In addition, as the punch descends into the surgical defect, the surrounding tissue retracts laterally and the tissue within the punch retracts medially; thus progressively less tissue in depth is obtained. Many cutaneous punches are made with outside sides that slope inward (see Fig. 7-25). Thus as the punch descends into the hole it produces, these outside sides tend to push the surrounding tissue to the side. This adds to the tapered appearance of tissue cut with a cutaneous punch.

The specimen should be removed from the cylindrical hole with the least possible trauma. One should keep from pinching the biopsy specimen with forceps, since this can cause artifacts seen in the histologic sections. A convenient tool for removing the plug of tissue is the needle on the syringe used to provide anesthetic. The biopsy plug is

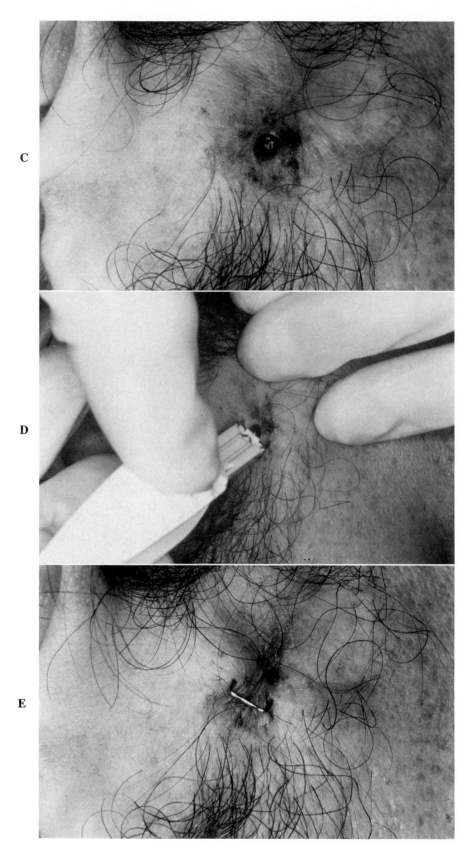

Fig. 14-6, cont'd. C, Elliptic defect after punch biopsy tissue removed. **D,** Insertion of staple perpendicular to long axis of ellipse. **E,** Staple in place.

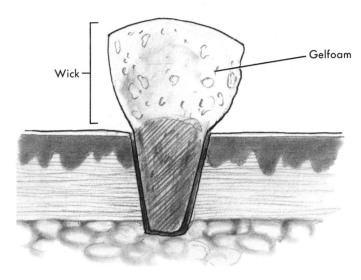

Wick

Gelfoam

Fig. 14-7. Gelfoam inserted into punch biopsy defect to control bleeding. Note that top half of Gelfoam is left as wick.

speared with the needle and lifted out of the hole while the pedicle base is transected with fine scissors or a scalpel blade.[1,21] Other suggestions for lifting a biopsy plug from the wound include the use of a skin hook (Fig. 14-4, *B*) and the use of a suture through the biopsy specimen.[23]

Usually bleeding from a punch biopsy site can be controlled by pressure or suture placement. If the wound is left open to heal by granulation, bleeding can usually be stopped by instillation of a styptic, such as aluminum chloride (35% in 50% isopropyl alcohol), or a caustic, such as ferric subsulfate (Monsel's solution). Ferric subsulfate, however, can result in pigmented tissue and destroys more dermis than less destructive methods do.[15]

Occasionally, bleeding from a punch biopsy site is profuse, because an artery has been transected by the cutaneous punch. If this occurs, a cotton-tipped applicator can be placed temporarily in the wound to stop the bleeding. As an alternative, an absorbable gelatin sponge (Gelfoam) can be placed in the hole (Fig. 14-7). However, the top half of the Gelfoam must be left out of the tissue as a wick; otherwise, the gelatin sponge is completely saturated with the blood. Bleeding then occurs around the Gelfoam.

Sometimes it is preferable to suture a punch biopsy site, especially on cosmetically apparent areas. If the wound is closed, it heals faster, and the scar produced is less apparent than if the biopsy site is allowed to heal by secondary intention. In addition, if there is considerable bleeding, suturing the wound will probably control the bleeding as well.

One of the main disadvantages of suturing a punch biopsy site is that the patient has to return for suture removal. If only one or two sutures have been placed and the patient must travel some distance, self-removable sutures can be placed.

Two methods for tying self-removable sutures have been described.[20,29] I prefer the technique termed "the looped square knot technique"[29] (Fig. 14-8). This is similar to the standard method of tying the knot at the end of a running continuous suture. One tail of the knot is left long, and the patient instructed simply to pull it on the day specified for suture removal. If nylon or polypropylene is used, there is little or no resistance as the suture is slipped through the wound. The patient is spared the unnecessary effort and needless time spent having to travel to the physician's office.

One disadvantage of the self-removable suture is that, theoretically, a contaminated part of the suture is being pulled through the wound. I have seen no infections to date from its use, however.

An alternative method of closing a punch biopsy site is by means of a small skin graft.[19] This technique is useful when direct closure of a punch biopsy site is difficult such as on the nose or in very porous cheek skin. The autograft is harvested from the donor site with a cutaneous punch approximately 0.5 mm larger than the recipient site. The larger punch is used to compensate for the retraction of the biopsy site and the contraction of the graft. The non–hair bearing skin from the ear (posterior lobule or helix) is an excellent donor area for the face. These grafts can be simply sutured or just taped in place (Fig. 14-9).

Some authors have advocated that the cutaneous punch be attached to an electric drill or motor.[9,36,38] This is said to produce a less distorted specimen, and the biopsy may even be obtained without anesthesia.[38] This technique has been used in Europe for almost 100 years, having been introduced soon after the cutaneous punch was first described.[7,35]

One disadvantage of a punch biopsy is that the punch can only descend in depth to a limited extent determined by the depth and size of the barrel. Therefore, for inflammatory conditions deep within the fat or below, a punch biopsy can

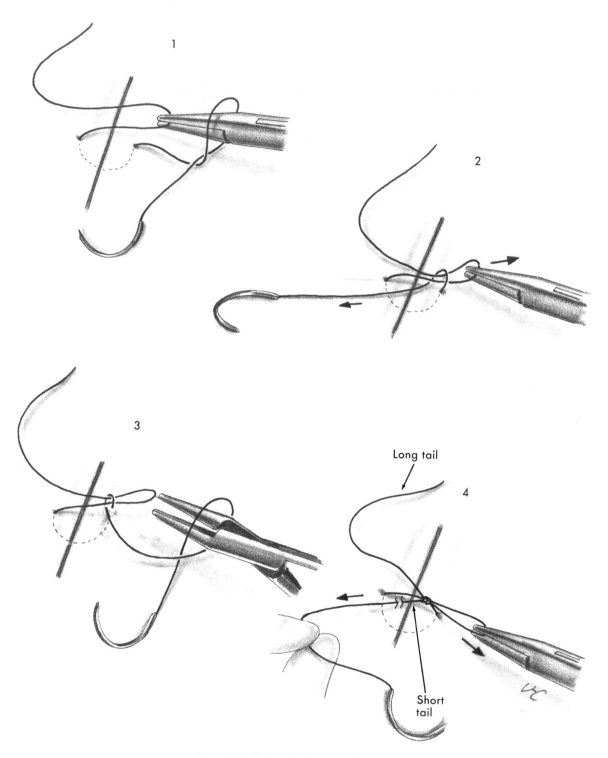

Fig. 14-8. Tying of self-removable suture.

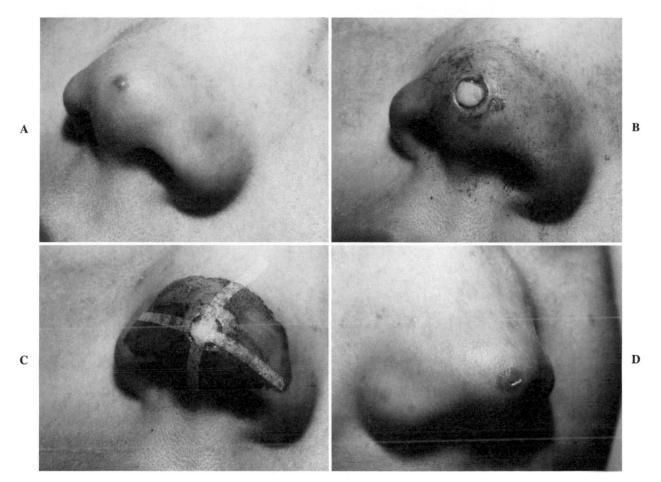

Fig. 14-9. Punch autograft for removal of nevocytic nevus on nose. **A,** Preoperative. **B,** Punch defect with donor plug in place. **C,** Autograft taped in place. **D,** Result 1 month later. Graft is still hyperemic.

be inadequate. For instance, it has been reported[39] that only 25% of punch biopsies in erythema nodosum provided enough tissue for diagnosis.

Punch biopsies into lesions such as basal cell carcinomas that later may be curetted can create difficulty. The skin punch creates a through-and-through defect of the dermis. After the wound is healed and a curettage is performed, the curette might descend through the hole created previously by the punch into the underlying fat where it flounders about.[18] This creates uncertainty in the mind of the treating physician regarding the actual extent of tumor penetration.

Curette biopsy

The dermal curette can be used to obtain tissue for biopsy. Even if curettage is truly excisional, it should be considered only incisional by the pathologist. He or she needs to be apprised of the fact that the specimen is the result of curettage, so that assessment of excision adequacy will not be stated in the pathology report.

The use of the curette for skin biopsy has been advocated

because it is fast, easy, and unlikely to cause cosmetically unacceptable scars.[34] The curette's efficacy is predicated on the theory that this instrument easily separates normal from abnormal tissue in situ. Once the specimen is removed, the surgical wound is compressed to stop bleeding. A styptic such as aluminum chloride can be used to provide hemostasis, and a bandage is applied.

The curette biopsy does not interfere with later therapy. In addition, if the lesion is superficial, the biopsy and the definitive treatment can often be performed simultaneously.[9]

The disadvantage of the curette biopsy is that sufficient tissue might not be obtained for the pathologist to make a diagnosis. In the case of malignancies, depth of invasion is usually impossible to assess properly with this biopsy technique. However, advocates of the procedure claim that sufficient tissue is obtained 90% of the time.[34] When this is not the case, a second biopsy can be obtained.

I have found the curette biopsy useful for superficial exophytic growths. Adequate specimens can be obtained most of the time.

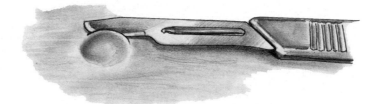

Fig. 14-10. Shave biopsy with scalpel blade.

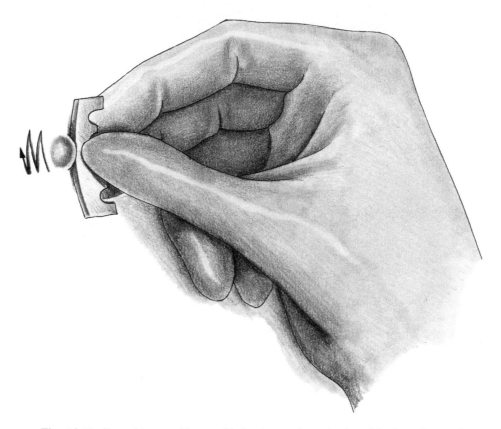

Fig. 14-11. Shave biopsy with razor blade. Arrow shows back-and-forth motion used.

Shave biopsy

The "shave biopsy" is a horizontal rather than vertical biopsy. Like the curette biopsy, this technique may be either incisional or excisional. When excisional, it is sometimes termed a "shave excision." For the shave biopsy, either a scalpel[18,30] or razor blade[5,32] is used to shave off, literally, an exophytic skin lesion. As with the curette biopsy, less depth is obtained by this technique than may be ideal for histopathologic purposes. Therefore pathologists prefer other methods of obtaining specimens[3]; but the shave biopsy can frequently obtain a wider specimen in the horizontal dimension than a cutaneous punch procedure.[32]

The shave biopsy is useful when a full-thickness biopsy is unnecessary[2] or cosmetically unacceptable. It is a tissue-sparing procedure that leaves the lower levels of the dermis

intact and therefore is ideal for removal of raised lesions that are strictly confined to the epidermis; but lesions that are flat, nonraised, and broad can also be removed with this technique. Melanomas or inflammatory lesions should not be biopsied by means of a shave.[2] The shave biopsy is useful for biopsies in areas, such as the lower extremities, that are notoriously slow to heal. The scar resulting from a shave biopsy is minimal compared to that resulting from deeper biopsy technique.

The use of the scalpel (No. 15) blade for a shave biopsy is shown in Fig. 14-10. The skin is immobilized by placing it on stretch between the thumb and index finger. The blade is held horizontal to the skin surface and brought through the base of the specimen in a sawing, back-and-forth manner. Frequently the specimen can be balanced on the

HISTOLOGIC ARTIFACTS IN BIOPSY SPECIMENS CAUSED BY SURGICAL MANIPULATION

Artifact	Cause
Holes in tissue	Dermojet used for instillation of anesthetic
Starch granules, talc	Powder from gloves, cosmetics
Epidermal invagination	Tissue cut by scalpel blade or teeth on forceps
Epidermal cell alteration	Heat
Basal cell carcinoma lying free	Compression
Curling of tissue	Compression
Marginal breaks	Freezing, vertical pressure (punch)

blade itself as it is removed and then placed into the fixative. Bleeding is controlled by pressure or a styptic, and the shallow wound is allowed to heal by epidermization.

An alternative to the use of the scalpel blade is the razor blade. The authors who initially described its surgical application advocated the Gillette Super Blue Blade because of its extremely sharp edge.[5] With such a sharp cutting edge, the blade can readily cut through a lesion, with little or no anesthetic needed. An injected local anesthetic has the disadvantage of ballooning the tissue under superficial cutaneous lesions, making it likely that more tissue will be removed than would happen with a shave biopsy without anesthesia (see Fig. 21-11). Most patients who are told that shaving the lesion *without anesthesia* eventuates in a better cosmetic result find this method acceptable.

The Gillette Super Blue Blade is a carbon steel blade with a cutting edge that is 1 millionth of an inch thick. It is coated with an anticorrosive oil that contains a bacteriostat, zinc naphthanate.[32] Although the theoretic possibility exists for wound infection caused by this nonsterile device, such an event is unlikely. Since the wound is left open, colonization by bacteria is more likely from the outside environment than from the razor blade.

The razor blade is broken in half lengthwise. The half blade is held in the hand as shown in Fig. 14-11, balanced between the index and middle fingers. The thumb is used to hold the blade in place as well as to adjust the curve of blade. The blade is gently bowed to match the visible edges of the lesion to be removed and is brought through the lesion in a steady back-and-forth sawing motion.[33]

Razor blades may also be held by hemostats or special razor blade holders (see Fig. 7-5). Special small miniblades are also available for shaving cutaneous lesions.

Scissors biopsy

The scissors biopsy technique is a variant of the shave biopsy. The specimen to be removed is elevated with pickups and is snipped at its base. Scissors with serrated edges (see Fig. 7-14) are particularly useful for this type of biopsy.

Vertical scalpel biopsy

A vertical scalpel biopsy is performed by basic excisional surgery, along the MaxSTLs, removing a cutaneous lesion in part or in toto. The surgical defect is then usually closed with the standard techniques described in Chapter 10. The specimen obtained by this method is usually ideal for histopathologic examination. If the physician wants the pathologist to assess the cut surgical margins for evidence of tumor, the specimen should be marked with either a dye or suture at one end.

HISTOLOGIC ARTIFACTS CREATED BY SURGICAL TECHNIQUE

As emphasized throughout this chapter, biopsy specimens should be handled gently to preclude the production of artifacts seen on histologic examination of the tissue (see box on this page). A pathologic artifact can be defined as a feature in tissue that did not originate in life but that might be mistaken as part of the intravital process.[22] The existence of artifacts should be appreciated so that they can be readily recognized.

Holes

Holes in tissue have been described after the Dermojet has been used for the instillation of local anesthesia.[11] These holes appear as rounded empty spaces both within the epidermis and between collagen bundles.

Starch granules

Starch granules appear as doubly refractile bodies under polarized light.[22] Such granules can be found in cosmetic preparations, topical medications, and sterile gloves. Therefore it is essential to cleanse the surface epidermis before biopsy not only to leave a surgical site with as few bacteria as possible but also to eliminate artifactual contaminants.

Epidermal invagination

The artifactual downward extension of the epidermis into the dermis can occur by compression of the surface of tissue with forceps, scissors, or scalpel blade. Sometimes this invagination of epidermis may simulate an intradermal cavity lined by epidermis.[22]

Epidermal cell elongation

Elongation of epidermal cells is produced with tissue heating, by either the high-frequency electrosurgery appara-

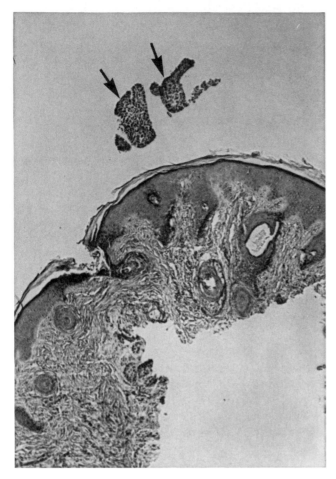

Fig. 14-12. Basal cell carcinoma, "floating" free *(arrows)* of tissue specimen.

tus (see Fig. 16-19), the electrocautery, or the laser that polarizes the cells. Dehydration and vacuolization can also occur. Therefore use of these devices on biopsy specimens is discouraged.[27]

Basal cell carcinoma lying free

Basal cell carcinomas are frequently not tightly bound to the surrounding tissue stroma. If tissue is pinched at the time of biopsy, the tumor might literally be squeezed out of the specimen.[22] On the histologic slide, masses of basal cell carcinoma can then be seen lying free from the main tissue specimen (Fig. 14-12). Such free floating masses of tumor can be overlooked by the pathologist as he or she reads the slide.

Tissue curling

Very thin tissue that is pinched at the time of removal might be curled, even to the point at which it may appear pedunculated when processed for histologic slides. Therefore it is important to prevent compression of tissue and to flatten out such curled specimens on paper or cardboard before placing them in the fixative solution.

Marginal breaks

Breaks in the continuity of the vertical margins of tissue specimens can occur. Such defects in the tissue usually do not cause a problem of histopathologic misinterpretation. Marginal breaks are commonly seen when tissue is frozen in situ for local anesthesia at the time of removal.[31] Manual cutaneous punches can produce vertical breaks, but breaks are much less common when punches attached to drills are used. Therefore the latter technique might be superior for harvesting less distorted tissue plugs to be used for hair transplantation.

REFERENCES

1. Ackerman, A.B.: Biopsy: why, where, when, how, J. Dermatol. Surg. **1**:21, 1975.
2. Ackerman, A.B.: Shave biopsies: the good and right, the bad and wrong [editorial], Am. J. Dermatopathol. **5**:211, 1983.
3. Ackerman, A.B.: Dermatologic surgery: better training of residents is needed [editorial], Am. J. Dermatopathol. **6**:211, 1984.
4. Ackerman, L.V., and Rosai, J.: The pathology of tumors. II. Biopsy and diagnostic cytology, CA **21**:220, 1971.
5. Arthur, R.P., and Shelley, W.B.: The epidermal biopsy: its indications and technique, Arch. Dermatol. **80**:95, 1959.
6. Beerman, H., and Wood, M.G.: Taking a biopsy. In Skin surgery, Epstein, E., and Epstein, E., Jr., editors: Springfield, Ill., 1982, Charles C Thomas, Publisher, Inc.
7. Busch, F.: Ueber die Exstirpation kleiner runder Geschwulste der Haut durch schnell rotirende Locheisen, Berl. Klin. Wochenschr. **21**:306, 1884.
8. Caro, M.R.: Diagnostic pitfalls of dermal pathology, Arch. Dermatol. Syph. **67**:18, 1953.
9. Caro, M.R.: Skin biopsy technique, Arch. Dermatol. **76**:9, 1957.
10. Caro, M.R.: The pathologist is not infallible in the diagnosis of skin lesions, Chicago Med. **64**:7, 1961.
11. Carpenter, Jr., C.L., Jolly, Jr., H.W., and Reed, R.J.: Dermojet hisopathological artifacts, Arch. Dermatol. **92**:304, 1965.
12. Editorial: Biopsy of skin—an underutilized laboratory "test," N. Engl. J. Med. **277**:49, 1967.
13. Epstein, E., Bragg, K., and Linden, G.: Biopsy and prognosis of malignant melanoma, J.A.M.A. **208**:1369, 1969.
14. Goodman, H.: Eponyms of dermatology, Series II. Arch. Dermatol. Syph. **17**:23, 1928.
15. Harris, D.R., and Youkey, J.R.: Evaluating the effects of hemostatic agents on the healing of superficial wounds. In Maibach, H.I., and Rovee, D.T., editors: Epidermal wound healing, Chicago, 1972, Year Book Medical Publishers.
16. Harris, M.N., and Gumport, S.L.: Biopsy technique for malignant melanoma, J. Dermatol. Surg. **1**:24, 1975.
17. Keyes, E.L.: The cutaneous punch, J. Cutan. G.U. Dis. **5**:98, 1887.
18. Kopf, A.W., and Popkin, G.L.: Shave biopsies for cutaneous lesions, Arch.Dermatol. **110**:637, 1974.

19. Loewenthal, L.J.A.: Punch biopsy with autograft: a cosmetic office procedure, Arch. Dermatol. Syph. **67:**629, 1953.
20. Lucid, M.L.: The interlocking slip knot, Plast. Reconstr. Surg. **34:**200, 1964.
21. Macy-Roberts, E., and Ackerman, A.B.: A critique of techniques for biopsy of clinically suspected malignant melanoma, Am. J. Dermatophathol. **4:**391, 1982.
22. Mehregan, A.H., and Pinkus, H.: Artifacts in dermal histopathology, Arch. Dermatol. **94:**218, 1966.
23. Patkin, M.: Skin lesion biopsy with transfixing suture, Med. J. Aus. **2:**536, 1974.
24. Piffard, H.G.: Histological contribution, Am. J. Syph. Dermatol. **1:**217, 1870.
25. Popkin, G.L., et al.: A technique of biopsy recommended for keratoacanthomas, Arch. Dermatol. **94:**191, 1966.
26. Roses, D.F., et al.: Assessment of biopsy techniques and histopathologic interpretations of primary cutaneous malignant melanoma, Ann. Surg. **189:**294, 1979.
27. Royster, H.P.: Selection of skin lesions for removal, Gen. Pract. **17:**121, 1958.
28. Sachs, W., Sachs, P.M., and Atkinson, S.C.: Peripheral, or five point, method of skin biopsy, J.A.M.A. **142:**902, 1950.
29. Sasaki, A., and Fukuda, O.: The looped square knot: a useful suture method, Plast. Reconstr. Surg. **67:**246, 1981.
30. Schellander, F., and Fritsch, P.: Eine einfache methode der Hautbiopsie, Kurtzmitteilung. Dermatol. Monatosschr. **157:**370, 1971.
31. Serup, J.: Punch biopsy of the skin: effect of temperature and local anesthesia with ethyl chloride freezing, J. Dermatol. Surg. Oncol. **9:**558, 1983.
32. Shelley, W.B.: The razor blade in dermatologic practice, Cutis **16:**843, 1975.
33. Shelley, W.B.: Epidermal surgery, J. Dermatol. Surg. **2:**125, 1976.
34. Traenkle, H.L., and Burke, E.M.: Curettement technic for biopsy: use in the detection of cutaneous cancer, J.A.M.A. **143:**429, 1950.
35. Urbach, E., and Fantl, P.: Methoden zur Quantitativ—Chemischen Analyse der Haut, I. Biochem. Ztschr. **196:**471, 1928.
36. Urbach, F., and Shelley, W.B.: A rapid and simple method for obtaining punch biopsies without anesthesia, J. Invest. Dermatol **17:**131, 1951.
37. Watson, B.A.: Gunpowder disfigurement, St. Louis Med. Surg. J. **35:**145, 1878.
38. Williams, J.P.G., Tomashefski, J.F., and Pavkov, K.L.: High-speed biopsy punch for electron microscopic studies of human skin [letter], Arch. Dermatol. **106:**595, 1972.
39. Winkelmann, R.K.: Skin Biopsy. In Techniques in Skin Surgery, Epstein, E., and Epstein, E., Jr., editors. Philadelphia, 1979, Lea and Febiger.

15

Curettage

The dermal curette is an instrument well known to dermatologists but not to other surgical specialists, so it is probably greatly underutilized.[41] Although this instrument is uniquely suited to remove (by curettage) a variety of superficial skin growths, skilled use of it requires training and experience to achieve consistently good results. This chapter explores the indications for and techniques of curettage.

HISTORICAL BACKGROUND

The dermal curette was developed by dermatologists specifically for the treatment of dermatologic lesions. Originally it was adapted from a uterine curette. The first dermal curette, introduced by Volkmann in 1870 and initially recommended for curettage of lupus vulgaris, was cupped-shaped and became known as Volkmann's sharp spoon.[43,74] However, it was soon appreciated that the curette had wide therapeutic application for a variety of dermatologic conditions. The early popularity of this instrument was the result of enthusiastic reports by notable dermatologists[14,74] who realized that curettage was an inexpensive, easy, and fast method for treatment of skin tumors. Additional historical information on the curette can be found in Chapters 1 and 7.

The ability of the curette to separate diseased tissue from normal surrounding tissue was written about as early as 1876.[74] It is because of this capability that it is so useful in the treatment of malignant neoplasms and benign lesions of the skin. With the curette, the maximal amount of normal tissue is preserved.

Early workers with curettage, however, remained unconvinced that curettage alone could cure carcinomas of the skin. Therefore other destructive methods were combined with curettage. These methods included the use of caustics such as acid nitrate of mercury (the Sherwell technique),[57] radiation,[16,19,44] electrodesiccation or electrocoagulation,[9,44,46] and, more recently, liquid nitrogen.[1,21,59] Some of these techniques are discussed more fully later in this chapter.

Modern dermatologists frequently uses the term D&C to describe curettage followed by electrodesiccation. Therefore the term D&C is actually a misnomer, particularly since the curettage normally precedes the electrodesiccation. Also, electrocoagulation is often used rather than electrodesiccation—so D&C should be replaced by C&E; that is, curettage and electrodesiccation (or electrocoagulation).

The origin of the misnomer D&C actually is rooted in an early described technique in which the electrodesiccation preceded the curettage.[9,54,74] Although this technique is little used today, some physicians as late as 1981 advocated its use[73] on the basis of their belief that high-frequency electrosurgery (electrodesiccation or electrocoagulation) was more important than the curette in the D&C procedure. However, others[5] think that, if electrodesiccation is the initial procedure, the subtle differences between tumor and normal structures will become obliterated; or that use of electrodesiccation first might needlessly destroy more tissue than necessary.[29]

Despite controversies over indications for usage or problems associated with its application, the curette is probably the instrument most frequently used by dermatologists today. Its utility has stood the test of at least 100 years and will undoubtedly continue to be appreciated in the future.

INSTRUMENTS

The dermal curette has a handle and a circular or oval, fenestrated head with a cutting edge that is sharp enough to cut through friable tissue but not normal skin. Therefore the dermal curette is most accurately described as a semisharp rather than a sharp cutting instrument. It removes superficial cutaneous lesions such as seborrheic keratoses without penetrating the surrounding epidermis or underlying dermis. This results in minimal disturbance to normal tissue and often produces the least apparent scar. Although a non-fenestrated, cup-shaped curette, the bone curette, can also be used,[51,73,76] the fenestration of the dermal curette allows soft tissue to be displaced easily through the opening during the curettage process.

The large- and medium-sized dermal curettes are of the Piffard or Fox type. The Fox curette (see Fig. 7-20) has a thin handle, whereas that on the Piffard curette (see Fig. 7-21) is larger and bulkier. Most commonly, 3 or 4 mm curettes are used.

Also available are the little curettes, which are useful to probe small extensions of tumors.[7,29] These little curettes measure 1 to 2 mm across their cutting surfaces. The most commonly used small curettes (see Fig. 7-22) are the Skeele, the Meyhoefer, or the Heath. These three small curettes are actually eye curettes. The Skeele curette is cup-shaped with sharp toothlike ridges on the cutting edge. The Meyhoefer curette is also cup-shaped, but without ridges on the cutting edge. The Heath curette is similar to a miniature Fox curette.

Curettes need to be kept reasonably sharp and free of nicks for efficient use. This may be accomplished either by the instrument manufacturer, who will resharpen the instrument, or with the use of a cone-shaped whetstone, such as soapstone.

INDICATIONS FOR CURETTAGE

Curettage is indicated for removal of small superficial growths on the cutaneous surface. Such growths would include actinic keratosis, seborrheic keratosis, warts, superficial basal cell carcinomas and superficial squamous cell carcinomas. These types of growths all have in common the fact that they are superficial and usually not associated with fibrous (scar) tissue. If fibrous tissue is a component of a skin growth such as morphealike basal cell carcinoma[61,63] or an angiofibroma, the curette does not work as well, since it cuts through fibrous tissue with difficulty. Therefore selection of lesions on which to use a curette is just as important to its successful use as the proper technique.

Because the curette has a moderately sharp cutting edge, yet is not sharp enough to cut into normal tissue like a scalpel blade, it is particularly useful for separating a soft skin growth from the firm surrounding dermis and intact epidermis.[26,46,72] It causes as little damage as possible to the skin, and a good cosmetic result is obtained. For example, warts "shell out" easily with this instrument.

Perhaps one of the most common uses for the curette is in the eradication of skin malignancies. This modality of treatment is commonly taught and recommended by standard dermatologic textbooks.[3,12,27] In one large teaching center with every modality of therapy available, 55.6% of all basal cell carcinomas were treated by this method in the dermatology clinic.[27] Both basal and squamous cell carcinomas, if reasonably small (less than 1 cm on the head or neck and less than 2 cm on the trunk) and superficial, can be removed simply by means of a curette.[13,28,62] As just emphasized, the curette helps differentiate between normal and abnormal tissue. When it is used properly on selected tumors, the curette affords the patient an excellent chance of cure and a high likelihood of an excellent cosmetic result.

The curette can be used to provide tissue for biopsy, the so-called "curette biopsy."[65] Used for this purpose, the curette scoops a sample of friable tissue and does not necessarily eradicate the lesion. Because the curette has a characteristic "feel" as it comes through tumorous tissue, the physician's suspicion that a malignancy is present is heightened. Thus in a sense the curette becomes a diagnostic tool,[26] although a tissue sample still needs to be submitted for confirmation. Such curette biopsies usually provide tissue adequate for diagnosis, although the pathologist may have difficulty orienting the specimen and is unable to assess the deep or lateral margins for penetration by the tumor.

CURETTAGE FOR NONMALIGNANT LESIONS
Technique

The mastery of curettage requires practice and experience. To maximize the efficiency and accuracy of the curette's cutting surface, it is very important to provide tension on the skin where the lesion to be curetted exists and to stabilize the hand that holds the curette. As is true for other types of surgery discussed in this book, stabilization of the hands as well as of the skin being operated on is very important.

Before curettage, the skin is cleansed with an aqueous antiseptic (for example, iodophor), since alcohol, which is inflammable, is a fire hazard if electrodesiccation or electrocoagulation is used. Curetting can be done with or without a local anesthetic. For small superficial lesions on stoic individuals, it may be less painful to not use a local anesthetic, since the anesthetic injection might hurt more than the procedure itself. For extensive curettage or if the electrosurgical apparatus is additionally used, a local anesthetic is necessary.

The curette is held in the hand like a pencil (Fig. 15-1). One balances and steadies the hand holding the curette with the little finger, which rests on the patient's skin. The thumb and index fingers of the opposite hand stretch the skin on which the curette is to be used. Thus three-point traction to the skin on which the lesion is to be curetted is achieved. This traction creates tension and a firm surface, which allow the physician to curette more easily through soft tissue. The firmer the surface, the better the curette works. Thus it works well on the forehead, which overlies bone, whereas it is difficult or impossible to curette on the eyelid unless a firm surface is provided, as with a chalazion clamp.

Once tension on the skin is attained, the curette is drawn through the lesion and toward the physician with a steady yet firm downward scooping motion (*inset,* Fig. 15-1) that literally scrapes the lesion from the adjacent normal tissue. If the lesion is raised, one hooks the curette over its distal side before pulling the instrument toward oneself. The

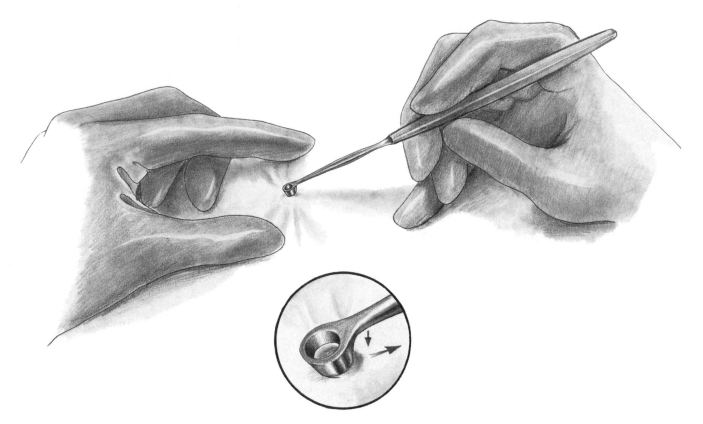

Fig. 15-1. Three-point traction, which places tension on skin for curettage.

scraping motion is repeated as many times as necessary to free the lesion completely from the surrounding stroma. Both the base and margin of the lesion should be scraped well. For most lesions treated with a curette, the bulk of the pathologic tissue "shells out" easily. A definite difference can be felt between the firm normal skin and the friable lesion. Normal dermis is relatively resilient. This ability to differentiate between normal and abnormal tissue is developed with experience. It is difficult to describe or to measure. It is thus the gestalt of curettage that leads to its success.

It is important that the physician press neither too firmly nor too gently to remove lesions adequately. The most common error made by a novice with a curette is to hold the instrument too loosely or to fail to press firmly when coming across the skin lesion. Like riding a bicycle, the use of the curette is learned with time. Once one has the feel for the most appropriate pressure to remove the skin lesion, one becomes very confident with this instrument.

It is important that the first relatively intact tissue removed by curettage be submitted for histologic examination if a previous biopsy has not been obtained, since relatively benign-appearing lesions might in fact be malignancies or precursors of malignancy.

Bleeding almost always occurs after curettage and is stopped with pressure, electrodesiccation (or electrocoagu-

lation), a styptic, or a caustic. The safest but the slowest way to stop bleeding is with pressure. This does not destroy additional tissue, perhaps unnecessarily. Styptic such as aluminum chloride (hydrous), 35%, in isopropyl alcohol, 50%; or ferric subsulfate (Monsel's solution) can also be useful. Ferric subsulfate seems to work well. However, it should be used sparingly, since it might leave pigment in the dermis that could lead to noticeable pigmentation of scar tissue—a potentially confusing situation for the dermatopathologist.[8,45]

An alternative method of stopping bleeding is electrocoagulation or electrodesiccation. Heat generated in the tissue stops bleeding, but it also destroys some additional tissue. Electrocoagulation or electrodesiccation is sometimes necessary when bleeding is so intense that caustics, styptics, or pressure alone does not control bleeding. In addition, sometimes one wants to destroy a little more tissue (for example, with warts); in this case electrocoagulation might be advantageous.

Application with pressure of oxidized cellulose (Oxycel) has been recommended to stop bleeding after curettage.[40] This substance which is discussed in Chapter 9, is used as a hemostatic material but has little direct effect on clotting. The good cosmetic results reported with oxidized cellulose[40] might in reality be caused by the pressure rather than by the Oxycel itself.

Specific nonmalignant lesions

Seborrheic keratoses are superficial growths, usually brownish, occurring on the trunk, face, or extremities of individuals as they grow older. Their cause is unknown, but they are extremely common. Sometimes patients have hundreds of such lesions. Since they are exophytic and above the dermis, seborrheic keratoses can be easily removed with a curette.

Seborrheic keratoses can generally be removed without anesthesia unless they are particularly large or in sensitive areas such as the eyelids.[41] These lesions can be "flicked off" so rapidly that the patient has only a slight, short-lived sensation of pain that is usually less than that caused by the injection of anesthetic. Hundreds of lesions can be removed in this manner within 20 minutes.

The wounds that result from removal of seborrheic keratoses are usually only superficial abrasions. The normal underlying dermis is not readily cut with the curette, so there is little danger of curetting too deeply, and the scars are almost imperceptible. Bleeding usually occurs following removal of seborrheic keratoses. This is best controlled with pressure or a mild styptic, such as aluminum chloride. Cottonlike oxidized cellulose with momentary pressure can also be used. Rarely is electrocoagulation necessary. The least destructive method to stop bleeding leads to the best cosmetic result.

Some physicians advocate freezing a seborrheic keratosis with ethyl chloride, liquid nitrogen, or dichlorotetrafluoroethane spray (Frigiderm) before removal with the curette.[4,12] This has been termed "cryocurettage."[55] Cryocurettage has the advantage of providing some anesthesia and at the same time hardening the lesion so that the curette is somewhat more effective. This works particularly well when the patient has many lesions to remove. However, patients have stated that the freezing spray is particularly painful.

Seborrheic keratoses should be submitted for histologic examination. Although this procedure may seem to be somewhat cautious when lesions have the "typical" appearance of seborrheic keratoses, cases of malignancies appearing within or beneath such lesions have been documented (see Fig. 14-1). Basal cell carcinoma,[38] squamous cell carcinoma,[30] and even melanoma[77] have all been described as appearing in association with seborrheic keratoses.

Actinic keratoses are also ideal lesions to remove with the curette. Like seborrheic keratoses, these are superficial growths. Generally they occur in sun-exposed areas and thus on solar-damaged skin. Histopathologically, actinic keratoses are composed of atypical epidermal cells that are confined to the epidermis. Although these lesions can be treated solely by liquid nitrogen, curettage has two advantages. First, there appears to be less recurrence of keratoses after curettage, because the curette helps to delineate the atypical epidermis, whereas with the liquid nitrogen the border of tissue frozen is estimated only by visual assessment. Second, curettage offers the opportunity to submit tissue for microscopic examination. If lesions are multiple, curettage might be less expeditious, but it can still be used. (Fig. 15-2, *A* through *C*)

Warts, particularly those that are filamentous, can also be easily curetted. Warts are caused by a number of papilloma viruses and, unlike seborrheic keratoses, can extend into the dermis. Therefore, with curettage, a deeper surgical defect and consequently more brisk bleeding results, frequently requiring the use of electrodesiccation or electrocoagulation. The latter are sometimes recommended on the premise that there is more tissue destruction and therefore a greater likelihood of cure. However, curettage and electrodesiccation of warts can result in scarring. Warts can be easily treated with liquid nitrogen, which, for deep warts, appears to result in less scarring.

Perhaps one area in which curettage may be expeditious in removing warts is the periungual area. In this location warts defy all forms of treatment. Sometimes curettage with removal of part or all of the nail plate is indicated. One of the little curettes might be of particular value in removing wart tissue along the crevices formed by the lateral nail folds.[29]

Molluscum contagiosum, another virally induced lesion, can also be easily curetted.[3] Other miscellaneous conditions reported to be amenable to curettage are cherry angiomatosis,[4] leishmaniasis,[11] dermatosis papulosa nigra,[24] and calcinosis cutis. In one study fifty patients with a total of 120 lesions of cutaneous leishmaniasis (caused by *Leishmania tropica*) were treated with curettage only.[11] The majority of the lesions healed within 4 weeks, but no long-term follow-up results were given. Compared to more expensive and complicated local or systemic medications, curettage might be a reasonable form of therapy, particularly for cutaneous leishmaniasis, which is known to lead to considerable scarring.

A series of 20 patients with dermatosis papulosa nigra were treated by curettage.[24] Of the 20 patients, 16 reported good or excellent results. The authors of this study emphasized that, rather than total removal of these lesions by the curette, only light abrasive curettage is needed. This makes the use of local anesthesia unnecessary and limits trauma. The latter is particularly important, since this condition occurs particularly in blacks, who are more prone to pigmentary changes, either hyperpigmentation or hypopigmentation, following surgery. It has been postulated that the light curettage causes involution of these lesions by way of an inflammatory cell exocytosis and subsequent epidermal degeneration.

At the Mayo Clinic, a study was performed[36] with a series of 11 patients (seven with scleroderma and four with dermatomyositis) with calcinosis cutis of the upper extrem-

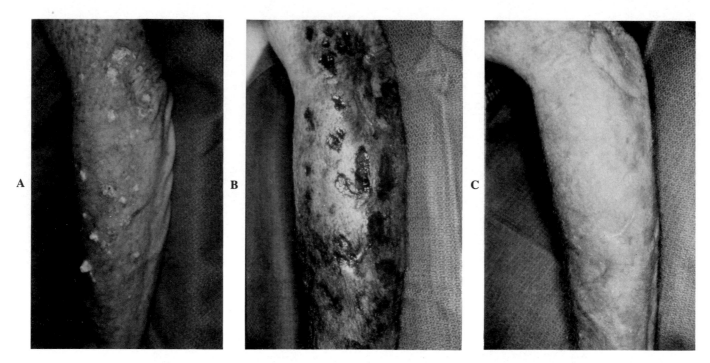

Fig. 15-2. A, Multiple keratoses, many of which are hyperkeratotic, of forearm. **B,** Immediately following curettage with patient under local anesthesia. Bleeding was controlled by pressure and aluminum chloride, 35%, in isopropyl alcohol. All wounds healed by secondary intention within 3 to 4 weeks. **C,** Healed result 6 months after curettage.

ities. The lesions were incised and then curetted, excised, or irrigated. All patients except one were satisfied, although redeposition of calcium occurred in 4 to 5 years. Complications such as difficulty with wound healing did not occur.

Epidermal inclusion cysts[29] or lipomas[22] have been reported to be amenable to removal by the curette, once a hole is created for passage of the curette. For epidermal inclusion cysts, the little curette, particularly the Skeele curette with its multiple sharp teeth that may help to locate and extract tiny cyst wall fragments, is said to be effective. For lipomas, the curette serves to free the lipoma from the surrounding tissues, and the lipoma is squeezed out. However, it is my experience that the use of curettes for removal of cysts or lipomas is less exacting than other methods, and lesions removed in this way are more prone to recurrence.

CURETTAGE FOR MALIGNANT LESIONS

Curettage for ablation of cutaneous malignancies has been widely used by dermatologists for at least a century, and this method provides an excellent likelihood of cure for certain selected tumors. In addition, curettage provides a simple, convenient, inexpensive, efficient, and fast method of treatment that usually results in good to excellent cosmetic results. Although curettage for removal of skin cancer is frequently criticized by physicians unfamiliar with either the instruments or the technique, there is no doubt that, properly used on appropriate lesions, this kind of removal is an

important method of treatment. Curettage is established in surgical oncology. Osborne[46] was one of the early enthusiastic proponents of curettage for cutaneous malignancies. He believed the curette was superior to other treatment methods because it afforded the operator knowledge by tactile sense of the depth and lateral extensions of tumor not provided by other methods. However, we now know the curette has limitations in its ability to delineate tumor margins accurately.

The use of C&E for either basal or squamous cell carcinomas has been questioned by some physicians, because it is a superficial and seemingly crude technique. Even though basal cell carcinomas[71] and squamous cell carcinomas[17,26,31] rarely metastasize, both kinds of tumor are capable of local destruction if left untreated or inadequately treated. Although metastases have been reported after C&E of squamous cell carcinoma, they appear with perhaps equal frequency after other forms of therapy such as excisional surgery or radiation.[25] Therefore, for appropriately selected tumors, C&E can be considered a safe form of therapy.

Commonly used technique

Although the principles of curettage are well established, there is no one standard curettage technique used by all physicians on malignancies. Still, there seems to be a general consensus of opinion in the literature as to a recommended method.

A

B

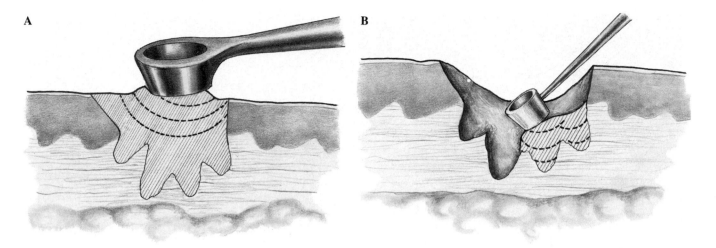

Fig. 15-3. A, Large or medium curette used to debulk soft basal cell carcinoma away from epidermis and dermis. **B,** Small curette used to dig small tumor extensions out from deeper stroma.

The skin tumor and surrounding skin are first cleansed with an aqueous antiseptic and then anesthetized. Care should be taken not to insert the needle (on the anesthetic-containing syringe) directly into the lesion itself. The tumor is then removed by means of a curette. Usually a 3 or 4 mm Fox curette is used for this purpose (Fig. 15-3, *A*). The method of holding the curette and establishing three-point traction has already been described and is illustrated in Fig. 15-1. Curettage must be vigorous and forceful. The bleeding is stopped with either electrodesiccation or electrocoagulation, which provides heat and is therefore destructive to tissue. Both the wound bed and a small (< 1 mm) rim of normal tissue beyond that removed by the curette should be seared. After sufficient electrodesiccation or electrocoagulation, the treated area appears dry, sunken, and contracted. The wound is then curetted a second time and electrodesiccated or electrocoagulated. If there is any doubt concerning the removal of the tumor, the curettage and electrodesiccation is repeated a third time. Frequently the third curettage and electrodesiccation (or electrocoagulation) is performed for good measure. At the end of the procedure, a 2 to 4 mm margin of surrounding normal tissue will have been destroyed.

Several physicians advise using magnification during the C&E procedure.[73] This can readily be provided by means of a Beebe Loupe (American Optical Corp., Southbridge, Mass.) or the OptiVisor (Donegan Optical Co., Lenexa, Kan.). These magnifiers supposedly aid in more accurate visual assessment of the borders of tumorous tissue. I have found that if such a delineation cannot easily be made with the naked eye, magnification is not very beneficial.

Occasionally, strands of tumor are so small that they are missed by a medium curette. As the tumor is curetted, these small strands are cut off from the main tumor mass and left behind. If these strands are not removed, persistence of tumor is inevitable, and recurrence of tumor is

likely. Some physicians believe that, because of the possibility of these small strands, a much smaller curette is necessary[7,29,57,66] (Fig. 15-3, *B*). Either a small 2 mm curette or even smaller little curettes (the Skeele, Meyhofer, or Heath) can be used.[66] Because the heads on these little curettes are much smaller than that on the medium curette, they are more likely to penetrate the anfractuosities down which fine extensions of malignancy penetrate. The base of the wound should be probed with a small curette to seek for soft spots that are probably pseudopod-like extensions especially typical of basal cell carcinomas. Most often the smaller curette is used after the larger curette or after the base of the wound has been electrodesiccated once or twice.

Occasionally, when one probes with a curette, the head of the instrument extends deeply into the fat. If this should occur, one can reasonably assume that malignant cells extend deeply and cannot be adequately extracted by means of curettage. Under such circumstances, curettage should be abandoned, and an alternative form of therapy (such as excision) should be chosen that will more likely remove or treat the malignant cells.

In treating basal cell carcinomas with a curette, the theoretic assumption is made that the tumor can be easily dislodged from the surrounding stroma. Basal cell carcinomas do tend to fall out of tissue easily when histologic sections are prepared. Since these tumors are frequently surrounded by acid mucopolysaccharides,[18,42] it has been hypothesized that this substance allows the curette to separate tumor cells more easily from the surrounding stroma.[48]

After treatment by C&E, a dry, whitish-appearing eschar results. Although some physicians feel that this should be left uncovered to allow reepithelialization to take place underneath the scab, I think it is best to keep the wound's environment moist. Twice daily dressings with hydrogen peroxide and an antibiotic ointment are recommended. A

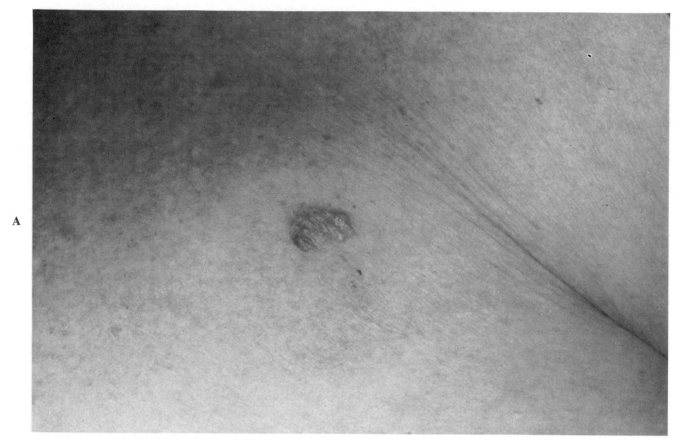

Fig. 15-4. A, Basal cell carcinoma of upper back near axilla.   *Continued.*

dressing should be worn until wound healing is complete.

A typical basal cell carcinoma amenable to treatment by C&E is shown in Fig. 15-4, *A.* This is a lesion less than 2 cm in its widest diameter on the trunk (upper back). In Fig. 15-4, *B,* the curette separates the lesion from the surrounding normal epidermis and underlying dermis. The base of the curetted wound is touched with an electrocoagulation electrode and completely singed (Fig. 15-4, *C*). The process of curettage followed by electrocoagulation was repeated twice more, resulting in a wound (Fig. 15-4, *D*) larger than both the preoperative size of the lesion (Fig. 15-4, *A*) and the wound after the first C&E (Fig. 15-4, *C*). Following C&E three times, the wound was allowed to heal by granulation and epidermization. In the case shown, a good cosmetic result has been obtained (Fig. 15-4, *E*).

Variations in technique

There are various techniques for removal of cutaneous tumors with the curette, as shown by the following:
- A. Curette alone[34,35,49,50,51,52]
- B. Curette followed by:
  1. Electrocautery plus acid nitrate of mercury (Sherwell technique)[57]
  2. Electrodesiccation and x-radiation (modified Sherwell technique)[16]
  3. Electrocoagulation and x-radiation[19]
  4. Electrodesiccation and radium[44]
  5. Electrocautery[33,44]
  6. Electrodesiccation[39,46,60,63]
  7. Electrodesiccation and curettage[66]
  8. Electrodesiccation and (curettage plus electrodesiccation) $\times$ 1[3,20,25,26,27,60]
  9. Electrodesiccation and (curettage plus electrodesiccation) $\times$ 2[5,27,60]
  10. Electrodesiccation and (curettage plus electrocoagulation) $\times$ 1[47]
  11. Cryosurgery (liquid nitrogen)[1,21,59]
  12. Excision[6,67,68]
- C. Electrodesiccation followed by:
  1. Curettage and electrodesiccation[9,54]
  2. (Curettage and electrodesiccation) $\times$ 2[76]
- D. Electrocoagulation followed by:
  1. (Curettage and electrocoagulation) $\times$ 1[72,73]

Many of these techniques have been abandoned and are mentioned only for historical interest. Others bear some discussion.

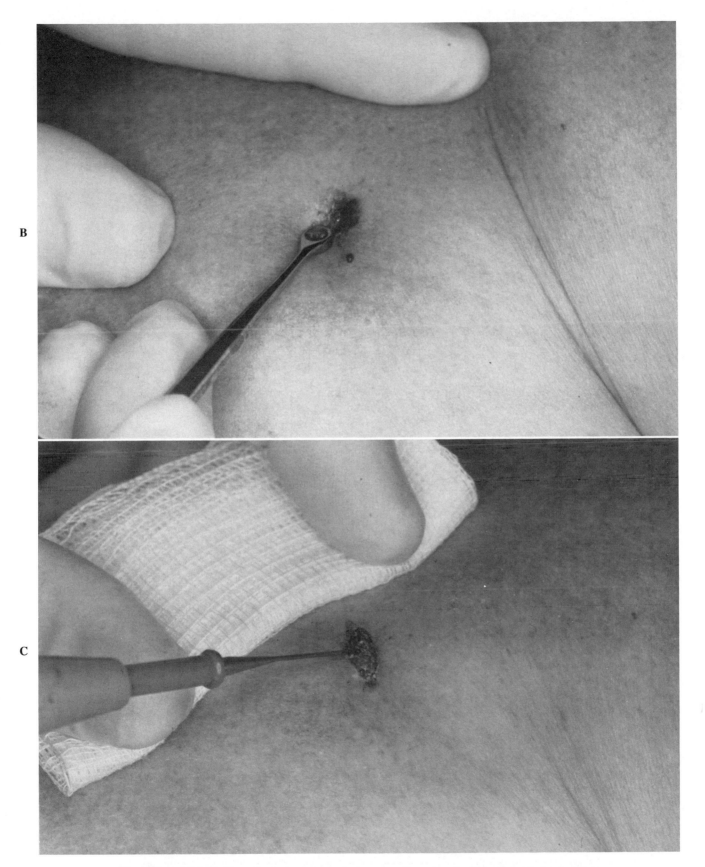

Fig 15-4, cont'd. B, Use of curette to scrape lesion away from dermis. Note that skin is placed on stretch by three-point fixation. **C,** Electrocoagulation of base of curetted wound.   *Continued.*

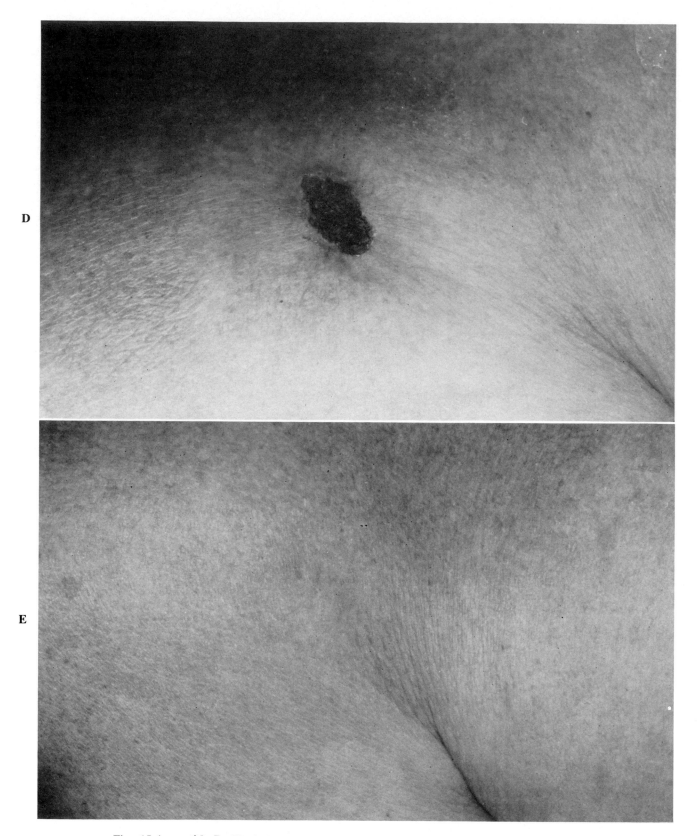

Fig. 15-4, cont'd. D, Final size of curetted and electrocoagulated wound after curettage and electrocoagulation has been performed three times successively. Note final size of this wound compared to initial size of lesion in **A. E,** Healed surgical site with imperceptible scar 6 months later. Actual healing took 2 weeks.

Curettage alone. The use of the curette alone without adjunctive destructive methods has had its advocates. In two studies, for patients with only a few lesions, comparable cure rates—90.3% and 91.5% for a 5-year follow-up—have been reported.[35,52] However, the cure rates apparently are much higher if patients have multiple lesions. In this circumstance, a 98.5% cure rate was reported.[49] It is important to stress that, in all of these studies, selected tumors that are small (usually less than 1.5 cm), in easy-to-cure sites (trunk, extremities), and histologically amenable to curettage (nonmorphealike) are being treated.

Many physicians believe that curettage alone is insufficient to cure basal or squamous cell carcinomas. Knox et al.[26] showed microscopically that curettage alone may not completely remove basal cell carcinoma. However, this was in only one case, and it may have been a difficult lesion to cure under any circumstances.

The rationale of using curettage alone on skin cancers is that the subsequent scarring is less than if a more destructive form of therapy (for example, electrocoagulation) is used adjunctively with curettage. However, in one study by Reymann[49] using curettage alone some depigmentation and scar hypertrophy, but no keloids, were noted. Since statistics are not given for cosmetic results in the published series in which curettage alone is used, it is impossible to draw any firm conclusion or to compare the cosmetic results with those of other studies.

One location on which it would seem reasonable to use curettage alone is the trunk, especially for small (less than 1 cm) histologically superficial basal cell carcinomas there. On the upper back and shoulders scars tend to hypertrophy and can be a nuisance to patients. Therefore anything that is done to minimize the depth of wounds in these areas leads to fewer problems. But, unfortunately, in one study, 14.5% of lesions removed from the back and shoulders with the curette alone recurred.[35] Therefore it is suggested that perhaps this method of treatment should not be used in this area.

Sherwell technique. At the beginning of the twentieth century Sherwell[57] recommended the use of 60% solution of acid nitrate of mercury on wounds after curettage and cautery of cutaneous malignancies. This technique enjoyed a certain popularity and became known as the Sherwell technique. When radiation became widely available and practiced, x-radiation replaced the escharotic paste.[16] The use of the curette followed by electrodesiccation followed in turn by radiation became known as the modified Sherwell technique. As late as 1960 Ferrara[19] reported a 100% cure rate using the modified Sherwell technique on basal and squamous cell carcinomas, whereas with curettage and electrocoagulation alone he obtained a 94.9% cure rate and with x-radiation alone a 93.9% cure rate. Therefore, although neither technique is currently used, the combined use of curettage and x-radiation might be beneficial under some circumstances.

Curettage followed by electrodesiccation (or electrocoagulation). The use of high-frequency electrosurgery combined with curettage is fairly standard practice. Curettage, removing the bulk of the tumor, is performed first, since it is the primary part of the treatment. Electrosurgery is also thought to be essential in the treatment of malignancies, since it destroys an extra layer of tissue that may contain tumor cells.[5,26] However, differences in technique have arisen with this seemingly simple combination that deserve some discussion.

The use of the curette and the electrodesiccation electrode have been likened to—and even elevated to—an art form by some C&E enthusiasts.[46,61] They discuss it almost in metaphysical terms. The repeated phraseology of the "feel" of the curette and "developing a feel" for abnormal tissue is mentioned. It is doubtful that such a feel or lack of it actually accounts for success or failure; rather, case selection is of much greater importance and relevance.

Both electrodesiccation and electrocoagulation produce heat in tissues surrounding the needle tip. However there are some differences. Electrodesiccation is monoterminal and uses a current of relatively high voltage and low amperage (see Fig. 16-9). Electrocoagulation, on the other hand, is biterminal and uses a current of relatively low voltage but high amperage (see Fig. 16-8). It destroys more tissue deeply than electrodesiccation.

The use of electrodesiccation or electrocoagulation on tissue results in dehydration destruction. The epidermal cells become condensed and elongated (see Fig. 16-19). In the dermis, thrombosis of small blood vessels occurs. The heat spreads in tissue some distance from where the tip of the electrosurgical electrode actually touches the wound. Therefore malignant cells theoretically are destroyed at a short distance away from the electrode tip both at and below the wound surface.

Electrodesiccation is less destructive than electrocoagulation, and some physicians prefer its use, since they think it causes less tissue loss and ultimately leads to a better cosmetic result. However, cosmetic results are difficult to quantitate, and therefore such assumptions, although reasonable, are difficult to prove.

Even more interesting is the variation in the number of times the C&E should be repeated to yield the best cure rates and yet still achieve optimal cosmetic results. Some authors advise C&E once,[25,39,46,60,63] twice,[3,14,25] or thrice.[5,60] Some think the number of times should vary with the circumstances,[27,60] whereas others propound variations in the method itself.[47,61]

Edens et al. reviewed excised tissue for remaining basal cell carcinoma following C&E once and C&E three times.[15] Although basal cell carcinoma was found in a large percentage of specimens after C&E once (45% to 49%), after C&E three times the percentage was only slightly smaller (35% to 37%). Therefore the additional number of times the C&E is carried out apparently makes only a small, perhaps insignificant difference in destroying or removing tumor. However, the additional C&E's might incite an enhanced inflammatory reaction that could help to destroy tumor cells and thus ultimately lead to higher cure rates.

There do not appear to be any studies that compare recurrence rates with C&E once versus C&E three times. However, in one report it was stated that, in a series of 90 lesions, of three recurrences 5 years after C&E, all occurred following treatment by one individual physician whose technique was to C&E once.[26] The other physicians in the study performed C&E twice.

Curettage followed by cryotherapy. Cryotherapy (liquid nitrogen delivered to the treatment area by either spray or probe apparatus) has been recommended following curettage for treatment of cutaneous malignancies. When used with cryotherapy, the curette can assume either a primary or secondary role. If it plays a primary role, the cryotherapy is viewed as "insurance" against the possibility that malignant tissue might have escaped mechanical removal by the curette.[1] In this case liquid nitrogen is sprayed on the curetted wound for good measure without strict adherence to freeze-thaw times. If the curette plays a secondary role, it functions to debulk the tumor so that the cryotherapy is more effective in reaching the deepest or widest portions of the tumor. In this instance, curettage allows better visualization of the deep and lateral extensions of tumor and thus helps delineate the field to be treated by cryotherapy. Following curettage, the wound containing the tumor is frozen with liquid nitrogen with adherence to freeze-thaw time measurements for adequacy of therapy.

Graham and Clark[21] think that curettage followed by cryotherapy is superior to curettage followed by electrodesiccation by three to four percentage points. In their study cure rates are reported as 97.2% for basal cell carcinomas and 98.2% for squamous cell carcinomas if curettage is followed by a single freeze-thaw cycle of liquid nitrogen spray. With a double freeze-thaw cycle, the percentage of cure was increased to 98.12% for basal cell carcinomas and 100% for squamous cell carcinomas.

It should be stressed that curettage followed by cryotherapy is used with the best results only on selected lesions. For example, in one report by Abadir[1] using this method on four patients with recurrent basal cell carcinomas, there were recurrences in three of four. In another study a cure rate of 98% for lesions less than 1 cm with this technique was reported[59]; however, for lesions 1.5 to 2 cm in diameter, the cure rate dropped to 90.7%.

Curettage followed by excision. Use of the curette to help delineate the gross extent of tumor can be followed by excision. In this case, the curette is used to help establish the margins of tissue that must be excised to ensure a cure. The tissue margins can then be checked by a pathologist with routine random vertical sections,[68] horizontal sections,[67] or by Mohs sections.[2] Mohs sections include the whole under surface and skin edge by a straight oblique cut through tissue specially oriented to accept such a cut.

Brooks[6] implies that curettage followed by horizontal frozen sections by a pathologist is the equivalent of Mohs surgery (fresh tissue technique) as described by Tromovitch and Stegman.[69] However, his pathologist was uncertain that tumor was present in 19 of 100 cases. Such uncertainty undoubtedly arose from inexperience in reading frozen sections horizontally rather than vertically.

Abide et al.[2] interviewed 11 pathologists concerning their understanding of how to perform margin examination of elliptically excised skin specimens.[2] No pathologist interviewed used the Mohs sectioning technique; no pathologist could even define what it entails. It has been my experience that once tissue is given to pathologists to section, they will do what they have been trained to do. This is particularly true when a large number of sections would be required to examine all the cut margins adequately.

Although curettage followed by excision with subsequent examination of tissue by pathologists might approximate Mohs surgery, it does not constitute the equivalent technique. There are many fine points in the grossing, dyeing, staining, and cutting of tissue that have been developed for Mohs surgery and that are not duplicated by most pathologists. Currently physicians who have taken fellowship training approved by the American College of Chemosurgery are best prepared to oversee the processing of tissue and the histopathologic interpretation of the specially dyed frozen sections.

Curettage followed by excision with immediate examination of the margins by random frozen sections can nevertheless be useful for uncomplicated tumors. It might also be of value for difficult tumors for which a Mohs surgeon is not readily available. However, cure rates with this technique will fall short of those for which the proper Mohs surgical and pathologic technique is used.

Scissors excision and curettage. Skin cancers can be removed in part by scissors, which provide a good specimen. The base is then curetted, and this is usually followed by electrodesiccation. Alternatively, where the skin is thin (for example, the back of the hand), scissors alone may be used.

Electrodesiccation (or electrocoagulation) followed by curettage. Some physicians[9,54,73,76] recommend electrosurgical destruction of a malignancy before removal by the curette and report excellent cure rates with this technique. The use of electrodesiccation before curettage is undoubtedly the origin of the term "D&C" as applied to removal of cutaneous malignancies. The rationale is that a small zone (2 to 3 mm) of seemingly normal tissue beyond the tumor is destroyed and is then removed by the curette as insurance. In addition, the malignant cells are thought to be more susceptible to the desiccating or coagulating current than are normal cells, and the current seals blood vessels and lymph spaces.[54]

Other physicians, however, do not advocate use of electrosurgery before use of the curette. Krull argues that to do so would destroy tissue needlessly.[29] Baer and Kopf[5] feel that initial electrodesiccation of tissue destroys the delicate differences in the feel of tumor tissue compared with the feel of normal tissue.

Experience of the physician

It has been said that C&E is a deceptively simple technique for removal of skin tumors.[10] Excellent cure rates are believed by some to be a function of how well a physician adheres to the techniques of C&E and performs this form of treatment *lege artis* (according to the rule of the art). In one report it was noted that residents in training who were not well supervised tended to have relatively high recurrence rates (18.8%) compared to dermatologists in practice (5.7%).[28] With more supervision, the resident group improved and subsequently demonstrated a lower recurrence rate (9.6%). However, it should be pointed out that the residents in this study were performing C&E on a greater percentage of tumors of the head and neck and a lesser percentage on the trunk and extremities than the "more experienced" attending dermatologists. Thus case selection might have been just as important as experience or the lack of it. Other studies have also demonstrated that residents or poorly trained physicians have lower cure rates,[76] which tend to improve with closer supervision.[23]

Cure rates for basal and squamous cell carcinomas

Although in the end cure rate statistics alone do not necessarily determine which method of therapy to choose for any given malignancy, such statistics do provide a crude method of comparison among several treatment possibilities. The published 5-year cure rates for squamous cell carcinomas and basal cell carcinomas treated by C&E are listed in Table 15-1. As can be seen, these vary from 74% to 100%, depending on the published series. It is difficult to compare studies of cure rates, since the criteria for case selection are not always clear, the precise technique of C&E is not always stated, and usually not all the tumors in one study are treated by one individual but by several different physicians. In studies for which multiple modalities of treatment are available, physicians tend to select C&E for easy-to-cure tumors (small, nonrecurrent, situated in low-recurrence areas) and other treatment methods for lesions that are more difficult to cure. This tends to inflate favorably the cure rate statistics for C&E. In addition, several studies present composite cure rate statistics for basal and squamous cell carcinomas without separately analyzing their data for each of these two types of malignancies.[16,19,72,73] Although at times it might be difficult to distinguish basal cell carcinomas from squamous cell carcinomas, since some overlap may exist,[70] usually this is not a problem. Since the growth pattern and potential seriousness of squamous cell

TABLE 15-1

Cure rates (5-year) for C&E of skin tumors

Type	Variables	Percentage
Basal cell carcinoma*		
Knox et al. (1960)[26]		96.43
Sweet (1963)[63]		87.70
Freeman, Knox, and Heaton (1964)[20]	< 2 cm	97.00
	> 2 cm	100.00
Tromovitch (1965)[66]		96.00
McCallum and Kinmont (1966)[33]		84.40
Simpson (1966)[58]		93.00
Knox et al. (1967)[25]	< 2 cm	97.50
	> 2 cm	100.00
Shanoff, Spira, and Hardy (1967)[56]		96.00
Kopf et al. (1977)[28]	group A†	81.20
	group B‡	90.40
	group C§	94.30
Dubin and Kopf (1983)[13]		74.00
Spiller & Spiller (1984)[60]		97.00
Squamous cell carcinoma		
Knox et al. (1960)[26]		97.06
Freeman, Knox, and Heaton (1964)[20]	< 2 cm	96.00
	> 2 cm	100.00
Tromovitch (1965)[66]		96.60
Knox et al. (1967)[25]	< 2 cm	99.50
	> 2 cm	100.00

*Mostly small (unless specified) nonrecurrent, nonmorpheaform tumors.
†Dermatology residents loosely supervised.
‡Dermatology residents closely supervised.
§Practicing dermatologists.

carcinomas are different from those of basal cell carcinoma, I have not listed in Table 15-1 studies that lump these two malignancies together.

What does emerge from the data in Table 15-1 is that cure rates for C&E for either basal or squamous cell carcinoma are generally quite high; in the range of 90% to 95%. Since case selection obviously is the most important factor that determines cure rates, this should be discussed.

Criteria for selection

No one treatment method is ideal for all malignancies. Theoretically the best method is one that completely eradicates the lesion with the best cosmetic result and the least amount of discomfort, inconvenience, and expense to the patient.[19] Ideally, in a setting in which most alternative forms of therapy besides C&E are available, including cold steel surgery, radiotherapy, cryosurgery, and Mohs surgery, cure rate statistics on the basis of size, type, and location should be the guide to appropriate management. In

**VARIABLES DETERMINING WHEN C&E
IS UNSUITABLE FOR BASAL CELL CARCINOMA**

1. *Size:* BCCs > 2 cm in diameter in general or > 1 cm on nasal tip
2. *Site:* BCCs occurring in high recurrence sites (for example, nasolabial fold, canthus of the eye, vermilion, postauricular sulcus)
3. *Histopathology:* Morphealike BCCs or infiltrating BCCs
4. *Previous treatment:* Recurrent BCCs
5. *Borders:* Ill-defined BCCs
6. *Invasion:* BCCs penetrating tumors into fat, muscle, bone, or cartilage

Modified from Crissey, J.T.: J. Surg. Oncol **3:**287, 1971 and Wilkinson, J.D.: Clin. Exp. Dermatol. **7:**75, 1982.

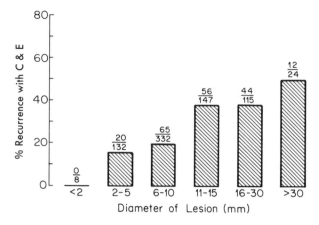

Fig. 15-5. Increased percentage of recurrences after curettage and electrodesiccation of basal cell carcinomas as preoperative lesion diameters increase. (Data from Dubin, N., and Kopf, A.W.: Arch. Dermatol. **119:**373, 1983.)

reality, other considerations such as the skill of the physician, the availability of a given treatment method, patient compliance, and economic pressures usually take precedence. Some of the adverse variables associated with the selection of cases for C&E are shown in the box above. Therefore, on the basis of the literature, certain criteria emerge that one needs to take into account.

In the 1956 edition of *Dermatology,* a major textbook on the subject, Pillsbury, Shelley, and Kligman[47] made the following suggestions (based on clinical impression) for selection of basal cell carcinomas amenable to C&E: (1) select tumors up to 1 cm; (2) avoid the nasolabial fold, tip of the nose, and ears; and (3) avoid recurrent lesions. Following publication of this book, their advice was largely unheeded and not adhered to by most dermatologists; however, the data available at this time support their beliefs.

Size. Cure rates with C&E vary with the size of skin cancers. Most commonly, skin cancers present to dermatologists as small, well-defined tumors, and therefore C&E can safely be used. In an important study by Dubin and Kopf,[13] it was shown that the recurrence rate for a basal cell carcinoma increases as the size (greatest diameter) of the lesion increases (Fig. 15-5). Above 3 cm in size, the likelihood of cure is only 50%.

Spiller and Spiller[60] likewise noted a decreased cure rate with increased size. These authors noted a 16% recurrence rate for lesions greater than 2 cm and a 1.23% recurrence rate for lesions less than 1 cm. Also, if the lesions over 2 cm were recurrent, the recurrence rate after C&E was even greater—33.3%. In other words, these two adverse factors (large lesion size, recurrent lesion) appear to be at least additive.

Good clinicians have known for some time that tumor

size is an important determinant of cure rates with C&E. Some opinions are as follows: (1) this technique is suitable for lesions up to 1 cm[12,47]; (2) on the nose, 1 cm is the upward limit appropriate for C&E[10]; (3) C&E is acceptable to 2[26] or 2.5[75] cm; and finally (4) for very small lesions (less than 0.5 cm) C&E is considered to be the treatment of choice, since it has even higher cure rates than conventional excisional surgery.[56] The last recommendation is, ironically, from a group of plastic surgeons.

Another way of assessing the relevance of tumor size to removal with C&E is to look for the *microscopic persistence* of tumor after C&E has been performed. In one study[62] the percentage of cases in which basal cell carcinoma is seen microscopically to be left behind microscopically after C&E increases with lesion size and at a rate similar to the *recurrence rates* found in the Dubin and Kopf study.[13] In other words, the larger the tumor is, the less likely it is that curettage and electrodesiccation (or electrocoagulation) will remove the whole tumor.

Knox and co-workers[20,25] analysed their cure rates with C&E on squamous cell carcinomas with respect to size. They found a very high rate of cure for lesions both less and greater than 2 cm (Table 15-1). However, very aggressive lesions or lesions on the mucous membranes were selected out for other forms of therapy and were not included in their study groups. Another factor contributing to the high cure rates with C&E for squamous cell carcinoma is the fact that many of the lesions treated in reported studies are superficial and perhaps noninfiltrating squamous cell carcinomas. More data are needed with C&E for squamous cell carcinoma before a valid assessment of this technique for this tumor can be made.

Site. It is a well-known clinical fact that basal and squamous cell carcinomas that occur in certain anatomic locations are prone to recurrence regardless of which treatment modality is used, including C&E. These sites include the nasolabial fold, the inner canthus, and the ear (especially the postauricular sulcus). The scalp, temple, and lips may also be areas on which tumors are difficult to cure. Locations where tumors are less prone to recurrence include the neck, trunk, and extremities.[13]

In one study tissue was examined microscopically for persistence of basal cell carcinomas in different locations after C&E.[62] This study showed that on the head, 46.6% of tumors persisted whereas only 8.3% on the trunk and extremities persisted. In a similar study,[53] a 30% incidence of microscopically residual tumor on and around the nose after C&E was seen. Therefore C&E works fairly well in completely removing tumors (in this case, basal cell carcinomas) from the trunk and extremities.

Why basal cell carcinomas are more difficult to eradicate in certain areas is unknown. It has been speculated that the seams of the embryonic fusion planes of the face tend to allow tumor to penetrate more deeply and thus out of the reach of the curette. In addition, the dense fibrous stroma of the nose and scalp can be a difficult tissue in which to curette; scar tissue presents the same difficulty.

For curettage to be adequate, the surface must be firm and in general not yield greatly underneath the curette. The eyelids and the vermilion of the lips in particular are two sites on which the softness of the tissue makes it difficult for the curette to separate adequately the tumorous tissue from normal tissue. Both these areas can be immobilized to a large extent by a chalazion clamp that overcomes the inherent softness of the underlying tissue.

Histopathology. The pathology of basal cell carcinoma might affect the rate of cure with C&E. Morphealike basal cell carcinomas recur frequently after C&E. In one report nine morphealike basal cell carcinomas were curetted and electrodesiccated, and eight recurred.[63] In another study two morphealike basal cell carcinomas were treated with C&E, and in one case persistence of tumor was found microscopically in tissue that was later removed.[62]

A less well-known and well-discussed pathologic pattern that may be associated with high recurrence rates with C&E is "infiltrative" or "invasive" basal cell carcinoma.[63] Edens et al.[15] excised tissue after C&E and examined it histologically. They found that tumors with an infiltrative pattern tended to persist microscopically after this form of treatment. These authors postulated that nonmorphealike tumors could be grouped into two patterns, well-circumscribed or invasive, a concept actually proposed many years previously.[64] Well-circumscribed basal cell carcinomas tend to have abundant mucopolysaccharide surrounding well-defined, large (nodular) clumps of tumor. Infiltrative ones, however, have less surrounding mucopolysaccharide, and the cells are arranged in small nests or strands. Sometimes these small strands are seen coming off large nodular tumor masses (see Fig. 20-8). Spiller and Spiller noted that all their recurrent tumors greater than 2 cm were invasive histologically.[60]

Although a morphealike basal cell carcinoma usually has a distinctive clinical appearance, an infiltrative basal cell carcinoma does not. Therefore preoperative biopsy of even clinically typical basal cell carcinomas seems to be warranted to detect the latter variety of basal cell carcinoma that may require a more definitive form of therapy than C&E.

Previous treatment. Recurrent tumors are not well suited for C&E. Usually such tumors are embedded in scar tissue through which the curette cannot cut easily. Therefore, cure rates with C&E on recurrent tumors are unacceptably high.[13] For example, in one report[37] the recurrence rate following retreatment of basal cell carcinomas with C&E, regardless of the initial type of treatment, was 59%; and in another study a 33.3% recurrence rate was obtained with the use of C&E on recurrent basal cell carcinomas.[60]

Borders. Ill-defined tumors are those with borders that are not clearly discernible clinically. Usually these tumors arise in locations such as the nose or ear, where the subcutaneous tissue and dermis are tightly bound to the underlying cartilage. Because the affected tissue is not loose, the tumor may not appear to be exophytic and thus may be larger than visually apparent. Such ill-defined tumors may progress insidiously. Ill-defined tumors may appear histologically as "infiltrative" basal cell carcinomas, discussed previously.

Invasion. Tumors that infiltrate deeply into fat or beyond are not amenable to curettage. Within fat, the curette tends to swirl and cannot easily bring out the tumor. Also when tumors are in fat, they are frequently embedded within scar tissue, which blocks the action of the curette. The endophytic basal cell carcinoma described in Chapter 20 is an example of a deep-penetrating tumor.

Curettage for other malignancies

Bowen's disease. Bowen's disease is a type of squamous cell carcinoma characterized by a scaly, erythematous patch that slowly enlarges with time. Histopathologically, Bowen's disease is confined to the epidermis, which is thickened and contains atypical cells as well as cells showing individual cell keratinization. However, Bowen's disease can progress slowly over time to invasive squamous cell carcinoma as the atypical cells infiltrate the dermis. Unlike actinic keratoses, Bowen's disease frequently extends down hair follicles. Therefore, theoretically at least, this particular malignancy is ineffectively treated by means of a curette, since the atypical cells within hair follicles are inaccessible to the curette.

The data in the literature on cure rates with C&E for Bowen's disease are scarce. It is my impression that these

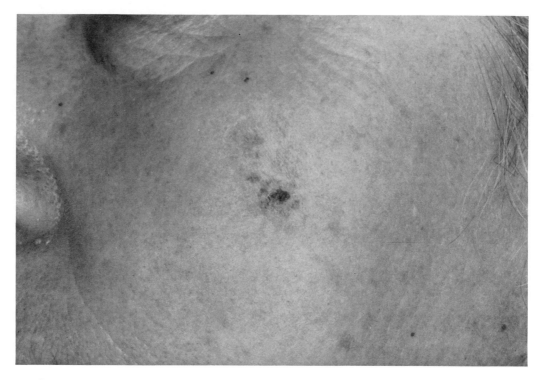

Fig. 15-6. Recurrence of lentigo maligna of cheek following curettage. Note that recurrence areas are small separate macules. These can be predicted if recurrence arises from persistence of tumor cells in hair follicles.

malignancies commonly recur after C&E and that surgical extirpation is necessary to remove them totally, especially in depth, and most especially in hair-bearing areas. Both McDaniel[34] and Reymann[49] treated Bowen's disease by curettage alone. Their cure rates were 60% and 83.4%, respectively, which are far below the cure rates of 93% to 97% reported by these same authors for basal cell carcinoma.

Lentigo maligna. Lentigo maligna is an unevenly pigmented macular lesion that occurs in sun-exposed areas and gradually expands peripherally. This lesion is an in situ melanoma. Although it is very slow growing and may not become invasive for many years, it does deserve adequate treatment, since one cannot predict when such an event will occur.

Histopathologically lentigo maligna is characterized by atypical melanocytes that are elongated, spindle-shaped, pleomorphic, and confined to the epidermis. Like Bowen's disease, this disease process extends down hair follicles (see Fig. 21-14).

Curettage has been recommended and used as a form of therapy for lentigo maligna, because curettage is hardly destructive. Since most lesions of lentigo maligna occur on the face, especially the cheek, cosmetic considerations are particularly important. However, curetting lentigo maligna is likely to lead to recurrence (Fig. 15-6). Although the curette can indeed remove the epidermis with its atypical melanocytes, it fails to remove totally atypical melanocytes that extend down the hair follicles. Therefore the curette is theoretically a poor choice for adequate treatment of lengito maligna.

PROBLEMS FOLLOWING CURETTAGE

Curettage usually cures the lesion treated and results in a good to excellent cosmetic result. However, like any surgical technique, curettage is not perfect and thus can be associated with certain problems. In fact, for treatment of basal cell carcinomas, it has been found that C&E had a higher complication rate (23%) than other forms of treatment such as cold steel surgery, radiation, or Mohs surgery.[5] It should be emphasized that such problems after C&E for malignancies can be minimized by careful case selection. For benign lesions, which are usually superficial, complications or problems following curettage are unusual.

Hypertrophic scar

The most common problem occurring after C&E of cutaneous malignancies is hypertrophic scarring, occurring in about 10% to 15% of wounds subsequent to treatment of basal cell carcinomas by C&E.[5,28] These scars are raised, pruritic, erythematous and commonly occur on the upper back and shoulders after C&E twice or C&E three times. Usually such scars soften, flatten and become white with time (6 months to 2 years). However, this process may be

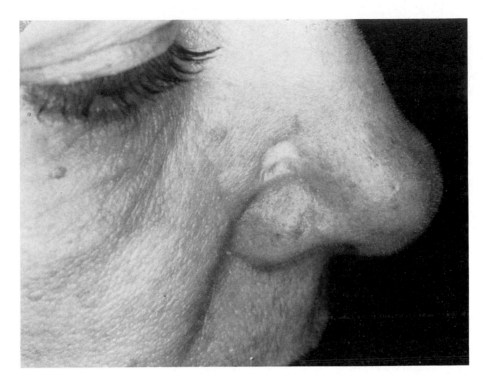

Fig. 15-7. Depressed smooth scar on nose following curettage and electrodesiccation of basal cell carcinoma.

hastened by injection with triamcinolone acetonide (Kenalog), 2.5 mg/ml to 10 mg/ml. Because of the frequency of this complication on the back or shoulders, I favor curettage once without electrodesiccation for small (less than 1 cm) histologically superficial basal cell carcinomas in these areas.

Depressed scar

A depressed (atrophic) scar, frequently hypopigmented, occurs rarely after C&E.[28] Fig. 15-7 shows such a depressed scar on the side of the nose. Such an unbecoming scar usually occurs after a lesion is removed into the deep dermis and the surrounding tissue cannot heal by contraction but mostly by granulation and epidermization. In other words, the scar does not "flatten out," because the surrounding tension forces do not allow the surrounding skin to move centripedally to help close the defect. The nose is a common place for this to occur, particularly if its skin is very porous and oily. Any other skin with a similarly porous texture may also heal in this manner.

Contracture

Distortion of adjacent structures, such as the upper lip or inner canthus can occur after C&E (Fig. 15-8). Fig. 15-8, *A,* shows an ill-defined, superficial basal cell carcinoma of the right upper lip. Fig. 15-8, *B* is the wound resulting from C&E three times of the basal cell carcinoma. The wound was allowed to heal by granulation, contraction, and epidermization. The resultant scar is hypertrophic and results

in upward retraction of the vermilion border (Fig. 15-8, *C*). Injections of triamcinolone acetonide were given. Although the scar flattened, the contracture could not be corrected in this way and persisted. Subsequent surgery was necessary to correct the lip retraction.

Hypopigmentation or hyperpigmentation

Often there is no pigmentary problem after curettage, especially for superficial seborrheic keratoses, and the treatment sites are thus difficult to detect. However, pigmentary changes following curettage can occur. Usually a slight loss of pigment occurs, resulting in hypopigmentation. This is more noticeable if the patient has a ruddy complexion or porous skin. The smooth-textured new epidermis that grows to replace that which has been curetted is particularly prominent next to skin with large pores. This new epidermis is at first erythematous, but this fades with time, and a more permanent hypopigmentation becomes apparent.

Hyperpigmentation is possible after curettage but is rare except in blacks. Usually this fades with time.

Recurrence of tumor

Patients treated by any modality, including C&E, for cutaneous malignancies should be carefully followed-up for signs of recurrence. Usually a recurrence occurs during the first year after treatment and appears as a small crusted area at the peripheral margin of the healed C&E scar (Fig. 15-9). Rarely tumors can recur deeply to the C&E scar. Certainly

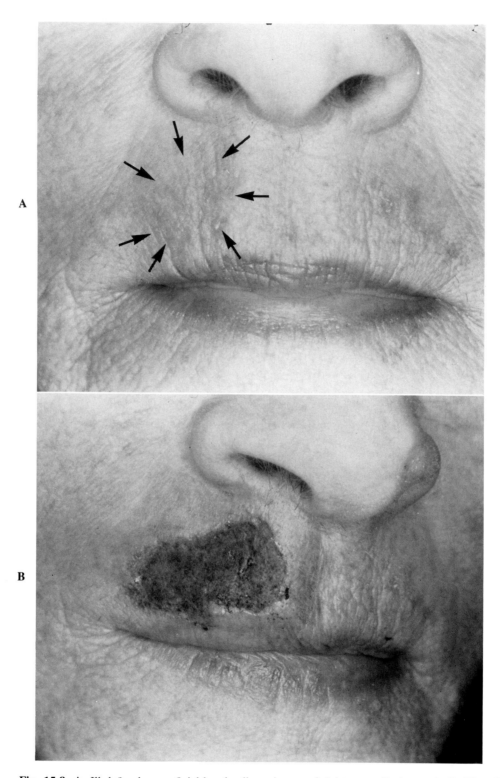

Fig. 15-8. A, Ill-defined, superficial basal cell carcinoma of right upper lip *(arrows).* **B,** Wound following curettage and electrodesiccation. **C,** Hypertrophic scar and distortion (contracture) of upper lip (3 months following curettage and electrodesiccation). Although the hypertrophic scar resolved with intralesional triamcinolone acetonide, contracture of vermilion persisted and required surgical correction.

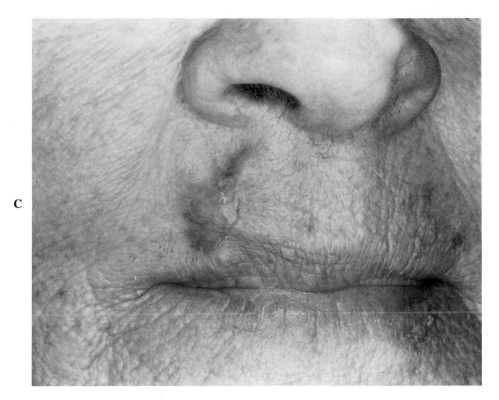

C

Fig. 15-8, cont'd. For legend, see opposite page.

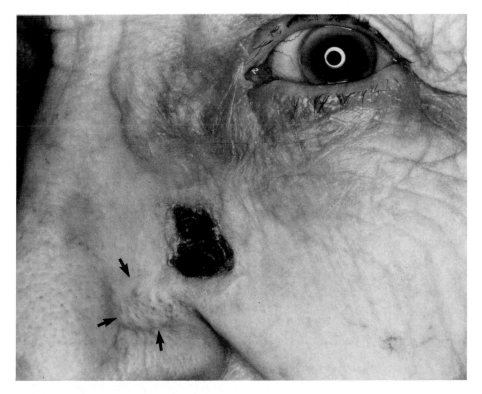

Fig. 15-9. Recurrent basal cell carcinoma (crusted area on nasofacial angle) at peripheral margin of previous C&E site *(arrows)* on nose.

any suspicious-looking lesion near a C&E scar deserves to be biopsied so that it can be assessed histologically. Because basal cell carcinomas are slow-growing malignancies, no one knows the proper length of time for adequate follow-up. Five years is suggested, but 10 years may give a more accurate assessment for true recurrence.

Even though some physicians[25,58,63] found that most of their recurrences of basal cell carcinoma appeared in 2.5 to 3 years after C&E, others[39] found that a significant number of their recurrences (38.5%) appeared 5 years or more after treatment. This seems to support follow-up periods longer than 5 years for slow-growing malignancies.

The most likely location for a recurrence of basal or squamous cell carcinoma after C&E is at the periphery of the treated area. C&E does not result in tissue rearrangement, and thus some physicians have stated that tumor recurrences with this treatment modality will be more easily detected than if they occur after, for example, conventional excisional surgery.[27] One physician found that 90% of his recurrences appeared at the periphery.[63] However, recurrences can still occur in the center of treatment sites. I have seen "hypertrophic scars" after C&E treated as such; later they were found to be growing because of the presence of tumor. Therefore one should consider obtaining a biopsy of a hypertrophic scar after C&E that fails to respond to intralesional steroids.

If a malignancy occurs at the periphery of a C&E site, the question arises, whether this is a new lesion or a persistence of the original tumor. This question is not so easily answered. Some authorities, particularly those in the surgical specialties, discuss the concept of multicentric tumors. By this they mean that tumors developed independently within a certain anatomic region (field) and are not microscopically interconnected. However, except when multiple tumors occur in a radiation field, this concept is probably spurious. Madsen has carefully mapped out extensions of basal cell carcinomas and concludes that for these tumors multicentricity does not exist.[32]

Metastases

Although metastases are rare with basal cell carcinomas,[71] they can occur after C&E of a squamous cell carcinoma, even with squamous cell carcinomas arising on the nonmucosal, sun-exposed skin.[17,31] Knox et al.[25] reported one case of a squamous cell carcinoma that metastasized after C&E. However, in his series, metastases of squamous cell carcinomas after C&E were no more frequent than after excisional surgery or radiation.

Delayed healing

Wounds resulting from C&E are allowed to heal by granulation and epidermization, and usually this process is complete in 2 to 4 weeks. However, if these wounds occur on the lower extremities in patients with poor vascular sup-

ply, healing can be delayed and much longer than if an excision had been performed. Occasionally hypergranulation can occur in a curetted wound and may impede wound healing. If this happens, the hypergranulation tissue should be curetted away so that wound healing can then progress.

REFERENCES

1. Abadir, D.M.: Combined curettage and cryosurgery for treatment of epithelial cancers of the skin, J. Dermatol. Surg. Oncol. **6:**633, 1980.
2. Abide, J.M., Nahai, F., and Bennett, R.G.: The meaning of surgical margins, Plast. Reconstr. Surg. **73:**492, 1984.
3. Arndt, K.A.: Manual of dermatologic therapeutics with essentials of diagnosis, ed. 3, Boston, 1983, Little Brown & Co.
4. Aversa, A.J., Miller, O.F., III: Cryo-curettage of cherry angiomas, J. Dermatol. Surg. Oncol. **9**(11):930, 1983.
5. Baer, R.L., and Kopf, A.W.: Complications of therapy of basal cell epitheliomas. In Baer, R.L., and Kopf, A.W. editors: Year book of dermatology, Chicago, 1964-1965, Year Book Medical Publishers.
6. Brooks, N.A.: Curettage and shave excision, J. Am. Acad. Dermatol. **10:**279, 1984.
7. Burns, R.E.: The "little curette": a useful adjunct in the treatment of epitheliomata, Arch. Dermatol. **84:**662, 1961.
8. Camisa, C., and Roberts, W.: Monsel solution tattooing, [Letter], J. Am. Acad. Dermatol. **8:**753, 1983.
9. Cipollaro, A.C.: Electrosurgery for the treatment of cutaneous neoplasms, Arch. Phys. Med. Rehabil. **34:**621, 1953.
10. Crissey, J.T.: Curettage and electrodesiccation as a method of treatment for epitheliomas of the skin, J. Surg. Oncol. **3:**287, 1971.
11. Currie, M.A.: Treatment of cutaneous leishmaniasis by curettage, Br. Med. J. **287:**1105, 1983.
12. Domonkos, A.N., Arnold, Jr., H.L., and Odom, B.: Andrews' diseases of the skin, ed. 7, Philadelphia, 1982, W.B. Saunders Co.
13. Dubin, N., and Kopf, A.W.: Multivariate risk score for recurrence of cutaneous basal cell carcinomas, Arch. Dermatol. **119:**373, 1983.
14. Duhring, L.A.: A practical treatise on diseases of the skin, Philadelphia, 1887, J.B. Lippincott Co.
15. Edens, B.L., et al.: Effectiveness of curettage and electrodesiccation in the removal of basal cell carcinoma, J. Am. Acad. Dermatol. **9**(3):383, 1983.
16. Elliot, J.A., and Welton, D.G.: Epithelioma: report on 1,742 treated patients, Arch. Dermatol. Syph. **53:**307, 1946.
17. Epstein, E., et al.: Metastases from squamous cell carcinoma of the skin, Arch. Dermatol. **97:**245, 1968.
18. Fanger, H., and Barker, B.E.: Histochemical studies of some keratotic and proliferating skin lesions. I. Metachromasia, Arch. Pathol. **64:**143, 1957.
19. Ferrara, R.J.: The private dermatologist and skin cancer: a clinical study of 226 epitheliomas derived from five dermatologic practices, Arch. Dermatol. **81:**225, 1960.
20. Freeman, R.G.: Knox, J.M., and Heaton, C.L.: The treatment of skin cancer, Cancer **17:**535, 1964.

21. Graham, G.F., and Clark, L.C.: Statistical update in cryosurgery for cancers of the skin. In Zacarian, S., editor: Cryosurgery for skin cancer and cutaneous disorders, St. Louis, 1985, The C.V. Mosby Co.
22. Hardin, F.F.: A simple technique for removing lipomas (surgical gem), J. Dermatol. Surg. Oncol. 8(5):316, 1982.
23. Jackson, R.: The treatment of basal cell carcinoma, Cutis 5:1231, 1969.
24. Kauh, Y.C., et al.: A surgical approach for dermatosis papulosa nigra, Int. J. Dermatol. 22:590, 1983.
25. Knox, J.M., et al.: Treatment of skin cancer, South. Med. J. 60:241, 1967.
26. Knox, J.M., et al.: Curettage and electrodesiccation in the treatment of skin cancer, Arch. Dermatol. 82:197, 1960.
27. Kopf, A.W.: Therapy of basal cell carcinoma. In Fitzpatrick, T.B., et al., editors: Dermatology in general medicine, New York, 1971, McGraw-Hill Book Co.
28. Kopf, A.W., et al.: Curettage-electrodesiccation treatment of basal cell carcinomas, Arch. Dermatol. 113:439, 1977.
29. Krull, E.A.: Surgical gems: the "little" curet, J. Dermatol. Surg. Oncol. 4:656, 1978.
30. Kwittken, J.: Squamous cell carcinoma arising in seborrheic keratosis, Mt. Sinai J. Med. 48:61, 1981.
31. Lund, H.Z.: How often does squamous cell carcinoma of the skin metastasize? Arch. Dermatol. 92:635, 1965.
32. Madsen, A.: The histogenesis of superficial basal-cell epitheliomas, Arch. Dermatol. 72:29, 1955.
33. McCallum, D.I., and Kinmont, P.D.C.: Basal cell carcinoma: an analysis of cases seen at a combined clinic, Br. J. Dermatol. 78:141, 1966.
34. McDaniel, W.E.: Surgical therapy for basal cell epitheliomas by curettage alone, Arch. Dermatol. 114:1491, 1978.
35. McDaniel, W.E.: Therapy for basal cell epitheliomas by curettage only: further study, Arch. Dermatol. 119:901, 1983.
36. Mendelson, B.C., et al.: Surgical treatment of calcinosis cutis in the upper extremity, J. Hand Surg. 2:318, 1977.
37. Menn, H., et al.: The recurrent basal cell epithelioma: a study of 100 cases of recurrent, re-treated basal cell epitheliomas, Arch. Dermatol. 103:628, 1971.
38. Mikhail, G.R., and Mehregan, A.H.: Basal cell carcinoma in seborrheic keratosis, J. Am. Acad. Dermatol. 6:500, 1982.
39. Mitchell, J.C., and Hardie, M.: Treatment of basal cell carcinoma by curettage and electrosurgery, Can. Med. Assoc. J. 93:349, 1965.
40. Mohs, F.E.: Seborrheic keratoses, scarless removal by curettage and oxidized cellulose, J.A.M.A. 212:1956, 1970.
41. Mohs, F.E.: The versatile curet, J. Dermatol. Surg. Oncol. 4:106, 1978.
42. Moore, R.D., Stevenson, J., and Schoenberg, M.D.: The response of connective tissue associated with tumors of the skin, Am. J. Clin. Pathol. 34:125, 1960.
43. Neisser, A.: Chronic infectious diseases of the skin. In Von Ziemssen, H., editor: Handbook of diseases of the skin. New York, 1885, Wm. Wood.
44. Newland, H.: Rodent ulcer: its development on the limbs, Med. J. Aust. 2:221, 1936.
45. Olmstead, P.M., et al.: Monsel's solution: a histologic nuisance, J. Am. Acad. Dermatol. 3:492, 1980.
46. Osborne, E.D.: Treatment of malignant cutaneous lesions, J.A.M.A. 154:1, 1954.
47. Pillsbury, D.M., Shelley, W.B., and Kligman, A.M.: Dermatology, Philadelphia, 1956, W.B. Saunders Co.
48. Popkin, G.L.: Curettage and electrodesiccation, N.Y. State J. Med. 68:866, 1968.
49. Reymann, F.: Treatment of basal cell carcinoma of the skin with curettage, Arch. Dermatol. 103:623, 1971.
50. Reymann, F.: Treatment of basal cell carcinoma of the skin with curettage. II. A follow-up study, Arch. Dermatol. 108:528, 1973.
51. Reymann, F.: Multiple basal cell carcinomas of the skin: treatment with curettage, Arch. Dermatol. 111:877, 1975.
52. Reymann, F.: Basal cell carcinoma of the skin: recurrence rate after different types of treatment [editorial], Dermatologica 161:217, 1980.
53. Salasche, S.J.: Curettage and electrodesiccation in the treatment of midfacial basal cell epithelioma, J. Am. Acad. Dermatol. 8:496, 1983.
54. Schmidt, W.H.: The surgical uses of high frequency current, Arch. Phys. Med. Rehabil. 34:686, 1953.
55. Schoch, Jr., E.P.: Cryocurettage, Schoch Letter 27(3):5, 1977.
56. Shanoff, L.B., Spira, M., and Hardy, S.B.: Basal cell carcinoma: a statistical approach to rational management, Plast. Reconstr. Surg. 39:619, 1967.
57. Sherwell, S.: Further observations on the technique of an efficient procedure for the removal and cure of superficial malignant growths, J. Cutan. Dis. 28:487, 1910.
58. Simpson, J.R.: The treatment of rodent ulcers by curettage and cauterization, Br. J. Dermatol. 78:147, 1966.
59. Spiller, W.F., and Spiller, R.F.: Treament of basal-cell carcinomas by a combination of curettage and cryosurgery, J. Dermatol. Surg. Oncol. 3:443, 1977.
60. Spiller, W.F., and Spiller, R.F.: Treatment of basal cell epithelioma by curettage and electrodesiccation, J. Am. Acad. Dermatol. 11:808, 1984.
61. Sturm, H.M., and Leider, M.: An editorial on curettage, J. Dermatol. Surg. Oncol. 5:532, 1979.
62. Suhge d'Aubermont, P.C., and Bennett, R.G.: Failure of curettage and electrodesiccation for removal of basal cell carcinoma, Arch. Dermatol. 120:1456, 1984.
63. Sweet, R.D.: The treatment of basal cell carcinoma by curettage, Br. J. Dermatol. 75:137, 1963.
64. Thackray, A.C.: Histological classification of rodent ulcers and its bearing on their prognosis, Br. J. Cancer 5:213, 1951.
65. Traenkle, H.L., and Burke, E.M.: Curettement technic for biopsy: use in the detection of cutaneous cancer, J.A.M.A. 143:429, 1950.
66. Tromovitch, T.A.: Skin cancer: treatment by curettage and desiccation, Calif. Med. 103:107, 1965.
67. Tromovitch, T.A.: The C and D check for skin cancer, Cutis 11:210, 1973.
68. Tromovitch, T.A., and Allende, M.: Curette-excision techniques for skin cancer, Cutis 6:1349, 1970.
69. Tromovitch, T.A. and Stegman, S.J.: Microscopic-controlled excision of cutaneous tumors, Cancer 41:653, 1978.
70. Welton, D.G., Elliot, J.A., and Kimmelstiel, P.: Epithelioma: clinical and histologic data on 1025 lesions, Arch. Dermatol. Syph. 60:277, 1949.
71. Wermuth, B.M., and Fajardo, L.F.: Metastatic basal cell carcinoma: a review, Arch. Pathol. 90:458, 1970.

72. Whelan, C.S., and Deckers, P.J.: Electrocoagulation and curettage for carcinoma involving the skin of the face, nose, eyelids, and ears, Cancer **31:**159, 1973.

73. Whelan, C.S., and Deckers, P.J.: Electrocoagulation for skin cancer: an old oncologic tool revisited, Cancer **47:**2280, 1981.

74. Wigglesworth, E.: The curette in dermal therapeutics, Bost. Med. Surg. J. **94:**143, 1876.

75. Wilkinson, J.D.: Current treatment of epitheliomas of the skin, Clin. Exp. Dermatol. **7:**75, 1982.

76. Williamson, G.S., and Jackson, R.: Treatment of basal cell carcinoma by electrodesiccation and curettage, Can. Med. Assoc. J. **86:**855, 1962.

77. Yakar, J.B., et al.: Malignant melanoma appearing in seborrheic keratosis, J. Dermatol. Surg. Oncol. **10**(5):382, 1984.

16

Electrosurgery

Modern cutaneous surgery uses both electrical and light energy to cut tissue or to stop bleeding. Electrical energy is commonly produced by an electrosurgical apparatus, whereas light energy is produced by a laser. Both types of energy are transformed into heat within tissue, resulting in cell injury or cell death, depending on the amount of heat produced.

The physics of electrosurgical apparatuses is poorly understood, even by physicians who use such machines on a daily basis. Their experience and knowledge gained largely from personal trial and error, are limited to the practical application of these machines. Electrosurgical machines have certain disadvantages: for instance, the actual extent of tissue damage cannot be assessed visually at the time of operation. Moreover, serious surgical complications may arise from use of these machines simply because they convey electricity. In-depth knowledge of the basic theory of such machines helps to prevent such complications from occurring and makes one more cognizant of the actual extent of tissue destruction occurring. Furthermore, a deeper understanding of such devices allows physicians to select more intelligently the optimal machine for their practice and to apply the appropriate electric current for the problem at hand.

Surgeons have over the centuries been wedded to the knife and suture, so there has always been some skepticism regarding other methods of cutting tissue and stopping bleeding. The distrust of and prejudice against electrosurgery are further compounded by the fact that electrical theory is not easy to understand and is based on the *effects* of electricity rather than on observation of electricity itself. In addition, since the tissue destruction produced by heat from an electrosurgical apparatus is always greater than that produced by a scalpel, wound healing is impaired. Nevertheless, electrosurgery is indispensable because it is fast, easy, efficient, and inexpensive. It may also be inherently antiseptic.

DEFINITIONS

The term *electrosurgery* is somewhat nonspecific and includes three different procedures (electrocautery, electrolysis, and high-frequency electrosurgery), all of which employ electricity during the performance of surgery. In *electrocautery* a heated element is brought into contact with tissues to transfer heat to them. The electric current flows only within the heated element—not through the patient. With electrolysis and high-frequency electrosurgery a current passes through the patient. *Electrolysis* requires direct current, and its results are caused by a chemical reaction at the tip of an electrode. In *high-frequency electrosurgery,* a high-frequency alternating current at the electrode tip cuts, coagulates, or desiccates tissue. This chapter discusses each of these three types of electrosurgery separately.

Diathermy is another term used occasionally in medical literature. This word means the passage of heat through some substance. It is specifically applied, however, to the heat generated when current from a high-frequency electrosurgical apparatus, which then passes into tissue. There are two types of diathermy: medical and surgical. Medical diathermy utilizes low current of very high frequency between two large electrodes. This produces a deep heat without a concentrated current or subsequent tissue necrosis. With surgical diathermy, on the other hand, there is a lower high-frequency current at the tip and sides of a small active electrode, usually with one distant, large indifferent electrode. Therefore the current is concentrated to a small point, and tissue necrosis results. Surgical diathermy is thus synonymous with high-frequency electrosurgery.

HISTORICAL CONSIDERATIONS
Cautery

The use of heat on tissue dates back to the earliest physicians caring for wounds. Heated metal used as a cautery iron is one of the oldest surgical tools. The word *cautery* comes from the Greek καυτήριον, meaning a branding iron. Undoubtedly some of the earliest cautery instruments were warriors' swords. By cautery I mean thermal cautery, as distinguished from chemical cautery. Thermal cautery is based on the conduction of heat from a heated instrument to tissue when the instrument touches the tissue; chemical cautery, on the other hand, produces its effects by means of the direct action of a caustic chemical, such as phenol, on tissue. Heat does not normally contribute significantly toward cell destruction when chemical cautery is used. The application of heat to wounds is mentioned in medical literature since the earliest written medical records. The Egyptians used heat to treat tumors in 3000 BC. They used a "fire drill," an instrument twirled back and forth to start fires.[8] Hippocrates used heat to open a suprapubic abscess, and Celsus used heat to control bleeding.[75]

In 1876 a special type of cautery was introduced as the Paquelin cautery.[38] In this device a flame was created from a mixture of benzene and air to heat tissue; it was like a blowtorch. Unna added a small wire tip (the Mikrobrenner) to control the effect of heating better.[10]

In the late 1800s battery current or electrical outlet current was used to heat metal. Metal becomes hot by resistance to the passage of current. An instrument based on this principle was similar to a soldering iron and became known as electrocautery, or galvanic cautery.[9] Hemostats were even developed with tips that heated to provide hemostasis.[101] Electrocautery became popular with dermatologists to remove small benign and malignant skin growths. Such instruments are still in use.

The latest addition to the surgeon's armamentarium of electrocautery instruments is the Shaw scalpel, invented by Robert Shaw in the 1970s. It is a heated scalpel blade that thermally cauterizes tissue as it cuts.[35]

Electricity

The therapeutic value of electricity (electrotherapeutics) on diseased tissues has been accepted for centuries. Mothers in western Africa dip their sick children into waters inhabited by an electric fish, the torpedo.[41] This same fish had been used by the Romans in the treatment of patients, and its generation of animal electricity was investigated in 1773 by the great surgeon John Hunter.[38] Strengths of more than 200 volts and 2000 watts have been recorded in the torpedo.[96]

Two natural phenomena known for years are that the black mineral magnetite (lodestone) attracts only iron and that rubbed amber attracts almost everything. The observation that a rubbed piece of amber attracts bits of straw is attributed to Thales of Miletus (639-544 BC). The attraction powers of both these materials were used for healing. William Gilbert (1540-1603), chief physician to Queen Elizabeth and later to James I, investigated these two phenomena and clearly distinguished the first one as a magnetic phe-

nomenon and the second as electric. Gilbert gave us the word *electricity* (from the Greek ἤλεκτρον, meaning amber) and related the pointing of the compass needle to the earth's magnetic field at the north pole. His book, *De Magnete,* is considered by many to be one of the most important scientific books ever published[58]; it is interesting to note that although the "father of electricity" was a physician,[40] most physicians today know very little about electricity.

The electricity first used widely in medicine was static electricity. Benjamin Franklin (1706-1790) used this form of electricity to treat paralysis in 1757, and its use medically became known as franklinism. The early machines used to produce static electricity were hand turned, and sometimes the charge was stored in Leyden jars. These glass jars were coated on the inside and outside with a metallic conductor; when the inner conductor came in contact with a metal hook, a spark could be produced. Static electricity was used to treat nervous disorders and spasmodic and convulsive diseases. Early static electricity machines were installed in England at Middlesex Hospital in 1767 and at St. Bartholomew's in 1777. Static electricity was also employed at Guy's Hospital in London around 1837 by Thomas Addison (1793-1860).[38] Unfortunately, the voltage and currents on these machines were difficult to control. Franklin electrocuted a turkey with such a device, and apparently some early investigators in Europe suffered fates similar to that of the turkey.[10]

In 1791 Luigi Galvani (1737-1798), an Italian anatomist in Bologna, reported a series of experiments detailing the contraction of a frog's leg when the frog was placed on an iron balustrade and a brass hook connected between a nerve in the frog's leg and the iron. Thus a complete circuit was produced. Galvani thought he had discovered animal electricity. Alessandro Volta (1745-1827) of Pavia was intrigued by Galvani's work. He interpreted these experiments as showing that a continuous flow of electricity took place whenever two different metals were in contact with each other and a moist conductor. In 1800 he introduced a "pile" of two dissimilar metals, with zinc connected to copper. This voltaic pile became known as a battery.

Galvanic, or direct, current was soon substituted for static electricity in medicine for treating nervous disorders. When the two ends of a battery were placed in water, hydrogen gas was produced at one end and oxygen at the other. Thus electrolysis was born. Galvanic electrolysis was first used for urethral stricture in 1839 by a Swede, Gustav Crusell.[38] In 1875 C.E. Michel in St. Louis used electrolysis for removal of eyelashes in trichiasis and districhiasis, and superfluous hairs in the glabellar area.[72] Dermatologists, especially W.A. Hardaway, were then instrumental in further refining electrolysis for hair removal and for use in removing superficial growths, especially nevi.[44] It is interesting that Hardaway was editor of the *St. Louis Clinical Record,* which published Michel's original article.

The relationship between magnetism and electricity became clarified during the nineteenth century and resulted in scientific investigations that led to significant advances in electricity. Hans Christian Oersted (1777-1851) published his observations in Copenhagen in 1820, which confirmed the influence of direct electric current on the magnetic compass needle. This work stimulated Michael Faraday (1791-1867) in England to suspect that the reverse may also be true; that a magnetic field could induce a current in a wire. Indeed, Faraday showed that *moving* a wire in a magnetic field or *moving* of the magnetic field relative to the wire produced an electric current. This became known as electromagnetic induction. At about the same time Joseph Henry (1787-1878) made the same discovery in the United States.

Electromagnetic induction led to discoveries of induction of currents in nearby wires and induction of higher voltages, which is discussed later. Electromagnetic induction is of immense value because nearly all the world's electrical power is produced by it. To produce electric power, a wire loop is rotated within a magnetic field. This results in a relative magnetic flux within the loop, which constantly changes and produces an electrical potential difference in the wire, thus causing current to flow. Because the current changes direction with the rotation of the wire loop, an alternating current is produced. This alternating current became known as the faradic current.

Initially, induced currents were applied not only for treatment but also for diagnosis of nervous disorders.[77] Guillaume-Benjamin-Amand Duchenne (1806-1875) and Wilhelm Erb (1840-1921) were early pioneers in the use of this current.

The next major discovery of value to medical science was made by d'Arsonval (1851-1940) in France in 1891. The alternating current at 10,000 cycles per second (cps) or above was found to pass through the human body without pain or muscle stimulation but also to produce heat. At less than 10,000 cps, patients experience intense muscle contraction. These high-frequency currents—greater than 10,000 cps—were then used for their heat production in medical treatment.[78]

Thus the use of electrical current for medical purposes evolved, with three types of electricity: static electricity, direct current, and alternating current. Static electricity (franklinism) was difficult to control and quantitate, and direct (galvanic) current also had limited applicability because of the limited voltages and currents obtained; however, alternating (faradic) current offered enormous variations of voltage and current, and moreover, because this type of current (above a certain frequency) could be passed through the human body without obvious harm, its effects were more easily controlled. Faradic current was used in the development of high-frequency electrosurgery units—one of the most important developments in surgery in this century; its history can be found later in this chapter.

ELECTRICAL THEORY

An electric current is the flow of electric charge from one place to another. In a metal the electric charge is composed of electrons that carry a negative charge. These electrons have been dislodged from the outer shell of the atoms comprising the metal. Therefore electric current (i) can be defined as the net negative charge (q) that flows through any cross section of a conductor in time (Δt).

$$i = \frac{q}{\Delta t}$$

The i is expressed in amperes (or amps), q in coulombs, and t in seconds. In a metal wire, 1 a (ampere) results from the movement of 6.242×10^{18} electrons per second.

In a given conductor the current i is the same for all cross sections of a conductor, regardless of the cross-sectional area at different points. Therefore, like water moving through a nozzle, the current flow is faster if the cross-sectional area is smaller, and the current flow is slower if the cross-sectional area is larger.

The volt is a unit of electrical force (electromotive force), which, when applied to a conductive substance, results in movement of electrons. It is generated by the potential difference between two ends of a subtance, which is the result of differences in electric charges.

When a potential difference is applied to a wire, the electrons drift toward the more positive pole. By convention, however, current is depicted to flow from positive to negative. The formulation of this notion is ascribed to Franklin, who proposed that current flows in this direction many years before the discovery of electrons and their charges. However, because a flow of negative electrons in one direction relativistically equals a "flow" of positive charges in the opposite direction, this misinterpretation of current direction was not corrected. *Conventional* current therefore flows from positive to negative, but *real* current flows in the opposite direction, from negative to positive (Fig. 16-1).

Two other useful concepts regarding current are current density and electron drift speed. The *current density (j)* is the current (i) per cross-sectional area (A) of the material through which a current flows. Thus

$$j = i/A$$

Since i (defined as the number of electrons moving past a given point in a unit of time) will be the same in all parts of a circuit, the current density increases or decreases as the cross-sectional size of the conductors in the circuit decreases or increases, respectively. Thus with a thinner electrosurgical electrode tip the current remains the same, but the current density increases.

Electron drift speed (Vd) is the average speed at which electrons move along a wire producing a current. Usually this speed is very slow, literally at a snail's pace. An electron taking 30 seconds to drift 1 cm is not uncommon. But

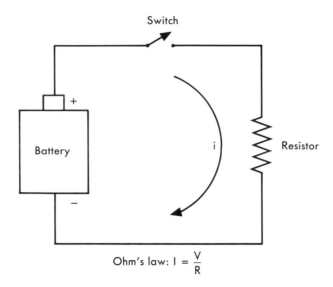

$$\text{Ohm's law: } I = \frac{V}{R}$$

Fig. 16-1. Direct-current circuit generated by battery. Shown here is direction of conventional current *(i)*, which flows from positive pole to negative pole.

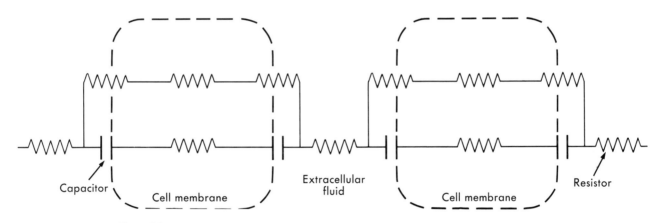

Fig. 16-2. Human tissue acting as both resistor and capacitor to flow of electric current.

this should not be confused with the speed at which the electromagnetic waves are produced along the wire. These waves travel near the speed of light.

Not all materials carry electric charges equally. Some materials are good *conductors*. Such materials, usually metals, have their electrons loosely bound to their atoms. Other materials are poor conductors or *nonconductors* because their outer shell electrons are tightly bound to their atoms. These materials are known as *insulators*. Rubber, as found in surgical gloves, is a good insulator. Materials that are intermediate in their conduction ability are known as *semiconductors;* two common examples are silicon and germanium. Semiconductors may be coated with various materials to enhance their conductivity. Semiconductors are also important in fashioning transistors, discussed later.

Resistance is the ability of a material to impede the passage of an electric current. It is defined as the ratio of the

potential difference at the ends of a material to the current that flows. For instance, if a wire has a potential difference *(V)* applied across its ends, a current *(i)* will flow. This current can be measured and is related mathematically to the resistance *(R)* and the voltage *(V)* by the following formula:

$$R = V/i$$

If *V* is in volts and *i* in amperes, *R* will be in ohms (Ω). Pertinent to the application of current to the human body is the resistance encountered. It was realized over a century ago that this resistance is colossal.[89] Dry skin has a resistance to direct current of 100,000 Ω (Fig. 16-2).

Related to resistance is *resistivity* (ρ), which is characteristic of the material itself rather than the amount of material. The body is not a homogeneous electrical conducting medium but is composed of various tissues, each with a different resistivity. For instance, fat has a high resistivity and muscle a low resistivity. Skin has a variable resistivity, depending on whether it is wet or dry. If wet, the resistivity is low, whereas if dry the resistivity is high. The resistivity of wet skin is about 200 ohm-cm.[46] Resistance is related to both the resisitivity of the substance and the amount of material through which a current flows. This is expressed by the following:

$$R = \rho \frac{l}{A}$$

An increase in the resistivity gives an increased resistance. Resistance may also be increased by increasing the length *(l)* of a substance or decreasing its cross-sectional area *(A)*. Consider two electrodes (an active and an indifferent) from an electrosurgical apparatus applied to a human body. The distance between the electrodes changes the resistance in the circuit in which the body is a part. If the electrodes are far apart, the resistance is greater than if they are closer together.

Current may be either direct current (DC) or alternating current (AC). Direct current is usually produced from a battery and is unidirectional—that is, the current produced flows only in one direction (Fig. 16-1). Direct current is used therapeutically in medicine for electrolysis, iontophoresis, and sometimes electrocautery. Alternating current is produced in power stations and is available at electrical outlets. Alternating current, in which the current flow continuously switches direction, is used in electrocautery and high-frequency electrosurgery (Fig. 16-3).

A battery is a unit that produces a potential difference between two electrodes. The dry-cell battery produces energy on its own, whereas the secondary-cell battery (such as an automobile battery) needs to be charged from without. Dry-cell batteries are usually made with a carbon core and a zinc casing. Electrons migrate from the zinc to the carbon to produce the potential difference, the carbon being positive and the zinc negative. A battery may also be made from copper and zinc electrodes immersed in sulfuric acid and water; the zinc becomes strongly negative and the copper positive. On connection of the two terminals to a circuit, a steady flow of electrons takes place.

If one brings a compass near a wire carrying a current that is moving in one direction (DC), the magnetized compass needle is deflected. Thus an electric current generates a magnetic force. Alternatively a magnet may induce in a wire a current that *moves* within its magnetic field; this phenomenon is known as *electromagnetic induction*. For this phenomenon to occur the wire must be moving, or the current must be increasing or decreasing. One means of producing a constantly increasing and decreasing current is by means of alternating current.

An alternating current from an electrical socket in the United States carries an average voltage of 120 V. Its alternation in current flow is 60 cps (cycles per second); in other words, its current changes direction 120 times a second

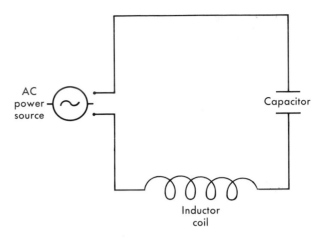

Fig. 16-3. Alternating-current circuit.

(each cycle requires two direction changes). The unit of frequency, cps, is commonly referred to as hertz. One kilohertz (kHz) is 1000 cps, and 1 megahertz (mHz) is 1,000,000 cps. Typically, electrical discharges of 500 to 2000 kHz (2 mHz) are used in an electrosurgical unit.

Consider a wire that is coiled rather than straight. The magnetic field generated by this wire is within the coils and at the ends of the coil. The coil of wire thus acts as a magnet when a changing current is put through the wire coil. The changing current induces a magnetic field flux that in turn induces a current. Thus the coil acts as an *inductor*. The more windings, the greater the voltage and the less the resultant current.

Next, consider a *capacitor*. A capacitor consists of a system, usually two conductive surfaces separated by an insulator (such as air or waxed paper). This insulator is known as the dielectric. In an electrical circuit, the separation of the plates keeps current from flowing across the gap. Therefore if a capacitor is placed in a DC circuit, the current compels negative changes to accumulate in one place and positive charges (really an absence of negative charges) to accumulate in the other plate. Thus a capacitor is a device that stores electric charges. In an AC circuit, a capacitor builds up and discharges charge with the reversal of current direction. Thus a capacitor blocks the flow of direct current but permits alternating current to flow.

Note, however, that the current (defined as movement of electrons) does not actually flow from one plate of the capacitor to the other. Nevertheless, because the plates of the capacitor are charged, a magnetic field in the dieletric is produced, which alters the charges and results in a displacement "current."

Electric current can pass through the human body either as DC or AC. If the current is direct, the human body can be thought of as a resistor with great resistance. This has already been discussed. If an alternating current passes through the body, resistance to current flow also occurs, but

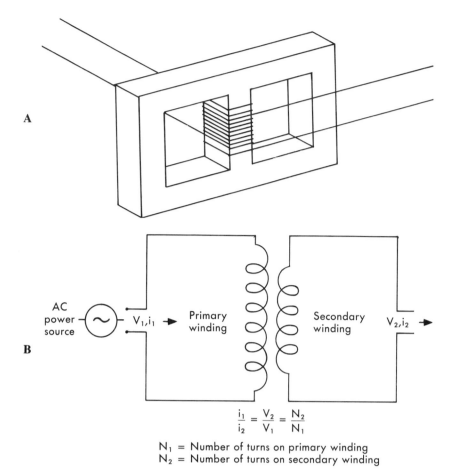

$$\frac{i_1}{i_2} = \frac{V_2}{V_1} = \frac{N_2}{N_1}$$

N_1 = Number of turns on primary winding
N_2 = Number of turns on secondary winding

Fig. 16-4. A, Transformer produced by winding wires in oposite directions around iron core. **B,** Relationship of primary and secondary winding to voltage and current.

with this type of current it is known as *impedance*. AC flow depends not only on the resistors in the circuit but also on other elements (such as capacitors) that impede the flow of current. Human tissue cells act as both resistors and capacitors in series[69,75] (Fig. 16-2). Therefore biologic impedance incorporates this concept and has greater meaning than simply resistance or resistivity, as it was defined previously.

Then consider a circuit in which the coil is connected in series with a capacitor (Fig. 16-3). Alternating current is provided that charges the capacitor. When the current is cut off, the stored charge is discharged into the coil. The coil current induces a magnetic field, which induces a current. The current flows back to the capacitor and charges it up. Again the capacitor discharges back to the coil. Since the current supplied is alternating, this "swinging" current will continue to oscillate. The coil and capacitor allow the oscillations in the current to be increased or amplified. The unit of a coil and capacitor in series is referred to as a resonator.

Imagine taking a wire and coiling it down a cylinder of wood or iron. Then take a second wire and wind it concen-

trically up the cylinder of wood or iron in the opposite direction, so these two wires wind in opposite directions but are intercalated between each other (Fig. 16-4, *A*). Each wire coil is connected to a separate circuit: one circuit is connected to an electrical outlet, and the other is connected to some other device. As the alternating current flows in the first wire, known as the *primary winding*, it induces a magnetic field, which induces a current to flow in the second wire, known as the *secondary winding*. This arrangement produces a transformer, which is a fancy inductor (Fig. 16-4, *B*). The number of turns *(N)* of these windings is related to the total voltage produced according to the following formula:

$$\frac{V_1}{V_2} = \frac{N_1}{N_2}$$

When N_2 has more turns than N_1, the voltage (V_2) is increased. This type of arrangement therefore gives a step-up transformer. Alternatively, when N_2 has fewer turns than N_1, the V_2 is decreased, giving a step-down transformer. Therefore a transformer is a device that uses alternating current to produce a voltage (either increased or decreased) and thus a current in a secondary circuit. In an ideal transformer the power input equals the power output. This can be expressed as the following:

$$P_1 = P_2$$

or

$$i_1 V_1 = i_2 V_2$$

so

$$\frac{i_1}{i_2} = \frac{V_2}{V_1} = \frac{N_2}{N_1}$$

As can be seen, increasing the number of turns in N_2 increases the voltage (V_2) but decreases the amperage (i_2).

Besides changing the voltage or current, transformers serve to separate electrical circuits from the main power supply, so that current cannot flow directly to the ground through the patient. This can be used to advantage in electrosurgical devices as an extra safety feature.

It should be emphasized that the coils of the transformer are quite different from a coil connected to a capacitor, described previously. The coil connected to a capacitor induces a current by the magnetic field it produces. This is sometimes called *self-inductance,* and the coil referred to as a *self-inducting coil.* The inductance that occurs with a transformer is different: one coil induces a current in a second coil.

HEAT PRODUCTION IN TISSUE

Electrosurgical units work in tissue by heat production. Therefore an understanding of heat and its production is essential to understanding how these surgical devices affect tissues and how tissue responds to these devices with the production or conveyance of heat.

Heat may be thought of as a quantity whose presence is associated with an increase in a substance's internal molecular energy. Heat is measured by a thermometer and is expressed in centigrade (Celsius) degrees (C) or Fahrenheit degrees (F). In the former scale 0° is the freezing point of water and 100° C the boiling point; the scale is divided into 100 equal segments in between. The *calorie* is the amount of heat necessary to raise the temperature of 1 g of water by 1° C. Heat may also be expressed in terms of the work done to raise the temperature by 1° C. One calorie equals 4.185 joules of work.

Not all substances subjected to a specified amount of heat have the same degree of temperature increase; some substances resist temperature change more than others. This inertia to temperature change is known as *specific heat,* which is defined as the amount of heat necessary to add to 1 g of a substance to raise its temperature by 1° C. For water this value is high, about 1 cal/g in centigrade.

Water does not necessarily remain fluid but may freeze into ice or may vaporize into steam. These changes in state occur at certain temperatures. To get water to vaporize requires bringing it to the boiling point and then adding more heat to make it vaporize. The amount of heat beyond what is necessary for boiling and which makes water vaporize completely is known as the *heat of vaporization.* For water this requires 540 cal/g (cm³).

Consider that we have 1 g (cm³) of water at body temperature—about 37° C. This amount of water would require 63 cal to raise its temperature to 100° C, the boiling point. An additional 540 calories would then be required to vaporize the water completely. Therefore the vaporization of 1 g of water at body temperature would require 63 cal + 540 cal, equalling 603 cal. This is the equivalent of 2524 joules of work.

Heat can be transferred from one body to another by direct contact (conduction), convection current (flow of matter such as warmed air or liquid), or by radiation. For instance, a true electrocautery (a heated metal) in direct contact with tissue will increase the heat of the tissue by transferring heat from the hotter body (the heated metal) to the colder body (the tissue).

When thermal energy is added to tissue, the local tissue temperature increases. This results in an acceleration of many biochemical reactions, and if this acceleration is great enough, cell death ensues. The cellular changes that take place include cell wall damage, RNA and DNA destruction, and enzyme deactivation. At 100° C, as heat continues to be added to tissue, the water content of cells vaporizes. A vapor seal is then produced, which protects deeper tissue from the further effects of intense heat.

Although H_2O begins to vaporize at 100° C, fats and proteins do not. Triglycerides vaporize at 300° to 400° C and proteins at 600° C. Therefore before fats and proteins dissociate, higher temperatures than 100° C are required. The dissociation of cell structure by heat is known as pyrolysis. Since this requires the falling apart of all cell components, it occurs over a range of 100° to 600° C.

The critical factors that determine cellular damage caused by heat include both the actual temperature and the time for which it is applied.[87] Henriques and Moritz[45] studied the production of thermal injury in pigskin. Irreversible cell damage could be produced with heat as low as 44° C, but the heat had to be applied for 6 hours. As the temperature was increased, the time required for cell injury decreased. These investigators also studied the thermal conductivity of various tissues. Muscle and dermis had the highest and fat the lowest. The heat conductivity of epidermis was also low, almost as low as fat.

With high-frequency electrosurgery, heat is generated within tissue. The electrode tip is not heated enough to cause observable tissue damage—in contrast to electrocautery (already described), in which the electrode tip is heated. Heat within tissues occurs with high frequency electrosurgery because electrical or mechanical energy is converted to heat energy. This conversion can take place in one of three ways. First, the resistance of the tissue to electric current flow causes an increase in the temperature of the tissue itself. The electrical energy is absorbed and converted to thermal energy. This increase in temperature (also known as ohmic heat[19]) is related to the resistance of the specific tissue (resistivity), the method of application of the electric current, the current density (the cross-sectional area of application of the current per unit time), the duration of application of the current, and the type of current. For instance, fat has a high resistance (about 2200 Ω) and muscle a low resistance (about 110 Ω).[75] Skin has a variable resistance, which is high when it is dry and low when it is wet. Therefore fat heats more than muscle, given equal current for an equal length of time. Another factor related to resistance of tissue is the method of current application. If two electrodes are placed 1 cm apart on tissue, the intervening tissue offers a certain resistance. If the same two electrodes are then placed a meter apart, the amount of intervening tissue is increased, and the resistance is subsequently increased. If only one electrode is used, as is common with electrodesiccation, the resistance is increased dramatically.

A high-frequency electrosurgical machine produces a concentrated current in a small needle type of electrode. This results in a high current density. The tissue heat produced, as shall soon be seen, is proportional to the square of the current and to the current density;[19] current density is inversely proportional to the area of application of the current.[28] As the current spreads out over the human body, it is conducted over a much larger surface area. This effectively reduces the current density, and no significant heating occurs. If an indifferent electrode is used, the current completes its path back to the electrosurgery unit via this pathway. Since the indifferent electrode is relatively large, it also serves to keep the current density low, and no significant heating occurs where it touches the patient's skin—assuming that a large area of adequate contact exists. Any heating that does occur is readily dissipated by the blood stream.

It is important to remember that with high-frequency alternating current, as produced by an electrosurgical unit, the current is flowing both into and out of the human body. The body acts as a capacitor, storing and discharging charge. If an indifferent electrode is not used, the earth forms the other plate of the capacitor, with air as the dielectric. If an indifferent electrode is used, then the circuit is primarily resistive. In either case the heat produced in tissue is a reflection of the work done to move this current in *both* directions.[48]

The second way a high-frequency electrosurgical apparatus can increase the heat in tissue is by the dissipation of electrical and thermal energy from the spark. When a current jumps across an air gap to tissue, a bright light (a *spark*) is produced in the air gap. The actual physics of sparks is poorly understood; they are presumed to be the result of ionization of gases that carry the current in the air. Spark size and temperature are related to the voltage of the machine. The greater the voltage, the greater the spark and the more its thermal energy. The temperature of an electric spark can be as high as 1000° C.[26] The electrodesiccation current is a relatively low current associated with a high voltage. Therefore production of heat with this current is mainly by the spark ("convective sparks"[15]) and secondarily by the current. Tissue destruction occurs mainly at the surface, where the spark energy is dissipated.

The third way in which a high-frequency electrosurgical apparatus can produce heat is by means of mechanical energy.[10] These machines produce at the active electrode tip electromagnetic waves that oscillate, and the waves result in a force that may produce disruption of cells and the production of some heat energy.

The amount of energy—heat, electrical, mechanical—that passes through a given space is expressed as the power density. At the tissue level the power density (PD) expresses the amount of energy (power) produced within a specified quantity of tissue. Therefore where P is power (expressed in watts or joules/second) and the unit of tissue is a cubic centimeter *(cm³)*,

$$PD = \frac{P}{cm^3}$$

Power is defined as the amount of work *(Δw)* per unit of time *(Δt)*, or

$$P = \frac{w}{\Delta t}$$

Power density at the point of tissue contact with an electrode tip is different than it is at a distance away from that point. The power density falls off rapidly as one moves away from the power source and is inversely related to the square of the distance.

$$PD \propto \frac{1}{r^2}$$

In this case r is the radial distance from an electrode tip.

In electrical terms power is defined as the work done in moving a current *(i)* over a voltage difference *(V)*.

$$(1)\ P = iV$$

In this instance i is in amperes, and V is in volts. Since in skin the resistance is constant, one can use Ohm's law (V = iR) and substitute into this equation. Therefore one gets the following:

$$(2) \ P = i(iR) = i^2R$$

$$(3) \ P = \left(\frac{V}{R} \right) V = \frac{V^2}{R}$$

The heating effects of electric currents are proportional to the square of the current (formula 2) or the square of the voltage (formula 3). Since the power delivered to tissue is proportional to the square of the current, then as the current is doubled, the power (which results in heat energy) is quadrupled. Thus the greater heat is produced where the current or the voltage is increased. Also note that since the resistance is constant, a greater increase in power (tissue heating) is achieved by an increase in current than by an increase in voltage.

Since joules can be related to calories (4.186 joules equals 1 cal), power density can then be related to temperature rise (ΔT) in tissue by converting joules into calories by the following formula:

$$\Delta T = \frac{PD}{4.186}$$

Honig calculated the PD for tissue at the point of contact of an electrode tip to be 3300 watts/cm^3 if the electrosurgical unit has a power output of 15 watts.[46] If the power output is 150 watts, the PD is 33,000 watts. These power densities give rise to approximate temperature increases (per second) of 830 cal/cm^3 (¼ × 3300 watt/cm^3) or 8300 cal/cm^3 (¼ × 33,000 watt/cm^3), respectively.

The heat of vaporization of water is the heat in calories that is necessary to produce water vapor once water is boiling. For water this is 540 cal/cm^3. Since epithelial tissue is mostly water, we can use the heat of water vaporization to approximate the heat necessary to vaporize this tissue. At 15 watts of power, there is enough heat (830 cal/cm^3) generated to vaporize tissue, since 603 cal/cm^3 is required to vaporize tissue at body temperature (540 cal/cm^3 + 63 cal/cm^3 = 603 cal/cm^3). At 150 watts of power there is certainly enough heat (8300 cal/cm^3 to cause vaporization. Most electrosurgical units operate in a range between these two extremes of wattage.

It should be appreciated that the foregoing calculations are only approximations. In the conversion of mechanical or electrical energy to heat energy some heat is lost, so this process is not 100% efficient; some heat is lost to the surrounding air or is swept away by blood vessels if it is applied to human tissue. However, such calculations do give us a means with which to compare different instruments that purportedly accomplish the same goal.

ELECTROLYSIS

Electrolysis is the destruction or decomposition of tissues with the negative pole of a galvanic (DC) current.[11]

The conduction of direct current through tissues is electrolytic—that is, this type of electric current results in chemical changes. The cell membranes, which are semipermeable, become polarized, and this polarization leads to cell death.

Equipment

A typical electrolysis circuit is shown in Fig. 16-5. A 22.5 V battery is connected to a variable resistor and a milliammeter. The patient holds the positive electrode in the hand, and the treatment is performed with the negative electrode.

The current that flows in this circuit ionizes the tissue solutions with which it comes in contact. At the negative pole the sodium ions (which have positive charges) accumulate and react with water. This produces sodium hydroxide and hydrogen gas. The sodium hydroxide destroys cells adjacent to the needle and produces very slight pain. At the positive pole the chloride ions (which have negative charges) accumulate and also react with water. This produces hydrochloric acid and oxygen gas. The hydrochloric acid causes pain and coagulation of proteins. In addition, ferrous ions (Fe^{++}) are repelled into the tissue, causing tattooing (the ferrous ion is probably oxidized by the readily available oxygen produced at this electrode to colloidal iron oxide, which is black). These reactions may be expressed as follows:

$$2 \ NaCl + 4 \ H_2O \overset{-}{\underset{+}{\Large\diagup\!\!\!\!\diagdown}} \begin{array}{l} \longrightarrow 2 \ NaOH + 2H_2 \uparrow \\ \longrightarrow 2 \ HCl + O_2 \uparrow \end{array}$$

Because tattooing and needless tissue destruction are undesirable, the negative pole is always the treatment electrode, and the positive pole is always the "indifferent," or nontreatment, electrode. The nontreatment positive electrode is large and is not inserted into tissue, so that any effects it might have are completely dispersed.

The current used for successful electrolysis varies from ¼ to 2 ma. Usually ½ to 1 ma is recommended.[11] At 2 ma the patient experiences significant pain. To achieve this low current, the variable resistor is used in the circuit, since innate body resistance to direct current is relatively low (2000 to 4000 ohms).

Using Ohm's Law for current,

$$I = \frac{V}{R}$$

we get

$$1 \ ma = \frac{22.5 \ volts}{R}$$

Electrolysis circuit

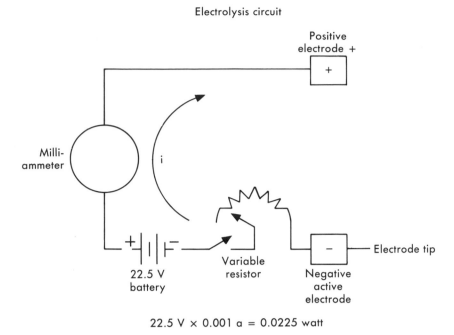

$$22.5 \text{ V} \times 0.001 \text{ a} = 0.0225 \text{ watt}$$

Fig. 16-5. Electrolysis unit circuit. Conventional current *(i)* is shown traveling from positive to negative pole. Actual electron flow is in opposite direction from negative to positive pole.

Solving this equation for *R*, we find that 22,500 ohms of resistance is necessary to provide 1 ma of current in the circuit in Fig. 16-5. To provide a ½ ma of current would then require 50,000 ohms of resistance. The resistor is invaluable in achieving such a low current with this circuit. Thus the electrolysis circuit is low amperage, low voltage.

Faraday investigated electrolysis in chemical solutions in the 1830s and showed that a fixed amount of charge always liberated a fixed amount of gas at each electrode. More specifically, he showed that 96,500 coulombs (a measure of electrical charge) in water evolved 1 g of H_2 gas at the negative electrode and 8 g of O_2 gas at the positive electrode. This unit—96,500 coulombs—became known as a faraday (F).

In an electrolysis circuit at the negative electrode, hydrogen gas is produced. If 1 ma is used for 60 seconds, approximately 0.06 coulombs is used, based on the following:

$$i = \frac{q}{\Delta t}$$

The current in amperes is *i*, *q* is the charge in coulombs, and *t* is the time in seconds.

$$0.001 \text{ amp} = \frac{q}{60 \text{ sec}}$$

$$q = 0.06 \text{ coulomb}$$

If 96,500 coulombs (96,500 Q) yields 1 g of H_2 gas, 0.06 Q yields the following:

$$\frac{96,500 \text{ Q}}{0.06 \text{ Q}} = \frac{1 \text{ g } H_2\uparrow}{x \text{ g } H_2\uparrow}$$

$$x \text{ g } H_2\uparrow = 1 \text{ g } H_2\uparrow \times \frac{0.06Q}{96,500Q} = 6 \times 10^{-7} \text{ g } H_2\uparrow$$

Clinical applications

The performance of electrolysis requires practice, patience, and time. It is useful for destroying hair papillae and telangiectasias but has been supplanted to a large extent by other techniques. Nevertheless, its proper performance probably leads to excellent results. Machines made specifically for electrolysis (for instance, Gal Tel-18, manufactured by Galvanic Medical Instruments, Inc., Paramus, N.J. 07652) are available commercially and should be used.

Hair removal. The technique of electrolysis for hair removal is as follows. The patient is placed supine on either an examining table or a reclining chair. The operator is usually behind the patient. The positive electrode is grasped by the patient and held in the palm. The skin is cleansed first with soap and then with a disinfectant. The active (negative) electrode is introduced into the follicular ostium and directed parallel to the hair shaft, which usually is tangential to the skin surface. Ideally the needle slides to the bottom of the hair follicle (approximately 3 to 5 mm below the skin surface), where slight resistance is felt. It may be best then to advance the needle an additional half millimeter to get to the hair bulb.[10] The current is *slowly* turned on until about 1

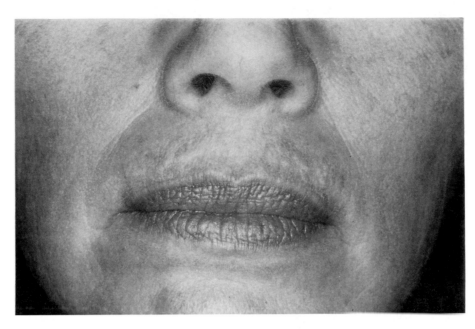

Fig. 16-6. Scarring of upper lip subsequent to electrolysis.

ma of current is flowing. After 30 to 60 seconds, small white bubbles, which appear as a white froth, arise at the ostium of the follicle. The bubbles are hydrogen gas bubbles (H_2). If the hair papilla has been acted upon sufficiently by the galvanic current, a slight tug on the hair itself will slide the hair easily out of the follicle. The current then is *slowly* turned off. Abrupt changes in current, which produce power surges, cause pain. *The needle is not removed until after the current has been turned off.*

It is recommended that contiguous hairs not be treated at the same sitting, since this may set up a mild inflammatory reaction. Improper placement of the treatment electrode needle may result in pain, bleeding, or edema. If resistance to entrance of the needle occurs, the needle should be repositioned. The smallest amount of current that can effectively and permanently remove hair should be selected.

Regrowth of hair from a follicle that has been subjected to electrolysis is not uncommon. This can occur because not enough current was produced for a long enough period of time to the area immediately adjacent to the papilla. It may also occur if multiple hairs with their papillae have a common follicular orifice. The patient is reseen at intervals to retreat the regeneration of hair in treated follicles.

The problems or complications from electrolysis include scars (Fig. 16-6) and pits (caused by too much current or improperly positioned needles), infection, edema, ecchymoses, pain, hypopigmentation, and keloids. Treating a small test area is therefore recommended.[11] Endocarditis has also been reported after electrolysis.[17]

Electrolysis produces a small (100 μm) zone of destruction around hair follicles.[32] This zone is cylindrical and extends from the base of the follicle to the skin surface. Some investigators mention a cone-shaped zone of destruction, with the skin surface representing the base of the cone; however, the cylindrical zone is more common. Whatever the shape, the necrosis of tissue leads inevitably to a small scar (microscar), which is frequently inapparent. Insulated treatment needles for electrolysis are available, which theoretically minimize surface scarring. The insulation may be Teflon, silicone or some other synthetic polymer. The insulation in the needle reaches to within 1 mm of the tip, thus concentrating the current at this point. Electrolysis needles may be tapered and have a rounded (or bulbous) tip to keep them from penetrating tissue. Insulated needles supposedly cause less pain on increasing the current and less tissue destruction above the area of the papilla. Theoretically this should result in less inflammation and less scarring.

Permanent removal of hair may also be achieved with a high-frequency electrosurgical apparatus (discussed later).

Most electrolysis is currently performed by properly trained electrologists, who in many states must be licensed.[105] Although Cipollaro[11] in 1938 advised that this technique be used only by physicians, most physicians currently refer their patients to nonphysicians for this treatment. Since the technique is time consuming and requires an experienced touch, this is probably acceptable; however, the relinquishment of electrolysis to nonmedical personnel has resulted in a lack of recent research on this technique.

Telangiectasias. Telangiectasias of the face may be treated successfully with electrolysis. This is accomplished by vertical insertion of the electrolysis needle at intervals along the vessel's course[11] or horizontal insertion of the electrode

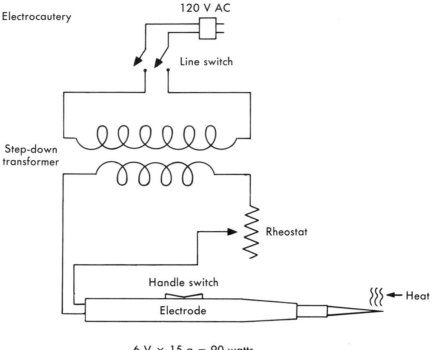

6 V × 15 a = 90 watts

Fig. 16-7. Electrocautery unit circuit.

needle into the vessel. The latter technique is more difficult and may lead to more scarring. The amperage used for treatment of telangiectasias is about 2 ma and is given until color change or blanching of the vessel is visible. Electrolysis is not recommended for treatment of telangiectasias on the legs, since it may lead to significant scarring in this area—probably caused by the difference in the types of vessels (venous rather than arterial), which are dilated on the lower extremities compared to the face (see Chapter 18).

Miscellaneous uses. Electrolysis was used more than a hundred years ago for removal of small nevi, warts, papillomas, and superficial carcinomas.[9,44] The multiple-needle technique, with several small negative electrodes which were inserted crisscross in the lesion, was once used for this purpose. However, the modern high-frequency electrosurgical apparatus is currently used almost exclusively for this purpose because it is faster. Whether less scarring occurs with electrolysis versus the other electrosurgical techniques has not been systematically investigated and may be worthy of future inquiry.

ELECTROCAUTERY

Electrocautery is the use of heated metal in direct contact with tissue to effect heating of the tissue. It results in tissue desiccation, coagulation, or necrosis. It should be emphasized that no electric current is passed to the patient; the destructive effects are caused solely by heat transference.

Equipment

A typical electrocautery circuit is shown in Fig. 16-7. A step-down transformer is used, so that the 120 V outlet current is decreased to 6 V or less. As we have seen, this occurs with a proportional increase in amperage. Thus the amperage produced is high: about 15 a. The resultant wattage will be 15 a × 6 V = 90 watts (P = i × V).

The treatment tip of the electrocautery unit is usually made of a wire of relatively high resistivity, such as a platinum alloy, that can also withstand high temperatures. The high current flowing through this wire increases its temperature. Thus the electrocautery unit is a medical toaster or soldering iron.[10] When this heated tip is applied to tissues, its heat is transferred to the tissue with subsequent destructive effects.

The heat transferred by electrocautery is limited in the extent of penetrance. Most of the heat is dissipated at the epidermis and papillary dermis, from which the cutaneous vasculature carries away heat. Thus the amount of tissue destruction with electrocautery is limited but also easily seen and controllable.

There is no temperature readout that determines the actual temperature of the electrocautery unit's tip. Resistance to the current flowing through the tip determines the temperature of the tip. The rheostat controls the circuit resistance. Decreasing the resistance increases the current (as given in Ohm's law V = iR). The color of the tip is roughly related to the temperature. When the tip is dull red it is ready to use. A bright cherry red is hotter, and white is hottest. Heating with a white-hot tip is to be avoided, since this destroys more tissue than necessary. Skene[101] determined the heat required for desiccation of tissue with electrocautery and found that it ideally occurs at 83° to 88° C. This is hot enough to cook tissue effectively without charring or burning. However, the duration of heat application was not recorded by this investigator—but, as we have discussed, it is critical in determining tissue destruction.[45]

A relatively new device, the Shaw scalpel (Oximetrix, Inc., Mountain View, Calif.) was introduced in the early 1980s.[35] It is a heated sharp scalpel blade and thus a true electrocautery device, which mechanically cuts and at the same time stops bleeding by thermal transference of heat. This device is highly sophisticated, with special sensors in the scalpel blade that automatically adjust the blade to whatever temperature the physician selects within the given range, 120° to 270° C.

The temperature-control mechanism of the Shaw scalpel compensates heat loss that varies depending on the vascularity of the tissue being cut and the rate at which the blade traverses the tissue. When more heat is desired for a short period of time for easy coagulation, a special switch on the handle automatically increases the blade temperature to 270° C. The blade is Teflon coated to keep tissue from sticking and may be obtained in either the No. 11 or the No. 15 scalpel blade configuration. An advantage of electrocautery is that there is no electric current passing through the patient and thus less danger in the surgical environment. In addition, the amount of tissue destruction is minimal and more easily controllable than with high-frequency electrosurgical devices.

Clinical applications

The electrocautery unit is useful in removing superficial exophytic skin growths.[10,101] Unlike high-frequency electrosurgery (discussed later), the amount of tissue damage is easily controllable and more readily apparent. In addition, electrocautery works in a bloody field to a greater extent than high-frequency electrosurgery does.

After the administration of a local anesthetic, the tip of the electrocautery unit (which is dull red) is stroked through the lesion to be removed. The handle is held at an angle to the skin, and the lesion is removed in layers. If deeper heating is required for greater tissue destruction, the current is turned up in the machine, and the tip on the handle becomes cherry red.

The Shaw scalpel is useful in excising tissue in very vascular areas, such as the scalp. Therefore I use it for scalp reductions or tumor excisions in this area. Because it coagulates tissue as it cuts, blood vessels are sealed as the scalpel traverses tissue, resulting in less blood loss at the time of surgery and less additional effort to seal these blood vessels

once the excision has been performed. Therefore this device saves time and drudgery during surgery.

Another use for the Shaw scalpel is in patients with pacemakers. Since no current flows to the patient, a significant electromagnetic field is not produced in the tissue being cut. Thus there is no interference with the sensing unit on a pacemaker.

I usually cut with the Shaw scalpel at 150° C. I have found empirically that this temperature usually gives adequate hemostasis with minimal tissue destruction. If any significant bleeding is encountered that is not controlled by this temperature, the temperature can be almost instantaneously elevated to 270° C by a switch on the handle. Occasionally arterial bleeding is not controlled even by 270° C, because the depth of heat penetration by contact transference is limited. In such a case I simply tie off the bleeders, or I may use high-frequency electrosurgery.

HIGH-FREQUENCY ELECTROSURGERY

High-frequency electrosurgery is the use of a high-frequency AC apparatus to destroy, cut, or coagulate tissue. The apparatus produces heat by allowing electric current to pass directly into tissue; an electrocautery apparatus, on the other hand, transfers heat to tissue by contact transference. With electrocautery, current does not flow directly to tissue, so its effects are indirect. The electrode tip of a high-frequency electrosurgical unit does not get hot enough from current flow to produce a significant effect on tissues.

Equipment

A typical spark-gap machine is shown in Fig. 16-8. The current from an AC wall outlet is fed into a step-up transformer. This increases the voltage from 120 V to 550 V. This high voltage is necessary to overcome the air gap between the two sides of a spark gap. The wider the spark gap is set, the higher the voltage must be to bridge it. When the spark jumps across the spark gap, it discharges the current into the coil and the capacitor. This current, being AC, produces electromagnetic waves that have a certain wavelength and frequency (explained later). The frequency of these waves is correlated with the AC frequency that is amplified in the coil and capacitor by the current swinging back and forth between them. The active treatment electrode is attached to one end of the coil; the indifferent electrode is attached somewhere between the coil and capacitor.

With high-frequency electrosurgery an alternating current flows through the patient. The patient's tissues act as a network of resistors and capacitors connected in parallel as well as in series[69] (Fig. 16-2). Therefore voltage differences arise when this current flows.

High-frequency electrosurgical machines may be either monoterminal or biterminal. In the biterminal arrangement the patient is grounded by a relatively large indifferent electrode, which does not concentrate current but diffuses it

Electrocoagulation

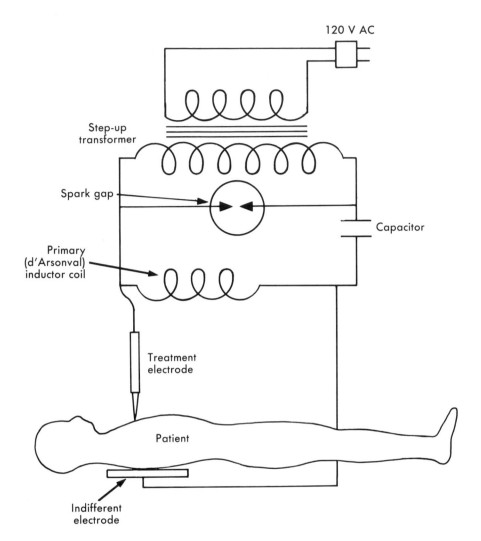

120 V AC

Step-up
transformer

Spark gap

Capacitor

Primary
(d'Arsonval)
inductor coil

Treatment
electrode

Patient

Indifferent
electrode

Fig. 16-8. High-frequency electrosurgical unit for electrocoagulation. Note that apparatus uses spark gap and is biterminal, having indifferent electrode as well as active treatment electrode.

harmlessly and carries it back to the machine and then to ground. In the monoterminal arrangement the patient does not have an indifferent electrode. The patient acts as a capacitor with ground, shedding free electrons to the air, walls, floors or any object contacting him (Fig. 16-9). One should note that the terms "monopolar" and "bipolar," which are often used instead of monoterminal and biterminal, are not entirely clear terms, since current does not flow continuously from one fixed positive electrode to a negative electrode, as in a DC circuit. The terms "monopolar" and "bipolar" should thus be eliminated when referring to a high-frequency electrosurgical unit outlet or its current.

A modern electrosurgical unit has a plug with three prongs. One prong carries the line current, whereas the other, similar prong is a neutral line that connects the unit

to ground. A third, usually round prong, is the safety ground line. This line is connected to the casing of the unit and carries any stray (leakage) currents that may be present back to ground. This prevents a current from flowing through any grounded individual who happens to touch the machine if a leakage current exists. Large leakage currents may cause a shock.

Waveforms and electromagnetic radiation. When alternating electric current flows, electromagnetic fields are generated. These fields produce electromagnetic radiation, which travels through space in waves at the speed of light and therefore behaves like other types of radiation—including visible light and x-rays. Electromagnetic radiation is a nonionizing form of energy, the basic unit of which is the photon. The energy of these photons is very low (10^{-6} elec-

Electrofulguration and
electrodesiccation

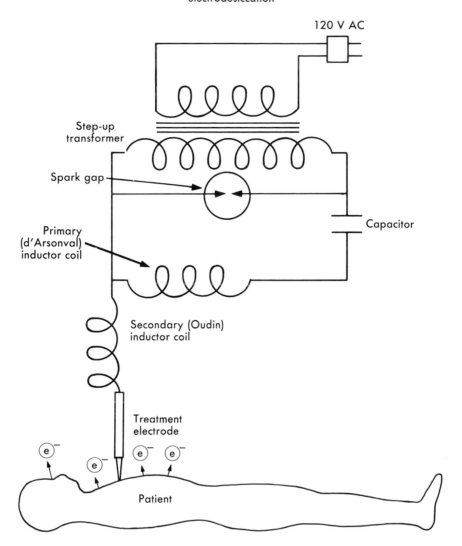

Fig. 16-9. High-frequency electrosurgical unit for electrodesiccation or electrofulguration. Note that apparatus uses spark gap and is monoterminal, having active treatment electrode only. Free electrons are thus shed into air and onto surrounding objects.

tron volts) compared with that of ionizing radiation (such as x-rays), which have a value of 10^3 electron volts, or a billion times more energy than nonionizing radiation.[88] Electromagnetic waves have a wavelength, frequency, and amplitude. Let us consider a sinusoidal wave (Fig. 16-10). It has a regular, even displacement above and below the horizontal axis. Its wavelength (λ), which can be measured as the distance between two peaks (or crests) on one side of the horizontal axis, is also regular. Its frequency (ν) is a measure of how many waves pass a given point within a specified period of time, usually a second. Since the waves travel at the speed of light *(C)*, the frequency (ν) is related to the wavelength (λ) by the following formula:

$$\lambda = \frac{C}{\nu} = \frac{300,000,000 \text{ meters/sec}}{\nu}$$

In electrosurgery, very frequent alternations of current (500,000 to 3,000,000 cps) produce electromagnetic waves with commensurate frequencies and wavelengths of 600 m to 100 m, respectively. These fall within the range of medium-frequency (MF) radio wavelengths. Low-frequency (LF) and very-low frequency (VLF) alternating currents below 100 kHz produce electromagnetic wavelengths that, when applied to the human body, result in tetany. Such currents are used in electroshock treatment for mental depression. Higher frequencies in the range 10,000,000 to 100,000,000 cps (wavelengths of 30 m to 3 m, respectively) result in high-frequency (HF) and very–high frequency (VHF) radio wavelengths and are used in medial diathermy. VHF radiowaves are 30 to 100 MHz. An AM radio receives radiowaves between 525 and 1610 kHz and thus will be

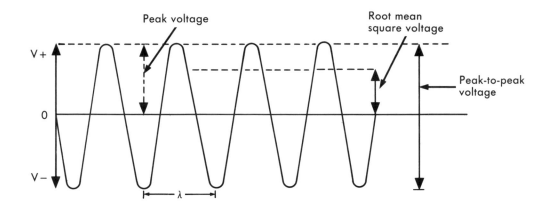

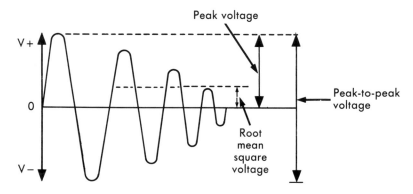

Fig. 16-10. Undamped *(top)* and damped *(bottom)* sinusoidal wavetrain configurations.

interfered with by a high-frequency electrosurgical unit. An FM radio, on the other hand, receives radiowaves between 88 and 108 MHz and is thus above the range for electromagnetic wave frequencies put out by such units.

Electromagnetic waves also have an amplitude, which is the measured deflection above or below the horizontal axis. This deflection is not related to wavelength or frequency. It is, however, determined by the voltage: the higher the voltage, the greater is the electromagnetic wave amplitude.

A damped sinuoidal wavetrain configuration (Fig. 16-10) is a strong primary wave followed by similar waves with amplitudes that diminish over time. A damped nonsinusoidal wavetrain is more regular and produced by a spark jumping across an air gap, which is found in a spark-gap high-frequency electrosurgical apparatus. The spark transmits the current to the resonator (coil and capacitor), which resonates the current, and the current produces diminishing electromagnetic waves like echoes. An undamped sinusoidal wavetrain configuration contains undamped waves that result from current movement in a vacuum tube, where there is no air resistance. Both damped and undamped waves can also be produced from current flow in transistors and diodes found in modern solid-state high-frequency electrosurgical apparatus.

Wavetrains may also be characterized by their continuity

(Fig. 16-11). An uninterrupted wavetrain is continuous. An interrupted wavetrain is discontinuous. Both undamped sinusoidal and damped wavetrains may be continuous or discontinuous.

Empirically it was found that a current associated with a continuous sinusoidal wavetrain is best for cutting, whereas a damped wavetrain is best for fulguration or coagulation. If damped wavetrains are discontinuous, less heat is produced because the current does not act continuously. If damped wavetrains of the same amplitudes are continuous, more heat is produced. In solid-state circuits the coagulation current may be associated with damped wavetrains and the cut-coagulation current (blended current) produced by an undamped discontinuous sinusoidal wavetrain.

Returning to Fig. 16-10, if we try to determine the average wave amplitude (average peak-to-peak voltage) of a sinusoidal wavetrain we arrive at a figure of 0 because the deflection is equal in both directions. This will be true of any wavetrain produced by AC. Therefore, another figure has been determined, known as the root mean square (RMS) amplitude which expresses the average effective amplitude (corresponding to the average effective voltage) for a wavetrain. The RMS amplitude may be close to the maximal amplitude of the wavetrain, or it may be far removed from it. The more irregular and damped the wavetrain, the less

Continuous undamped

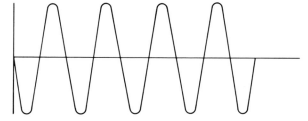

Continuous damped

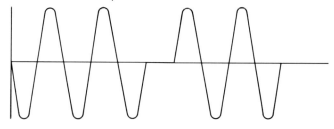

Discontinuous undamped

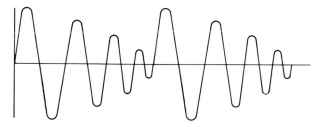

Discontinuous damped

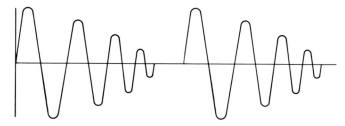

Fig. 16-11. Comparison between continuous and discontinuous wavetrains, which are either damped or undamped.

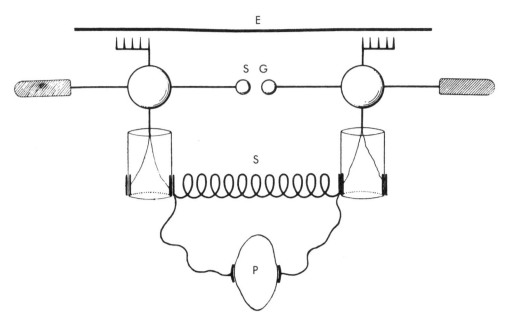

Fig. 16-12. Early device for medical diathermy. (From Morton, W.J.: Arch. d'Elect. Med. **16**:163, 1908.)

likely it is that the RMS amplitude will be near the maximal amplitude. Also, the more discontinuous the wavetrains, the lower the RMS voltage. For an electrical outlet the standard voltage in the United States (120 V) represents RMS voltage. The true peak voltage is about 170 volts, and the peak-to-peak voltage is 340 volts.

Consider a damped wavetrain with a very high-amplitude initial wave followed by waves of successively lower amplitudes. The RMS amplitude may be fairly low. The peak amplitude represents the highest or lowest power (or voltage) and occurs at the beginning portion of the damped wavetrain. With an undamped continuous wavetrain the RMS amplitude is closer to the peak amplitude, because the amplitude of the first wave is followed by waves with similar amplitudes. One way in which a damped wavetrain can have the same effective power (expressed as RMS voltage as an undamped wavetrain is to have an extremely high peak voltage. Such a high peak voltage results in longer sparks at the site of the treatment electrode. Thus the peak voltage is proportional to how far a spark jumps in the air.

The ratio of the maximal amplitude to the RMS amplitude may be expressed as a numerical value known as the *crest factor*. The higher this value, the greater is the coagulation effect on tissue because the peak voltage is increased compared with the RMS voltage. The lower the crest factor, the less is the coagulation effect of the current because the peak voltage is probably lower.[68]

High-frequency electrosurgery and its historical development

Various authors distinguish between electrofulguration, electrodesiccation, electrocoagulation, and electrotomy currents produced by high-frequency electrosurgical units. As with many electrosurgical terms, the best way to understand the meaning of these designations is to view the historical development of the modern electrosurgical machine.

After it was discovered, alternating current was tried on patients for a variety of ailments, mostly nervous disorders. However, at the low frequencies initially used it led to spasmodic contractions of muscles and pain. Around 1890 Jacques Arséne d'Arsonval introduced higher-frequency alternating currents by means of a special tightly wound coil (a solenoid), which became known as the d'Arsonval coil. Used with a capacitor, this coil could generate electromagnetic waves with frequencies greater than 10,000 cps. D'Arsonval demonstrated that with more than 10,000 cps, there were no muscular contractions and no pain for patients.[21,28] In other words, here was a form of electricity that did not have any apparent untoward effects on patients. D'Arsonval later demonstrated that he could illuminate a light bulb by passing his high-frequency current through two persons.[23]

Another important investigation by d'Arsonval was the effect of voltage on tissues when the average voltage was varied. With constant current a high voltage resulted in decomposition of cells, whereas a low voltage resulted in vaporization of water in tissues only.[22] This study was a prelude to the development of different types of high-frequency electrosurgical currents. It is worth remembering that a direct current passing through tissue is electrolytic and polarizes cell membranes, resulting in cell death. An alternating current, however, by reversing its direction of flow reverses any cell membrane polarity produced. The net effect is little tissue damage at low current densities.

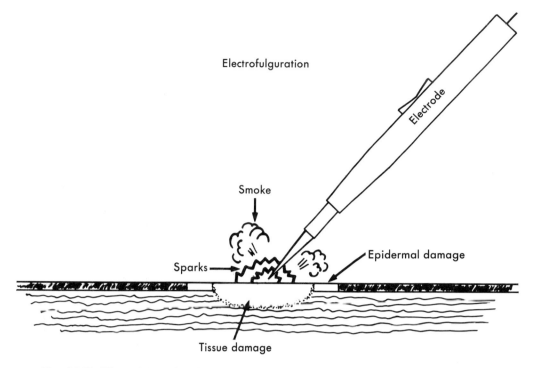

Fig. 16-13. Electrofulguration. Note long, thick sparks. Electrode tip does not touch tissue.

The high-frequency apparatus of d'Arsonval was used to treat a number of disorders (Fig. 16-12). Although no muscular contraction occurred, deep heat did occur. This heat was used successfully by Nagelschmidt as early as 1907 to treat joint and circulatory diseases.[78]

Around the turn of the century, A.J. Riviére treated a lesion (probably a squamous cell carcinoma) on the back of a musician's hand with such an apparatus.[93] The treatment electrode was large, so as to not concentrate the current, and by accident Riviére touched one of the circular wires in the d'Arsonval coil. This generated a spark, which was harmless but gave him the idea to use a spark to treat the patient's lesion, which he did. The lesion healed and high-frequency electrosurgery was born.

The next advance came with the use of the Oudin "resonator": an additional coil attached to the d'Arsonval coil (really a solenoid, or tightly wound coil). This effectually raised the voltage of the apparatus and produced a very fine spraylike series of sparks. (Remember that increasing the number of turns in an inductor coil increases the voltage but decreases the amperage.)

DeKeating-Hart in 1908 or earlier is credited with introducing the term *fulguration* (from the Latin *fulgur,* meaning lightning), referring to the use of the spark from the Oudin coil[15,16,24,91] (Fig. 16-13). He claimed that this method (sparking from a distance) was effective in the cure of deep-seated malignancies, and that the spark from the Oudin coil selectively destroyed tumor cells. Pozzi confirmed the work of deKeating-Hart and used the same type of apparatus successfully for tumors.[91] The sparks produced by these early machines were quite long, up to 3 inches.[49] In addition, the tissue destruction produced was erratic because the sparking to the tissue could not be easily controlled.

In 1909 Doyen introduced the term *coagulation* (from the Latin *coagulare,* meaning to curdle). He added an indifferent electrode at the other end of the Oudin coil and thus produced a biterminal device.[15,29] Doyen realized that using the Oudin or d'Arsonval coil without the indifferent electrode resulted in giving the surgeon or other bystanders shocks. This occurred because the electrosurgical device acted to charge the patient statically. The indifferent electrode gave this charge a path on which to flow back to the machine. In addition, since it increased the voltage difference in the current pathway, the current itself was increased (remember that V = iR, or i = V/R). Moreover, the quantity of heat produced in tissue was more easily controlled.[49]

Doyen measured the temperature of tissue at the surface and deeper. He measured temperatures of 500° to 600° C at the skin surface if the electrode was separated from the tissue, but only 65° to 70° C within the coagulation zone if the electrode touched the skin (Fig. 16-14). Doyen realized that the biterminal arrangement allowed a stronger current with the electrode in contact with the tissue; it penetrated more deeply and coagulated the tissue, whereas if the electrode was separated from the tissue, carbonization occurred, mostly on the surface. In other words, fulguration severely cooks the tissue at the skin surface with little depth destruction, whereas coagulation is produced by contact with the tissue of an electrode with a high current. Doyen claimed that his more deeply penetrating current was more likely to

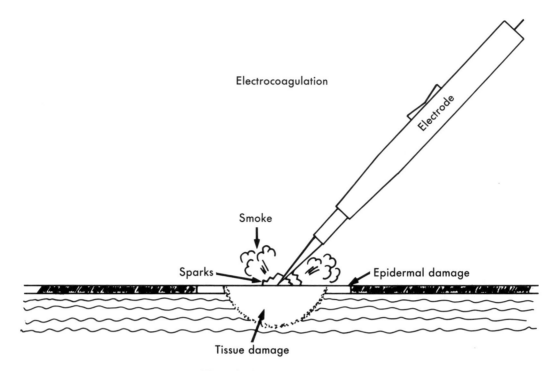

Fig. 16-14. Electrocoagulation.

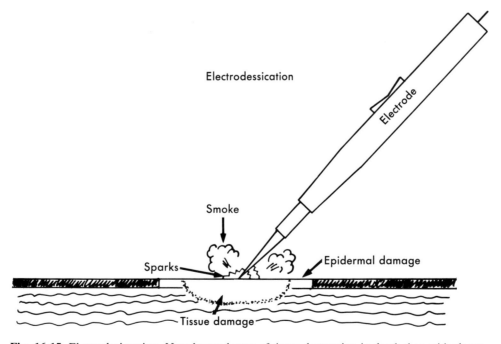

Fig. 16-15. Electrodesiccation. Note lesser degree of tissue destruction in depth than with electrocoagulation. Sparks may not occur initially with electrodesiccation.

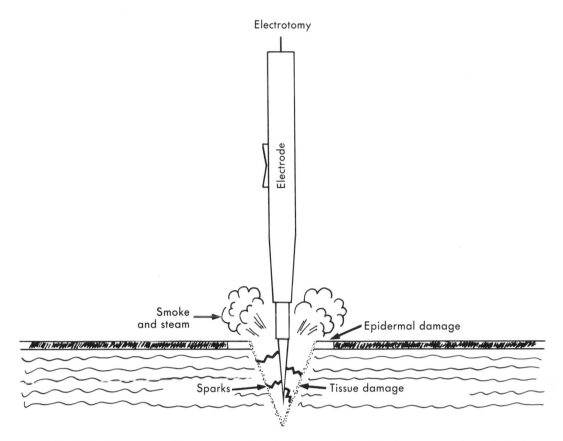

Fig. 16-16. Electrotomy. Note presence of sparks and steam. Steam barrier separates electrode *(top)* from tissue.

destroy tumor cells. DeKeating-Hart also realized the stronger effects of a biterminal apparatus.[24] The biterminal apparatus was soon applied by other physicians to other surgical problems, such as abscesses in body cavities.[25]

A variation of the biterminal approach is to use the two electrodes, an active and an "indifferent" electrode, both with needlelike tips set into the tissue to be treated. The current density and thus the heat in the tissue is great at both electrode tips, and hence coagulation occurs at the tips and between them if the tips are close enough. Pfahler described this method for treating skin cancers and keratoses in 1914.[84,85] It works on the same principle as "bipolar" forceps, described later. Jackson[50] calls this form of electrocoagulation "biactive coagulation" and states that the electrodes need to be about 1 cm apart. Biactive coagulation is not routinely used on the skin any more.

The term *desiccation* (from the Latin *desiccare,* meaning to dry out) originated in 1910 with one of the earliest pioneers in electrosurgery, W.L. Clark of Philadelphia.[13,14] In his early descriptions of this type of electrosurgical method, a monoterminal Oudin current is used, giving a high voltage and low amperage. To make the current smoother, he substituted a multiple spark gap for a single one. The tissue is heated by fine sparks just hot enough to cause dehydration

but not carbonization (Fig. 16-15). Because electrodesiccation caused less tissue destruction and less subsequent scar formation, Clark felt that it was preferable in the treatment of skin malignancies.

Almost forgotten in the early history of electrosurgery is Piffard, a dermatologist from New York City. This physician devised his own coil in place of the Oudin coil to step up the voltage from the electrosurgical apparatus.[86] Piffard was involved early on with investigations of the effects of high-frequency current on the metabolic rate. As early as 1906 he described an indifferent electrode. Initial use of the electrosurgical apparatus was mainly confined to the cutaneous surfaces. MacKee[65] was also an early worker and advocate for the use of electrosurgery within the practice of dermatology.

In 1910 Czerny introduced the term *diathermy,* meaning the passage of heat through tissues.[20] He described the formation of the electric arc that cut through tissues—the earliest description of electrocutting.

The first use of sinusoidal waves for cutting was introduced by G.A. Wyeth in 1924. His term for the instrument that produced these waves was the *endotherm.*[112] It utilized the deForest vacuum tubes, which were the same tubes Lee deForest used in the first radios.

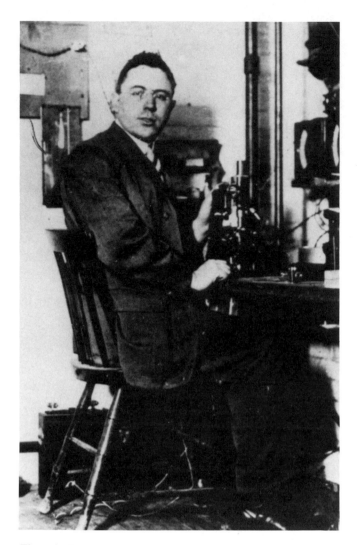

Fig. 16-17. W.T. Bovie. (From Goldwyn, R.M.: Bovie: the man and the machine, Ann. Plast. Surg. **2**(2):135-153, 1979.)

Discussion of the historical development of high-frequency electrosurgical machines would not be complete without mention of the Bovie machine. Bovie (1882-1958), a Ph.D., was director of the Biophysical Laboratories of the Cancer Commission of Harvard University[18] (Fig. 16-17). Synthesizing the knowledge previously described, he developed a machine for major surgical procedures, which had both a coagulation and a cutting current. It was first used clinically by Cushing, a famous neurosurgeon, at many of his neurosurgical procedures; Bovie manned the machine's controls. The loop electrode was first used by Cushing to scoop out a brain tumor. In a 1928 paper Cushing publicized to the surgical world the advantages of high-frequency electrosurgery, which until that time had been kept out of operating rooms.[19] Cushing described using the Bovie machine for coagulating bleeding vessels and cutting through tissue. He also noted that electrical burns could

occur from under the indifferent patient electrode if it was not properly positioned. Bovie gave freely of his time to be with Cushing during long neurological operations, which sometimes lasted 12 or more hours. In addition, Liebel of the Liebel-Flarsheim Co. of Cincinnatti, enthusiastically helped Bovie financially to produce his machine. In return for this Bovie sold his patent for $1.00. Unfortunately, Bovie was denied tenure at Harvard University on the basis of his poor publication record. Disgruntled, he left Boston and assumed a professorship at Northwestern University; subsequently he left that institution and went into obscurity in Maine.[41] His name, however, lives on and is generically applied to high-frequency electrosurgical units.

To summarize, the four types of high-frequency electrosurgical devices are compared in Table 16-1. *Electrofulguration* is produced by a relatively high-voltage, low-amperage current. The active electrode tip is not held in contact with the tissue surface but some distance away, so that a spark traverses the electrode-tissue air gap. This sparking results in superficial dehydration of tissue. The circuit for electrofulguration is monoterminal. The patient's body becomes charged and discharged with each alternation of the current. The net current flow over the body may actually be zero, but an adequate amount of current passes into and out of the tissue at the active electrode.

Electrodesiccation is similar in many respects to electrofulguration, except that the active electrode tip is held in contact with the skin. Sparks are still produced with electrodesiccation but are finer than with electrofulguration.

Electrocoagulation is produced by a low-voltage, high-amperage current. The electrode may or may not be in contact with the tissue, although sparks are still produced.[15] Tissue destruction is greater with electrocoagulation than with electrodesiccation or electrofulguration because the current is greater. If the electrode tip is not in contact with the tissue, the current goes to the tissue by means of convective sparks and the coagulation is superficial. If the active electrode tip contacts the tissue, heat is produced deep in tissue with sparks and the tissues are deeply coagulated. The patient is always in the circuit, so electrocoagulation is biterminal. This effectively lowers the voltage necessary to provide current flow to the patient and thereby increases current flow.

It should be appreciated that these terms may be defined primarily in view of the tissue effects and only secondarily by the circuitry involved. *That is, although electrodesiccation usually is produced by a monoterminal circuit and electrocoagulation by a biterminal circuit, it does not hold true that desication means treatment with a monoterminal circuit and tissue coagulation with one that is a biterminal circuit.*[107] One may obtain tissue electrodesiccation with an electrocoagulation apparatus by turning down the current; alternatively, one may obtain tissue electrocoagulation from an electrodesiccating apparatus by maintaining contact with the tissue for an excessive period of time.

TABLE 16-1

High-frequency electrosurgery currents

	Circuit	Active electrode tip	Voltage	Amperage	Wavetrain	Sparks	Tissue destruction
Electrofulguration	Monoterminal	Does not contact tissue	High >2000 V	Low 100 ma	Damped	Long, thick	Superficial necrosis
Electrodesiccation	Monoterminal	Does contact tissue	High >2000 V	Low 500 ma	Damped	Short, fine	Superficial mummification, necrosis
Electrocoagulation	Biterminal	Does contact tissue	Low <1500 V	High 600 ma	Damped or undamped discontinuous	Short, thick	Deep necrosis with hyalinized appearance
Electrotomy	Biterminal	Does contact tissue	Low <2000 V	High 700 ma	Undamped continuous	Short, thick	Fine-line destruction of cells

Another viewpoint of the definition of electrocoagulation is that it is composed of both electrofulguration and electrodesiccation.[68] That is, since some sparks are produced with biterminal electrocoagulation, electrofulguration also occurs. In addition, since some tissue desiccation occurs, electrodesiccation similarly occurs with electrocoagulation. Electrofulguration, then, is the heating of tissue with sparks, whether by a monoterminal or biterminal apparatus. Electrodesiccation is the heating of tissue by means of tissue resistance to current (ohmic heat).

Electrotomy (from the Greek τέμνω, meaning to cut) is, like electrocoagulation, produced by a low-voltage, high-amperage current. The active electrode tip is in contact with the tissue and the patient is always in the circuit (see Fig. 16-16). The tissue separates with movement of the active electrode through it. Pure electrotomy currents are associated with low-amplitude continuous sinusoidal wavetrains. The resistance of tissues to these currents may be less than to currents associated with high-amplitude damped or undamped discontinuous wavetrains. Therefore more current per unit time is produced in the tissues with cutting current than with electrofulguration, electrodesiccation or electrocoagulation, all of which utilize currents associated with damped or undamped discontinuous wavetrains. Other terms synonymous with electrotomy are electrocutting and electrocision.

The blended cutting current is a combination of a pure cutting and coagulation current. It may be associated with waves that are discontinuous high-amplitude sinusoidal wavetrains or slightly continuous or discontinuous wavetrains. By increasing the voltage amplitude, increased coagulation or desiccation may be produced.

The term *diathermy* means the passing of heat through tissues. Two types of diathermy are generally distinguished: medical diathermy and surgical diathermy (Fig. 16-18). *Medical diathermy* utilizes very high frequency currents, which are applied to tissue by means of large active and indifferent electrodes. Because the surface areas of the electrodes are large, the current density is low, and local tissue effects directly under the electrodes are minimal or undetectable. Deep heat is generated within the tissues by this current. In contrast, *surgical diathermy* utilizes an active electrode with a small surface that concentrates the current to a small point at the electrode tip. This results in significant tissue destruction because of local tissue resistance to the resultant high-density current flow. Since most of the energy transfer occurs near the tip of the electrode, very little deep heating of tissue occurs. In addition, surgical diathermy utilizes alternating current frequencies that are lower than those used in medical diathermy. The term *endothermy* may be used as a synonym for diathermy.

Effects on tissue

The immediate and delayed effects of high-frequency electrosurgical currents on tissues must be appreciated for optimal surgical results. The most important variables to consider in this regard include the power (related to voltage and current) and the duration of application of a given power.

The effect of high-frequency electrosurgical currents is to produce heat in tissue. This heat is probably the result of three factors previously discussed: ohmic heat, convective sparks, and mechanical energy. Ohmic heat is the heat produced from tissue resistance to current flow (which is related to current density). The greater the current and the current density that can be induced, the greater is the tissue destruction. Therefore electrocoagulation with a greater current destroys more tissue than does the lower-current flow of electrodesiccation with equal duration of current application. The voltage controls the sparking and the current. The sparking from the electrode also heats tissue. Therefore, with the high-voltage low-amperage currents of electroful-

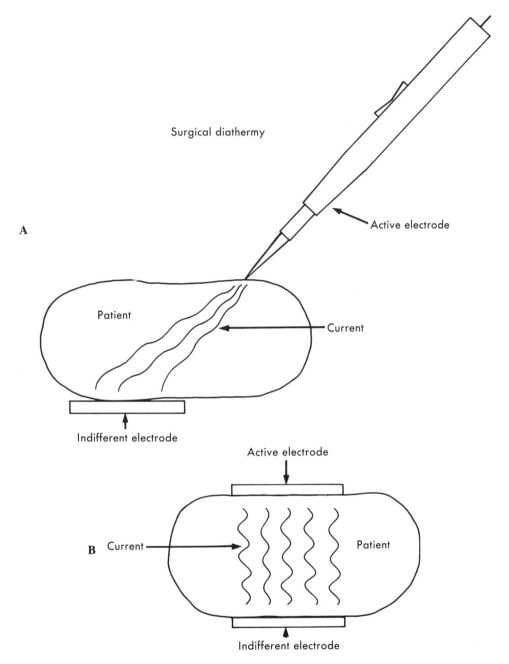

Fig. 16-18. A, Surgical diathermy has point on active electrode that concentrates current. **B,** Medical diathermy with large, active electrode and indifferent electrode.

guration, tissue is heated by heat dissipated from sparks and to a lesser extent by current. Mechanical disruption of tissue is poorly understood, but it has been theorized that it plays some role due to alternating electromagnetic field forces.[10]

The heat produced near the electrode tip of a high-frequency electrosurgical apparatus is very concentrated. Therefore the three mechanisms (already outlined) by which heat is produced in tissue with this machine are very powerful and are capable of exploding cells and destroying tissue. The heat production varies with a number of factors, includ-

ing (1) voltage, (2) amperage, (3) tissue resistivity and resistance, (4) current density (which is related to the electrode contact area), (5) local blood flow, (6) wavetrain continuity, (7) wavetrain configuration (damped or undamped), and (8) length of time the current flows. Voltage is related to the spark heating, and current amperage to the ohmic heating. Both tissue resistance and current density are related to the amount of current flowing per unit area, so these factors are also related to the ohmic heat produced. Local blood flow, which helps to dissipate heat, may be important in determining heat production in tissue. For instance, electrocoagulation of lesions on the lower extremities may result in more tissue destruction than electrocoagulation of comparable lesions on the face because the lower extremities have a relatively low blood supply, whereas the face has a relatively high supply that will help to dissipate any heat produced within the tissues. Wavetrains that represent AC voltage changes, as previously described, may be continuous or discontinuous. A discontinuous wavetrain leads to less heating of tissue, compared with a continuous wavetrain of the same amplitude and configuration. Less heat occurs because the current flows for a shorter length of time. A damped wavetrain leads to more heating in tissue than an undamped wavetrain. This is thought to be caused by the greater hindrance of tissue to currents whose peak voltages vary. The amount of time the electrode tip contacts the tissue also affects the heat production. Thus hemostasis and tissue destruction are affected by the speed of the electrode tip's movement.

Paver et al.[82] applied current at various power settings from the Birtcher Hyfrecator to rat skin and calculated the amount of tissue damage that resulted. They found that with a constant power the tissue destruction increased linearly with increasing time of application. If the power settings were increased but the time of application remained constant, then the tissue destruction also increased. Therefore both factors—power and time—are important determinants of tissue destruction.

The effect of pure electrotomy current in producing division of tissues is not well understood.[110] There are two basic theories to explain this phenomenon. The first is that the heat generated by this current produces vaporization of water within cells, exploding ("volatilizing") cells by the explosive escape of steam ahead of the electrode tip.[19] The heating occurs so rapidly that steam bubbles are generated, helping to rupture tissue.[46] Some of the heat produced is caused as well by small sparks that bridge the gap from the electrode tip to the tissues (Fig. 16-16). The water vapor produced cases a vapor seal that prevents deeper heat penetration and thus continues heat damage to the surface of the cut tissues. The second theory proposes that the electromagnetic sinusoidal wavetrains generated at the electrode tip mechanically disrupt cells.[10] This could be likened to an army troop marching across a bridge in regular step. At a certain point the bridge swings up and down at intervals synchronous with the overlying interval force of the march step; the amplitude increases with each swing, and at a certain point the bridge mechanically breaks; if the soldiers march out of step, no synchronous swinging of the bridge is produced. In a similar manner, cell membranes may mechanically rupture with regular amplitude of the sinusoidal wavetrains (acting like the regular step of soldiers).[10] In support of this latter theory is a study showing an individual mast cell on electron microscopy, which had been cleaved

in two by an electrotomy current.[30] This event would have been unlikely with vaporization of cells.

Cutting of tissues with a high-frequency electrosurgical apparatus may occur not only with a current producing a continuous undamped sinusoidal wavetrain, but with a current producing a continuous damped sinusoidal wavetrain. Since the common factor in these two currents is the continuity of the wavetrain, this may relate to the cutting action. Elliot[31] thinks that continuity leads to continuous ionization in the airgap of the electrode-tissue interface. Ionization leads to increased temperatures important for cutting.

A high-frequency electrosurgical current or spark that heats the tissue produces a small thermal burn. Burn wounds have three well-defined zones, both laterally and in depth: the zone of coagulation, the zone of vascular stasis, and the zone of hyperemia.[59] The zone of hyperemia is commonly seen clinically as an erythematous halo around superficial wounds, which results from curettage and electrocoagulation of skin cancers.

Doyen realized as early as 1909 that sparks from a high-voltage spark-gap machine (electrofulguration) resulted in carbonization at the wound surface.[29] This can be likened to heating a piece of meat quickly in an open fire: the surface is blackened, but the middle is still rare. Moreover, the carbonization of tissue provides insulation, which prevents deeper heating of tissue.

An early comparative histologic study of tissue that had been electrodesiccated or electrocoagulated was performed in 1924.[15] With electrodesiccation the water content of cells evaporates, which causes the cells to shrink and shrivel, and the nuclei to condense and elongate, especially in the epidermis (Fig. 16-19). The tissue is said to have a mummified appearance. Some blood vessels are thrombosed. With electrocoagulation not only do cells dehydrate, but cell protoplasm coagulates. This latter effect is the result of the more intense heat produced by electrocoagulation. The cell outlines are lost, and the tissue elements are fused. The tissue becomes a structureless homogeneous mass resembling hyalinized tissue. Thrombosis of blood vessels occurs as well. Fibrous tissue was found in this study to form in greater amounts with electrocoagulation than with electrodessication.

Electrodesiccation and electrocoagulation were shown early on to be successful on carcinomas. Investigators claimed that successful treatment resulted from the heat from these currents, which selectively destroyed tumor cells while leaving normal healthy tissue unaffected.[15,24] Thus the maximal amount of normal healthy tissue could be salvaged. Electrocoagulation, because it produced heat more deeply, was said to be more likely to destroy cancer cells.[29] In addition, it was also stated that both electrodesiccation and electrocoagulation sealed blood vessels and lymphatics, thereby preventing the spread of tumor cells by these routes to sites remote from the primary focus.[15] Although the suc-

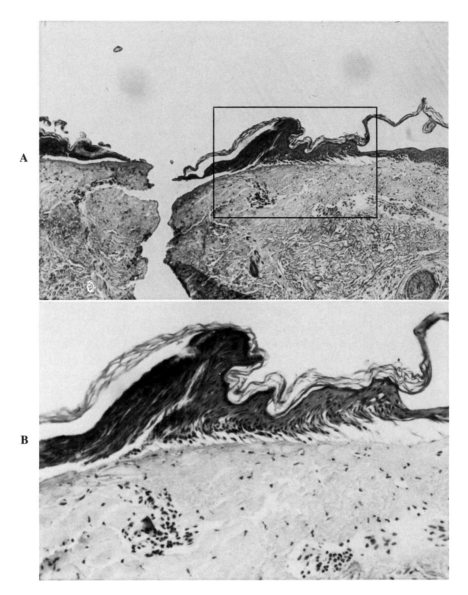

Fig. 16-19. A, Appearance of epidermis and dermis after electrotomy of human skin. **B,** Enlargement of portion of **A.** Note elongated spindle-shaped cells with nuclei, which are condensed. Such elongation of epidermal cells occurs with heating of skin by any device, including laser, electrocautery, and high-frequency electrosurgery. (Hematoxylin and eosin × 40 in **A** and × 100 in **B.**)

cessful management of cutaneous neoplasms with these treatment modalities has been reported up to modern times, the selective action of electrosurgical currents on tumor cells has not been investigated scientifically.

Epidermal cell damage is greater with a damped current (electrodesiccation or electrocoagulation) than with an undamped cutting current.[37] This is possibly caused by the high-voltage spikes that commonly occur with the damped wavetrains; with undamped wavetrains such high voltages are unnecessary to give the same average wave amplitude. The damped waveform has a high ratio (crest factor) of peak amplitude to root mean square amplitude.

Various studies have been made of wound heating after use of high-frequency electrosurgical currents. In general, electrosurgery always impairs wound healing more than excision with a scalpel blade does.[40] This is true whether electrodesiccation, electrocoagulation, or electrocutting currents are used.[90,104] This effect is probably caused by two factors. Electrosurgery seals blood vessels at the time of surgery. Since the blood vessels are the main avenue for inflammatory cells and other important modulators of wound healing, wound healing is necessarily slowed. Electrosurgery also results in necrotic tissue, which acts as a foreign body in wounds. Elimination of this foreign body takes energy, which must be diverted from the primary process of wound repair. The necrotic tissue also acts as a physical barrier between the site of incision and the site of the inflammatory response. Moreover, it may serve as a nidus for infection, since wounds produced by electrosurgery are easier to infect experimentally than wounds produced by a scalpel blade.[66] Parenthetically, wounds produced by the laser also are more susceptible to infection than are electrosurgical wounds.[66]

Thus the thermal damage done by electrosurgery impairs wound healing. It is therefore logical that the more tissue destruction and charring that occurs, the more impaired wound healing will be. Other tools that produce heat in tissues for surgical purposes—the laser and the plasma scalpel (which uses ionized gases)—also result in impaired wound healing compared with wounds made by the scalpel alone.[40,64]

In an early study in 1931 by Ellis, incisions on dogs were made with either a scalpel or cutting current.[33] Only 60% of electrosurgically produced skin wounds healed completely by primarily intention, compared with 97.5% of wounds made by the scalpel alone. Furthermore, the wounds that did heal primarily after electrosurgical cutting were initially weaker than the comparable scalpel wounds.

The differences seen in wound healing after heat damage as reflected in tensile or breaking strengths occur before maximal wound strength occurs. For instance, with the cutting current the main impairment in wound strength occurs within 40 days after wounding. No differences are seen after 50 days.[40]

On closer inspection, during the immediate postwounding period (within less than 4 days), the tensile strength of electrosurgically made wounds can be actually increased over that of similar wounds made by the scalpel. It is only after this time that these effects are reversed.[104] Such an early increase in tensile strength is reminiscent of the so-called tissue welding that occurs with lasers.

It is interesting to compare the effects of heat from electrosurgical currents with those produced by electrocautery. The latter, it should be remembered, heats tissues by thermal transfer. The ensuing damage is very superficial, much more so than with electrodesiccation or electrocoagulation. The initial char produced by electrocautery actually acts as an impediment to further heat transfer and thus limits deeper tissue destruction. The breaking strength of wounds was shown at 21 days and later in rats to be less if the wounds had been made with electrosurgical cutting current than if they had been made with the Shaw scalpel.[62] This probably reflects the lesser tissue damage made by the electrocautery than by high-frequency electrosurgery.

Types of units

Many models of high-frequency electrosurgical units are available and are constantly being updated. These units can be divided into spark gap and solid state (Table 16-2). Unfortunately, innovations in these machines are usually based on the manufacturers' ideas rather than the experience of physicians.

The spark-gap unit consists of a spark gap, which generates the current surge necessary for the resonant current between the coil and capacitor. These machines emit a loud buzzing noise when the active electrode is activated. The advantage of a spark-gap machine is that the spark gaps are excellent in producing high peak voltages for fulguration or desiccation. However, the points on the spark gap wear out with time.

Some modern spark-gap units have a preset spark distance (for instance, the Bantam Bovie), whereas in other, older units (such as the Bovie) the spark gaps can be set by the physician. The older units are excellent machines, since one can deliberately set the spark-gap distance and thus alter the current frequency and voltage. As one increases the distance between the spark gap electrodes, the distance in air that the spark must traverse increases, resulting in an increased voltage needed to bridge this gap and a decreased frequency of the discharge. Moreover, the damping is greater. One obtains a greatly damped wave with a high-voltage initial amplitude, which results in greater superficial tissue destruction. If increased hemostasis is desired, this type of current is maximally effiacious. When the spark is narrowed, the air-gap distance is decreased. This produces a lower voltage and a current associated with continuous wavetrains, which lead to less superficial tissue destruction and less hemostatic effect.[10]

The older Bovie units also produced a cutting current by use of a triode vacuum tube. The circuits were adjusted so that currents could also be produced partially from the triode tube and partially from the spark gap.

The more modern spark-gap units have preset spark gaps that can be selected either by choosing the outlet terminal (which may be labeled for electrodesiccation or electrocoagulation) or by turning a dial from "coagulation" to "cutting." However, the vacuum tubes may be absent, and the cutting current is actually associated with less damped wavetrains.

A popular electrosurgical unit among dermatologists is the Hyfrecator (Birtcher Corp.). This unit produces a low voltage spark, which results in a minimal amount of heat.[52] It is often used in a monoterminal arrangement. However, for cutaneous surgery in which there is extensive bleeding, this unit is inadequate.

Solid-state machines are rapidly replacing the spark-gap machines. The former are smaller and quieter and thus less frightening to patients. The variations in electric current are produced through diodes and transistors, which are small, solid blocks of laminated semiconductor material (hence the name "solid state"), pieced together to act as a spark gap or triode tube. Transistors do the same job as vacuum tubes, and diodes function as spark gaps but with less energy and lasting longer. The current produced in these units is not as

TABLE 16-2

Electrosurgical units

Unit	Manufacturer	Monoterminal desiccation	Biterminal coagulation	Cutting	Switch	Wattage (maximum)*
Spark gap						
Bantam Bovie†	Clinical Technology, Rochester, N.Y.	−	+	+	Foot	46
Birtcher Hyfrecator†	Birtcher Corp., El Monte, Calif.	+	+	−	Foot	30
Blentome†	Birtcher Corp., El Monte, Calif.	+	+	+	Foot	20
Cameron-Miller Electrosurgery Unit 26-230	Cameron Miller, Chicago	−	+	+	Foot	60
Cameron-Miller Electrosurgery Unit 26-0345	Cameron Miller, Chicago	+	+	+	Foot	95
Coagulator	Clinical Technology, Rochester, N.Y.	+ / +	+ / +	− / −	Hand / Foot	16
Solid state (coagulation) and triode tube (cutting)						
Surgitron FFPF	Ellman, Hewlett, N.Y.	+	+	+	Foot or hand	140
Spark gap (coagulation) and solid state (cutting)						
Hyfrecutter†	Birtcher Corp., El Monte, Calif.	−	+	+	Foot	15
Solid state						
Birtcher Hyfrecator 733	Birtcher Corp., El Monte, Calif.	+	+	−	Foot or hand	22
ESU-30	Elmed, Inc., Addison, Ill.	+	+	+	Foot	30
ESU-SU-60	Elmed, Inc., Addison, Ill.	+	+	+	Foot or hand	60
Bovie Specialist	Clinical Technology, Rochester, N.Y.	+	+	+	Foot or hand	36
Cameron-Miller 80-1983	Cameron Miller, Chicago	−	+	+	Foot or hand	80
Surgistat	Valley Lab. Corp., Boulder, Colo.	−	+	+	Foot or hand	25

*For coagulation mode only.
†Discontinued model.

susceptible to the large-voltage spikes characteristic of spark-gap machines. The less erratic current results in a smoother coagulation effect on tissue. The actual power is related to the crest factor, which for these machines may be similar to that from the spark-gap machines. Effective coagulation is provided but with lower peak voltage amplitudes. Therefore solid state machines are more efficient in that they produce similar tissue heating with less spark heat. This leads to greater smoking at the time of tissue destruction. Consequently, solid-state units may produce more of an odor, which may be unpleasant for both the patients and the staff.

Technique

The use of an electrosurgical device requires some practice and experience. One generally uses the lowest possible power setting to accomplish the task at hand. This minimizes tissue destruction and subsequent wound healing problems or scar formation.

Each machine is different. The numbered calibrations on the control knobs do not conform to a standard power output in watts. They represent only a range of power, which varies from manufacturer to manufacturer and from one machine to another. Therefore one learns what each machine does only by using it.

For electrodesiccation or electrofulguration with some

low-power units in dermatology (such as the Birtcher Hyfrecator) it is unnecessary to ground the patient. With electrofulguration the active electrode is held a distance from the skin surface. Fairly strong sparks are produced which dance circumferentially around the needle tip to the skin. With electrodesiccation the electrode tip is placed in contact with the tissue. This does not preclude sparks from flying to the sides of the electrode. With either electrofulguration or electrodesiccation the tissue damage is superficial but the surface area of damage is somewhat uncontrollable (Figs. 16-13 and 16-15). The patient is not connected back to the machine by means of an indifferent electrode (Fig. 16-9). Therefore electrons passed to the patient are shed into the air or to nearby objects: to grounded metal the patient may touch or even to the surgeon or assistants. Therefore the patient forms a capacitor with ground.

With electrocoagulation an indifferent electrode is used (Fig. 16-8). This allows the electrons shed to the patient to flow back to the machine. Since this electrode represents a ready source of current drain-off, the potential difference between the machine and the patient in this circuit is greater than if the plate were not present. Lower machine voltages are therefore required with electrocoagulation while the current flow is increased.

If a patient is touched by a bystander without rubber gloves when the active electrode of the electrosurgical device is active, a tingling will be felt by the bystander. This is caused by the building of greater electrical charge (and therefore electrical potential) on the patient than on the person touching the patient. If a monoterminal unit is used, this tingling is quite pronounced. If a biterminal unit is used, it may be minimal, since the current drains off down the path of least resistance (the indifferent electrode). However, if this latter electrode is broken or in poor contact, the tingling will increase. If the person touching the patient simultaneously touches an earthed object when the indifferent electrode is disconnected, the tingling increases even more.

A common problem that may occur when using electrocoagulation is that the power of the unit may suddenly appear to be greatly lessened. When this occurs, the indifferent electrode should be checked to ensure that good contact has been made. If good contact has not been made, the electrons flow to the patient without the current drain-off into the indifferent electrode. This results in increasing the electrical potential of the patient, which decreases the voltage difference between the machine and the patient. The voltage on a patient's body is about 50 V during electrosurgery when the indifferent electrode plate is connected, but it increases to as high as 100 V if the plate is disconnected.[26] In effect there is less force to move the current across the electrode-patient interface, and the machine appears to be working poorly.

Whatever the use or the high-frequency electrosurgery device employed, a few simple rules are in order. The active electrode tip should be clean. Adherent coagulum makes it less effective and allows sparks to jump to tissue out of the treatment area. Special adherent patches with a rough surface may be purchased (Surgikos Corp.), which help to clean the electrode tip during surgery. The problem of tissue sticking to the electrode tip is more common with higher voltages, which cause more sparking. Sticking therefore occurs more frequently with electrofulguration currents than with electrocoagulation currents. If a sterile field is desirable, the electrode tip, handle, and cord should all be sterilized. Placing the electrode tip into a sterile glove as I have seen residents do is unsound surgically. If a sterile tip alone is desirable, it may be purchased separately and sterilized; a special adapter also is available, on which a 25-gauge needle can be mounted (Bernsco, Seattle, Wash.).

It is interesting to note that most dermatologists do not routinely employ a sterile electrode tip with each surgery. Instead, the same electrode tip is used day after day on one patient after another without intervening sterilization or even cleansing with an antiseptic. There have not, to my knowledge, been any instances of infection directly linked to this practice; the high-frequency electric current at the electrode tip may be bactericidal as well as virucidal. Nevertheless, for extensive surgery that requires the laying open of tissue planes that will then be closed over, a sterile electrode tip and handle are probably preferable.

Most machines offer a foot switch or hand switch for activation of the active electrode. I prefer the hand switch control, since the foot switch is more tiresome to use and is more likely to be accidentally activated.

The heat produced in tissue at the electrode tip can be very high, and dangerous temperatures can be generated for several millimeters. Production of such temperatures can be minimized by using short applications of current and moving the electrode during application of the current. As already mentioned, one should use as little current for as short a time as possible to accomplish the task at hand. This minimizes tissue destruction.

A number of different electrode tips are available with various sizes and shapes. The two I have found most useful are the needle electrode and the loop electrode. The former is used almost exclusively to stop bleeding. The latter is used in paring tissue—for instance, with a rhinophyma. One company (Ellman) makes a scalpel blade attachment for their electrosurgery unit. This blade is claimed to cut mechanically while at the same time coagulating tissue. I prefer the paddle electrode or the wire loop electrode for cutting. The larger the surface of the cutting electrode the less efficient the electrocutting will be.[46] The wire electrode needs less power to cut and produces less tissue damage at its sides than a blade electrode does. With the cutting current there exists some small arcing (sparking) to tissue. The rate at which the cutting electrode progresses through tissues is controlled by the intensity and concentration of the arc and not by any pressure exerted by the surgeon.[71]

Another device that can be used as an accessory on electrosurgery machines is the "bipolar" forceps or "bipolar" coagulators. These are in fact not bipolar; each tip of the forceps simply represents at different times either a small active or a small indifferent electrode. Therefore the current flows between the tips, but because the current is alternating, there are no true persistent positive and negative poles. These forceps are discussed later, in the section on coagulation of blood vessels.

If an indifferent electrode is used, make sure that adequate contact is made between the patient and the electrode surface. Finally, make sure there are no cracks in the wires or loose connections. If sparks or shocks are being felt by the personnel, cracks in the wires may be shedding electrons to the air.

Selected clinical applications

The suggested applications of high-frequency electrosurgery currents in surgery are myriad and make fascinating reading. Such currents have been suggested for the removal of almost all cutaneous growths, from mundane warts to skin cancers to superficial hemangiomas. The claims of successful application almost exactly duplicate similar claims in the current medical literature for laser therapy (another form of electromagnetic radiation).[31,86] At the turn of the century electricity was a hot topic, whereas space age lasers are currently in vogue. Whether the ultimate tissue effects from these two forms of electromagnetic energy are any different will be decided only by time. The advantages of electrosurgical currents are the speed, efficacy, and low cost.

Skin cancers. A common use of electrosurgery is to destroy tissue after removal of a superficial skin cancer—either a basal cell or a squamous cell carcinoma. The technique for doing this and the indications have been discussed in Chapter 15.

Early investigators believed that the electric current from electrodesiccation or electrocoagulation in some way damaged or killed tumor cells. In 1910 Clark stated, "In disfiguring neoplastic blemishes of the skin, we have a potent weapon."[13] Explanations for the success of electrosurgery on skin cancer were of course offered and included the sealing of blood and lymph channels or the sensitivity of tumor cells to the current or heat.[13,113] It is interesting to note that Strauss et al. in 1962 showed partial regression of mammary carcinomas using electrocoagulation alone.[102] They speculated that breakdown products of the necrotic tumor have an antigenic effect and thus stimulate an immune response. Another possible explanation is the local anesthesia used before electrocoagulation. Local anesthesia has been shown to potentiate the destructive effects of heat on tumors.[114] Whatever the explanation, there is no doubt that electrosurgical currents result in high cure rates for *selected* skin tumors.

Dermatologists who use curettage and electrodesiccation (or electrocoagulation)—C & E—on skin tumors place great emphasis on the curettage portion of the procedure. They view removal of the bulk of the tumor by the curette as the primary part of the treatment; electrosurgery has a secondary role in obliterating small, undetected pockets of tumor and in hemostasis.[74]

Cure rates with curettage followed by electrodesiccation are high. Knox and coworkers reported cures in excess of 97% for basal and squamous cell carcinomas using curettage followed by electrodesiccation and repeated once.[36,53,54] These results have been duplicated by others.[74] Kopf recommends that the curettage and electrodesiccation be performed two or even three times.[55] In contrast, some dermatologists—for instance, McDaniel[70]—report excellent cure rates with curettage only, seeming to support the contention of many dermatologists that the curette is of primary importance in the cure of skin tumors.

The surgical oncologist who uses electrosurgery to treat skin cancers places great emphasis on the electrosurgical portion of the therapy and a lesser emphasis on the curettage portion.[98] That technique (E & C) is to electrocoagulate or electrodesiccate the tumor first and then to curette.[111] Using this method, Whelan and Deckers[108,109] achieved cure rates exceeding 96% for squamous and basal cell carcinomas. In their 1981 paper they concluded that electrocoagulation is an effective method of eradicating skin cancer.[109]

The reason why there is a difference between the technique of dermatologists (curettage followed by electrodesiccation or electrocoagulation) and that of surgical oncologists (electrodesiccation or electrocoagulation followed by curettage) is unknown but seems to have been deeply implanted from the time these techniques were first used. In 1909 MacKee, a dermatologist, recommended curettage first and electrodesiccation second.[65] This seems to have been followed by subsequent generations of dermatologists. One exception was the dermatologist Cipollaro, who advised electrodesiccation followed by curettage.[12] The early workers in electrosurgery (which at that time was closely associated with radiotherapy)—for instance, Clark in 1910[13] or Ward in 1925[107]—recommended electrodesiccation or electrocoagulation of tumors first and curettage second. Regardless of the reasons or the rationalizations, both techniques (C & E or E & C) have been shown to have high cure rates.

Nevocytic nevi and melanomas. Electrosurgery used to be used to burn off moles. This could be accomplished with electrolysis,[9] electrocautery,[10] electrodesiccation,[106] electrocoagulation, or even electrocutting current. When any of these techniques is employed alone, there is destruction of tissue, making pathologic examination difficult and frequently impossible. Therefore it is recommended that none of these techniques be used by itself. Although there is no evidence that such removal could provoke malignant change,[106] it is possible that diagnostic error may lead to overlooking a melanoma whenever one is dealing with a pigmented lesion. Therefore an adequate biopsy is recommended on all pigmented lesions.

Does electrodesiccation or electrocoagulation of a melanoma tend to be ineffective and cause this malignancy to spread into lymphatics or other vascular structures? The concept that it does seems to be entrenched in the surgical literature, apparently based on a paper by Amadon in 1930.[1] This report attested to the dangers of electrocoagulation for melanomas based on five patients. However, experimental evidence to support Armadon's contention is lacking. Therefore the premise that heat from electrosurgery causes melanomas to spread may have little scientific basis.

One occasionally encounters a patient who had a lesion removed by electrocoagulation (or electrodesiccation) with or without curettage, which later proved to be a melanoma—either by biopsy of the lesion at the time of treatment or regrowth of the lesion at the primary site with subsequent biopsy or metastasis. Since the lesion may already have metastasized at the time of the original treatment, it is impossible to conclude that electrosurgery by itself played a role in the dissemination of this tumor.

Coagulation of blood vessels. Another major use of high-frequency electrosurgery is for the coagulation of blood vessels at the time of surgery; this readily produces hemostasis and thus reduces the loss of blood. This application was described in 1928 by Cushing,[19] who was responsible for the introduction of electrosurgery into the operating theater. He noted that blood vessels could be picked up and occluded by means of dehydration with electrocoagulation and electrodesiccation and also noted that the active electrode did not work in a bloody field—an observation that is quite correct, since blood dissipates the heat produced by electrosurgical currents.

Electrosurgery to stop bleeding is usually performed in one of two ways: (1) the active electrode is applied directly to the blood vessel or tissue; or (2) a hemostat or pickup is applied to the blood vessel, which isolates the vessel and compresses its sides mechanically. With biterminal electrocoagulation current the active electrode is touched to the metal instrument, which conducts the current to its tip and then to the vessel, where heat is produced. The vessel is then sealed by heat generated within its wall by the passage of current. This technique is known as coaptive vessel coagulation.[99] With monoterminal electrodesiccation the active electrode touches the vessel itself and not the hemostat or pickups, because the current is very low.[52]

With coaptive vessel coagulation the tissues on opposite walls of the blood vessel bond together due to a fusion of collagen and elastic fibers. Mechanical pressure is at the moment of heating necessary for coalescence of these fibers.[99] Just the right amount of heat results in a strong bond with minimal tissue destruction. The goal is to see

retraction of tissue with a white color change. Too much heat produces a popping sound from the tissues, and coagulation necrosis results. Too little heat gives a weak bond, and rebleeding may occur if the arterial pressure is great enough.

I restrict electrocoagulation to small vessels. For larger vessels (larger than 1mm) that are spurting blood under significant pressure, I frequently choose ligation with dissolvable suture. Larger vessels have a greater chance of rebleeding after electrocoagulation; furthermore, some necrotic tissue develops with vessel coagulation. In general I agree with Johnson, who states that if the vessel has a name, one should tie it.[52]

A few points of technique help to minimize the amount of electrosurgical power used to stop bleeding. First, the field should be free of blood. Blood diffuses the current flowing from the electrode tip, rendering the apparatus less effective. Second, as little tissue as possible should be grasped by the hemostat. This minimizes tissue destruction.

An interesting accessory for electrocoagulation of vessels is the "bipolar" forceps[67] or "bipolar" coagulator.[40] As mentioned previously, each tip of this forceps functions at different times as an active and an indifferent electrode. The current flow is mainly from tip to tip. However, neither tip is continuously the positive or negative pole, since the current is alternating. Therefore it is not really bipolar; biterminal forceps is a preferable name. A distant indifferent electrode can still be used, even when the bipolar forceps are used to pick up any additional stray currents on the patient.

Bipolar forceps are usually insulated, which helps to eliminate inadvertent burns caused by contact with nearby tissues or instruments in the operative field. The tissue damage is thus confined to the tissue between the tips of the forceps. Since both tips are small, the current density is great at each tip and results in considerable heat damage. Because the distance between the active and return electrodes is small, the voltage necessary to produce tissue coagulation is much reduced—as low as 0.6V.[97] (One should remember that Ohm's law states i = V/R. By shortening the distance between electrode tips, resistance is decreased, so voltage is also decreased to produce the same current.) Decreased voltage results in less, more controllable sparking and thus helps to minimize unwanted tissue damage. It is interesting to note that deaths caused by thermal bowel injuries have occurred during tubal ligations where standard biterminal electrocoagulation has been used, but such complications and deaths are almost nonexistent if "bipolar" forceps are used.[76,83] Although this may seem somewhat irrelevant to cutaneous surgery, it points out that inadvertent tissue damage from conventional electrocoagulation may be greater than is commonly appreciated and documented.

Hair removal. Excess hair may be removed permanently by electrodesiccation or electrocoagulation, a technique sometimes referred to as thermolysis.[105] Heat is generated near the active electrode tip, which destroys the hair bulb papilla. Use of diathermic currents for this purpose was introduced by Bordier in 1924.[7] Needles with small diameters are used to concentrate the current. The current may be further concentrated if the needle is insulated.

Two techniques are used in thermolysis, the flash and the manual techniques.[105] The flash technique uses a high current for a short period of time ($1/20$ to $1/2$ second), which produces slight pain for the patient. The manual technique uses a lower current for 3 to 20 seconds. The end point of both these methods is when the hair is easily extracted from the follicle. The effects of thermolysis (or electrolysis) depends on the *total amount of current* applied. This is a function of current and time. If one uses a little current and a lot of time, one gets a great deal of destruction: if one uses a little amount of time but a lot of current, one still gets a great deal of destruction.

Ellis[32] studied the comparative effects of electrolysis, electrodesiccation, electrocoagulation, and electrocutting current on hair follicles. His experiments indicated increased tissue destruction and scarring with diathermy machines, compared with that from true electrolysis. Moreover, regrowth of hair was more frequent with diathermy machines. Robinson[95] also noted increased tissue destruction, but more so with biterminal (electrocoagulation) than with monoterminal (electrodesiccation) currents.

Two other devices for removal of superfluous hairs are the electronic tweezers and the electric pencil. Electronic tweezers (for instance, Depilatron or Permatron) use high-frequency current applied to the portion of the hair shaft that is above the surface of the skin. This high-frequency current is supposed to be carried via the hair shaft down to the papilla. There is no evidence that such a device permanently epilates hair. The electric pencil is a battery-powered, direct-current device for removal of hair. Its limitation is that the patient himself or herself must position the tip into a tiny hair follicle.

In general I have been unhappy using high-frequency electrosurgical instruments for permanent hair removal. Such devices are made to stop bleeding, not for thermolysis. The current flow that results from their use is excessive for hair removal and is likely to leave a scar. Although special electrodes that pinpoint the current for thermolysis can be purchased, I refer patients needing permanent hair removal to the individuals with the proper equipment and training.

Telangiectasias. Telangiectasias can be treated by touching the overlying skin surface with a fine-treatment electrode. The wattage output on the machine should be turned to its lowest setting. I have found that electrocoagulation is preferable to electrodesiccation for this procedure. The active electrode tip is touched to the vessel; it is then activated at the same time that one lifts it away from the tissue. This way, less tissue damage occurs. Alternatively, one may use a sterile, 30-gauge needle, and either touch its tip to or insert its tip slightly into the superficial dilated vessel, and then touch the needle with the treatment electrode (Fig. 16-20). For this technique the electrosurgery machine should be on the coagulation mode.

Telangiectasias on the face, particularly in the perinasal area, respond well to electrocoagulation. On the lower extremities, vessels treated with this modality are likely to scar, hyperpigment, or form depressed tracts. Therefore microsclerotherapy is preferable in this area (see Chapter 18).

Warts. Warts can be readily treated by electrosurgery. After local anesthesia has been obtained, the wart may be burned with electrodesiccation or electrocoagulation and then scraped away with a dermal curette. If a wart is large, hard, and verrucous, the active electrode may be plunged into the substance of the wart itself. When current is applied, the wart glows and turns white as it bubbles. The softened wart is then removed with the curette, which more easily establishes a plane of cleavage between the "cooked" wart tissue and the surrounding normal skin.

Warts are not uniform entities but arise in different locations, in different numbers, and with different histologic appearances (see Chapter 22). Several alternative treatment modalities may be useful for each type of wart. Besides electrosurgery these treatment methods include cryosurgery, laser therapy, and topical or intralesional chemotherapy. The method chosen should have the highest likelihood of cure with the least amount of scarring. The major problems with wart treatment are scarring and recurrence.

If warts are superficial and flat, electrosurgery may lead to more scarring than that found with other treatments. All physical methods tend to scar warts on the hands.

Laser therapy has to some extent replaced the electrosurgical treatment of warts. Although cure rates with this newer form of heat production are encouraging, controlled studies are needed. For instance, Billingham and Lewis compared electrosurgery to laser therapy for condylomata acuminata of the anus.[6] Half the patients were treated by a CO_2 laser and half with electrosurgery. In this series there was less pain and less recurrence with electrosurgery than with the laser. Therefore electrosurgery may be advantageous under certain circumstances, especially where scar tissue will be minimal, as in the anus.

Rhinophyma. Tumorous proliferation of sebaceous glands on the nose is readily removed by the cutting current of a high-frequency electrosurgical apparatus.[43] After nerve and field block anesthesia of the nose is obtained (Fig. 6-12), the electrode is used to cut through the excess tissue. I have personally found that the loop electrode is the most efficacious electrode to use for this purpose. If one is conservative and careful, the excess tissue filled with hypertrophied sebaceous glands can be pared down without resultant scarring. Scarring occurs if one goes too deeply.

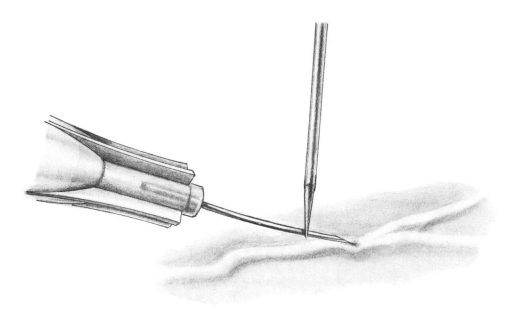

Fig. 16-20. Insertion of 30-gauge needle tip into vessel. As needle is touched with electrode tip of activated electrosurgery machine, vessel is coagulated.

Neurofibromas. Neurofibromas are protuberant soft tumors easily removeable by means of high-frequency electrosurgery with a cutting current. I have found, like other investigators,[94] that the wire loop electrode is best for removing neurofibromas. The neurofibroma is brought through the loop electrode and picked up with forceps, and then the cutting current is activated. The loop electrode sweeps through the base of the neurofibroma, sectioning the tissue and providing some hemostasis (see Fig. 25-1). Although slow regrowth of some neurofibromas removed in this way is probable, the immediate cosmetic result is excellent.

Problems with high-frequency electrosurgery

With any electrical device harm may come to the patient from either defects in the machine or human error. No machine is foolproof under all circumstances. Although fortunately adverse incidents are rare, it is beneficial for all physicians to be aware of potential problems and dangers to prevent their occurrence.

Burns. Burns from the different electrode are well described in the surgical literature and almost always occur in patients under general anesthesia.[61,75] These burns are usually caused either by faulty application of the indifferent electrode or by failure to isolate the patient from a metal surface if the return electrode is not used or its cables are faulty. A burn under the indifferent electrode occurs because the usually dispersed current load on the wide surface of this electrode is concentrated. The patient's skin is then in contact with only a small area of the electrode or perhaps only a small edge. Too much current flows through too little an area for too long a time. The current becomes concentrated (high current density) and results in a burn. If the patient is conscious he will always complain of pain before a burn ensues; however, if the patient is under general anesthesia, complaints to the physician are impossible.

Most indifferent electrodes are currently designed to minimize patient burns. Many are made of metal, which is a good electrical conductor, with the edges rounded to keep the current from concentrating at sharp points. Electrode paste is useful on metallic plates as an intermediary conductor to decrease resistance to current flow between the patient and the electrode plate. The wet-skin resistance is only $\frac{1}{5}$ to $\frac{1}{10}$ that of dry-skin resistance.[5] Many new indifferent electrodes conform to the body contour and have a protective interface gel.[60] To keep the current from being too concentrated, about 20 square inches is adequate contact area for the indifferent electrode.

Another source of burns on patients is a broken indifferent electrode or one that is not in contact with the patient. In either case there is no return route provided for the current distributed to the patient by the active electrode. The indifferent electrode is the route of least resistance for the electrosurgical current; however, if the indifferent electrode is in poor contact with the skin or is broken, the current follows any other available alternative low-resistance pathway from the patient to ground.[3] Should the patient touch a metal object that is grounded, current flows from the patient through the metal object. A painful sensation may occur if the patient is conscious. If the patient is under general anesthesia, a burn may occur. The seriousness of the injury depends on the area of contact and the current density achieved. Therefore any piece of equipment that makes

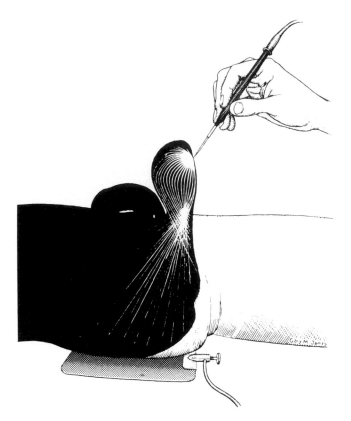

Fig. 16-21. Channeling of high-frequency electrosurgical current. Current flows over expanded surface and concentrates at base, as shown here with scrotum. (From Mitchell, J.P., and Lamb, G.N.: A handbook of surgical diathermy, Bristol, U.K., 1978, John Wright and Sons, Ltd.)

contact with the patient should be considered a possible hazard during electrosurgery.

With the high-frequency current generated by an electrosurgical apparatus, one does not have much indication of where the current is at all times. It is possible for current to concentrate in a small area as it flows. Consider the electrosurgical electrode as it is used on a large papilloma. The current flows over the papilloma and may concentrate at its base, causing a burn. The same concentration of current may occur on any structure with an expanded mass but relatively thin base or stalk. This channeling of current has been reported on the scrotum with subsequent necrosis[75] (Fig. 16-21).

Inadvertent activation of the treatment electrode may burn tissue. This could accidentally occur with foot switch activation or activation of the hair-trigger hand switch that has been left on a patient. Therefore the active electrode should not be left on the patient when it is not being used.

The surgeon may experience burns through surgical gloves if there are puncture holes.[75] High-voltage currents may also burn through the gloves while the surgeon is hold-

ing forceps.[103] Such high voltages (6000 V) are almost never used in cutaneous surgery—but if thin disposable gloves are used, burning through gloves may occur more easily and at lower voltages.

Inadvertent burns may also occur to surgeons through metal objects that carry current from the patient directly to the surgeon. Such problems, again, are of only theoretical interest in cutaneous surgery.

Ignition. Electrosurgical devices are the leading cause of fires in the operating room.[79] Early on it was realized that such devices should not be used around inflammable anesthetics, such as nitrous oxide or ethyl chloride, since explosive ignition could occur. Most spark ignitions do not involve anesthetics because most modern anesthetics are noninflammable; however, alcohol and skin disinfectants with alcohol (such as chlorhexidine [Hibitane]) can ignite with the spark from an electrosurgery unit.[34,55] Second- and third-degree burns have subsequently occurred on patients.[81] Alcoholic disinfectants may contaminate plastic or paper drapes, which may then be ignited.[39]

Ignition may also occur with bowel gas if the electrosurgery unit is used around the rectum—for instance, to remove warts. Bowel gas may contain high concentrations of methane or hydrogen gas, both of which are combustible if ignited by a spark. To prevent such an event, one may use cotton in the rectum at the time of the procedure.

Fatty tissue may be ignited with the sparks from an electrosurgical apparatus. Although I have occasionally seen a flame produced in this tissue, I have never seen any untoward effects.

Pacemaker interference. The electromagnetic field generated by a high-frequency electrosurgical device theoretically can interfere with cardiac pacemakers.[100] Although reports of such interference are virtually unknown among dermatologists using electrosurgical equipment for cutaneous surgery,[57,92] other specialists have noted adverse interactions.[27,42,115] Ventricular fibrillation and inhibition of demand pacemakers have been reported as complications of electrosurgery. Because these complications could occur even during small procedures, some knowledge in this area is necessary for using high-frequency electrosurgery safely. It is wise to remember that those patients with permanent pacemakers have significant underlying cardiovascular disease.

Pacemakers come in two types: fixed rate (continuous and asynchronous) or demand (noncontinuous and synchronous). Fixed-rate pacemakers emit impulses even when the patient has a physiologic heartbeat. Demand pacemakers, on the other hand, are either triggered or inhibited by heartbeats. The demand pacemaker has both a sensing function and a pulse-generating function. The sensing function may pick up electromagnetic radiation from an electrosurgical apparatus, and this radiation interferes with proper pacemaker function. The fixed-rate pacemaker has only a pulse-generating function, so it is resistant to electromagnetic radiation (EMR).

The most common demand pacemaker is the ventricular inhibited type, VVI (ventricle-paced, ventricle-sensed, inhibited). Other types of demand pacemakers are the QRS synchronous, atrial synchronous, and the bifocal demand. The VVI is inhibited each time the patient has a ventricular beat. The electromagnetic radiation from the electrosurgery unit may be picked up by the sensing function of this pacemaker and be interpreted as a cardiac muscle myopotential. Theoretically this could inhibit the generator function if the R wave sensitivity is exceeded. Patients subject to asystole or bradycardia may have their pacemaker put into the standby mode by EMR. If this interference lasts long enough, persistent bradycardia or asystole could result in syncope or even death.

Pacemakers are programmed to fire at a certain rate. This programming is achieved with high-frequency waves similar to the electromagnetic waves emitted by an electrosurgical unit. Therefore an electrosurgical unit could reprogram a pacemaker, converting it to an asynchronous pacing mode, or increasing or decreasing the pace rate. Such phantom reprogramming is much more likely with continuous electromagnetic waves than with discontinuous ones. Most ventricular inhibited pacemakers are designed to revert automatically to a fixed-rate pacing as a result of EMR.

Applying a magnet over the demand pacemaker generator usually converts it to a fixed-rate pacemaker, which practically eliminates inhibition of the pacemaker to EMR. However, a few pacemakers are put into the programming mode by a magnet, and when EMR appears from an electrosurgical unit, reprogramming to a different rate occurs.[27]

The reason why EMR from electrosurgery units does not commonly cause problems with pacemakers is that the pacemaker design has kept pace with the known theoretical problems, such as this type of EMR. Modern pacemakers have a metallic covering (usually titanium) for shielding and filters to screen out stray EMR. Interference from microwaves, electric shavers, or other EMR pollution is rare; modern pacemakers have certain although not infallible safeguards against stray EMR.

What does one do, practically speaking, when surgery is to be performed on a pacemaker patient? Based on the foregoing and on my experience, I would offer the following suggestions:

1. Avoid electrosurgery if possible. Consider using electrocautery or the Shaw scalpel, in which a current does not pass to the patient.
2. Discuss the case in advance with the patient's cardiologist. It may be wise to convert a demand pacemaker to fixed-rate mode before surgery.
3. Place the indifferent electrode as far from the heart but as close to the active electrode as is feasible. This helps confine the EMR between the two electrodes

and decreases current flow severalfold elsewhere.[4] However, one should remember that current flow from the active electrode takes the *route of least resistance* to the indifferent electrode. This is not necessarily the shortest distance but depends upon the resistivities of the tissue through which the current might flow. Bipolar forceps are useful in limiting current flow.

4. Use short bursts (less than 5 seconds).
5. Be sure all the apparatuses connected to electrical outlets have a safety ground line on their plugs.
6. Consider use of a cardiac monitor in a hospital setting.
7. Do not use electrosurgical units on patients with direct lines to the heart from external sources unless in a full operating room setting within a hospital and with anesthesiologists in attendance.
8. Do not use an active electrosurgery electrode in the skin overlying the heart of a pacemaker patient or in the skin overlying the pacemaker power source.

Interference with patient-monitoring devices. The EMR from electrosurgical units may interfere with cardiac monitors. This usually is not a problem, since the physician knows when the electrosurgery unit is in operation. The farther distal any monitoring device leads are from the indifferent electrode plate, the less current spreads to them.[4]

Small metal electrodes from ECG machines should not be used at the same time as electrosurgery, because they may attract the current preferentially to the indifferent patient electrode of the electrosurgery machine, especially if the latter is broken or is in inadequate contact with the patient. If this occurs, the current will be concentrated and may burn the patient at the monitoring electrodes.

Ventricular fibrillation. Ventricular fibrillation has been reported with use of an electrosurgical apparatus.[47] In all reported cases, however, the patients were "electrically susceptible." That is, either pacemaker wires or catheters were placed in contact with the heart and with external connections outside the body. These connections provide electrically conductive routes directly to the heart.[61] Therefore if such patients need surgery, monitoring equipment should be used in a hospital setting.

Electric shock. Painful stimuli from the flow of electrons is perceived as electric shocks. Such shocks can occur from a patient to those in the nearby vicinity if the patient is not in contact with an indifferent electrode. The patient acts as a receptacle for static charge, which can easily be discharged to casual onlookers if they are grounded.

Electrocution. The worst catastrophe that can occur with an electrosurgical unit is electrocution. Electrocution is caused by ventricular fibrillation, which results from an electric current passing through the body, usually for longer than a second. Because the body offers considerable resistance to current (unless it is wet), a large voltage is required to produce a significant current flow through the body.[80] Although unlikely, electrocution is theoretically possible with any electrical device. Modern machines are well grounded and isolated from the main power source by transformers, so the possibility of such an event occurring is minimized.

Effects on operating personnel. Electrosurgical equipment emits EMR at the active electrode. This radiation is thought to be harmless to those in the vicinity because it penetrates tissues poorly. Although the issue of an increase in cancer among electrical workers has been raised,[70,73] genuine liability has not been substantiated.[63] Experts in the field feel that there is no evidence of decreased longevity or increased risk for either cancer or congenital defects from continuous long-term exposure to high-frequency radiation.[88]

REFERENCES

1. Amadon, P.D.: Observations on the malignant melanoma, J. Mich. State Med. Soc. **29:**713, 1930.
2. Bassett, C., Mitchell, S.N., and Gaston, S.R.: Treatment of ununited tibial diaphyseal fractures with pulsing electromagnetic fields, J. Bone Joint Surg. **63A:**511, 1981.
3. Battig, C.G.: Electrosurgical burn injuries and their prevention, J.A.M.A. **204:**1025, 1968.
4. Becker, C.M., Malhotra, I.V., and Hedley-Whyte, J.: The distribution of radiofrequency current and burns, Anesthesiology **38:**106, 1973.
5. Billin, A.G.: Patient safety and electrosurgery, A.O.R.N.J. **14**(2):62, 1971.
6. Billingham, R.P., and Lewis, F.G.: Laser versus electrical cautery in the treatment of condylomata acuminata of the anus, Surg. Gynecol. Obstet. **155:**865, 1982.
7. Bordier, H.: Noveau traitement de l'hypertrichose par la diathermie, Vie Méd. (Paris) **5:**561, 1924.
8. Breasted, J.H.: The Edwin Smith surgical papyrus, vol. 1, Chicago, 1930, University of Chicago Press.
9. Bryant, T.: Clinical lectures on bloodless operating and bloodless operations as illustrated by the use of the galvanic cautery, Lancet **1:**469, 1874.
10. Burdick, K.H.: Electrosurgical apparatus and their application in dermatology, Springfield, Ill., 1966, Charles C Thomas, Publisher, Inc.
11. Cipollaro, A.C.: Electrolysis: a discussion of equipment, method of operation, indications, contraindications, and warnings concerning its use, J.A.M.A. **111:**2488, 1938.
12. Cipollaro, A.C.: Electrosurgery for the treatment of cutaneous neoplasms, Arch. Phys. Med. Rehabil. **34:**621, 1953.
13. Clark, W.L.: Oscillatory desiccation in the treatment of accessible malignant growths and minor surgical conditions, J. Am. Med. Assoc. **55:**1224, 1910.
14. Clark, W.L.: A preliminary report upon the destruction of surface and cavity neoplasms by desiccation, N.Y. Med. J. **93:**1131, 1911.
15. Clark, W.L., Morgan, J.D., and Asnis, E.J.: Electrothermic methods in the treatment of neoplasms and other lesions, with clinical and histological observations, Radiology **2:** 233, 1924.
16. Cook, F.R.: The high-frequency metallic discharge—a new treatment: its possibilities, Med. J. Rec. **72:**1017, 1907.
17. Cookson, W.O.C., and Harris, A.R.C.: Diphtheroid endocarditis after electrolysis, Br. Med. J. **282:**1513, 1981.
18. Cushing, H.: Meningiomas arising from the olfactory groove and their removal by the aid of electro-surgery, Lancet **1:** 1329, 1927.
19. Cushing, H.: Electro-surgery as an aid to the removal of intracranial tumors; with a preliminary note on a new surgical-current generator by W.T. Bovie, Surg. Gynecol. Obstet. **47:**751, 1928.
20. Czerny, V.: Ueber Operationen mit dem elektrischen Lichtbogen und Diathermie, Dtsch. Med. Wochenschr. **36:**489, 1910.
21. d'Arsonval, J.A.: Action physiologique des courants alternatifs, Compt. Rend. Soc. Biol. **43:** 283, 1891.
22. d'Arsonval, J.A.: Influence des variations de la force electromotrice sur les effets physiologiques du courant continu, Compt. Rend. Soc. Biol. **43:**286, 1891.
23. d'Arsonval, J.A.: Production des courants de haute fréquence et de grand intensité; leurs effets physiologiques, Compt. Rend. Soc. Biol. **45:**122, 1893.
24. deKeating-Hart, W.V.: La fulguration dans le traitement du cancer, Arch. d'Electricité Médicale **16:**371, 1908.
25. DeKraft, F.: High frequency currents, J.A.M.A. **55:**1223, 1910.
26. Dobbie, A.K.: The electrical aspects of surgical diathermy, Biomed. Eng. **4:**206, 1969.
27. Domino, K.B., and Smith, T.C.: Electrocautery-induced reprogramming of a pacemaker using a precordial magnet, Anesth. Analg. **62:**609, 1983.
28. Dornette, W.H.L.: An electrically safe surgical environment, Arch. Surg. **107:**567, 1973.
29. Doyen, E.: Sur la destruction des tumeurs cancéreuses, accessibles par la méthode de la voltäisation bipolaire et de l'électrocoagulation thermique, Arch. Electricité Médicale **17:** 791, 1909.
30. Eisenmann, D., Malone, W.F., and Kusek, J.: Electron-microscopic evaluation of electrosurgery, Oral Surg. Oral Med. Oral Pathol. **29:**660, 1970.
31. Elliott, J.A., Jr.: Electrosurgery: its use in dermatology with a review of its development and technologic aspects, Arch. Dermatol. **94:**340, 1966.
32. Ellis, F.A.: Electrolysis versus high frequency currents in the treatment of hypertrichosis: a comparative histologic and clinical study, Arch. Dermatol. Syph. **56:**291, 1947.
33. Ellis, J.D.: The rate of healing of electrosurgical wounds as expressed by tensile strength, J.A.M.A. **96:**16, 1931.
34. FDA Drug Bulletin: Burns with Hibitane tincture, **15**(1):9, 1985.
35. Fee, W.E., Jr.: Use of the Shaw scalpel in head and neck surgery, Otolaryngol. Head Neck Surg. **89:**515, 1981.
36. Freeman, R.G., Knox, J.M., and Heaton, C.L.: The treatment of skin cancer: a statistical study of 1341 skin tumors comparing results obtained with irradiation, surgery, and curettage followed by electrodesiccation, Cancer **17:**535, 1964.
37. Friedman, J., Margolin, J., and Piliero, S.: A preliminary study of the histological effects of three different types of

electrosurgical currents, N.Y. State Dent. J. **40**(6):349, 1974.

38. Garrison, F.H.: An introduction to the history of medicine, Philadelphia, 1929, W.B. Saunders Co.

39. Gibbs, J.M.: Combustible plastic drape [letter], Anaesth. Int. Care **11**(2):176, 1983.

40. Glover, J.L., Bendick, P.H., and Link, W.J.: The use of thermal knives in surgery: electrosurgery, lasers, plasma scalpel, Curr. Probl. Surg. **15**:1, 1978.

41. Goldwyn, R.M.: Bovie: the man and the machine, Ann. Plast. Surg. **2**:135, 1979.

42. Greene, L.F., and Merideth, J.: Transurethral operations employing high-frequency electrical currents in patients with demand cardiac pacemakers, J. Urol. **108**:446, 1972.

43. Gurdin, M., and Pangman, W.J.: A simple electrosurgical treatment of rhinophyma, Cal. Med. **73**:171, 1950.

44. Hardaway, W.A.: Some further observations on electrolysis in diseases of the skin, J. Cutan. G.U. Dis. **15**:399, 1897.

45. Henriques, F.C., and Moritz, A.R.: Studies of thermal injury. I. The conduction of heat to and through skin and the temperatures attained therein: a theoretical and an experimental investigation, Am. J. Pathol. **23**:531 & 695, 1947.

46. Honig, W.M.: The mechanism of cutting in electrosurgery, I.E.E.E. Trans. Biomed. Eng. **22**:58, 1975.

47. Hungerbuhler, R.F., Swope, J., and Reves, J.G.: Ventricular fibrillation associated with the use of electrocautery: a case report, J.A.M.A. **230**:432, 1974.

48. Huntoon, R.D.: Tissue heating accompanying electrosurgery: an experimental investigation, Ann. Surg. **105**:270, 1937.

49. Iredell, C.E., and Turner, P.: The treatment of malignant disease by diathermy and fulguration, Proc. R. Soc. Med. **12**:23, 1919.

50. Jackson, R.: Basic principles of electrosurgery: a review, Can. J. Surg. **13**:354, 1970.

51. Johnson, C.C., and Guy, A.W.: Nonionizing electromagnetic wave effects in biological materials and systems, I.E.E.E. Proc. **60**:692, 1972.

52. Johnson, H.: The hyfrecator—a useful device for conserving time in surgery: a point of surgical technique, Plast. Reconstr. Surg. **34**:630, 1964.

53. Knox, J.M., et al.: Curettage and electrodesiccation in the treatment of skin cancer, Arch. Dermatol. **82**:197, 1960.

54. Knox, J.M., et al.: Treatment of skin cancer, South. Med. J. **60**:241, 1967.

55. Kopf, A.W.: Therapy of basal cell carcinoma. In Fitzpatrick, T.B., et al., editors: Dermatology in general medicine, New York, 1971, McGraw-Hill Book Co.

56. Kromann, N., Hyer, H., and Reymann F.: Chondrodermatitis nodularis chronica helicis treated with curettage and electrocauterization: follow-up of a 15-year material, Acta Derm. Venereol. **63**:85, 1983.

57. Krull, E.A., Pickard, S.D., and Hall, J.C.: Effects of electrosurgery on cardiac pacemakers, J. Dermatol. Surg. **1**(3):43, 1975.

58. Krusen, F.H.: William Gilbert, the father of electrotherapy, Arch. Physical Therapy **12**:737, 1931.

59. Lawrence, J.C.: The perinecrotic zone in burns and its influence on healing, Burns **1**:197, 1975.

60. Lawson, B.N.: A nurse's guide to electrosurgery, A.O.R.N. J. **25**:314, 1977.

61. Leonard, P.F.: Characteristics of electrical hazards, Anesth. Analg. **51**:797, 1972.

62. Levenson, S.: Studies with a heated scalpel for "bloodless surgery," 1 Oct. 1978—30 Oct. 1979: data on file at Oximetrix Inc., Mt. View, Calif. 94043.

63. Liburdy, R.P.: Carcinogenesis and exposure to electrical and magnetic fields [letter], N. Engl. J. Med. **307**:1402, 1982.

64. Link, W.J., Incropera, F.P., and Glover, J.L.: Plasma scalpel: comparison of tissue damage and wound healing with electrosurgical and steel scalpels, Arch. Surg. **111**:392, 1976.

65. MacKee, G.M.: Fulguration—the local application of a current of high frequency by means of a pointed metallic electrode: its use in dermatology, J. Cutan. Dis. Syph. **27**:245, 1909.

66. Madden, J.E., et al.: Studies in the management of the contaminated wound. IV. Resistance to infection of surgical wounds made by knife, electrosurgery, and laser, Am. J. Surg. **119**:222, 1970.

67. Marino, H., and Marino, H., Jr.: Bipolar coagulation of vessels in aesthetic plastic surgery, Aesth. Plast. Surg. **2**:163, 1978.

68. McCarthy, J.: Electrosurgery. In McAinsh, T.F., editor: Physics in medicine and biology encyclopedia, New York, 1986, Pergamon Press.

69. McClendon, J.F.: Colloid properties of the surface of the living cell: electric impedance and reactance of blood and muscle to alternating currents of 0-1,500,000 cycles per second, Am. J. Physiol. **82**:525, 1927.

70. McDaniel, W.E.: Therapy for basal cell epitheliomas by curettage only: further study, Arch. Dermatol. **119**:901, 1983.

71. McLean, A.J.: The Bovie electrosurgical current generator: some underlying principles and results, Arch. Surg. **18**:1863, 1929.

72. Michel, C.E.: Trichiasis and districhiasis; with an improved method for their radical treatment, St. Louis Clin. Rec. **2**:145, 1875.

73. Milhan, S., Jr.: Mortality from leukemia in workers exposed to electrical and magnetic fields [letter], N. Engl. J. Med. **307**:249, 1982.

74. Mitchell, J.C., and Hardie, M.: Treatment of basal cell carcinoma by curettage and electrosurgery, Can. Med. Assoc. J. **93**:349, 1965.

75. Mitchell, J.P., and Lumb, G.N.: A handbook of surgical diathermy, Bristol, U.K., 1978, John Wright and Sons, Ltd.

76. Morbidity and Mortality Weekly Report: Deaths following female sterilization with unipolar electrocoagulating devices, **30**:149, 1981.

77. Morton, W.J.: Le wave current et les courants de haute frequence, Arch. d'Elect. Med. **16**:163, 1908.

78. Nagelschmidt, F.F.: Zur Indikation der Behandlung mit Hochfrequenzströmen, Dtsch. Med. Wochenschr. **33**:1025, 1907.

79. Neufeld, G.R.: Principles and hazards of electrosurgery, including laparoscopy, Surg. Gynecol. Obstet. **147**:705, 1978.

80. Noordijk, J.A., Oey, F.T., and Tebra, W.: Myocardial elec-

trodes and the danger of ventricular fibrillation, Lancet **1:** 975, 1961.

81. Ott, A.E.: Disposable surgical drapes: a potential fire hazard, Obstet. Gynecol. **61**(5):667, 1983.

82. Paver, K., et al.: Power and time factors in electrocautery and diathermy, Cutis **29:**497, 1982.

83. Peterson, H.B., et al.: Deaths associated with laparoscopic sterilization by unipolar electrocoagulating devices, 1978 and 1979, Am. J. Obstet. Gynecol. **139:**141, 1981.

84. Pfahler, G.E.: Electrothermic coagulation and Röntgen therapy in the treatment of malignant disease, Surg. Gynecol. Obstet. **19:**783, 1914.

85. Pfahler, G.E.: Electrocoagulation or desiccation in the treatment of keratoses and malignant degeneration which follow radiodermatitis, Am. J. Roentgenol. **13:**41, 1925.

86. Piffard, H.G.: The d'Arsonval and other high-frequency currents, what they are and what they will do, N.Y. Med. J. **83:**1218, 1906.

87. Pincus, G., and Fischer, A.: The growth and death of tissue cultures exposed to supranormal temperatures, J. Exp. Med. **54:**323, 1931.

88. Pollack, H.: Medical aspects of exposure to radiofrequency radiation including microwaves, South. Med. J. **76:**759, 1983.

89. Poore, G.V.: Electro-therapeutics, Lancet **1:**471, 1874.

90. Pope, J.W., et al.: Effects of electrosurgery on wound healing in dogs, Periodontics **6:**30, 1968.

91. Pozzi, S.J.: Remarques sur la fulguration, Bull. Assoc. Franc. pour l'Étude du Cancer **2:**64, 1909.

92. Ricchiuti, J.F.: Urologic electrosurgery doesn't disturb pacemakers, nor does a Bovie, Schoch Letter **32:**88, 1982.

93. Riviére, J.A.: Action des courants de haute fréquence et des effluves du résonnateur Oudin sur certaines tumeurs malignes et sur la tuberculose, Gaz. de Gynéc. **15:**241, 1900.

94. Roberts, A.H.N., and Crockett, D.J.: An operation for the treatment of cutaneous neurofibromatosis, Br. J. Plast. Surg. **38:**292, 1985.

95. Robinson, M.M.: Removal of superfluous hair by monopolar coagulation, Med. Ann. D.C. **15:**531, 1946.

96. Romer, A.S.: The vertebrate body, Philadelphia, 1962, W.B. Saunders Co.

97. Rosenberg, V.I.: A new fingertip-controlled bipolar forceps for electrocoagulation, Plast. Reconstr. Surg. **54:**228, 1974.

98. Schmidt, W.H.: The surgical uses of high frequency current, Arch. Phys. Med. Rehabil. **34:**686, 1953.

99. Sigel, B., and Dunn, M.R.: The mechanism of blood vessel closure by high frequency electrocoagulation, Surg. Gynecol. Obstet. **121:**823, 1965.

100. Simon, A.B.: Perioperative management of the pacemaker patient, Anesthesiology **46:**127, 1977.

101. Skene, A.J.C.: Electro-haemostasis in operative surgery, New York, 1899, D. Appleton & Co.

102. Strauss, A.A., Appel, M., and Saphir, O.: Electrocoagulation of malignant tumors, Am. J. Surg. **104:**37, 1962.

103. Taylor, K.W., and Desmond, J.: Electrical hazards in the operating room, with special reference to electrosurgery, Can. J. Surg. **13:**362, 1970.

104. Tipton, W.W., Jr., Garrick, J.G., and Riggins, R.S.: Healing of electrosurgical and scalpel wounds in rabbits, J. Bone Joint Surg. **57A:** 377, 1975.

105. Wagner, R.F., Tomich, J.M., and Grande, D.J.: Electrolysis and thermolysis for permanent hair removal, J. Am. Acad. Dermatol. **12:**441, 1985.

106. Walton, R.G., Sage, R.D., and Farber, E.M.: Electrodesiccation of pigmented nevi: biopsy studies—a preliminary report, A.M.A. Arch. Dermatol. **76:**193, 1957.

107. Ward, G.E.: Value of electrothermic methods in the treatment of malignancy, J.A.M.A. **84:**660, 1925.

108. Whelan, C.S., and Deckers, P.J.: Electrocoagulation and curettage for carcinoma involving the skin of the face, nose, eyelids, and ears, Cancer **31:**159, 1973.

109. Whelan, C.S., and Deckers, P.J.: Electrocoagulation for skin cancer: an old oncologic tool revisited, Cancer **47:**2280, 1981.

110. Williams, V.D.: Electrosurgery and wound healing: a review of the literature, J. Am. Dent. Assoc. **108:**220, 1984.

111. Williamson, G.S., and Jackson, R.: Treatment of basal cell carcinoma by electrodesiccation and curettage, Can. Med. Assoc. J. **86:**855, 1962.

112. Wyeth, G.A.: The endotherm, Am. J. Electrother. Radiol. **42:**186, 1924.

113. Wyeth, G.A.: The evolution and present status of electrosurgery in the treatment of cancer, Radiology **17:**1028, 1931.

114. Yatvin, M.B., Clifton, K.H., and Dennis, W.H.: Hyperthermia and local anesthetics: potentiation of survival of tumor-bearing mice, Science **205:**195, 1979.

115. Zaidan, J.R.: Pacemakers, Anesthesiology **60:**319, 1984.

17

Collagen Implantation

Soft tissue augmentation for scars and wrinkles has been practiced for years with silicone and fibrin foam. But silicone is difficult to obtain and can be responsible for long-lasting and disfiguring reactions; and fibrin foam probably does not result in long-lasting corrections of scars and is not reproducibly successful in all physicians' hands.

In 1981 the FDA approved for use the Zyderm collagen implant (Collagen Corp., Palo Alto, Calif.), an injectable sterile device derived from bovine collagen. This was the first time a product for soft tissue augmentation became legally available in the United States, and it is currently in wide usage. By 1984 it had been used in over 130,000 patients for correction of soft tissue deformities with relatively few problems.[6] Subsequently other forms of injectable collagen have become available (Table 17-1). Since these are all composed of similar collagen, I will refer to them as injectable atelopeptide collagen (IAC).

PREPARATION

IAC is a sterile injectable form of bovine dermal collagen derived from calf hide. It is thus a xenogeneic material. The collagen is selectively hydrolyzed by pepsin so that the end (telopeptide) regions are removed and thus the collagen is rendered less likely to induce immune reactions. Thus a monomeric, telopeptide-poor (atelopeptide) collagen is produced. It should be pointed out that the helical region of collagen is left intact and that this portion of the collagen molecule can induce antibody formation. Perhaps as high as 20% of antibodies directed against collagen are directed against this helical region.[7]

Although the collagen in IAC is mainly type I collagen, small amounts of type III collagen are also present. The purified, hydrolyzed product is then dispersed in physiologic saline and 0.3% lidocaine.[12]

Zyderm is packaged in syringes and is fluid enough to allow injection through fine needles (27- to 30-gauge). It is sterile and nonpyrogenic. The dispersion of collagen fibers remains fluid at low temperatures (about 4° C or 39° F); but, on warming to 37° C, or 98.6° F, the collagen fibrils precipitate, and a cohesive mass forms. Therefore Zyderm must be kept refrigerated until ready for use.[14]

There are currently three different forms of injectable collagen for patient use (Table 17-1). These differ either in the concentration of collagen fibrils or in their cross-linking. Zyderm I has approximately 35 mg/ml of collagen fibrils, whereas Zyderm II has approximately twice this concentration (65 mg/ml). The more concentrated dispersion supposedly gives a longer-lasting correction. Zyplast has about the same concentration of collagen fibrils as Zyderm I but is cross-linked with glutaraldehyde. The cross-linkage helps the Zyplast to persist for a longer period of time compared with Zyderm I or Zyderm II.

FATE OF IAC ON INJECTION

Normally Zyderm does not induce a marked inflammatory reaction. Within hours after implantation, the collagen fibrils condense out of the dispersion into a cohesive implant, and the carrier saline is thus extruded and then absorbed. This process is known as *syneresis,* the contraction of gel particles (the dispersion phase) that separates and extracts the liquid component particles (the dispersed phase). Unlike silicone, Zyderm is assimilated by the host tissue. It is thought that the collagen implant forms a latticework into which host fibroblasts and capillaries can grow.[12] This latter process, however, does not occur for a few weeks after implantation. Before that time IAC might migrate from the dermis to the subdermis.[9]

HISTOLOGY

Histologically IAC can be differentiated from normal collagen in routine hematoxylin and eosin preparations. IAC stains lighter, and the bundles are thicker and more amorphous than host collagen. Masson's trichrome stain can be helpful in differentiating IAC from host collagen if doubt exists.[3,25] With this stain IAC appears pale blue compared to the medium blue of normal collagen. A colloidal iron stain counterstained with nuclear fast red or van Gieson's solution may also be useful in better defining IAC.

TABLE 17-1

Types of injectable atelopeptide collagen (IAC)

	Concentration	Cross-linked	Recommended level of placement	Typical uses
Zyderm I	35 mg/ml	No	Superficial dermis Mid dermis	Superficial wrinkles Superficial dermal defects
Zyderm II	65 mg/ml	No	Mid dermis Lower dermis	Furrows Deeper dermal defects
Zyplast (Carrigan)*	35 mg/ml	Yes	Lower dermis Subdermis	Atrophy, furrows Deep contour defects

*Trade name marketed to podiatrists.

TREATMENT VARIABLES
Patient selection

Before use of IAC, a medical history should be taken. Patients with a personal history of autoimmune disease, joint disease, or immunologic disorders should not receive IAC. Also patients with a history of reacting to lidocaine (Xylocaine) should be excluded. A family history of these disorders can also contraindicate IAC treatment, but such patients have been treated without untoward reactions (assuming a negative skin test).[12]

All patients should be skin tested initially with 0.1 ml of Zyderm I. This is given in the volar forearm, placing about half of the test dose in the dermis and half subdermally. A typical positive test site reaction is an erythematous nodule that appears days to weeks after implantation. Such a positive response might be pruritic and can persist for months.

Positive test site reactions occur in about 3% of patients.[12,25] These reactions can be false-positive as well as false-negative. False-positive reactions can be precipitated by alcohol or trauma, although this phenomenon has not been well studied. False-negative reactions can occur if the test site is not observed for a long enough period of time. Cases in which the skin test sites did not become positive for 6 weeks after implantation have been reported.[7,15] Other false-negative reactions can occur in which test sites show an equivocal reaction.[10] In addition, less than 1% of patients may show a negative test site response but a positive reaction to therapeutic IAC.[18,25] Medical history and negative test site responses do not eliminate all persons who will show a reaction at the treatment site to IAC.

On the basis of the preceding information, some physicians advise a second skin test with Zyderm I at 1 month following the first skin test. This repeat test will probably more accurately define the small percentage of patients who develop reactions to IAC after an initial negative skin test.

An alternative explanation for a false-negative reaction to IAC is that in some individuals 1 month is too short a time to see a reaction.[15] Therefore, rather than perform a second skin test, one may wait 6 to 8 weeks after the test site implantation to ensure that the patient does not react to IAC.

The histopathology of the skin from the positive test site shows a pattern of necrobiotic granulomas similar to those seen in necrobiosis lipoidica diabeticorum or granuloma annulare.[3] However, foreign body granulomas have also been described.[4,15] An amorphous center of wavy, homogeneous, eosinophilic material surrounded by lymphocytes, histiocytes, plasma cells, and giant cells can be seen.[2] Whether this reaction is allergic or nonallergic and similar to other types of granuloma formation is unknown.[21]

The positive test site reactions to IAC frequently persist for months before resolution. Usually the patient is not too bothered by the reaction. Because such reactions tend to resolve in time by themselves, injection of steriods or excision is not recommended unless the patient is very symptomatic or the reaction does not resolve itself within one year. Topical steroids may be useful in the treatment of positive test site reactions.

Lesion selection

Although any depression in the skin from superficial wrinkles to deep depressions can theoretically be treated by injection of IAC, in reality IAC benefits very few such depressions to a significant degree for one or more of the following reasons: (1) IAC is mostly water and thus any immediate benefit is soon lost; (2) there is probably some migration of this material[9]; (3) after IAC implantation the normal stresses on tissue are still present and alter the location of the implant; and (4) where IAC is used in or under significant scar tissue, little benefit can be expected, since the scar tissue is relatively nondistensible.

The studies that have been done attesting to the efficacy of this material are not double-blind or even comparative (saline versus IAC). It has been my experience that the

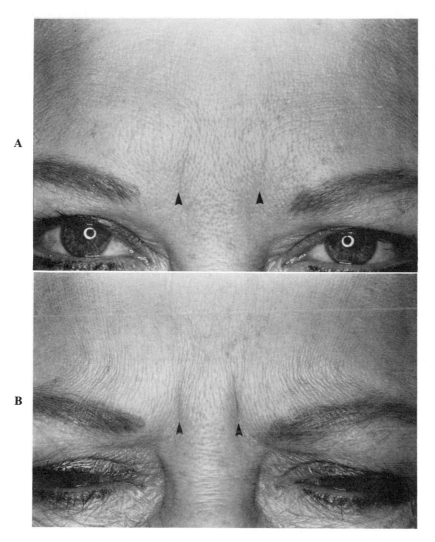

Fig. 17-1. A, Glabellar creases and, **B,** glabellar furrows. *Continued.*

successful use of IAC has a large psychologic overlay by patient and physician. Nevertheless, in a small percentage of lesions treated, reasonably persistent improvement occurs that can be photodocumented. Proper lesion selection and technique are the keys to successful correction with IAC.

IAC is recommended for acne scars, viral pox scars, depressed postsurgical scars, traumatic scars, and age-related wrinkles. However, IAC works best on superficial wrinkles and on superficial soft scars with smooth margins. The superficial wrinkles or creases on the glabella (Fig. 17-1, *A* through *D*) and just lateral to the angles of the mouth seem to respond the best. Crow's feet lateral to the eyes are also said to respond to IAC,[25] but I have no experience in this area. Those with experience advise against overcorrection in this location because the skin is thin. Mature, shallow (saucerlike) acne scars show moderate improvement. Deeper "ice pick" scars do not respond to IAC injections.

Viral pox scars are also difficult to distend with IAC.

Neither furrows (that is, depressions caused by direct muscle insertions), including the melolabial crease and the nasolabial crease, nor the sunken cheek appearance caused by malar prominence is significantly corrected for any length of time by IAC. One exception is the glabellar furrows (Fig. 17-1, *B*), which possibly respond better because of the firm underlying surface provided by the frontal bone. An interesting use of IAC is to correct angular cheilosis (perlèche) by injection into the grooves extending inferolaterally from the sides of the mouth.[5]

Small dermal contour deficiencies caused by trauma, surgery, or disease might respond to IAC injections. For example, depressed scars following secondary wound healing after Mohs surgery are said to be improved with IAC.[1] The newer cross-linked IAC (Zyplast) or the higher concentration IAC (Zyderm II) might result in even better, longer-lasting correction of these deep scars.

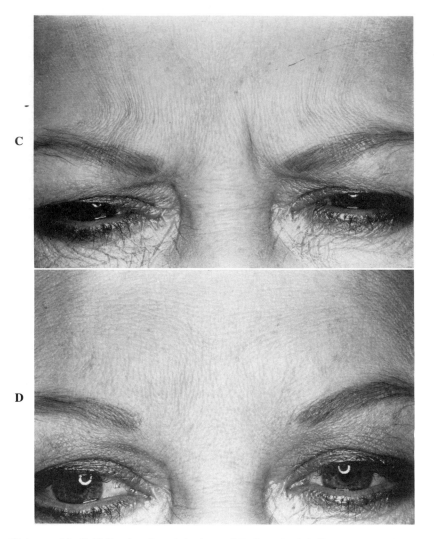

Fig. 17-1, cont'd. C, Following three injections of Zyderm I, glabellar creases are inapparent. **D,** Furrow on patient's right has disappeared after three injections of Zyderm I. Subsequent injections flattened out furrow on patient's left. There was no recurrence of these creases or furrows for 2 years after injection.

Technique of injection

Besides lesion selection, injection technique is the other critical factor that influences results with IAC. Injection technique involves a number of variables that need to be considered. These include (1) injection volume, (2) level of injection, (3) injection intervals, (4) needle gauge, and (5) concentration and relative cross-linking of IAC.

An important concept to understand is that at the time of injection, only a limited volume of IAC can be accommodated per injection site. With Zyderm I, one should try to overcorrect by 1.5 or 2.0 times normal (150% to 200%). This is known as the overcorrection technique and is necessary because IAC is mostly water that is subsequently absorbed. As a rule of thumb, one should expect a semipermanent correction roughly equal to one-fourth the per-

centage of correction at the time of treatment.[12] For example, an initial 200% correction ultimately yields within a few days a semipermanent 50% correction.

Zyderm I is placed in the superficial or mid dermis. Dermal placement replaces tissue where it has been lost from scarring, aging, or trauma; that is, in the dermis itself. To ensure this, it is recommended that Zyderm I be injected with the needle bevel down and the skin tented up.[13] The multiple puncture technique is also recommended because it appears to be superior to the tracking or fanning technique. The multiple puncture technique requires several separate injections of small amounts of collagen to be placed along a wrinkle or crease line. These separate injection sites are between 2 and 3 mm apart. In contradistinction is the tracking or fanning technique in which collagen is placed intradermally for several millimeters in a given direction. The multiple puncture technique allows the maximal amount of IAC to be located in the dermis, whereas tracking or fanning tends to implant some IAC deep to the dermis. The beneficial effect of IAC is lost by such deeper placement in the subdermal tissue. The value of the multiple puncture technique has been substantiated by experiments in pigs.[9] In this animal model 0.1 ml of Zyderm leads to the maximal amount of correction possible per injection site. Larger volumes injected are lost as they are forced down into the subdermis. It has been stated that perhaps large volumes injected tend to open up channels between the collagen bundles, which facilitate passage of excess collagen into the subdermal fat.[9] It was also found that use of a 30-gauge needle affords more superficial placement of IAC than is possible with a 22-gauge needle.[9] Following overcorrection of the defect, the area should be massaged to help evenly disperse the collagen and to eliminate the excess elevation.

For superficial acne scars or other depressions, it is helpful to outline before injection the areas to be injected with a skin marker such as gentian violet. Also, patients should be in the sitting position when injected under a good light source that throws a tangential light. This helps to accentuate wrinkles and depressions so that proper overcorrection can be achieved.

It is important to realize that restoration of contour with Zyderm I or Zyderm II is obtained from incremental improvements from several injections. Normally injections are given at 2- to 4-week intervals until maximal correction is obtained. This usually requires two to five injections sessions at each treatment site. I usually see the patients back after 1 month to assess the degree of correction made. If more correction is needed, additional injections are then given. These sessions are repeated until the desired degree of correction is achieved or until the maximal possible correction is obtained. Once this point is reached the patient might need "touch-up" injections 6 months or more later. The persistence of correction is variable, and in many patients there is a 30% loss of correction within a year. Therefore the patient should be informed that uncertainties exist regarding the degree and persistence of correction possible with IAC and that supplemental injections might be necessary. I have occasionally seen corrections that lasted more than 2 years to date, although these are exceptions.

Recent data in pigs imply that more frequent (weekly) injections with smaller amounts of IAC result in more IAC being retained within the dermis.[9] More studies must be done on the value of frequent injections in humans.

To circumvent the problem of inadequate correction of deep scars, Zyderm II and Zyplast have recently been made available. The actual benefits, advantages, and disadvantages of these products need to be determined by carefully controlled studies. Theoretically Zyderm II, which has

almost twice the IAC concentration of Zyderm I, is expected to provide a faster, longer-lasting correction. Zyplast is less likely to disperse into smaller masses because it is slightly cross-linked and might last longer than Zyderm I.

The injection techniques with these newer products differ somewhat from those with Zyderm I. Zyderm II should be placed in the mid or lower (reticular) dermis, and Zyplast is ideally placed in the deep dermal or subdermal tissue. If placed in the superficial dermis, Zyplast can result in a beading effect similar to that produced by silicone. It is recommended that Zyplast not be used around the vermilion or periorbital areas, because Zyderm has been slow to resolve here. With Zyplast it is preferable to aim for an initial 100% correction rather than the 150% to 200% for Zyderm I, because Zyplast might not be as forgiving as Zyderm I.

ADVERSE TREATMENT SITE REACTIONS TO IAC

Despite having negative test site reactions, some patients have either localized reactions at treatment sites (Fig. 17-2), systemic reactions, or even both. Presumably these patients become sensitized to IAC at some point during the treatment course. The incidence of such treatment site reactions is anywhere from 0.3% to 6.2%.[9,12,22] Usually localized reactions include swelling and induration of treatment sites. These localized reactions may appear only intermittently and can be precipitated by alcohol or minor trauma. Although most localized reactions regress within 6 months, some occasionally take longer. In a report published in 1980 all localized reactions eventually resolved.[23] Topical steroids and watchful waiting are recommended for these reactions.

A small percentage of patients (0.5%) might develop more severe reactions to IAC injections characterized by a serum sicknesslike reaction or migrating giant hives.[23] Acute arthritis[11] and malaise and flulike syndromes[8] have also been reported. However, such patients usually have had positive skin test reactions.

The histologic picture of reactions at treatment sites is similar to that at test sites and shows a palisading granuloma.[24] Both the time course and the histologic picture seem to imply a delayed type of hypersensitivity reaction.

The number of exposures to IAC before a patient has a reaction varies. Although most have their reactions after the first or second treatment session, one study found that 18.9% of patients who develop a treatment site reaction do so after the third session, 8.1% after the fourth, and 2.7% after the fifth.[8] Therefore, if a patient does not develop a reaction at IAC implant sites early in the course of treatment, this may still eventually occur.

Humoral antibody responses to IAC are possible and have been investigated.[22] In a group of 61 patients prospectively studied,[7] two patients experienced localized inflammatory responses at treatment sites despite negative reactions at skin test sites at 4 weeks. In both of these patients a

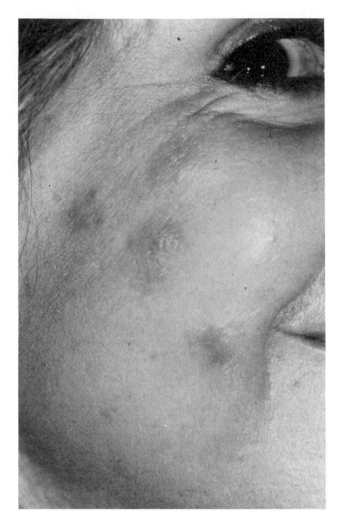

Fig. 17-2. Adverse treatment site reaction to Zyderm I. Erythematous nodules at injection sites. Within a year these nodules disappeared with no treatment. (Courtesy Victor D. Newcomer, Los Angeles.)

greater serum level of IAC antibodies was found than in 59 patients without localized reactions to IAC. Also, in both patients the antibodies did not cross-react with human collagen, and immune complexes were not increased. In another study elevated levels of circulating antibody to IAC in patients with treatment site reactions were also found.[22] Thus there appears to be a correlation between elevated antibody levels to IAC and adverse treatment site reactions.

In a further study,[8] the same authors of the prospective study (just mentioned) retrospectively examined 72 patients. Thirty-five had generalized symptoms without implant test site reactions, 31 had implant site reactions alone, and six had implant site reactions along with generalized symptoms. Elevated levels of anti-IAC antibodies correlated with positive implant site reactions but not with generalized symptoms.

The precise role antibodies to IAC play in localized reactions to this material is unclear. First, some patients have detectable antibodies to IAC before their initial exposure. Second, systemic symptoms (achiness, nausea, flulike syndrome) do not correlate with antibody titers. Third, the clinical response of the patients who do react reminds one of a delayed hypersensitivity type of reaction rather than an antigen-antibody type reaction. However, antigen-antibody reactions can modulate delayed hypersensitivity reactions.

The long-term consequences of deposition of IAC or continuous exposure to repeated injections over time are unknown. There must be some concern over chronic exposure to a foreign antigen. However, late reactions have not been reported to date, and the problems encountered may be analogous to those seen with chronic exposure to insulin, another foreign protein.

There has been one documented case of blindness caused by injection of Zyderm I in the periorbital area.[6] It is

TABLE 17-2

Comparison between silicone and injectable atelopeptide collagen (Zyderm collagen implant)

	Silicone	IAC
Source	Mineral	Animal
Purity	Questionable	Pure
Histology	Honeycomb appearance	Tinctorially different collagen
Overcorrection	Can be permanent; Might see beading, peau d' orange appearance	Not permanent
Migration	Yes	No or minimal
Indications	Similar to those for IAC	Similar to those with silicone
Treatment site reactions		
Incidence	0.12%-14%	0.3%-6.2%
Time of onset after injection	Months to years	Weeks
Clinical appearance	Intermittent erythema and/or granulomas	Erythema, induration
Histologic appearance	Foreign body type	Necrobiotic granuloma

thought that this occurred because of inadvertent injection of Zyderm I into a vascular space with subsequent migration to the retinal arteries producing vascular occlusion. Parenthetically, similar cases of blindness have also been reported with the use of silicone or steroid injections in the central face.[16,19,20]

COMPARISON OF IAC TO SILICONE

Some dermatologists, plastic surgeons and other physicians involved in cosmetic surgery prefer silicone to elevate depressions in the skin. Silicone is not approved for general medical use by the FDA, and therefore this product has not been widely studied. Table 17-2 contrasts silicone with Zyderm collagen implant.

Liquid silicone is of mineral origin and is related to sand and glass, whereas IAC is of animal origin. Medical-grade silicone is used for implantation by injection in man, but it is not easy to ascertain the purity of this product. Normally, on injection silicone results in a mild inflammatory cell reaction with a round cell infiltrate. One also sees multiple cysts resembling a honeycomb.

After implantation by injection, silicone has a tendency to migrate from the site of injection, especially around the eyelids and lips. It should not be used below the neck because of this problem with migration. There is also a tendency for shrinkage of up to 30% within 3 weeks of injection.[17]

The indications for use of silicone are similar to those of IAC. However, on injection, silicone is not as forgiving as IAC. If placed superficially, silicone can give a beaded

effect and even produce a peau d'orange (orange peel) appearance to the skin, since the dermis is elevated around hair follicles.

The development of treatment site reactions to silicone has prevented its approval by the FDA and led investigators to prefer other substances for injection such as IAC. The incidence of such reactions is between 0.12% and 14%, depending on the study and the grade of silicone used.[17,26] These treatment site reactions are usually of the foreign body type in contrast to IAC reactions, which appear as necrobiotic granulomas. With silicone reactions, one sees foreign body giant cells and mononuclear cells. In some giant cells, silicone can be seen. Cystlike spaces are present amidst the reaction.[26]

The most distressing aspects of silicone reactions are the clinical appearance and the long time interval before such reactions occur. Silicone reactions can appear either as firm nodular granulomas[17] (Fig. 17-3) that are unsightly or as intermittent erythema.[26] Unlike IAC reactions, which usually appear within a few weeks after implantation, silicone reactions can take years to develop. By that time large quantities might have been used on an individual patient, and thus severe or widespread cutaneous reactions may appear. In one study 13 reactions to silicone were reported.[26] Six of the 13 reactions occurred after 1 year following placement, and one reaction occurred 7 years later. Such delayed reactions are analogous to silica reactions, which occur after a period of time in association with breakdown of silica particles. Thus silicone reactions are probably a foreign body reaction rather than an allergic phenomenon. Although

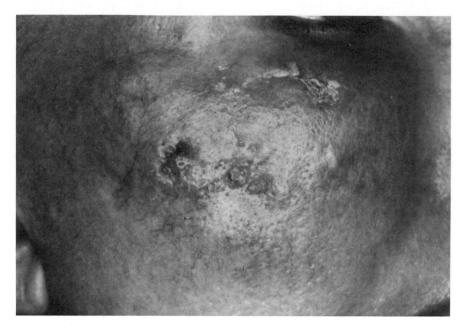

Fig. 17-3. Granulomatous nodules on cheek, the site of silicone injections 10 years previously. Reaction did not occur until 8 years after injections.

many of the silicone reactions are blamed on impurities, these types of reactions can be seen with a high frequency even where the source is known and checked and the material is "the high-grade medical silicone."[17]

Despite the foregoing, silicone offers distinct advantages compared to IAC for correction of tissue loss. Silicone might be more successful in correcting deeper defects, both immediately and permanently. Unfortunately, the silicone used in the past has been difficult to test for impurities and to standardize. One hopes these difficulties can be overcome in the future, and prospective clinical trials will be conducted, particularly in cases in which IAC has been unsuccessful.

REFERENCES

1. Bailin, P.L., and Bailin, M.D.: Correction of depressed scars following Mohs surgery: the role of collagen implantation, J. Dermatol. Surg. Oncol. **8**:845, 1982.
2. Barr, R.J., et al.: Necrobiotic granulomas associated with bovine collagen test site injections, J. Am. Acad. Dermatol. **6**:867, 1982.
3. Barr, R.J. and Stegman, S.J.: Delayed skin test reaction to injectable collagen implant (Zyderm), J. Am. Acad. Dermatol. **10**:652, 1984.
4. Brooks, N.: A foreign body granuloma produced by an injectable collagen implant at a test site, J. Dermatol. Surg. Oncol. **8**:111, 1982.
5. Chernosky, M.E.: Collagen implant in management of perlèche (angular cheilosis), J. Am. Acad. Dermatol. **12**:493, 1985.
6. Collagen Corporation: Annual report 1984, Palo Alto, Calif., 1984, Collagen Corporation.
7. Cooperman, L. and Michaeli, D.: The immunogenicity of injectable collagen. I. A 1-year prospective study, J. Am. Acad. Dermatol. **10**:638, 1984.
8. Cooperman, L. and Michaeli, D.: The immunogenicity of injectable collagen. II. A retrospective review of seventy-two tested and treated patients, J. Am. Acad. Dermatol. **10**:647, 1984.
9. Grosh, S.K., et al.: Variables affecting the results of xenogenic collagen implantation in an animal model, J. Am. Acad. Dermatol. **13**:792, 1985.
10. Hanke, C.W., and Robinson, J.K.: Injectable collagen implants, Arch. Dermatol. **119**:533, 1983.
11. Jarrett, M.P., and Roguska-Kyts, J.: Collagen-induced arthritis in a human [letter], Arthritis Rheum. **25**:1024, 1982.
12. Kaplan, E.N., Falces, E., and Tolleth, H.: Clinical utilization of injectable collagen, Ann. Plast. Surg. **10**:437, 1983.
13. Klein, A.W.: Implantation technics for injectable collagen: two and one-half years of personal clinical experience, J. Am. Acad. Dermatol. **9**:224, 1983.
14. Knapp, T.R., Kaplan, E.N., and Daniels, J.R.: Injectable collagen for soft tissue augmentation, Plast. Reconstr. Surg. **60**:398, 1977.
15. Labow, T.A., and Silvers, D.N.: Late reactions at Zyderm skin test sites, Cutis **35**:154, 1985.
16. McGrew, R.N., Wilson, R.S., and Havener, W.H.: Sudden blindness secondary to injections of common drugs in the head and neck. I. Clinical experiences, Otolaryngology **86**:147, 1978.
17. Milojevic, B.: Complications after silicone injection therapy in aesthetic plastic surgery, Aesth. Plast. Surg. **6**:203, 1982.
18. Ruiz-Esparza, J., Bailin, M., and Bailin, P.L.: Necrobiotic granuloma formation at a collagen implant treatment site, Cleve. Clin. Q. **50**:163, 1983.

19. Schorr, N., and Seiff, S.R.: Central retinal artery occlusion associated with periocular corticosteroid steroid injection for juvenile hemangioma, Ophthalmic Surg. **17:**229, 1986.

20. Selmanowitz, V.J., and Orentreich, N.: Cutaneous corticosteroid injection and amaurosis, Arch. Dermatol. **110:**729, 1974.

21. Shelley, W.B., and Hurley, H.J.: The pathogenesis of silica granulomas in man: a non-allergic colloidal phenomenon, J. Invest. Dermatol. **34:**107, 1960.

22. Siegle, R.J., et al.: Intradermal implantation of bovine collagen: humoral immune responses associated with clinical reactions, Arch. Dermatol. **120:**183, 1984.

23. Stegman, S.J., and Tromovitch, T.A.: Implantation of collagen for depressed scars, J. Dermatol. Surg. Oncol. **6:**450, 1980.

24. Swanson, N.A., et al.: Treatment site reactions to Zyderm collagen implantation, J. Dermatol. Surg. Oncol. **9:**377, 1983.

25. Watson, W., et al.: Injectable collagen: a clinical overview, Cutis **31:**543, 1983.

26. Wilkie, T.F.: Late development of granuloma after liquid silicone injections, Plast. Reconstr. Surg. **60:**179, 1977.

18

Sclerotherapy for Telangiectasias and Superficial Veins

Telangiectasias are tiny, dilated superficial vessels of the skin that are visible to the naked eye. Individually they measure 0.1 to 1 mm in diameter and represent either an expanded venule, a capillary, or an arteriole. Telangiectasias that originate from arterioles or the arterial side of a capillary loop tend to be small and bright red and do not protrude above the skin surface. Telangiectasias that originate from venules or the venous side of a capillary loop, on the other hand, are blue, raised, and wider. Sometimes telangiectasias, especially those from the mid capillary loop, are at first red but with time become blue, probably because of a worsening hydrostatic pressure and backflow from the venous side of a capillary loop. Varicose veins are dilated veins arising in vessels larger than venules and measuring more than 1 mm in diameter.

Telangiectasias are quite common and have a variety of causes, including genetic (for example, ataxia telangiectasia), collagen vascular disease, hormonal, physical damage (for example, trauma or radiodermatitis), or venous hypertension. In addition, a variety of primarily cutaneous diseases such as poikiloderma atrophicans vasculare or basal cell carcinoma can also be associated with telangiectasias (see Fig. 21-1, *B*).

Telangiectasias clinically have been classified into four patterns simple linear, arborizing, spider (or star), and papular (or mats)[42] (Fig. 18-1). Papular telangiectasias are frequently part of genetic syndromes such as Osler-Weber-Rendu syndrome, or collagen vascular disease. Spider telangiectasias are red and arise from a central filling vessel of arteriolar origin. If one puts pressure on the feeding vessel, the branching ''arms'' of the spider blanch. Red linear telangiectasias of the face (especially the nose) or legs and blue linear or arborizing telangiectasias of the legs most commonly are presented for treatment. Since the patho-genesis of these types of telangiectasias vary, it must be understood so that the choice of therapy is more rational.

Telangiectasias of the face are probably caused by persistent active arteriolar vasodilation (for example, from chronic alcohol consumption) or weakness in the vessel wall resulting from elastotic change from chronic sun exposure. These telangiectasias most often arise from arterioles; they are seen frequently in individuals with fair complexions and are most often located on the nose, especially on the ala and nasolabial crease. Rosacea can be present along with telangiectasias in this location.

Telangiectasias on the legs are usually different from those on the face both in pathogenesis and vessel type. The former mostly arise in venules and are caused by persistent passive venous vasodilation and weakness in the vessel wall, probably related to hormones or heredity.[4] Such telangiectasias are common in females between the ages of 30 and 50, many of whom have been pregnant or have taken birth control pills. This suggests a direct hormonal influence on the pathogenesis of telangiectasias in this location. Although they might appear at first as erythematous streaks, with time they turn blue. Often these vessels are directly associated with underlying varicose veins so that the distinction between telangiectasias and varicose veins becomes blurred.[4]

Two common patterns of telangiectasias on the legs of women besides singular red or blue streaks are the parallel linear pattern, especially found on the medial thigh, and the aborizing or radiating cartwheel pattern, especially seen on the lateral thigh.[1,25] These two subsets of telangiectasias seem to run in families and might form anastomizing complexes that can be as large as 15 cm square and are known as ''venous stars'' or ''sunburst venous blemishes.''

Varicose veins of the lower legs are thought to be caused

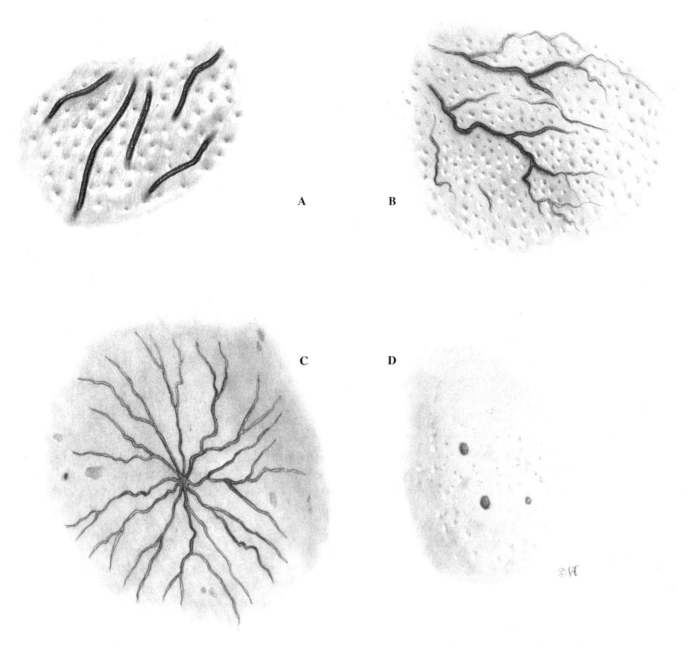

Fig. 18-1. Four common patterns of telangiectasias. **A,** Simple linear. **B,** Arborizing. **C,** Spider. **D,** Papular (mats).

mainly by incompetent perforating veins.[45] These veins connect the deep venous system to the superficial veins in the lower extremities. When the leg muscles relax, deep vein pressure falls below that in the superficial veins. Blood then flows from the superficial to the deep venous system. With muscle contraction, the blood in the deep veins is forced up toward the heart. The valves in the deep and perforating veins help keep the blood from being pushed into the superficial veins with muscle contraction. If these valves are incompetent, venous backflow occurs, resulting in venous hypertension, chronic venous insufficiency, stasis

dermatitis, ulceration due to tissue edema, and local tissue anoxia. Incompetent valves can occur as a result of local trauma, thrombophlebitis, familial weakness in vein structure, increased blood volume, or hormonal influences.

Telangiectasias of the face are usually asymptomatic, but on the legs they can cause a burning discomfort in warm weather and preceding or during menses. Large varicose veins are more symptomatic, causing most patients to complain of tiredness in the legs and throbbing pain.[45] Itching, dermatitis, night cramps, and ulceration with bleeding can also occur.

HISTOPATHOLOGY

Histopathologically simple telangiectasias are seen as blood channels with a single endothelial lining and no muscularis.[42] Therefore many telangiectasias evolve from dilated capillaries. However spider telangiectasias can arise in terminal arterioles.[37] Bluish arborizing telangiectasias of the lower legs are probably dilated venules, possibly with intimate and direct connections to underlying larger veins from which they are direct tributaries. In two reports, such "telangiectasias" have been found on biopsy to be ectatic veins.[7,14]

TREATMENT

Patients seek therapy for telangiectasias or varicose veins because of discomfort or the unsightly appearance. However, treatment is frequently difficult to obtain because, except for surgical venous stripping, other forms of therapy are largely untaught in surgical programs in medical schools. This is at least in part because of the perennial battle between the cutters who would strip every vein and the medically oriented injectors.[13] For smaller telangiectasias on the legs, patients are told they must live with their problem. Forms of therapy such as sclerotherapy are either not discussed or mentioned disparagingly. However, the available evidence would indicate that safe, effective forms of treatment (other than surgery) are possible and mostly successful.[1,7,22,43] The following discussion excludes the medical forms of treatment such as hormones or tetracycline; the discussion confines itself to the surgical or sclerosing types of treatment for telangiectasias. Sclerosing therapy and surgical therapy for large varicose veins are beyond the scope of this textbook.

Electrosurgery

Electrosurgery has been used for many years for telangiectasias, especially those on the face. If high-frequency electrosurgery is used, very low amperage current is used, as in electrolysis.[29] The vessel is penetrated by the electrode tip, or the skin overlying the vessel is touched without penetration.[41] With the machine on and the tip of the electrode on or in the telangiectasia, the switch is gently tripped to provide a short, quick current burst. The vessel rapidly disappears, and the current is switched off. Alternatively, one can use a small, 30-gauge needle, which is either touched to or inserted slightly into the vessel; the needle is then in turn touched with the electrode tip as the electrosurgery machine is activated (Fig. 16-20). This latter technique is useful, especially on telangiectasias that are small. It is ideal for spider telangiectasias on the face. The current is directed to the central feeding vessel. Once obliteration of this vessel occurs, the surrounding vessels disappear. The problem with electrodesiccation and electrocoagulation is that some superficial necrosis almost always occurs. In addition, subcutaneous tissue coagulation might be necessary to produce vascular sclerosis.[8] Thus scarring is a definite possibility. On the face one may notice that small whitish scars appear with time, and on the legs linear depressions may result. New types of equipment with special needles and more controlled current that cause less heat destruction are being made and hold promise for the future.[8,10]

Laser therapy

Laser therapy for telangiectasias is currently being recommended by those with lasers. The CO_2 laser destroys the tissue overlying the vessel and thus is of no advantage over high-frequency electrosurgery. However, the argon laser is theoretically better suited for treating telangiectasias. The blue-green light (488 to 514 nm) that is emitted from this machine passes relatively unabsorbed through the skin surface and is mostly selectively absorbed by the red-purple oxygenated hemoglobin located in the superficial dermal ectatic blood vessels. Light energy is transformed into heat, and dermal damage ensues. Vessel thrombosis occurs and lesions lighten. However, the argon laser light is not entirely hemoglobin specific, and the pulse duration necessary results in radial heat diffusion and nonselective thermal destruction. Nevertheless, excellent results have been reported with the argon laser on facial telangiectasias and venous lakes.[3,30] The latter lesions are dilated veins on the vermilion of the lower lip. However, other investigations with the laser have produced depressed trenchlike scars and hypopigmentation, especially around the ala and nasolabial folds.[17] Vessels in these areas require a relatively large amount of energy from the laser for obliteration. Telangiectasias or superficial varicosities on the legs also respond poorly to laser treatment. Not only do telangiectasias here frequently recur, but scarring and hyperpigmentation are more noticeable than was the original telangiectatic vessel.[3,16] Thus the laser is currently a satisfactory method for the treatment only of selected telangiectasias of the face in nonalar areas. In the future, the tunable dye laser, with its ability to be adjusted to produce highly selective vascular damage, might become the laser of choice for treating vascular lesions. When the laser is tuned to 577 nm (corresponding to the α-band of oxyhemoglobin), its light energy penetrates the dermal blood vessels with little interferring absorption of melanin. Thus highly specific vessel damage occurs.

Dermabrasion

Dermabrasion can be used successfully for telangiectasias of the face, especially for those found over the bridge of the nose.[31] This modality of therapy removes many telangiectasias at one time. However, if such telangiectasias are associated with an underlying cause—for instance, rosacea or cortisone therapy—they will recur within a few years.

Microsclerotherapy

Microsclerotherapy is a popular method of obliteration of both telangiectasias and small varicose veins that is widely practiced in Europe. The term *sclerotherapy* is derived from the Greek word σκληρός, meaning hard. It refers to the introduction of a foreign substance into the lumen of a vessel that subsequently thromboses and fibroses and thus becomes firm. Performed on telangiectasias, this procedure is called *microsclerotherapy*.[25] Such small vessels usually "disappear" after injection and cannot be found by palpation. Thus they do not become palpably hard, fibrous cords after injection, as larger veins may become.

Indication. Theoretically, microsclerotherapy can be used on any small telangiectatic vessel on the cutaneous surface. Best results are obtained on superficial linear or radiating vessels on the lower extremities. Telangiectasias of the face are less reliably responsive to microsclerotherapy, although they can still be successfully injected. Such variable results occur in this location because telangiectasias here probably have more of an arteriolar component and are caused by active vasodilation. Some sclerosants affect arteries in a different manner from veins. Although thrombosis may occur, intimal damage might not.[34] The blood flow in arterioles is faster than that in venules, providing faster dilution of the sclerosant and less chance for prolonged contact with the endothelium. In addition, prolonged compression cannot be placed easily on facial vessels after microsclerotherapy to minimize recanalization. Therefore recurrences or poor results might be expected on the face within injection of sclerosants.

Mechanism of action. Few studies have been done on the injection of sclerosants in man with serial biopsies at intervals. However, it is generally held that most sclerosants irritate the vascular endothelium and thus result in inflammation as well as spasm of vessel walls.[49] Ideally, the inflamed contracted walls of the vessel adhere together permanently. The damaged intima normally provokes clotting of blood, which forms a thrombus. Most likely the clotting is largely caused by the intrinsic clotting pathway, which is stimulated by exposure of blood to the basement membrane collagen underlying or between damaged endothelial cells.[33] This thrombus becomes fibrotic, causing "endosclerosis"; but it may recanalize. Enlarged clots are minimized by compression and emptying of the veins by gravity. Compression also minimizes clot retraction away from vessel walls. Such areas of retraction can provide avenues for reestablishment of the circulation through the vessel.[36] For small telangiectasias, clinically noticeable thrombosis and fibrosis are usually not present, even if minimal or no compression is used.

In one study hypertonic saline was injected into veins, and the injection sites were biopsied in six patients.[36] By 24 to 48 hours some degree of exudative reaction was found in all vessels with mild diffuse scattering of polymorphonuclear leukocytes and mononuclear leukocytes in the muscularis and adventitia. In every specimen the intima was found to be severely injured at the point of attachment of the thrombus. Organization of the thrombus began by the fifth day and was complete in 2 months; however the vessels were tremendously shrunken because of sclerosis.

Following injection with a sclerosing agent, the vessel turns blue as a thrombus is formed and then gradually disappears as the thrombus organizes into a fibrous band. However, recanalization of the thrombus can occur with recurrence of the vessel clinically if the recanalized lumen is large enough. Whether this occurs depends at least partially on the type and concentration of the sclerosing agent used. One study found that in the rabbit ear model 0.5% Sotradecol, 23.4% hypertonic saline, and 1% polidocanol (Aethoxysclerol) all produced sclerosis of vessels with clinical disappearance.[24] However, recanalization did take place within the fibrosed thrombus formed after Sotradecol injection, but not after injection of hypertonic saline or Aethoxysclerol. In addition, sclerosis following a thrombus did not occur with 0.5% Aethoxysclerol. The thrombus formed with this lesser concentration recanalized and the vessel clinically reappeared.

On the basis of the foregoing, a successful sclerosing agent would be both an irritant to the endothelium and a hemolytic agent. The hemolysis of red blood cells assists in minimizing extensive thrombosis. In this regard it is interesting to note that Sotradecol causes in vitro hemolysis and inhibits blood coagulation,[19] probably because this substance interferes with the cell surface lipids, not only on the surface of endothelial cells, but also on red blood cells by detergent action. Aethoxysclerol and morrhuate sodium act by a similar mechanism. Hypertonic saline probably causes dehydration of endothelial cells and hemolysis of red blood cells by an osmotic gradient. It thus extracts water from cells in the injected areas. Whether damaged vessels that are dilated are more susceptible to the action of sclerosants than undamaged vessels is unknown. Certainly, in experiments sclerosants appear to work well on undamaged vessels.

Contraindications. Patients with a history of thrombophlebitis or pulmonary embolism are generally excluded from microsclerotherapy.[43] Most authorities do not advise performing sclerotherapy on pregnant patients,[21,43] although one believes it is safe to use Aethoxysclerol during pregnancy.[20] Allergy to a sclerosant is a contraindication to its further use but not to the use of other sclerosing agents. Although allergic reactions to injected medications seem to be more likely in those with a history of multiple drug allergies, such a history does not in itself exclude sclerotherapy. Small amounts of the sclerosant can be used as a test dose, or a nonallergenic sclerosing solution such as hypertonic saline may be chosen. One investigator[12] has used Aethoxysclerol in patients on anticoagulants without excessive ecchymoses or other problems.

Available sclerosing agents. The ideal sclerosant should

TABLE 18-1

Sclerosing agents for telangectasias and small dilated veins

Name	Active ingredient	Allergic reactions	Necrosis	Hyper-pigmentation	Pain on injection
Morrhuate sodium*	Fatty acids in cod liver oil	Occasional	Frequent	Occasional	Mild
Sotradecol* (or Trombovar)	Sodium tetradecyl sulfate with benzyl alcohol	Occasional but severe	Frequent	Frequent	Mild
Hypertonic saline	18%-30% hypertonic saline	None	Occasional	Occasional	Mild
Hypertonic saline and heparin (Heparasal)	20% hypertonic saline, 100 U/ml heparin, 1% procaine	None	Occasional	Rare to occasional	Mild
Sclerodex†	10% sodium chloride and 25% dextrose	None	Occasional	Occasional	Mild
Aethoxysclerol† (Aethoxysklerol or Aetoxisclerol)	Hydroxypolyethoxydo-decane (polidocanol)	Rare	Rare	Rare to occasional	Minimal

*Approved for use by FDA in the United States.

†Not approved for use by FDA in the United States.

be nontoxic, efficient as an endothelial irritant, nonpainful on injection, and incapable of inducing necrosis or slough formation. In addition it should be chemically pure, easily standardized, and easily available.[5] No one sclerosing solution currently available meets all these criteria, and therefore one needs to know the relative advantages and disadvantages of each agent. Table 18-1 lists the solutions currently used for sclerotherapy.

The treatment of telangiectasias was largely ignored until the 1930s when the microinjection technique with the use of extremely fine needles of 32- or 33-gauge was developed by Biegeleisen.[6] This investigator used morrhuate sodium and injected not only intravascularly into telangiectasias and varicose veins, but also extravascularly either intradermally or subdermally. The extravascular injections resulted in tissue necrosis with little effect on the telangiectasia.

Morrhuate sodium is a mixture of sodium salts of saturated and unsaturated fatty acids found in cod liver oil. It is still available and approved for use by the FDA for injection of varices. However, injection of this substance is associated with occasional allergic reactions.[5]

Sodium tetradecyl sulfate (STS) is the other sclerosing agent approved for use in the United States by the FDA. Besides the active ingredient (STS), it contains benzyl alcohol and is marketed as Sotradecol in the United States and Trombovar in Europe. STS is a synthetic, surface-active agent (a long-chain, fatty-acid salt of an alkali metal) and thus has properties of a soap. In one series the use of 1% STS for injection of superficial telangiectasias on the lower extremities was reported, and only one episode of necrosis occurred in 600 treatments.[43] However, Mantse[35] reported frequent necrosis when 1% STS was used to sclerose tel-

angiectasias even when extravasation did not occur (Fig. 18-2). The frequent necrosis caused by STS was also shown experimentally using the rabbit ear vein model.[24] STS has also been reported to cause allergic reactions, including anaphylaxis.[40] Therefore, the manufacturer recommends allergy testing with 0.5 ml intravenously before injection of varices. However, some authorities do not feel this is necessary for microsclerotherapy when small quantities of STS are injected into small telangiectasias.[43] Hyperpigmentation following injection can occur in up to one third of patients.[46] This hyperpigmentation probably represents hemosiderin deposits and disappears usually within 3 to 4 months[43] (Fig. 18-3). The abundant hemosiderin deposits may be related to the hemolytic action of STS. Thus STS has a measurable but small incidence of allergic reactions, a risk for epidermal and dermal necrosis with inadvertent extravasation, and hyperpigmentation after sclerosis occurring in a significant number of patients.

The use of *hypertonic saline* for injection into telangiectasias and small veins was introduced by Foley in 1965.[22] He advocated a solution composed of 20% hypertonic saline with 100 units/ml of heparin and 1% procaine, which he patented and termed Heparsal. (Isotonic saline is 0.9% sodium chloride.) He advised the addition of heparin to prevent excessive thrombosis in injected vessels; that had been a problem seen with other sclerosants on larger vessels. He also advised placing about 0.1 cc of air in the syringe before injection. When the air was injected, the blood rushed out of the vessel before infusion of his solution, and this helped to visualize that one was truly within a vessel lumen. In over 1000 treatments in more than 100 patients, Foley reported no allergic reactions and only minor pigmentary

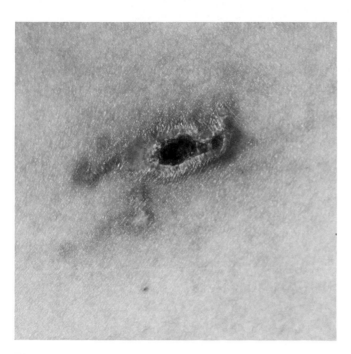

Fig. 18-2. Necrosis with Sotradecol caused by inadvertent extravasation.

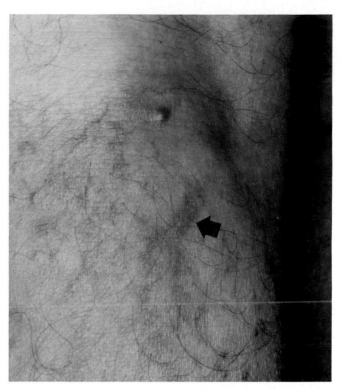

Fig. 18-3. Hyperpigmentation *(arrow)* following microsclerotherapy. Note that hyperpigmentation follows course of blood vessels injected.

problems. However, he did note necrosis if this solution leaked from the vessel or was inadvertently injected extravascularly. In another study small blebs were noted that could occur with hypertonic saline extravasation[1] (Fig. 18-4). The problem with necrosis has also been confirmed experimentally in rabbits.[23,24] But good results have been obtained by using varying concentrations of hypertonic saline, depending on the difficulty in sclerosing various vessels.[1] Use of 18% to 20% saline for venous lesions, 22% to 25% for arterial lesions, and 30% for vessels unresponsive to lower concentrations was recommended by Alderman. In 150 cases he reported 100% patient satisfaction. Another recommendation[35] is use of solution, Sclerodex (manufactured by Laboratoire Ondée Limitée, Longueuil, Quebec) containing 10% sodium chloride and 25% dextrose with 0.8% phenylethyl alcohol as a local anesthetic.

Excellent results have been reported by Bodian using hypertonic saline (23.4%) for dilated venous telangiectasias of the legs.[7] In a comparison of hypertonic saline with and without heparin, it appears that the addition of heparin is not necessary for effective sclerosis.[7] Bodian's technique is to inject into the vessel 0.5 to 1 ml of hypertonic saline after a small air bolus. The injection of air serves several purposes. First, it helps to establish that the needle is within the vessel. As air is forced into the vessel, the blood is forced out and injection can then proceed without likelihood of inad-

vertent extravasation. Second, the empty vessel becomes a receptacle for undiluted hypertonic saline. This solution thus provides maximal irritation to the endothelium of the vessel wall. Third, the lessening of contact between the blood within the vessel and the hypertonic saline minimizes hemolysis of red blood cells. This hemolysis produces brownish pigmentation caused by hemosiderin if extravasation occurs.[22]

The amount of air that can be safely injected into humans is unknown. One authority[22] recommended 1 cc of air for 4 ml of solution, whereas another[1] used 0.25 cc of air per a 1 ml syringe injecting between 3 and 8 ml of solution per treatment session. To date no adverse side effects have been reported with such small quantities of air injected at one treatment session.

The amount of hypertonic saline that can be safely injected at one treatment session is unknown. One source advised 0.2 g of NaCl (about 1 ml of his 23.4% NaCl solution),[7] whereas another used from 3 to 8 ml of 18% to 30% NaCl without problems.[1] Treatment sessions were every 1 to 4 weeks.

On injection, either intravenously or extravascularly, hypertonic saline stings.[1,11] This stinging or burning is more pronounced when inadvertent extravascular injection occurs, probably partially because of tissue expansion. Bodian[7] believes that the burning associated with hyper-

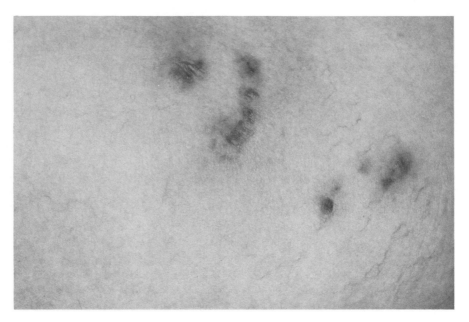

Fig. 18-4. Blebs (small bullae) caused by extravasation of hypertonic saline.

tonic saline injection occurs on withdrawal of the needle, at which time small quantities of saline are inadvertently deposited underneath the skin. To minimize this discomfort, one authority[22] recommended adding procaine (1%) to the injection solution and another[1] advised adding lidocaine (to a 0.4% concentration). However, because these local anesthetics by themselves sting, this addition probably does little good.

Another problem occasionally associated with hypertonic saline injection is muscle cramping deep to the area of injection.[11] Cramping occurs for 3 to 5 minutes and is relieved by gentle massage or walking.[7] It is frequently present after injections around the lower legs and ankles.

A further problem encountered with hypertonic saline injection is inadvertent extravascular injection. Should this occur, immediate pressure should be placed on the area of extravasation to minimize any blebs that may occur[1,7] (Fig. 18-4). In addition, if injection is being done on the legs, gauze and tape should be placed on the areas, and the legs should be wrapped with elastic bandages. However, sometimes blebs occur anyway, and this extravasation frequently leads to brownish macules.[11]

In summary, hypertonic saline injection, compared with other sclerosing solutions, is a useful and safe method of obliterating telangiectasias or small, dilated veins of the legs. However, it stings, is associated with some postinjection pigmentation, and may lead to blebs and necrosis. These adverse reactions may be minimized by experience and careful attention to proper injection techniques (discussed later).

Polidocanol was initially developed in the 1950s as a local anesthetic. It is an aliphatic molecule composed of a hydrophilic chain of polyethylene glycolic ether and a liposoluble radical of dodecylic alcohol.[15] Although its systemic toxicity is similar to that of procaine or lidocaine,[44] polidocanol was abandoned as a local anesthetic because of its peculiar tendency to cause sclerosis of blood vessels on intravascular or even intradermal installation.

Polidocanol was first successfully used as a sclerosant in the 1960s in Germany by Eichenberger.*[18] Some favorable reports appeared from other European countries (for example, Austria,[26] Denmark,[27] France,[28,38] and Italy.[9]) Concentrations of 0.4% to 0.7% were adequate for telangiectasias, whereas varicose veins required 1% to 3% AES. The success is high for small vessels and telangiectasias, whereas larger vessels do not respond as dramatically.[2,18,38]

AES has some advantages over other sclerosing agents. It is painless on injection, virtually without toxicity, and its allergenicity is low.[2,48] In one study, no allergic reactions were reported in over 19,000 patients.[27] However, rare allergic reactions have been reported,[27] including one case of nonfatal anaphylactic shock.[20] Therefore, as with other sclerosants or local anesthetics (like AES), such reactions are possible.

Superficial necrosis can occur rarely with AES, but it is probably related to the concentration used.[28] Experimentally in the rabbit ear model, AES was found to produce cutaneous necrosis on intravascular injection rarely at 0.5% or 1% concentration and not at all at 0.25% concentration.[24] If

---

*It was marketed in Germany under the trade name Aethoxysklerol. The anglicized spelling of this is Aethoxysclerol (AES), which is the form used in this text. Other trade names for this substance in Europe include Aetoxisclerol (France) and Atossisclerol (Italy).

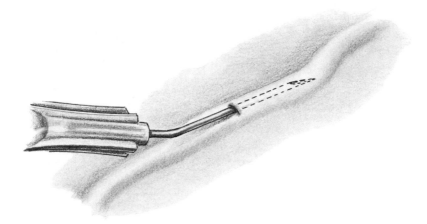

Fig. 18-5. Injection technique in microsclerotherapy. Needle with bevel up is bent 45 degrees to facilitate entry into vein.

extravasation occurs, AES is less likely to cause cutaneous necrosis than either hypertonic saline or Sotradecol.[23] In a series of 458 cases, necrosis was noted in 2.9% of patients using 0.25% to 0.5% AES.[9] However, this relatively high incidence of necrosis has not been noted by other authors, even those who purposely or accidentally inject AES intradermally.

Hyperpigmentation following injection of AES can occur.[7,9] However, Hofer[26] did not note hyperpigmentation even with intradermal injection of 0.5% AES. Perhaps some of the pigmentation problem is related not only to extravascular hemosiderin deposits but to hyperpigmentation of the overlying epidermis as well. Those patients with dark complexions will then be more likely to have hyperpigmentation. Fortunately in almost all cases this hyperpigmentation resolves in from 6 months to 1 year.[9]

AES, therefore, is a very useful agent for microsclerosis. Compared with other available sclerosants, it has low allergenicity, is painless on injection, and rarely causes cutaneous necrosis or pigmentation. Although not available in the United States, it can be obtained in Europe (Laboratoires Pharmaceutiques DEXO S. A., 31 Rue D'Arras, 92000 Nanterre, France, or Kreussler & Co., Gmbh D-6200, Wiesbaden-Biebrich, W. Germany).

Injection technique. Regardless of the sclerosant used, microsclerotherapy is performed with a standard technique. The patient is placed into the supine or prone position. It can be argued (if the vessels to be injected are on the leg) that the leg should be elevated so the vessels are above the heart[22]; this allows gravity to assist in immediate drainage and lessens the likelihood of excessive thrombosis after injection. I have not found this to be necessary for telangiectasias or small dilated veins. Before injection the skin is wiped liberally with alcohol to make the telangiectasias or dilated venules more visible by indirect lighting. The glistening effect of the alcohol is due to heightened light reflection. Alcohol also helps to clean the injection site. In contrast with treatment of large varicose veins, treatment of telangiectasias does not require first marking them with the patient standing, although on occasion this can be useful. A loupe for magnification might also be helpful to visualize tiny vessels.

Ideally, the goal of microsclerotherapy is to canulate small vessels so that the sclerosant is deposited within and not outside the vessel wall. To do this, a small needle on a tuberculin syringe should be used. Usually a 30-gauge needle is sufficient, although some physicians,[6,43] feel that a 32-gauge needle is less likely to result in extravasation. It is helpful if the needle is bent 45 degrees with the bevel side up, so that one can enter the vascular lumen at a small angle (Fig. 18-5), with the needle almost parallel to the vessel, and thus lessen the likelihood of vessel wall transection.

When the vessel is entered, aspiration is usually not possible because of the small caliber of the lumen. Therefore placement of the needle in the vessel lumen is largely by "feel." On injection, the vessel and its tributaries blanch. If hypertonic saline is used, one recommendation might be to inject a small amount of air to clear the vessel before injection of the sclerosant.[1,7,22] Its use with other sclerosants has not been studied; and, because clearing vessels might expose the vascular endothelium to undiluted concentrations of sclerosants, air injection may be unwise with sclerosants other than hypertonic saline

One starts by injecting the largest telangiectasias or the largest portion of the telangiectasia to be treated and then progresses gradually to the smallest ones. Usually only 0.1 to 0.25 ml of sclerosant is used at each treatment site. If extravasation occurs, immediate pressure is placed on the area for a few minutes. Then gauze and adhesive tape are placed on the area of extravasation. Following a treatment session at which usually 1 to 3 ml of sclerosant is used, pressure is usually placed over the injected areas. This is done with gauze, cotton balls or a sponge directly on the skin, followed by gum adhesive tape, followed by an elastic

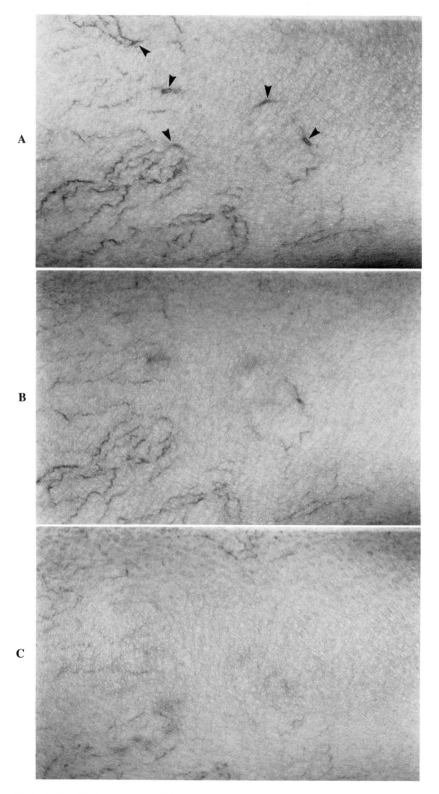

Fig. 18-6, A, Small dilated veins of legs. Arrowheads show sites of injections with 1% Aethoxy-sclerol. **B,** Fading of dilated veins at sites of injection 1 month after first injection. Some veins reinjected. **C,** Further fading of veins 1 month after second injection with Aethoxysclerol.

wrap. Graded-tension stockings (prescribed to give 30 to 40 mm Hg of compression) such as Sigvaris, Medi Strumpf, or Jobst, can be useful and more convenient.[32] The wraps or stockings should be placed on the patient while he or she is still supine, and they should be worn at least overnight before being changed, and then ideally for 1 to 2 weeks.[39] The patient is instructed to walk immediately after the injection session to help minimize significant thrombosis.

Elastic leg wraps or stockings placed after injection of vessels serve a number of purposes. First, they help to provide isotonic compression that minimizes venous stasis and will thus help prevent new ectasias from forming. Second, the pressure provided helps to seal irritated vascular lumina shut. Third, the pressure helps decrease the likelihood of recanalization of sclerosed vessels.[26] Fourth, the possibility of clinical and symptomatic thrombosis is minimized. Should extensive thrombosis occur, hyperpigmentation and necrosis can result.[47] Although some physicians[7,11,18,43] do not advocate wrapping extremities after injection of telangiectasias the procedure is so simple and the benefits theoretically so great that its routine use is recommended. Recurrence of individual telangiectasias has not been carefully studied, but on the basis of the foregoing, compression after injection might help prevent recurrences. Certainly for larger venules (larger than 0.5 cm), compression is mandatory. Rarely, an extensive thrombosis can occur even with use of careful injection technique followed by wrapping the extremity. Should this occur, it is recommended that an incision be made and the clot evacuated so as to minimize hyperpigmentation.[38]

The treatment sessions are usually given every 3 to 4 weeks until satisfactory improvement has occurred. This time interval between sessions is necessary, because complete venous obliteration usually takes from 1 to 3 weeks.

Fig. 18-6, *A,* shows a number of dilated veins on the lateral thigh of a middle-aged woman. The arrowheads point to the main sites of injection. After two injection sessions 4 weeks apart with 1% Aethoxysclerol (Fig. 18-6, *B* and *C*), the small dilated venules disappear.

REFERENCES

1. Alderman, D.B.: Therapy for essential cutaneous telangiectasia, Postgrad. Med. **61:**91, 1977.
2. Amblard, P.: Our experience with aethoxyskerol, Phlebologie **30:**213, 1977.
3. Apfelberg, D.B., and McBurney, E.: Use of the argon laser in dermatologic surgery. In Ratz, J.L., editor: Lasers in cutaneous medicine and surgery, Chicago, 1986, Yearbook Medical Publishers, Inc.
4. Bean, W.B.: Vascular spiders and related lesions of the skin, Springfield, Ill. 1958, Charles C Thomas, Publisher, Inc.
5. Biegeleisen, H.: The evaluation of sodium morrhuate therapy in varicose veins: a critical study, Surg. Gynecol. Obstet. **57:**696, 1933.
6. Biegeleisen, H.I.: Telangiectasia associated with varicose veins; treatment by a micro-injection technic, J.A.M.A. **102:** 2092, 1934.
7. Bodian, E.L.: Techniques of sclerotherapy for sunburst venous blemishes, J. Dermatol. Surg. Oncol. **11:**696, 1985.
8. Bolliger, A., and Holzer, J.: The problem of electrocoagulation of the smallest telangiectasias, Zentralbl. Phlebol. **5:**185, 1966.
9. Cacciatore, E.: Experience of sclerotherapy with aethoxysclerol, Minerva Cardioangiol. **27:**255, 1979.
10. Capurro, S.: Timed diathermocoagulation for the treatment of microtelangiectasias of the face: first impressions, Minerva Chir. **38:**947, 1983.
11. Chrisman, B.B.: Treatment of venous ectasias with hypertonic saline, Hawaii Med. J. **41:**406, 1982.
12. Dastain, J.Y.: Sclerotherapy of varices when the patient is on anticoagulants, with reference to two patients on anticoagulants, Phlebologie **34:**73, 1981.
13. Dee, R., and Finkelstein, J.E.: Treatment of varicose veins: sclerotherapy with compression or stripping with multiple ligations? Angiology **28:**223, 1977.
14. De Faria, J.L., and Moraes, I.N.: Histopathology of the telangiectasia associated with varicose veins, Dermatologica **127:**321, 1963.
15. DEXO, S.A.: Aethoxisclerol for venous insufficiency, Nanterre, France, Laboratoires Pharmaceutiques.
16. Dixon, J.A., Rotering, R.H., and Huether, S.E.: Patient's evaluation of argon laser therapy of port wine stain, decorative tattoo and essential telangiectasia, Lasers Surg. Med. **4**(2):181, 1984.
17. Dolsky, R.I.: Argon laser skin surgery, Surg. Clin. North Am. **64**(5):861, 1984.
18. Eichenberger, H.: Results of phlebosclerosation with hydroxypolyethoxydodecane, Zentralbl. Phlebol. **8:**181, 1969.
19. Fegan, G.: Varicose veins; compression sclerotherapy, London, 1967, Wm. Heinemann Medical Books Limited.
20. Feuerstein, W.: Anaphylactic reaction to hydroxypolyaethoxydodecan, Vasa **2:**292, 1973.
21. Foley, W.T.: Office treatment of varicose veins and ulcers, G.P. **31:**90, 1965.
22. Foley, W.T.: The eradication of venous blemishes, Cutis **15:** 665, 1975.
23. Goldman, M.P., et al.: Extravascular effects of sclerosants in rabbit skin: a clinical and histologic examination, J. Dermatol. Surg. Oncol. **12:**1085, 1986.
24. Goldman, M.P., et al.: Sclerosing agents in the treatment of telangiectasia: a review of the literature and comparison of the clinical and histological effects of intravascular aethoxysclerol, sotradecol, and hypertonic saline in the dorsal rabbit ear vein. (In press).
25. Green, A.R., and Morgan, B.D.G.: Sclerotherapy for venous flare, Br. J. Plast. Surg. **38:**241, 1985.
26. Hofer, A.E.: Aethoxysklerol (Kreussler) in the sclerosing treatment of varices, Minerva Cardioangiol. **20:**601, 1972.
27. Jacobsen, B.H.: Varicesklerosering med hydroksypolyaetoksy-dodekan Aethoxysklerol, Ugeskr. Laeger **136:**532, 1974.
28. Jaquier, J.J., and Loretan, R.M.: Clinical trials of a new sclerosing agent, aethoxysklerol, Phlebologie **22:**383, 1969.
29. Kirsch, N.: Telangiectasia and electrolysis [letter], J. Dermatol. Surg. Oncol. **10:**9, 1984.

30. Landthaler, M., et al.: Laser therapy of venous lakes (Bean-Walsh) and telangiectasias, Plast. Reconstr. Surg. **73:**78, 1984.

31. Lapins, N.: Dermabrasion for telangiectasia, J. Dermatol. Surg. Oncol. **9:**470, 1983.

32. Lewis, M.R.: Management of varicose veins by surgery and by injection, J. Tenn. Med. Assoc. **75:**11, 1982.

33. Lindemayer, H., and Santler, R.: The fibrinolytic activity of the vein wall, Phlebologie **30:**151, 1977.

34. MacGowan, W.A.L., et al.: The local effects of intra-arterial injections of sodium tetradecyl sulphate (S.T.D.) 3%: an experimental study, Br. J. Surg. **59:**101, 1972.

35. Mantse, L.: A mild sclerosing agent for telangiectasias, J. Dermatol. Surg. Oncol. **11:**855, 1985.

36. McPheeters, H.O., and Anderson, J.K.: Injection treatment of varicose veins and hemorrhoids, Philadelphia, 1938, F.A. Davis Co.

37. Merlen, J.F.: Red telangiectasias, blue telangiectasias, Phlebologie **23:**167, 1970.

38. Ouvry, P., Chaudet, A., and Guillerot, E.: First impressions of aethoxysklerol, Phlebologie **31:**75, 1978.

39. Ouvry, P.A., and Davy, A.: Le traitement sclerosant des telangiectasies des membres inferieurs, Phlebologie **35:**349, 1982.

40. Passas, H.: One case of tetradecyl-sodium sulfate allergy with general symptoms, Phlebologie **25:**19, 1972.

41. Recoules-Arché, J.: Breakdown of telangiectasia by electrocoagulation, Phlebologie **35:**885, 1982.

42. Redisch, W., and Pelzer, R.H.: Localized vascular dilatations of the human skin: capillary microscopy and related studies, Am. Heart J. **37:**106, 1949.

43. Shields, J.L., and Jansen, G.T.: Therapy for superficial telangiectasias of the lower extremities, J. Dermatol. Surg. Oncol. **8:**857, 1982.

44. Soehring, K., and Frahm, M.: Studies on the pharmacology of alkylpolyethyleneoxide derivatives, Arzneimitt: Forsch **5:**655, 1955.

45. Tolins, S.H.: Treatment of varicose veins: an update, Am. J. Surg. **145:**248, 1983.

46. Tretbar, L.L.: Spider angiomata: treatment with sclerosant injections, J. Kans. Med. Soc. **79:**198, 1978.

47. Wenner, L.: Sind endovariköse hämatische ansammlungen eine normalerscheinung bei sklerotherapie? Vasa **10:**174, 1981.

48. Wesener, G.: Morphology and modern therapy of small varicose dilatations of cutaneous veins and essential telangiectasias, Berufsdermatosen **17:**273, 1969.

49. Williams, R.A., and Wilson, E.: Sclerosant treatment of varicose veins and deep vein thrombosis, Arch. Surg. **119:**1283, 1984.

19

Ear Piercing

Pierced ears appear to be fashionable not only in primitive societies but also in the more "enlightened" modern world. Women as well as men currently have their ear lobes or other portions of the pinna pierced for reasons of fashion. Although this is usually performed by nonphysicians, physicians may be asked to perform this simple procedure.

PROCEDURE

The patient is instructed to bring a pair of earrings for pierced ears to the office or clinic. Before initial placement, the earrings are soaked in alcohol for 30 minutes. Sterilization is unnecessary, in my experience. The front and back of the lobule are cleansed with an antiseptic, and the point on the anterior portion of the lobule where the earring is to be placed is marked with gentian violet. Usually one double-checks with the patient to make sure that he or she desires the location marked. The lobe is then anesthetized with a local anesthetic. A 14- or 16-gauge needle is inserted from the posterior to anterior skin surface of the lobe (Fig. 19-1, B). The site of insertion posteriorly is approximately behind the previously marked exit point anteriorly. The needle tip is directed anteriorly to exit at the marked point on the anterior lobe. The thin post attached to the earring stud is then inserted into the barrel of the needle (Fig. 19-1, D). The needle with the post inserted is then drawn back through the ear lobe (Fig. 19-1, E). The needle is withdrawn from the post, and the clasp attached (Fig. 19-1, F).

The patient is instructed to leave the earrings in place until the newly created channels have fully epidermized. Usually this occurs within 1 to 2 weeks. During this time the earrings are turned once or twice a day by about 180 degrees to keep small adhesions from forming.

An alternative method of ear piercing is to use one of the "ear piercing kits" available [for example, Debut (H&A Enterprises, Inc., Whitestone, N.Y. 11357)]. Although they are convenient, they offer no advantage over the method previously described.

Problems

Ear piercing can be associated with certain problems of which the physician needs to be aware. Infection can occur after ear piercing. In one study,[2] 24% of individuals surveyed stated they had infections with pus after ear piercing. Cases of hepatitis, tuberculosis, or staphylococcal sepsis have also occurred after ear piercing. Another group reported a case of acute poststreptococcal glomerulonephritis following ear piercing performed with an unsterilized safety pin.[1] Although one might think that complications are more common with amateur practitioners, infection appears to be equally common with physicians, regardless of the instruments used to pierce the ear.[2,3]

Other problems associated with ear piercing include bleeding, cyst formation, keloids, or tears. A patient might develop an allergy to one of the metallic components of the earring post, usually nickel. If an allergy does develop, stainless steel posts can be used in place of gold posts. Because the nickel component is less in 18-carat gold than in 14-carat gold, I usually recommend that patients begin with 18-carat gold posts to minimize any allergic sensitization that may occur.

Elongated slits can occur following ear piercing if downward trauma occurs on the earrings (Fig. 19-2). Occasionally the earlobe slit completely transects the lobule, resulting in a split earlobe (Fig. 19-3, A).

The repair of elongated slits is simply to excise circumferentially the epidermis of the slit and and suture side-to-side the resulting surgical defect (Fig. 19-2). Although a new earring tract can be created at the time of this surgery, I usually prefer to let the wound heal first and then at a later time recreate the tract if the patient desires.

The split earlobe is more difficult to repair. If the epidermal surface of the split is simply excised and sutured side-to-side, a slight dimple in the inferior lobe results (Fig. 19-1, A). Dimpling occurs because the scar formed by the side-to-side closure contracts; the shortened scar pulls up on

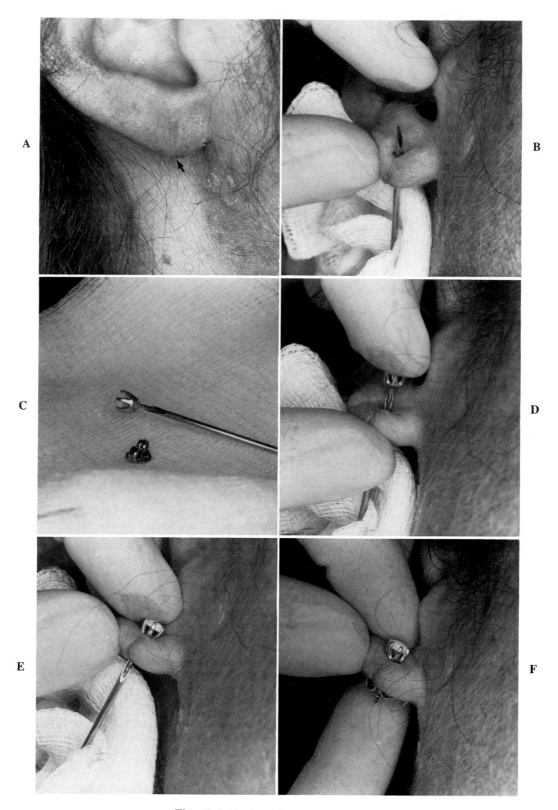

Fig. 19-1. For legend, see opposite page.

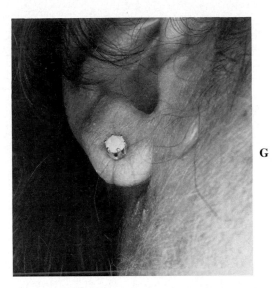

G

Fig. 19-1, cont'd. A, Earlobe before placement of pierced earring. Note small notch at lower end of lobule *(arrow)*. This resulted from prior repair of split earlobe by incorrect simple linear excision. **B,** Sixteen-gauge needle from posterior to anterior aspect of lobe. Note small amount of gentian violet that was used to mark anterior position of lobe, where patient prefers placement of earring. **C,** Earring post fits easily into 16-gauge needle shaft. Clasp lying off to side. **D,** Post placed into needle. **E,** Earring post is completely through earlobe. Needle is then withdrawn. **F,** Clasp attached to earring post. **G,** Final placement of earring, anterior view.

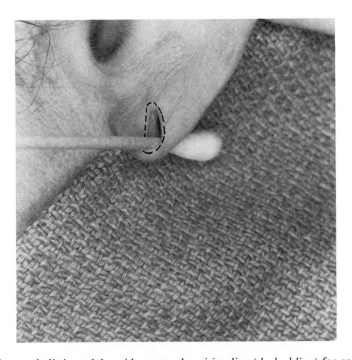

Fig. 19-2. Elongated slit in earlobe with proposed excision line *(dashed line)* for correction.

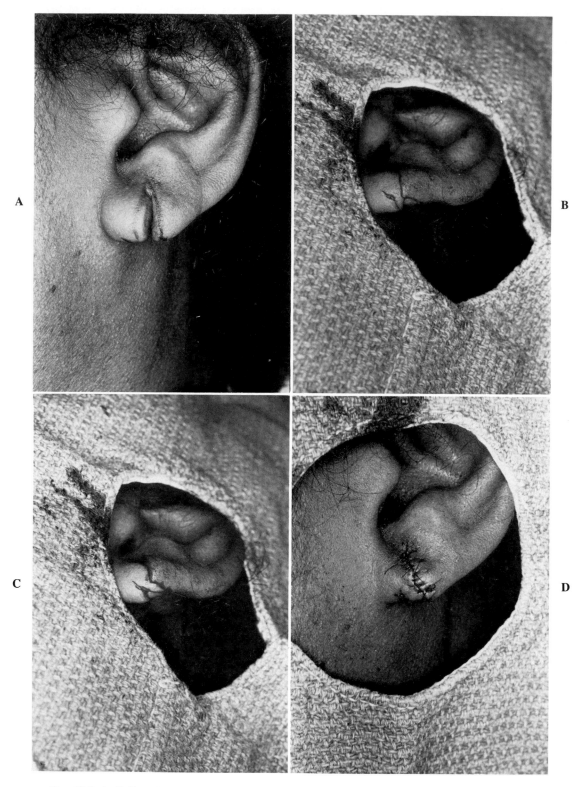

Fig. 19-3, A, Split earlobe secondary to earring trauma. Planned lines of excision plus Z-plasty (not completely visible). **B,** Small triangles at inferior aspect of each side of excised split lobule. **C,** Triangles rotated to interdigitate so as to form Z-plasty. **D,** Sutured lobule with Z-plasty at end.

the inferior surface of the lobe. To prevent this contracture, the scar can be modified at the inferior surface of the lobe by a small Z-plasty (Fig. 19-3). This effectually lengthens the scar and changes the direction of contraction. As with the elongated slit repair, I usually totally close the surgical defect created and only later repierce the earlobe, should the patient so desire.

REFERENCES

1. Ahmed-Jushuf, I.H., Selby, P.L., and Brownjohn, A.M.: Acute post-streptococcal glomerulonephritis following ear piercing, Postgrad. Med. J. **60:**73, 1984.
2. Biggar, R.J., and Haughie, G.E.: Medical problems of ear piercing, N.Y. State J. Med. **75:**1460, 1975.
3. Cockin, J., Finan, P., and Powell, M.: A problem with ear piercing [short report], Br. Med. J. **2:**1631, 1977.

P A R T

V

SURGICAL MANAGEMENT OF SELECTED CUTANEOUS LESIONS

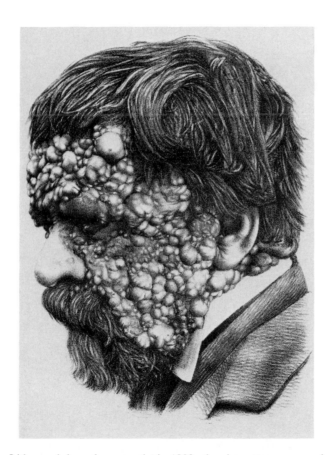

Lithograph by unknown artist in 1893, showing extreme example of multiple neurofibromas on face. At that time condition was known as molluscum fibrosum. (From Hutchinson, J.: Arch. Surg. [London] **4:**Plate LXIV, 1893.)

Non-Melanoma
Skin Cancers

BASAL CELL CARCINOMA

Skin cancers are the most common form of cancer. In the United States, it is estimated that there are 300,000 to 370,000 new cases (basal and squamous cell carcinomas) per year and that this figure is equal to about half the total of all other forms of cancer combined.[75,121] Since approximately 66% to 80% of all skin cancers are basal cell carcinomas, this means that about 200,000 to 300,000 new basal cell carcinomas occur each year.

In an evaluation of over 2000 skin cancers treated at the University of Michigan, 71.3% of the lesions treated were basal cell carcinomas, whereas 27.9% were squamous cell carcinomas.[57] The other 0.8% was composed of lesions referred to as basosquamous cell carcinomas. Men were affected more often than women, and more than 80% of lesions occurred after the age of 50 years.

Most basal cell carcinomas (BCCs) occur on the head and neck, especially those areas with abundant sebaceous glands.[146] Broders reported that 96% occurred above the clavicle.[12] This figure is similar to data from other authors[60,122,130]; however, most of these studies were done in surgical departments and probably exclude many superficial BCCs of the trunk. In contrast, in one dermatology department only 78.4% of BCCs occurred on the head and neck. This lower figure, which is more recent, may also reflect a difference in sun-exposure habits (such as sunbathing) from those prevailing at the time of earlier studies. BCCs infrequently develop on the extremities.[146]

Cause

Chronic sun exposure is usually accepted as the most common cause of BCCs.[146] Patients of fair complexion are at a high risk, since their inability to tan and susceptibility to sunburn maximize the potential for damage from the sun. The association with cumulative ultraviolet exposure over a lifetime is underscored by an increase in the incidence of BCC with age. With each decade after the fifth, the incidence increases by approximately one third.[75] Other important causes of BCCs include previous radiation exposure[2] and arsenic ingestion. Rarely, BCCs are associated with genetic syndromes, such as basal cell nevus syndrome or xeroderma pigmentosum. These syndromes are discussed later. More complete information regarding the carcinogenesis of skin may be found in reviews by Epstein[38] and Lang.[85]

Rate of growth

A BCC is a slow-growing malignancy.[139] One estimation on the basis of patient history was that this tumor increases at a rate of about 1 cm a year for the first 2 years of growth.[122] After that time the investigators felt that the growth rate is unpredictable and may become accelerated: morphealike and superficial BCCs are relatively slow growing, whereas nodular basal cell carcinomas grow at a faster rate.[71] This has been my experience as well.

Clinical appearance

There are four types of clinically distinguishable BCCs, nodular, superficial, morphealike, and inverted. Nodular BCCs typically appear as raised nodular lesions with translucent pearly borders (Fig. 20-1, A). Usually a few small telangiectatic vessels occur on the surface of the tumor (Fig. 20-1, B). Nodular BCCs are sometimes pigmented and may resemble melanomas (Fig. 20-2). When they attain a size of approximately 1 cm, the lesions may ulcerate centrally, giving rise to the term "rodent ulcer" (Fig. 20-3). As these tumors insidiously expand, they may destroy structures in their path, giving rise to considerable tissue destruction.

Superficial BCCs appear initially as almost flat erythematous macular areas. With time the involved tissue increases, and the tumor eventuates into a scaly patch (Fig.

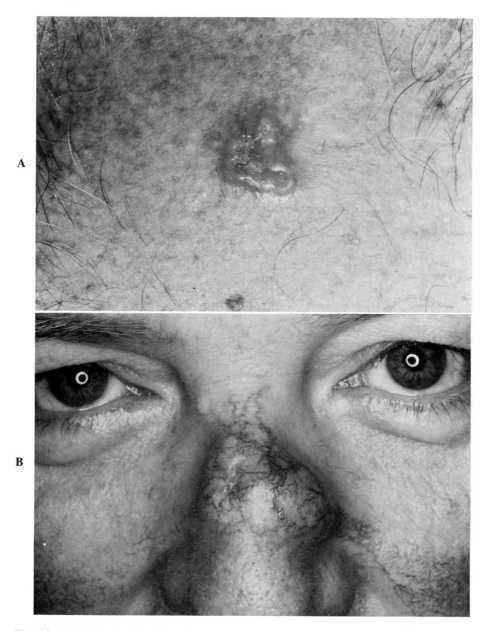

Fig. 20-1. Nodular basal cell carcinoma. **A,** Lesion on chest. Note translucent surface, smooth "pearly" border, and surface ulceration. Telangiectasias not well seen here. **B,** Lesion on nose with marked telangiectasias and no ulceration despite extensive growth. **C,** Microscopic appearance of nodular basal cell carcinoma. (Hematoxylin and eosin × 40.) Tumor masses contain basaloid cells with peripheral palisading. Note retraction spaces.

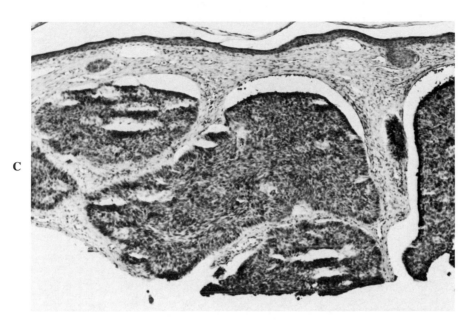

C

Fig. 20-1. For legend, see opposite page.

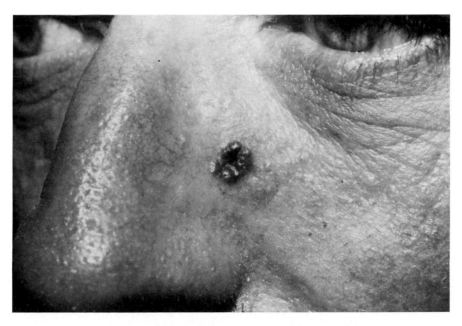

Fig. 20-2. Pigmented basal cell carcinoma.

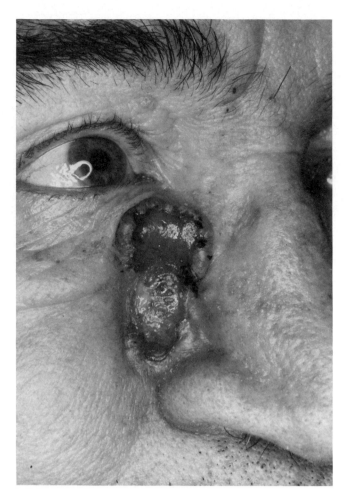

Fig. 20-3. Ulcerated basal cell carcinoma ("rodent ulcer").

20-4, *A*). Sometimes these patches have a fine threadlike pearly border and may show areas of ulceration. This type of BCC usually occurs on the trunk and extremities.

Morphealike BCCs appear as waxy indurated plaques (Fig. 20-5). Usually such lesions occur on the face and appear to be more common in individuals with a history of keloids or other diseases of fibrous tissue, such as Dupuytren's contractures. The borders of morphealike BCCs are notoriously difficult to determine with certainty by visual inspection alone.

Inverted BCCs are unusual. This tumor appears as a pit or shelf-like crater, without ulceration in the skin (Fig. 20-6). Tumor cells invade the dermis and usually subcutaneous tissue without a visibly apparent exophytic growth. Thus these lesions are purely endophytic.[47] Although a mostly nodular growth pattern is seen with this morphologic type of BCC, an infiltrative growth pattern may also be seen.

Despite the "typical" clinical appearance of the BCCs just described, many BCCs have an atypical appearance. They may appear as small pimples, papules, cysts, scaly patches or nondescript crusts. They may also occur as a true nevus (linear basal cell nevus) or in association with sebaceous nevus of Jadassohn. Therefore any persistent lesion, particularly in a patient already known to have had skin cancer, should be biopsied.

Histopathology

BCCs are traditionally divided into a number of histopathologic types. For the sake of simplicity, I usually recognize five types: nodular, superficial, adenoid, morphealike, and infiltrative. It is important to differentiate among these five histopathologic variants to select the proper treatment modality that affords the highest cure rate. An additional type of BCC—the basosquamous cell carcinoma—is discussed in the section on squamous cell carcinomas because this variant behaves more like a squamous carcinoma than a BCC.

The nodular BCC has masses of basaloid-appearing cells in the dermis or below (Fig. 20-1, *C*). The edges of these nests of cells are smooth and rounded. Retraction of the nests from the stroma may be present on paraffin sections. Sometimes in nodular BCCs one may see keratin

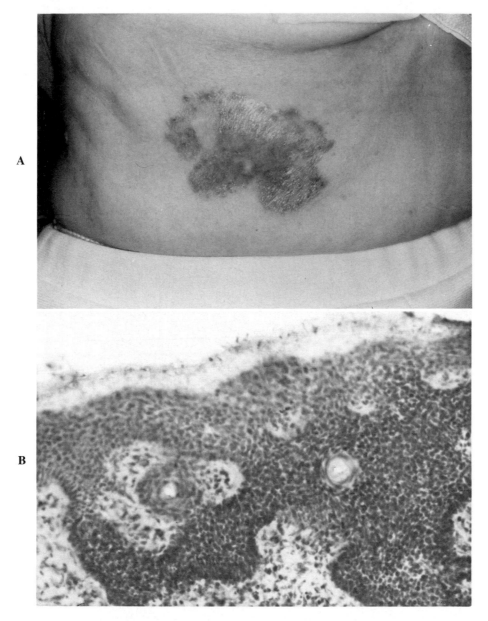

Fig. 20-4. A, Superficial basal cell carcinoma. Note resemblance to patch of psoriasis. **B,** Microscopic appearance of superficial basal cell carcinoma. (Toluidine blue × 100.) Note cells proliferating down from epidermis.

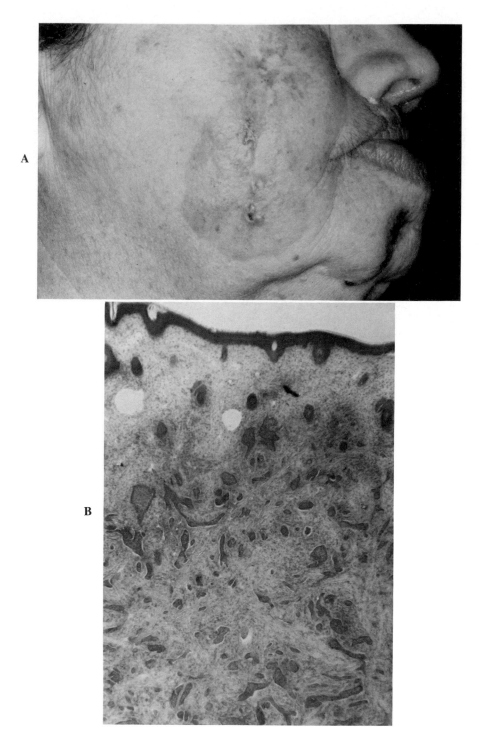

Fig. 20-5. A, Morphealike basal cell carcinoma on cheek. Previous excision attempt in center of lesion can be seen. **B,** Microscopic appearance of morphealike basal cell carcinoma. (Toluidine blue × 40.) Multiple small islands of cells are seen within dermis.

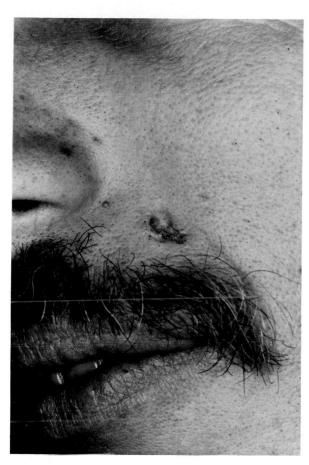

Fig. 20-6. Inverted basal cell carcinoma on upper lip with shelflike defect.

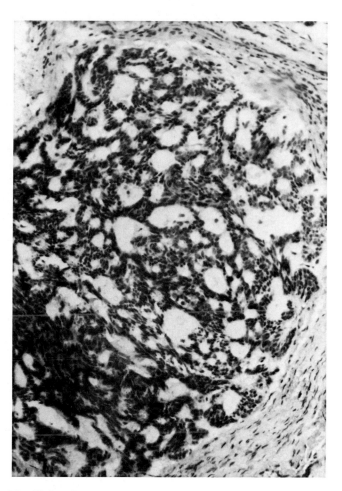

Fig. 20-7. Adenoid basal cell carcinoma. Pseudoglandular appearance with lacelike appearance of cellular strands. (Hematoxylin and eosin × 100.)

production (keratotic BCCs), cyst production (cystic BCCs), or calcification. These features probably do not influence invasiveness of tumors or recurrence rates.

A superficial BCC occurs as small superficial buds of tumor from the epidermis (Fig. 20-4, *B*). Usually these small buds of cells show peripheral palisading. It has been shown that the buds are actually interconnected if careful horizontal sections are performed.[94]

An adenoid BCC is a peculiar and distinctive histopathologic variant of basal cell carcinoma; clinically it resembles a nodular BCC. The cell nests are arranged in a lacelike or pseudoglandular pattern with multiple pseudolumina surrounded by tumor cells (Fig. 20-7). Thus adenoid BCC has a glandular appearance, which is referred to as pseudoglandular. This type of BCC tends to be infiltrative.

A morphealike BCC is characterized by multiple small strands of tumor, usually embedded in a fibrous stroma (Fig. 20-5, *B*). Often these strands are only one or two cells thick. On careful searching larger masses of nodular BCC are frequently found in some sections.

An infiltrative BCC is a type of nodular BCC, in which the nests of tumor have projections of infiltrative cords of cells (Fig. 20-8). Some of the cell nests are small (micronodular) or angulated with spikelike advancing edges. In addition, poor palisading of the peripheral cells within the tumor islands also exists. This histologic appearance is associated with aggressive BCCs.[86]

It should be emphasized that these descriptions and classifications are idealized and somewhat arbitrary. Frequently, some overlap exists. For instance, superficial BCCs may show areas of nodular BCC. However, the major portion of the tumor can usually be histopathologically classified into one of these five types. Ideally the treating physician should review the histopathology before treatment of the patient, so that the most appropriate treatment method is chosen.

Pretreatment biopsy

Biopsy before selection of therapy is advisable, if possible, for all malignancies of the skin and especially for

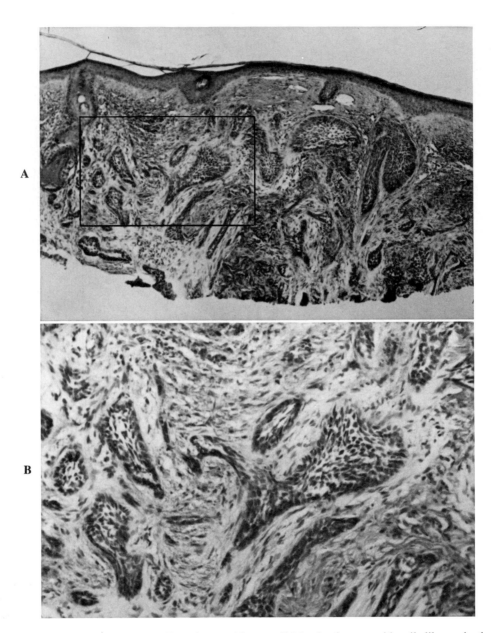

Fig. 20-8. Infiltrative basal cell carcinoma. Note small islands of tumor with spikelike projections (A). (Toluidine blue × 40.) **B,** Close-up of box in A. (Toluidine blue × 100.)

BCCs.[20,63] With these tumors, there is approximately a 17% error rate in making the correct diagnosis from clinical grounds alone.[90] When a procedure might lead to some disfigurement, a pretreatment biopsy is wise. There are two other advantages in establishing the diagnosis before treatment. First, the physician can speak with more authority to the patient regarding the precise type of tumor present, its known biologic behavior, and the most appropriate form of therapy. Second, not all BCCs show the same histopathologic growth pattern. Since the most appropriate therapy is partially determined by the growth pattern, the patient is best served by having this information available. For example, certain histopathologic types of BCC (infiltrative

and morphealike) tend to recur more frequently after routine excision than do other types.[45] Should a biopsy prove that a tumor is one of these two types, one should anticipate removing larger margins of normal tissue or obtaining frozen-section analysis of the margins at the time of removal, either by Mohs surgery or less ideally by standard surgical pathologic technique. Saving the patient an office visit does not justify immediate treatment.

The method of biopsy for BCCs is probably of little importance. Some physicians advise always doing a punch biopsy on the theoretic grounds that tumor may be missed on a superficial biopsy; in addition, deeper more invasive elements not apparent in more superficial aspects of the tumor may be seen.[45] Some dermatopathologists specify on their reports the depth of tumor penetration in millimeters if provided with a punch biopsy.

I prefer to take a superficial curetted specimen or even a superficial shave biopsy for obvious BCCs, because if the lesion is superficial, only superficial treatment is indicated. Punch biopsies have not been demonstrated to yield more information than simple shave or curette biopsies when the tumor is obvious. In addition, punch biopsies create a defect through the whole dermis, which is perhaps needless when the tumor penetrates only a small distance into the dermis. This may make further treatment more difficult and give rise to slightly more scarring. When the diagnosis of a skin tumor is not obvious, or if the presence of a tumor is suspected within scar tissue, a punch biopsy is preferable.

Treatment

There are six methods of therapy for BCC: (1) curettage with or without electrodesiccation or electrocoagulation, (2) excisional surgery with or without closure by primary repair (complex closure, skin graft, or skin flap), (3) cryosurgery, (4) radiotherapy, (5) topical chemotherapy (5-fluorouracil or dinitrochlorobenzene [DNCB]), and (6) Mohs surgery. All these methods have advantages, disadvantages, and cure rates, which must be weighed with each individual lesion and with each patient.

It should be emphasized that treatment of BCC has three goals: to provide the highest chance of cure, to give the best cosmetic result, and to provide the maximal degree of function. All three of these goals must be kept in mind. However, the first and foremost goal is to provide the patient with the highest likelihood of cure. To do less is to jeopardize the patient's welfare. Recurrences in the future may lead to disfigurement, disability, and even death. Warren and Lulenski[137] described this situation well: "Ineffective initial treatment often means dreary unprofitable hours in office or clinic and endurance of slowly increasing deformity which after years may end in death." Certainly the physician who initially treats a patient with a BCC has the best opportunity to eradicate the tumor.

The use of curettage for BCCs is explored in great detail in Chapter 15. Certainly for many basal cell carcinomas this is an ideal technique. Cryosurgery, radiotherapy and Mohs surgery are also excellent techniques but require special experience and training. Therefore these techniques are not discussed in any detail here.

5-Fluorouracil. Topical chemotherapy can be used on certain selected BCCs.[80] It is thought that 5-fluorouracil (5-FU) selectively destroys tumor cells through specific inhibition of DNA during the S (synthesis) phase of the cell cycle. The inflammatory reaction induced by this agent may also play a role in tumor destruction.

5-FU should be used for curative treatment *only* on small superficial BCCs. Such tumors usually occur on the trunk and extremities but rarely above the clavicle. When 5-FU is used, patients should be firmly instructed to apply the cream twice a day for at least 4 to 6 weeks. Patients need to be counseled that application of the cream leads to marked redness and some pain. If little or no inflammation occurs at 4 weeks, patients should continue to use the cream an additional 2 weeks. When treatment has been adequate (producing erythema) and has lasted for the prescribed time, therapy is discontinued. Patients may then be given a topical steroid cream to decrease more rapidly any inflammation that has occurred.

Fig. 20-9, *A,* shows a patient with a biopsy-confirmed superficial BCC of the forehead immediately above the eyebrow. After all the treatment options were explained to the patient, she chose to have the area treated with 5-FU. Since this was a primary lesion of relatively small size and the precise histologic appearance of the tumor (superficial), was known, I felt that 5-FU would afford her the best cosmetic result. Surgery in this location would have resulted in an obvious scar. The patient applied 5-FU for 4 weeks and a good response was obtained (Fig. 20-9, *B*). The patient was seen in a follow-up examination 6 months later, at which time the erythema had faded and the cosmetic result was excellent (Fig. 20-9, *C*).

In general I feel that 5-FU should be used cautiously as a definitive method of therapy for BCCs. Only on small superficial BCCs can it be considered a curative form of treatment. On nodular BCCs, larger lesions, or recurrent tumors, 5-FU is frequently an ineffective therapy. Klein et al. treated 36 nodular basal cell carcinomas with 20% 5-FU in a hydrophilic base for 1 month. This resulted in only a 50% cure rate.[80] Thus on common nodular BCCs, 5-FU should be considered palliative. Nevertheless, such palliative therapy may have a place in the treatment of BCCs when the patient is elderly or ill. When 5-FU is used for palliation, the patient and the patient's family should understand the lessened likelihood of cure compared with that from other treatment methods.

A characteristic problem that may occur with the use of topical 5-FU on nonsuperficial BCCs is that it may appear to cure the cancer on the skin surface but in reality allow deeper tumor extensions to persist and extend. Several cases have been reported in which indiscriminate use of 5-FU had placed patients in a holding pattern; that is, it prevented early definitive treatment for their neoplasms because the lesions appeared to be getting better.[98] Such a delay in definitive treatment undoubtedly leads to needless tissue destruction.

The advantages of 5-FU are that it is relatively inexpensive, convenient, leaves an excellent cosmetic result, and requires no surgery. On areas prone to hypertrophic scarring (shoulders, back, lips) or in patients with multiple lesions, 5-FU frequently gives the best cosmetic result. The disadvantages are that it may cure only a select few BCCs

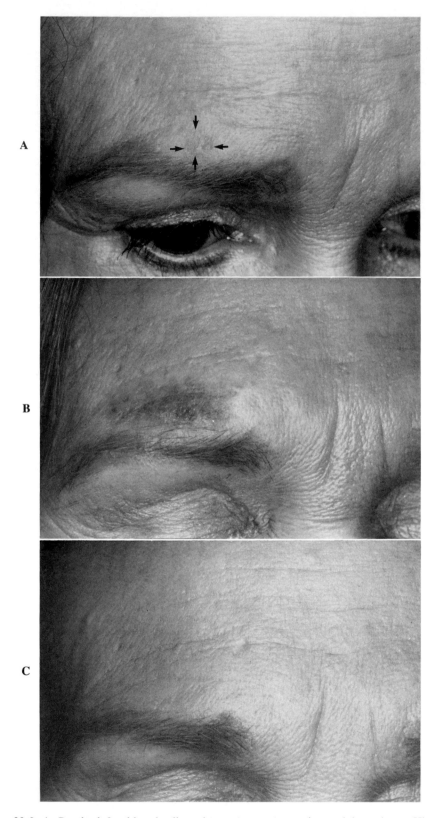

Fig. 20-9. A, Poorly defined basal cell carcinoma *(arrows)* superior to right eyebrow. Histopathologically this was shown to be superficial type of basal cell carcinoma. **B,** Erythema of basal cell carcinoma and surrounding area subsequent to 4-week application of 5-fluorouracil. **C,** Healed result at 6 months following completion of 5-FU treatment for 4 weeks. No recurrence of tumor after 2 years.

and causes irritation for the patient. Nevertheless, used under the appropriate circumstances 5-FU can be an excellent treatment modality.

Excisional surgery. Scalpel excision is a very common method of therapy for BCCs. For certain select tumors this seems to be an ideal method of providing the patient with a high likelihood of cure and an excellent cosmetic result. However, I disagree with those who think that the surgeon's method alone has no limitation to its application.[130] Certainly such an attitude is foolhardy and unwise.

After the lesion and surrounding areas are anesthetized and cleansed, I prefer first to use a curette to scrape the lesion. This gives good delineation of the tumor border, better than can be obtained by visual assessment alone.[133,134] The lesion is then removed with a 2 to 3 mm margin on all sides of the border produced by the curette, and the resultant wound is closed in the manner described in Chapters 10, 11, and 12. As pointed out in previous chapters, it is best to excise the lesion in a circular manner first and then close the circular defect along the maximal skin tension lines (Max-STLs). The inevitable dog-ears at both ends are then repaired so as to extend the incision line into the natural creases of the skin or along the MaxSTLs. If the lesion cannot be closed by means of a simple or complex closure, a skin graft or skin flap must be used or the wound may be allowed to heal by granulation and epidermization. Usually, however, it is preferable to repair a surgical defect immediately. Unless one has considerable experience, it is difficult to predict how a wound will heal and what distortion will ensue. Skin flaps and skin grafts are discussed in subsequent volumes.

Complications. The problems associated with excisional surgery for BCC, besides persistence of tumor, include problems that occur with any surgical excision. The resultant scars may be hypertrophic, keloidal, atrophic, or spread. Moreover, areas of hypopigmentation or hyperpigmentation can occur. Overall such problems can be expected in about 10.5% of cases.[6]

Advantages. The advantages of excisional surgery over other methods of treating BCCs are that the wound heals rapidly, tissue is provided for histopathologic examination, and the cosmetic result is usually excellent. If excision and closure are performed properly, a narrow, almost imperceptible scar should be produced most of the time.

Disadvantages. The disadvantages of excisional surgery are that it is time consuming and sacrifices normal tissue to provide a closure. Also, routine excisional surgery with simple closure has its limitations if the tumor is very large, deep, or in an area that is difficult to treat. In these circumstances grafts, flaps, or special reconstructive techniques may be necessary.

Margins necessary. The margin of clinically normal-appearing skin surrounding a BCC that must be excised to provide a cure is unknown. Various authors have offered suggestions that usually range from 0.5 to 1 cm on all sides of the lesion.[7,82] Such ideal margins are, however, in reality rarely adhered to [60] and may in fact be unnecessary.

Epstein studied the accuracy of visual assessment of the borders in basal BCCs.[35] He found that most tumors extended only 1 to 2 mm beyond the borders seen, and that therefore excision of such a margin of normal tissue cures 98% of tumors. The problem with the Epstein study is that he selected out the more difficult (such as the morphealike) tumors for Mohs surgery. In addition, the 2 mm margin was insufficient to excise his larger tumors totally, some of which were superficial. This is one of the reasons why I recommend curetting a tumor before excision, to define the borders more accurately.

In a study of tumors excised with small margins (2 to 3 mm) compared with those excised with larger (10 mm) margins, the recurrence rates were the same.[60] However, in this study the average size of lesions was relatively small, and the histologic types of tumors were not mentioned. As is discussed later, both of these variables are important in determining the margin necessary for cure.

Assessment of cut margins. Several papers have appeared in which the significance of "positive" or "negative" cut margins at the time of BCC excision is investigated* (Table 20-1). In general these studies suggest that if a margin is positive—that is, a BCC extends to the cut tissue edge examined histopathologically—a recurrence can be expected within 5 years in about 25% to 33% of cases, provided that no further therapy is given. This has led many surgeons simply to wait and hope that a given patient will not have a recurrence in the future.[1] This attitude is generally but not uniformly accepted.[4,63,83]

In contrast to the teaching in surgery, the teaching in dermatology has been to reexcise immediately if margins are involved with tumor.[4] It is felt that tumor masses left behind frequently lie deep in the lower dermis or subdermal tissue rather than in the upper dermis. Because of their location, deep recurrences are not readily apparent; they may appear as deep nodules or cysts without affecting the skin surface.

How does one make sense of the paradox that positive margins infrequently (about a third of the time) result in recurrence of tumor? Various explanations have been proposed such as inflammation, immune response, tumor trapped in scar tissue, or artifacts of fixation.[55,56,70] However, these are merely rationalizations to explain facts and not facts in themselves. More pertinent is the fact that in most studies the patients are not carefully followed-up. Although some studies state that their follow-up duration has been 5 or even 10 years, frequently this is only an average follow-up period. Furthermore, the patients are not systematically seen back and examined by one or two investigators; usually records are retrospectively reviewed. It is

---

*References 56, 66, 88, 106, 122, 130.

TABLE 20-1

Recurrence rates after incomplete excision of basal cell carcinoma

	Recurrence rate			
Author	Margins positive	Margins close	Margins clear	Follow-up
Gooding et al.[56]	34.8%	—	—	5 years
Hayes[66]	16%	—	13.8%	1-20 years
Pascal et al.[106]	33%	12%	1.2%	10 years
Shanoff et al.[122]	19%	67%	5.5%	Not stated
Taylor and Barisoni[130]	24.4%	—	5.7%	2 years (average)

sometimes assumed that if the patient does not return in follow-up, there has been no recurrence.

New data suggest that such watchful waiting is perhaps dangerous. One group correlated the type of histologic appearance of BCC with possible recurrence in the future if the margins at the time of surgery were positive.[26] The investigators found that if the margins were positive and the tumor histologically had large numbers of irregularities in the peripheral palisade and invasive elements, then 93% of these patients had a recurrence. In contrast, if the margins were positive and these irregularities were minimal, none of the patients had a recurrence in the future.

Pathologists occasionally use the term *close* to describe the proximity of a tumor to the cut surgical margin. Unfortunately there is no uniform definition of this term.[1] Some pathologists mean one high-power field, whereas others mean only a few cell diameters. Thus "close" is a rather subjective term.

Another study found the rate of a BCC recurrence with positive margins to be 19%[122] (Table 20-1); however, if the margins were "close," the recurrence rate increased to 67%. The authors were at a loss to explain these incongruous data. However, several explanations are possible. Perhaps with positive margins reexcision was more likely, whereas with close margins the surgeons were more likely not to reexcise. Whatever the reason, *close margins* may be practically synonymous with and carry the same significance as *positive margins*.

Before one can understand the significance of these data one needs to explore the implication of the term *margin* as meant by the pathologist. By this term the pathologist means the margin histologically examined. Usually this is only a very small portion of the total specimen. The standard method to assess a surgical specimen is the cross method, shown in Fig. 20-10. Note that only a small portion of each of the two axes is actually grossly cut and placed into cassettes. Of the tissue then placed into cassettes, only a small portion is actually examined histologically. When pathologists speak of tumor extending to the margin, then,

they actually refer only to the relatively small sample of the cut margin actually examined histologically.

There are other techniques for histopathologic examination of tissue that examine a greater proportion of the cut margins. They are the breadloaf method (Fig. 20-11) and the margin method (Fig. 20-12). Although both of these methods examine more of the cut margins, a significant amount of tissue still remains unexamined. In the breadloaf method, most tissue within each slice is unexamined. In the margin method, the undersurface of the tissue is largely unexplored.

The ideal method to examine *cut* margins would be to examine every cell along both the lateral and deep cut margins in the search for tumor extension. There are two techniques for doing this. One is to perform the margin method combined with a horizontal section across the base.[116] In a typical fusiform excision of 2 to 3 cm, this yields 5 pieces of tissue (the 4 sides and 1 bottom section) to be placed (properly oriented) into cassettes for processing. The other method is the Mohs method (Fig. 20-13).[1] This method uses tissue removed in a saucerized fashion, so that sections are made of the sides and bottom of the tissue at one time.

The need for such thorough examination of the cut margins is not universally accepted. In interviews with 11 pathologists, Abide et al. found that most favored the cross method of examining tissue.[1] The methods to examine *all* of the cut margins were not performed by any of the pathologists questioned.

Necessity of frozen sections at the time of excision. Most BCCs can be readily excised and cured without the necessity of frozen-section analysis of the cut surgical margins. Only in a minority of circumstances are frozen sections recommended. The major indications are listed in the box on p. 633; they include recurrent tumors, tumors with aggressive or difficult pathology, large tumors, and tumors that occur in anatomic locations where cure is difficult. Discussed later is the evidence that these factors influence cure to a large extent and thus make frozen-section analysis advisable.

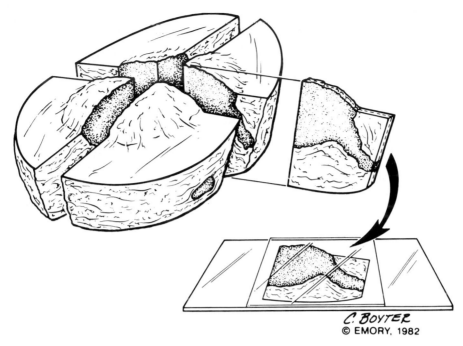

Fig. 20-10. Cross method used routinely by most pathologists to grossly section excised tissue containing tumor. Note that tumor extends to cut surgical margin, which will be undetected in histologic section. (From Abide, J.M., Nahai, F., and Bennett, R.G.: The meaning of surgical margins, Plast. Reconstr. Surg. **73:**492, 1984.)

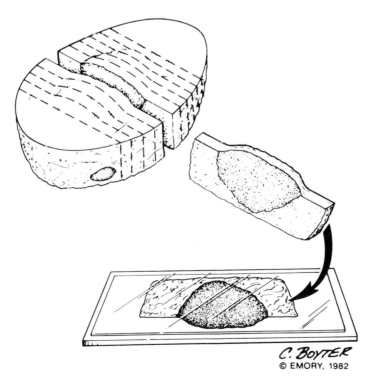

Fig. 20-11. Breadloaf method of sectioning excised tissue containing tumor. From each grossed slice only a thin tissue section is placed on slide. Note that tumor can still extend to cut surgical margin and be undetected in prepared pathologic sections. (From Abide, J.M., Nahai, F., and Bennett, R.G.: The meaning of surgical margins, Plast. Reconstr. Surg. **73:**492, 1984.)

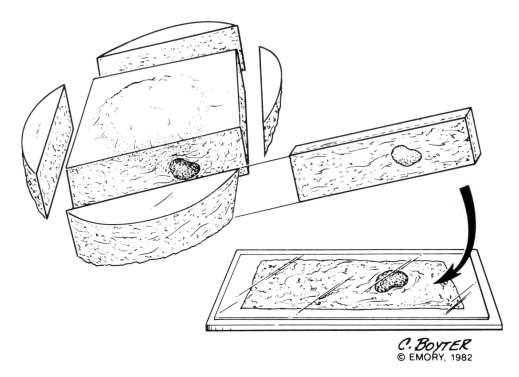

C. BOYTER
© EMORY, 1982

Fig. 20-12. Margin method of sectioning excised tissue containing tumor. Although outermost cut margins are totally examined, bottom is not completely examined unless horizontal section is taken across whole undersurface. (From Abide, J.M., Nahai, F., and Bennett, R.G.: The meaning of surgical margins, Plast. Reconstr. Surg. **73:**492, 1984.)

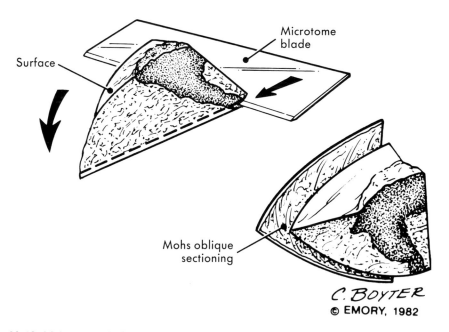

C. BOYTER
© EMORY, 1982

Fig. 20-13. Mohs method of sectioning excised tissue containing tumor. Tissue is oriented at time of sectioning so that *both* whole skin edge and whole undersurface are cut at one time. This is surest method to examine all cut margins of tissue. (From Abide, J.M., Nahai, F., and Bennett, R.G.: The meaning of surgical margins, Plast. Reconstr. Surg. **73:**492, 1984.)

INDICATIONS FOR FROZEN SECTIONS AT TIME OF EXCISION OF BASAL CELL CARCINOMA

A. Recurrent lesions
B. Lesions with aggressive or difficult pathology
   1. Morphealike basal cell carcinoma
   2. "Infiltrative" basal cell carcinoma
   3. Adenoid basal cell carcinoma
C. Large basal cell carcinomas
   1. Larger than 2 cm on face
   2. Larger than 4 cm on trunk
D. Difficult-to-cure anatomic locations
   1. Nose, periorbital, lips, ears, perineum

TABLE 20-2

Variables influencing recurrence rates with nonMohs excision of basal cell carcinoma

Variable	Recurrence rate
Recurrent	
From prior excision	46%[6] to 62%[95]
From any prior treatment method	8.8%[6] to 39%[95]
Histopathology	
"Invasive"	30%[124]
Margins positive (Table 20-1)	19%[122] to 34.8%[56]
Margins positive and "invasive"	93%[26]
Size	
Less than 2 cm	4.3%[82]
More than 2 cm	8%[82]
Anatomic Location	
Trunk and extremities	Less than 1%[122]
Head (site unspecified)	15%[122]
Scalp	10.5%[6]
Periocular	13%[6]
Nose	14%[106]
Lips	40%[6]
Ears	33.3%[6]

Most of the time routine frozen sections performed by pathologists are available. As previously discussed, these types of sections (Fig. 20-10) are less than ideal but are better than no frozen sections at all. Mohs frozen sections are ideal and should be cut if possible in selected cases; however, the preparation and interpretation of such sections requires proper equipment, personnel, training, and experience, which frequently are not readily available.

A concept has arisen that routine frozen sections taken at the time of surgery are equivalent to Mohs sections. However, most pathologists grossly cut tissue for frozen sections in much the same way as the cross method shown in Fig. 20-10.[1] In other words, routine frozen sections do not have a greater proportion of the margins histologically examined than do permanent sections. One can get a faster report but only on the same small fraction of the margin.

Of course with a relatively small piece of tissue, full assessment of all cut margins is within the ability of most pathologists. Still, once the tissue is larger than 2 or 3 cm, to do this requires a progressively larger number of sections, soon outstripping the facilities normally at hand. Therefore Mohs surgical units, which are well equipped for this purpose, are the most suitable for large excisions.

If frozen sections are necessary, an additional reason why tissue assessment of the whole cut margin is best performed within Mohs surgical units is that the average pathologist usually does not have a large amount of experience in interpreting frozen sections, particularly those cut on an oblique or horizontal plane. In a study of 100 cases of basal cell and squamous cell carcinoma removed by a dermatologist and examined by pathologists using Mohs method of sectioning, the pathologists were unsure of the presence or absence of tumor in 19% of cases.[14] This is in my opinion an inordinately high percentage of equivocation, but it simply suggests a lack of experience.

Cure rates following excisional surgery. The great majority of carcinomas of the skin can be cured with any of the standard treatment methods, including excisional surgery, cryosurgery, radiotherapy, and curettage and electrodessication.[24] However, no prospective controlled studies are available regarding cure rates for these different modalities of treatment. Almost all studies are biased in one of two ways. First, the reported method is frequently the only method chosen for treatment. Second, when several methods are reported, the way cases are selected for the separate treatment methods is not random but usually by vote of a tumor committee or, more commonly, unstated. Nevertheless, certain concepts have emerged with respect to treatment of BCCs, largely from the cases in which treatment was inadequate and recurrence with tumor extension and even death occurred.

Published cure rates with excision of BCCs range from 75.8%[11] to 98.6%,[60] although most studies report cure rates ranging between 90% to 95% at 5 years.[6,24,82] At first glance it therefore seems that excisional surgery is an excellent method of therapy. However, several variables need to be taken into account that markedly increase or decrease the likelihood of recurrence with excision (Table 20-2). These are (1) the tumor's status—primary or recurrent, (2) the histopathology, (3) the size, and (4) the anatomic location.

Recurrent BCCs are more difficult to cure by excision than are primary BCCs.[6,66] In one study 39% of recurrent

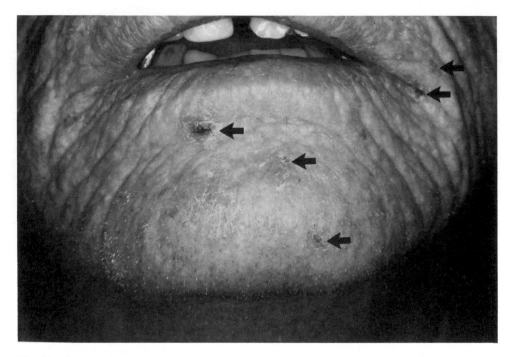

Fig. 20-14. Multiple basal cell carcinomas *(arrows)* occurring as separate tumors within previously irradiated field. Radiotherapy of face was given for acne 35 years earlier.

BCCs recurred by 5 years if excision was used regardless of the types of previous treatment.[95] Interestingly in this same study the recurrence rate rose to 62% if the prior form of treatment was excision. Undoubtedly tumor becomes embedded in scar tissue with previous excision and bits of tumor are discontinuous. Thus "blind" reexcision may have a poor chance of successful cure.

The histologic appearance of BCC influences the likelihood of cure with excision. For instance, morphealike BCCs are known to be more extensive than their perceptible borders.[17] Since one does not know the direction they will spread, one ideally should recommend Mohs surgery to remove such tumors. Adenoid BCCs also tend to go very deeply and to spread insidiously in my experience, and therefore Mohs surgery is a logical choice of therapy. Superficial BCCs, not being invasive, can be cured by almost any treatment modality if the lesion is less than 1 to 2 cm. Nodular BCCs can also be treated by almost any modality (except 5-FU) if the lesions are well defined and smaller than 2 cm.

A histopathologic concept commonly unappreciated but in the literature is the "invasive" or "infiltrative" basal cell carcinoma, which implies a basal cell carcinoma with nodular masses of tumor but with small strands extending from the nodular masses and appearing to invade the surrounding stroma[34] (Fig. 20-8). These small strands are frequently described as spiky.[74] As early as 1951 the invasive

pattern of basal cell carcinomas was recognized as a distinct histopathologic entity associated with a high chance of recurrence after treatment.[131] This has subsequently been confirmed by others,[34,45,86] who state that the likelihood of recurrence of "invasive" basal cell carcinomas is two to three times that of other basal cell carcinoma patterns.[57,124] Recently Dellon et al. recognized this pattern in most of their recurrent tumors that on previous surgery had been found to extend to the histologic margins of the excised tissue.[26]

The concept of multifocal BCC is used repeatedly in the medical literature with little documentation that such a clinical entity exists. Indeed, such a designation is usually not based on factual data but is more often a rationale for treatment failure. In one study it was shown that many so-called multifocal (separate) BCCs actually had small superficial connections.[94] Thus it seems that if multifocal BCCs exist at all, they are extremely rare except in certain situations. One situation in my own experience in which a true multifocal BCC may occur is in a previously irradiated field of skin (Fig. 20-14). Here multiple separate and clinically unconnected BCCs may occur that are histologically unconnected although occurring in close proximity. A second situation in which true multifocal BCCs may appear is in basal cell nevus syndrome or xeroderma pigmentosum. The usual patient with multiple basal cell carcinomas does not fit into either of these two latter categories.

The size of BCCs may also influence the cure rates with excision but less so than the other variables mentioned.[31,57,72] In most studies this variable is ignored. When attempts have been made to assess its influence, only crude estimates of size are used because precise measurements are frequently not available, since most studies are performed retrospectively, with analysis of patient charts. In a 1941 hospital study[137] the likelihood of cure was less for larger BCCs when either surgery or radiation was used for treatment. The investigators found a recurrence rate of 9% for lesions smaller than 1 cm, 30% for lesions 1 to 2 cm, and 65% for lesions larger than 5 cm. In contrast, two dermatology studies[6,82] found that cure rates varied little with the sizes of the lesions; however, the majority of tumors studied were small (less than 2 cm). For small tumors of a certain size (perhaps less than 2 cm), size might not be an important factor influencing cure rates. For larger lesions size is an increasingly important variable related to cure.

Perhaps the most important variable influencing cure rates with excisions is anatomic location of the BCC. In one study 15% of all facial lesions and 13% of neck lesions recurred.[122] In contrast, less than 1% of lesions treated on the trunk and extremities recurred. A reason for lower recurrence rates on the trunk and extremities may be that it is easier to excise a greater amount of tissue in these locations than in the more cosmetically conspicuous locations of the face. Another possible reason may be that the growth pattern of BCC is different in these two areas. Some evidence for this is suggested in a study in which BCCs were found histologically to extend less deeply on the trunk than on the face or scalp, leading to more complete removal with the curette.[128]

On the head BCCs in certain anatomic locations are particularly prone to recur or extend to the cut tissue margins. An area where this frequently occurs is the nose. In one study 41% of lesions with marginal extension were situated on the nose, although only 27% of the total lesions in that study occurred on the nose.[56] This has been confirmed by others.[106]

Other areas of high recurrence on the head include the ears, eyelids, lips, and scalp. Bart et al.[6] found BCC recurrence rates in these areas following excision of 33.3%, 13%, 40%, and 10.5%, respectively, compared to an overall recurrence rate of 6.8%

BCCs adjacent to any orifice are particularly difficult to treat and are likely to recur. Such sites include the external ear canal, nasal vestibule, mouth, vagina, and anus.

Clinical appearance of recurrences. Usually a recurrent BCE appears as a scaly macular or papular area adjacent to the treatment site. Sometimes the recurrent tumor appears to be similar to the primary lesion. Occasionally, however, recurrent basal cell carcinomas appear as cysts. Therefore any cystic lesion appearing in an area of previous treatment should be biopsied.

Time of recurrence. BCCs are relatively slow-growing neoplasms, and therefore an adequate length of time is necessary to follow up patients for possible recurrence after excision. Recurrences have been documented anywhere from weeks to 10 years or longer after treatment.[137] In one study, all 23 recurrences occurred between 1 month and 4 years, with the mean time of recurrence at 15.6 months.[56] However, patients in this study were followed-up for only 5 years. In other studies in which patients have been followed-up for longer periods of time, up to 10 years, some later recurrences have been noted.[117] Lauritzen et al. found that about 10% of their recurrences occurred 6 to 8 years after excision.[88] Hayes found that 44% of his recurrences appeared more than 5 years after excision.[66] Therefore to catch this significant number of recurrences, a 10-year follow-up period is advised after excision or other treatment of BCCs.

Other treatment modalities. Ideally the patient with a skin cancer is given the opportunity for treatment with one of several different modalities. For complicated lesions, patients may be presented at tumor conferences, where physicians representing a number of different disciplines meet. Although the participating physicians do not always agree, the opinion of each is solicited and respected.

The cure rates with curettage and electrodesiccation are presented in great detail in Chapter 16. Excisional surgery and 5 FU are discussed earlier in this chapter.

Cryosurgery cure rates are difficult to assess since so few studies have been performed. Graham and Clark[58] report a cure rate for BCCs of 95.57% overall[5]; for recurrent BCCs their cure rate fell to 89.5%. The cure rate for morphealike BCCs was 94.3%. They do not think that either site or size make much of a difference in cure rates.

Cryosurgery is a deceptively simple technique that requires special equipment and experience. The cure rate achieved by Graham and Clark on unselected cases certainly compares favorably with those of other treatment modalities. However, confirmatory studies by others are needed.

Radiotherapy is another useful treatment for BCCs. Cure rates range from 87.4%[31] to 94%[103] in relatively unselected cases. In a series of 500 lesions the highest recurrence rates occurred for BCCs on the nose, perinasal areas, and scalp.[5] The cosmetic results deteriorated with time and were only fair or poor in most patients 9 to 12 years after treatment. Three patients developed squamous cell carcinomas in the treatment sites (presumably from the radiotherapy), one of which metastasized and caused the death of the patient. Ten patients developed radiation ulcers or erosions. The authors recommend excluding lesions on the trunk or extremities from radiotherapy because healing is slow and the cosmetic results particularly poor in these locations. In addition, patients less than 40 years old are excluded to prevent late radiation sequelae (radiodermatitis and radiation-induced carcinomas).

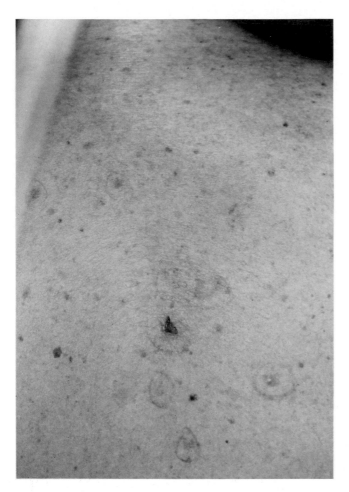

Fig. 20-15. Multiple separate basal cell carcinomas of back. These lesions appear somewhat clustered. Patient had undergone multiple chest fluoroscopic procedures 30 years previously for tuberculosis.

Mohs surgery is the specialized technique for excision of BCCs first described by Frederic Mohs in 1941.[97] Basically it is a staged procedure for removal of tumors that allows the physician to scan the whole cut surgical margin under a microscope. Sections are cut as shown in Fig. 20-13. This requires a special pathology laboratory. The cure rates for certain selected BCCs with Mohs surgery are higher than those with excisional surgery. These selected tumors include those that are recurrent, have an aggressive histopathologic pattern (such as a morphealike BCC), have a large size, or occur in areas difficult to cure. For such difficult lesions Mohs surgery has consistent cure rates of about 95%, compared with those of excisional surgery (38% to 99%) (Table 20-2).

Special considerations

A few special considerations regarding BCCs should be addressed since they directly influence treatment beyond what has already been discussed.

Basal cell carcinomas in children. BCCs occur rarely in children, but when they do they are frequently associated with sebaceous nevus of Jadassohn (described later) or basal cell nevus syndrome. These two conditions must therefore be searched for. Rahbari and Mehregan found that 36% of BCCs in children occur in association with one of these two conditions.[110] In addition, some cases diagnosed as BCCs in children may be misdiagnosed and actually be trichoepitheliomas. These same investigators reclassified 4 such cases out of 85 examined.[110] Otherwise the pathologic picture and clinical behavior of BCCs are no different in children than in adults. Every attempt should be made to provide definitive treatment for this group of patients, so that progression of the tumor does not occur.

Basal cell carcinomas in young women. Robins and Albom[112] emphasized that in their practice of Mohs surgery, they were referred an inordinately higher number of young women than young men with recurrent BCC. They thought that this lack of proportion was caused by prior surgical conservatism because of cosmetic concerns. Therefore they emphasize the necessity for objective assessment of the whole cut surgical margin, especially in young women, to ensure cure and conserve normal tissue. Doing so leads to less tendency to consider cosmetic result before cure.

Basal cell carcinomas in a radiation field. Patients who have had previous radiotherapy may develop multiple BCCs 15 to 30 years later within or near the field of radiation[2] (Fig. 20-14). Such tumors are likely to be multifocal. These patients should be followed-up closely for the likelihood of recurrences or more lesions within the radiation field. I do not recommend excision of the entire radiation-damaged area unless multiple carcinomas exist there. Excisions in radiation-damaged skin on the face heal with better cosmetic results (less perceptible scarring) than in normal skin.

In patients with multiple radiation-induced BCCs, the most common reason for prior radiotherapy was for treatment of acne (Fig. 20-14). These patients typically develop multiple BCCs mostly on the central face, especially the nose. However, other unusual patterns of BCCs should alert the physician to inquire about previous radiation exposure. Fig. 20-15 shows a patient with many separate BCCs of the back; 30 years before the development of these lesions he had received multiple chest fluoroscopies for tuberculosis. This association of previous multiple fluroscopies with BCCs has been noted by others.[2]

Multiple basal cell carcinomas in one patient. Patients may have multiple separate BCCs, either de novo or associated with a hereditary condition such as basal cell nevus syndrome. Many of these patients have been treated by numerous physicians with every method of therapy available. Occasionally some of the lesions are allowed to progress. Such patients need to be dealt with in a consistent but compassionate manner. All recognizable BCCs should be adequately treated and the patient advised to return at 3- to 6-month

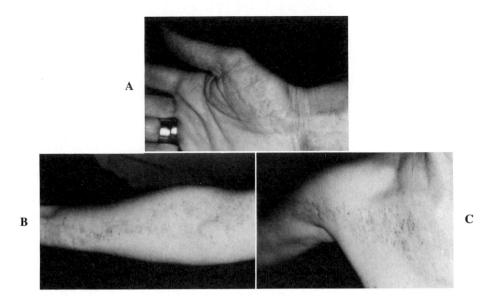

Fig. 20-16. Linear basal cell carcinoma extending from, **A,** palm and thumb to **B,** forearm to, **C,** anterior chest.

intervals so that any additional BCCs can be detected and more easily treated. If skin cancers in these patients are allowed to progress, patients tend to get discouraged and depressed. Once most of the skin cancers are treated, these patients can cope with life in a more productive fashion.

Unusual locations. BCCs can occur in unusual locations such as digits, perineum, vulva, and rectum. In these situations the recurrence rates with routine excisional surgery are high and Mohs surgery should be considered.[97,147]

Linear basal cell carcinoma nevus. BCCs occur rarely in a linear fashion associated with a nevoid growth similar to nevus comedonicus (Fig. 20-16). BCCs developing in this growth pattern are superficial for the most part and may be treated with topical 5-FU or DNCB.

Hereditary conditions. A few hereditary conditions are associated with the development of BCCs. Basal cell nevus syndrome is inherited as an autosomal dominant trait and is characterized by numerous BCCs that begin at an early age, usually adolescence.[67] Moreover, patients have pitting of their palms (Fig. 20-17), odontogenic jaw cysts, and skeletal abnormalities such as bifid ribs. Calcifications of the falx cerebri and basal ganglia may also exist (Fig. 20-17, *B*).

Xeroderma pigmentosum is an autosomal recessive condition in which patients from a very young age develop multiple skin cancers, including BCCs, squamous cell carcinomas, and melanomas. These patients are exquisitely sensitive to sunlight; they have a defective DNA repair mechanism, so that they are unable to excise abnormal DNA damaged by exposure to ultraviolet light.

BCCs that occur in both basal cell nevus syndrome and xeroderma pigmentosum behave and histologically appear as typical BCCs. If allowed to persist, these tumors show relentless growth and destroy structures in their path.

Metastatic BCCs have been reported with basal cell nevus syndrome.[102] Therefore every attempt should be made to treat these lesions definitively. One should not be deluded into thinking that BCCs that are part of a syndrome are less aggressive than other BCCs.[71]

Albinism may also be associated with the development of BCCs. This condition is transmitted as a simple recessive trait, often with consanguinity. The cutaneous pigment-forming cells, melanocytes, are present in adequate numbers but are defective in the synthesis of melanin. Thus the pure white skin of albinos provides inadequate protection against the harmful carcinogenic effects of sunlight.

Basal cell carcinomas associated with other abnormal cutaneous pathology. BCCs may be found in association with other pathologic conditions, such as sebaceous nevus of Jadassohn and dermatofibromas.[51] Usually the finding with a dermatofibroma is incidental and inconsequential. A BCC developing within sebaceous nevus of Jadassohn is not uncommon. Frequently such a basal cell carcinoma extends into the normal-appearing adjacent skin (Fig. 20-18). The whole sebaceous nevus, in addition to the basal cell carcinoma, must then be removed.

Basosquamous cell carcinoma. Basosquamous cell carcinoma, also known as metatypic basal cell carcinoma, is an ambiguous term because it apparently means different things to different pathologists. Supposedly this type of tumor has histopathologic features of both a BCC and a squamous cell carcinoma. It is important to distinguish a basosquamous cell carcinoma because such a tumor is more aggressive than a pure BCC and is as likely to metastasize as a squamous cell carcinoma is.[11] A more complete discussion of basosquamous cell carcinoma is found in the section on squamous cell carcinoma.

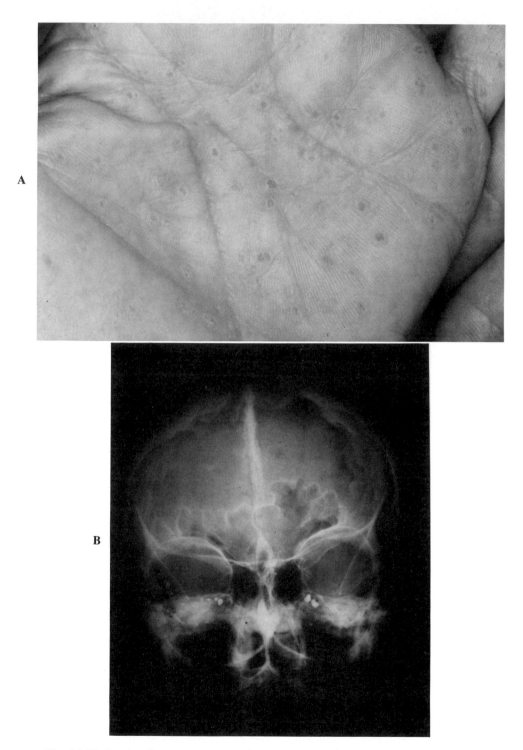

Fig. 20-17. Basal cell nevus syndrome. **A,** Pits on palm. **B,** Calcification of basal ganglia.

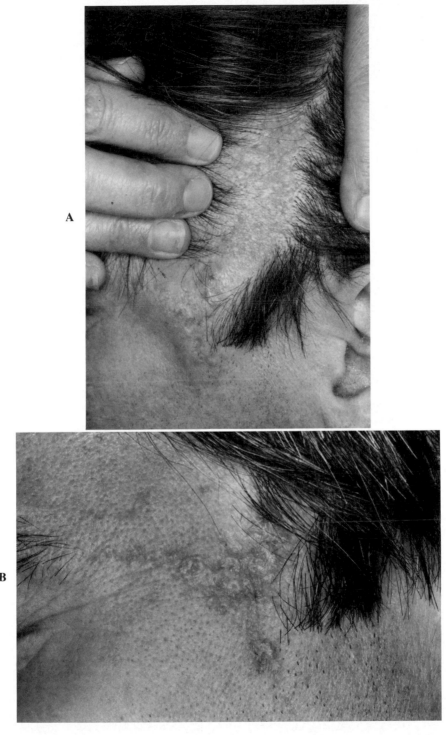

Fig. 20-18. A, Basal cell carcinoma within sebaceous nevus of Jadassohn in 35-year-old man. **B,** Close-up of **A**. Tumor extends onto adjacent skin uninvolved by nevus.

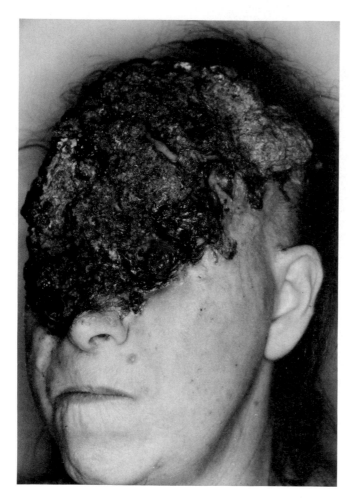

Fig. 20-19. Extensive basal cell carcinoma, which progressed over 10-year period. Only treatment was injection with 5-FU.

Metastatic basal cell carcinoma

BCCs may rarely become metastatic. As of 1984 there were 205 reported cases in the medical literature.[30] The exact incidence of metastatic BCC is unknown but is estimated to be less than 0.01% and is related to the complexity of the cases in a given series. In a large chemosurgery practice or plastic surgery referral center that handles many patients with aggressive and large BCCs, the metastatic rate is high and has been reported to be 0.1%.[30,84] In a general dermatology practice, which typically treats small, uncomplicated BCCs, the incidence is much lower, about 0.0028% or 1 in 36,000.[107,138]

In a study by Farmer and Helwig[40] of 17 cases of metastatic BCC, all lesions except four occurred on the head. Ten of the 17 lesions began before the age of 50, and 13 of the 17 lesions were recurrent. Where tissue was available for study, 8 out of 10 cases showed metatypic features (keratinizing squamous cells mixed with basal cells) in the initial biopsy. Recurrent tumors showed a progressively more metatypic appearance. Most cases (9) metastasized to the lung, followed by bone (5 cases), and lymph nodes (3 cases). Therefore unlike squamous cell carcinomas—which metastasize, through the lymphatics—BCCs metastasize by either lymphatics or blood vessels. Mean survival time after metastases was only 1.6 years, with only 4 patients surviving beyond 1 year. 5-FU was the only chemotherapeutic agent associated with patient survival beyond 2 years.

Most authors do not note perineural or blood vessel invasion with the primary basal cell carcinomas before metastases; however, Domarus and Stevens did note such invasions in three of their five cases.[30] Probably this event occurs more commonly than is appreciated because of the usually limited amount of tumor tissue actually examined histologically.

In every case of metastatic BCC I have seen, the primary lesion was very large and had been treated unsuccessfully a number of times previously. Moreover, in most cases there seemed to be some dispute as to the pathology. Commonly metastatic basal cells appeared to be basosquamous cell carcinomas (also called metatypic basal cell carcinomas).[11,25]

Death

Inadequate excision or nontreatment of BCCs may lead to disfigurement (Fig. 20-19) and even death. In a study of 2900 BCCs, 0.14% resulted in the death of the patient, usually by direct extension and subsequent meningitis.[88] Of the 101 patients with recurrent tumors in this study, 4 (3.9%) died from BCCs. Therefore recurrence of tumor places the patient at 28 times greater risk for this event to occur. In my experience patients who die of BCC have the initial development of their lesion at a relatively young age (usually twenties or early thirties). The anatomic location is usually the central face, and radiation has been used at least once early in the course of tumor treatment.

Follow-up examinations

After treatment of a BCC, every patient should return for examination of the treatment site at intervals for at least 5 years and preferably 10 years to detect possible recurrence. During the first year, follow-up visits need to be more frequent, since this is the time when most recurrences become apparent. After that time the patient needs to return only once a year. Every office or clinic should maintain its own follow-up system to ensure that patients are reexamined at intervals. For patients who find it impossible or inconvenient to return, a family physician may be helpful in obtaining follow-up information.

Follow-up examinations of patients treated for skin cancer are also useful to detect additional separate skin tumors. One study reported that 20% of patients treated previously for a BCC were found to have a new skin cancer (usually

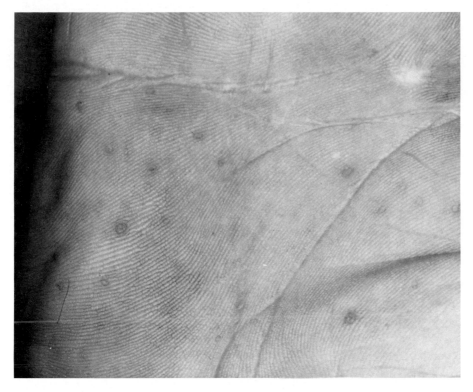

Fig. 20-20. Multiple raised keratoses of palms in patient with previous history of arsenic exposure.

BCC) within 1 year study period.[36] In addition, of those patients treated for two or more BCCs, 41% developed a new skin cancer; if treated for three or more BCCs, 56% developed a new skin cancer within the same study period.

Prophylaxis

Patients who have developed a basal cell carcinoma are at risk to develop additional lesions in the future. Since sunlight is probably the main potentiating factor in the production of this neoplasm, patients should be instructed to be cautious regarding further sun exposure. Although I do not advocate a change in life-style, patients should keep from *burning* in the sun. Sunscreens, hats, clothing, and avoidance of the sun at midday are all helpful.

BOWEN'S DISEASE

Bowen's disease is an intraepidermal epidermoid carcinoma that occurs on the skin or mucous membranes. It spreads locally by radial diffusion within the epidermis and with time may become invasive within the dermis. It sometimes then metastasizes. The likelihood of Bowen's disease becoming invasive probably varies with the size, location, and duration of the lesion. In one study of black patients 26% of lesions became invasive and 15.8% developed metastases that resulted in death.[101]

Cause and association with other malignancies

Usually Bowen's disease appears as a solitary lesion on the sun-exposed portion of the body, and thus solar damage is thought to be an etiologic factor. It may nevertheless also appear on non–sun exposed areas. In either location a history of arsenic exposure, either medicinal or environmental, is occasionally present.[115] The patient with Bowen's disease should be examined for palmar or plantar keratoses (Fig. 20-20). These are a clue to prior arsenic exposure. Patients with *both* arsenical keratoses and Bowen's disease are at higher risk for the presence or development of internal malignancies, especially of the genitourinary and gastrointestinal tracts.

When palmar-plantar arsenical keratoses or a prior history of arsenic is absent, the association of Bowen's disease with a separate noncutaneous internal malignancy is controversial. Since the initial report, which proposed this association between Bowen's disease and internal malignancy,[59] other reports have appeared that dispute such an association. One study of patients with Bowen's disease found no greater incidence of internal malignancy than in suitable controls.[3] Callen and Headington compared the incidence of internal malignancy in patients with Bowen's disease to those with non-Bowen's carcinoma in situ; they found no difference in the incidence of malignancy in these two groups.[19] However, in certain locations such as the

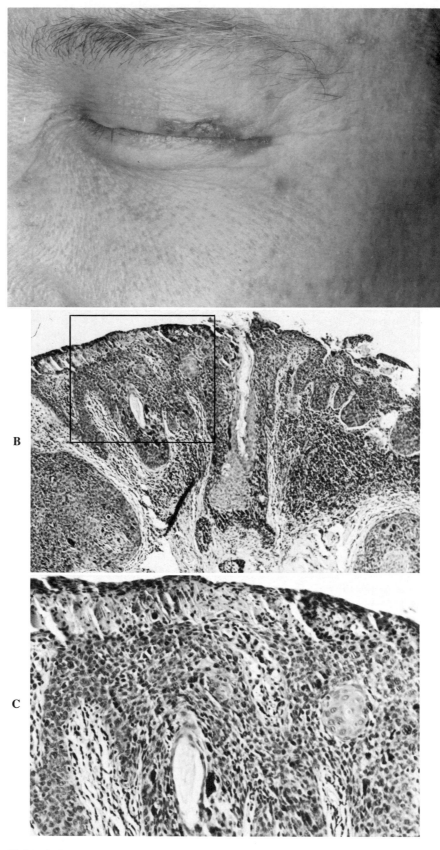

Fig. 20-21. A, Bowen's disease on upper eyelid and outer canthus. **B,** Histopathologic appearance of Bowen's disease. Note atypical epidermis involving external root sheath. (Hematoxylin and eosin × 40.) **C,** High-powered view of **A.** (Hematoxylin and eosin × 100.)

vulva, the association of Bowen's disease with underlying cacinomas of the genital tract may be frequent.[91]

One widely held contention is that Bowen's disease located on non–sun exposed areas carries an increased risk of internal malignancy. However, Callen and Headington found that there was no difference in the malignancy rate if the Bowen's disease occurred on non–sun exposed areas versus sun-exposed sites.[19] Rosen et al. were also unable to establish such an association.[115] In contrast is a study of 19 black patients with Bowen's disease, 5 of whom also had a noncutaneous malignancy.[101] All 5 patients had their Bowen's disease on non–sun exposed areas.

Despite the foregoing, it has been my impression, as stated earlier, that patients with Bowen's disease *and* multiple keratoses on the palms or soles are at greater risk of developing internal malignancies.

Clinical appearance

Bowen's disease appears as a slowly enlarging erythematous, scaly patch (Fig. 20-21, *A*). It varies in size from a few millimeters to several centimeters. The border is often indistinct but may be sharp and irregular. In blacks, Bowen's disease may be pigmented brown or black. When the lesion becomes invasive, it becomes nodular.

Bowen's disease may also occur on the mucous membranes including the glans penis, vulva, oral mucosa, nasal mucosa, and conjunctiva. Lesions in the first three sites are referred to as erythroplasia of Queyrat—a red, velvety macular area that with time becomes elevated and may ulcerate.

Histopathology

The epidermis is thickened with a parakeratotic, horny layer. The cells within the epidermis above the basal cell layer lie in disarray. These cells are atypical, and some of them have large hyperchromatic nuclei. Occasionally multinucleated epidermal cells are present. Individual epidermal cell keratinization may also exist. Keratinized cells appear with a round, homogeneous, eosinophilic, stained cytoplasm and a pyknotic nucleus.

Characteristic of Bowen's disease is involvement of the cutaneous appendages by the dysplastic epidermis (Fig. 20-21, *B*). The external root sheath and sweat ducts are usually involved as extensions of the surface epidermis. This is in contrast to carcinoma in situ from actinic keratoses or de novo, which tends to spare the cutaneous appendageal structures.[44]

Under low power, intraepidermal Bowen's disease shows a relatively sharp line of demarcation from the surrounding normal epidermis. Thus this carcinoma is thought to spread by radial diffusion within the epidermis.

Treatment

Surgical excision is the treatment of choice for Bowen's disease, since it usually involves the underlying appenda-

geal structures to an unpredictable extent. Curettage and electrodesiccation may also be used on small lesions or for palliation. However, recurrences are frequent with this form of therapy because it might not destroy the atypical epidermis within the depths of the follicular or sweat duct structures (see Chapter 15).

Topical therapy with 5-FU is recommended by some as adequate therapy.[127] A twice-a-day application of 5% cream usually produces a brisk erythema in 1 to 2 weeks. Therapy must be continued for at least 4 and ideally 8 weeks. However, I have seen recurrences with this form of therapy. Limmer reported recurrences within 3 years in 4 of 13 cases treated with 5-FU for Bowen's disease in the nongenital areas and 3 of 5 cases in the genital area.[91]

Erythroplasia of Queyrat on the glans penis may also be treated with 5-FU cream.[53] If it is used, occlusion with a condom should be used to ensure penetration and to keep the cream from coming into contact with the scrotum, where it causes irritation. Failure of 5-FU may occur with erythroplasia of Queyrat; these patients, like other skin cancer patients, should be followed closely.

In the vulvar and perirectal areas Bowen's disease tends to be quite extensive despite appearances. In the cases I have personally traced in these areas using microscopically controlled Mohs surgery, Bowen's disease frequently extends great distances. Therefore on the mucous membrane areas Mohs surgery is the treatment of choice for this tumor.

Bowen's disease may recur despite proper and judicious use of any of the foregoing forms of therapy. When this happens, Mohs surgery should be considered so as to microscopically and histographically trace out the remaining atypical epidermis.

BOWENOID PAPULOSIS

Bowenoid papulosis is a fairly recently recognized entity which occurs in the genital areas of young men and women.[135] Usually multiple, small (1 to 2 mm), flesh-colored or slightly hyperpigmented papules appear which are asymptomatic but may be pruritic (Fig. 20-22). About one third of the patients have a history of warts or herpes simplex in the area.

Whether bowenoid papulosis is benign or malignant is currently a subject of debate. There have been at least two cases reported that became invasive squamous cell carcinomas.[28,78] In addition, an oncogenic human papillomavirus (HPV-16) has been identified in some cases of bowenoid papulosis.[61] This seems to imply that bowenoid papulosis is a malignant process that might be capable of invasion if left untreated; however, the majority of cases follow a benign course despite recurrences.

Histopathology

The microscopic appearance of bowenoid papulosis is similar to that of Bowen's disease.[125] There are no histopathologic features to distinguish these two entities reliably

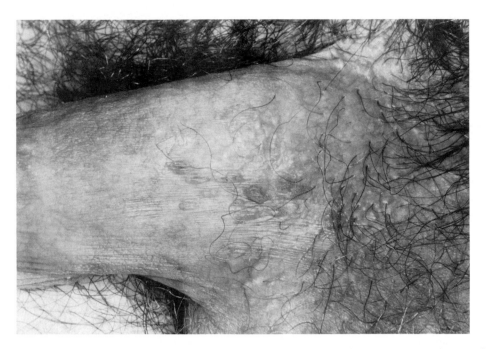

Fig. 20-22. Bowenoid papulosis. Note multiple small, flesh-colored and slightly hyperpigmented papules clustered on one side of penis.

except that the cells may not quite so atypical in bowenoid papulosis. Thus the diagnosis is based on both the clinical and the histologic appearance of the lesions.

Treatment

Bowenoid papulosis may be treated by a number of different methods. Cryosurgery, curettage and electrodesiccation, and 5-FU have all been tried, but recurrences are frequent.[78] Surgical excision with closure by simple suturing or skin grafting has also been tried. Some cases regress spontaneously, so many authorities do not advise aggressive treatment.[135] However, as previously mentioned, there have been cases reported to progress to invasive squamous cell carcinoma.

I have treated two cases of bowenoid papulosis with Mohs surgery. Both cases extended much further than could be appreciated by visual inspection alone. There have been no recurrences to date with a 4- to 5-year follow-up period.

KERATOACANTHOMA

A keratoacanthoma is a rapidly growing skin tumor that usually occurs on sun-exposed areas in patients over the age of 40. It arises within a short period of time, usually a few weeks to 2 months, and if left to observation it often completely and spontaneously regresses. Because they are characterized by spontaneous involution and an absence of metastases, keratoacanthomas are considered benign neoplasms. However, it has been reported that rapidly destructive growth and even metastases may occur rarely.

Keratoacanthomas usually are solitary but may be multiple. Two types of multiple keratoacanthomas are recognized, the Gryzbowski type and the Ferguson-Smith type. The latter type is ulcerating and found in atypical distributions (for example, on the oral mucosa), whereas the former is found in sun-exposed and hair-bearing areas. Although Kingman and Callen did not find any association of internal malignancy with keratoacanthomas,[79] patients with multiple keratoacanthomas should be investigated for immunologic impairment.

Only since about 1950 has the keratoacanthoma been accepted as a true clinical entity distinguishable from squamous cell carcinoma, which it may resemble both clinically and histologically.[114] Nevertheless, the keratoacanthoma was probably described by Hutchinson over a hundred years ago.[68] Before it was apparent that this lesion is different from a squamous cell carcinoma, many keratoacanthomas were considered squamous cell carcinomas. Therefore early cure rates for squamous cell carcinomas undoubtedly included keratoacanthomas, and this inclusion skewed the cure rate statistics to falsely high levels.

Clinical appearance

A keratoacanthoma is a firm, smooth, dome-shaped nodule or tumor, usually 0.5 to 2 cm in diameter, which is either flesh colored or slightly erythematous and sharply demarcated from the surrounding skin (Fig. 20-23). In its center is a crater filled with a keratin plug. Left alone, keratoacanthomas often involute in 2 to 6 months. If self-

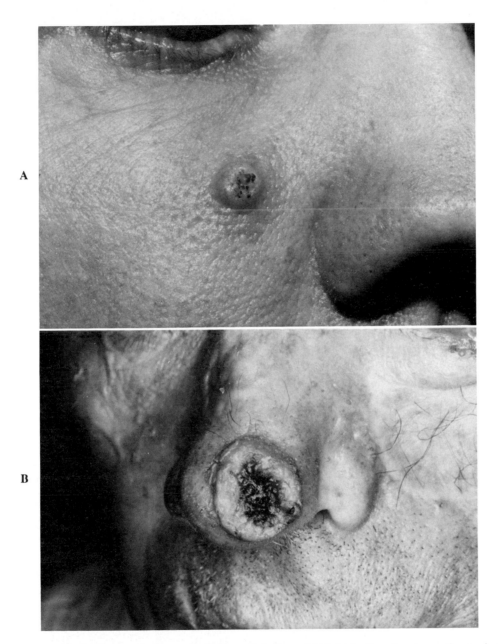

Fig. 20-23. A, Keratoacanthoma. **B,** Lesion clinically and histologically a keratoacanthoma, but tumor grew over 3 months and was found to invade through nose **(C).**

Continued.

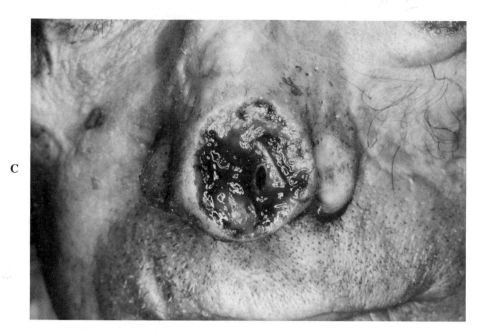

C

Fig. 20-23, cont'd. For legend, see previous page.

healing is allowed to take place, a depressed scar usually results. Sometimes keratoacanthomas reach a very large size—5 cm or larger—particularly in the central face or on the lip. These giant keratoacanthomas may become destructive in this location before undergoing regression and have thus been called *mutilating keratoacanthomas*.

Histopathology

The differentiation of a keratoacanthoma from a low-grade squamous cell carcinoma is not absolutely possible by histopathologic criteria alone. The clinical appearance and biologic behavior must be taken into account and correlated with the histologic appearance before a diagnosis of keratoacanthoma can be entertained. Only if a lesion completely involutes can one be secure in the diagnosis of keratoacanthoma.

On low power a keratoacanthoma has a characteristic craterlike appearance with overlapping epidermal margins at the sides. This overall architecture is necessary to establish a diagnosis of keratoacanthoma, and therefore it is essential to have available a full cross-sectional view of the lesion. The tumor projects both above the surface and deeply into the dermis. The crater is filled with dense parakeratotic horny material with many horn pearls. At the base and sides of the crater, acanthosis of the epithelium occurs. This acanthosis resembles pseudoepitheliomatous hyperplasia with minimal cellular atypia. The cells have an eosinophilic glassy appearance caused by the fairly advanced degree of keratinization. This keratinization is extensive, and only at the outer margins of the epithelium are the cells smaller, basophilic, and nonkeratinized. Beneath and toward the

sides of the tumor is a dense, inflammatory infiltrate. Loculated masses of inflammatory cells may be seen within the proliferating epidermis.

Squamous cell carcinomas are distinguished by the presence of cellular atypia and mitotic activity, both of which are uncommon in keratoacanthomas. In addition, invasion with anaplasia is a feature of squamous cell carcinomas. It is important to stress, however, that many tumors may be histopathologically borderline between keratoacanthoma and squamous cell carcinoma.[77] There are no reliable histopathologic criteria to differentiate keratoacanthomas from squamous cell carcinomas in all instances. Therefore some clinicians prefer to group keratoacanthomas within the category of well-differentiated squamous cell carcinomas.[54]

Treatment

Many different forms of treatment have been recommended for keratoacanthomas and include observation,[125] surgical excision,[118,125] curettage,[79] blunt dissection,[64] cryosurgery, radiotherapy, and intralesional injections of such agents as 5-FU,[52,104] bleomycin, or steroids. In addition, topical 5-FU has also been advocated.[33,50,62] If the keratoacanthoma is small (less than 1 cm), nonrecurrent, and not on a mucous membrane, then almost any form of therapy is successful because this lesion probably would have regressed by itself anyway. Furthermore, any form of treatment on such small lesions yields excellent cosmetic results.

The use of topical or injectable 5-FU is currently a popular form of therapy. Although topical 5-FU has been reported to be highly successful, with cure rates ranging from

93%[50] to 100%,[33] it is important to point out that almost all the lesions treated were small. For instance, in a series of 15 patients treated successfully with topical 5-FU, the lesions ranged in size from 4 to 16 mm.[50] In another series of 41 cases of keratoacanthoma, 40 of which were successfully treated by intralesional injections of 5-FU (50 mg/ml), the sizes of the lesions were not given.[52] I suspect that the majority of these lesions also were small. One cannot extrapolate these excellent results to lesions that are large (more than 2 cm) or recurrent. In addition, it is fair to point out that in these studies histopathologic confirmation was not given in the majority of lesions treated topically or by injection. Such information is necessary to establish valid cure rates. For instance, Grupper successfully treated 12 of 15 "keratoacanthomas" with 2% to 5% topical 5-FU.[62] Histopathologic examination of two tumors in which this treatment method failed showed a spindle cell carcinoma.

Small keratoacanthomas (less than 1 or 2 cm) may be easily curetted or excised and primarily closed. Cure rates are high under such circumstances, and the cosmetic results are excellent. Such therapeutic intervention may be considered preferable, since the resultant scar from such procedures is less noticeable than that occurring after spontaneous involution. In addition, the patient does not need to live with an unsightly tumor for up to 6 months, and material for pathologic examination is obtained.

Radiotherapy may be considered for keratoacanthomas when surgical excision would be particularly destructive, such as on tumors that deeply involve the nasal ala.[39] However, the cosmetic results following radiation to the skin may be poor and can include noticeable atrophy.

Lesions that are large (more than 2 cm), recurrent, or occurring on the mucous membranes should be totally excised, preferably by microscopically controlled surgery (Mohs surgery), because the possibility of metastases is probably relatively high in such circumstances (Fig. 20-23, *B* and *C*). I have seen at least one patient die from a "keratoacanthoma" on the lip unresponsive to injections of 5-FU given by other physicians. Although such cases are rare, the initial treating physician should be aggressive in the management of such tumors. Even though there have been isolated case reports of very large lesions (5 cm or more) that have been allowed to regress spontaneously,[144] the patient's life may be put in jeopardy by such watchful waiting.

Special considerations

Invasive and metastasizing keratoacanthomas. Some tumors originally thought to be keratoacanthomas have been reported to have metastasized.[108,118] Keratoacanthomas have also been reported to invade muscle and nerve.[87] The question thus arises as to whether such growths are true keratoacanthomas initially but become more aggressive and dangerous entities—or alternatively, whether such lesions are squamous cell carcinomas from the beginning.

Pathologists invariably argue, when retrospectively reviewing histopathologically such metastasizing tumors that significant cellular atypia was present but not appreciated at the time of the original biopsy; therefore these tumors were erroneously misdiagnosed as keratoacanthomas instead of squamous cell carcinomas.[77,144] In one study histopathologic misdiagnosis of squamous cell carcinomas as keratoacanthomas occurred 20% of the time.[77] Since the clinician has the final responsibility for care of the patient, such a high rate of misinterpretation should make every practicing physician suspicious of the diagnosis of keratoacanthoma, especially if the tumor continually grows or recurs.

In one study of 18 cases of keratoacanthoma with perineural invasion, none recurred or metastasized.[87] The authors posit that perineural invasion, although disturbing, does not affect the prognosis. In support of their contention that this is a banal event, they cited the fact that some cancers, such as prostatic or cervical carcinomas, can show perineural invasion without affecting the prognosis. The problem with this study is that the extent of resection was not given. If the authors were looking at perineural invasion in "keratoacanthomas" that were excised widely and deeply, then the prognosis would be good. If, on the other hand, perineural invasion was seen in "keratoacanthomas" that were inadequately excised, the prognosis would not be good. In addition, evidence of perineural invasion may have led to more aggressive treatment, which resulted in less likelihood of recurrence or metastases, whereas less complete therapy (for instance, by curettage or intralesional 5-FU) may have led ultimately to deeper invasion and serious consequences.

My own experience with perineural invasion in "keratoacanthomas" is that when this event occurs, the tumor has been followed clinically as a keratoacanthoma but it continues to progress relentlessly. At the time of tumor removal, extensive tissue involvement is found histologically. Since the nerve involvement with keratoacanthoma is indistinguishable from that found with squamous cell carcinoma, one needs to be very cautious by totally extirpating such tumors and closely following up such patients.

Case reports of keratoacanthomas that metastasize continue to be recorded. Schnur and Bozzo report two cases on the lip,[118] and Piscioli et al. report one case on the back of the hand in an immunoincompetent patient.[108] In all cases these tumors recurred after initial treatment. All were clinically and histopathologically considered keratoacanthomas. The great potential problems with recurrence of keratoacanthomas on the dorsum of the hand and the lip (or mucosal surfaces) has been pointed out by others.[114,144] Immunologically impaired patients may also be more prone to the "transformation" of keratoacanthomas into invasive squamous cell carcinomas.[109]

Recurrent keratoacanthomas. Stranc and Robertson rightly called a keratoacanthoma "a wolf in sheep's clothing.''[125] The concept that the biologic behavior of a tumor is ultimately the deciding factor in choosing treatment cannot be stressed enough. *Any recurrent keratoacanthoma should be treated as an aggressive squamous cell carcinoma.* Since the reported cases of ''metastatic keratoacanthoma'' all occurred in recurrent keratoacanthomas, these recurrent lesions deserve careful attention.

In a series of 90 keratoacanthomas 8% were recurrent after initial therapy.[79] These 8% of cases were more difficult to cure than the original lesions were. One of the cases was incurable by the methods available to the authors.

SQUAMOUS CELL CARCINOMA

Squamous cell carcinoma (SCC) is the second most common malignancy of the skin next to BCC. In the United States, there are about 60,000 to 100,000 new cases every year: about 20% to 33% of the number of BCCs.[121] Although the incidences of melanoma and BCC appear to be increasing, the incidence of SCCs does not.[41] This may have certain implications regarding the pathogenesis and latency interval necessary for development.

The average age of onset for an SCC is slightly higher than for a BCC. One study found that the average age of onset for SCCs was 66.2 to 69.8 years, about 8 to 9 years later than the average age of patients who developed BCCs.[120] The authors also found that before the age of 40, 80% of cutaneous tumors were BCCs, whereas after the age of 85, 80% of tumors were SCCs. This supports the concept of a longer latency period for an SCC to develop compared with a BCC.

The most common anatomic locations of an SCC are somewhat different than those for a BCC. SCCs are most common (in order of decreasing frequency) on the ears, hands, and upper face, whereas BCCs are most common on the upper face, nose, ears, and lower face. A carcinoma of the ear or an extremity is thus more likely to be an SCC than a BCC. Although men overall have a greater incidence of SCC, in certain locations (the scalp, legs, and trunk) the incidence in women is higher.[119]

Rate of growth

The growth rate of SCCs is faster than that of BCCs. This is supported by a study that found that patients waited 1.2 years before presenting for treatment with an SCC but waited 3.5 years if they had a BCC, despite the fact that both tumors were the same size at presentation.[120] Thus by history alone the average SCC probably grows about twice as fast as the average BCC.

Cause

Clinical and experimental evidence exists that SCCs are usually related to unprotected exposure to the sun. An Argentinian study in the 1930s showed that SCCs could be produced on the naked ears of white mice with either natural sun exposure or mercury vapor light sources.[113] The production of these carcinomas was found to be blocked by ordinary window glass, which filters out the rays of the sun below 320 nm (nanometers) in wavelength. Freeman later showed more specifically that SCCs could be produced in albino mice with monochromatic light at wavelengths of 300, 310, and 320 nm.[43] Since these are also the wavelengths that are known to produce erythema in the animal model and sunburn in humans, the tumor-producing spectrum has been said to parallel the erythema-producing or sunburn-producing spectrum.

Individuals with fair complexions and light-colored eyes and hair appear to be particularly prone to develop SCCs. Blacks, on the other hand, have pigment protection within the epidermis and only uncommonly develop SCCs.[100] Outdoor workers are ten times more likely to develop SCCs than those with indoor jobs.[129] Women, who traditionally have had indoor jobs, have a lesser incidence of squamous cell carcinoma.[13,119,136] However, on unexposed surfaces, the sex differential disappears[76] or is even reversed.[119] Other environmental factors, such as increased temperature or wind, may also influence the subsequent sun damage to the skin and the development of tumors.[105]

SCCs may be associated with predisposing factors other than ultraviolet radiation. Broders found that 24% of his patients gave a history of previous injury, of which about 25% were from burns and 20% from x-radiation.[13] SCCs in scars most commonly occur in old scars on the scalp, trunk, and extremities[16,119] and develop about 23 years after the initial injury[126] (Fig. 20-24, *A*). X-radiation may also induce SCCs, especially on the hands (Fig. 20-24, *B*), whereas on the face BCCs are the tumor type more commonly produced by x-radiation. The average lag period of malignancy development with x-radiation is, like that with burn scars, from 20 to 25 years.[49] Chronic trauma may also be associated with squamous cell carcinoma, for instance in epidermolysis bullosa dystrophica (Fig. 20-24, *C*).

Some rare genetic disorders predispose individuals to SCCs. Xeroderma pigmentosum is a rare genetic disease associated with a defective repair mechanism for ultraviolet light–induced DNA damage.[21] SCCs, BCCs, and melanomas occur in such individuals (beginning at an early age) and are usually the cause of death. SCCs also commonly occur in albinos.

Immunosuppression may also give rise to the development of an SCC. Renal transplant recipients on immunosuppressives commonly develop SCCs. In one study 7.25% of such patients developed neoplasms, mostly SCCs on sun-exposed skin.[29] This was calculated to be 16 times the predicted rate of skin cancers in the normal population. The authors observed that patients showing fewer signs of kidney rejection (and therefore perhaps more immunosuppression) were more likely to develop SCCs. SCCs that occur in immunosuppressed individuals may resemble keratoacanthomas; however, the biologic behavior of such lesions may

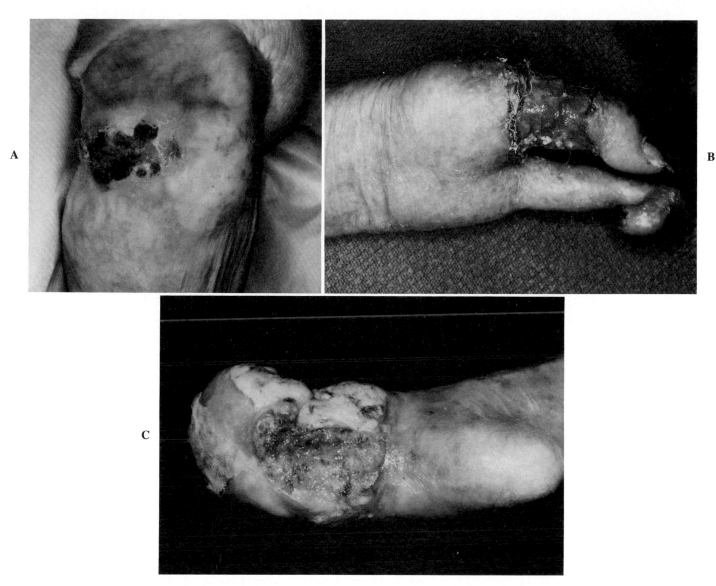

Fig. 20-24. A, Squamous cell carcinoma developed in skin graft for thermal burn 68 years previously. **B,** Squamous cell carcinoma of hand subsequent to radiation given for supposed eczema 40 years previously. Other fingers have been amputated for other squamous cell carcinomas. **C,** Squamous cell carcinoma of foot in 23-year-old patient with epidermolysis bullosa dystrophica.

be that of an SCC.[109] An oncogenic human papillomavirus (HPV-5) has been detected in cutaneous squamous cell carcinomas from such individuals, suggesting a pathogenic role along with sunlight as the cause of these lesions.

SCCs may also be associated with arsenic ingestion or cutaneous exposure to tars or other chemicals. A more complete discussion of the carcinogenesis of SCC is found in the reviews by Epstein[38] and Lang.[85]

Clinical appearance

An SCC on the skin usually appears as a scaly macular or papular area, which may become nodular and then frequent-

ly ulcerates. Once ulceration occurs, the border is indurated, and the ulcer is covered by a crust (Fig. 20-25). Unlike a BCC, an SCC frequently does not have a typical appearance. Therefore it is difficult to diagnose by clinical appearance alone, and a histologic examination is mandatory.[142] Occasionally an SCC resembles a keratoacanthoma, already described.[54,77,118] On the mucosal surfaces (conjunctival nasal, oral, vaginal, and rectal mucosae) an SCC appears different than it does on the nonmucosal surfaces. In the former locations an SCC manifests itself initially as an erythematous or whitish macular area, which with time becomes papular, nodular, or even verrucous.

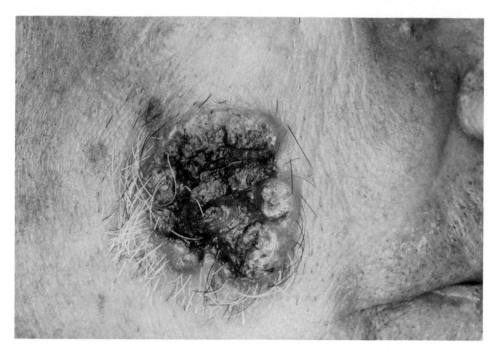

Fig. 20-25. Squamous cell carcinoma.

**ADVERSE FACTORS AFFECTING CURE RATES
OF CUTANEOUS SQUAMOUS CELL CARCINOMA**

Size of more than 3 cm
Duration of longer than 1 year
Previous treatment
Histopathology
    Poorly differentiated
    Acantholytic
    Neural invasion
Anatomic location
    Mucous membranes
    Ear
Occurrence in chronic scar (such as a burn scar)
Occurrence in irradiated skin

Variables that affect treatment results

The most effective treatment of an SCC, like that for other cutaneous neoplasms, is related to certain variables that must be understood so that appropriate therapy can be selected. These variables include size, duration, previous treatment, histopathology, anatomic location, and occurrence in a chronic scar or irradiated skin (see box above).

Size. The size of the SCC influences the 5-year cure rate. Larger lesions are more likely to recur locally, become in-

vasive, or metastasize, resulting in death.[12,69,96] Mohs reported a 99.5% cure rate for lesions smaller than 1 cm but only a 59% cure rate for lesions larger than 3 cm.[97] In all cases Mohs surgery had been performed. Similarly, Warren and Hoerr thought that the initial lesion size had the greatest influence on the overall prognosis.[136] They reported a mortality of 82% for lesions larger than 5 cm but only a 7% mortality for lesions smaller than 1 cm.

Duration. The duration of an SCC is sometimes mentioned as a variable that influences its prognosis. For instance, one study states that a duration of longer than 1 year is associated with an increased chance of local recurrence, metastasis, and death.[9] Certainly duration and size are interrelated, since tumors of a longer duration will almost undoubtedly attain a larger size.

Previous treatment. Previous unsuccessful treatment is an extremely important variable regarding prognosis. Once an SCC recurs, its chances of further recurrence or metastasis increase. For instance, Mohs reported a 5-year cure rate of 94% for all SCCs but only a 76.3% cure rate if previous surgery or radiation therapy had been performed.[97] Modlin found that 58% of patients with SCCs who developed lymph node metastases had been given some form of previous treatment.[96]

Specific forms of therapy for SCCs, if unsuccessful, may decrease the likelihood of ultimate cure. For instance, in one study prior treatment by radiation decreased the 5-year cure rate compared with that if prior treatment by surgery had been given.[136] However, this may reflect the selection of radiotherapy for initial larger, more difficult-to-manage lesions and the choice of surgery as the initial form of treatment for smaller lesions.

Histology. Histopathology may be influential in helping the physician determine the overall prognosis.[9,45] In 1921 Broders described a classification system for SCC based on the degree of differentiation of the tumor.[13] If a tumor was well differentiated—that is, readily recognizable as composed of squamous cells by the presence of keratinization and horn pearls—it was designated grade I. If a tumor was composed of very undifferentiated cells, it was classified as grade IV. Grades II and III were intermediate. Broders found that no grade I SCCs caused patients to die, but 100% of grade IV SCCs did.[13] For the intermediate grades II and III, 61.3% to 86% of cases died from SCCs. Mohs also found such classification to be useful[97]; in his series, grade I tumors had a 98.9% cure rate, whereas grade IV had only a 45.2% cure rate. Warren and Hoerr found that even when the size of the lesion was allowed for, undifferentiated tumors carried a 5% to 20% greater mortality than that of well-differentiated tumors.[136]

Other histopathologic features may also be important in determining the degree of an SCC malignancy. They incude the presence of mitotic figures, the degree of nuclear variation and atypia, and the depth of penetration by the tumor. Multiple sections should be examined, since on some sections only atypia within the epidermis may be seen, whereas in other sections from the same tumor a penetration of the dermis is apparent.

Some dermatologists have the mistaken impression that histopathologic differentiation has little to do with the prognosis of a cutaneous squamous cell carcinoma. Such an impression undoubtedly has arisen because the majority of squamous cell carcinomas arising on the skin are well differentiated. In Broders' original paper, 78% of tumors were grades I or II, whereas only 22% were grades III or IV.[13] Statements in the surgical literature have also resulted in the lack of appreciation for the importance of tumor histopathology. For instance, Brown et al. state that "in 75% of cases histologic differentiation did not affect recurrence or survival."[15] They mean to say that histologic differentiation does not make a difference most of the time because most of the tumors are well differentiated. Poor differentiation of tumors certainly leads to an extremely poor prognosis.[93]

SCCs can be classified as in situ or invasive. The former are confined totally to the epidermis, whereas the latter show invasion of malignant cells into the dermis, and the basement membrane is then frequently indistinct. With invasive SCCs Broders' classification system is in modern times commonly modified from the original four groups to three: well differentiated, moderately well differentiated, and poorly differentiated. Well differentiated implies obvious cell keratinization and the presence of horn pearls, which are collections of keratin produced by surrounding squamous cells. A poorly differentiated SCC shows little, if any, evidence of keratinization. Frequently such tumors contain spindle cell tumors, such as malignant melanomas. Moderately well-differentiated SCCs are somewhere in between the two extremes just described. This type of SCC shows keratinizing cells but no horn pearls.

Occasionally an invasive SCC contains cells with a lack of cohesion. Such acantholytic collections of cells, if the tumor extends deeply, are associated in my experience with an extremely poor prognosis (Fig. 20-26). Cox and Becker have labeled this the adenoid variant of SCC.[23] However, the acantholytic aspect is more important than the adenoid collections of cells. Cells that do not adhere are probably more likely to spread locally or break off and metastasize.

An SCC may invade a perineural nerve sheath and spread proximally along this conduit (Fig. 20-27). In addition, an SCC may metastasize to local or even distant lymph nodes. When these events occur, the prognosis becomes much worse.

SCCs are at times difficult to distinguish from keratoacanthomas.[77] Cellular atypia and mitotic activity are rare in keratoacanthomas but common in SCCs. A more complete discussion of this controversial subject is found in the section on keratoacanthomas.

The concept of basosquamous cell carcinoma (BSCC) as a distinct entity bears some discussion. Darier and Ferrand in 1922 originally proposed a special classification of BCCs with features of SCC.[25] They described two types of these special BCCs: the metatypic mixed type and the metatypic intermediate type. The former is composed of masses of basaloid cells with transitional areas to typical keratinizing cells seen in SCCs; the latter is composed of large atypical basaloid cells. Both types are sometimes referred to today as metatypic basal cell carcinomas. BCCs that contain keratotic masses (so-called keratotic basal cell carcinomas) are not considered to be BSCCs.

It has been recognized for years that some cutaneous tumors resist clear-cut classification as either a BCC or a SCC.[140] Such tumors were categorized as basosquamous carcinomas in some series.[42,49,57] This ability of squamous differentiation seems consistent with the embryologic potential of the basal cell layer of the skin. However, the concept of BSCC as a distinct entity has been doubted.[89] Freeman, for instance, feels that a BSCC is either a small-cell SCC interpreted as a basal cell carcinoma, squamous metaplasia overlying a basal cell carcinoma, or even pseudoepitheliomatous hyperplasia.[44]

Nevertheless, the concept of the BSCC may be valid and important from a prognostic point of view. Borel followed 35 cases classified as BSCC for an average of 6.8 years.[11] Of these lesions 8.6% metastasized and 45.7% recurred. The author compared this to over 1000 cases of BCC and 600 cases of SCC at the same institution. The rate of metastases from SCCs was 7.9% and from BCCs was 0.09%. In addition, the local recurrence rate for SCCs was 21.9%—

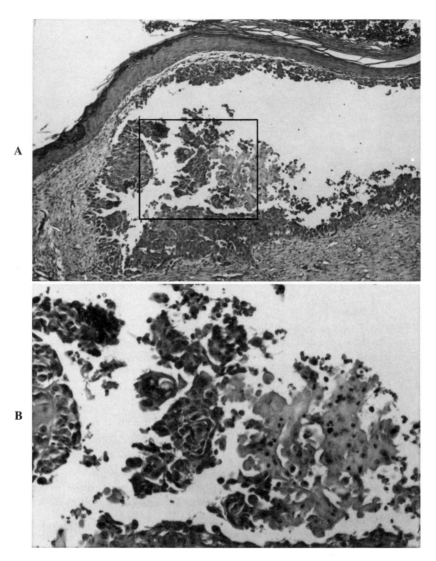

Fig. 20-26. A, Acantholytic squamous cell carcinoma. (Hematoxylin and eosin × 40.) Note lack of cell cohesion. **B,** Close-up of **A.** (Hematoxylin and eosin × 400.)

half that of BSCCs. This higher recurrence rate for BSCCs may have been caused by less aggressive treatment of BCCs than of SCCs. Thus a BSCC clearly behaves more like an SCC than a BCC, indicating that treatment of a BSCC should be similar to that of an SCC and not of a BCC. Patients should be followed-up at closer intervals with careful evaluation of lymph nodes.

SCCs occasionally arise from a cyst wall[145] (see Fig. 26-11). Such tumors should be treated as SCCs and not regarded as any less likely to behave in a malignant fashion. This is discussed more fully in the section on epithelial cysts.

Anatomic location. An SCC can occur on either mucous membrane or non–mucous membrane areas. The likelihood of metastases and recurrence is higher on the mucous membranes than on the skin. However, on the skin itself (except possibly the ear) the site has little to do with prognosis.[97]

SCCs of the mucous membranes of the lip can and do kill, either by metastases with subsequent extensive neck disease or by spreading along the perineural nerve sheaths to the middle cranial fossa. In a series of 62 well-differentiated tumors of the lower lip in mostly elderly patients, there was an 11% metastatic rate and an 11% death rate.[15] When tumors were poorly differentiated, the metastatic rate was 100% and the death rate 50%.

An SCC may occur on the lip in patients under the age of 40.[10] When it does, a special effort should be made for definitive therapy. In a series of 97 patients in this category, the determinate mortality was 22%, and thus the overall death rate appeared to be higher than it was for SCCs in the same location in older patients.[10]

An SCC of the external ear may be more likely to metastasize than those from other sites[136] (Fig. 20-28). Unlike

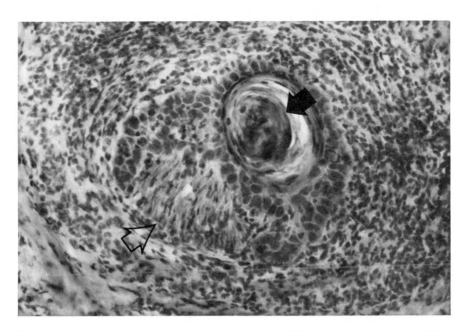

Fig. 20-27. Perineural invasion by squamous cell carcinoma. (Hematoxylin and eosin × 100.) *Open arrow,* Nerve; *closed arrow,* keratin pearl.

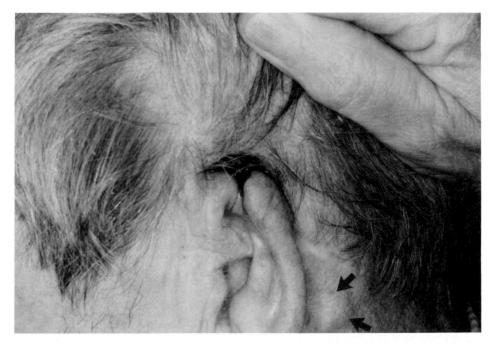

Fig. 20-28. Lymph node metastasis *(arrow)* from squamous cell carcinoma of ear. Wound on superior helix is site of primary tumor removal.

other sites, where large lesions are most likely to metastasize, SCCs on the ear may metastasize even if small.[18] One report shows an overall recurrence rate of 14% in this area;[18] Mohs reports an 8.3% recurrence rate,[97] higher than his overall recurrence rate (6%) of all SCCs of the skin.

Other sites of occurrence of SCC (scalp,[111] nose,[9,22] trunk and extremities[123]) appear to have about the same overall 5-year cure rates, ranging from 75% to 90%. At these sites the other factors previously mentioned (size, duration, previous treatment, and histopathology) all influence the prognosis rather than the site itself. There are a few exceptions, however, even within these sites. For instance, SCCs of the nasal columella are more likely to extend locally or metastasize than lesions elsewhere on the nose.[22]

Occurrence in chronic scar. SCCs that occur in old scars are stated to be particularly prone to local recurrence or metastases.[93,123] Stromberg et al. reported 31 cases of "scar carcinoma."[126] The average time period between the injury and the development of the SCC was 23 years. If the tumors were well differentiated, the 3-year survival rate was 94%, but only 38% if they were poorly differentiated. These figures are not different from those of other studies of survival with SCC with similar differentiation.[16,97,136] Mora and Perniciaro found an only slightly increased mortality of 24.3% compared with an overall mortality of 18.4% if the SCC occurred in association with scars or other predisposing processes in blacks.[100] Thus the overall statistics do not uniformly support a worse prognosis of SCC developing in scars. However, because there may be more delay in recognizing an SCC within a scar, the tumors at the time of treatment are probably larger than those occurring de novo.

Occurrence in irradiated skin. An SCC that develops in skin which had been previously irradiated may be more aggressive. Conley reported 456 patients with BCCs, SCCs, or both of the nose, 80 of whom having had previous radiotherapy.[22] Seven patients developed an SCC in the irradiated area, and six of these seven patients died from the tumor. This same study reported nine patients whose SCC metastasized from the nose. Five of these nine patients had undergone full-face irradiation, usually for acne, 15 to 20 years previously. Therefore an SCC that occurs in irradiated tissue, especially in certain locations such as the nose, should be treated carefully and aggressively.

Treatment

The treatment of an SCC should be predicated on the previously mentioned factors that affect the prognosis (see box on p. 650). As with other forms of skin cancer, no one form of therapy is uniformly successful in all instances; ideally therapy should be individualized for each patient. As previously emphasized with BCC, a pretreatment biopsy is advisable, particularly because errors can be made in the diagnosis of SCCs from clinical appearance alone.[142]

Surgical excision is the most commonly used method to treat SCCs of the skin or mucous membranes. Recommendations regarding the margins of normal-appearing skin that should be excised vary from 0.5 cm[82] to 2 cm,[111] depending on the size of the lesion and the degree of differentiation. Certainly for lesions with one or more of the adverse factors listed in the box on p. 650, a greater surgical margin should be chosen. Unfortunately no good systematic study of these variables has yet been done with SCCs, as has been done with melanomas and BCCs.

It is extremely difficult to determine the 5-year cure rate for excisions of SCCs, since so many variables affect the prognosis. Dermatologists are more prone to have their statistics skewed toward high cure rates by inclusion of many small tumors, whereas surgical specialists in general treat larger and more complicated tumors, and thus have lower cure rates. For instance, two dermatology studies[20,82] report cure rates of 93% to 100% with excisional surgery. On the other hand, reports by surgeons include cure rates of 87%,[96] 80%,[69] and only 74%.[9] When one is more specific about size, the reason for these differences in cure rates become apparent. For instance, one dermatology series reports an 83% 5-year cure rate for lesions larger than 2 cm but a 96% cure rate for lesions smaller than 2 cm.[46]

Sometimes after seemingly adequate excision, the pathology report states that the SCC extends to the surgical margins. Most surgeons perform a reexcision of the treatment area if this occurs.[1] Glass et al.[48] followed-up 44 patients whose surgical margins were positive for SCC. Six lesions were immediately retreated and only one recurred, giving a cure rate of 83%. Thirty-four lesions were watched and 16 recurred, giving a cure rate of 53%. Four lesions of carcinoma in situ at the time of initial excision were watched and one lesion recurred, as an invasive SCC. Of the 16 patients with invasive SCCs that recurred, 4 (25%) developed metastases with an uncontrolled primary lesion. Therefore a positive margin on an excised SCC dictates immediate retreatment.

Curettage and electrodesiccation (C&E) is mentioned mostly by dermatologists as an adequate method for treatment of SCC.[81] Again, the dermatology series report cure rates of 96%[46,132,142] to 100%,[46] but these include tumors that are undoubtedly mostly small (less than 1 cm) and well differentiated. Larger lesions have also been reported to be successfully treated by C&E, but valid cure rate statistics are not stated.[141] Metastases may occur after C&E as with any form of therapy, but they do not appear to be more frequent after C&E than after excision or radiotherapy.[82]

Cryosurgery is another method of treatment of an SCC. A cure rate of 97.7% has been reported with SCCs overall but only 86.7% for recurrent SCCs.[58] The authors thought that size and site did not make a difference in cure rates. However, most of these lesions undoubtedly were small and uncomplicated.

Mohs surgery offers a consistently high rate of cure for SCCs. Mohs reported an overall 5-year determinate cure rate of 94%[97]; however, this cure rate dropped if other adverse factors, listed in the box on p. 650, were present. Most have been discussed.

The metastatic rate of SCCs on the lips after Mohs surgery is about half the rate for cases treated by conventional surgery, so it may thus be the treatment of choice for lip carcinomas.[97]

Radiotherapy is an alternative treatment method for SCCs. This form of therapy is chosen for selected cases, especially if the other, previously mentioned treatment methods cannot be used. Indications for radiotherapy include inoperable tumors or tumors occurring in those who would be jeopardized by surgery. When an unselected series of cases treated with radiotherapy was compared with a later series treated with surgery at the same institution, there were approximately twice as many recurrences with radiotherapy and six times the number of complications.[9] Overall cosmetic results subsequent to radiotherapy are poor or only fair.[65] Therefore cases need to be selected carefully for this form of therapy.

On SCCs 5-FU may be used topically. However, the reported cure rates are about 80%, which is less than cure rates with other modalities.[92] It should be stressed that if 5-FU is to be used, the patient needs to apply it for 6 to 8 weeks, longer than for actinic keratoses. It can be useful for palliation in circumstances where other forms of therapy cannot be used.

Metastases

Unlike BCCs, SCCs of the skin occasionally metastasize. The rate of metastasis varies between sites (see box on this page) and with the degree of differentiation of the tumor,[15] size,[9,15,96] and previous treatment.[96]

Several studies done by dermatologists have estimated the likelihood of metastases from SCCs to be from 0.1%[93] to 3.3%,[99] excluding lesions of the mucous membranes. The often quoted study by Lund estimated a metastatic frequency of 0.1% to 0.5%.[93] Most of his metastatic tumors were from nonactinic SCCs. This study was performed with questionnaires and therefore can be considered only a crude estimate at best. The study by Epstein et al. is also widely quoted[37]; it was done by review of the California Tumor Registry. The authors found a 2% incidence of metastases and emphasized that 74% of their metastatic primaries occurred on the head and neck. This seems to be consistent with the notion that actinic causation does not mean that a SCC is less likely to metastasize. The previous studies quoted find some support from Knox et al. (0.3% metastatic rate),[82] Grabb et al. (2% metastatic rate),[57] Katz et al. (2.6% metastatic rate),[76] Mohs (3.7% metastatic rate),[98] and Møller et al. (3.3% metastatic rate).[99] Older studies from surgical services give higher overall metastatic rates

---

METASTATIC RATE OF CUTANEOUS SQUAMOUS CELL CARCINOMA

Mucosal surfaces

Lip	6.7%[97]*
	10%[99]†
	12%[15]*

Non-mucosal surfaces

Overall	0.1% to 0.5%[93]†
	0.3%[80]†,[48]*
	2%[37]†,[57]*
	2.6%[76]†
	3.3%[99]†
	3.7%[97]*
	11%[96]*
	16%[119]*
Ear	12%[18]†
	14%[119]*
Nose	8%[9]*
	18.5%[22]*
	25%[119]*
Arm	8%[129]‡
Hand	2.3%[129]‡
Lower limb	12.6%[129]‡
Trunk	14.0%[129]‡

*Surgical series
†Dermatologic series
‡Combined Dermatologic and Surgical Series

(11%[96] and 16%[119]); undoubtedly these studies were biased toward larger, more neglected lesions.

The metastatic potential of an SCC varies with the site. Lesions of the mucosal surfaces are prone to metastasize. Estmates of metastases from the lip vary between 6.7%[97] and 12%.[15] Metastatic rates on other anatomic areas are listed in the box above; however, it is difficult to compare these statistics to overall rates and to those in the dermatologic literature. Undoubtedly, high rates are caused by selected problem lesions being referred for treatment to referral centers, whose figures are thus skewed toward larger, more aggressive lesions. The study by Swanbeck and Hillström[129] (see the box above), although from the dermatologic literature, was done with statistics from Sweden that included lesions treated by dermatologists and by surgeons. It is more accurate not only because it includes large and small lesions but also because of the centralized record keeping done within that country. Thus these metastatic rates are probably more accurate and reflect the real metastatic potential better than purely dermatologic or purely surgical studies.

The likelihood of patient survival after metastasis is less than if metastasis does not occur. In one study all patients with metastases died within a few years; only two patients survived more than 2 years.[99] Similarly dismal results have also been noted by other authors.[9,15,22] The survival rate is also worse if more than one lymph node is involved.[18]

Death

Death from skin cancer is uncommon but does occur. The incidence of death caused by a cutaneous SCC has been estimated to be between 1%[32] and 22%.[96] The higher figures are from earlier studies—1939[136] and 1954.[96] Perhaps the better prognosis from more recent studies reflects more aggressive and earlier therapy. Although only about 20% to 30% of all non-melanoma skin cancers are SCCs, this tumor accounts for 75% of all skin cancer deaths.[32] Thus SCCs can be considered more serious than the more common BCCs. Interestingly the number of deaths caused by BCCs is about 10% to 12% of that from SCCs and this percentage has not changed over the years.[32,65,73] This is also consistent with the notion that all types of skin cancers (including BCCs and SCCs) are currently being treated earlier and more carefully.

Follow-up examinations

Once a patient with an SCC has been treated, careful follow-up examinations should be required as part of the overall treatment plan. Usually examination of the primary site and lymph node drainage areas is performed every 3 months for the first year and then every 6 months for the next 4 years. Early detection of local recurrences or metastases is essential to survival. SCCs tend to recur or metastasize within 3 years after treatment.[49,76] (It should be remembered that BCCs recur even after 5 years in some cases.)

An additional reason for careful follow-up examinations of skin cancer patients is that subsequent separate lesions occur in a high percentage of such patients. From 22%[8] to 38%[96] of such patients develop additional BCCs or SCCs in the future.

Prophylaxis

Patients who have developed a cutaneous SCC related to sun exposure should be educated on the harmful effects of chronic sun exposure and its probable causative role in their skin cancer. They should use common sense regarding sun exposure in the future—limiting the time they are directly exposed to the sun and keeping the sunlight itself from irradiating the skin, which is best achieved by avoiding the sun during the middle of the day (when the sunlight is strongest) and wearing appropriate clothing (including a hat) and sunscreens.

REFERENCES

1. Abide, J.M., Nahai, F., and Bennett, R.G.: The meaning of surgical margins, Plast. Reconstr. Surg. **73:**492, 1984.
2. Allison, J.R., Jr.: Radiation-induced basal-cell carcinoma, J. Dermatol. Surg. Oncol. **10:**200, 1984.
3. Anderson, S.L.C., Nielsen, A., and Reymann F.: Relationship between Bowen disease and internal malignant tumors, Arch. Dermatol. **108:**367, 1973.
4. Baer, R.L., and Kopf, A.W.: Complications of therapy of basal cell epitheliomas (based on 1,000 histologically verfied cases). In Baer, R.L., and Kopf, A.W., editors: 1964-1965 Year book of dermatology Chicago, 1965, Year Book Medical Publishers, Inc.
5. Bart, R.S., Kopf, A.W., and Petratos, M.A.: X-ray therapy of skin cancer: evaluation of a "standardized" method for treating basal-cell epitheliomas. In Sixth National Cancer Conference Proceedings (1968), p. 559, Philadelphia, 1970, J.B. Lippincott Co.
6. Bart, R.S., et al.: Scalpel excision of basal cell carcinomas, Arch. Dermatol. **114:**739, 1978.
7. Beirne, G.A., and Beirne, C.G.: Observations on the critical margin for the complete excision of carcinoma of the skin, A.M.A. Arch. Dermatol. **80:**344, 1959.
8. Bergstressor, P.R., and Halprin, K.M.: Multiple sequential skin cancers: the risk of skin cancer in patients with previous skin cancer, Arch. Dermatol. **11:**995, 1975.
9. Binder, S.C., Cady, B., and Catlin, D.: Epidermoid carcinoma of the skin of the nose, Am. J. Surg. **116:**506, 1968.
10. Boddie, A.W., Fischer, E.P., and Byers, R.M.: Squamous carcinoma of the lower lip in patients under 40 years of age, South. Med. J. **70:**711, 1977.
11. Borel, D.M.: Cutaneous basosquamous carcinoma: review of the literature and report of 35 cases, Arch. Pathol. **95:**293, 1973.
12. Broders, A.C. Basal cell epithelioma, J.A.M.A. **72:**856, 1919.
13. Broders, A.C.: Squamous-cell epithelioma of the skin, Ann. Surg. **73:**141, 1921.
14. Brooks, N.A.: Curettage and shave excision: a tissue-saving technic for primary cutaneous carcinoma worthy of inclusion in graduate training programs, J. Am. Acad. Dermatol. **10:**279, 1984.
15. Brown, R.G., et al.: Advanced and recurrent squamous carcinoma of the lower lip, Am. J. Surg. **132:**492, 1976.
16. Browne, H.J., Coventry, M.B., and McDonald, J.R.: Squamous carcinoma of the extremities, Staff Meetings, Mayo Clin. **28:**590, 1953.
17. Burg, G., et al.: Histographic surgery: accuracy of visual assessment of the margins of basal-cell epithelioma, J. Dermatol. Surg. **1**(3):21, 1975.
18. Byers, R., et al.: Squamous carcinoma of the external ear, Am. J. Surg. **146:**447, 1983.
19. Callen, J.P., and Headington, J.: Bowen's and non-Bowen's squamous intraepidermal neoplasia of the skin, Arch. Dermatol. **116:**422, 1980.
20. Chernosky, M.E.: Squamous cell and basal cell carcinomas: preliminary study of 3,817 primary skin cancers, South. Med. J. **71:**802, 1978.

21. Cleaver, J.E.: Defective repair replication of DNA in xeroderma pigmentosum, Nature **218**:652, 1968.

22. Conley, J.: Cancer of the skin of the nose, Ann. Otol. **83**:2, 1974.

23. Cox, F.H., and Becker, F.F.: Metastatic potential of biologic variants of skin squamous cell carcinoma, J. Fla. Med. Assoc. **69**:516, 1982.

24. Crissey, J.T.: Curettage and electrodesiccation as a method of treatment for epitheliomas of the skin, J. Surg. Oncol. **3**:287, 1971.

25. Darier, J., and Ferrand, M.: L'epithéliome pavimenteux mixte et intermédiaire: forme metatypique du cancer malpighien de la peau et des orifices muqueux, Ann. Dermatol. Syph. **3**:385, 1922.

26. Dellon, A.L., et al.: Prediction of recurrence in incompletely excised basal cell carcinoma, Plast. Reconstr. Surg. **75**:860, 1985.

27. Dercum, F.X.: Three cases of a hitherto unclassified affection resembling in its grosser aspects obesity, but associated with special nervous symptoms: adiposis dolorosa, Am. J. Med. Sci. **104**:521, 1892.

28. De Villez, R.L., and Stevens, C.S.: Bowenoid papules of the genitalia: a case progressing to Bowen's disease, J. Am. Acad. Dermatol. **3**:149, 1980.

29. Disler, P.B., et al.: Neoplasia after successful renal transplantation, Nephron **29**:119, 1981.

30. Domarus, H.V., and Stevens, P.J.: Metastatic basal cell carcinoma: report of 5 cases and review of 170 cases in the literature, J. Am. Acad. Dermatol. **10**:1043, 1984.

31. Dubin, N., and Kopf, A.W.: Multivariate risk score for recurrence of cutaneous basal cell carcinomas, Arch. Dermatol. **119**:373 1983.

32. Dunn, J.E., Jr., et al.: Skin cancer as a cause of death, Cal. Med. **102**:361, 1965.

33. Ebner, H., and Mischer, P.: Lokalbehandlung des Keratoakanthoms mit 5-Fluorouracil. II. Universitäts-Hautklinic Wien, Hautarzt **26**:585, 1975.

34. Edens, B.L., et al.: Effectiveness of curettage and electrodesiccation in the removal of basal cell carcinoma, J. Am. Acad. Dermatol. **9**:383, 1983.

35. Epstein, E.: How accurate is the visual assessment of basal carcinoma margins? Br. J. Dermatol. **89**:37, 1973.

36. Epstein, E.: Value of follow-up after treatment of basal cell carcinoma, Arch. Dermatol. **108**:798, 1973.

37. Epstein, E., et al.: Metastases from squamous cell carcinomas of the skin, Arch. Dermatol. **97**:245, 1968.

38. Epstein, J.H.: Photocarcinogenesis, skin cancer, and aging, J. Am. Acad. Dermatol. **9**:487, 1983.

39. Farina, A.T., et al.: Radiotherapy for aggressive and destructive keratoacanthomas, J. Dermatol. Surg. Oncol. **3**:177, 1977.

40. Farmer, E.R., and Helwig, E.B.: Metastatic basal cell carcinoma: a clinicopathologic study of seventeen cases, Cancer **46**:748, 1980.

41. Fears, T.R., and Scotto, J.: Changes in skin cancer morbidity between 1971-72 and 1977-78, J. Natl. Cancer Inst. **69**:365, 1982.

42. Ferrara, R.J. The private dermatologist and skin cancer: a clinical study of 226 epitheliomas derived from five dermatologic practices, A.M.A. Arch. Dermatol. **81**:225, 1960.

43. Freeman, R.G.: Data on the action spectrum for ultraviolet carcinogenesis, J. Natl. Cancer Inst. **55**:1119, 1975.

44. Freeman, R.G.: Histopathologic considerations in the management of skin cancer, J. Dermatol. Surg. **2**:215, 1976.

45. Freeman, R.G., and Duncan, W.C.: Recurrent skin cancer, Arch. Dermatol. **107**:395, 1973.

46. Freeman, R.G., Knox, J.M., and Heaton, C.L.: The treatment of skin cancer: a statistical study of 1,341 skin tumors comparing results obtained with irradiation, surgery, and curettage followed by electrodesiccation, Cancer **17**:535, 1964.

47. Fuchs, G.H., and Braun, M.: Primary endophytic nodular basal cell carcinoma, Cutis **29**:453, 1982.

48. Glass, R.L., Spratt, J.S., Jr., and Perez-Mesa, C.: The fate of inadequately excised epidermoid carcinoma of the skin, Surg. Gynecol. Obstet. **122**:245, 1966.

49. Gliosci, A., Hipps, C.J., and Diehl, J.J.: Cancer of the skin: an analysis of 238 cases, Internatl. Surg. **48**:290, 1967.

50. Goette, D.K.: Treatment of keratoacanthoma with topical fluorouracil, Arch. Dermatol. **119**:951, 1983.

51. Goette, D.K., and Helwig, E.B.: Basal cell carcinomas and basal cell carcinoma-like changes overlying dermatofibromas, Arch. Dermatol. **111**:589, 1975.

52. Goette, D.K., and Odom, R.B.: Successful treatment of keratoacanthoma with intralesional fluorouracil, J. Am. Acad. Dermatol. **2**:212, 1980.

53. Goette, D.K., et al.: Erythroplasia of Queyrat: treatment with topically administered fluorouracil, Arch. Dermatol. 110, 271, 1974.

54. Goldenhersh, M.A., and Olsen, T.G.: Invasive squamous cell carcinoma initially diagnosed as a giant keratoacanthoma, J. Am. Acad. Dermatol. **10**:372, 1984.

55. Goldwyn, R.M., and Kasdon, E.J., The "disappearance" of residual basal cell carcinoma of the skin, Ann. Plast. Surg. **1**:286, 1978.

56. Gooding, C.A., White, G., and Yatsuhashi, M.: Significance of marginal extension in excised basal-cell carcinoma, N. Engl. J. Med. **273**:923, 1965.

57. Grabb, W.C., et al.: Statistical evaluation of the treatment of basal cell and squamous cell carcinoma, U. Mich. Med. Ctr. J. **35**:205, 1969.

58. Graham, G.F., and Clark, L.C.: Statistical update in cryosurgery for cancers of the skin. In Zacarian, S., editor: Cryosurgery for skin cancer and cutaneous disorders, St. Louis, 1985, The C.V. Mosby Co.

59. Graham, J.H., and Helwig, E.B.: Bowen's disease and its relationship to systemic cancer, A.M.A. Arch. Dermatol. **80**:133, 1959.

60. Griffith, B.H., and McKinney, P.: An appraisal of the treatment of basal cell carcinoma of the skin, Plast. Reconstr. Surg. **51**:565, 1973.

61. Gross, G., et al.: Bowenoid papulosis: presence of human papillomavirus (HPV) structural antigens and of HPV 16-related DNA sequences, Arch. Dermatol. **121**:858, 1985.

62. Grupper, C.: Treatment of keratoacanthomas by local applications of 5-fluorouracil (5-FU) ointment, Dermatologica **140**(Suppl. I):127, 1970.

63. Gumport, S.L.: Surgical treatment, N.Y. State J. Med. **68**:869, 1968.

64. Habif, T.P.: Extirpation of keratoacanthomas by blunt dissection, J. Dermatol. Surg. Oncol. **6:**652, 1980.

65. Hansen, P.B., and Jensen, M.S.: Late results following radiotherapy of skin cancer, Acta Radiologica [Ther.] (Stockholm) **7:**307, 1968.

66. Hayes, H.: Basal cell carcinoma: the East Grinstead experience, Plast. Reconstr. Surg. **30:**273, 1962.

67. Howell, J.B., and Caro, M.R.: The basal-cell nevus: its relationship to multiple cutaneous cancers and associated anomalies of development, Arch. Dermatol. **79:**67, 1959.

68. Hutchinson, J.: The crateriform ulcer (acute epithelial cancer), Arch. Surg. (Lond.) **1:**241, 1889.

69. Immerman, S.C., et al.: Recurrent squamous cell carcinoma of the skin, Cancer **51:**1537, 1983.

70. Jackson, R.: Why do basal cell carcinomas recur (or not recur) following treatment? J. Surg. Oncol. **6:**245, 1974.

71. Jackson, R.: Observations on the natural course of skin cancer, Can. Med. Assoc. J. **92:**564, 1965.

72. Jackson, R.: The treatment of basal cell carcinoma, Cutis **5:**1231, 1969.

73. Jackson, R.: Hutchinson's Archives of Surgery revisited, Arch. Dermatol. **113:**961, 1977.

74. Jacobs, G.H., Rippey, M.B., and Altini, M.: Prediction of aggressive behavior in basal cell carcinoma, Cancer **49:**533, 1982.

75. Johnson, M.L., and Roberts, J.: Prevalence of dermatologic disease among persons 1 to 74 years of age: United States, Advance data No. 4, Washington, D.C., 1977, U.S. Department of Health and Welfare.

76. Katz, A.D., Urbach, F., and Lilienfeld, A.M.: The frequency and risk of metastases in squamous-cell carcinoma of the skin, Cancer **10:**1162, 1957.

77. Kern, W.H., and McCray, M.K.: The histopathologic differentiation of keratoacanthoma and squamous cell carcinoma of the skin, J. Cutan. Pathol. **7:**318, 1980.

78. Kimura, S.: Bowenoid papulosis of the genitalia, Int. J. Dermatol. **21:**432, 1982.

79. Kingman, J., and Callen, J.P.: Keratoacanthoma: a clinical study, Arch. Dermatol. **120:**736, 1984.

80. Klein, E., et al.: Tumors of the skin. VI. Study on effects of local administration of 5-fluorouracil in basal cell carcinoma, J. Invest. Dermatol. **47:**22, 1966.

81. Knox, J.M., et al.: Curettage and electrodesiccation in the treatment of skin cancer, Arch. Dermatol. **82:**197, 1960.

82. Knox, J.M., et al.: Treatment of skin cancer, South. Med. J. **60:**241, 1967.

83. Koplin, L., and Zarem, H.A.: Recurrent basal cell carcinoma: a review concerning the incidence, behavior, and management of recurrent basal cell carcinoma, with emphasis on the incompletely excised lesion, Plast. Reconstr. Surg. **65:**656, 1980.

84. Kord, J.P., Cottell, W.I., and Proper, S.: Metastatic basal-cell carcinoma, J. Dermatol. Surg. Oncol. **8:**604, 1982.

85. Lang, P.: Nonmelanoma skin cancer. In Thiers, B.H., and Dobson, R.L., editors: Pathogenesis of skin disease, New York, 1986, Churchill Livingston.

86. Lang, P.G., Jr., and Maize, J.C.: Histologic evolution of recurrent basal cell carcinoma and treatment implications, J. Am. Acad. Dermatol. **14:**186, 1986.

87. Lapins, N.A., and Helwig, E.B.: Perineural invasion by keratoacanthoma, Arch. Dermatol. **116:**791, 1980.

88. Lauritzen, R.E., Johnson, R.E., and Spratt, J.S.: Pattern of recurrence in basal cell carcinoma, Surgery **57:**813, 1965.

89. Lever, W.F.: Histopathology of the skin, Philadelphia, 1967, J.B. Lippincott Co.

90. Lightstone, A.C., Kopf, A.W., and Garfinkel, L.: Diagnostic accuracy: a new approach to its evaluation, Arch. Dermatol. **91:**497, 1965.

91. Limmer, B.L.: Bowen's disease: treatment with topical 5-fluorouracil, Cutis **16:**660, 1975.

92. Litwin, M.S., et al.: Proceedings: use of 5 fluorouracil in the topical therapy of skin cancer: a review of 157 patients, Proc. Natl. Cancer Conf. **7:**549, 1973.

93. Lund, H.Z.: How often does squamous cell carcinoma of the skin metastasize? Arch. Dermatol. **92:**635, 1965.

94. Madsen, A.: De l'épithélioma baso-cellulaire superficiel: études histologiques de l'architecture de l'épithelioma en coupes horizontales en série, Acta Dermatoven. **22**(7):1, 1941.

95. Menn, H., et al.: The recurrent basal cell epithelioma: a study of 100 cases of recurrent, retreated basal cell epitheliomas, Arch. Dermatol. **103:**628, 1971.

96. Modlin, J.J.: Cancer of the skin: surgical treatment, Mo. Med. **51:**364, 1954.

97. Mohs, F.E.: Chemosurgery: microscopically controlled surgery for skin cancer, Springfield, Ill., 1978, Charles C Thomas, Publisher.

98. Mohs, F.E., Jones, D.L., and Bloom, R.F.: Tendency of fluorouracil to conceal deep foci of invasive basal cell carcinoma, Arch. Dermatol. **114:**1021, 1978.

99. Møller, R., Reymann, F., and Hou-Jensen, K.: Metastases in dermatological patients with squamous cell carcinoma, Arch. Dermatol. **115:**703, 1979.

100. Mora, R.G., and Perniciaro, C.: Cancer of the skin in blacks. I. A review of 163 black patients with cutaneous squamous cell carcinoma, J. Am. Acad. Dermatol. **5:**535, 1981.

101. Mora, R.G., Perniciaro, C., and Lee, B.: Cancer of the skin in blacks. III. A review of nineteen black patients with Bowen's disease, J. Am. Acad. Dermatol. **11:**557, 1984.

102. Murphy, K.J.: Metastatic basal cell carcinoma with squamous appearances in the naevoid basal cell carcinoma syndrome, Br. J. Plast. Surg. **28:**331, 1975.

103. Nevrkla, E., and Newton, K.A.: A survey of the treatment of 200 cases of basal cell carcinoma (1959-1966 inclusive), Br. J. Dermatol. **91:**429, 1974.

104. Odom, R.B., and Goette, D.K.: Treatment of keratoacanthomas with intralesional fluorouracil, Arch. Dermatol. **114:**1779, 1978.

105. Owens, D.W., and Knox, J.M.: Influence of heat, wind, and humidity on ultraviolet radiation injury, Natl. Cancer Inst. Mongr. **50:**161, 1978.

106. Pascal, R.R., et al.: Prognosis of "incompletely excised" versus "completely excised" basal cell carcinoma, Plast. Reconstr. Surg. **41:**328, 1968.

107. Paver, K., et al.: The incidence of basal cell carcinoma and their metastases in Australia and New Zealand [letter], Australas. J. Dermatol. **14:**53, 1973.

108. Piscioli, F., et al.: A giant, metastasizing keratoacanthoma: report of a case and discussion on classification, Am. J. Dermatopathol. **6:**123, 1984.

109. Poleksic, S., and Yeung, K.-Y.: Rapid development of keratoacanthoma and accelerated transformation into squamous cell carcinoma of the skin, Cancer **41:**12, 1978.

110. Rahbari, H., and Mehregan, A.H.: Basal cell epithelioma (carcinoma) in children and teenagers, Cancer **49:**350, 1982.

111. Ratzer, E.R., and Strong, E.W.: Squamous cell carcinoma of the scalp, Am. J. Surg. **114:**570, 1967.

112. Robins, P., and Albom, M.J.: Recurrent basal cell carcinoma in young women, J. Dermatol. Surg. **1**(1):49, 1975.

113. Roffo, A.H.: Cutaneous cancer and the sun: a clinical and experimental study, Urol. Cutan. Rev. **43:**411, 1939.

114. Rook, A., and Whimster, I.: Keratoacanthoma: a thirty-year retrospect, Br. J. Dermatol. **100:**41, 1979.

115. Rosen, T., Tucker, S.B., and Tschen, J.: Bowen's disease in blacks, J. Am. Acad. Dermatol. **7:**364, 1982.

116. Sachs, W., Sachs, P.M., and Atkinson, S.C.: Peripheral, or five-point, method of skin biopsy, J.A.M.A. **142:**902, 1950.

117. Sakura, C.Y., and Calamel, P.M.: Comparison of treatment modalities for recurrent basal cell carcinoma, Plastic Reconstr. Surg. **63:**492, 1979.

118. Schnur, P.L., and Bozzo, P.: Metastasizing keratoacanthomas? The difficulties of differentiating keratoacanthomas from squamous cell carcinomas, Plast. Reconstr. Surg. **62:**258, 1978.

119. Schrek, R.: Cutaneous carcinoma. III. A statistical analysis with respect to site, sex, and pre-existing scars, Arch. Pathol. **31:**434, 1941.

120. Schrek, R., and Gates, O.: Cutaneous carcinoma. I. A statistical analysis with respect to the duration and size of the tumors and the age of the patients at onset and at biopsy of tumor, Arch. Pathol. **31:**411, 1941.

121. Scotto, J., Kopf, A.W., and Urbach, F.: Non-melanoma skin cancer among caucasians in four areas of the United States, Cancer **34:**1333, 1974.

122. Shanoff, L.B., Spira, M., and Hardy, S.B.: Basal cell carcinoma: a statistical approach to rational management, Plast. Reconstr. Surg. **39:**619, 1967.

123. Shiu, M.H., Chu, F., and Fortner, J.G.: Treatment of regionally advanced epidermoid carcinoma of the extremity and trunk, Surg. Gynecol. Obstet. **150:**558, 1980.

124. Sloane, J.P.: The value of typing basal cell carcinomas in predicting recurrence after surgical excision, Br. J. Dermatol. **96:**127, 1977.

125. Stranc, M.F., and Robertson, G.A.: Conservative treatment of keratoacanthoma, Ann. Plast. Surg. **2:**525, 1979.

126. Stromberg, B.V., et al.: Scar carcinoma: prognosis and treatment, South. Med. J. **70:**821, 1977.

127. Sturm, H.M.: Bowen's disease and 5-fluorouracil, J. Am. Acad. Dermatol **1:**513, 1979.

128. Suhge, d'Aubermont, P.C., and Bennett, R.G.: Failure of curettage and electrodesiccation for removal of basal cell carcinoma, Arch. Dermatol. **120:**1456, 1984.

129. Swanbeck, G., and Hillström, L.: Analysis of etiological factors of squamous cell skin cancer of different locations. 4. Concluding remarks, Acta Derm. Venereol. **51:**151, 1971.

130. Taylor, G.A., and Barisoni, D.: Ten years' experience in the surgical treatment of basal-cell carcinoma: a study of factors associated with recurrence, Br. J. Surg. **60:**522, 1973.

131. Thackray, A.C.: Histological classification of rodent ulcers and its bearing on their prognosis, Br. J. Cancer **5:**213, 1951.

132. Tromovitch, T.A.: Skin cancer: treatment by curettage and desiccation, Calif. Med. **103:**107, 1965.

133. Tromovitch, T.A.: The C and D check for skin cancer, Cutis **11:**210, 1973.

134. Tromovitch, T.A., and Allende, M.: Curette-excision technique for skin cancer, Cutis **6:**1349, 1970.

135. Wade, T.R., Kopf, A.W., and Ackerman, A.B.: Bowenoid papulosis of the genitalia, Arch. Dermatol. **115:**306, 1979.

136. Warren, S., and Hoerr, S.O.: A study of pathologically verified epidermoid carcinoma of the skin, Surg. Gynecol. Obstet. **69:**726, 1939.

137. Warren, S., and Lulenski, C.R.: End results of therapy of epithelioma of the skin, Arch. Dermatol. Syph. **44:**37, 1941.

138. Weedon, D., and Wall, D.: Metastatic basal cell carcinoma, Med. J. Aust. **2:**177, 1975.

139. Weinstein, G.D., and Frost, P.: Cell proliferation in human basal cell carcinoma, Cancer Res. **30:**724, 1970.

140. Welton, D.G., Elliott, J.A., and Kimmelstiel, P.: Epithelioma: clinical and histological data on 1025 lesions, Arch. Dermatol. Syph. **60:**277, 1949.

141. Whelan, C.S., and Deckers, P.J.: Electrocoagulation for skin cancer: an old oncologic tool revisited, Cancer **47:**2280, 1981.

142. Williamson, G.S., and Jackson, R.: Treatment of squamous cell carcinoma of the skin by electrodesiccation and curettage, Can. Med. Assoc. J. **90:**408, 1964.

143. Wojcieszek, Z.: Five-year surgical cure rate in carcinoma of the skin, Pol. Przegl. Chir. **39:**994, 1967.

144. Wolinsky, S., et al.: Spontaneous regression of a giant keratoacanthoma, J. Dermatol. Surg. Oncol. **7:**897, 1981.

145. Yaffe, H.S.: Squamous cell carcinoma arising in an epidermal cyst [letter], Arch. Dermatol. **118:**961, 1982.

146. Zaynoun, S., et al.: The relationship of sun exposure and solar elastosis to basal cell carcinoma, J. Am. Acad. Dermatol. **12:**522, 1985.

147. Zerner, J., and Fenn, M.E.: Basal cell carcinoma of the vulva, Int. J. Gynaecol. Obstet. **17:**203, 1979.

21

Lesions Derived from Melanocytes or Nevus Cells

ACTINIC LENTIGO

Actinic lentigo (also called lentigo senilis) is a discrete, hyperpigmented, macular lesion occurring on sun-exposed areas, particularly on the face and the dorsum of the hands. Although the hyperpigmented areas are most commonly multiple, actinic lentigo can also occur as a solitary lesion. Since its development is associated with cumulative sun exposure, it usually is found in the elderly. Most elderly individuals have such lesions. Actinic lentigo can also develop in patients in their thirties—especially on the face, where it becomes a cosmetic problem. In this circumstance, "lentigo senilis" is perhaps a poor choice of terms.

Actinic lentigo is a macular, noninfiltrated lesion that has a uniform brownish color and a slightly irregular outline. The size can vary from a few millimeters to 1 cm or more.

Histopathology

Actinic lentigo is characterized by elongation and tortuosity of the rete papillae and increased pigmentation of the basal cell layer. In addition, an increased number of melanocytes are also present.

Treatment

Although bleaching creams containing hydroquinone can be tried, I have not been impressed by the ultimate results. Another approach is to peel the epidermis by means of any of a variety of peeling agents. Trichloroacetic acid, phenol, light electrodesiccation, and even cryosurgery have all had their advocates. Unfortunately, none of these methods consistently produces total removal and excellent cosmetic results.

I have personally found that Baker's formula[85] (3 ml of full strength phenol [about 88% USP], 2 ml water, 3 drops of croton oil, and 8 drops of liquid soap), when it is unoccluded, results in complete removal of an actinic lentigo with excellent cosmetic results. It is important to stress that Baker's formula should be mixed fresh and applied without occlusion if used for actinic lentigo. The occluded Baker's formula destroys tissue more deeply than the unoccluded Baker's formula.[102,103] Such deep destruction of tissue is unnecessary to remove an actinic lentigo.

Fig. 21-1, *A*, shows a patient with an actinic lentigo on the upper eyelid. Baker's formula is applied without occlusion. Soon after application a frost appears (Fig. 21-1, *B*). I usually apply tap water by means of a cotton-tipped applicator to dilute further the concentration of the material and to make the patient more comfortable. A bandage is not applied. The patient keeps the area clean by daily cleansing with hydrogen peroxide and moist by application of an ointment. The epidermis sloughs off and an excellent cosmetic result is obtained when reepithelization takes place (Fig. 21-1, *C*).

CONGENITAL NEVOCYTIC NEVUS

Congenital nevocytic nevi (CNNs) are pigmented lesions that usually are present at birth or shortly thereafter. On biopsy such lesions are seen to be composed mostly of nevus cells. These lesions are considered separately from acquired nevocytic nevi (those occurring after the age of 1 or 2), because the risk of malignant degeneration is different, and the management will thus be altered.

Classification

CNNs are usually classified as either large or small. Large CNNs, also commonly known as giant CNNs, are usually

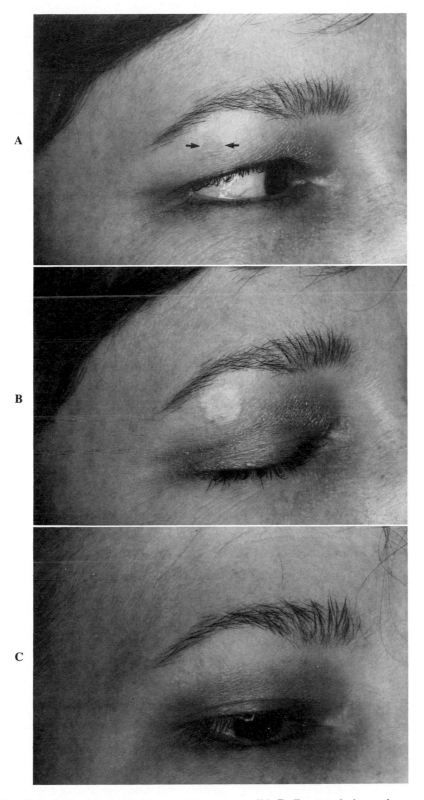

Fig. 21-1. A, Actinic lentigo *(arrows)* on upper eyelid. **B,** Frost on lesion and surrounding skin immediately after application of Baker's formula. **C,** Eyelid 3 months later. Actinic lentigo has totally disappeared, and scar is imperceptible.

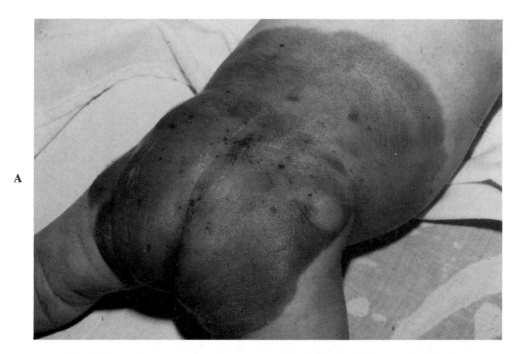

Fig. 21-2. A, Large congenital nevocytic nevus. Note bathing trunk distribution.

defined as lesions that cannot be easily excised and closed by means of a simple or complex repair in a single operation.[60,82] Thus large CNNs require skin grafting or skin flaps for immediate closure. This definition is rather pragmatic and open to question, but it does seem to have wide acceptance.[89] Large CNNs measure several centimeters and are frequently extensive, covering a large portion of the surface of an anatomic location such as the back or extremities. Frequently, when a large CNN is present, many smaller scattered satellite nevi are also present.[99] Small CNNs are usually considered to be lesions less than 1.5 to 3.0 cm in larger diameter; such lesions can be easily excised and closed.

An alternative suggestion[54] for classifing CNNs by largest diameter is as follows: small, less than 1.5 cm; medium, 1.5 to 19.9 cm; large (giant), larger than 20 cm. However, this classification system is not widely used. Although most investigators agree on the definitions of small and large, few are comfortable with an arbitrary definition of medium based on measurements alone.

Incidence

The incidence of CNNs was estimated to be 1.3% by one group of authors after an examination of 1058 newborn infants.[108] These authors noted 41 pigmented lesions. Biopsies were performed on 34 lesions, but only 11 of 34 were confirmed histologically to be CNNs. Thus only about one third of congenital pigmented lesions are of nevus cell origin. Five of the 41 lesions were greater than 1.5 cm, but only two of these contained nevus cells. Thus the incidence of large CNNs (defined as larger than 1.5 cm in this study) was 0.2% (2 of 1058 patients), and the incidence of small CNNs was 1.1% (9 of 1058). On the basis of estimates of 3 million babies born each year in the United States, approximately 6000 additional CNNs and 33,000 small CNNs would be expected annually.

Clinical appearance

CNNs are pigmented, slightly raised (softly infiltrated) lesions. In small lesions, the border is fairly regular, as is the pigmentation (see Chapter 4, Fig. 4-8, *A*). Large CNNs also have regular borders but are more irregularly pigmented, often with areas of nodularity. Frequently many small satellite lesions are present in the vicinity of a large CNN. The distribution can be anywhere on the skin surface, including the scalp. Large CNNs usually have a dermatomal distribution.[84] In one study of 67 large CNNs, it was found that about 66% occurred on the head and neck, 13% on the trunk, 4% on the upper extremities, and 16% on the lower extremities.[60] The trunk, the back, and the buttocks are favored sites. In the latter location, a large CNN is known as a "bathing trunk nevus" (Fig. 21-2). The term "garment nevus" is used in referring to CNNs that cover large anatomic areas, including the bathing trunk area.

Small CNNs are usually oval, their long axes frequently directed along the maximal skin tension lines. Both large and small CNNs often have coarse hair growing within the boundary of the lesion, and the surface can be very thick-

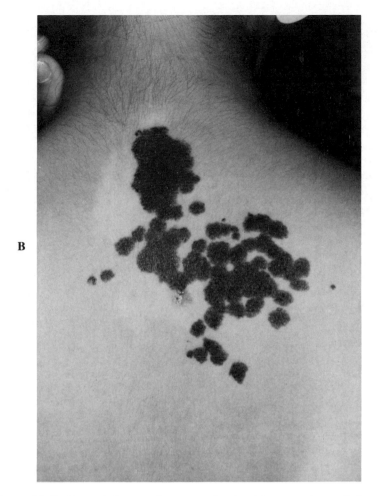

Fig. 21-2, cont'd. B, Congenital nevocytic nevus on back, with progressive evolution of pigmented lesions and areas of regression (hypopigmentation). Several biopsies showed only benign-appearing nevus cells.

ened, even verrucous (Fig. 21-3). As patients age, the pigmentation of the lesions can fade in much the same way as in acquired nevocytic nevi. Usually large CNNs are asymptomatic, although pruritus occurs in a minority of patients.[80]

Large CNNs that are situated on the head and neck can be associated with leptomeningeal melanocytosis.[84] Such involvement can be associated with epilepsy, mental retardation, and leptomeningeal melanoma.

Malignant degeneration

Malignant degeneration of a large or small CNN is of ultimate concern to those caring for patients. The large number of reported cases of a melanoma occurring within a large CNN seems to confirm beyond a reasonable doubt the propensity for these lesions to undergo malignant degeneration. Melanomas can also arise in small CNNs, although the actual rate at which such an event occurs has not been well studied.[74] In this regard it is interesting to note that relatively few melanomas have histopathologic features of a CNN.

In one histopathologic study, 18.4% of melanomas had evidence of acquired nevocytic nevi, whereas only 1.1% had evidence of CNNs.[54]

The high likelihood for malignant change in a large CNN is probably the result of the large number of nevus cells present rather than other pernicious factors. Therefore patients with multiple separate small or medium-sized CNNs should be considered to have the same probability of malignant degeneration occurring as patients with one large CNN.

In one report it is estimated that the likelihood of developing a cutaneous melanoma in a small CNN is approximately three to 21 times greater than the overall risk of developing a melanoma, depending on whether one is relying on history alone or history as well as histology to confirm the presence of a CNN.[88] Since the overall risk of developing a melanoma by age 80 is about 0.4%,[55] conservatively the risk of malignant degeneration within a small CNN is about 1% but can be as high as 8% or 9%.

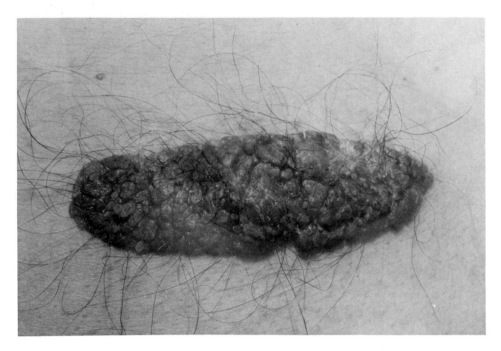

Fig. 21-3. Verrucous type of congenital nevocytic nevus.

Therefore some authorities recommend prophylactic excision of all small CNNs.[41,101]

Malignant degeneration within large CNNs has been better studied. When this event occurs, usually the nevus develops nodules within the lesion, and the skin surface becomes lobulated or hypertrophic. Ulceration in particular should be considered an ominous sign. Darkening of the surface pigmentation frequently occurs, but occasionally lightening might also occur, perhaps because of nevus regression or decreased melanin synthesis.

The most accurate studies made to estimate malignant degeneration in large CNNs come from Scandinavia, where a reasonably small homogeneous population is cared for within a national health service that maintains careful records and follow-up data. One author reported a series of 110 cases of large CNN in Denmark followed for an average of 17.3 years.[80] Only two patients developed malignancy associated with the nevus. Thus the incidence of malignant degeneration in this study was 1.8%. A later extension of this study reports malignant degeneration in three of 151 patients (2.0%) followed to an average age of 31.2 years.[62] However, if one assumes that the average life span is about 72.8 years, the probability of developing melanoma becomes 4.6%. If one further takes into account the fact that patients were not registered until about 8 years of age, the observation period falls to 23 years, and the estimated lifetime probability rises to 6.3%. If one further assumes that about half of the melanomas in large CNNs would have developed before the age of registration (8 years) in this study, which is reasonable from other cases reported,[52] the

TABLE 21-1

Published rates of melanoma developing in large CNN

Reference	Percentage
Pack and Davis (1961)[78]	10/57 = 18%
Reed et al. (1965)[84]	17/55 = 31%
Greeley et al. (1965)[43]	6/56 = 11%
Lanier et al. (1976)[60]	5/72 = 7%
Lorentzen et al. (1977)[62]	3/151 = 2.0%
Others[52]	20/100 = 20%
TOTAL	61/491 = 12.4%

probability increases to 8.7%. Several reported series have been published and are listed in Table 21-1. The probability of a melanoma developing in association with a large CNN in these series varies greatly—from 2.0%[62] to 31%[84]; still, the average of these reports is 12.4%. It should be stressed that many of these reported patients have had prophylactic surgery, which probably influences to an unknown extent the calculated probability figures. Nevertheless, assuming a normal lifetime risk of 0.4% for the development of a melanoma, the risk of development of a melanoma within a large CNN is probably between 22 and 31 times normal.

The age of onset of malignant transformation in large CNNs has been studied[52] (Fig. 21-4). Of the cases reported,

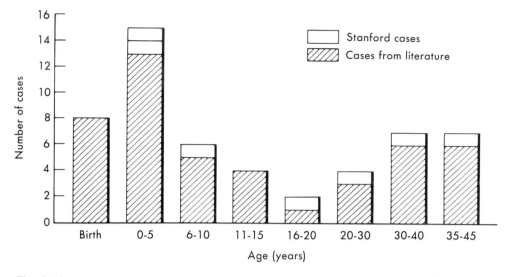

Fig. 21-4. Age of development of malignant melanomas within large congenital nevocytic nevi. (From Kaplan, E.N.: The risk of malignancy in large congenital nevi, Plast. Reconstr. Surg. **53:**421, 1974.)

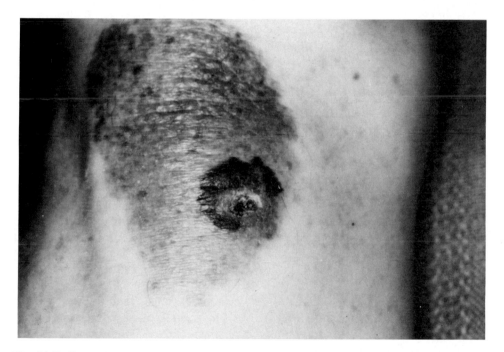

Fig. 21-5. Congenital nevocytic nevus on knee with development of level IV melanoma (darker area) in 80-year-old patient.

60% of melanomas developed during the first decade, mostly before the age of 6. Another 10% appeared between ages 10 and 20. However, other authors believe that overdiagnosis of melanomas within CNNs is common in children.[65] Therefore careful study of the pathology in such cases through several opinions is advisable. I have personally seen a melanoma appear in a medium-sized CNN as late as age 80 (Fig. 21-5).

Histopathology

The microscopic appearance of CNNs is somewhat variable. Nevus cells are always present in the upper dermis. Often such nevus cells extend into the lower dermis or below and tend to involve adnexal structures. In addition, large CNN can contain spindle nevus cells found in a blue nevus or in a neural nevus. These latter spindle nevus cells might closely resemble the cells seen in a neurofibroma.[84]

The depth of penetration of nevus cells within the dermis and their tendency to surround or infiltrate cutaneous appendages is thought by some to be specific for a CNN. One can see nevus cells as single cells or in "Indian file" within sebaceous glands, nerves, vessels, hair follicles, or arrectores pilorum muscles, and in the lower dermis these cells are sometimes present within eccrine ducts as well as lymphatics.[54] Nevus cells can also be found in the subcutaneous tissue in many if not most CNNs.[67]

However, one group of authors has found that some acquired nevi that develop by history after age 2 also contain nevus cells in these same locations.[97] Therefore the use of depth of invasion or infiltration of appendages is not necessarily specific for CNN.

In one report the pattern of nevus cells in 38 CNNs excised to subcutaneous fat and skin grafted was studied.[104] These lesions can be considered large or at least medium-sized CNNs (larger than 1.5 to 3 cm). The patterns of nevus cell groups were described as either patchy or diffuse, sometimes confined just to the upper dermis and sometimes to both upper and lower dermis. In only 37% of cases were nevus cells seen to extend into the deep dermis, and the depth of penetration of nevus cells was not correlated with CNN size. In contrast, small CNNs are perhaps more likely to have nevus cells distributed only in the superficial dermis.[114]

On the basis of the foregoing, it is difficult to generalize concerning the specific histologic picture of a CNN, whether large or small. One should therefore be encouraged to biopsy lesions whenever they are suspicious or whenever one contemplates therapy.

The development of a malignant melanoma within a CNN is of ultimate concern, as has been previously discussed. Unlike sporadic cases of melanoma or those associated with acquired nevocytic nevi, many of those associated with large CNNs arise from nevus cells deep within the dermis or lower.[84] This has certain implications for treatment, which are discussed later.

The histologic picture of melanoma within a large CNN can be confusing. Twenty-six cases labeled as melanoma in children under the age of 14 were reviewed in a study by Malec and Langerlöf.[65] These authors considered only one case to be a bona fide melanoma. The other cases proved to be either a Spitz nevus (juvenile melanoma), blue nevus, compound nevus, or neurofibroma. Therefore one should be cautious in accepting a diagnosis of melanoma in a large CNN in the very young.

Treatment

The treatment of a CNN, whether large or small, is excision because of the high probability of malignant degeneration that was discussed previously.[101] In addition, large CNNs are a cosmetic handicap. Because of emotional suffering, a majority of adults with a large CNN who have been polled would desire removal of such a nevus were it to occur in their children.[80] Therefore treatment should be offered to patients with a large CNN, and an aggressive approach should be taken early in the patient's lifetime, especially before he or she goes to school. It is best to inform patients and their families that malignant change has been known to occur in CNN but that its frequency in small lesions is unknown.

Excision is the surest method of removing all potentially lethal cells. However, excision does carry an aesthetic price. Fortunately in infants the skin is excessive and has excellent elasticity and healing properties. Therefore fairly large amounts of skin can be excised, especially in areas such as the abdomen where a large "abdominoplasty" can be easily performed in young infants.[66] Such large excisions can be performed at an early age but become more difficult as the child grows older.

Excision of a small CNN poses little problem. Because of the possibility of hospital-acquired infection and the relatively immature immune system of newborns, excisions are usually delayed until a few months following discharge from the hospital (see Chapter 4, Fig. 4-8). Frequently, small oval CNNs are situated with their long axes along the maximal skin tension lines, thereby facilitating closure.[36] For moderately large CNNs that measure greater than 1.5 to 3.0 cm, closure after excision may be difficult. Staged excision is recommended whenever feasible for these lesions, since this usually leads to an excellent cosmetic result with little morbidity.[41,73] Skin grafting and skin flaps can thus be avoided.[26] Staged excisions are successive excisions repeated at variable intervals, usually from 3 to 6 months, that result in the progressive reduction of the size of a lesion that could not otherwise be excised and easily sutured in one stage. Staged excisions are based on the premise that normal skin has a tremendous capacity to stretch, especially when the stretching is done slowly over time.

The recommended method for staged excisions of CNNs is illustrated in Fig. 21-6.[113] Note that the first and second excisions in this example are on the lateral sides of the lesion, leaving the last excision for the middle. This sequence helps to minimize the number of resultant scars, since the last excision includes the scars from the previous two excisions. An alternative to excision and side-to-side closure for a large CNN is skin grafting or skin flaps. Both of these procedures usually require general anesthesia in young children and thus result in some morbidity and mortality.[89] The decision to perform such an extensive procedure is based on the relative risks to the infant, taking into consideration his or her general health. The risk of death from general anesthesia is much less than the risk of development of melanoma within a large CNN, and thus excision would seem to be justfiable.[89] In general, the cosmetic results with skin grafts are poor. However, there are situations in which this is the most reasonable approach. For very

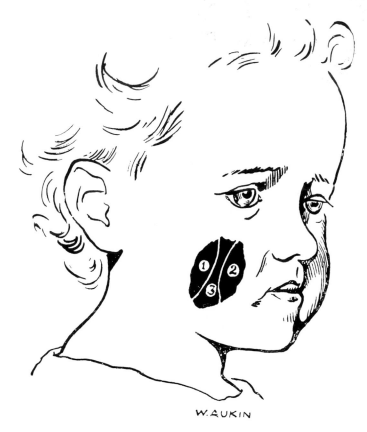

W. AUKIN

Fig. 21-6. Staged excision method of removal of congenital nevocytic nevus of cheek. Note that first and second stages of excision are on lateral sides of lesion. (From Wilson, J.S.P.: Br. J. Plast. Surg. **1:**117, 1948.)

large lesions on the trunk, segmental excisions followed by split-thickness skin grafting in several operative sessions might be the only way to achieve total excision and coverage of the resultant wound. On the scalp extensive staged excisions early in life are probably unwise, because the bones of the cranium have not yet fused and the skull continues to expand until age 7 (see Chapter 3). Therefore, ideally, excisions on the scalp should place little tension on the surrounding scalp—to accommodate the expanding skull. Skin grafting with or without skin flaps allows normal development of the bony vault in young children.

Skin grafting does not necessarily imply that all nevus cells in depth have been removed. The decision of how deeply to remove tissue containing a CNN is usually based on functional and cosmetic considerations rather than histologically determined depth of penetration of nevus cells. Therefore, it is not surprising that recurrences of CNN[104] or even development of melanomas within skin grafts[89] have been reported. Nevertheless, lowering the total number of total nevus cells present probably lessens the likelihood of malignant transformation in the future.

Some authors suggest that instead of grafting surgical defects from large CNN, strips of skin be excised and the resultant wounds be allowed to heal by secondary inten-

tion.[107] At a later time, intervening strips of skin containing remaining CNN are removed, and again the wound is allowed to heal secondarily. This method gradually replaces the lesion with a scar. Multiple skin punches can also be used instead of strips of skin.

Perhaps the most controversial method of treatment for large CNNs is dermabrasion. In a seminal report by Johnson,[50] four children with CNNs had their lesions dermabraded. Three were dermabraded early in life, two at 2 months and one at 5 months; the fourth was dermabraded at 11 months. The pigment recurred in the last case but not in the other three cases. Equally encouraging results were subseqently reported by other authors.[16,69] It is emphasized by those with experience that, if dermabrasion is to be successful, it must be performed early and deeply. Some authors state that they dermabrade until no more pigment is seen.[16] Others dermabrade immediately after a dermatome excision to achieve a very deep wound.[69] The authors of the studies just mentioned[16,69] believe that nevus cells descend in depth as the infant ages, so the earlier the dermabrasion the better. However, there is no objective proof that this supposition is correct.

In another study the healed skin after dermabrasion of four CNNs was biopsied.[114] One had been dermabraded at 2 weeks, two at 4 weeks, and one at 6 weeks of age. In all cases remaining nevus cells were found beneath the level of dermabrasion, although the CNN was cosmetically improved. The authors of this study suggest that dermabrasion is inadequate to remove totally a large CNN, because in such a lesion some nevus cells extend deeply. In addition, since a melanoma arising in a large CNN often originates from these deeper nevus cells, the risk of malignant degeneration might not be lessened by dermabrasion alone.

Excision of CNNs with the dermaplaning rather than dermabrasion has also been advocated. However, as could be predicted, complete removal is not obtained with this method, and recurrences are the rule.[78]

It is generally assumed that excision to fat eradicates the nevus cells in a CNN. However, nevus cells can extend deeply into fat, muscle fascia, and even muscle itself. As stated previously, it is likely that a melanoma that develops in a large CNN does so in association with these deeper elements rather than with the more superficially situated nevus cells.[84] Therefore histopathologic examination of all cut margins, lateral and deep, is necessary to ensure total extirpation.

Deep excision of CNNs extending to and perhaps including muscle fascia should be considered. One group of authors reported a case of a boy who at the age of 3 had had a split-thickness skin graft to the chest for a large CNN.[89] Seventeen years later a melanoma appeared as a deep nodule in the skin graft. A mastectomy was performed, and, in addition to the melanoma, benign nevus cells were seen within the pectoralis muscle. Therefore, theoretically at the time of initial excision, a portion of the superficial pectoralis muscle would need to have been removed to have excised the CNN completely.

Before any extensive procedure for removal of a large CNN, multiple biopsies should be obtained and studied. Nevus cells do not necessarily always extend into the deep dermis. On the other hand, they frequently do so, going deeply into subcutaneous tissue and rarely even into muscle. More aggressive therapy needs to be planned for more deeply extending lesions; otherwise the risk of recurrence is great, and the potential for the development of melanoma is still present.

Patients with a large CNN should be followed closely at intervals of 6 months to 1 year. Suspicious new areas of growth or any persistent ulcerations should be biopsied. If questions arise concerning proper management, the patient can be referred for advice or treatment to tumor conferences or pigmented lesion clinics that are available at most medical centers.

ACQUIRED NEVOCYTIC NEVUS

The common mole or acquired nevocytic nevus (ANN) is a lesion frequently presented to the physician for removal. Sometimes the patient is concerned regarding recent growth or change in appearance of the mole, but commonly requests for removal are based on the desire for cosmetic improvement or repeated traumatization by clothing such as a bra or pants. Several factors influence the advisability of removal or biopsy, and therefore some background on the nature of this lesion is necessary.

Although they occasionally resemble each other, ANNs are usually clinically distinguishable from CNNs (congenital nevoctic nevi). The latter appear at or shortly after birth, whereas the former usually appear after the age of 1 or 2. Other distinctions between these two types of lesions are discussed later.

Incidence

A 1952 report states that whites have an average of 15 ANNs per person.[79] However, more recent studies indicate that the number of ANNs per individual is increasing. For example, in a study published in 1985 an average of 39 moles per individual was found.[24]

The number of ANNs also varies with age and sex. The average number of moles has been found to be maximal at age 15 in men and at ages 20 through 29 in women. At these ages the averages are 43.23 moles for men and 27.13 moles for women.[75] The number of ANNs declines after the age of 30 and decreases to a very low figure in persons 80 years old.[24]

Etiology

Sun exposure probably plays a significant role in the development of ANN, and thus the number of moles varies with the anatomic location. On sun-protected parts of the body, development of moles is delayed, whereas on the face moles evolve more rapidly, appearing in the first or second decade of life.[75] Men have a higher incidence of moles on their back and chest than women, possibly related to relative sun exposure. ANNs are more common on the lateral (sun-exposed) surfaces of the arms than the medial (sun-protected) aspects.[56] Fewer ANN also appear in the axilla, another relatively sun-protected area, than in the posterior thoracic area.[57] Of interest in this regard is the fact that just as the incidence of skin cancers is increasing because of frequent sun exposure and outdoor activity, so too is the incidence of ANN rising.[24]

Clinical appearance

ANNs are either flat or raised. A flat ANN is pigmented and is known as a junctional nevus (Fig. 21-7, *A*). A raised ANN is either flesh-colored or hyperpigmented. It represents either a compound or intradermal nevus (Fig. 21-8). A junctional nevus has nevus cells either singly or in nests confined to the lower epidermis. A compound nevus has nevus cells within both the epidermis and the dermis. An intradermal nevus contains groups of nevus cells in the upper and lower dermis with little junctional activity. Compound and

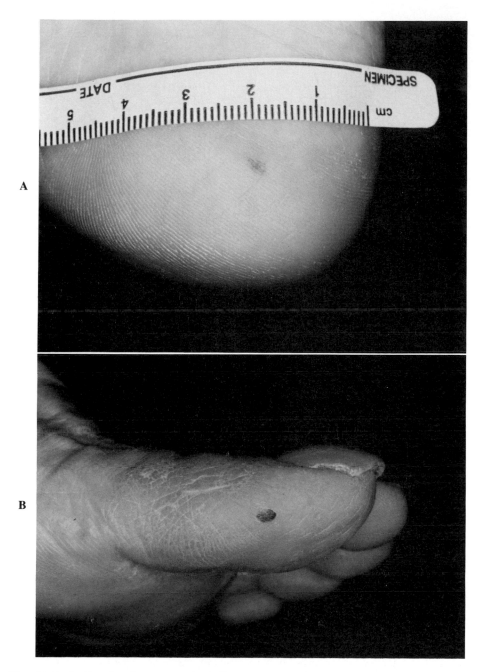

Fig. 21-7. A, Junctional nevus on heel. **B,** Hemorrhage into stratum corneum on toe. Rapid development of lesion, caused by trauma, was alarming to patient.

intradermal nevi are often clinically indistinguishable.

The ANN is not a stable lesion; that is, it has periods of growth and regression.[33] It usually develops in infancy or early childhood but it can appear at any age—however, it rarely appears after the age of 40 years. An ANN commonly appears at first as a flat junctional nevus. With time, usually during adolescence, the nevus cells proliferate and become predominant in the upper dermis and the epidermis, thus forming a compound nevus. The last stage of maturity before involution is an intradermal nevus with all nevus cells lying deep within the dermis. Intradermal nevi are common in middle-aged adults. These concepts of ANN growth are based on observations of nevi at various ages rather than on observed changes in individual nevi.

There are a few exceptions to the preceding scenario. On the palms, soles, and genital areas, ANNs are usually the

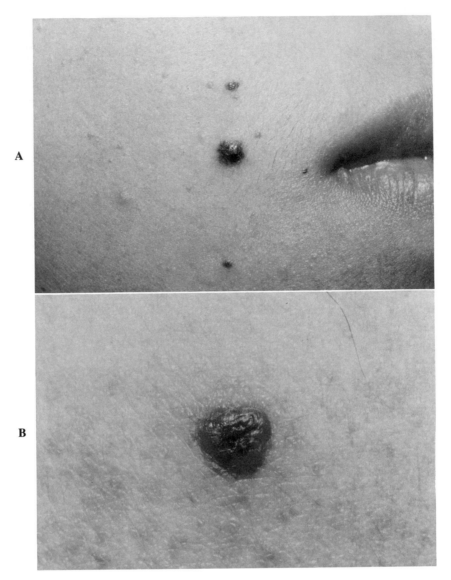

Fig. 21-8. A, Compound nevus. **B,** Hemorrhage into compound nevus. When this occurs, patient and physician might be concerned about development of a melanoma.

junctional type with little change into intradermal nevi with age. In these locations junctional nevi might also appear later in life. Although few conditions are known that influence the growth of an ANN, pregnancy is an exception. Showers of ANNs might appear during pregnancy, and existing moles might darken. Such changes are common enough to be expected.

Most ANN are pigmented light brown to black. This pigmentation is relatively uniformly distributed. In addition, the borders of the lesion are fairly well demarcated and regular. ANNs vary in size from 1 mm to 5 mm; they are rarely larger. Occasionally ANNs have hairs protruding from their surfaces. These hairs are common on the face with compound or intradermal nevi but are unusual with junctional nevi.

Occasionally hemorrhage (Fig. 21-8, *B*) or an infected pustule may arise within an ANN. When either of these events occurs, it may be alarming to patient and physician alike. Hemorrhage into normal stratum corneum may also occur subsequent to minor trauma (as in tennis) on the ventral feet and toes (Fig. 21-7, *B*). The resulting lesion may mimic a junctional nevus or a melanoma.

Dysplastic nevus

A special type of ANN, the dyplastic nevus (DN), has been recently described and characterized.[37] This lesion is believed to have special biologic significance, since it may be a precursor of melanoma and serves as a marker for familial melanoma. The term *dysplasia* means abnormal development of tissue. It here applies to both the clinical

TABLE 21-2

Comparison between ANNs, DNs, and melanomas

	ANN	DN	Melanoma
Size	1 to 5 mm	>6 mm; frequently >10 mm but <15 mm	>6 mm
Distribution	Sun-exposed areas above the waist	Sun-exposed and non–sun exposed areas (for example, scalp, pubic areas)	Sun-exposed and non–sun exposed areas
Color	Uniform tan or brown	Irregular mixtures of tan, brown, black, red, or pink	Irregular mixtures of tan, brown, black, red, or pink
Borders	Regular, sharp	Irregular, indistinct	Irregular, sharp
Number	20 to 40 (in adults)	Sometime > 100 (but sometimes normal number of nevi present)	One
Surface configuration	Smooth uniform macular papular	Macular and papular, "fried egg," "pebbly"	Irregular macular, macular and papular, macular and nodular, or nodular
Age of appearance	Usually in childhood; unusual after age 40	Anytime, but usually after puberty	Anytime, but usually after adolescence

and the histopathologic appearance of lesions. DNs are "funny-looking" moles both on the skin and under the microscope.

Clinically, DNs may superficially resemble ANNs, but several features serve to distinguish these two lesions[44] (Table 21-2). In addition, some of the features of a DN are also found with melanomas. This has led some investigators to believe that the DN represents a middle ground between a common ANN and a fully developed melanoma. A DN is usually larger than an ordinary ANN, frequently measuring 6 to 15 mm in greatest diameter (Fig. 21-9). It has an irregular border with indistinct margins that fade imperceptibly into the surrounding skin. The color is also variegated. Mottled brown hues often predominate; but areas with haphazard mixtures of tan, black, red, or pink often appear. The surface characteristics of a DN are also somewhat distinctive. Whereas common ANNs have a smooth uniform macular or papular surface configuration, DNs are frequently "pebbly" or papular in one area and macular in another. Often this mixture gives a fried egg appearance (central or eccentric papules surrounded by nearly macular pigmentation).

In patients with several DNs, there is great variability from one lesion to the next. DNs are mainly found on the trunk and arms, but they are also found on skin that is seldom exposed to the sun and on areas such as the scalp, pubic area, or women's breasts. Although DNs can occur in individuals with a normal number of moles (usually 20 to 40), frequently they appear in those with many more moles than normal; sometimes there are as many as 100 dysplastic

lesions. The characteristic changes of DNs usually do not appear until after puberty: somewhat later than the time of appearance of normal moles but somewhat earlier than that of most melanomas.

The belief that DNs are precursors of melanomas is predicated on several pieces of evidence. Approximately 2% to 6% of whites without melanomas have DNs; however 30% to 37% of patients with cutaneous melanoma have DNs.[91] In other words, the likelihood of the appearance of a DN in patients with a melanoma is 6 to 15 times that in normal patients. A significant number of patients (7.5%) with sporadic (nonfamilial) melanomas clinically have DNs.[37] Up to 57% of these sporadic melanomas have histopathologic evidence of a DN,[59] although the true figure is probably lower, as is discussed shortly. In cases of multiple DNs followed over time, development of melanomas from lesions thought to be DN has been documented photographically.[37] Finally, the occurrence of melanomas is greater in patients with DNs whose family members have either or both DNs and melanomas.[45]

Patients with DNs are a heterogeneous group in which there are several subsets of patients that have different likelihoods of lifetime risk for development of a melanoma.[59,91] At one end of the spectrum is the patient with one or a few DNs but no relatives with either DNs or melanomas. This individual has *sporadic dysplastic nevi,* and the lifetime risk of developing a melanoma is low and perhaps not much different from that of the general population without DNs. At the other end of the spectrum is the patient with multiple DNs, who has at least two blood relatives

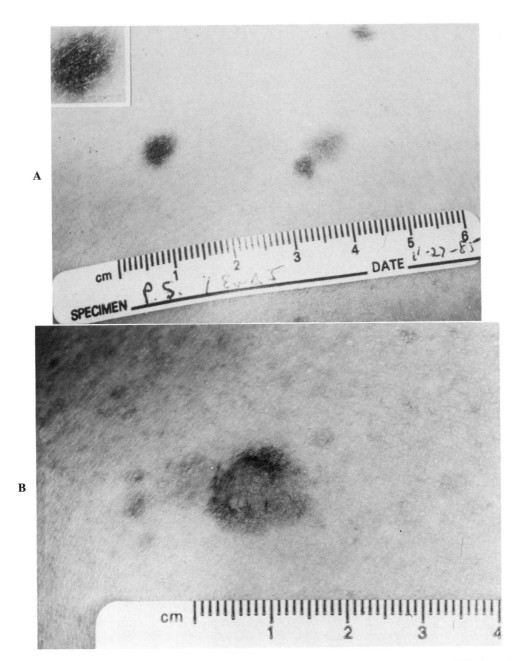

Fig. 21-9. A, Dysplastic nevocytic nevus *(inset).* **B,** Dysplastic nevus, papular with diffusion of pigment. Note that size is greater than 6 mm.

with DNs and with melanomas. An individual with this familial background is said to have the *familial dysplastic nevus syndrome,* which appears to be dominantly inherited. This person has a lifetime risk for developing a melanoma that approaches 100%.[59] Many patients with multiple DNs fit somewhere between these two extremes and have a risk of about 18% for developing a melanoma (the lifetime risk of melanoma development in normal patients in the United States in 1980 was 0.4%[55]). These patients have DNs, but their blood relatives either have no DNs but do have mela-

nomas or have DNs but no melanomas. The last group has *familial dysplastic nevi* that, like dysplastic nevus syndrome, appears to be inherited as an autosomal dominant trait. Categorizing patients with DNs is difficult and complicated by the fact that classification is made on the basis of family history, which can be unknown, inaccurate, or incomplete.

One group of authors has followed 401 members of 14 families with hereditary melanomas for 8 years.[45] A total of 39 new melanomas was detected in 22 participants, but only in family members with DNs, most of whom had had a previous melanoma. Of 77 participants with DNs but no personal history of melanoma, four developed melanomas. Some of these lesions were photographically shown to progress from what appeared to be a DN to a melanoma.[37] The 5% chance of developing melanoma in this 8-year period compares with a risk of 0.04% of expected cases, or 125 times the normal risk. Thus DNs are clinical markers for a relatively high risk of melanoma development in certain individuals. It should be pointed out that, although hereditary melanomas comprise only 3% to 8% of melanomas, most of these are associated with DNs.[59]

Histopathology

The microscopic appearance of ANNs has already been partially described. In the typical ANN, the nevus cells are clustered into groups, or thèques. These cells are small and oval or cuboidal with a homogeneous cytoplasm. The nucleus is large and rounded. However, there can be some variation in the appearance of these cells in the lower dermis, where the nevus cells tend to be more elongated. The origin of the nevus cell is unclear, but it is most likely derived from a melanocyte or nevoblast.

The pathologic appearance of a DN has the following features: (1) epidermal melanocytic hyperplasia both within the lesion and to the sides (shoulders) with elongation of the rete ridges; (2) nuclear atypia (size or density) of melanocytes; (3) nevus cells, either spindle-shaped or epithelioid, in nests of variable size and distribution; (4) dermal fibroplasia; (5) a patchy dermal infiltrate of lymphocytes; and (6) telangiectasia. The histopathologic distinctions between a DN, a melanoma in situ, and a nevocytic nevus are subject to interpretation and are not always clear-cut. Unfortunately this ambiguity has given rise to different histologic interpretations of the same specimen by different dermatopathologists.

To qualify as a DN histopathologically, the lesion should have at least nuclear atypia present within the nevus cells' epidermal melanocytes. Therefore it might be difficult to conclude with certainty that a given lesion is a DN or an early melanoma. Some authors believe that many histopathologically interpreted DNs are in fact melanomas in situ associated with an intradermal nevus.[1]

The pathologic evolution of melanomas from DNs is thus a subject of some debate and open to speculation. In one study it is reported that 20% to 35% of all primary melanomas have remnants of DN.[44] Others believe that this figure is an exaggeration and that melanomas rarely develop from DNs.[1]

Further confusing the issue of evolution of melanomas from DNs is the relationship between DNs and ANNs or CNNs. One group reports that 21.8% of 225 level II melanomas they have studied have features of DN.[90] However, some 45% of these melanomas with features of DN also have features of ANN (29%) or CNN (16%). This is thus consistent with the concept that DNs are a stage in the progression to malignancy of some nevocytic nevi, whether acquired or congenital.

Treatment

ANNs can be removed in one of two ways: (1) complete removal by deep excision, or (2) partial (incisional) removal by a superficial method. Complete removal is usually accomplished by scalpel excision and closure by sutures. The advantages of complete excision are that a total specimen is obtained for histologic examination, and regrowth of the nevus does not occur. The disadvantage is that occasionally the cosmetic result is inferior to that obtained by partial removal. The methods of partial removal include an incision parallel to and at the same level as the skin surface ("shave"), electrocautery, or electrodesiccation. One of the advantages of partial removal is that the cosmetic result is frequently superior to that obtained by total excision. The disadvantages are that since the lesion is usually not totally removed,[109] complete histologic examination is not obtained and the lesion is likely to regrow. If electrodesiccation or electrocautery is used alone, either no tissue or severely damaged tissue is available for pathologic examination; but the cosmetic results obtained might be superior to those resulting from any other treatment method. Since a small percentage of "clinically normal" ANNs can be either DNs, or melanomas, it is preferable to obtain a tissue specimen at the time of treatment, so that a dermatopathologist can be consulted. If the ANN contains hairs, they will regrow if the lesion is merely shaved. However, these hairs can be removed by electrolysis after removal of the lesion.

When an ANN recurs after partial removal, it can reappear either as an area of pigmentation or an elevation at the site of previous removal. Usually the recurrence is in the center of the removal site, although the lesion might regrow as a ring around the periphery. It is thought that the regrowth is caused by nevus cells migrating from the periphery and from the external hair root sheaths in the same manner as regenerating epidermis.[93] In this period of regrowth the nevus can be reliving an earlier part of its history, appearing first as a junctional nevus and then as a compound nevus.

One important problem seen occasionally with ANNs that are shaved is that if a recurrence develops and is excised, subsequent histopathologic examination is more difficult. The remaining nevus cells embedded in scar tissue or associated with pigmentation following use of ferric subsulfate (Monsel's solution) can create confusion with melanoma under the microscope.[58]

Fig. 21-10 shows a shave excision of an ANN. If possible, an infiltrative anesthetic is not used. This is because an anesthetic tends to elevate the ANN (Fig. 21-11). As the scalpel blade comes through an anesthetized ANN, a great-

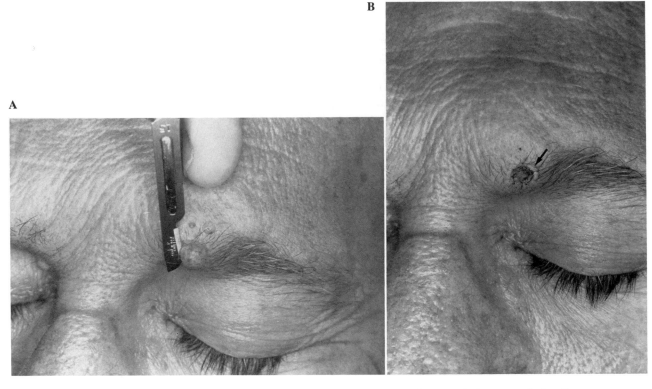

Fig. 21-10. A, Incisional (''shave'') removal of intradermal nevus. **B,** Wound after removal. Small portion of nevus still remains *(arrow),* which was subsequently shaved off.

er portion of skin and ANN may be removed than is necessary. When the anesthetic is subsequently absorbed, one is left with a slightly depressed scar at the site of the removal. To further minimize excessive tissue excision at the time of nevus removal, a fine razor blade can be useful.

An alternative method of removal of ANNs that are elevated is to freeze the lesion with Frigiderm followed by a shave parallel to the skin surface.[8] This prevents the problem of elevation from an infiltrative anesthetic but at the same time provides adequate anesthesia. Because the lesion becomes hard, it is easily removed. The method, however, does not work well for relatively flat moles and is not as precise (due to tactile differences) as shaving with a razor blade without an anesthetic.

After shave removal of an ANN, the bleeding is either controlled by a styptic such as aluminum chloride, 35% in isopropyl alcohol, or electrodesiccation. The latter method may help to destroy slightly more nevus cells and thus result in less chance of recurrence.[109] The use of ferric subsulfate (Monsel's solution) as a styptic should be avoided. If the lesion regrows and needs to be removed in the future, iron deposits from the ferric subsulfate can be misconstrued as melanin pigment within dermal macrophages, leading to confusion of these cells with melanoma cells.[35]

DNs should be excised totally so that full histopathologic examination can be obtained. Unfortunately, most DNs oc-

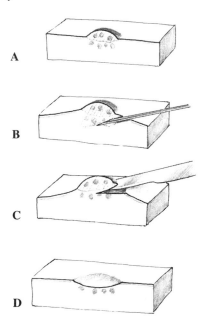

Fig. 21-11. Explanation for depressed scar following ''shave'' removal of nevocytic nevus. **A,** Nevocytic nevus with both exophytic (cross-hatched area) and endophytic elements. **B,** Injection of local anesthetic, causing skin to balloon up. **C,** Horizontal incision with scalpel blade. Because of swelling caused by local anesthetic, more tissue than the exophytic (cross-hatched) area is removed. **D,** Healed result. Depression appears when swelling from local anesthetic recedes.

cur on the trunk, where excisions result in a poor cosmetic appearance. Shave "excisions" of DNs, like those of regular ANNs, can lead to recurrences, and histopathologic interpretation of recurrent DNs can be more difficult than that of primary DNs that are excised in toto to begin with.[35]

The skin of patients with multiple DNs should be closely scrutinized.[44] Complete cutaneous examination and excisional biopsies of a few representative lesions should be performed to establish the diagnosis. Complete cutaneous examination of parents, siblings, and first-degree relatives should also be done to determine whether family members have DNs. A complete cutaneous examination includes examination of the hair-covered areas, especially the scalp and pubic areas, where lesions can often be missed. It is recommended that lesions in these areas be excised, since they are difficult to follow.

Individuals with DNs and relatives with either melanomas or DNs need to be followed very closely. Photographs of all pigmented lesions should be obtained. These photographs need to be updated periodically, should new lesions occur or old lesions progress. Full cutaneous examination needs to be performed twice a year. Instructions should be given to avoid sunburning and excessive sun exposure and to use a sunscreen. Sunlight probably induces both ANNs and DNs in patients with DNs.[57]

Indiscriminate prophylactic removal of DNs is to be avoided if possible to prevent scarring. Only lesions that are clinically most suspicious need to be removed. Other lesions that are documented to change over time also should be removed.

Women of childbearing age with multiple DNs need close observation if they become pregnant. These patients should be seen monthly, and lesions that enlarge or change should be biopsied. In addition, it is probably best for women with multiple DNs to keep from using oral contraceptives.

The wisdom of removing ANNs on the acral or mucosal areas is controversial. One authority advocates removal of all nevocytic nevi on the plantar surfaces because of the possible role of trauma in causing melanomas in this area.[100] He also advises removal of all ANNs greater than 7 mm on the palmar surface and all pigmented lesions of the mucous membranes. However, these recommendations are not uniformly accepted by all physicians.[100]

MELANOMA
Incidence

Melanoma is the most common deadly tumor arising in the skin. The rate of melanoma has been rising worldwide during the latter half of this century.[55] Currently it is estimated that approximately one in 250 people (0.4%) will develop a melanoma in his or her lifetime. If this trend continues, the probability risk will further increase to one in 150 individuals (0.7%) by the year 2000. In 1974 it was estimated that in the United States with a population then of about 210,000,000, there were approximately 9000 new melanomas annually, 300,000 other skin cancers and 600,000 cancers of other organs.[95] Thus melanomas comprise about 1% of all cancers.

Cause

The cause of melanomas is not completely known. Sunlight is thought to play an important role. Unlike basal or squamous cell carcinomas, however, which are associated with chronic solar ultraviolet exposure, melanoma is probably more closely associated with acute, infrequent, and high-intensity sun damage.[94] The incidence of melanoma is higher in the southern United States and lower in the northern United States,[95] which correlates with the greater intensity and quantity of sunlight per year in the sun belt. In addition, individuals with fair complexions (light eyes, light hair) appear to be more likely to develop melanomas. In particular, persons with red hair early in life (age 5) are most susceptible to the later development of melanoma. This increased risk is three times normal and twice the risk of individuals with blond hair.[7] Persons with xeroderma pigmentosum and albinos are more susceptible to the development of not only basal and squamous cell carcinomas, but melanomas as well.

Melanomas can arise in association with ANNs, CNNs, or DNs. However, the majority of melanomas probably arise de novo, unassociated with other lesions. Only 10% to 28% of all melanomas have histopathologic evidence of contiguous ANNs.[18,21,54-90]

Cutaneous melanomas occasionally can be familial and inherited. In the animal kingdom genetically inherited melanomas have been studied in fish, mice, snakes, and several other creatures. Familial ocular melanomas have been known in humans since the nineteenth century; however, it was not until a 1952 report that familial cutaneous melanoma was first recognized.[15] This was a study of a father with melanoma who had three children, two of whom also developed a melanoma (one son and one daughter). No mention was made in these cases of multiple ANNs.

The incidence of familial melanomas is approximately 3% to 8% of all melanomas.[59,63] The predisposition for their development appears to be inherited as an autosomal dominant trait and can be associated with other tumors such as cancers of the breast, lung, or gastrointestinal tract.[63] Thus patients with familial melanomas have a cancer diathesis. Their melanomas frequently begin early and are multiple.

A special type of hereditary melanoma syndrome is the familial dysplastic nevus syndrome (F-DNS), which is characterized by the presence of multiple (10 to 200) atypical (dysplastic) moles in individuals with a personal and family history of melanoma. In addition, at least two blood relatives also have dysplastic nevi (DNs). Like familial melanomas, F-DNS is thought to have an autosomal dominant

TABLE 21-3

Major categories of invasive melanomas

		LMM	SSM	NM
Ulceration		None	Infrequent	Frequent
Surface		Flat	Slightly raised	Nodular
Border		Very irregular	Irregular	Slightly irregular
Size		Large	Medium	Small
Colors		Brown	Variegated	Black-variegated
Regression		Common	Unusual	Rare
Common locations		Head and neck	Leg and upper back	Any location, especially leg
Age (average)*		70	52.9	51.8
Mortality (5-year)*		10.3%	31.5%	56.1%
Relative incidence*		13.9%	54.5%	31.6%
Progression		Slow (10-15 years)	Intermediate	Fast
Melanocytes		Spindle-shaped	Epithelioid	Epithelioid

*Data from Clark et al.: Cancer Res. **29**:705, 1969.

mode of inheritance. However, sporadic DNs (S-DNs) can also occur in which the patient has multiple DNs and melanoma but no family history of DNs or melanoma. The moles in individuals with F-DNs or S-DNS might be precursors of malignant melanomas.[19] Originally F-DNS was known as the B-K mole syndrome (the initials of the first two families described by Clark et al.[19]) or the FAMMM (familial atypical multiple mole-melanoma) syndrome, as described by Lynch et al.[42,64] Further discussion of the DNS is found earlier, in the section on acquired nevocytic nevi.

Classification

Cutaneous melanomas are usually classified into one of three main clinicopathologic types: lentigo maligna melanoma (LMM), superficial spreading melanoma (SSM), or nodular melanoma (NM).[18] These three varieties of melanoma each evolve at a different rate, which affects the prognosis in terms of metastasis and mortality (Table 21-3). In addition, three other rare varieties of cutaneous melanoma are usually separately classified because of their unusual behavior patterns. These are acral lentiginous melanoma, mucosal melanoma, and polypoid melanoma.

Lentigo maligna melanoma. LMMs are fairly large, flat, brown-black lesions that occur almost exclusively on the faces of elderly individuals (Fig. 21-12). The average age of patients with LMMs is 70 years compared to 52.9 years for patients with SSMs.[17,23,83] Of all types of melanomas, LMM has the best overall prognosis and survival rate.

An LMM was originally described by Hutchinson in 1894,[49] when the progression of a lesion was observed over a 2-year period from a few lentigos on the lower eyelid and malar eminence of a woman to a larger coalescence of these

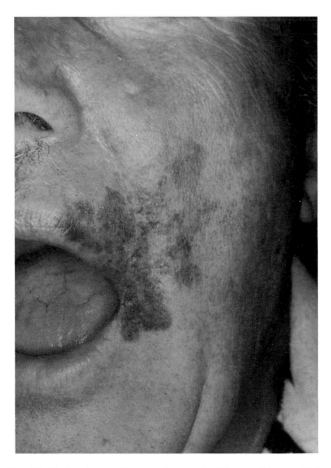

Fig. 21-12. Lentigo maligna melanoma in 55-year-old man. Note involvement of oral mucosa.

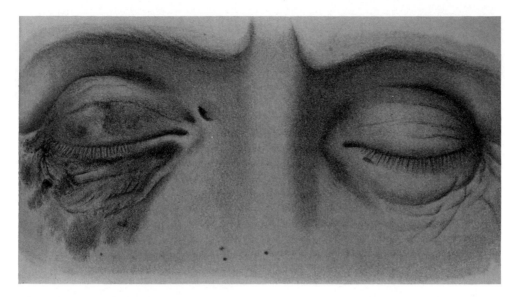

Fig. 21-13. Patient of Hutchinson with lentigo maligna melanoma of right eyelids. (From Hutchinson, J.: Arch. Surg. (London) **5:**253, 1894. Copyright 1984, American Medical Association.)

lesions and the development of a nodule (Fig. 21-13). Hutchinson also noted that an LMM could occur on the lip or prepuce, perhaps an early reference to a mucosal melanoma that can histologically resemble LMM. At about the same time that Hutchinson first described lentigo maligna (LM) and LMM, a series of similar cases was also published in France by Dubreuilh.[34]

It is important to understand that LM and LMM are actually different phases of the same disease process. The early noninvasive stage of LMM (confined only within the epidermis) is properly referred to as LM, whereas the later invasive stage (malignant cells within the dermis) is LMM. The terms *Hutchinson's melanotic freckle* and *circumscribed precancerous melanosis of Dubreuilh* are sometimes used synonomously for LM.

LMMs are found on the heavily sun-exposed parts of the body, usually the face, although they can occur elsewhere. The lesion begins as a small tan macular area with slightly irregular edges that on biopsy contains melanocytic dysplasia confined to the epidermis. At that point the lesion is considered an LM. With time the lesion slowly progresses by spreading centrifugally and changes color. It turns brown; and, as more abnormal melanocytes coalesce, reticulated, black macular areas appear as small flects. As these dark areas continue to grow, nodules might appear that herald frank invasion. With invasion the lesion becomes an LMM. The border of the lesion is usually very irregular. The evolution of an LM into an invasive neoplasm (LMM) can take as long as 50 years, although usually this process occurs over 10 to 20 years.[17,112]

The surface of an LM or LMM is flat except where the areas of invasion occur in the latter. In contradistinction, other types of melanoma are at least slightly raised. It should be pointed out, however, that the flat surface of a lesion considered clinically to be an LM can overlie histologically invasive tumor, and therefore the lesion may be a true LMM.[46] In one study it was found that 53% (45 of 85) of LMs had evidence of invasion unappreciated clinically.[112] The color of an LMM is usually light to dark brown with black areas of tumor progression. Rarely this lesion can be erythematous and amelanotic. Signs of regression such as whitish or grey areas can also frequently be present. Sometimes an LM can reach a very large size before actual invasion begins. Therefore these lesions tend to be larger than SSMs.

The histopathology of LMs and LMMs is characterized by an increased number of atypical melanocytic cells that are palisaded or clustered in the basal cell layer of the epidermis. These cells do not extend above the basal cell layer, in contradistinction to those of other types of melanomas, which frequently invade the upper epidermis. The atypical melanocytes in LMs and LMMs also extend down the external root sheath (Fig. 21-14). Therefore these lesions might not be easily cured by superficial types of therapy. The dermis underlying LMs and LMMs contains abundant evidence of solar damage, such as elastotic material and collagenous degeneration. A marked inflammatory infiltrate is also usually present. When the atypical melanocytes bud off the epidermis and invade the dermis, usually in clusters, the lesion becomes a truly invasive melanoma and is referred to as an LMM.

The importance of distinguishing an LMM from other melanomas is that the overall prognosis in terms of likelihood of metastasis and survival is much better. In one study it was found that four of 45 cases (9%) of LMM developed regional or systemic metastases and that the 5-year survival

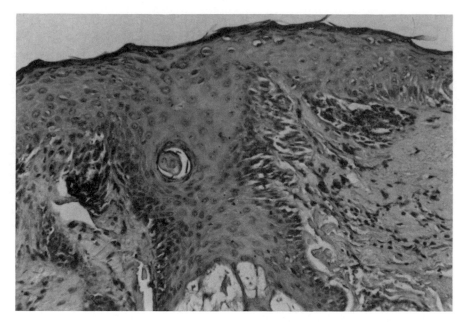

Fig. 21-14. Atypical spindle melanocytes in lentigo maligna. Note involvement of the external root sheath. (× 100.)

rate was 73%.[112] Another study reported a 27% determinate rate of metastases for 22 cases and a 4-year survival rate of 86%.[17]

Superficial spreading melanoma. SSM occurs in younger patients than those with LMM, with the average age being 52.9.[18] An SSM can occur anywhere on the cutaneous surface but is more frequently found on the legs of women or the trunk of both sexes. Its surface is slightly raised with a moderately irregular border. The color of an SSM can be brown or black, but frequently it is variegated with mixtures of bluish, reddish, or whitish hues (Fig. 21-15). Normally an SSM is not as large as an LMM and frequently measures only 1 to 2 cm. Rarely it can measure several centimeters (Fig. 21-16).

The evolution of an SSM begins with a proliferation of melanocytic cells in the epidermis. These cells are usually epithelioid; they invade the upper epidermis and proliferate along the basal cell layer. This proliferation within the epidermis (mainly within the basal cell layer) and parallel to the surface of the skin is known as the horizontal (or radial) growth phase. Clark et al.[20] consider that melanoma cells are incapable of metastasis while in this phase. If the proliferation of atypical melanocytic cells is confined entirely to the epidermis, the lesion is properly termed a melanoma in situ. Pathologists may sign out such a lesion as "atypical melanocytic hyperplasia" or as "melanoma in situ, superficial spreading type." The latter term is preferred, since it is more specific and differentiates such a lesion from an LM, which is also a melanoma in situ but of the lentigo maligna type. With time, the atypical melanocytic cells invade the

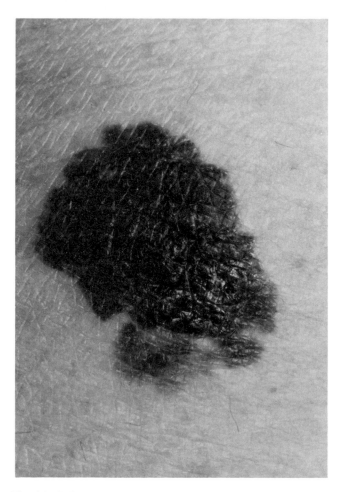

Fig. 21-15. Superficial spreading melanoma. Note irregular border and irregular pigmentation.

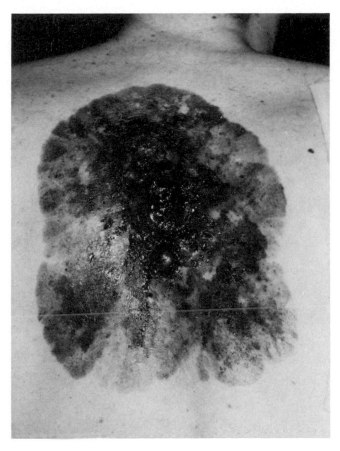

Fig. 21-16. Large superficial spreading melanoma of back with nodular melanoma in center. (Courtesy Paul Hartman, M.D., San Francisco.)

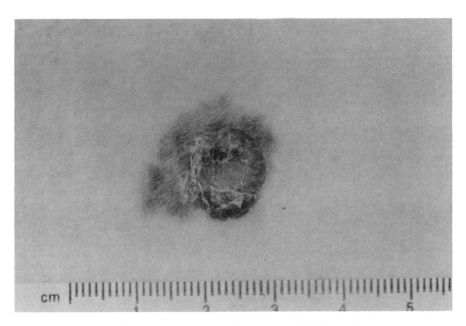

Fig. 21-17. Nodular melanoma with small, flat, superficial spreading component.

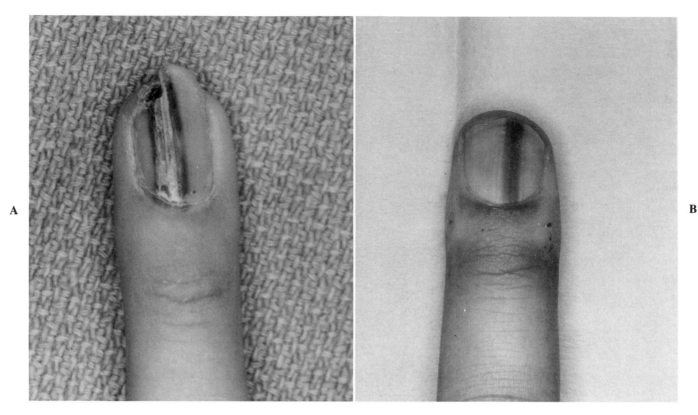

Fig. 21-18. A, Melanoma of nail bed and nail matrix. Note pigmentation of posterior nail fold (Hutchinson's sign). **B,** Acquired nevocytic nevus of nail matrix. Hyperpigmentation of posterior nail fold caused by rubbing.

dermis, either singly or in clusters. This downward growth of cells is known as the vertical growth phase. Clinically, papules or nodules appear in the vertical growth phase.

Nodular melanoma. NM appears rapidly as a nodule or papule with little surrounding flat SSM component (Fig. 21-17). Therefore, almost from the beginning, the tumor cells are rapidly growing and invasive, producing a vertical growth phase and a minimal or absent horizontal growth phase. Such lesions are frequently ulcerated and bleed. An NM is likely to metastasize and cause death. Thus it is the most feared type of melanoma.

Acral lentiginous melanomas. Acral lentiginous melanomas occur on the palms, soles, or digits, especially under the nail plate (Fig. 21-18). In this last location, melanomas can be very difficult to interpret histologically. It is not unusual for several biopsies to be performed to establish the true diagnosis. The overall prognosis with such lesions is regarded as poor, but it is difficult to know whether this occurs because of delay in establishing the diagnosis or because of metastases that can occur from even very superficially invasive lesions of the nail bed.[110] When a melanoma arises underneath the nail plate, the proximal nail fold is almost invariably hyperpigmented, a clinical clue to the diagnosis known as Hutchinson's sign. However, rarely hyperpigmentation may be found in association with an ANN (Fig. 21-18, *B*).

Mucosal melanomas. Mucosal melanomas (mucosal maligna melanomas) are more common in non-whites and tend to be difficult to treat effectively. These lesions are usually similar histologically to LMMs.

Prognostic variables

Melanoma overall has a poor 5-year survival rate. However, the death rate from this cancer is declining. Older studies in the 1960s or earlier quote around 34% to 45% survival figures,[18,51,61] whereas more recent studies are more encouraging, with figures as high as 58% to 69% for 10-year survival.[14,106] The reason for the improved survival at 5 and 10 years is probably earlier detection rather than improved treatment techniques, since the surgical management of this tumor has changed very little over the years. A relative increase in low-risk melanomas and a decrease in high-risk melanomas at the Lahey clinic between 1955 and 1979 were noted[3]; this trend probably testifies to earlier detection and patients seeking treatment earlier.

Several factors influence the overall prognosis for the individual melanoma patient (see the box on p. 682). Although each variable is important by itself, some of these

PROGNOSTIC VARIABLES WITH MELANOMA

Clinical variables

Age
Sex
Anatomic site
Ulceration
Lesion type
Lesion diameter
Satellitosis
Palpable lymph nodes

Histological variables

Level of invasion (Clark)
Thickness (Breslow)
Volume (thickness × surface diameter or area)
Regression
Mitotic rate
Inflammatory infiltrate
Nodal metastases
Association with ANN or CNN

prognostic variables have come to be recognized as more important than others.

Clinical variables

Age. Most melanomas in men occur between the ages of 50 and 59 years, whereas in women the age of onset is somewhat earlier (40 to 49 years).[39,51] Older men seem to have a poorer prognosis than women of all ages or younger men.[51]

Sex. Most studies show a slight female predominance among melanoma patients. Moreover women almost invariably have a better prognosis than men.[9,51,61,81,92] This may be because women are more likely to have melanomas on the lower legs, which prognostically is a favorable site. In addition, women develop melanomas at a younger age and tend to have thinner, less invasive tumors. Other studies dispute the sex advantage of women over men with melanoma.[39,106]

Anatomic site. Melanomas do not occur with the same frequency in all anatomic locations. The prognosis may be more favorable in some locations than in others.[30] Most melanomas occur on the lower extremities in women, whereas in men the trunk appears to be the most frequent site of occurrence.[9,39] The prognosis appears to be best on the upper and lower extremities, excluding the feet[5,9]; next best on the head and neck[92]; and worst on the trunk and feet.[32,39,51] The concept that thicker lesions (0.76 to 1.69 mm) carry a worse prognosis if they occur in the BANS location (back, posterolateral arm, posterior neck, and pos-

terior scalp) has been proposed.[112] However, this concept is disputed.[9]

Within certain anatomic locations the prognosis of melanoma can vary tremendously. For example, melanomas of the foot (especially the sole) carry a worse prognosis than melanomas that occur elsewhere on the leg. Therefore it is unwise to generalize about the prognosis within anatomic regions.

Ulceration. Ulceration of a melanoma is a poor prognostic variable.[5,21,39,61] Whether it occurs depends partially on the size of the tumor and the degree of malignancy. A large protruding tumor is more likely to be traumatized than a small one. When tumors are small, deep, or associated with metastatic nodes, ulceration is a particularly bad prognostic sign.[6,30] One author studied 52 nodular melanomas, half of which (26) had ulceration and half of which (26) did not.[81] Sixteen of 26 patients (61.5%) with ulcerated melanomas died, whereas only two of 26 patients (7.7%) without ulceration died.

Lesion type. The general clinicopathologic categories of melanomas (LMM, SSM, NM) have been previously discussed. In a cross-sectional profile the LMM is mostly flat (or macular), the SSM is convex or slightly raised, and the NM appears as a markedly raised mass or nodule. Each of these three categories carries with it a separate prognosis.[68] In one study, the 5-year mortality rate for LMM was 10.3%, whereas for SSM it was 31.5%.[18] SSM is the most frequent type of melanoma, accounting in one series[39] for 56.5% of cases; whereas LMM accounted for 14.2% and NM for 28.4% of cases (0.9% of cases were unclassified).

One special variety of melanoma that is rare and eludes the foregoing classification system is the *polypoid melanoma.* Superficially it may resemble a pyogenic granuloma, a skin tag, or an ulcerated fibroepitheliomatous polyp.[76,96] This tumor grows fast and is highly malignant but is unable to invade the reticular dermis as readily as a nodular melanoma. Polypoid melanoma uniformly carries a very poor prognosis; therefore some authorities believe that it should be designated at least a level III (defined later) melanoma, irrespective of actual depth of penetration seen under the microscope.[68] One study found that the 5-year survival rate for patients with polypoid melanomas was only 49.1%, whereas that for patients with flat melanomas was 91.9%.[39]

Lesion diameter. The greatest measured cross-sectional diameter of a melanoma on the surface of the skin can affect the prognosis.[39] For instance, the results of one study showed that patients with melanomas measuring less than 3 cm had a 49% 5-year survival, whereas patients with lesions measuring greater than 3 cm had only a 9% 5-year survival.[51] However, the actual lesion diameter is usually not taken into account for prognostic purposes for two reasons. First, it is only a rough guide to the actual surface area, since the border of melanomas is usually irregular. Second, where lesion diameter has been used in conjunction with

Clark's levels   **Breslow's measure**

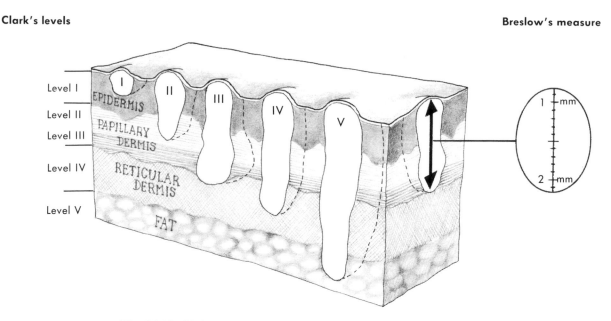

Fig. 21-19. Clark's levels and Breslow's measure of melanoma thickness.

tumor thickness to calculate the cross-sectional area of melanomas,[10] it has been found that tumor thickness alone is just as good a prognostic indicator as cross-sectional area. Thus the measurement of lesion diameter is little emphasized today.

Satellitosis. Small pigmented macules or papules in the near vicinity of a primary melanoma are referred to as satellite lesions. On the basis of the studies of Handley,[48] it appears that such lesions arise from metastatic emboli in the lymphatics rather than from direct extensions of the primary focus. Thus lesions that present with satellites have already metastasized and carry a poor prognosis. Such initial presentations are currently rare, probably because of earlier therapeutic intervention.

Palpable lymph nodes. The presence of palpable lymph nodes in the drainage area of a melanoma frequently means that the melanoma has metastasized at least to these nodes and perhaps even beyond to other organs and thus carries a poor prognosis.[111] Palpable lymph nodes serve to stage melanoma. Stage I melanoma is defined as the presence of a primary lesion alone. The draining lymph nodes are clinically negative. Stage II melanoma consists of the primary lesion and clinical involvement of draining nodes. Stage III melanoma refers to the presence of a primary lesion with widespread disease, irrespective of whether the draining nodes are involved. About 75% to 80% of patients present with stage I melanoma, 20% with stage II, and fewer than 1% with stage III.[51]

The probability that nonpalpable lymph nodes contain tumor is small but still exists.[98] One study was conducted of 380 patients with clinically negative nodes on whom a "prophylactic" node dissection had been carried out.[71] It

was found that in about 5% of patients there was microscopic evidence of tumor within nodes, even though this had not been clinically suspected. The survival in this group was twice that of the group with clinically palpable nodes. This is probably best explained on the basis of tumor burden rather than to imputed benefits of lymph node dissection. Patients with a larger tumor burden have palpable lymph nodes, whereas those with a smaller tumor burden do not.

Histologic variables

Level of invasion. Before 1969 the level of invasion of melanoma within skin was known to correlate with survival,[21] but no widely accepted method of classifying the level of invasion had been well worked out. Clark developed a grading system for melanomas that is based on the actual level of invasion within the dermis[18] (Fig. 21-19). A level I lesion is confined entirely to the epidermis above the basement membrane and is thus an in situ melanoma. A level II melanoma extends *into the papillary dermis only but not to the reticular dermis.* A level III lesion infiltrates the whole papillary dermis and extends *to—but not into—the reticular dermis.* A level IV melanoma infiltrates the reticular dermis, and a level V melanoma extends throughout the whole dermis and into subcutaneous tissue. This grading system is used to help define better the clinical types of melanoma that have been discussed. For example, most LMMs are found to be level II or III; most SSMs level II, III, or IV; and most NMs levels III, IV or V. In addition, on the basis of a study of 209 patients, Clark also showed that his grading system correlated well with the determinant survival at 5 years. The survival rates he calculated were as follows: level II, 89.6%; level III, 56.9%; level IV, 40.6%;

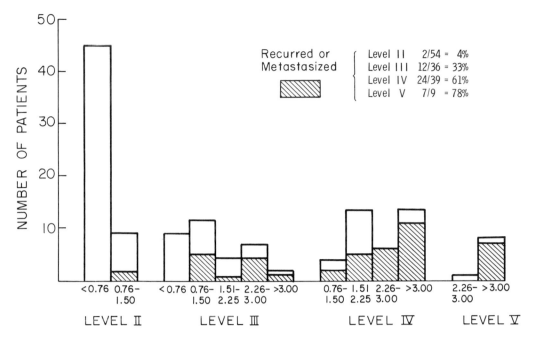

Fig. 21-20. Correlation between Clark's levels and Breslow's measured thickness intervals. Note that at Clark's levels II and V the number of Breslow's thickness intervals is small, and therefore at these levels there is greater congruence of these two assessments of melanoma invasion. However, at level III or IV, the number of Breslow's intervals is larger. (From Breslow, A.: Ann. Surg. **182:**572, 1975.)

and level V, 18.7%. Also, as can be expected, the rate of metastasis increases with the greater depth of melanoma penetration.[98] For example, in another study, the metastatic rate was 7% for level II, 49% for level III, 55% for level IV, and 80% for level V.[92] This correlation of survival and metastatic rate with Clark's levels has been confirmed by others.[111]

Thickness. Perhaps the most important single variable in assessing the prognosis of a melanoma is the thickness of the melanoma. In 1970 Breslow described a retrospective study of 98 melanomas (excluding LMM) in which he measured the tumor thickness under a microscope with an ocular micrometer.[10] This measurement extends from the *top of the granular layer* in the epidermis to the *deepest portion of tumor invasion* (Fig. 21-19). If the tumor is ulcerated and a granular layer is thus not present, the measurement is made from the base of the ulcer over the deepest portion of the tumor to the deepest tumor extension. Breslow found that the measured tumor thickness by itself, regardless of other variables, is the best prognostic indicator of metastasis and survival. This has been subsequently confirmed by others.[4,5,32]

Breslow[10] applied his measurements and designated certain thickness intervals in millimeters that correlated with the patient's subsequent course. These intervals were as follows: less than 0.76 mm, from 0.76 mm to 1.50 mm, from 1.51 mm to 2.25 mm, from 2.26 mm to 3 mm, and

greater than 3 mm. He determined that all patients with lesions less than 0.76 mm survived more than 5 years without recurrence, whereas one third of patients with lesions from 0.76 to 1.50 mm subsequently developed recurrences or metastases.[11] It is interesting to note that some of the patients in this latter study with lesions less than 0.76 mm had lesions that would be considered Clark's level II or III.

The importance of Breslow's thickness intervals and Clark's levels is that these determinations of tumor penetration point out that anatomic differences exist within the dermis that are critical to the natural progression of melanoma. The sharp differences in metastatic rate and survival between each of Breslow's measured intervals or Clark's levels exist because microscopic anatomic boundaries must exist that help impede or allow tumor spread.

The correlation between Clark's levels and Breslow's thickness intervals is shown in Fig. 21-20. Note that for each of Clark's levels, there might be several different Breslow measurement intervals. The range of the Breslow measurements is larger for Clark's levels III and IV but much less for levels II or V. Thus there is greater congruence of Clark's levels with Breslow's thickness intervals at these latter two levels. This would be expected because of the great variation in thickness of the dermis, especially the reticular dermis in different areas of the body. Note also that some level III melanomas are less than 0.76 mm.

Both Clark's level of invasion and Breslow's thickness

measurements are subject to error. The skin in various parts of the body is of different thickness (see Fig. 2-4). For example, a Clark level IV lesion (into the reticular dermis) might be much thinner on the eyelid than a Clark level IV lesion on the back. In addition, Clark's levels of invasion are based on the pathologist's ability to distinguish between the papillary and the reticular dermis. Although in most instances this is not a problem, in some locations the interface can be vague and indistinct. Thus Clark's levels can be somewhat subjective.

Like Clark's levels, Breslow's measurements are also subject to error. Sampling error of tumor can make a difference in measurement of depth of invasion. Breslow thus recommends that all melanomas be step-sectioned at 1 to 2 mm intervals.[12] Measuring the thickness of a melanoma by inspection of only one or two slides gives less than optimal information. For example, in one study if specimens were not step-sectioned, 32.9% were measured to be less than 0.76 mm.[105] However, when lesions were carefully step-sectioned, only 21.1% were less than 0.76 mm. Thus with careful and extensive sectioning and examination of multiple slides, areas of invasion can be found that are not evident on only a few sections.

Other sources of error can also occur in determining the thickness of melanomas. The embedded tissue must be cut perpendicular to the surface to get an accurate measurement. If epidermal hyperplasia occurs over the melanoma, the measured thickness can be falsely high. Areas of regression can also change the measured degree of invasion.

Because of these problems, most melanomas today are graded by both Clark's and Breslow's classification systems so that the maximal amount of information is available for patient management. Many physicians consider these two classification systems to be somewhat complimentary.[98] The measured depth of microinvasion adds prognostic insight to each of Clark's levels.

Perhaps the most important contribution of the Breslow thickness measurements is the finding that lesions less than 0.76 mm rarely metastasize. This has been confirmed by others.[5,92] Thus for this group of patients only local conservative excision is indicated, and node dissection probably would be fruitless.

Although the level or stage of invasion can indicate the likelihood of metastases and survival, once metastases have occurred, these indicators become less important in determining 5-year survival. At that point, the number of nodes containing tumor and the presence of ulceration are the most important prognostic indicators.[6] Therefore Clark's and Breslow's classification systems are not totally predictive under all circumstances.

Since the introduction of the Breslow thickness measurement, other physicians have attempted to define their own thickness intervals in millimeters, which they feel hold more prognostic insight than Breslow's intervals. For example, one author feels that <0.85 mm is a better indicator of survival than Breslow's <0.76 mm.[29] These variants have not, however, been widely tested and accepted.

Tumor volume. Theoretically tumor volume at the primary site can be calculated by multiplying the surface area by the depth of invasion. Since there are irregularities in the borders of melanomas and in depth of invasion, exact measurements are difficult to compute. Breslow,[10] however, calculated a representative cross-sectional area by multiplying the largest surface diameter by the greatest depth of tumor invasion. Since the values he obtained were of no greater prognostic value than the depth of tumor invasion alone, this method of calculation has been abandoned.

Regression. Melanomas are unusual tumors in that they are known to undergo spontaneous regression. Sometimes this regression is complete, but more often it is incomplete. Because completely regressed melanomas can produce metastases, it is reasonable to assume that incompletely regressed tumors can likewise be a source of metastases.

Regression in a melanoma appears as a whitish or gray area within the borders of the lesion. Histologic examination of these areas shows fibrosis, frequently without tumor. Such areas of regression are not uncommon in LMMs or SSMs but are rare in NMs.[105] In one investigation 121 thin melanomas (<0.76 mm) were studied[47]: 19% (23 in 121) showed areas of regression, and 22% of these (5 of 23) metastasized. On the other hand, 81% (98 of 121) showed no areas of regression, and only 2% (2 of 98) of these lesions metastasized. The authors concluded that thin melanomas with areas of regression are likely to metastasize. But in another study, on careful step sectioning, 41 thin melanomas were defined, and only 1 metastasized.[105] Although this one had histologic evidence of regression, so did about one fourth of all the thin melanomas. Therefore the concept that regressing thin melanomas are more likely to metastasize cannot be fully accepted.

Mitotic rate. Tumors with a high mitotic rate are usually more aggressive. Therefore it would seem reasonable that this would be the case with melanomas as well. It has been found that melanomas with less than 1 mitosis per high-power field (HPF) have a significantly better prognosis than tumors with greater than 1 mitosis per HPF.[21] Other investigators as well have found that mitotic rate is correlated with survival or metastases.[30,32,39,68] One group calculated what they term a "prognostic index" by multiplying the thickness of tumor by the number of mitoses per square millimeter.[92] In their hands, the prognostic index appears to be as good a prognosticator as Breslow's measured thickness or Clark's levels for stage I melanoma. Unfortunately the value of the prognostic index has not been confirmed by others.[32]

Inflammatory infiltrate. Since melanomas are tumors to which the body responds immunologically, one could expect an inflammatory infiltrate to have some bearing on the prognosis. The more intense the infiltrate, the larger the response. However, most dermatopathologists do not believe, except in a general way, that the inflammatory infiltrate can be correlated with tumor prognosis. One investigator believes that the larger the tumor and longer the duration, the less the inflammatory infiltrate.[21] However, one group states that the inflammatory infiltrate is difficult to quantitate,[68] and yet another notes no difference in the inflammatory infiltrate between tumors that metastasized and those that did not.[92]

Association with nevocytic nevus. Normal nevocytic nevi can be found in association with melanoma from 10% to 28% of the time.[18,21,54,90] Although Cochran[21] thinks that local recurrence is less likely when this association is seen, his assertion has not been well studied.

Nodal metastases. The presence of nodal metastases seen microscopically alters the prognosis. When this event occurs, the number of positive nodes is helpful in determining the prognosis.[6]

One basic problem that occurs with metastases to lymph nodes is that lymph nodes with few melanoma cells can be overlooked on routinely stained sections, whereas lymph nodes that are replaced by melanoma cells or contain significant amounts of tumor are easily seen. One new approach to detecting the lymph nodes with a small number of melanoma cells is by use of S-100 protein. This substance is an acidic protein named for its solubility in saturated ammonium sulfate. Its function is unknown, although its presence has been demonstrated in glial cells of the brain, Schwann cells of the peripheral nervous system, melanocytes, and Langerhans' cells. Thus S-100 protein is not a specific marker for melanocytic cells. Recently one group of authors retrospectively studied a number of nodes from melanoma patients that previously had been stained by routine methods.[22] When these nodes were stained with S-100 protein, additional positive nodes were determined in several patients, especially in those who subsequently became poor survivors. This supports the concept that nodal tumor burden is a major prognostic factor in survival. It also helps to explain the small subset of patients with thin melanomas (less than 0.76 mm) who are almost invariably negative at the time of node dissection, yet 5 to 10 years later do develop metastatic disease. The sensitivity of routine stains might not be great enough to pick up small occult melanoma cells in nodes from these patients, and thus S-100 protein may be helpful here.

Treatment

The treatment of the melanoma is individualized on the basis of foregoing prognostic variables. Previous dogma regarding treatment that frequently resulted in mutilating surgery is giving way to more moderate management of melanoma patients. Therefore, in light of our current knowledge, careful examination of the data available is beneficial to proper management.

Incisional versus excisional biopsy. Surgical dogma in the past has advised against incisional biopsy of melanomas on the basis of the premise that tumor cells can be implanted or seeded into lymphatics during the biopsy procedure. In addition, if an incisional biopsy is obtained, an inadequate or unrepresentative sample may result. Data can be cited to suggest that trauma to melanoma, caused by incomplete removal for biopsy or treatment with cautery, is associated with a high likelihood of local recurrence, metastases, or death.[81] However, these cases have not been analyzed for depth of invasion or compared to controls. Therefore one wonders whether these melanomas might have been highly invasive from the beginning.

In contrast to the just-mentioned study, other investigators have concluded that there is no decrease in survival or increase in metastases in patients who had an incisional biopsy of a melanoma compared with patients who had an excisional biopsy.[40,51] Perhaps the most salient and relevant study was carried out by a group of investigators who performed an incisional biopsy with a dermal punch in 22 patients.[3] The biopsy was performed in the thickest portion of the lesion. Even though lesions were analyzed by thickness, there was no difference in survival between those patients who had such incisional biopsies and those who had excisional biopsies irrespective of depth of penetration. Thus an incisional biopsy of a melanoma probably does no harm.

Lateral excision margins. The amount of normal-appearing surrounding skin that needs to be removed when excising a melanoma is a matter of some debate and has troubled surgeons for years. However, as with incisional biopsy, data are available to make an informed judgment.

The concept that large (5 cm) margins of surrounding normal tissue need to be removed when excising a melanoma dates back to 1907.[48] In a lecture at that time, Handley concluded that melanoma is primarily disseminated via the lymphatics, particularly in the subdermal and papillary dermal locations. Although his studies were based on a single autopsy specimen of a metastatic tumor with several satellites, he recommended the initial skin incision to be "about an inch from the edge of the tumor." He further recommended removing the underlying fat, fascia, and superficial muscle within the incision and for 2 inches laterally. Thus Handley actually recommended removal of 3 inches (7.62 cm) of tissue around the tumor (1 inch of skin, fat, fascia, and muscle vertically and 2 more inches of fat, fascia, and muscle below the skin laterally). Unfortunately Handley had not studied a primary melanoma before his lecture.

Until recently, the surgical dictum was that excision of a melanoma should include a border of normal tissue measuring 5 cm.[77] Some authors have even recommended margins as great as 15 cm, because recurrences were seen within that range in some patients.[81] Other authors felt comfortable with a 3 to 5 cm margin but in continuity with the draining lymph nodes, since recurrences or metastases more frequently arose in that direction.[61] Additional data seemed to support the concept of higher cure rates with wider excision. In one study patients whose melanomas were widely excised and the subsequent wounds covered with grafts seemed to have a higher survival rate than those who had only a local excision and closure.[61] Although exact measurements were not made, it was presumed that those lesions requiring a graft were more widely excised than those closed primarily. Furthermore, these data were published before the significance of the depth of melanoma penetration was known, and the details regarding placement of patients into these two treatment groups were not given. It is quite possible that deeply invasive nodular melanomas were probably excised and closed primarily, whereas less invasive superficial spreading melanomas were excised and the surgical defect grafted.

The most suitable margin for excision of a melanoma is probably related to the depth of penetration by the tumor.[38] Breslow studied the excision margins of 62 primary melanomas whose depth of penetration was less than 0.76 mm (excluding LMM).[13] These were excised with margins ranging from 0.10 to 5.15 cm (14 cases with margins less than 0.5 cm) (Fig. 21-21). All patients survived for 5 years without a recurrence. Thus for thin melanomas (less than 0.76 mm in thickness), a margin of 0.5 cm seems adequate.

Another study that supports the idea of conservative excision margins for most superficial melanomas is that of Cascinelli et al.,[14] in which a group of 593 patients with stage I melanomas were followed-up. Some patients (36) had resection margins of 1 cm or less, whereas others had resection margins of greater than 1 cm up to more than 5 cm. There was no difference in survival, although there were more local recurrences in the group with excisions of less than 2 cm. However, when corrected for thickness of lesion (greater than 2 mm), this difference in local recurrence disappeared.

It should be emphasized that such a small excision margin (0.5 to 1.0 cm) is probably not adequate for all thin melanomas. Subungual melanomas perhaps should be excised with more of a margin, as should LMMs (which were excluded from the study just cited by Breslow).

Another exception to small excision margins for thin melanomas may be for those occurring in the BANS region. Cosimi et al.[25] studied a group of 49 patients with low-risk melanomas (less than 0.85 mm or between 0.85 and 1.69 mm, not in the BANS area). Excisions of 0.7 to 4 cm were performed. In two of the 49 patients (4%) residual invasive tumor was found on reexcision after the primary excisional biopsy was interpreted to be free of tumor. An additional eight patients (16%) had atypism (probably in situ melanoma) but no invasive melanoma. Therefore 20% (10 of 49) of presumed tumor-free excisional specimens can contain potentially malignant cells even with these low-risk melanomas. Conservative reexcisions were performed. Two patients subsequently developed metastases, one of whom had

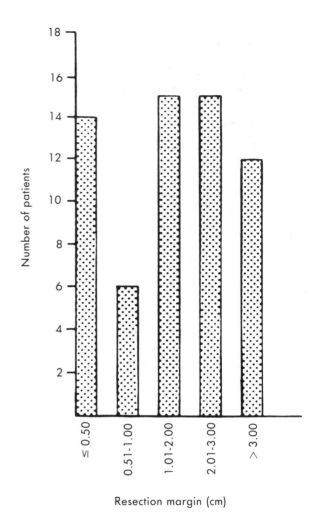

Fig. 21-21. Range of resection margins for thin (<0.76 mm) melanomas. All patients survived 5 years without recurrence, regardless of margin of normal tissue excised. (From Breslow, A.: Surg. Gynecol. Obstet. **145**:691, 1977. By permission of SURGERY, GYNECOLOGY, & OBSTETRICS.)

a 0.5 mm melanoma on the neck and the other a 1.2 mm melanoma on the back. However, because no patients had local recurrences of their melanomas, the authors recommend conservative surgical excision for low-risk melanomas except in the BANS area. Yet, in the BANS area, a larger excision may not have changed the probability of metastases anyway.

The 5 cm margin as commonly proposed by many surgeons is thus unjustified, since it is arbitrary and based on very weak data. On the basis of the foregoing studies, I recommend a margin of from 0.5 to 1 cm for all thin (<0.76 mm) stage I melanomas (except subungual melanomas or LMMs or possibly melanomas in the BANS area). How much tissue is taken is at least partially based on the anatomic location. When the wound can be closed easily, a 1 cm margin should be chosen. For thicker melanomas (0.76 to 1.50 mm), except in areas of high recurrence (the trunk and sole of foot), a margin of 1 to 1.5 cm appears to be adequate. For all other melanomas, a margin of 3 cm in all directions from the edge of the lesion should be taken.[31] The 3 cm margin for thick melanomas is at least as good as the 5 cm margin and represents a reasonable compromise that is less mutilating.

It is important to emphasize that careful assessment of the cut surgical margins should be performed on all excised melanoma specimens. This is supported by the study[25] cited earlier, which found a high (20%) persistence of atypical cells in reexcision specimens after initial excisions previously reported to have margins free of tumor. Even leaving in situ melanomas will probably lead to recurrences.[2]

The method that will assess the cut surgical margins most accurately is that described by Mohs. It is adaptable as an alternative form of therapy for melanomas.[72] Basically this step-by-step removal of tumor-containing tissue should be considered when maximal preservation of normal tissue is desirable or when there is doubt concerning total extirpation of the tumor. Cure rates with Mohs surgery for melanomas compare favorably with those of the standard surgical series.[72]

Deep excision margins. The depth of an excision for removal of melanomas has been little studied. Although removal of deep fascia and even superficial muscle with the melanoma has been recommended,[48] at least one study shows that removal of deep fascia does not appear to affect survival.[51] Most authorities recommend excision at least to the deep fascia.

Metastases from thin melanomas. Thin melanomas (<0.76 mm) almost never recur locally but can metastasize, although this event is rare. When it does occur, the initial tumor usually arose in locations where thickness measurements are difficult to perform, such as in the subungual area or on the genitalia, although metastases from thin melanomas in other locations such as the back have been reported.[5,25,111] There is no evidence that the rare metastases that do occur from thin melanomas could be prevented by larger excisions than those just recommended. Metastases from thin melanomas not infrequently occur more than 5 years after initial treatment, so patients should be carefully followed-up for at least 10 years. In contrast, local recurrences or metastases of thick melanomas (greater than 3 mm) almost always occur within 6 years after treatment.[70]

Lentigo maligna and lentigo maligna melanoma. LMs and LMMs are slowly evolving melanomas whose therapy should be considered separately from that of the other types of melanomas. The relative lack of aggressiveness of LMs and LMMs and the fact that they almost always occur on the face has frequently led to more conservative management than should otherwise be used. Although these tumors are at first superficial and confined to the epidermis, the physician should treat aggressively to destroy a potentially invasive neoplasm before it becomes life-threatening.

Besides excision, other methods of treatment of an LM or LMM recommended by various authors include topical 5-fluorouracil, radiotherapy, cryosurgery, curettage, electrodesiccation, and even dermabrasion. As discussed previously, the melanocytic dysplasia of an LM or LMM involves the epithelium of cutaneous appendages. Therefore, since these dysplastic melanocytes are deeper in the skin than the epidermis, they may escape destruction by superficial methods. In addition, as pointed out previously, a clinical LM can have histologic areas of invasion so that in actuality it is an LMM.[46]

In comparisons of different treatment modalities for LM and LMM, surgical excision seems to offer overall the highest likelihood of cure (that is, 91% for LM and LMM).[23,83] Other treatment modalities do not appear to be nearly as effective. For example, in one study by Pitman et al.,[83] 50% of LMs recurred with cryosurgery, 25% with curettage and electrodesiccation, and 37% with radiotherapy. For LMMs the cure rates with treatment other than excisional surgery were particularly dismal. Five cases were treated by either cryosurgery, curettage and electrodesiccation, or radiotherapy. Of these five cases, four recurred locally, and three cases metastasized. In a study by Coleman et al.,[23] when 5-fluorouracil was used as a form of treatment, three of three LMs and one of one LMM all recurred. These studies seem to argue strongly against treatment methods other than excisional surgery for LM or LMM.

For recurrent LM or LMM, Mohs surgery (fresh or fixed tissue technique) is an alternative method of excisional therapy.[72] The cure rates using this method certainly compare favorably with those of other forms of excisional treatment. In addition, in cosmetically important areas Mohs surgery helps to preserve normal tissue.

Lymphadenectomy. Perhaps no aspect of melanoma surgery is as emotionally discussed as is the advisability of "prophylactic" or elective lymph node dissection (ELND). Removal of microscopically invaded lymph nodes purportedly results in elimination of a tumor that may metastasize further, resulting in death of the patient. However, this procedure is not without complications. One report states that 29% of patients undergoing ELND had lymphedema.[98]

Three prospective randomized studies seem to agree that survival is not improved by elective lymph node dissection (ELND) for stage I melanoma.[9,98,106] Other studies that are nonprospective or nonrandomized purport to show that ELND is useful, especially for tumors of intermediate thickness (0.76 to 3.99 mm).[5,71,86,111] With all these studies there are notable flaws such as exclusion or inclusion of patients with certain types of melanomas (for example, LMM) or melanomas in certain locations (for example, head and neck). Such variables can greatly affect the prognosis.

Breslow[13] has criticized even his own earlier statistics[11] that demonstrated the benefits of ELND for melanoma patients with lesions of thicknesses greater than 1.5 mm. Only later did he discover that his surgeons were more likely to perform ELND for melanomas of the leg, which carry a more favorable prognosis, and avoid ELND for lesions of the trunk, which are more prone to metastasize. This is because the lymphatic drainage is not as apparent on the trunk as on the leg. Also, the need for ELND was also precluded for level V lesions, which also carry a much worse prognosis.

Taken together, all studies of ELND seem to agree on a few points. ELND is of no benefit for patients with thin lesions (less than 0.76 mm) or for patients with very thick (4 mm or greater) lesions. The former lesions rarely metastasize, which would outweigh any benefit of ELND.[10] The latter lesions have probably already widely metastasized, which negates any possible benefit of ELND.

Lesions with thickness between 0.76 and 3.99 mm can possibly be benefited by ELND. All of the nonrandomized, nonprospective studies show a small but significant benefit to this procedure.[5,71] One randomized prospective study also shows a benefit of ELND for this group, but it is not statistically significant.[106] Balch et al.[5] believe that the benefits (increased survival) of ELND are not seen for at least 5 to 10 years after the initial surgery. Unfortunately few studies give survival data beyond 5 years from the time of initial treatment. One hopes that these statistics will be available in the future. For an excellent review of elective lymph node dissection for melanoma, one should consult the paper by Day and Lew.[27]

Melanoma and pregnancy. During pregnancy, melanogenesis occurs, resulting in hyperpigmentation in most women, as well as a darkening and increase in size of existing nevi. This presumably is caused by increased systemic levels of estrogen, progesterone, and melanin-stimulating hormone. Melanomas frequently appear during pregnancy, probably related to the same hormonal influences. The prognosis of melanoma during pregnancy is probably no worse than if the patient is not pregnant, although literature can be cited on both sides of this issue. One recent study investigated 58 women who developed melanoma during pregnancy and 43 women who became pregnant within 5 years after the appearance of a melanoma.[87] The authors showed that if a melanoma develops during pregnancy, there is an increased risk of recurrence after treatment, especially during the first 2 years after pregnancy. Thus they advise against oral contraceptives or a subsequent pregnancy for 2 years. Patients should have frequent follow-up visits during this time. Although the likelihood of recurrence in this group is higher than in nonpregnant controls, survival appears to be no different. For the group of women who had had a melanoma and subsequently became pregnant, the pregnancy had no effect on recurrence or survival.

Pregnancy itself is not considered a contraindication for definitive treatment of melanoma. Any suspicious nevi arising during pregnancy should be removed immediately rather than postponing this surgery until after delivery. If a melanoma is found and a lymph node dissection indicated, this should also be performed as soon as possible, unless the patient is near term, in which case it is advisable to wait until after delivery.[87]

Workup and follow-up. Patients with melanomas need to have a workup and be followed-up closely. The extent of the workup, treatment, and follow-up care depends on the depth of tumor penetration. Patients with melanomas unlikely to metastasize (less than 0.76 mm or 0.76 to 1.49 mm in areas of low aggressiveness, especially in women) can undergo a conservative excision according to the guidelines previously discussed. In addition, each patient needs a complete history (including a review of systems) and physical examination, a CBC, SMA-12, and chest x-ray film. These patients should be seen at 3-month intervals for the first year after the primary excision. After the first year, follow-up visits should occur once a year for patients with lesions less than 0.76 mm thick and every 6 months for patients with lesions that are 0.76 through 1.49 mm thick.[53] At the time of each follow-up visit, examination of the primary treatment site and lymph nodes is performed. In addition, a review of systems is obtained. A repeat chest x-ray film should be taken at 6- to 12-month intervals. Current studies suggest that a significant number of melanomas recur or metastasize 5 years after initial therapy. Ironically, this seems to be particularly true of thin melanomas (<0.76 mm).[5,70] In addition, long-term follow-up after 5 years is currently determining the benefits of ELND not seen in earlier studies.[5] Therefore careful follow-up of melanoma patients is warranted for 10 years after initial treatment of the primary lesion or subsequent treatment of any recurrence.

Patients with melanomas of intermediate (1.5 to 3.99 mm) or deep (greater than 4 mm) thickness or those with obvious lymphadenopathy should be referred for treatment ideally to a comprehensive cancer center that is organized for the management of such patients.

REFERENCES

1. Ackerman, A.B., and Mihara, I.: Dysplasia, dysplastic melanocytes, dysplastic nevi, the dysplastic nevus syndrome, and the relation between dysplastic nevi and malignant melanomas, Hum. Pathol. **16:**87, 1985.
2. Alper, J.C., et al.: The surgical management of "in situ" melanoma, J. Dermatol. Surg. Oncol. **8:**771, 1982.
3. Bagley, F.H., et al.: Changes in clinical presentation and management of malignant melanoma, Cancer **47:**2126, 1981.
4. Balch, C.M., et al.: A multifactorial analysis of melanoma: prognostic histopathological features comparing Clark's and Breslow's staging methods, Ann. Surg. **188:**732, 1978.
5. Balch, C.M., et al.: A comparison of prognostic factors and

surgical results in 1,786 patients with localized (Stage I) melanoma in Alabama, USA, and New South Wales, Australia, Ann. Surg. **196:**677, 1982.

6. Balch, C.M., et al.: A multifactorial analysis of melanoma. III. Prognostic factors in melanoma patients with lymph node metastases (stage II), Ann. Surg. **193:**377, 1981.

7. Beral, V., et al.: Cutaneous factors related to the risk of malignant melanoma, Br. J. Dermatol. **109:**165, 1983.

8. Biro, L., and Price, E.: Cryogenic anesthesia and hemostasis, J. Dermatol. Surg. Oncol. **6:**608, 1980.

9. Blois, M.S., et al.: Judging prognosis in malignant melanoma of the skin, Ann. Surg. **198:**200, 1983.

10. Breslow, A.: Thickness, cross-sectional areas and depth of invasion in the prognosis of primary cutaneous melanoma, Ann. Surg. **172:**902, 1970.

11. Breslow, A.: Tumor thickness, level of invasion and node dissection in stage I cutaneous melanoma, Ann. Surg. **182:**572, 1975.

12. Breslow, A.: In search of thin lethal melanomas [editorial], Surg. Gynecol. Obstet. **143:**799, 1976.

13. Breslow, A., and Macht, S.D.: Optimal size of resection margin for thin cutaneous melanoma, Surg. Gynecol. Obstet. **145:**691, 1977.

14. Cascinelli, N., et al.: Stage I melanoma of the skin: the problem of resection margins, Eur. J. Cancer **16:**1079, 1980.

15. Cawley, E.P.: Genetic aspects of malignant melanoma, A.M.A. Arch. Dermatol. **65:**440, 1952.

16. Chait, L.A., White, B., and Skudowitz, R.B.: The treatment of giant hairy naevi by dermabrasion in the first few weeks of life: case reports, S. Afr. Med. J. **60:**593, 1981.

17. Clark, W.H., Jr., and Mihm, M.C., Jr.: Lentigo maligna and lentigo-maligna melanoma, Am. J. Pathol. **55:**39, 1969.

18. Clark, W.H., Jr., et al.: The histogenesis and biologic behavior of primary human malignant melanomas of the skin, Cancer Res. **29:**705, 1969.

19. Clark, W.H., Jr., et al.: Origin of familial malignant melanomas from heritable melanocytic lesions: "the B-K mole syndrome," Arch. Dermatol. **114:**732, 1978.

20. Clark, W.H., Jr., et al.: A study of tumor progression: the precursor lesions of superficial spreading and nodular melanoma, Hum. Pathol. **15:**1147, 1984.

21. Cochran, A.J.: Histology and prognosis in malignant melanoma, J. Pathol. **97:**459, 1969.

22. Cochran, A.J., Wen, D.-R., and Herschman, H.R.: Occult melanoma in lymph nodes detected by antiserum to S-100 protein, Int. J. Cancer **34:**159, 1984.

23. Coleman, III, W.P., et al. Treatment of lentigo maligna and lentigo maligna melanoma, J. Dermatol. Surg. Oncol. **6:**476, 1980.

24. Cooke, K.R., Spears, G.F.S., and Skegg, D.C.G.: Frequency of moles in a defined population, J. Epidemiol. Community Health **39:**48, 1985.

25. Cosimi, A.B., et al.: Conservative surgical management of superficially invasive cutaneous melanoma, Cancer **53:**1256, 1984.

26. Davis, J.S.: The removal of wide scars and large disfigurements of skin by gradual partial excision with closure, Ann. Surg. **90:**645, 1929.

27. Day, C.L., Jr., and Lew, R.A.: Malignant melanoma prognostic factors 7: elective lymph node dissection, J. Dermatol. Surg. Oncol. **11:**233, 1985.

28. Day, C.L., Jr., et al.: Prognostic factors for melanoma patients with lesions 0.76 to 1.69 mm in thickness: an appraisal of "thin" level IV lesions, Ann. Surg. **195:**30, 1982.

29. Day, C.L., Jr., et al.: The natural break points for primary-tumor thickness in clinical stage I melanoma [letter], N. Engl. J. Med. **305:**1155, 1981.

30. Day, C.L., Jr., et al.: Prognostic factors for patients with clinical stage I melanoma of intermediate thickness (1.51-3.99 mm), Ann. Surg. **195:**35, 1982.

31. Day, C.L., Jr., et al.: Narrower margins for clinical stage I malignant melanoma, N. Engl. J. Med. **306:**479, 1982.

32. Day, C.L., Jr., et al.: A prognostic model for clinical stage I melanoma of the lower extremity: location on foot as independent risk factor for recurrent disease, Surgery **89:**599, 1981.

33. Domonkos, A.N., Arnold, H.L., Jr., and Odom, R.B.: Andrews' diseases of the skin: clinical dermatology, ed. 7, Philadelphia, 1982, W.B. Saunders Co.

34. Dubreuilh, W.: Lentigo malin des vieillards, Bull. Soc. Fr. Dermatol. Syph. **5:**460, 1894.

35. Duray, P.H., and Livolsi, V.A.: Recurrent dysplastic nevus following shave excision, J. Dermatol. Surg. Oncol. **10:**811, 1984.

36. Eade, G.G: The long axis of facial nevi: fortuitous fact? or coincidence? [letter], Plast. Reconstr. Surg. **47:**184, 1971.

37. Elder, D.E., et al.: Dysplastic nevus syndrome: a phenotypic association of sporadic cutaneous melanoma, Cancer **46:**1787, 1980.

38. Elder, D.E., et al.: Optimal resection margin for cutaneous malignant melanoma, Plast. Reconstr. Surg. **71:**66, 1983.

39. Eldh, J., Boeryd, B., and Peterson, L.E.: Prognostic factors in cutaneous malignant melanoma in stage I: a clinical, morphological and multivariate analysis, Scand. J. Plast. Reconstr. Surg. **12:**243, 1978.

40. Epstein, E., Bragg, K., and Linden, G.: Biopsy and prognosis of malignant melanoma, J.A.M.A. **208:**1369, 1969.

41. Feins, N.R., Rubin, R., and Borger, J.A.: Ambulatory serial excision of giant nevi, J. Pediatr. Surg. **17:**851, 1982.

42. Frichot, B.C., et al.: New cutaneous phenotype in familial malignant melanoma [letter], Lancet **1:**864, 1977.

43. Greeley, P.W., Middleton, A.G., and Curtin, J.W.: Incidence of malignancy in giant pigmented nevi, Plast. Reconstr. Surg. **36:**26, 1965.

44. Greene, M.H., et al.: Acquired precursors of cutaneous malignant melanoma, N. Engl. J. Med. **312:**91, 1985.

45. Greene, M.H., et al.: High risk of malignant melanoma in melanoma-prone families with dysplastic nevi, Ann. Intern. Med. **102:**458, 1985.

46. Gromet, M.A.: Treatment of lentigo maligna [letter], Arch. Dermatol. **113:**1128, 1977.

47. Gromet, M.A., Epstein, W.L., and Blois, M.S.: The regressing thin malignant melanoma: a distinctive lesion with metastatic potential, Cancer **42:**2282, 1978.

48. Handley, W.S.: The pathology of melanotic growths in relation to their operative treatment, Lancet **1:**927, 1907.

49. Hutchinson, J.: Lentigo-melanosis: a further report, Arch. Surg. (London) **5:**253, 1894.

50. Johnson, H.A.: Permanent removal of pigmentation from giant hairy naevi by dermabrasion in early life, Br. J. Plast. Surg. **30:**321, 1977.

51. Jones, W.M., et al.: Malignant melanoma of the skin: prognostic value of clinical features and the role of treatment in 111 cases, Br. J. Cancer **22:**437, 1968.

52. Kaplan, E.N.: The risk of malignancy in large congenital nevi, Plast. Reconstr. Surg. **53:**421, 1974.

53. Kelly, J.W., Blois, M.S., and Sagebiel, R.W.: Frequency and duration of patient follow-up after treatment of a primary malignant melanoma, J. Am. Acad. Dermatol. **13:**756, 1985.

54. Kopf, A.W., Bart, R.S., and Hennessey, P.: Congenital nevocytic nevi and malignant melanomas, J. Am. Acad. Dermatol. **1:**123, 1979.

55. Kopf, A.W., Rigel, D.S., and Friedman, R.J.: The rising incidence and mortality rate of malignant melanoma, J. Dermatol. Surg. Oncol. **8:**760, 1982.

56. Kopf, A.W., et al.: Prevalence of nevocytic nevi on lateral and medial aspects of arms, J. Dermatol. Surg. Oncol. **4:**153, 1978.

57. Kopf, A.W., et al.: Relationship of nevocytic nevi to sun exposure in dysplastic nevus syndrome, J. Am. Acad. Dermatol. **12:**656, 1985.

58. Kornberg, R., and Ackerman, A.B.: Pseudomelanoma: recurrent melanocytic nevus following partial surgical removal, Arch. Dermatol. **111:**1588, 1975.

59. Kraemer, K.H., et al.: Dysplastic naevi and cutaneous melanoma risk [letter], Lancet **2:**1076, 1983.

60. Lanier, V.C., Jr., Pickrell, K.L., and Georgiade, N.G.: Congenital giant nevi: clinical and pathological considerations, Plast. Reconstr. Surg. **58:**48, 1976.

61. Lehman, J.A., Jr., Cross, F.S., Richey, D.G.: Clinical study of forty-nine patients with malignant melanoma, Cancer **19:**611, 1966.

62. Lorentzen, M., Pers, M., and Bretteville-Jensen, G.: Incidence of malignant transformation in giant pigmented nevi, Scand. J. Plast. Reconstr. Surg. **11:**163, 1977.

63. Lynch, H.T., et al.: Family studies of malignant melanoma and associated cancer, Surg. Gynecol. Obstet. **141:**517, 1975.

64. Lynch, H.T., et al.: Familial cancer: implications for surgical management of high-risk patients, Surgery **83:**104, 1978.

65. Malec, E., and Lagerlöf, B.: Malignant melanoma of the skin in children registered in the Swedish Cancer Registry during 1959-1971, Scand. J. Plast. Reconstr. Surg. **11:**125, 1977.

66. Marchac, D., and Weston, J.: Abdominoplasty in infants for removal of giant congenital nevi: a report of three cases, Plast. Reconstr. Surg. **75:**155, 1985.

67. Mark, G.J., et al.: Congenital melanocytic nevi of the small and garment type: clinical, histologic, and ultrastructural studies, Hum. Pathol. **4:**395, 1973.

68. McGovern, V.J., et al.: The classification of malignant melanoma and its histologic reporting, Cancer **32:**1446, 1973.

69. Miller, C.J., and Becker, Jr., D.W.: Removing pigmentation by dermabrading naevi in infancy, Br. J. Plast. Surg. **32:**124, 1979.

70. Milton, G.W., et al.: Tumour thickness and the site and time of first recurrence in cutaneous malignant melanoma (stage I), Br. J. Surg. **67:**543, 1980.

71. Milton, G.W., et al.: Prophylactic lymph node dissection in clinical stage I cutaneous malignant melanoma. Results of surgical treatment in 1,319 patients, Br. J. Surg. **69:**108, 1982.

72. Mohs, F.E.: Chemosurgery for melanoma, Arch. Dermatol. **113:**285, 1977.

73. Morestin, H.: La réduction graduelle des difformités tégumentaires, Bull. Mem. Soc. Chir. **41:**1233, 1915.

74. Myhre, E.: Malignant melanomas in children, Acta Pathol. Microbiol. Scand. **59:**184, 1963.

75. Nicholls, E.M.: Development and elimination of pigmented moles, and the anatomical distribution of primary malignant melanoma, Cancer **32:**191, 1973.

76. Niven, J., and Lubin, J.: Pedunculated malignant melanoma, Arch. Dermatol. **111:**755, 1975.

77. Olsen, G.: The malignant melanoma of the skin: new theories based on a study of 500 cases, Acta Chir. Scand. suppl. **365:**1, 1966.

78. Pack, G.T., and Davis, J.: Nevus giganticus pigmentosus with malignant transformation, Surgery **49:**347, 1961.

79. Pack, G.T., Lenson, N., and Gerber, D.M.: Regional distribution of moles and melanomas, A.M.A. Arch. Surg. **65:**862, 1952.

80. Pers, M.: Naevus pigmentosus giganticus: indikationer for operativ behandling, Ugeskr. Laeger **125:**613, 1963.

81. Petersen, N.C., Bodenham, D.C., and Lloyd, O.C.: Malignant melanomas of the skin: a study of the origin, development, aetiology, spread, treatment, and prognosis, Br. J. Plast. Surg. **15:**49, 1962.

82. Pilney, F.T., Broadbent, T.R., and Woolf, R.M.: Giant pigmented nevi of the face: surgical management, Plast. Reconstr. Surg. **40:**469, 1967.

83. Pitman, G.H., et al.: Treatment of lentigo maligna and lentigo maligna melanoma, J. Dermatol. Surg. Oncol. **5:**727, 1979.

84. Reed, W.B., et al.: Giant pigmented nevi, melanoma, and leptomeningeal melanocytosis: a clinical and histopathological study, Arch. Dermatol. **91:**100, 1965.

85. Rees, T.D.: Aesthetic plastic surgery, Philadelphia, 1980, W.B. Saunders Co.

86. Reintgen, D.S., et al.: Efficacy of elective lymph node dissection in patients with intermediate thickness primary melanoma, Ann. Surg. **198:**379, 1983.

87. Reintgen, D.S., et al.: Malignant melanoma and pregnancy, Cancer **55:**1340, 1985.

88. Rhodes, A.R., and Melski, J.W.: Small congenital nevocellular nevi and the risk of cutaneous melanoma, J. Pediatr. **100:**219, 1982.

89. Rhodes, A.R., et al.: Nonepidermal origin of malignant melanoma associated with a giant congenital nevocellular nevus, Plast. Reconstr. Surg. **67:**782, 1981.

90. Rhodes, A.R., et al.: Dysplastic nevi in histologic association with 234 cutaneous melanomas [abstract], Lab. Invest. **46:**69A, 1982.

91. Roush, G.C., et al.: Diagnosis of the dysplastic nevus in different populations, J. Am. Acad. Dermatol. **14:**419, 1986.

92. Schmoeckel, C., and Braun-Falco, O.: Prognostic index in malignant melanoma, Arch. Dermatol. **114:**871, 1978.
93. Schoenfeld, R.J., and Pinkus, H.: The recurrence of nevi after incomplete removal, A.M.A. Arch. Dermatol. **78:**30, 1958.
94. Schreiber, M.M., Moon, T.E., and Bozzo, P.D.: Chronic solar ultraviolet damage associated with malignant melanoma of the skin, J. Am. Acad. Dermatol. **10:**755, 1984.
95. Scotto, J., Kopf, A.W., and Urbach, F.: Non-melanoma skin cancer among caucasians in four areas of the United States, Cancer **34:**1333, 1974.
96. Shapiro, L., and Bodian, E.L.: Malignant melanoma in the form of pedunculated papules, Arch. Dermatol. **99:**49, 1969.
97. Silverman, R.A., et al.: The histology of congenital nevi [abstract], J. Invest. Dermatol. **78:**353, 1982.
98. Sim, F.H., et al.: A prospective randomized study of the efficacy of routine elective lymphadenectomy in management of malignant melanoma: prelminary results, Cancer **41:**948, 1978.
99. Slaughter, J.C., et al.: Neurocutaneous melanosis and leptomeningeal melanomatosis in children, Arch. Pathol. **88:**298, 1969.
100. Sober, A.J., Mihm, M.C., and Fitzpatrick, T.B.: Guidelines for removal of acral and mucosal nevi [letter], J. Am. Acad. Dermatol. **3:**206, 1980.
101. Solomon, L.M.: The management of congenital melanocytic nevi, Arch. Dermatol. **116:**1017, 1980.
102. Spira, M., et al.: Chemosurgery—a histological study, Plast. Reconstr. Surg. **45:**247, 1970.
103. Stegman, S.J.: A study of dermabrasion and chemical peels in an animal model, J. Dermatol. Surg. Oncol. **6:**490, 1980.
104. Stenn, K.S., Arons, M., and Hurwitz, S.: Patterns of congenital nevocellular nevi: a histologic study of 38 cases, J. Am. Acad. Dermatol. **9:**388, 1983.
105. Trau, H., et al.: Metastases of thin melanomas, Cancer **51:**553, 1983.
106. Veronesi, U., et al.: Stage I melanoma of the limbs: immediate versus delayed node dissection, Tumori **66:**373, 1980.
107. Vilain, R., Glicenstein, J., and Latouche, X.: Treatment of giant nevi. In Goldwyn, R.M., editor: Long-term results in plastic and reconstructive surgery, vol. 1, Boston, 1980, Little, Brown, & Co.
108. Walton, R.G., Jacobs, A.H., and Cox, A.J.: Pigmented lesions in newborn infants, Br. J. Dermatol. **95:**389, 1976.
109. Walton, R.G., Sage, R.D., and Farber, E.M.: Electrodesication of pigmented nevi, A.M.A. Arch. Dermatol. **76:**193, 1957.
110. Wanebo, H.J., et al.: Selection of the optimum surgical treatment of stage I melanoma by depth of microinvasion: use of the combined microstage technique (Clark-Breslow), Ann. Surg. **182:**302, 1975.
111. Wanebo, H.J., Woodruff, J., and Fortner, J.G.: Malignant melanoma of the extremities: a clinicopathologic study using levels of invasion (microstage), Cancer **35:**666, 1975.
112. Wayte, D.M., and Helwig, E.B.: Melanotic freckle of Hutchinson, Cancer **21:**893, 1968.
113. Wilson, J.S.P.: Serial excision (as applied to a naevus of the cheek), Br. J. Plast. Surg. **1:**117, 1948.
114. Zitelli, J.A., et al.: Histologic patterns of congenital nevocytic nevi and implications for treatment, J. Am. Acad. Dermatol. **11:**402, 1984.

Lesions of the
Surface Epidermis

ACROCHORDONS AND PAPILLOMAS

Acrochordons (skin tags) occur as small (1-2 mm), soft papules (Fig. 22-1, *A*), usually located on the neck or intertriginous areas such as the axilla. Larger growths, known as fibroepitheliomatous polyps (cutaneous papillomas), may also grow in the same locations and in addition are commonly found in the perineum or groin. These latter growths frequently have a baglike end and a narrow stalk (Fig. 22-1, *B*). Occasionally fibroepitheliomatous polyps become twisted or outgrow their blood supply. When this occurs, they may become gangrenous.

Histopathology

Both skin tags and papillomas are histopathologically classified fibromas, with a connective tissue stalk composed of loose collagen fibers and numerous capillaries. The epidermis is slightly hyperplastic with both acanthosis and hyperkeratosis.

Treatment

Most patients seek removal of these acrochordons or fibroepitheliomatous polyps because of irritation or because in the neck area they tend to get caught in jewelry.

Excision is a simple matter (Fig. 22-1, *A*). The lesion is picked up with forceps and cut across the base. Many lesions (20 to 100) can be removed at one sitting. I have found serrated scissors to be of particular value in snipping these tiny growths, since the small notches in the scissor blades keep the stalk from slipping as the blades are closed. Usually a local anesthetic is unnecessary and is in fact more painful than the procedure itself. Bleeding is stopped by means of pressure or a styptic, such as 35% aluminum chloride in 50% isopropyl alcohol.

Acrochordons and fibroepitheliomatous polyps, like other cutaneous lesions that are removed, should be submitted for histopathologic examination. Melanomas occasionally arise as pedunculated lesions that can resemble skin tags or fibroepitheliomatous polyps.[29,32]

CALLUSES AND CORNS
Callus

A callus (also known as a callosity) is a circumscribed area of thickened skin that results from prolonged pressure. Calluses appear on areas subjected to pressure and where the stratum corneum is normally thick, especially on the palms and soles. On the hands, calluses usually are fairly well circumscribed, whereas on the feet, they are poorly demarcated, blending in with the peripheral skin. The usual location of calluses on the feet is beneath the metatarsal heads, around the heel, and on the inframedial side of the great toe.

Histopathologically a callus is composed of hyperkeratosis, a thickened granular layer, and flattening of the dermal papillae.

Clavus (corn)

A corn is an area of thickened skin more well-defined than a callus. Like a callus, it results from intermittent pressure, but the pressure is usually confined to a small area. A corn is composed of a cone-shaped wedge of compressed stratum corneum with the base of the cone toward the surface of the skin. The apex of the cone is pointed directly inward and causes pain by impingement on subadjacent structures, including nerves. The patient often describes a sensation like "a stone in the shoe." Corns are localized almost exclusively to the feet and are usually found on the dorsolateral side of the fifth toe and the ball of the foot.

Histopathologically a corn is composed of compressed stratum corneum appearing denser than the surrounding

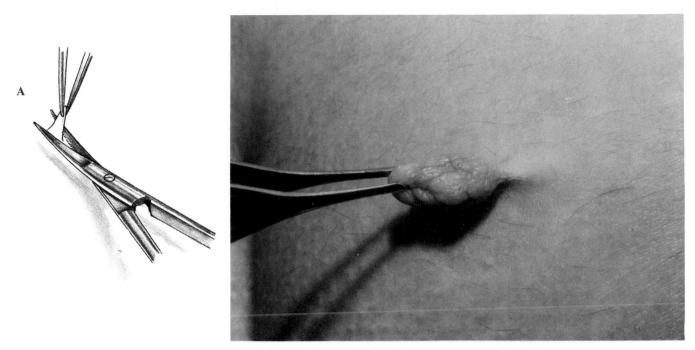

Fig. 22-1. A, Acrochordon (skin tag) being cut with serrated scissors. **B,** Fibroepitheliomatous polyp (cutaneous papilloma).

stratum corneum. As with calluses, the dermal papillae are flattened by chronic pressure.

Corns can be classified as hard corns (heloma durum) or soft corns (heloma molle). Hard corns occur on the exposed portions of the feet and have a translucent, firm surface (Fig. 22-2, *A*). Soft corns are soft because of maceration and are typically found between the toes, especially in the fourth interspace between the fourth and fifth toes (Fig. 22-2, *B*). In this location bony projections from the bases of the proximal phalanges give rise to underlying pressure.

Usually the diagnosis of a callus or corn is obvious— they are rarely confused with other entities. However, a wart may be embedded in a callus. This becomes obvious as the thickened stratum corneum is pared away, revealing the tiny, dark, dotlike areas representing the thrombosed capillaries characteristic of warts.

Treatment

Calluses and corns result from pressure, either internal or external, on the skin. When the sources of pressure are eliminated, the thickened stratum corneum may spontaneously revert to normal thickness.

On the feet, underlying exostoses or other orthopedic problems seen with aging are the usual causes of calluses and corns. Padding and corrective footwear might help somewhat in relieving the problem, but resolution usually does not occur until the underlying problem is established and definitely corrected, usually with surgery. Podiatrists and orthopedic surgeons with special training in foot dis-

orders can be of great value in determining the underlying cause.

Reducing the thickness of calluses brings about temporary relief, which for many patients is all that is desired. Calluses can be partially removed by soaking them in water and then filing them with a pumice stone. Alternatively, the callus can be deeply pared by a razor or scalpel blade held parallel to the skin surface. Application of a keratolytic such as salicylic acid plaster (40%) helps soften the calluses and thus makes removal easier.

Hard corns are removed in a different fashion, known as enucleation[31] (Fig. 22-3). A No. 15 blade is angled parallel to the conical sides of the corn. I have found it easier to use the blade without the blade handle to angle the blade more precisely. The tip of the blade descends approximately to the depth of the apex of the corn. With a circular, clockwise (if right-handed) rotational motion, the sides of the cone are circumscribed with the blade, which is held slightly obliquely to the skin surface (Fig. 22-3, *A*). The corn is shelled out by lowering the blade and at the same time continuing the rotational motion (Fig. 23-3, *B*). Flexibility of the wrist, firm skin tension, and gentle handling of the blade are all essential for good results with enucleation.

If one goes too deeply with the scalpel tip, bleeding may be observed, and the patient invariably complains of pain. When this occurs, it is possible to continue, but more superficially. With practice, enucleation of corns should be painless and hemorrhage free.

In the elderly or those with known atherosclerotic vascu-

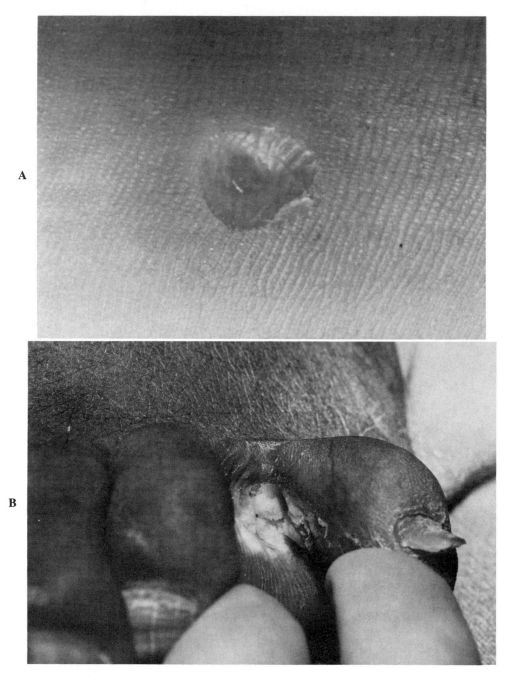

Fig. 22-2. A, Hard corn (heloma durum). **B,** Soft corn (heloma molle).

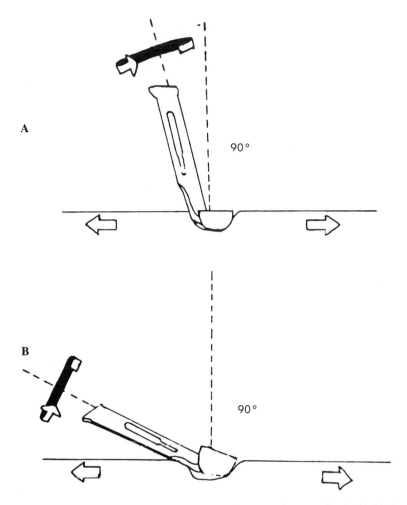

Fig. 22-3. Enucleation technique for corns. **A,** Sides of cone are circumscribed with blade. **B,** Corn is shelled out. (From Scullion, P.J.: Dermatologic review: scalpel technique in removing heloma and hyperkeratosis, J. Foot Surg. **23**(4):344-9, Copyright by Am. Coll. of Foot Surgeons, 1984.)

lar disease, the pedal and tibial arteries should be palpated before removing corns or calluses. I have personally seen a typical corn converted into a nonhealing ulcer on the ball of the foot following removal in a patient with severe arteriosclerosis of the femoral arteries.

Hard and soft corns can also be treated by the injection of silicone or bovine collagen (Zyplast or Carrigan), which acts as an internal cushion and distributes the pressure from a localized area. This is an alternative to corrective surgery, but too little experience exists at this point to know how long the injected collagen remains effective.

Padding can alleviate pain and resolve soft corns to a greater extent than it can for hard corns. Lamb's wool placed in the interspace helps distribute pressure from underlying bony prominences; it also allows aeration, thereby helping to clear up any maceration that is present. Soft cotton is too compressible for this purpose and should not be used.

SEBORRHEIC KERATOSIS

Seborrheic keratoses are common lesions occurring mainly on the trunk and face. Usually these lesions make their appearance in middle age. They are sharply demarcated, brownish, and raised above the surface of the skin. The surface is usually rough although occasionally it is smooth and covered with a greasy crust (Fig. 22-4, *A*). The average seborrheic keratosis measures 0.5 to 1 cm, but larger lesions may occur (Fig. 22-4, *D*). Although it frequently occurs as a solitary lesion, some patients may literally have hundreds of such lesions, especially on the trunk (Fig. 22-4, *B*). A seborrheic keratosis is an important lesion to recognize, since it can be confused with melanoma when very darkly pigmented (Fig. 22-4, *C*).

Histopathology

A seborrheic keratosis is a tumor that lies entirely above the surface of the skin. It is characterized by acanthosis, hyperkeratosis, and papillomatosis. The cells have a par-

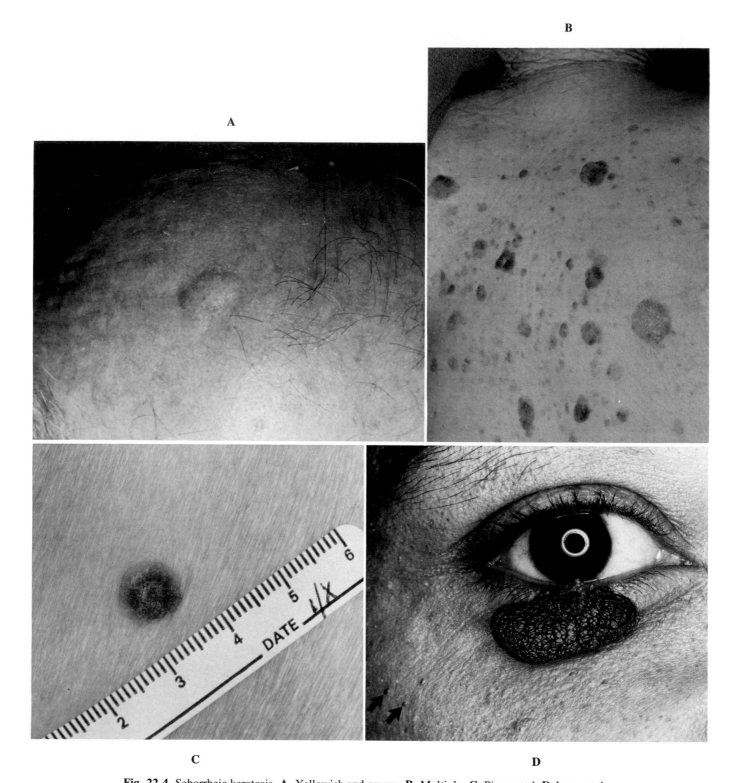

Fig. 22-4. Seborrheic keratosis. **A,** Yellowish and greasy. **B,** Multiple. **C,** Pigmented. **D,** Large and pigmented. Also shown are small lesions of dermatosis papulosa nigra.

ticularly basaloid appearance, and collections of horny material are frequently present. These are referred to as horn pseudocysts (if from invagination of the stratum corneum) or horn cysts (if no connection with stratum corneum).

An irritated seborrheic keratosis (see Fig. 25-2) is composed of keratinized epidermal cells, some of which are arranged in whorls or eddies. As in typical seborrheic keratoses, horn pseudocysts are also present. Despite a malignant appearance, such lesions are benign.

Treatment

The goals of treatment for a seborrheic keratosis are complete removal (to avoid recurrence) and at the same time creation of an excellent cosmetic result. Many methods of removal have been suggested; these include curettage (with or without electrodesiccation), shave excision, scissors excision, scalpel excision, electrodesiccation alone, cryotherapy, dermabrasion, laser, and application of trichloroacetic acid or other irritants. One author feels that recurrences are most likely with cryotherapy but least likely with any of the surgical methods.[11] Use of a piece of gauze wrapped around the index finger to scrape off seborrheic keratoses has been described.[7] I have tried this and found that it does not work well. Since occasionally skin tumors (for example, basal cell carcinoma) are found beneath seborrheic keratoses (see Fig. 14-1), it is preferable to have tissue to submit for pathologic examination.

I have found that the simplest method of removing seborrheic keratoses is curettage followed by a styptic (such as 30% aluminum chloride in 50% isopropyl alcohol). Frequently a local anesthetic is unnecessary. When it is required, either an injectable anesthetic or a cryospray (such as Frigiderm) may be used. The advantage of the latter is that in addition to providing local anesthesia by freezing the lesion, it also renders the lesion brittle, so that it can be curetted more easily.

Following removal of seborrheic keratoses, hypopigmentation may occur. This is more of a problem when the seborrheic keratosis is very large and occurs in an area devoid of hair follicles. Because treatment of a seborrheic keratosis effectually removes the epidermis with its melanocytes, repigmentation of the new epidermis that grows over the wound must come from the surrounding skin or the hair follicles below. If the seborrheic keratosis occurs in an area where hair follicles are sparse or absent, repigmentation may be slow or nonexistent, and hypopigmentation results. Also since repigmentation of the skin from follicles occurs only 1 to 2 mm from the follicle, hypopigmentation is a problem if removal sites are in an area with sparse hair and are larger than 3 or 4 mm in diameter.[11]

DERMATOSIS PAPULOSA NIGRA

Dermatosis papulosa nigra is a common condition that occurs exclusively in blacks and orientals. It is characterized by numerous smooth, small, hyperpigmented papules on the face, especially on the malar eminences and below the eyes (Fig. 22-4, *D*). As time goes on, these lesions usually increase in number and, slightly, in size.

Histopathology

Microscopically dermatosis papulosa nigra resembles a seborrheic keratosis. Irregular acanthosis and increased amounts of pigment are seen throughout all layers of the epidermis.

Treatment

Usually the lesions of dermatosis papulosa nigra can be snipped off with scissors or lightly electrodesiccated. Light curettage alone has also been described.[18] With this last method the whole lesion is not removed but only irritated enough by the curette to induce regression. This technique supposedly results in little or no hyperpigmentation.

EPIDERMAL NEVUS

An epidermal nevus is usually categorized into one of three types: (1) localized and papular, (2) localized and verrucous, or (3) systematized and verrucous. All three types appear at birth or in early childhood and may be linear.

The localized and papular epidermal nevus (Fig. 22-5) is composed of hyperpigmented papules. Histologically these show thickening of the epidermis (acanthosis) with extension of the dermal papillae (papillomatosis) and hyperkeratosis. Thus such lesions are indistinguishable from cutaneous papillomas.

The localized and verrucous epidermal nevus frequently occurs on the lower extremities and is pruritic. In addition to the histopathologic features mentioned for a papular epidermal nevus, the localized verrucous type has a chronic inflammatory infiltrate. This has led to it being called inflammatory linear epidermal nevus (ILEN).

The systematized and verrucous epidermal nevus is similar in appearance to the ILEN, except that it appears as many parallel linear lesions that are distributed widely on the body.

Treatment

Each epidermal nevus must be treated individually. The therapeutic dilemma imposed by these lesions is removal with the least amount of scarring. It is important to understand that epidermal nevi involve more tissue than merely the epidermis, although the underlying dermis appears to be clinically normal. Therefore simply shaving these lesions does not result in a long-term cure. Although some authors believe that electrodesiccation and cryosurgery are successful,[13] long-term follow-up and a series of patients are not offered. Other methods of treatment include deep shave excision, dermabrasion, and topical application of skin ir-

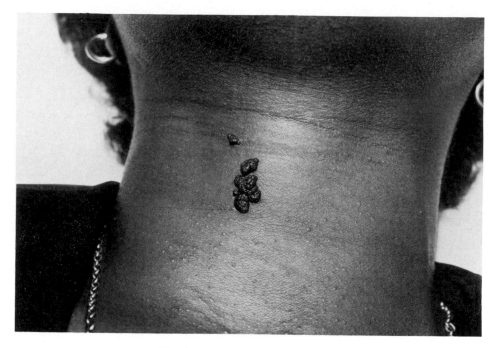

Fig. 22-5. Papular epidermal nevus.

ritants such as retinoic acid, chemical peeling agents, or even podophyllin ointment with occlusion.

Surgical excision, including underlying dermis, is the definitive method of cure. However, if the nevus is large, widespread, or located perpendicular to the maximal skin tension lines, excision may lead to a cosmetic result that is worse than the nevus itself. Laser excision offers some advantage in that the lesion may be vaporized with minimal injury to surrounding tissue. However, long-term follow-up data on patients who had laser excisions of epidermal nevi are not currently available.

ACTINIC KERATOSIS

An actinic (solar) keratosis can occur as a single lesion, but usually keratoses are multiple, appearing on the most sun-exposed areas of the skin in elderly individuals of fair complexion. One of every 15 individuals between the ages of 65 and 74 has actinic keratoses.[17] Although they usually appear past the age of 40 or 50, actinic keratoses may be seen in persons in their twenties or thirties, especially if prolonged and frequent sun exposure has occurred. Actinic keratoses usually appear on the face, especially the forehead, and the dorsum of the hands and forearms. In bald men, these lesions can also be seen on the top of the scalp because of the sun damage that occurs as a result of a lack of hair coverage.

The precise cause of actinic keratoses has not been investigated in great depth. Actinic damage undoubtedly plays a role. Individual susceptibility can also be important. Individuals with fair complexions and light-colored eyes

and hair are particularly prone to these keratoses. It has been shown that cells (peripheral lymphocytes) in patients with multiple actinic keratoses have decreased DNA repair activity in response to sunlight, compared with those in normal age-matched controls.[3] Similar results have been found with tissue fibroblasts in this same type of patient.

Actinic keratoses are usually small, measuring about 0.5 cm in diameter or less. They are erythematous and covered by an adherent scale that is of variable thickness (Fig. 22-6). On the dorsum of the hands, forearms, and top of the scalp this scale is thick, which makes medical treatment more difficult. Occasionally the scale is markedly thickened, giving rise to a cutaneous horn.

Actinic keratoses rarely eventuate into invasive squamous cell carcinomas. The physician should be alert to this possibility if on biopsy an "actinic keratosis" shows evidence of dermal invasion or if the lesion recurs despite several attempts at removal.

Histopathology

An actinic keratosis is characterized microscopically by the presence of atypical cells within and confined to the epidermis. These cells are in their earliest stages on the lower one third of the epidermis and appear as smaller-than-normal basal cells and prickle cells. The nuclei are dark, and the cells are crowded together. The prickle cells often show a disorderly arrangement and some premature keratinization. A fully evolved actinic keratosis shows atypia and premature keratinization of the whole epidermis.

The stratum corneum overlying an actinic keratosis usu-

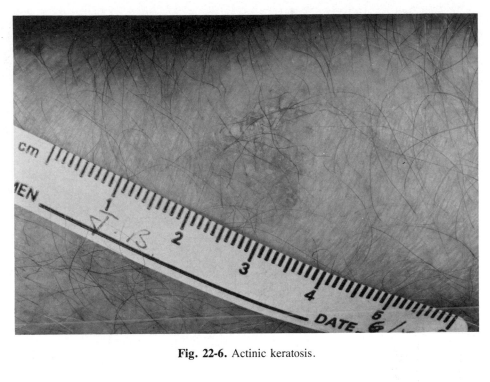

Fig. 22-6. Actinic keratosis.

ally shows parakeratosis. In addition, the atypical proliferation of cells within the epidermis frequently does not involve follicular or eccrine structures, in contradistinction to Bowen's disease, which usually involves the outer root sheaths and acrosyringia. The dermis underlying an actinic keratosis contains a chronic inflammatory infiltrate and evidence of solar damage (collagen degeneration and elastosis). When histopathologically evaluating an actinic keratosis, one should look for evidence of dermal invasion. When this exists, small buds of atypical epidermal cells are found lying free within the dermis, and the basement membrane of the epidermis is often indistinct. Such lesions should be regarded as invasive squamous cell carcinomas.

Treatment

Curettage and shave excision. If only a few lesions are present, actinic keratoses can either be curetted with a dermal curette or frozen with liquid nitrogen. The methods of curettage are discussed in Chapter 15. The advantage of curettage is that a biopsy specimen can be obtained at the time of treatment. In addition, in my experience the cure rate is higher than with other techniques, since the curette helps to define the extent of the atypical epidermis.

One group of authors studied 45 lesions removed and believed to be typical actinic keratoses.[10] On histologic examination two of the 45 proved to be invasive squamous cell carcinomas, and three of the 45 contained basal cell carcinomas. Thus about 11% of such lesions may contain more invasive elements. These authors recommend a "shave excision for keratoses" to obtain histopathologic

assessment. In addition, it is their belief and mine that a number of keratoses recur following other treatment methods, especially freezing with liquid nitrogen.

When actinic keratoses occur over thin skin, such as on the backs of the hands in the elderly, it may be preferable to remove them with scissors or shave excision. The use of the curette in such thin skin frequently results in needless tearing of the tissue.

Cryosurgery. Cryosurgery may be advantageous for actinic keratoses, particularly if there are several lesions that need treatment. Usually a hand-held liquid nitrogen spray apparatus is used. The lesions are frozen until white for about 15 seconds. The thaw time is about 15 to 20 seconds. This technique is rapid and results in few complications. For large actinic keratoses, best results are obtained if the spray is directed either centrifugally from the center of the lesion or transversely in a paintbrush pattern. In one study, a 98.8% cure rate was reported with a 1-year follow-up examination after cryotherapy was used for specific actinic keratoses.[23] This cure rate is higher than any in my experience or in that of others.[10]

5-Fluorouracil. The topical use of 5-fluorouracil (5-FU) for actinic keratoses evolved from serendipitous clinical observation of the drug's effect on cutaneous lesions when used systemically. In a study of 85 patients treated with systemic 5-FU for internal malignancies, it was observed that intense erythema developed around active actinic keratoses on the skin, and in 3 weeks the lesions cleared.[12] This led to further studies with this medication for cutaneous lesions.

5-FU is a fluorinated pyrimidine that acts as an antimetabolite. It inhibits thymidylate synthase activity and thus blocks the incorporation of thymidine into deoxyribonucleic acid (DNA). Topically applied (without occlusion) to actinic keratoses, 5-FU has been shown to block DNA synthesis for 2 hours.[9] In addition, 5-FU selectively penetrates actinic keratoses but not normal skin.

5-FU can be used either as a 1% cream (Fluoroplex) or a 5% cream (Efudex), or in propylene glycol as a 1% (Fluoroplex) or 2% (Efudex) solution. The cream may be less irritating than the solution. Although some investigators[8] believe that the 1% or 2% concentrations may be inadequate for treatment, others disagree.[33]

Simmonds[33] studied use of 1% 5-FU cream on 123 patients with actinic keratoses. Application twice daily for 2 weeks on the face, for 4 weeks on the scalp, and for 8 weeks on the dorsum of the hands or forearms was found to be necessary. Although in most patients rapid resolution of lesions took place with this regimen, in about 25% of patients new lesions appeared within 24 months, and in 50% of patients they appeared within 36 months. Men required retreatment twice as frequently as women. A significant relapse rate even with 5% 5-FU was found in another study,[8] in which 5 of 24 patients (21%) with facial actinic keratoses had recurrences by 11 months.

Topical 5-FU is useful in treating multiple actinic keratoses over large areas, where treating specific lesions is impractical. Many inapparent lesions ''light up'' with topical application of 5-FU, especially the lesions that are better felt than visualized and even lesions that cannot be detected at all. In a sense 5-FU then acts as a diagnostic and therapeutic modality, assuming that the lesions that react at least contain actinically damaged epidermis.

Ideally, topical 5-FU should be prescribed as soon as the earliest signs of actinic keratoses are noticed, so that individual lesions can be cured before growing larger and thus more difficult to eradicate. Usually twice-a-day application for 3 weeks is sufficient, but treatment may be extended to 4 weeks. If lesions are particularly thick, such as those on the backs of the hands or top of the scalp, adjunctive measures may be used to potentiate the effect of the 5-FU. These methods include wrapping the involved areas in a plastic wrap (for example, Saran Wrap) at night to aid in penetration of the cream or the concomitant use of a keratolytic such as salicylic acid or urea. 5-FU is excellent for eliminating many small keratoses but causes discomfort to patients.

The sequence of events that occurs with topical use of 5-FU for facial actinic keratoses is reasonably predictable. The patient gets an erythematous, scaly reaction within 4 to 5 days. This reaction increases in intensity by 9 to 11 days and peaks at 11 to 13 days. Treatment is usually terminated between 14 and 21 days, depending on the magnitude of the patient's reaction to 5-FU. For maximum benefit a full 21-

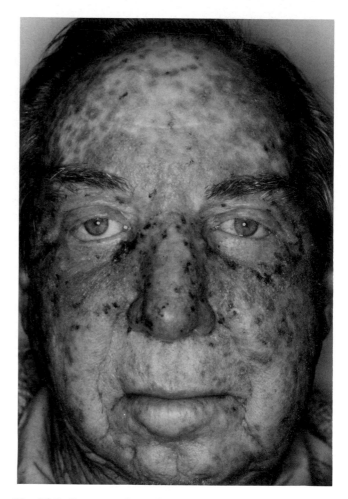

Fig. 22-7. Exaggerated reaction to topical 5-FU. Patient became febrile and developed temporary ectropions.

day treatment period should be completed. The patient then begins a ''cooling off'' period.[33] During this time, which lasts from 7 to 14 days, a topical nonfluorinated corticosteroid cream and lubrication of the crusting that normally occurs are helpful.

Certain areas of the face tend to be particularly sensitive to 5-FU. These include the eyelids, the vermilion of the lips, and the nasolabial creases. In addition, sun exposure tends to potentiate the inflammatory response to 5-FU. This can be lessened by the use of a sunscreen during the treatment period. During the ''cooling down'' period the sunscreen may also be useful in helping the reaction to abate more quickly.

Some patients appear to be exquisitely sensitive to 5-FU, particularly during retreatment at a later time, sometimes a year later. Swelling of the face and eyelids with extreme crusting can then be seen (Fig. 22-7). It has been proposed that this heightened sensitivity is caused by a contact dermatitis to the 5-FU. Indeed, some physicians[25] believe that 5-FU works by means of such an allergic reaction rather

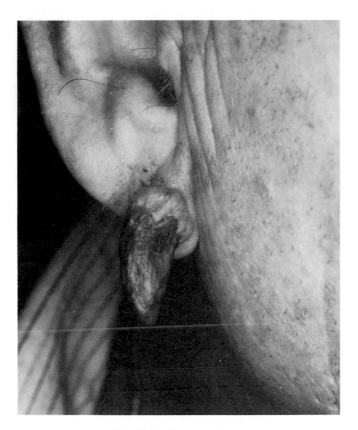

Fig. 22-8. Cutaneous horn.

than by a direct cytotoxic effect on atypical cells or by nonspecific irritation.

Occasionally one is confronted with a patient with severely sun-damaged skin and a plethora of lesions of different sizes and degrees of scaling seemingly blending together. Because some of these lesions may be basal or squamous cell carcinomas that are indistinct, it has been proposed by some physicians that one should give the patient a course (3 to 4 weeks) of 5-FU to eradicate first the actinic keratoses.[8] The remaining tumors are then more easily seen and can be biopsied. It is presumed by these physicians that any invasive neoplasm will not disappear from sight with a course of topical 5-FU; however, this concept is probably fallacious. Other authors report that use of 5-FU can result in growth of normal-appearing skin over carcinomas and thus give the false impression of having cured these tumors.[28] Certainly, any obvious basal or squamous cell carcinomas should be noted and biopsied before use of 5-FU.

Another group of authors proposed that 5-FU be used in combination with a topical steroid so that the redness and scaling produced by the 5-FU would be lessened or even eliminated during treatment.[5] With the application of 0.4% to 0.5% triamcinolone 10 to 15 minutes after 5-FU during a 3-week period of time, these investigators showed similar resolution and recurrence rates of actinic keratoses to those

shown with 5-FU alone. The inflammatory response was lessened considerably, although not totally eliminated; and the patients preferred to use 5-FU with a topical steroid rather than 5-FU alone. These authors thus concluded that the success of 5-FU in the treatment of actinic keratoses is not related to the degree of visible inflammation.

An abbreviated (10-day) course of 5-FU followed by cryotherapy to the lesions is recommended by one author.[1] She uses the 5-FU to ''light up'' the lesions. Since the 5-FU probably induces some damage within a short time to the epidermis, less intense freezing with liquid nitrogen is required for cure. This author thinks that with her technique she gets good cure rates with less discomfort and more patient compliance.

There is no doubt that the cosmetic results from the use of 5-FU are superior to those from other treatment methods. Curettage or cryotherapy can result in hypopigmented areas; although, if these are small, they eventually resolve. The areas treated with 5-FU frequently show recurrence of lesions within 1 to 2 years. Since individuals continue to be exposed to the sun, it is difficult to know if these ''new'' lesions are in reality persistent old lesions or newly induced actinic keratoses.

Dermabrasion. If they are multiple and resistant to other forms of therapy, actinic keratoses can be dermabraded. This method of therapy works especially well on the forehead or scalp, where thickened lesions are difficult to eradicate. The problem with dermabrasion is that it leaves a slightly hypopigmented epidermis; however, this is usually acceptable to patients. The regrowth of actinic keratoses after dermabrasion that is properly performed is minimal and does not occur for several years. This leads me to believe that the recurrences shortly after treatment with topical 5-FU are the result of the inability of 5-FU to eliminate atypical epidermis to the same extent that dermabrasion eliminates it.

Recurrent lesions. It cannot be stressed enough that, no matter what technique is used for treatment of actinic keratoses, should a single lesion continue to recur, a biopsy must be obtained. The clinical ''behavior'' of recurrent lesions should arouse one's suspicions that deeper invasive elements may be present.

CUTANEOUS HORN (CORNU CUTANEUM)

Cutaneous horns are hard hyperkeratotic excrescences 2 to 25 mm long that occur on the face, scalp, extremities, or penis. Usually the projection of horny material is conical, slightly curved, and faintly pigmented. The base may be mildly erythematous and slightly wider than its projection (Fig. 22-8).

Rarely do cutaneous horns reach enormous proportions, suggesting the horns of animals. Horns of animals that usually contain a bony core differ from cutaneous horns of man that are simply compacted keratin. An exception is the ''horn'' of the rhinocerous, which contains only compacted keratin and thus is similar to the human cutaneous horn.

Cutaneous horns can arise from and thus overlie a number of different pathologic processes. More than half of all cutaneous horns overlie benign processes, especially seborrheic or actinic keratoses.[4] Other pathologic processes that can give rise to cutaneous horns include warts, Bowen's disease lesions, squamous cell carcinomas, or basal cell carcinomas. Whenever a very large cutaneous horn occurs it is likely to overlie a squamous cell carcinoma.

Treatment

The cutaneous horn is either sliced off at the base or excised. Because most cutaneous horns overlie benign pathologic conditions, it might be preferable to perform a biopsy before definitive therapy. Since there may be potential carcinoma at its base, it is essential that all tissue be submitted for histopathologic examination. If carcinoma exists at its base and there is doubt that the lesion has been totally extirpated, a more definitive excision is mandatory.

MOLLUSCUM CONTAGIOSUM

Molluscum contagiosum occurs as one or several small (2 to 3 mm) papules that are round, smooth, and have an umbilicated center. These lesions are caused by a DNA poxvirus. Molluscum contagiosum commonly occurs on the face and genitals, but it can be widely distributed, especially in children.

Histopathology

The histopathology of molluscum contagiosum is characterized by a well-localized area of acanthosis. Many of the uppermost epidermal cells contain intracytoplasmic inclusion bodies.

Treatment

Curettage is a simple treatment for molluscum contagiosum. Usually a local anesthetic is unnecessary but may be used. For children with numerous lesions, nitrous oxide sedation can be useful during curettage. Occasionally molluscum contagiosum is secondarily infected with *Staphylococcus aureus* or *Streptococcus,* the latter giving rise to erythema surrounding the lesion. I prefer to treat such infected lesions with antibiotics before surgical removal.

VERRUCA

There are four common types of verruca: verruca vulgaris, verruca plana, verruca plantaris, and condyloma acuminatum. Athough all four types are caused by human papillomavirus (HPV), which is a DNA virus, several subtypes of this virus are now identified and are specific for each of the four types of warts.

Verruca vulgaris, also known as the common wart, is a firm, well-circumscribed, rough, hyperkeratotic growth elevated above the skin surface. It is thus commonly papular but may be papillomatous or filamentous. It can occur almost anywhere on the skin but is most common on the hands and is found mostly in children. Usually these warts are numerous when they do occur in children, whereas in adults only a few lesions may be present. When verruca vulgaris occurs around the nails (periungual wart), it can be particularly painful and difficult to treat.

Verrucae planae, or flat warts, are small (1 to 3 mm), slightly elevated, smooth papules with a flat surface. These warts are usually multiple. They often have a slight tan color but may also be so slightly pigmented that they blend in with the surrounding skin. When this occurs the warts might be so inconspicuous that good indirect lighting is necessary to see them more easily. Flat warts appear mostly on the face and dorsum of the hands. When verrucae planae are extensive and located over the trunk and extremities, a familial condition known as epidermodysplasia verruciformis may exist. Verrucae planae in epidermodysplasia verruciformis can undergo malignant change into Bowen's disease or squamous cell carcinoma. This transformation is associated with the presence of certain human papillomaviruses (HPV-3, HPV-5, HPV-8) that are believed to be oncogenic in this disorder.[24]

Verruca plantaris occurs on the soles of the feet, especially at points of pressure such as the ball of the foot. The patient usually complains of pain. The lesion appears as an area of thickened skin that may be slightly whitish or pink or may resemble a callus. When the superficial epidermis is removed, a few bleeding points or black dots become visible. The latter represent thrombosed capillaries in the papillary dermis. Sometimes plantar warts are grouped, or several warts fuse, so that when the surface is shaved off, multiple discrete whitish cores are seen. Such a coalescence of warts on the sole of the foot is known as a mosaic wart.

Condylomata acuminata occur on the genital area, perineum, and anus. In addition, these warts can be found within the mucosal surfaces in these areas extending up the urethra or into the vagina or anal canal. In one study 34 patients with anogenital warts were examined under general anesthesia.[15] Of 24 men, 33% had obvious intraanal extension of their warts. One man had warts seen above the dentate line. Of 10 women examined, 60% had warts not only perianally but also in the vulva and vagina. Therefore for patients with warts in these areas, full anoscopy (and pelvic examination for women) is necessary to detect all warts so that the treatment method chosen is more likely to be successful.

The lesions of condylomata acuminata are soft, pink, verrucous papules that can enlarge into cauliflower-like masses. Development of carcinomas in large condylomata acuminata of long standing have been reported.

Histopathology

The major histopathologic change in warts is in the epidermis, which is acanthotic. Verruca vulgaris shows prominent thickening of the horny layer caused by both parakeratosis and hyperkeratosis. Flat warts, on the other hand, show little change in the stratum corneum. Large vacuolated cells frequently exist in the upper epidermis including the granular layer. Papillomatosis with elongation of the rete ridges also exists.

Treatment

Most warts respond to initial therapy or even disappear spontaneously, whereas some persist despite many attempts at eradication. It has been found that in institutionalized children, two thirds of the 168 lesions observed without therapy involuted within 2 years.[26] Therefore, because scarring is always possible from vigorous therapy, one needs to balance the probability of cure from treatment against ultimate cosmetic results.

The forms of therapy for warts include almost anything from witchcraft to immunotherapy, but in general the following are used: cryosurgery (liquid nitrogen), curettage, curettage and electrodesiccation, electrodesiccation alone, elctrocautery excision, and laser-induced vaporization. The choice of therapy is determined by the location, size, number, age, and history of previous treatments. In addition, certain types of warts appear to be more amenable to certain special types of therapy. For example, 25% podophyllin in tincture of benzoin is used commonly for condylomata acuminata. In general surgical types of therapy have greater risk of scarring.

Cryosurgery. Cryosurgry is a popular method of therapy for warts. It is simple to learn and perform, the patient has little morbidity, and scar formation is minimal. A cotton-tipped applicator is dipped into liquid nitrogen and then applied to the wart long enough to whiten the wart and a small ring (approximately 1 to 2 mm) of surrounding tissue. For this procedure the small (6-inch) cotton-tipped applicator is less than satisfactory, since the cotton on the tip is too tightly bound. A more loosely woven rayon or cotton-tipped applicator (that is, the long proctoscopic applicator with a "jumbo" tip) is more efficient in providing a freeze. This procedure is repeated a few times, depending on the site and thickness of the wart and whether it has recurred from previous treatment. Care should be taken to freeze recurrent lesions for at least 30 seconds. Following treatment, the patient should be warned that a blister will form. The blister roof should be kept intact. Frequently the blister is hemorrhagic. Within a few weeks the blister dries and peels away, together with the wart.

Cure rates with cryosurgery for warts, like cure rates for other forms of therapy, are difficult to assess. In one study[6] the use of liquid nitrogen was compared with use of a simple topical cream (composed of a mixture of salicylic acid and lactic acid) for all types of warts. Both the liquid nitrogen and the topical preparation resulted in a similar cure rate (about 57%). However, when these two forms of therapy were used in combination, a 71.8% rate of cure was obtained.

Cryosurgery is an excellent method of therapy for warts on the face, hands, and genital areas (mucosal and nonmucosal). In one study, when cryosurgery was compared with electrocautery for anogenital warts, patients preferred the cryosurgery, although the success rate was about equal in both groups.[34] Periungual warts and plantar warts can also be cured with liquid nitrogen.[20] When this is used for plantar warts, the overlying thickened stratum corneum is first removed. One group of authors reported a 91% cure rate using liquid nitrogen spray on 89 plantar warts.[22] For the patients' comfort on the feet they advised debridement at 14 days of the bulla that forms. In contrast to this study is a report that compared acyclovir cream to either liquid nitrogen or placebo for plantar warts.[14] The findings were that all three forms of therapy gave about the same poor percentage of cure (28% for placebo, 39% for acyclovir cream, and 41% for liquid nitrogen) and that liquid nitrogen was not recommended because it was painful and unpleasant. The variance between these two studies is a classic example of variances commonly seen among many other studies on warts. Patient expectation and the physician's enthusiasm undoubtedly play a role in the success or failure of treatment methods for warts.

Electrodesiccation and curettage. Electrodesiccation and curettage of warts is a simple and expedient treatment method that provides a cure for most common warts but can lead to scarring. After appropriate anesthesia, the electrodesiccation current is applied to the wart. The heat in the tissue causes the wart to become white and puffy. The desiccated lesion is then curetted free. Use of the curette before electrodesiccation is more difficult unless the lesion is a filiform or papillomatous wart. Curettage may be an excellent treatment modality for recurrent periungal warts. After removal of the nail plate, the lesion is thoroughly curetted. The little curette can be very useful in this location to extract small extensions of wart tissue from under the lateral or proximal nail folds.[19]

Excision. Surgical removal of warts is performed either with a curette alone (previously discussed), with scissors, or by blunt dissection. Scissors removal of warts is highly successful in the anogenital areas or where warts are papillomatous.[15] If electrodesiccation is used in the perianal area either alone or combined with excision, care needs to be taken that the flatus from the bowel is not ignited by a spark from the electrodesiccating needle. To prevent this from happening, it is advisable to place some cotton into the rectum.

Blunt dissection. Blunt dissection for plantar warts was recommended in one study on the premise that warts are

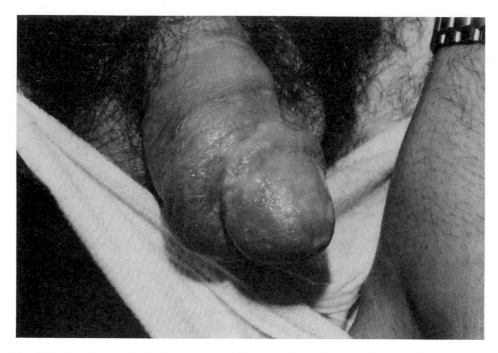

Fig. 22-9. Swelling and irritation of penis following self-application of podophyllin for condylomata acuminata.

solitary lesions that can be easily demarcated and separated from surrounding normal tissue, since cohesion is not very firm.[30] A blunt dissector can be fashioned from a scalpel handle tip. The superficial thickened stratum corneum is first removed by scissors or a scalpel blade. The scissors are then used to establish a plane of dissection between the wart and the surrounding normal tissue. The blunt dissector is then inserted and used to separate the wart completely—in a circular manner—figuratively shelling out the lesion. These authors claimed an 85% cure rate on 58 patients, 46 of whom had suffered from recurrent lesions. The average follow-up period was 10 months, and no scarring was noted. Recurrences were more common if the warts were long-standing (average 55 months) and located on the ball of the foot. Size of the lesions did not seem to affect cure rates. Blunt dissection has also been recommended for stubborn periungal warts.[16]

Laser vaporization. Laser treatment of warts is a newer treatment modality that is successful and becoming more widely available.[4] The carbon dioxide laser is both precise and effective. Those with experience claim that one can tell the difference between normal tissue and wart tissue when this instrument is used. Warts vaporize quickly and give the appearance of bubbling, whereas normal tissue does not. I have not been able to appreciate the differences seen by others in tissue heated with the CO_2 laser. In one study an 81% cure (at 6 months) was reported on all types of warts with one treatment.[27] The rest of the patients required a second or third treatment, but all patients were eventually cured with this modality. The disadvantages of CO_2 laser therapy are that it is expensive and can result in scarring. This latter problem is more common on the hands and almost absent on the bottom of the feet with this treatment modality. The CO_2 laser can be of particular benefit in treatment of warts of the mucous membrane areas, especially in the nose, mouth, vagina, cervix, urethra, and anus. Warts in these areas are difficult to treat because of their relative inaccessibility and the vascularity of the tissue.

Podophyllin. Podophyllin, 25%, in compound tincture of benzoin is an excellent topical preparation for treatment of warts in the genital mucous membrane areas. This substance must be carefully applied to minimize inadvertent application to the surrounding normal tissue. The patient is instructed to wash the area 3 hours after application to preclude significant systemic absorption and local tissue irritation. The podophyllin is applied weekly until the warts completely regress.

Sometimes warts in the genital areas are resistant to podophyllin application. Usually such warts are hyperkeratotic and not located on the mucous membranes. Those warts that are moist and on mucous membranes respond best. If moist warts in these areas fail to respond, the podophyllin can be applied more frequently, usually two or three times a week. Under no circumstance should patients be allowed to apply podophyllin to themselves, since serious tissue irritation can result (Fig. 22-9). In addition, as previously emphasized, anoscopy and vaginal inspection should be performed so that secluded warts can be treated as well.

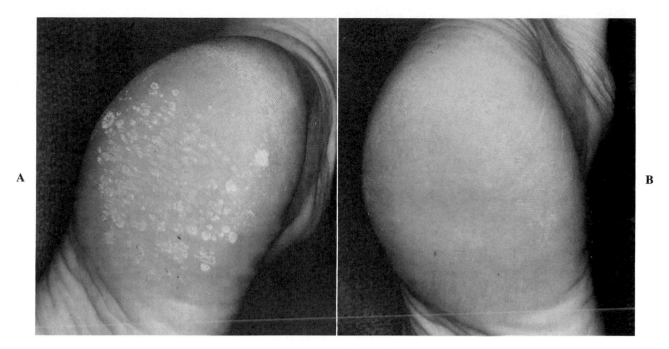

Fig. 22-10. A, Plantar warts before treatment with DNCB. **B,** After treatment.

Plantar warts can also be successfully managed with podophyllin. This substance is painted on after paring of the overlying hyperkeratotic stratum corneum. Gum adhesive tape is then applied. The patient is instructed to leave the tape in place for at least 1 week if possible. Two weeks later the same treatment is performed. This is repeated every 2 weeks until the wart disappears completely. With this method a cure rate of 81% for simple plantar warts was achieved in one study.[7]

Bleomycin. Bleomycin is a newer substance used to treat warts by injection. This substance is a complex glycopeptide with both antibiotic and antitumor properties. It binds to DNA, preventing thymidine incorporation and causing single strand scission in DNA. After intravenous injection, bleomycin tends to be found in high concentrations in the squamous epithelium particularly of the skin and lungs. Subsequent elimination from these sites is slow because of the relatively low concentration of the enzyme bleomycin hydrolase, which is normally in higher concentrations in other tissues.

One of the initial studies using bleomycin was by Abbott,[2] who reported in 1978 his experience injecting this substance into warts. A solution was made from 15 mg of bleomycin sulfate in 15 ml of distilled water. Only 0.2 ml of this solution was injected, and no more than 5 ml was used for all warts to preclude any possible systemic effects. This study reported a 50% cure rate on 61 warts within 78 days. The author stated that healing is scarless, although pain may result from injection. The use of bleomycin is too new for full assessment of its effectiveness and drawbacks.

Dinitrochlorobenzene. Dinitrochlorobenzene (DNCB) is a topical medication highly successful on those selected patients for whom other simple methods have failed to eradicate warts.[21] It is especially useful for warts on the palms and soles. The use of DNCB is based on the premise that some type of allergic response results in the resolution of warts. The patient is sensitized initially by using 0.15 ml of a 2% solution of DNCB in acetone placed on a 2 cm² area of the anterior forearm, allowed to evaporate, and then covered with a perforated bandage. The cover is removed in 24 hours. Two weeks later, after sensitization has occurred, the patient is challenge-tested with DNCB of different strengths in aquaphor. Usually 0.001%, 0.01%, and 0.1% concentrations are used. The concentration that results in slight redness is chosen as the treatment concentration. The patient is instructed to rub it into the wart twice a day. Usually the warts regress in 3 to 6 weeks. Fig. 22-10 shows before and after use of DNCB for recalcitrant plantar warts.

In one study using the just mentioned sensitization and treatment schedule, DNCB was successful in 70 of 77 patients (91%) followed-up for an average of 8 months.[21] Most of these patients had recurrent warts. Five patients developed an autosensitization reaction, and only one could not be sensitized.

It should be emphasized that the sensitization solution of DNCB in acetone should be mixed weekly and not allowed to sit for months between usage. When it is allowed to stand, the acetone evaporates and the actual DNCB concentration increases. In my experience, this has led to severe sensitization reactions.

REFERENCES

1. Abadir, D.M.: Combination of topical 5-fluorouracil with cryotherapy for treatment of actinic keratoses, J. Dermatol. Surg. Oncol. **9:**403, 1983.
2. Abbott, L.G.: Treatment of warts with bleomycin, Australas. J. Dermatol. **19:**69, 1978.
3. Abo-Darub, J.M., MacKie, R., and Pitts, J.D.: DNA repair in cells from patients with actinic keratosis, J. Invest. Dermatol. **80:**241, 1983.
4. Bart, R.S., Andrade, R., and Kopf, A.W.: Cutaneous horns: a clinical and histopathologic study, Acta Derm. Venereol. **48:**507, 1968.
5. Breza, T., Taylor, J.R., and Eaglstein, W.H.: Noninflammatory destruction of actinic keratoses by fluorouracil, Arch. Dermatol. **112:**1256, 1976.
6. Bunney, M.H., Nolan, M.W., and Williams, D.A.: An assessment of the methods of treating viral warts by comparative trials based on a standard design, Br. J. Dermatol. **94:**667, 1976.
7. Crile, G., Jr.: Thirteen shortcuts in office surgery, Surg. Clin. N. Am. **55:**1025, 1975.
8. Dillaha, C.J., et al.: Further studies with topical 5-fluorouracil, Arch. Dermatol. **92:**410, 1965.
9. Eaglstein, W.H., Weinstein, G.D., and Frost, P.: Fluorouracil: mechanism of action in human skin and actinic keratoses. I. Effect on DNA synthesis in vivo, Arch. Dermatol. **101:**132, 1970.
10. Emmett, A.J.J., and Broadbent, G.D.: Shave excision for keratoses [letter], Med. J. Aust. **2:**335, 1980.
11. Everett, M.A.: Treatment of seborrheic keratoses and related tumors, Ala. J. Med. Sci. **17:**47, 1980.
12. Falkson, G., and Schulz, E.J.: Skin changes in patients treated with 5-fluorouracil, Br. J. Dermatol. **74:**229, 1962.
13. Fox, B.J., and Lapins, N.A.: Comparison of treatment modalities for epidermal nevus: a case report and review, J. Dermatol. Surg. Oncol. **9:**879, 1983.
14. Gibson, J.R., et al.: A comparison of acyclovir cream virus placebo cream versus liquid nitrogen in the treatment of viral plantar warts, Dermatologica **168:**178, 1984.
15. Gollock, J.M., Slatford, K., and Hunter, J.M.: Scissor excision of anogenital warts, Br. J. Vener. Dis. **58:**400, 1982.
16. Habif, T.P., and Graf, F.A.: Extirpation of subungual and periungual warts by blunt dissection, J. Dermatol. Surg. Oncol. **7:**553, 1981.
17. Johnson, M.L., and Roberts, J.: Prevalence of dermatologic disease among persons 1-74 years of age: United States, Advance Data No. 4, Washington, D.C., 1977, U.S. Dept. of Health Education and Welfare.
18. Kauh, Y.C., et al.: A surgical approach for dermatosis papulosa nigra, Int. J. Dermatol: **22:**590, 1983.
19. Krull, E.A.: The "little" curet (surgical gems), J. Dermatol. Surg. Oncol. **4:**656, 1979.
20. Kuflik, E.G.: Cryosurgical treatment of periungual warts, J. Dermatol. Surg. Oncol. **10:**673, 1984.
21. Lewis, H.M.: Topical immunotherapy of refractory warts, Cutis **12:**863, 1973.
22. Limmer, B.L., and Bogy, L.T.: Cryosurgery of plantar warts, J. Am. Podiatry Assoc. **69:**713, 1979.
23. Lubritz, R.R., and Smolewski, S.A.: Cryosurgery cure rate of actinic keratoses, J. Am. Acad. Dermatol. **7:**631, 1982.
24. Lutzner, M.A.: The human papillomavirus: a review, Arch. Dermatol. **119:**631, 1983.
25. Mansell, P.W.A., et al.: Delayed hypersensitivity to 5-Fluorouracil following topical chemotherapy of cutaneous cancers, Cancer Res. **35:**1288, 1975.
26. Massing, A.M., and Epstein, W.L.: Natural history of warts: a two-year study, Arch. Dermatol. **87:**306, 1963.
27. McBurney, E.I., and Rosen, D.A.: Carbon dioxide laser treatment of verrucae vulgares, J. Dermatol. Surg. Oncol. **10:**45, 1984.
28. Mohs, F.E., Jones, D.L., and Bloom, R.F.: Tendency of fluorouracil to conceal deep foci of invasive basal cell carcinoma, Arch. Dermatol. **114:**1021, 1978.
29. Niven, J., and Lubin, J.: Pedunculated malignant melanoma, Arch. Dermatol. **111:**755, 1975.
30. Pringle, W.M., and Helms, D.C.: Treatment of plantar warts by blunt dissection, Arch. Dermatol. **108:**79, 1973.
31. Scullion, P.G.: Dermatologic review: scalpel technique in removing heloma and hyperkeratosis, J. Foot Surg. **23:**344, 1984.
32. Shapiro, L., and Bodian, E.L.: Malignant melanoma in the form of pedunculated papules, Arch. Dermatol. **99:**49, 1969.
33. Simmonds, W.L.: Management of actinic keratoses with topical 5-fluorouracil, Cutis **18:**298, 1976.
34. Simmons, P.D., Langlet, F., and Thin, R.N.T.: Cryotherapy versus electrocautery in the treatment of genital warts, Br. J. Vener. Dis. **57:**273, 1981.

23

Lesions of Fibrous Tissue

DERMATOFIBROMA

A dermatofibroma is a common lesion that appears as a firm, smooth, slightly hyperpigmented or reddish nodule usually on the lower legs in adults. In most cases, this lesion is solitary and measures about 5 mm, but occasionally it is larger. Typically dermatofibromas remain indefinitely and do not regress or increase in size. Other names for dermatofibroma based on variations in the histopathologic appearance include sclerosing hemangioma or histiocytoma. The cause is unknown, but some authorities believe dermatofibromas are caused by previous injury or insect bites. Dermatofibromas are benign.

Histopathology

Histopathologically, dermatofibromas consist of masses of collagen and fibroblasts that, although not circumscribed, are fairly well demarcated. The amassed collagen appears in whorls. Usually the collagen predominates, giving rise to "fibrous" dermatofibromas. When the fibroblasts predominate, the stroma contains only relatively small amounts of collagen. This latter type of dermatofibroma is known as the "cellular" dermatofibroma. When small capillaries are prominent within the fibrous or cellular stroma, this lesion is known as a *sclerosing hemangioma*. When histiocytes with or without pigment are prominent, the lesion may be referred to as a *histiocytoma*. Usually hyperplasia of the overlying epidermis is present. Rarely such hyperplasia resembles basal cell carcinoma.[19]

Treatment

A dermatofibroma usually requires no treatment unless the patient insists on removal. Simple local excision usually suffices to remove this lesion completely. However, because dermatofibromas are commonly situated on the lower legs, the cosmetic results after excision are poor.

DERMATOFIBROSARCOMA PROTUBERANS

Dermatofibrosarcoma protuberans (DFSP) is a malignant tumor of fibrous tissue best described as a low-grade sarcoma that originates within the dermis. Typically it appears as a raised, firm, multinodular, flesh-colored tumor on the trunk or proximal extremities, but it can occur on the face.

DFSP usually occurs in adults but may occur in children or the elderly. It usually grows slowly over time, but it can have a rapid growth phase that typically prompts the patient to seek medical attention. Initially it appears as a solitary nodule resembling a keloid. As it grows, the overlying epidermis expands while the tumor at the depths of the lesion infiltrates adjacent dermis, subcutaneous tissue, and other structures. During this expansion phase, other circumferentially located nodules might appear, and the tumor may become bulky and protuberant. Sometimes DFSP appears as a firm plaque rather than a multinodular tumor. As the overlying skin is thinned by the underlying expansile growth, it may be subject to ulceration.

Histopathology

Microscopically, DFSP is a well-differentiated fibrosarcoma composed of fibrocellular fascicles of spindle-shaped cells and collagen. These fascicles are arranged in stellate (cartwheel or whirligig) or whorled patterns with fibroblasts arranged radially about a small central hub of collagenous tissue; on low power these patterns may appear woven (storiform). Infiltration of the subcutaneous tissue is almost always present. Myxoid areas might also occur. Beneath the epidermis is a small (grenz) zone of apparently uninvolved dermis.

Treatment

The treatment of choice for DFSP is Mohs surgery (fresh tissue technique).[45] It is essential to realize that this tumor is insidious in its growth characteristics. Typically the fibrous extensions penetrate much farther than can be appreciated either visually or by palpation. In depth the tumor frequently invades underlying muscle fascia or even muscle fibers (Fig. 23-1). Therefore the Mohs technique affords the highest likelihood of cure, because the tumor is microscopically traced out in its entirety.

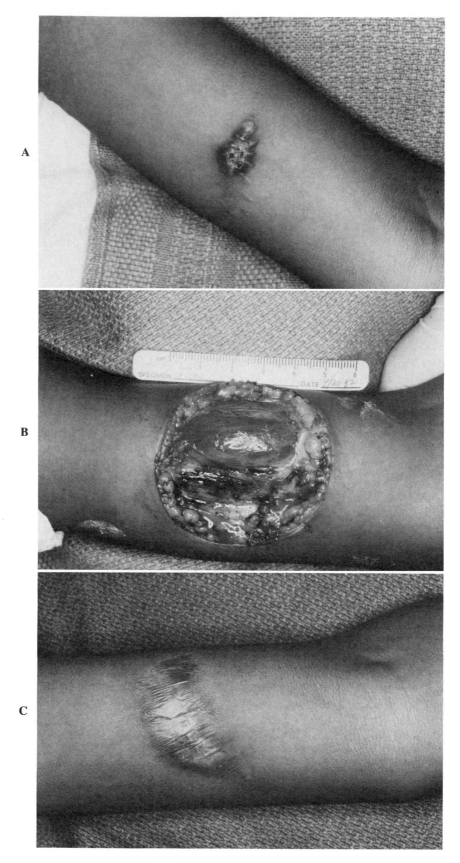

Fig. 23-1. A, Recurrent dermatofibrosarcoma protuberans on medial upper arm of 6-year-old girl. **B,** Wound following removal using Mohs surgery (fresh tissue technique). Note muscle fascia involved by tumor that has been removed. Wound healed by secondary intention within 6 weeks. **C,** Scar from healed wound 2 years after surgery. Arm had full function and there has been no recurrence 5 years after operation.

The recurrence rates with standard surgical extirpation of DFSP are high. One group of authors reported 63 recurrences in 82 patients,[32] and another reported 88 recurrences in 98 patients.[53] In the latter study only 51% of the patients studied were free of recurrence on long-term follow-up (more than 3 years for most patients). Rarely metastases may occur, but these usually happen after the DFSP has been present for many years and is very large. It is thought that the metastases occur by hematogenous dissemination rather than by lymphatic spread because palpable lymph nodes are usually not present. In one of the previously cited studies metastases occurred in 5 of 82 patients, and they did not seem to correlate with the number of mitoses per high-power field.[32] The metastases involved the brain, lungs, abdominal organs, or bones but not the lymph nodes.

KELOIDS AND HYPERTROPHIC SCARS

Keloids and hypertrophic scars are lesions composed of abnormal amounts of scar tissue, usually resulting from trauma. However, keloids may appear from no apparent injury and are then termed "spontaneous keloids." Usually this latter variety occurs on the chest or shoulders and may be related to the high skin tension in these areas.

Alibert is credited with the introduction of the term *keloid*. Originally he had referred to this lesion in 1806 as "le cancroïde" (cancerlike) but first used the name "chéloïde" (like a crab's claw) in 1816 because of the visible clawlike extensions of the lesions and their tendency to grow into surrounding normal tissue.[11]

Clinical appearance

Initially, both keloids and hypertrophic scars have a similar clinical appearance. Both are raised, erythematous, smooth, and firm. However, within months to years, a keloid continues to grow and extends beyond the boundaries of the original injury. A hypertrophic scar, on the other hand, is confined to the boundaries of the injury and tends to regress in time.

Keloids appear to have a particular affinity for development in certain anatomic locations (Fig. 23-2). The ears, sides of the neck, shoulders, chest, and upper back seem to be especially prone to keloids.[13] Keloids in the central face are rare if they occur at all.[35]

Both hypertrophic scars and keloids can be painful and pruritic, but keloids tend to produce these symptoms more often. In one study 27% of keloids (92 of 340) were pruritic, and 19% (65 of 340) were painful.[11] These symptoms may be related to the histamine content of keloids, which has been shown to be elevated above that in normal skin or scar tissue. Diphenhydramine (Benadryl) has been reported to alleviate these symptoms to some degree.[8] Histamine has also been shown to stimulate growth of some keloid fibroblasts and therefore might be a factor in the growth of these lesions.[54]

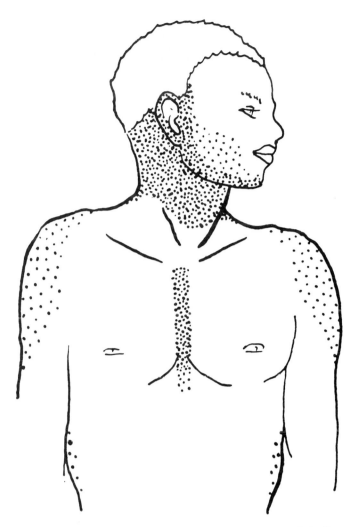

Fig. 23-2. Usual distribution of keloids. (From Crockett, D.J.: Br. J. Plast. Surg. **15:**408, 1962.)

Cause

The cause of keloids or hypertrophic scars is unknown. Heredity, age, previous trauma, sex, and endocrine function are all important predisposing factors. Keloids are much more common in blacks, Polynesians, and Chinese than in whites. In one study 5.4% of black patients questioned had a history of keloid formation.[35] Another group of authors found that of 340 lesions they studied, 76% occurred in blacks, 20% in whites, and 4% in others.[11] The average age of their patients was 25.8 years, although lesions were recorded from 1 year of age to age 73. However, in general, keloids appear rarely in the very young or very old. Trauma, surgery, infection or burns were initiating factors in almost all cases (98%). In the study just mentioned,[35] a family history of keloids was found in 68% (17 of 25) of patients with facial keloids. Women may be more affected than men, and pregnancy appears to hasten the growth of keloids. Although there have been several studies on the management of keloids, little basic research has been done on the cause of this problem. Since keloids mostly affect third world peoples, the issue of medical racism has been raised as a factor in lack of concern and funding for investigative work in this area.[43]

Histogenesis

In an important study, induction of scars and keloids in healthy human volunteers was investigated.[31] Some of the volunteers were known keloid formers, whereas others were normal scar formers. At 26 days after trauma, a critical deviation of fibroblastic growth occurred in lesions destined to be keloids. In normal scars the fibroblastic growth almost completely stopped, whereas in keloids it continued. Theoretically, this implies that any therapeutic intervention after excision to preclude development of keloids in keloid formers should be performed within 3 weeks or shortly thereafter.

Clinically and histologically keloids go through three phases.[31] The first phase is the fibroblastic phase, which lasts for a few months and is characterized by fibroblast and vascular proliferation and at which time the lesion appears red. With time, (months to years later), fibrous tissue is laid down, but the collagen is at first thin. This is the fibrous phase, at which time the lesion is less red (appearing pink) because of decreasing vascularity. After a longer time, usually years, a third and final phase is reached, the hyaline phase. At this point, the collagen is thick and in whorls. Clinically the keloid is white and hard.

The presence of the whorls of collagen (histologically seen as nodules) appears to be essential for keloid growth. These nodules seem to arise from fibroblasts that initially cuff blood vessels during wound healing.[36] Thus as the fibroblasts proliferate and lay down collagen, the early appearing blood vessels form a nidus for growth. Later these blood vessels are obliterated.

Compared to scars, keloids are more cellular and thus have an increased DNA content.[36] In addition, the rate of collagen synthesis per fibroblast appears to be increased[15] as it is in hypertrophic scars; however, the degradation rate is decreased.[9] This decreased degradation is not the result of collagenase deficiency because the collagenase level in keloids is actually elevated in keloids. Thus possibly the decreased collagen degradation is caused by inhibition of collagenase, for instance by α-globulins.

Additional discussion of keloids and hypertrophic scars can be found on pp. 72 to 75.

Histopathology

The microscopic appearance of mature keloids is characterized by large bands of collagen in the dermis. These bands often lie in a haphazard arrangement, or they can be arranged in nodules or whorls. Because of the expansile growth of keloid tissue, the overlying papillary dermis is thinned, and cutaneous appendages are atrophied.

The broad bands of collagen in keloids are usually associated with increased amounts of mucopolysaccharide ground substance. This association has been designated as "collagen bundle complexes" by two authors, who believe that such complexes are specific for keloids.[4] Lever, however, disagrees and thinks that keloids cannot be distinguished histologically from hypertrophic scars.[28] This author points out that both hypertrophic scars and keloids have nodules and whorls of collagen. However, in keloids these whorls persist, whereas in hypertrophic scars they flatten out and become aligned parallel to the surface of the skin.

Treatment

My preference is to excise keloids surgically. However, if excision is used to treat keloids, at least one other treatment modality must be used to ensure success. According to one study, there was a 38.5% recurrence rate for 244 lesions treated by excision alone and a higher recurrence rate (58%) if the patient had had pain or pruritus.[11] In addition, the success of surgical removal of keloids depends on creation of a wound with a lack of tension. Keloids arise spontaneously on the chest or shoulders, probably because of increased skin tension in those areas. If keloid tissue is autotransplanted to an area of low tension such as the inner thigh, the keloid mass atrophies.[6]

On excision of keloids, primary closure of the subsequent surgical defect results in tension on the wound edges. This occurs even if it appears as though one can simply excise a keloid along the maximal skin tension lines. Therefore some technique must be used to remove the ever-present tension.

One method of solving this problem is to use the epidermis and upper dermis overlying the keloid as a skin graft[1] or skin flap.[55] This tissue is usually unaffected by the underlying keloid collagen nodules. If used as a graft, the overlying epidermis with the upper dermis is carefully removed from the underlying keloid and any adherent firm tissue. Although removal may be difficult without perforating the epidermis, with patience and persistence it can be done. The separated normal tissue is then sutured into the surgical defect as a free full-thickness graft. One major advantage of this technique is that if a graft is mandatory because of the size of the surgical defect, a skin graft donor site can be avoided. Some physicians believe that total removal of keloidal tissue is unnecessary and that the recurrence rate is not increased if some is left behind.[12,44] Too few studies have been made to assess the recurrence rate when overlying keloidal epidermis is used to cover a partially excised keloid.

I prefer to use the overlying epidermis and upper dermis as a flap rather than a skin graft. Instead of initially removing the keloid totally, one makes an incision extending about halfway around the base. The keloid is then lifted back, and the fibrous tissue removed from the wound and

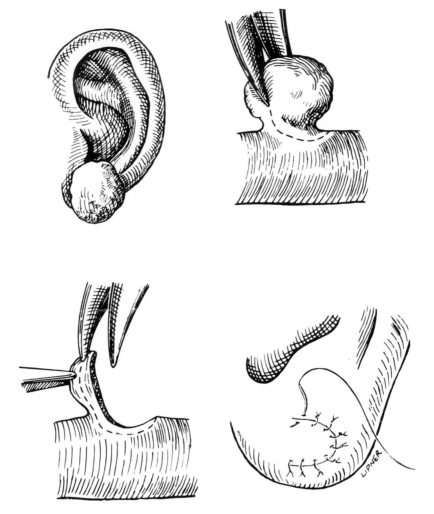

Fig. 23-3. Use of overlying skin (epidermis and dermis) to cover wound after removal of keloid. (From Weimer, V., and Ceilley, R.I.: J. Dermatol. Surg. Oncol. **5:**522. Copyright 1979, The Journal of Dermatologic Surgery and Oncology, Inc.)

from the underside of the upper dermis as much as possible without perforating the overlying tissue. One can ascertain that all the fibrous tissue has been removed by feeling the tissue. The epidermis with the upper dermis that is attached at one edge is then sutured into the surgical defect. My preference for this technique versus the free graft technique previously mentioned is that, by having one edge attached, one ensures a greater likelihood that the tissue will take and lessens the chance of necrosis.

The use of overlying epidermis and dermis is shown schematically in Fig. 23-3. Fig. 23-4, *A,* show a keloid of the posterior earlobe. The keloid is incised along one side and the nodular tissue underlying the epidermis and superficial dermis is removed (Fig. 23-4, *B*). The skin is then tailored to fit the surgical defect and used as a flap (Fig. 23-4, *C*). It is sutured into the surgical defect (Fig. 23-4, *D*). Note that the contour of the earlobe is preserved (Fig. 23-4, *E*), making this an ideal method in this location. Also note that the previously created tracts going through the

earlobe have been removed and sutured. Fig. 23-4, *F* and *G,* shows the patient at 6 months after surgery with no regrowth of the keloid. Postoperative steroid injections were given (Kenalog, 10 mg/ml at 1 week, 1 month, and 3 months).

A good pressure dressing is important when one uses this technique. Usually the dressing is left in place for at least 24 hours to preclude excessive bleeding into the wound. Should this occur, tension can be created in the wound edges, and the keloid may reform. A foam-padded aluminum finger splint, commonly used in emergency rooms for maintaining digits in the position of function, may be adapted for dressing the earlobe after keloid excision.[27] The aluminum splint is cut to the right length, and a double right-angle bend is fashioned to mold over the earlobe.

Steroid injections are an important adjunct to the surgical treatment of keloids. I usually inject into the wound edges triamcinolone, 10 mg/ml, 1 week after surgery at the time of suture removal. This is followed by subsequent injections

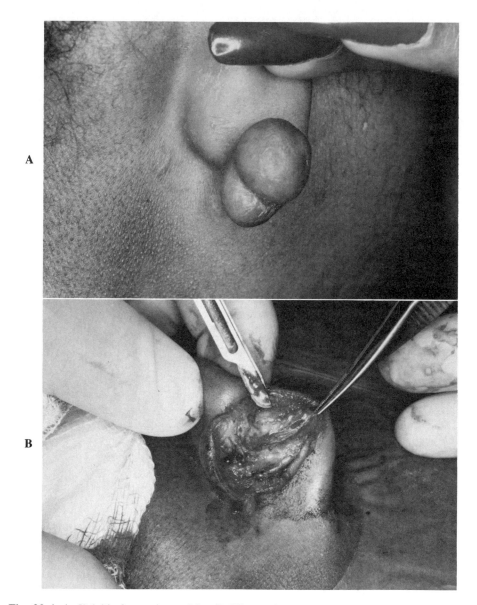

Fig. 23-4. A, Keloid of posterior earlobe. **B,** Fibrous tissue removed leaving overlying skin intact.

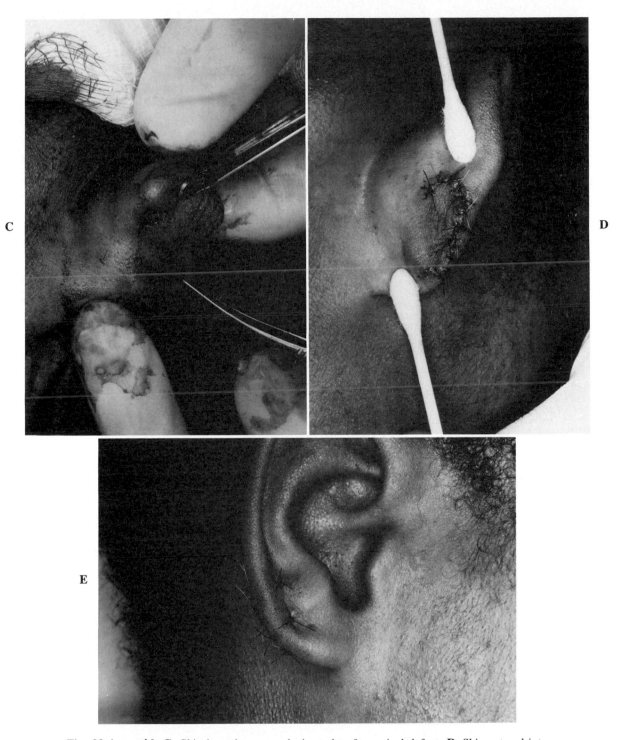

Fig. 23-4, cont'd. C, Skin brought over and trimmed to fit surgical defect. **D,** Skin sutured into surgical defect (posterior view). **E,** Anterior view. Note good contour and sutures in anterior portion of lobe at exit of fibrous tract. *Continued.*

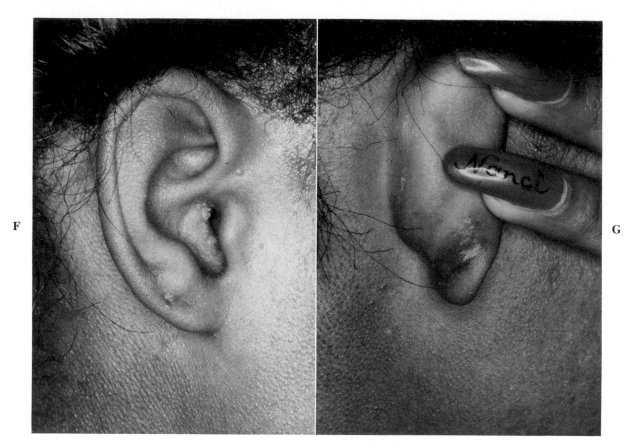

Fig. 23-4, cont'd. F and **G,** Healed wound 6 months postoperatively. Patient injected with triamcinolone acetonide (10 mg/ml) at time of suture removal, and 1 month and 3 months postoperatively.

of the same concentration at 3 to 4 week intervals for two or three sessions and then less frequently as required for 1 year after surgery. If the patient is doing well, the subsequent injections are given at 2- to 3-month intervals.

A reasonable time for injection of steroids seems to be 1 week after surgery, because immediate injection may lead to dehiscence.[37] Although this occurs in a small percentage of cases, it is best to avoid the problem if possible. Since the patient needs to return for suture removal anyway, injection at that time would be convenient. Because fibroblasts in future keloids do not appear to deviate from normal in their growth pattern for at least 3 weeks following surgery,[31] injection of steroids should be given before this time.

Some authors advise removing earlobe keloids in toto and suturing the resultant surgical defect side-to-side.[46] Although this may be performed successfully when the keloid is small, large keloids should not be removed in this manner. Fig. 23-5 shows an earlobe from which the keloid was simply removed and the surgical defect sutured. Note that the lobe is poorly contoured and almost absent.

Earlobe keloids sometimes occur simultaneously in front of and behind the earlobe. Usually the anterior keloid is smaller than the posterior keloid, and frequently there is only a small papule on the anterior portion of the earlobe. Because at one time when the ears were successfully pierced an epidermized tract extended through the earlobe, there is fibrosed tissue between these two keloids or between the small anterior papule and the posterior keloid. This fibrosed tract should be completely removed, since it can form a nidus for future keloids. Therefore, when removing earlobe keloids, one needs to remove the "core" of the keloid from posterior to anterior. Usually the anterior portion of the lobe can be sutured primarily, since the resultant surgical defect is very small and the posterior surgical defect can be sutured side to side. If the anterior and posterior keloids are both sizable, I usually operate on one side at a time and use the procedure shown in Fig. 23-3. Alternatively, both anterior and posterior keloids could be removed at the same time along with the connecting central fibrosed tract: the removed tissue then would be dumbbell-shaped.[23,46] Closure of the resultant defect is either performed side-to-side (horizontal in the front and vertical in

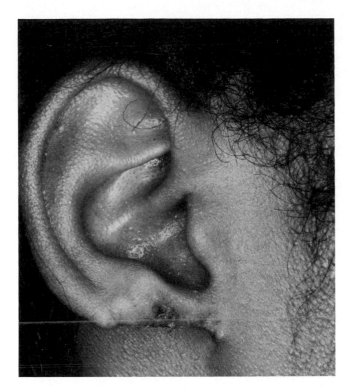

Fig. 23-5. Poorly contoured earlobe after large keloid removal and simple closure. Use of method in Fig. 23-4 would have resulted in naturally contoured earlobe.

TABLE 23-1

Treatment modalities for keloids

Modality	Published cure rates
Surgical excision alone (total or intra-keloidal removal)	
Clinically keloid	61.5%[11]
Clinically and histologically keloid	37%[14]-53%[11]
Steroid injection alone	73.8%[20]
Surgical excision + steroid injection	
All keloids	94%[20]-100%[35]
Earlobe keloids	88%[51]-100%[3]
Surgical excision + irradiation	79%[39]-88%[16]
Surgical excision + graft from keloid	60%[1]
Surgical excision + graft from distant site	None
Surgical excision + pressure	
Earlobe keloids	100%[5,33]
Cryosurgery alone	12%[49]
Cryosurgery + steroid injection	76%[22]
Laser	55%[21]
Retinoic acid (topical)	None[14]
Methotrexate	None[41]
Excision + BAPN or penicillamine + colchicine	100%[42]

the back)[46]; or the inferior portion of the lobe is excised, and the edges advanced.[23] In my opinion both of the latter two techniques lead to poorly contoured earlobes, especially if the keloids are large. This can be prevented by operating on one side at a time with the method previously outlined in Fig. 23-3.

Assessment of treatment methods

Many papers have addressed different methods of treatment of keloids (Table 23-1). In reviewing these publications it becomes clear that no single method of treatment ensures success. Each case must be assessed individually. In addition, most studies of keloid treatment contains two flaws: (1) histopathologic criteria are not used to confirm that the lesions under study are keloids, and (2) long-term (at least 2-year) follow-up examinations are not performed. Distinguishing a keloid histopathologically from a hypertrophic scar becomes important when assessing results of therapy, because it can sometimes be difficult to distinguish a keloid from a hypertrophic scar by clinical appearance alone. Ideally the initial and recurring histopathology of both should be correlated to long-term follow-up data. The importance of the histopathologic study of treated keloids was demonstrated by one group of authors who found that 63% of lesions recurred if labeled histopathologically as keloids, but only 10% recurred if labeled histopathologically

as hypertrophic scars.[4] Most keloids regrow by 2 years after treatment, so that this should be the ideal minimal time for follow-up examination.[24,39,51] In one study the median time of recurrence of keloids was 12.9 months.[11] The physician and patient need to realize that the treatment of a keloid is a long-term management problem.

It should also be stressed that keloids in different sites can respond differently to alternative forms of therapy. For example, earlobe keloids, which are frequently the result of infection, seem to respond well to all forms of therapy. However, keloids on the chest have a more variable response. Keloids that recur after therapy and those that occur in patients with multiple keloids have a poor prognosis.[11]

Excision alone. Excision of keloids alone yields a fairly high chance of recurrence, 38.5% in one study.[11] Interestingly, with this treatment there does not seem to be a correlation between the likelihood of recurrence and the completeness of keloid excision.[12,34]

Steroid injection alone. One of the earliest reports of steroid injection alone for treatment of keloids was a case of a 9-year-old black male with a very large keloid on the neck.[30] Triamcinolone acetonide (10 mg/ml) was injected at 4- to 6-week intervals. Review of the photographs shows some but not total resolution of the keloid. Therefore, although some response may occur with steroids, complete regression is usually not the rule.

A series of 95 patients with keloids (without histopathologic confirmation) was studied, 61 of whom were injected with triamcinolone acetonide alone and 34 of whom were injected with triamcinolone acetonide in addition to surgical excision.[20] Of those patients with keloids that were only injected, 26.2% (16 of 61) showed either no improvement or a recurrence after initial improvement. Ten of 61 developed atrophy, and two of 61 developed depigmentation of the surrounding skin. In most cases the depigmentation and atrophy disappeared within 1 year.

The lack of response to steroid injection into keloids or hypertrophic scars should arouse suspicion that an embedded foreign body may be present. One case was reported of an earlobe "keloid" that was the result of an earring clasp that had become buried in the tissue of the earlobe.[47] Wire suture in abdominal scars can also irritate the overlying tissues and result in hypertrophic scars or keloids. These conditions do not resolve completely until the underlying foreign body is removed.

The injection of steroids for keloids or hypertrophic scars is done intralesionally and not around or underneath the lesion. This requires a large amount of pressure to force the steroid into the tight fibrous matrix and may be facilitated by use of a tuberculin syringe with a Luer Lok. A 30-gauge needle is preferable, since it causes less pain on insertion into skin. The tuberculin syringe allows one to inject material more efficiently and easily (see Chapter 6). Usually only small amounts (0.05 ml) are injected in one area. The side effects of dermal atrophy and depigmentation occur in association with high steroid concentrations (40 mg/ml), indirect steroid spillage from the keloid or hypertrophic scar into the surrounding normal tissue, or direct injection into the surrounding skin. Spillage may occur, in part caused by the great force necessary to inject into the fibrous tissue. If the steroid is properly placed, the keloid or hypertrophic scar blanches superficially. Before injections, one should shake the syringe to keep the steroid from settling out and becoming more or less concentrated at the injection site.

The injection of keloids or hypertrophic scars is painful. This pain is probably mostly related to tissue expansion. Some physicians recommend the addition of lidocaine to the steroid mixture to lessen the pain. However, since the injection of a local anesthetic is itself painful, this probably is of little value in lessening the pain of injection.

The dosage and time intervals for injection of keloids vary somewhat with the response to treatment. These variables have not been well studied. Total dosages at one treatment session ranging from 5 to 10 mg[55] to as much as 120 mg[25] have been recommended. However, the higher dosages run the risk of producing systemic side effects as well as local atrophy and depigmentation. Systemic side effects and suppression of the endogenous corticoid production may be expected with dosages of 60 mg of triamcinolone acetonide every 30 days. For children, one needs to be mindful of the possible systemic effects at lower dosages. The usual dosage is 1 to 2 ml of 10 mg/ml of triamcinolone acetonide given at monthly intervals. The clinical course dictates the frequency and dosage of subsequent injections. For patients unresponsive to 10 mg/ml, increasing concentrations of up to 40 mg/ml may be considered.[17] Since the deposition of triamcinolone acetonide gives some effect in the tissue for 3 to 4 weeks, injections more frequently probably serve to increase the tissue dosage and thus may be unnecessary or at least no better than simply increasing the dosage at each treatment session. However, recurrent keloids, large keloids, or keloids in true keloid formers with multiple keloids may need the higher concentrations of steroid to produce regression.

Empirically triamcinolone acetonide (Kenalog) appears to be the steroid of choice for injection into keloids or hypertrophic scars. The fact that its effect lasts about 1 month makes it most suitable for this purpose. Other injectable steroids act for only a short time (few days)—for example, betamethasone sodium phosphate (Celestone)—or a long time (2 or 3 months)—for example, triamcinolone hexacetonide (Aristospan).

The mechanism of action of triamcinolone in keloids or hypertrophic scars is unknown. It does not appear to alter collagen formation or protein synthesis in keloids but may act by inhibiting histamine release or perhaps by removing a collagenase inhibitor such as an α-globulin.[9] Perhaps immune mechanisms that could be involved in keloid production and regression may also be modulated by steroids.

Surgical excision and subsequent steroid injection. Currently the most frequent treatment of keloids is undoubtedly surgical excision followed by steroid injection. For large keloids on the trunk (larger than 15 cm²) or any keloid on the face, this is the preferred method of treatment.[25] The injection of steroids for 1 to 2 months before excision and after excision is advocated by a few physicians,[55] but there are no data to substantiate that this works any better than steroid injections following excision.

One group[20] injected 34 keloids following excision. The recurrence rate was 6% (2 of 34). In 31 of these patients steroid was injected into the wound edges at the time of surgery and not subsequently. Only 2 of these 31 recurred. In three patients, steroid was injected not only at the time of surgery but at a later date as well. None of these three cases recurred. Similar results were reported on earlobe keloids with injection at the time of surgery and reinjection 1 week later.[3] Of 19 keloids thus treated, there were no recurrences, although one patient required two additional injections. One patient had dehiscence of the wound edges. Similarly good results with this method on earlobe keloids have been reported by others.[35,51]

The use of steroid injection 3 weeks postoperatively and twice thereafter at 1 month intervals but not at the time of surgery was reported.[50] The cure rate was 97%, which is comparable to that in the other studies cited, in which steroids were given at the time of surgery. Therefore there does not seem to be an advantage to steroid injection at the time of surgery, and in fact it may be disadvantageous because of the potential problem of wound dehiscence. Therefore, as previously stated, I prefer to wait at least 1 week before instituting postoperative steroid injections. As an alternative, some physicians advise leaving the sutures in place for 2 weeks before removal to prevent dehiscence when steroids are injected at the time of surgery.[44] This is probably unwise because of the known problem of suture tract epidermization with subsequent track marks.

Excision with subsequent skin graft and steroid injection. Excision of an ear keloid followed by a skin graft (full-thickness) followed by Kenalog-40 injection has been proposed on the basis of one successful case thus treated.[10] No study on this approach has been studied, so its efficacy in comparison with other methods is unknown.

Cryosurgery alone. Freezing keloids in an effort to produce regression has had its advocates.[38,56] The advantages of cryosurgery are that it is fast, easy, and results in no blood loss. Often cited as particular advantages of cryosurgery compared with other forms of surgery are the lack of scarring produced and the lessened likelihood of reformation of the treated keloids. Minimal scarring can be particularly advantageous for lesions on the chest or back. The disadvantages include loss of pigment, which may be a problem for blacks.

How well does cryosurgery alone work on keloids? A spray apparatus was used on 17 keloid scars.[49] Only two scars exhibited a decreased volume with one treatment. Furthermore, almost half of the 17 patients showed less than 50% improvement with additional cryosurgery. Therefore, compared with other methods, the technique does not seem to work particularly well.

Cryosurgery followed by steroid injection. The use of cryosurgery first to freeze the keloid followed by injection of triamcinolone was reported.[7] As the frozen keloid thaws, it becomes pink, softer, and edematous; swelling facilitates the injection of steroid. Steroid injection is also less painful for patients after cryosurgery, and even if cryosurgery and steroid together do not cause complete regression of the keloid, the combination makes subsequent surgery easier.[2]

A series of 58 patients on whom this technique was used was reported.[22] Seventy-one percent showed complete regression, 14% showed partial regression, and 15% regressed but then recurred. Earlobe keloids proved to be the most responsive, whereas keloids in the sternum or shoulders were the most resistant. This treatment response is also the case with all other forms of therapy.

Surgical extirpation followed by cryosurgery. Zacarian[57] advises surgical removal of keloid tissue followed by freezing the base of the surgical defect. This method does not require full removal of the keloid tissue; rather, the lesion may simply be "shaved off." After freezing, steroid injections can be given. He also suggests the use of cones if a spray device is used to extend the ice front in depth and prefers the cryoprobe over the cryospray apparatus for treatment of keloids.

Pressure. Continuous and even pressure on hypertrophic scars causes flattening.[18] On keloids, pressure is also beneficial if used after excision. However, pressure alone does not appear to work on keloids. The mechanisms of pressure on hypertrophic scars and keloids is unclear. One hypothesis is that pressure leads to tissue hypoxia with degeneration of fibroblasts and a decrease in collagen synthesis.

Pressure devices for use following earlobe keloid excision have been described. These include specially molded plastic devices with a spring ("oyster splints"),[33,48] buttons on each side of the earlobe that are sutured into place through the lobe,[52] and simple earrings with springs worn after surgery. A spring pressure earring is specially made for this purpose by the Padgett Instrument Co. (Kansas City, Mo. 64108). To be effective, the device should provide uniform adjustable compression and be easy to apply and clean. Caution should be exercised, since pressure necrosis can occur when a pressure device is applied immediately after surgery, particularly if intraoperative steroids have been used. Therefore it is recommended that, if these devices are used, their application should be delayed until about 2 weeks after surgery.[5]

The successful use of spring pressure earrings after excision of bilateral earlobe keloids in 5 patients was reported by Brent.[5] The pressure device was used on only one lobe in each patient. Three of five patients developed thickening on the earlobe on which the spring device was not used. Subsequent use of the spring device resulted in resolution of the thickening. In another study excellent results and high cure rates were also reported with a spring pressure device.[33]

Radiation following excision. X-radiation has been used after excision of keloids with good results.[16] Radiation works because it retards the growth of endothelial vascular buds, which are extremely radiosensitive. In addition, proliferation of new fibroblasts is decreased.

Good results with the use of radiation following excision of keloids have been reported by several investigators.[16,24,29] For example, in one study[39] 68 lesions in 40 patients were treated by intrakeloidal excision followed by x-radiation. A total dose of 1500 rad was given (using a 100 kV machine at 15 ma with 1 mm aluminum filtration) in three equal doses, beginning within 2 to 3 hours after surgery and then at 2- to 3-day intervals. The overall cure rate in this study was 79%, regardless of site. Complications following x-radiation of keloids included hyperpigmentation, telangiectasia, and atrophy.[16]

Laser. Excision of keloids with the CO_2 or argon laser is currently a popular method of removal. Theoretically, because the laser may slow the wound-healing process, it may be useful in keloid excision by preventing regrowth after removal. However, the published results to date are not any better than with other modalities and are worst than most. For example, one author reports good-to-excellent results in only 55% of patients.[21]

Miscellaneous pharmacologic agents. Retinoic acid was proposed for topical use on keloids because it is known to decrease DNA synthesis of fibroblasts in tissue culture. A favorable response was reported in 77% of keloids on which topical retinoid acid was used.[14]

The use of methotrexate on keloids has been proposed.[41] However, a preliminary report did not show this to be useful.[44] Nitrogen mustard combined with triamcinolone and hyaluronidase also has been suggested for injection of keloids.[40]

Two lathyrogenic agents, β-aminopropionitrile (BAPN) or penicillamine, combined with colchicine (as a tissue collagenase stimulant) have been tried in patients following excision of keloids.[42] Although the results are encouraging (no recurrences of keloids in 15 patients), this has yet to be confirmed by other authors.

REFERENCES

1. Apfelberg, D.B., Maser, M.R., and Lash, H.: The use of epidermis over a keloid as an autograft after resection of the keloid, J. Dermatol. Surg. **2:**409, 1976.
2. Babin, R.W., and Ceilley, R.I.: Combined modalities in the management of hypertrophic scars and keloids, J. Otolaryngol. **8:**457, 1979.
3. Barton, R.P.E.: Auricular keloids: a simple method of management, Ann. R. Coll. Surg. **60:**324, 1978.
4. Blackburn, W.R., and Cosman, B.: Histologic basis of keloid and hypertrophic scar differentiation: clinicopathologic correlation, Arch. Pathol. **82:**65, 1966.
5. Brent, B.: The role of pressure therapy in management of earlobe keloids: preliminary report of a controlled study, Ann. Plast. Surg. **1:**579, 1978.
6. Calnan, J.S., and Copenhagen, H.J.: Autotransplantation of keloid in man, Br. J. Surg. **54:**330, 1967.
7. Ceilley, R.I., and Babin, R.W.: The combined use of cryosurgery and intralesional injections of suspensions of fluorinated adrenocorticosteroids for reducing keloids and hypertrophic scars, J. Dermatol. Surg. Oncol. **5:**54, 1979.
8. Cohen, I.K., et al.: Histamine and collagen synthesis in keloid and hypertrophic scar, Surg. Forum **23:**509, 1972.
9. Cohen, I.K., and Diegelmann, R.F.: The biology of keloid and hypertrophic scar and the influence of corticosteroids, Clin. Plast. Surg. **4**(2):297, 1977.
10. Converse, J.M., and Stallings, J.O.: Eradication of large auricular keloids by excision, skin grafting, and intradermal injection of triamcinolone acetonide solution: case report, Plast. Reconstr. Surg. **49:**461, 1972.
11. Cosman, B., et al.: The surgical treatment of keloids, Plast. Reconstr. Surg. **27:**335, 1961.
12. Cosman, B., and Wolff, M.: Correlation of keloid recurrence with completeness of local excision: a negative report, Plast. Reconstr. Surg. **50:**163, 1972.
13. Crockett, D.J.: Colour, cancer, and keloids in the Sudan, Br. J. Plast. Surg. **15:**408, 1962.
14. De Limpens, A.M.P.J.: The local treatment of hypertrophic scars and keloids with topical retinoic acid, Br. J. Dermatol. **103:**319, 1980.
15. Diegelmann, R.F., Cohen, I.K., and McCoy, B.J.: Growth kinetics and collagen synthesis of normal skin, normal scar and keloid fibroblasts in vitro, J. Cell Physiol. **98:**341, 1979.
16. Enhamre, A., and Hammar, H.: Treatment of keloids with excision and postoperative x-ray irradiation, Dermatologica **167:**90, 1983.
17. Freeman, R.G.: Data on the action spectrum for ultraviolet carcinogenesis, J. Nat. Cancer Inst. **55:**1119, 1975.
18. Fujimori, R., Hiramoto, M., and Ofuji, S.: Sponge fixation method for treatment of early scars, Plast. Reconstr. Surg. **42:**322, 1968.
19. Goette, D.K., and Helwig, E.B.: Basal cell carcinomas and basal cell carcinoma-like changes overlying dermatofibromas, Arch. Dermatol. **111:**589, 1975.
20. Griffith, B.H., Monroe, C.W., and McKinney, P.: A follow-up study on the treatment of keloids with triamcinolone acetonide, Plast. Reconstr. Surg. **46:**145, 1970.
21. Henderson, D.L., Cromwell, T.A., and Mes, L.G.: Argon and carbon dioxide laser treatment of hypertrophic and keloid scars, Lasers Surg. Med. **3:**271, 1984.
22. Hirshowitz, B., Lerner, D., and Moscona, A.R.: Treatment of keloid scars by combined cryosurgery and intralesional corticosteroids, Aesth. Plast. Surg. **6:**153, 1982.
23. Howell, S., Warpeha, R., and Brent, B.: A technique for excising earlobe keloids, Surg. Gynecol. Obstet. **141:**438, 1975.
24. Inalsingh, C.H.A.: An experience in treating five hundred and one patients with keloids, Johns Hopkins Med. J. **134:**284, 1974.
25. Ketchum, L.D., Robinson, D.W., and Masters, F.W.: Follow-up on treatment of hypertrophic scars and keloids with triamcinolone, Plast. Reconstr. Surg. **48:**256, 1971.
26. Kischer, C.W., Shetlar, M.R., and Shetlar, C.L.: Alteration of hypertrophic scars induced by mechanical pressure, Arch. Dermatol. **111:**60, 1975.
27. Lapidus, S.M., and Davis, R.K.: A simple dressing for earlobes, Plast. Reconstr. Surg. **59:**287, 1977.
28. Lever, W.F., and Schaumburg-Lever, G.: Histopathology of the skin, ed. 6, Philadelphia, 1983, J.B. Lippincott Co.
29. Levy, D.S., Salter, M.M., and Roth, R.E.: Postoperative irradiation in the prevention of keloids, Am. J. Roentgenol. **127:**509, 1976.
30. Maguire, H.C., Jr.: Treatment of keloids with triamcinolone acetonide injected intralesionally, J.A.M.A. **192:**325, 1965.
31. Mancini, R.E., and Quaife, J.V.: Histogenesis of experimentally produced keloids, J. Invest. Dermatol. **38:**143, 1962.
32. McPeak, C.J., Cruz, T., and Nicastri, A.D.: Dermatofibrosarcoma protuberans: an analysis of 86 cases—five with metastasis, Ann. Surg. **166:**803, 1967.
33. Mercer, D.M., and Studd, D.M.M.: "Oyster splints": a new compression device for the treatment of keloid scars of the ear, Br. J. Plast. Surg. **36:**75, 1983.
34. Minkowitz, F.: Regression of massive keloid following partial

excision and post-operative intralesional administration of triamcinolone, Br. J. Plast. Surg. **20**:432, 1967.

35. Moreno, F.G., et al.: Facial keloids and their management, Ear Nose Throat J. **60**:519, 1981.

36. Murray, J.C., Pollack, S.V., and Pinnell, S.R.: Keloids: a review, J. Am. Acad. Dermatol. **4**:461, 1981.

37. Murray, R.D.: Kenalog and the treatment of hypertrophied scars and keloids in negroes and whites, Plast. Reconstr. Surg. **31**:275, 1963.

38. Muti, E., and Ponzio, E.: Cryotherapy in the treatment of keloids, Ann. Plast. Surg. **11**:227, 1983.

39. Ollstein, R.N., et al.: Treatment of keloids by combined surgical excision and immediate postoperative x-ray therapy, Ann. Plast. Surg. **7**:281, 1981.

40. Oluwasanmi, J.O.: Keloids in the African, Clin. Plast. Surg. **1**(1):179, 1974.

41. Onwukwe, M.F.: Surgery and methotrexate for keloids, Schoch Letter **28**:4, 1978.

42. Peacock, E.E., Jr.: Control of wound healing and scar formation in surgical patients, Arch. Surg. **116**:1325, 1981.

43. Pierce, H.E.: Keloids: enigma of the plastic surgeon, J. Natl. Med. Assoc. **71**:1177, 1979.

44. Pollack, S.V., and Goslen, J.B.: The surgical treatment of keloids, J. Dermatol. Surg. Oncol. **8**:1045, 1982.

45. Robinson, J.K.: Dermatofibrosarcoma protuberans resected by Mohs' surgery (chemosurgery): a 5-year prospective study, J. Am. Acad. Dermatol. **12**:1093, 1985.

46. Salasche, S.J., and Grabski, W.J.: Keloids of the earlobes: a surgical technique, J. Dermatol. Surg. Oncol. **9**:552, 1983.

47. Saleeby, E.R., et al.: Embedded foreign bodies presenting as earlobe keloids, J. Dermatol. Surg. Oncol. **10**:902, 1984.

48. Sela, M., and Taicher, S.: Prosthetic treatment of earlobe keloids, J. Prosthet. Dent. **52**:417, 1984.

49. Shepherd, J.P., and Dawber, R.P.R.: The response of keloid scars to cryosurgery, Plast. Reconstr. Surg. **70**:677, 1982.

50. Shons, A.R., and Press, B.H.J.: The treatment of earlobe keloids by surgical excision and postoperative triamcinolone injection, Ann. Plast. Surg. **10**:480, 1983.

51. Singleton, M.A., and Gross, C.W.: Management of keloids by surgical excision and local injections of a steroid, South. Med. J. **64**:1377, 1971.

52. Snyder, G.B.: Button compression for keloids of the lobule, Br. J. Plast. Surg. **27**:186, 1974.

53. Taylor, H.B., and Helwig, E.B.: Dermatofibrosarcoma protuberans: a study of 115 cases, Cancer **15**:717, 1962.

54. Topol, B.M., Lewis, V.L., Jr., and Benveniste, K.: The use of antihistamine to retard the growth of fibroblasts derived from human skin, scar, and keloid. Plast. Reconstr. Surg. **68**:227, 1981.

55. Weimar, V.M., and Ceilley, R.I.: Treatment of keloids on earlobes, J. Dermatol. Surg. Oncol. **5**:522, 1979.

56. Zacarian, S.A.: Cryosurgery of tumors of the skin and oral cavity, Springfield, Ill., 1973, Charles C Thomas Publisher.

57. Zacarian, S.A.: Discussion of Shepherd, J.P., and Dawber, R.P.R.: The response of keloid scars to cryosurgery, Plast. Reconstr. Surg. **70**:682, 1982.

24

Lesions of Vascular Tissue

CHERRY HEMANGIOMAS

Cherry hemangiomas (senile hemangiomas) are common lesions appearing as bright red papules of small size (1 to 6 mm) and usually occurring on the trunk. These papules tend to be dome-shaped. Microscopically, cherry hemangiomas are seen to be composed of dilated capillaries (Fig. 24-1).

Treatment

Usually treatment is unnecessary except for cosmetic purposes. The simplest method to remove these lesions is by means of a curette. One author[2] recommends the argon laser for these lesions, since the wavelength from this instrument is selectively absorbed by the color of the lesion.

PYOGENIC GRANULOMA

A pyogenic granuloma is a common vascular tumor appearing as a soft, red papule 0.5 to 1 cm in size (Fig. 24-2). The surface is smooth, but superficial ulceration and crusting may occur. If traumatized, the lesion bleeds easily. Most commonly pyogenic granulomas are found on the face and extremities.

Histopathology

Under the microscope a pyogenic granuloma appears as a well-circumscribed pedunculated lesion consisting of granulation tissue covered by a flattened epidermis. The granulation tissue consists of newly formed capillaries with endothelial cell proliferation. The capillary lumina are prominent. Also present is fibroblastic proliferation within an edematous stroma.

Treatment

Usually simple curettage with light electrodesiccation of the base cures a pyogenic granuloma. Laser treatment may also be of value and perhaps result in less potential for scarring.[1]

Rarely, a "pyogenic granuloma" may arise in response to an underlying foreign body (see Figs. 13-4 and 28-2). Therefore, if the pyogenic granuloma is persistent and recurrent, the underlying tissue should be probed for foreign substances, such as metal or wood splinters.

Melanomas also occasionally resemble pyogenic granulomas. Therefore submission of tissue for biopsy is mandatory on removal of pyogenic granulomas.

CONGENITAL HEMANGIOMAS

The common congenital hemangiomas usually occur in one of three forms: (1) the nevus flammeus, (2) the strawberry hemangioma, and (3) the cavernous hemangioma. All of these hemangiomas occur at birth or shortly thereafter.

The nevus flammeus is also called the port-wine stain. It appears as a flat pink or dark red patch with an irregular outline (Fig. 24-3, A). The most common variety occurs on the lower occipital scalp or posterior neck (the so-called "stork bite"). The less common variety is much larger and occurs away from the midline, usually on one side of the face or arm. In this location, with time, small papular hemangiomas may develop in adulthood. Occasionally a nevus flammeus may be associated with a deep underlying proliferation of blood vessels. For example, the Sturge-Weber syndrome is associated with ipsilateral retinal and meningeal angiomatosis. In the Klippel-Trenaunay-Weber syndrome, a nevus flammeus is associated with underlying hypertrophy of soft tissues and bone. Histopathologically one sees dilated capillaries but no apparent proliferation of vessels.

The strawberry hemangioma is a bright red papule or nodule that usually appears at about 1 month after birth (Fig. 24-3, B). It increases in size for the first 6 months or 1 year of life and then usually regresses spontaneously. Involution is characterized by whitish specks or streaks within

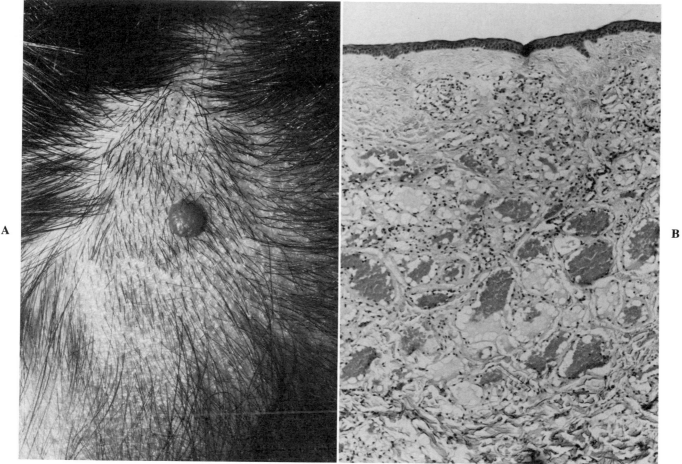

Fig. 24-1. **A,** Cherry hemangioma. **B,** Dilated capillaries within the dermis.

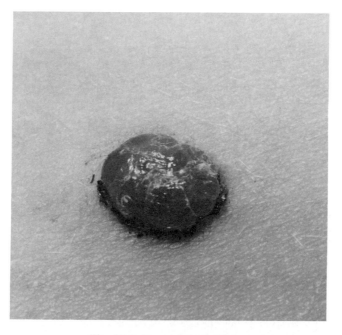

Fig. 24-2. Pyogenic granuloma.

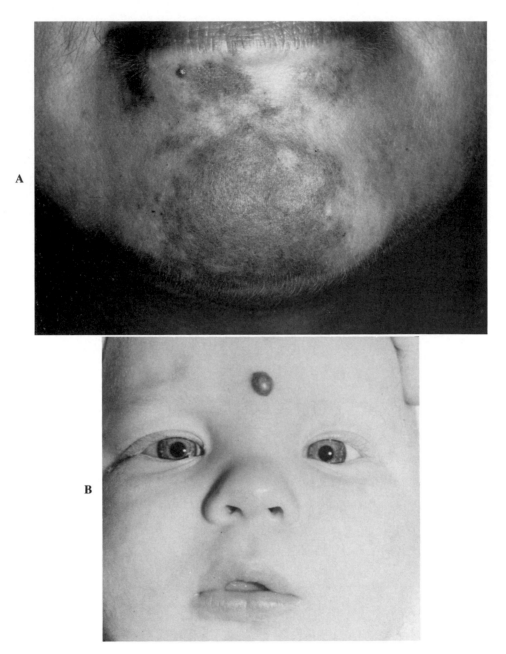

Fig. 24-3. A, Nevus flammeus in 30-year-old woman. **B,** Strawberry hemangioma in 3-month-old baby.

Continued.

the red lesion. Most strawberry hemangiomas regress by age 5, although a few may take longer. Little regression occurs after age 10. Histopathologically one sees proliferation of endothelial cells and also some dilated capillaries. With involution, the capillaries are replaced by fibrous tissue.

Cavernous hemangioma is a large mass that lies deeper than the other types of congenital hemangiomas. This type of hemangioma is red to deep purple and is spongy and compressible (Fig. 24-3, *C* and *D*). There is usually both a

superficial and a deep component. The cutaneous superficial portion is usually slightly elevated. The deep portion may be quite extensive and involve subdermal structures. A cavernous hemangioma may be associated with a nevus flammeus (Fig. 24-3, *D*) or strawberry hemangiomas. Large cutaneous cavernous hemangiomas can be accompanied by occult internal hemangiomas. Histopathologically one sees numerous large dilated vessels. The blue rubber-bleb nevus is a type of cavernous hemangioma characterized by numerous small (up to 3 to 4 cm in diameter) lesions

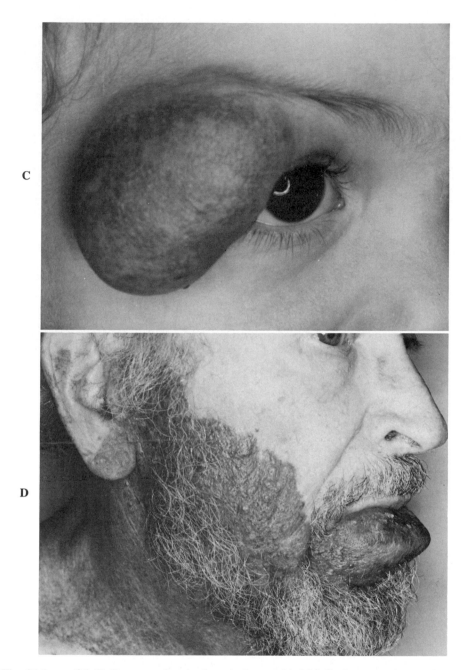

Fig. 24-3, cont'd. C, Cavernous hemangioma in 1-year-old child. **D,** Cavernous hemangioma with nevus flammeus component. Note protuberance of lower lip caused by infiltration by vascular tissue.

distributed widely on the skin surface and hemangiomas of the intestinal tract.

Treatment

The treatment of congenital hemangiomas is complex, and should be individualized. Underlying pathologic complications should be sought in all cases of nevus flammeus or cavernous hemangiomas.

A nevus flammeus usually requires no treatment except for cosmetic reasons. If treatment is desired, laser therapy should be considered. Camouflage by means of a tinted waterproof makeup may be satisfactory. Covermark (manufactured by Lydia O'Leary, New York City) or Dermablend (manufactured by Dermablend Corrective Cosmetics, Farmingdale, N.J.) might be useful.

A strawberry hemangioma is best treated by watchful waiting. Parents should be encouraged to avoid surgery, because the resultant scar is frequently worse than the result

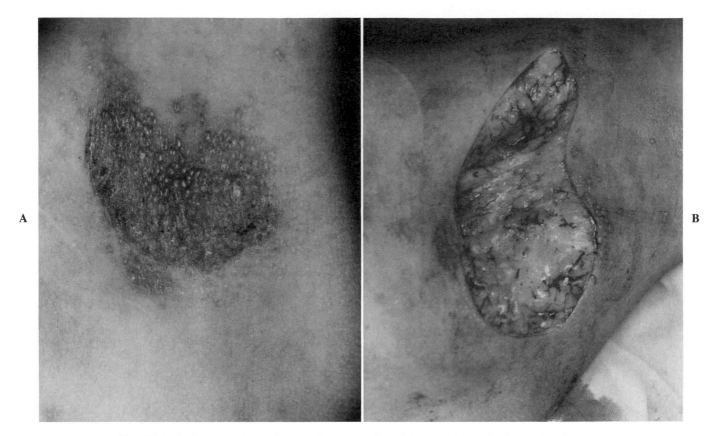

Fig. 24-4. A, Lymphangioma circumscriptum in axilla of 7-year-old boy. **B,** Subtotal excision.

from regression. However, under some unusual circumstances such as frequent bleeding or obstruction of vision, therapeutic intervention is required. Surgical excision is rarely required. Shrinkage of lesions can be facilitated by pressure (if on an extremity), systemic steroids, or local injection of steroids.[3,8] The latter needs to be done cautiously, since blindness can result from injection of steroids around the eyes.[4,6,7] Therefore injections of anesthetic mixtures combined with steroids should be avoided in the central face. Under experimental conditions, blindness with steroid injection is particularly apt to occur when the solution is mixed with an anesthetic containing epinephrine.[5] The epinephrine apparently induces vasospasm, which traps particles of the suspended steroid. Besides, the anesthetic itself is painful on injection, and thus it serves no purpose.

Many cavernous hemangiomas regress spontaneously despite their enormous size. The surgical treatment of cavernous hemangiomas is beyond the scope of this text. Systemic steroids may be useful to help shrink such lesions.[8]

LYMPHANGIOMA CIRCUMSCRIPTUM

Lymphangioma circumscriptum appears as grouped vesicle-like lesions resembling frog spawn. The lesions are clear or slightly yellowish and filled with lymph fluid. The grouping of lesions is usually localized to one region. Most often lymphangioma circumscriptum occurs on the trunk or axilla. The lesions may appear shortly after birth or in early life. Frequently, particularly in the axilla, there is diffuse swelling of the underlying tissue and the skin surface may appear verrucous (Fig. 24-4, *A*).

Histopathology

Dilated lymph vessels are present in the upper dermis and may extend into the subcutaneous fat.

Treatment

The treatment goal for lymphangioma circumscriptum is subtotal rather than total removal (Fig. 24-4, *B*). Even when extensive excisions are carried out for this condition, recurrences are the rule. Therefore one should balance the benefits of removal against considerations such as the appearance of the resultant scar. Usually subtotal excision gives the patient the best cosmetic result while achieving almost complete removal.

Fig. 24-4, *A*, shows lymphangioma circumscriptum in the axilla of a 7-year-old boy. Subtotal excision was performed with a lazy-S excision (Fig. 24-4, *B* and *C*). The

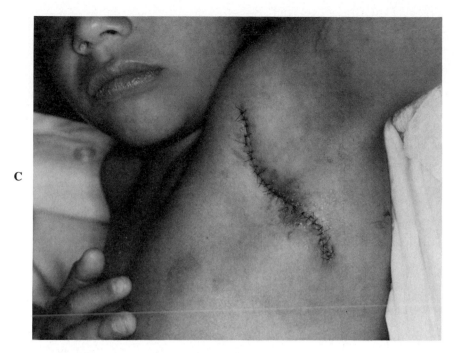

Fig. 24-4, cont'd. C, Wound sutured with lazy-S appearance. Patient has full range of motion in arm. Note remaining lymphangiomas.

final cosmetic result was acceptable, and the patient was pleased.

REFERENCES

1. Apfelberg, D.B., et al.: Efficacy of the carbon dioxide laser in hand surgery, Ann. Plast. Surg. **13:**320, 1984.
2. Arndt, K.A.: Argon laser therapy of small cutaneous vascular lesions, Arch. Dermatol. **118:**220, 1982.
3. Mazzola, R.F.: Treatment of haemangiomas in children by intralesional injections of steroids, Chir. Plast. **4:**161, 1978.
4. McGrew, R.N., Wilson, R.S., and Havener, W.H.: Sudden blindness secondary to injections of common drugs in the head and neck. I. Clinical experiences, Otolaryngology **86:**147, 1978.
5. McGrew, R.N., Wilson, R.S., and Havener, W.H.: Sudden blindness secondary to injections of common drugs in the head and neck. II. Animal studies, Otolaryngology **86:**152, 1978.
6. Selmanowitz, V.J., and Orentreich, N.: Cutaneous corticosteroid injection and amaurosis, Arch. Dermatol. **110:**729, 1974.
7. Shorr, N., and Seiff, S.R.: Central retinal artery occlusion associated with periocular corticosteroid steroid injection for juvenile hemangioma, Ophthalmic Surg. **17:**229, 1986.
8. Zarem, H.A., and Edgerton, M.T.: Induced resolution of cavernous hemangiomas following prednisolone therapy, Plast. Reconstr. Surg. **39:**76, 1967.

Lesions of Neural and Fat Tissue

NEUROFIBROMA

Neurofibromas usually appear as papules superficial tumors, which may arise sporadically or in association with multiple neurofibromatosis (von Recklinghausen's disease). The latter condition is dominantly inherited and characterized not only by multiple neurofibromas but also by cafe-au-lait spots and axillary freckling. In addition, several internal organs may be involved. Roughly 10% of patients with neurofibromatosis develop pheochromocytoma. Epilepsy, mental retardation, and tumors of the cranial nerves are also common.

Clinical appearance

Neurofibromas are flesh-colored, soft, smooth lesions varying in size from a few millimeters to several centimeters. Sometimes neurofibromas become very large and pendulous. With finger pressure, these tumors can usually be invaginated into the skin, but they spring back when the pressure is released. The multiple neurofibromas that occur in von Recklinghausen's disease appear in late childhood and gradually increase in size and number. Usually they are widely disseminated (see illustration on p. 617).

Histopathology

A neurofibroma consists of wavy collagenous fibrils that frequently occupy the whole dermis. Usually this mass of fibrils is fairly well demarcated but occasionally it infiltrates surrounding tissue and may extend into subcutaneous fat. Oriented parallel with these fibrils are small spindle cells.

Treatment

Patients with multiple neurofibromas have a significant cosmetic problem. No one method of therapy is totally satisfactory for all lesions. Excision is adequate but must be balanced against the ultimate cosmetic results. Certainly some lesions can be managed in this way.

For removal of many lesions I have found that the loop on the electrosurgical apparatus is most satisfactory. The loop is placed around the lesion, and the neurofibroma is grasped with forceps and elevated through the loop (Fig. 25-1). The cutting current on the electrosurgical apparatus is selected and the loop is drawn through the base of the lesion. This current cuts the tissue and stops the bleeding simultaneously. The subsequent wound is allowed to heal by secondary intention. Although this form of treatment does not totally remove in depth the neurofibroma, regrowth is slow and patients appear to be pleased by the cosmetic result. The advantages of this procedure are its speed and the fact that many lesions can be removed within a short period of time.[19]

LIPOMA

Lipomas are common benign tumors of mesenchymal origin characterized by fairly well circumscribed collections of fat cells. Most often lipomas are located in the fatty subdermal tissue but they sometimes occur in deeper tissues as well. Lipomas may penetrate deeply, invading muscle fascia, muscle, and even bone. Although lipomas can occur anywhere within the body (subdermal, intramuscular, or visceral), they are usually situated in periaxial locations (nape of the neck, trunk, proximal upper and lower extremities, and sometimes on the face, scalp, or distal extremities.[1,20]

Clinical appearance

Typically lipomas are rounded or ovoid tumors that protrude slightly above the surface of the skin. Although lipomas vary in size from minute to enormous (Fig. 25-2), most are less than 5 cm.[20] On palpation, lipomas have a characteristic soft, doughy feel. Lipomas are usually lobulated. This lobulation can be made out if the mass is compressed between the thumb and index finger of one hand, and the

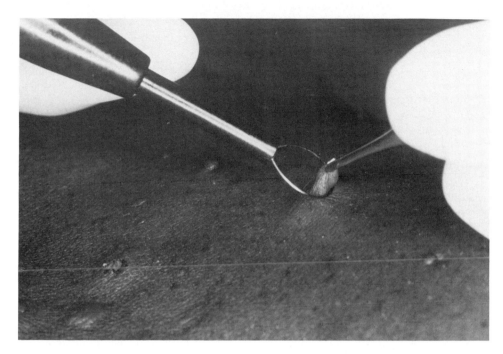

Fig. 25-1. Use of loop electrode on electrosurgical apparatus (set on cutting current) to remove neurofibroma.

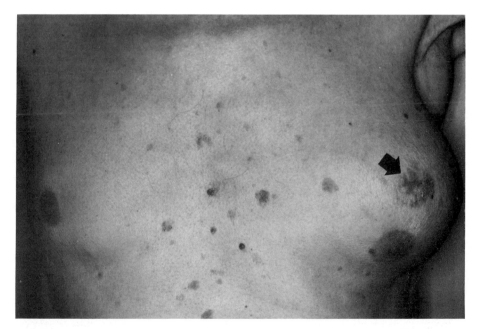

Fig. 25-2. Large lipoma of breast in man. Lesion *(arrow)* proved on biopsy to be irritated seborrheic keratosis.

surface—which is thereby made more prominent—is stroked by the index finger of the other hand.

One common entity sometimes confused with a lipoma is accessory breast tissue in women. Usually this appears in the axilla as a soft swelling and a history of enlargement with menses is usually obtained.

Incidence

A lipoma is one of the most common soft tissue tumors. Rydholm and Berg found that 1 out of 1000 patient visits per year were consultations for clinical lipomas.[20] Lipomas overall appear to be more common in women than in men,[1,20] although with multiple lipomas there is a strong male predominance.[20] Lipomas are rare in children and usually appear in early adulthood. The average age of patients with lipomas in one study was 41 years.[1]

Cause

The cause of lipomas is unknown but does not appear to be related to trauma. Patients with multiple lipomas often give a family history of similar lesions, so heredity undoubtedly plays some role. Multiple lipomas may be more common in diabetic persons. In an autopsy study there was a higher incidence of diabetes in patients with multiple lipomas of the gastrointestinal tract than in normal patients.[8] Lipomas themselves have also been found to have a metabolism different from that of normal subcutaneous fat in the same individual. Acetate incorporation occurs more rapidly in lipomas.[10]

Classification

Most lipomas may be clinically classified into four types: simple solitary, multiple, diffuse congenital, and diffuse symmetric in adults. In addition, lipomas may rarely occur in certain heritable disorders, for example Gardner's syndrome, which is also characterized by multiple cysts.

Simple solitary lipomas are the most common lipomas; they occur at any age and particularly when patients gain weight.[1] They are usually superficially located and small but may be deeper and larger.

Multiple lipomas in the same individual are also commonly seen and may represent a distinct clinical entity unrelated to solitary lipomas.[20] One study found that 6.7% of its patients had multiple lipomas, and the largest number in any subject was 160.[1] Frequently there is a family history of multiple lipomas[1]; Rydholm and Berg feel that this entity is transmitted in an autosomal dominant mode of inheritance with low penetrance.[20] There is a strong predominance for multiple lipomas in men, and many of these lesions tend to be angiolipomas, discussed later. The multiple lipomas are usually more or less symmetrically distributed.

Multiple lipomas can be associated with a few genetic syndromes. Dercum's disease (adiposis dolorosa) is a condition characterized by "obesity" and painful, multiple, symmetric, subcutaneous lipomas.[6] The obesity is really fairly well-defined collections of fat outwardly resembling obesity. Asthenia and psychologic disturbances (usually depression) may also be present. The family history is not usually relevant, but in some patients who have a family history, Dercum's disease appears to be transmitted as an autosomal dominant gene.[16] Other genetic syndromes associated with multiple lipomas include Gardner's syndrome (characterized by intestinal polyps, osteomas, fibromas, and multiple cysts in addition to lipomas) and multiple endocrine adenomatosis.[3]

Diffuse congenital lipomatosis occurs mainly on a baby's trunk as rolls of fat (the "Michelin tire" baby). Diffuse symmetric lipomatosis, usually of the neck, may appear in adult life, as described by Madelung; it may be familial.[5]

Differential diagnosis

Lipomas are always considered in the differential diagnosis of soft tissue neoplasms. Although the diagnosis of lipoma is usually readily apparent, one should consider a few other entities: besides liposarcoma there is a possibility of myxolipoma, hibernoma, and neurofibroma. Lipomas are associated rarely with neurofibromatosis and with cavernous hemangiomas, sometimes confusing the diagnosis.

Histopathology

Histopathologically lipomas are not much different from ordinary fat tissue except for the presence of increased fibrous tissue. Most lipomas are composed of mature lipocytes with eccentric nuclei and are categorized as either a lipoma or an angiolipoma. A lipoma is composed mostly of fat cells with little collagenous stroma, whereas an angiolipoma contains more fibrous tissue and a moderate to large number of blood vessels. This distinction may be somewhat arbitrary, however, because there is probably a continuum between these two histopathologic types. The difference in the blood vessels between angiolipoma and lipoma is purely quantitative. The typical angiolipoma also tends to be fairly well circumscribed by fibrous tissue, with extension of collagenous bundles into the tumor—producing incomplete fibrous septae and dividing it into lobular masses. Clinically an angiolipoma looks like a lipoma.

Howard and Helwig popularized the concept of angiolipomas.[13] Typically this histopathologic variant occurs in young patients shortly after puberty as painful, soft, subcutaneous lumps in the skin of the trunk or extremities.[4] These are followed by the development of 2 to 3 more each year for several years. Thus angiolipomas are the usual type of lipoma seen in the multiple lipoma lipomatosis just described, and a family history is obtained in about one third of patients.[4] Of the fatty tumors examined by Howard and Helwig, 17% were classified as angiolipomas.[13]

Angiolipomas are slightly painful; there is a vague tenderness on palpation. The cause of the pain is unknown. A suggestion has been made that an angiolipoma may compress neural structures and thus give rise to pain; however, when looked for, such envelopment was not readily apparent histologically.[4] Some investigators think that the pain is related to the amount of underlying vascular tissue,[13] but this is disputed by others.[4] The injection of various pharmacologic agents directly affecting blood vessels, such as histamine epinephrine, does not induce pain.[4]

Angiolipomas in general follow a benign course. However, there may be deeply infiltrating invasion into fibrocollagenous, neural, muscular, and even bony tissues.[15] Although the histopathology of such infiltrating angiolipomas is benign, such deep penetration may give rise to clinical suspicion of a malignant neoplasm.

Unusual variants. Lipomas may be very large, may occur in unusual anatomic locations, and may be unusually invasive. Fig. 25-2 shows a man with a large lipoma that resembles as a gigantic breast. Large lipomas of the vulva,[9] palm,[12] and foot[7] have also been described and may be confused with gigantism of these structures. When lipomas occur on the palm, fingers, or wrist, they may be attached to underlying tendons or nerves.[12,14,17] Therefore microdissection may be necessary at the time of removal.

Infiltrating lipomas are either simple lipomas or angiolipomas that infiltrate deeply and may be in a totally subfascial location. Lipomas are the most common subfascial tumors and histologically appear identical to superficial, non-subfascial lipomas or angiolipomas,[20] except that they may be relatively "unencapsulated".[4] Usually these deep-seated lipomas are slow growing and painless.

Infiltrating lipomas and angiolipomas may extend deeply into muscle. When this occurs, the individual muscle fibers may be separated by the lipoma. The lipoma becomes more readily palpable after contraction of the involved muscle group. Infiltrating angiolipomas are more firm and fixed than superficial lipomas because they have an increased amount of fibrous tissue. Sensory changes or muscle dysfunction may occur, caused by pressure on nerve trunks. An x-ray film may show a radiolucent mass that can be distinguished from bony structures.[2]

Malignant degeneration. Malignant change in lipomas or angiolipomas is rare if it occurs at all. Slow-growing lipomas may be confused with liposarcomas, which enlarge more quickly.[20] Since these two entities can clinically appear indistinguishable, histopathologic examination of removed lipoma tissue is recommended. In a surgical study from Sweden[20] it was not uncommon for patients to be referred for further surgery for a liposarcoma that had been clinically misinterpreted as a lipoma. Even in patients with multiple subcutaneous lipomas, malignant degeneration has been known to occur.[13] In one series, 4 of 134 "lipomas" (6.7%) were recurrent, and 1 of these 4 proved to be a liposarcoma.[1] Infiltrating "lipomas" greater than 10 cm on

the thigh have statistically been shown to be likely (much more likely than superficial lipomas of less than 5 cm in other locations) to be liposarcomas.[20] Therefore beware of large, deep "lipomas" located on the thigh and recurrent lipomas.

Treatment

The treatment of lipomas, should the patient desire this for cosmetic or psychologic reasons, is surgical removal. If the patient has multiple lesions, one or two may be removed to establish the diagnosis and to give the patient peace of mind; removal of many lesions inevitably leads to multiple scars, the undesirability of which must be weighed against the benefits to the patient.

Lipoma removal is based on the concept that these lesions are more or less circumscribed by fibrous tissue and therefore can be separated from the surrounding tissue with reasonable ease and certainty. When the fibrous "capsule" is delineated, lipoma extraction is simple, and the lipoma almost never recurs. However, this is usually the case only with small lipomas. Larger, more uncommon, infiltrating lipomas are more difficult to define and extract, and thus they more frequently recur because they have not been totally removed.[2] At the time of removal, lipomas may feel more firm than surrounding fat lobules because of the fibrous tissue component.

If lipomas are small, it may be possible to remove them by a small stab incision in the overlying skin, followed by mechanical pressure with a curette. Usually a small curette (2 mm) is used before expression of the lipoma to free the fibrofatty lobules from the surrounding tissue. The curette may also be used to help extract the lipoma.[11] My own experience with this technique is that it is useful only in a minority of lipomas and is certainly of less value if a large amount of fibrous tissue has surrounded and invaded the fat cells.

Most lipomas are removed by simple excision. One should always plan to remove more tissue than is apparent clinically, because lipomas usually insidiously extend well beyond their clinical borders. One thus should be prepared to spend considerable time in removal and repair.

Fig. 25-3, *A,* shows a lipoma of the back. Note the clinical palpable borders that are indicated. After an incision is made in the skin over the lipoma, the fibrofatty lobules are gently dissected away from the surrounding tissue. Usually undermining scissors, such as the Lahey or baby Metzenbaum, are useful for large lesions. As can be seen in Fig. 25-3, *B,* a large lipoma can be extracted through a relatively small incision if one has patience. Subsequent to removal, all bleeding should be controlled. This frequently requires a good light and a suction machine. The overlying wound is then closed and a pressure dressing is applied and kept in place for at least 24 hours. Dead space is inevitable even if the overlying skin is removed because of the great

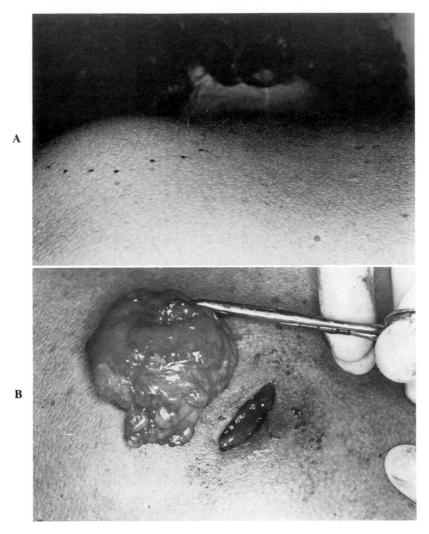

Fig. 25-3. A, Large lipoma of left upper back. Dotted line shows palpable extent. **B,** Extracted lipoma after considerable dissection. Note large size of lipoma compared to small incision. Also the relatively fibrous capsule which would preclude removal by other methods such as the curette.

lateral and deep extension that occurs with lipomas. One may use a few buried absorbable sutures to close this space partially. However, it is probably best not to be too vigorous in closing dead space, since not all of it can be closed anyway.

Despite a good pressure dressing, hematoma formation can occur after removal of a large lipoma, especially if located on the trunk. A drain may be used to prevent this. However, a drain is a two-way street, inviting infection; its use should be reserved only for large lesions or those in which hematomas have formed for unknown reasons.

If a hematoma forms, one may open the wound, express or suction the clots, control the bleeding, and resuture the wound. It is not necessary to trim the wound edges before resuturing if these steps are taken in 3 to 4 days from the time of surgery. It may be preferable to place a rubber drain

in such wounds to be removed gradually over 2 to 3 days.

An alternative method of removing lipomas that should be considered is excision from a distance.[18] With this technique one makes an incision not over the lipoma itself but at a distance from the lipoma, so that the incision scar will be inconspicuous. In Fig. 25-4, *A,* a lipoma of the temple is to be removed. Instead of making the incision overlying the lesion itself, the incision is camouflaged within the hairline. As previously emphasized, incisions in the scalp should be oblique to the skin surfaces, since the hair follicles descend obliquely from the surface of the skin. After undermining and tunneling toward the lesion, one visualizes the lipoma and carefully dissects it from the surrounding tissue (Fig. 25-4, *B* and *C*). The incised wound is then sutured (Fig. 25-4, *D*). Good hemostasis is mandatory after removal, and a pressure dressing is required for 24 hours. This technique

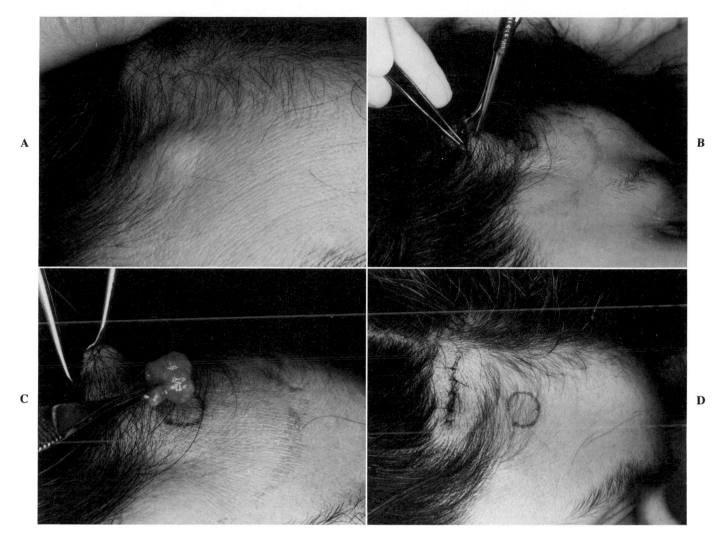

Fig. 25-4. A, Lipoma of temple in young woman. **B,** Incision within nearby hairline and lipoma being extracted through incision after tunnelling to site of lipoma. Gentian violet marks skin overlying original position of lipoma. **C,** Extracted lipoma, **D,** Sutured incision line. Future resultant scar will be less conspicuous than one placed directly over lipoma.

leads to superior cosmetic results but is time consuming. Moreover, it has the potential for nerve damage; still, with gentle tissue handling this should not be a problem.

Liposuction is another method of removing lipomas. For large superficial lipomas, this technique gives excellent cosmetic results with minimal morbidity. Lesions that in the past were considered inoperable are currently being liposuctioned.

XANTHOMAS

Xanthomas are firm, yellowish nodules or plaques that arise on the skin surface, usually the extensor surfaces, tendons, or eyelids. Clinically five types are recognized: eruptive xanthomas, tuberous xanthomas, tendon xanthomas, plane xanthomas, and palpebral xanthomas. All of these types may be associated with various hyperlipopro-

teinemias, a discussion of which is beyond the scope of this text. However, medical management of the underlying conditions, if determined, may be unsuccessful in bringing about a resolution of the cutaneous lesions.

Eruptive xanthomas occur as papules, most commonly on the buttocks and posterior thighs. Tuberous xanthomas are large nodules or plaques that occur on the elbows, knees, fingers, or buttocks. Tendon xanthomas usually are found on the Achilles tendon or the extensor tendons of the finger. Plane xanthomas are found in the palmar creases.

A plaque that occurs on the eyelid is known as a palpebral xanthoma, which is the commonest type of xanthoma. It is yellowish, oblong, slightly raised, and usually situated toward the medial side of the eyelid. These lesions are commonly seen in middle-aged women. Although palpebral xanthomas can be found in hyperlipoproteinemias,

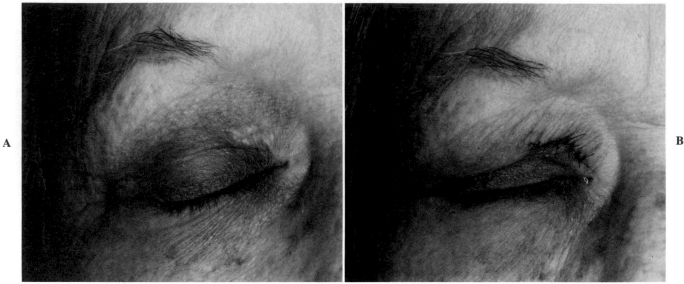

Fig. 25-5. A, Palpebral xanthoma. **B,** Wound after excision and placement of sutures.

this is rare. Most patients with this condition have normal lipid levels in their serum.

Histopathology

The microscopic appearance of a xanthoma is characterized by the presence of foam cells, which are macrophages that contain lipid droplets. In palpebral xanthomas the foam cells are located within the superficial dermis, whereas in the other types of xanthomas, the foam cells are deeper and associated with a chronic inflammatory infiltrate and fibrosis.

Treatment

The treatment for palpebral xanthomas is surgical excision (Fig. 25-5). After infiltration of local anesthesia, the xanthoma is excised, and then the wound is sutured. Undermining is unnecessary. The resultant wound may also be allowed to heal by granulation and epidermization, but this process requires 4 to 6 weeks of dressing changes for the patient.

Some physicians recommend topical application of trichloroacetic acid to a palpebral xanthoma every month to melt it away. I have not been impressed by this method.

The CO_2 laser may be used to vaporize xanthoma-containing tissue, including not only palpebral xanthoma but also other types of xanthoma. Because of its pinpoint accuracy and minimal tissue destruction, laser removal of xanthomas leads to excellent cosmetic results. Xanthoma-containing tissue can be easily seen at the time of laser removal, making total removal easier and thus lessening the likelihood of recurrence.

REFERENCES

1. Adair, F.E., Pack, G.T., and Farrior, J.H.: Lipomas, Am. J. Cancer **16:**1104, 1932.
2. Austin, R.M., et al.: Infiltrating (intramuscular) lipomas and angiolipomas, Arch. Surg. **115:**281, 1980.
3. Ballard, H.S., Frame, B., and Hartsock, R.J.: Familial multiple endocrine adenoma-peptic ulcer complex, Medicine **43:** 481, 1964.
4. Belcher, R.W., et al.: Multiple (subcutaneous) angiolipomas, Arch. Dermatol. **110:**583, 1974.
5. Carlsen, A., and Thomsen, M.: Different clinical types of lipomatosis: case report, Scand. J. Plast. Reconstr. Surg. **12:** 75, 1978.
6. Dercum, F.X.: Three cases of a hitherto unclassified affection resembling in its grosser aspects obesity, but associated with special nervous symptoms: adiposis dolorosa, Am. J. Med. Sci. **104:**521, 1892.
7. Erichsen, B., and Medgyesi, S.: Congenital lipoma imitating gigantism of a toe: case report, Scand. J. Plast. Reconstr. Surg. **17:**77, 1983.
8. Feldman, M.: An appraisal of associated conditions occurring in autopsied cases of lipoma of the gastrointestinal tract, Am. J. Gastroenterol. **36:**413, 1961.
9. Fukamizu, H., et al.: Large vulvar lipoma, Arch. Dermatol. **118:**447, 1982.
10. Gellhorn, A., and Marks, P.A.: Composition and biosynthesis of lipids in human adipose tissues, J. Clin. Invest. **40:**925, 1961.
11. Hardin, F.F.: A simple technique for removing lipomas [surgical gem], J. Dermatol. Surg. Oncol. **8:**316, 1982.
12. Hoehn, J.G., and Farber, H.F.: Massive lipoma of the palm, Ann. Plast. Surg. **11:**431, 1983.
13. Howard, W.R., and Helwig, E.B.: Angiolipoma, Arch. Dermatol. **82:**924, 1960.
14. Kalisman, M., and Dolich, B.H.: Infiltrating lipoma of the proper digital nerves, J. Hand Surg. **7:**401, 1982.

15. Lin, J.J., and Lin, F.: Two entities in angiolipoma: a study of 459 cases of lipoma with review of literature on infiltrating angiolipoma, Cancer **34:**720, 1974.

16. Lynch, H.T., and Harlan, W.L.: Hereditary factors in adiposis dolorosa (Dercum's disease), Am. J. Hum. Genet. **15:**184, 1963.

17. Paletta, F.X., and Senay, L.C.: Lipofibromatous hamartoma of median nerve and ulnar nerve: surgical treatment, Plast. Reconstr. Surg. **68:**915, 1981.

18. Peinert, R.A., and Courtiss, E.H.: Excision from a distance: a technique for removal of benign subcutaneous lesions, Plast. Reconstr. Surg. **72:**94, 1983.

19. Roberts, A.H.N., and Crockett, D.J.: An operation for the treatment of cutaneous neurofibromatosis, Br. J. Plast. Surg. **38:**292, 1985.

20. Rydholm, A., and Berg, N.O.: Size, site and clinical incidence of lipoma: factors in the differential diagnosis of lipoma and sarcoma, Acta Orthop. Scand. **54:**929, 1983.

26

Cystic Lesions

EPITHELIAL CYST

Epithelial cysts are cysts derived from the epidermis or its appendages. This category includes not only the common epidermal cysts, but also less common cysts such as pilar (trichilemmal) cysts, dermoid cysts, milia, cysts found in steatocystoma multiplex, and hydrocystomas.

Epidermal cyst

One of the most common lumps in the skin presented for treatment is the epidermal cyst, also known as a keratinous cyst. The epidermal cyst is the most frequently occurring cutaneous cyst, comprising about 80% of all cysts.[24] Formerly, epidermal cysts were erroneously called "sebaceous cysts," but this term has fallen into disuse as the pathogenesis of cysts has become better understood.[19]

Epidermal cysts are rounded elevations that slowly grow, reaching a size of 1 to 5 cm in diameter. Most often they are of several years' duration. Usually they occur on the head, neck, and trunk, although they may appear anywhere on the skin surface—even the palms or soles, where there are no hair follicles.[13] Epidermal cysts occur most frequently, after the face and scalp, on the genitalia.[22]

Epidermal cysts can be solitary or in groups of a few, but they are rarely multiple. They usually occur in middle age but can be seen at any age. Epidermal cysts are not painful unless they become infected; when they do so, patients complain of exquisite pain.

The diagnosis of epidermal cysts is usually quite obvious. The smooth lump is fluctuant, tense, and often slightly ballottable. Its hallmark is a small punctum overlying the cyst, which is almost always present. Frequently these cysts are freely moveable and occur within the dermis, the subcutaneous tissue, or both. The contents of epidermal cysts have a particularly foul-smelling odor. This can be noticed on expression of the contents and may be a clue that one has inadvertently incised a cyst wall while attempting to remove the cyst.

Cause. The cause of epidermal cysts is largely unknown.

Most appear to arise spontaneously, although trauma, follicular occlusion disease, and exposure to acnegenic agents (such as oils and hydrocarbons) may be predisposing factors. Since there are no follicles on the palms or soles, traumatic implantation of epidermis is probably the cause in these locations. Epstein and Kligman implanted excised pieces of skin into the skin of volunteers.[10] Epidermal cysts resulted in some subjects, which established that burial of epithelium may produce cysts.

The histogenesis of keratinous cysts is based on the concept that the epidermis is pluripotential. Under certain circumstances the epidermis, sweat ducts, or follicles are probably capable of producing cystic structures.

The most common cause of cysts is probably follicular occlusion or degeneration. In a study on the formation of cysts in hairless mice (mice that are particularly prone to cyst formation), the investigators found that the formed cysts were associated with fragmented or disoriented hair follicles and with imperfectly grown hair bulbs.[26] Thus degeneration of hair follicles or injury to normal follicular growth and development may predispose to keratinous cyst formation.

Multiple epidermal cysts are sometimes found with Gardner's syndrome. This rare inherited syndrome consists of (1) multiple intestinal polyps, (2) epidermal cysts, (3) osteomas and exostoses, (4) fibrous tissue tumors (either fibromas or dermoid tumors), and (5) lipomas.

Histopathology. An epidermal cyst is composed of a wall of true epidermis that surrounds horny material (stratum corneum); the horny material is usually arranged in laminated layers (Fig. 26-1). The keratinizing epidermis casts off stratum corneum into the sac-like space. Thus with time—as the epidermis survives, and the stratum corneum accumulates—the cyst grows. The thickness of the cyst wall may decrease, perhaps because of pressure buildup from within the cyst itself.

Epidermal cysts' walls may weaken with or without in-

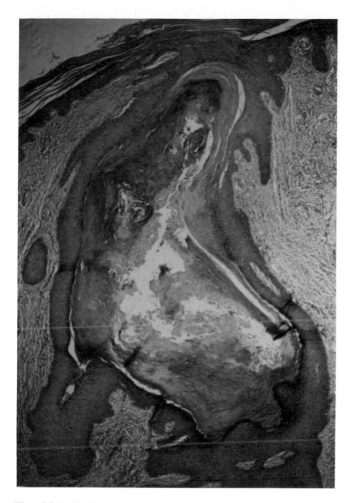

Fig. 26-1. Epidermal cyst. Note presence of granular layer and concentric keratin contents.

fection and subsequently rupture into the surrounding dermis. When rupture occurs, a foreign-body reaction characterized by numerous multinucleated giant cells results. The cyst may then persist, and fibrotic tissue may appear and attach to the wall, making treatment more difficult.

Treatment. Patients desire treatment of epidermal cysts because of inflammation, infection, or aesthetic concerns. Each of these problems has to be treated somewhat differently.

An inflamed cyst has presumably spilled its keratinous contents into the dermis and thus has incited an inflammatory reaction. Usually such cysts are on the face and have been manipulated by the patient. The erythematous lesions that result are reasonably small (less than 1 cm), of recent onset, and often associated with acne. Patients are concerned more about the appearance of these lesions than the pain. Inflamed cysts should be allowed to resolve on their own, or a small amount of triamcinolone acetonide (2.5 to 5 mg/ml) can be injected into the lesion to hasten resolution.

On resolution, this type of cyst usually does not recur in the same area.

The infected cyst is usually a good-sized cyst (larger than 1 cm) of long standing. Compared with the inflamed cyst, the infected cyst is much more painful and much more erythematous. The surrounding erythema can extend from the cyst itself for a few centimeters into the surrounding skin. The treatment of such cysts is drainage, systemic antibiotics, or both. Warm soaks, which help to increase the circulation in the area of the cyst, should be used because they help to concentrate the antibiotic in that location. In addition, the increased circulation helps in resolving the inflammation. Since the most common pathogen in infected epidermal cysts is *Staphylococcus aureus,* an appropriate antibiotic should be empirically chosen for this organism.

When the patient is in considerable pain from an infected epidermal cyst, drainage of the cyst contents gives immediate relief. Drainage may be achieved either through a large-bore needle (14 or 16 gauge) into an attached syringe or by means of a no. 11 scalpel blade. Drainage through a large-bore needle should be attempted first, since it leads to less scarring. This is important for lesions of the face. Frequently, however, such needles are not wide enough to drain off enough of the cyst contents to provide relief; in this case an incision should be made.

An incision into an infected cyst should be made along the maximal skin tension lines so that the healed scar is as inconspicuous as possible. Prior anesthesia, either with a skin refrigerant or a local anesthetic, is necessary. Because the pH of infected tissue is low, local anesthetics may work poorly; their activity is best in a slightly alkaline environment.[2] The blade is held perpendicular to the skin over the apex of the cyst and plunged firmly but gently into the cyst cavity. Usually the purulent contents stream out through the incision hole. A small hemostat can be inserted into the cyst cavity and spread to open up the cyst's often loculated contents further and thus provide easier access for the pus to drain to the outside. Once most of the pus is removed, the cyst cavity is packed with a gauze packing strip (for instance, Iodoform gauze), which is removed gradually by the patient or physician over a 2- to 3-day period. This gauze helps to provide a conduit for further evacuation of pus. The cyst is then allowed to heal spontaneously, which usually takes 2 to 3 weeks.

A few critical points need to be stressed concerning infected cysts. First, when the pus is either aspirated or drained, it should be cultured and sensitivities should be determined.[23] This is consistent with optimal patient care. Ideally both anaerobic and aerobic cultures should be obtained. Antibiotics are started before culture results are learned, but if the patient is not improving these results may be critical to the selection of an appropriate alternate antibiotic.

Second, one should not attempt to remove an infected

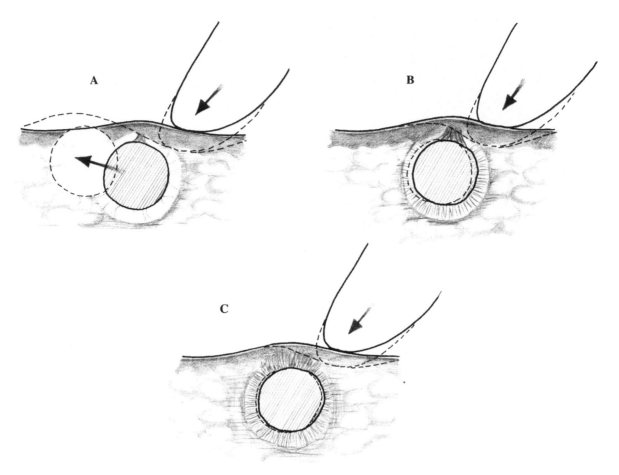

Fig. 26-2. Ballotement of, **A,** freely moveable cyst; **B,** slightly moveable cyst; **C,** nonmoveable cyst.

cyst. Usually a cyst wall is friable, and its attempted removal results only in further inflammation. In addition, inflammation itself tends to decrease collagen.[33] Deficient collagen leads to hemorrhage, possible dehiscence, and a poor cosmetic result. Therefore, if the patient, physician, or both think that a cyst should be removed, the operation should wait for 4 to 6 weeks after the infection or inflammation has subsided. This not only eventuates in a better chance of complete removal but also in a better final cosmetic result.

Third, infected cysts should not be injected with steroids. Steroids tend to weaken further the collagen surrounding cyst walls. If these cysts are to be removed in the near future, such weakened supporting stroma will lead, like inflammation, to wound hemorrhage, dehiscence, and unsightly scars.

The noninflamed, noninfected cyst can be treated in a number of different ways. However, I have found that all successful methods are predicated on *complete* removal or destruction of the cyst wall; otherwise recurrence is the rule. If the cyst is punctured and the contents merely expressed, the sac usually refills. Since epidermal cysts are almost always benign lesions, they should be removed so that the

least possible scarring results. It cannot be stressed enough, however, that after removal, cysts should be submitted for histopathologic examination. Not only are some cysts histopathologically interesting, but occasionally malignancies develop in cyst walls[39] (see Fig. 26-11).

Before attempting to remove an epidermal cyst, ballotement should be performed to ascertain how freely moveable the cyst is. This gives some indication of how firmly attached the cyst wall is to the surrounding connective tissue and thus helps one choose the method of removal. In general, I divide all cysts by ballotement into one of three types: (1) freely moveable (Fig. 26-2, *A*); (2) moderately moveable (Fig. 26-2, *B*); and (3) nonmoveable (Fig. 26-2, *C*). Freely moveable cysts commonly occur on the face. These cysts have well-defined walls with loose attachment to the surrounding connective tissue. They are suspended from the overlying epidermis and are usually found where the dermis is thin. In contrast, nonmoveable cysts are well attached to the surrounding dermis by a considerable amount of scar tissue. Usually they have been previously infected and are found where the dermis is thick, such as on the back. The previous infection has resulted in thick scar tissue formation that binds down the cyst wall and makes

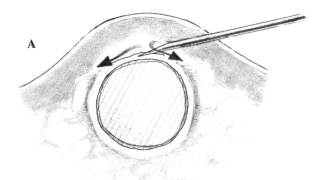

A

Fig. 26-3. A, Method of injection of local anesthetic before removal of epidermal cyst. When needle is placed between overlying skin and underlying cyst, anesthetic diffuses *(arrows)* in plane between cyst and surrounding tissue. This helps to separate cyst from surrounding tissue and thus facilitates surgical dissection. **B,** Immediate blanch with injection of local anesthetic and peripheral spread. Dotted line demarcates palpable extent of cyst.

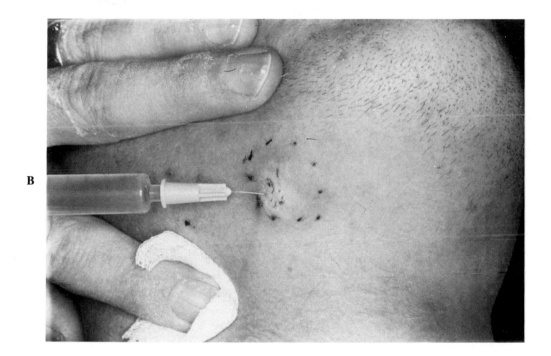

B

motion difficult. In between the freely moveable cysts and the nonmoveable cysts are other cysts, whose walls are less firmly attached to the surrounding tissue. I designate them moderately moveable.

Anesthesia. Before removal of an epidermal cyst, the overlying and surrounding skin must be anesthetized. This is best done as shown in Fig. 26-3, *A*. The needle is inserted bevel up into the skin overlying the cyst. Proper placement of the needle is between the skin and the cyst wall. As the local anesthetic is injected, it dissects around the cyst wall and separates it from the surrounding tissue. An immediate blanching occurs, which moves centrifugally (Fig. 26-3, *B*). Anesthetizing around a cyst in this way prevents puncturing the cyst before removal and helps to separate the cyst wall attachments from the surrounding tissue. Other supplemental injections may be necessary surrounding the cyst and deep to the cyst, depending on the complexity of surgery necessary for removal. However, usually such injections need not be given until absolutely necessary—when the patient experiences significant pain.

Freely moveable cysts. (Fig. 26-2, *A*) With palpation a freely moveable cyst moves easily underneath the skin surface (Fig. 26-2, A). This occurs because there is little attachment of the cyst wall to surrounding tissue. Removal of freely moveable cysts is shown in Fig. 26-4. After local anesthesia is obtained, the top of the cyst is incised with a no. 11 scalpel blade along the maximal skin tension lines (Fig. 26-4, *A*). If a punctum is present, I usually incise through it or just to one side of it and then trim it off. The punctum is the site of attachment of the underlying cyst to the skin above. Unless this punctum is removed, it will probably tend to persist; still, it may disappear spontaneously. The contents of the cyst are expressed manually (Fig. 26-4, *B*). Sometimes the cyst wall everts spontaneously with lateral pressure as the contents of the cyst are extruding. It then appears as glistening white tissue at the edge of the incision (Fig. 26-4, *C*). Often the cyst wall must be extracted manually by being grasped with a fine hemostat and turned inside out (Fig. 26-4, *D*). To accomplish this, one needs to use small, delicate hemostatic forceps to grab the cyst wall

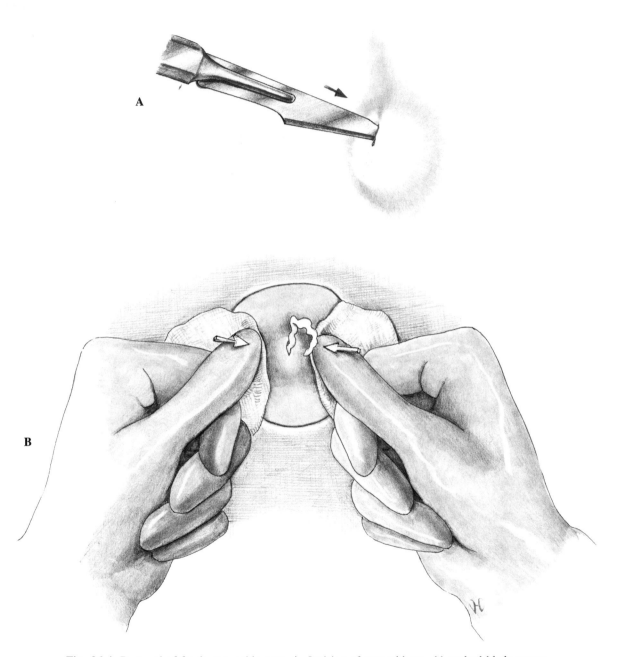

Fig. 26-4. Removal of freely moveable cyst. **A,** Incision of cyst with no. 11 scalpel blade across punctum. **B,** Manual expression of cyst contents.

C

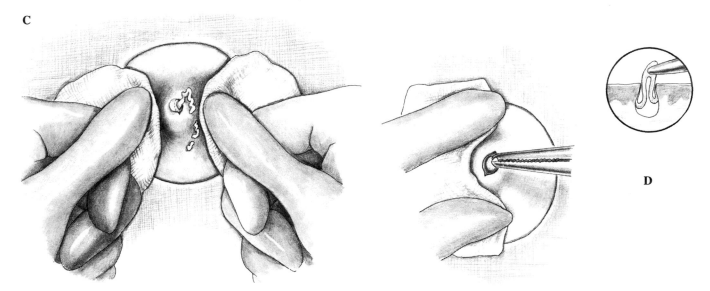

D

Fig. 26-4, cont'd. C, Expression of portion of cyst wall (seen at left side of incision). **D,** Removal of cyst wall with hemostatic forceps. *Inset,* Cyst wall everts as it is extracted.

and evert it manually. With a gentle, steady pull it usually comes free. A clinical example of this method of cyst removal is shown on Fig. 26-5. It is important to inspect the wound cavity to make sure no bits of cyst wall remain. If any cyst wall fragments do remain, they should be removed. A little curette, especially the Skeele curette, is of particular value in this regard, according to Krull.[20] It may also be more useful than fine forceps to remove the sac initially.[21] The small incision may then be closed by means of sutureless skin closures (for example, Steri-Strips), buried absorbable sutures, or a few fine percutaneous sutures. The resultant scar is normally imperceptible because of its small size. This method of removal was described in 1956[16] and 1972.[37]

Slightly moveable cysts. (Fig. 26-2, *B*) Slightly moveable cysts are removed by dissection if possible. A slightly curved incision is made to the one side in the skin overlying the cyst because the other half of a fusiform excision may become necessary (Fig. 26-6, *A*). As with all cutaneous incisions, it should be directed along the maximal skin tension lines. As stated before, if the punctum is off center, one should try to incise through it so that it can be trimmed off. Using a skin hook and blunt dissecting scissors, the cyst is separated from the surrounding tissue (Fig. 26-6, *B*). If significant fibrous tissue exists, this separation may be impossible without rupture of the cyst and prolongation of the procedure. If one can dissect totally around the cyst, it can be removed in toto (Fig. 26-6, *C*).

Sometimes during the dissection of the cyst from the surrounding tissue, the wall is inadvertently incised. The contents then invariably spill forth into the surrounding wound. These contents (keratin) have a characteristic foul-smelling odor. This odor by itself may be a clue that one has punctured the cyst wall and that the contents are leaking out. Often, if one continues to be patient, gentle, and careful, the remaining cyst can be dissected and extracted without further appreciable spillage. Sometimes it is best to empty the contents of the cyst before going further. Each case should be evaluated separately.

After removal in toto of fairly large cysts by dissection two problems occur: the presence of dead space and the expanded, excessive skin that previously had overlayed the cyst. The dead space can be almost closed by interrupted buried absorbable sutures; but, as discussed in previous chapters, one should not be overly vigorous in doing this because more harm than good can come from burying too much suture. An alternative I have found to be quite useful is to employ the deep figure-eight suture (see Fig. 11-21). This suture closes in one stitch the dead space and the overlying skin. Because it puts considerable tension on the skin, it is useful in locations where the sutures have little influence on the final cosmetic appearance of the scar: for instance, on the back, neck, and scalp. My experience with the excessive skin overlying cysts is that with time it shrinks back to normal if left intact. Since trimming away the excess tissue puts more tension on the skin with sutures, I prefer to leave this tissue for a slightly better cosmetic result.

A clinical example of dissection of an epidermal cyst is shown in Fig. 26-7. In Fig. 26-7, *A*, note that the incision line laid to one side of the cyst is directed so as to be camouflaged in the melolabial crease.

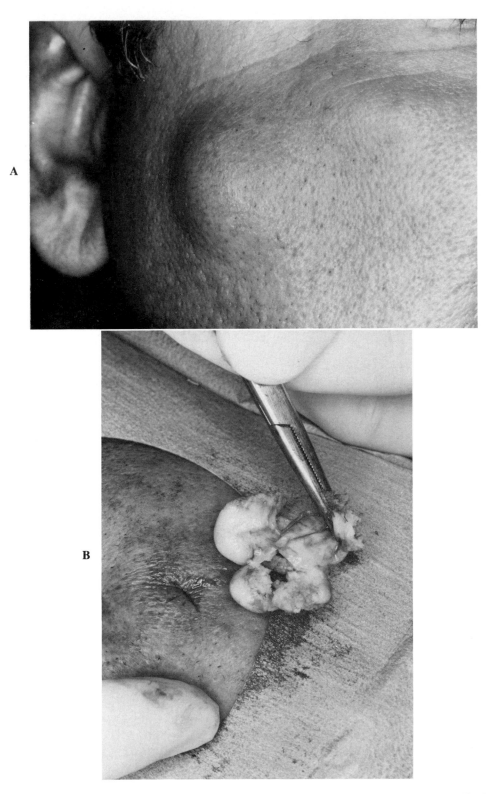

Fig. 26-5. A, Large but freely moveable epidermal cyst on cheek. **B,** Epidermal cyst wall with keratin immediately after removal (as shown in Fig. 26-4, *D*) through relatively small incision. Wound was closed with few interrupted sutures, leading to excellent cosmetic result.

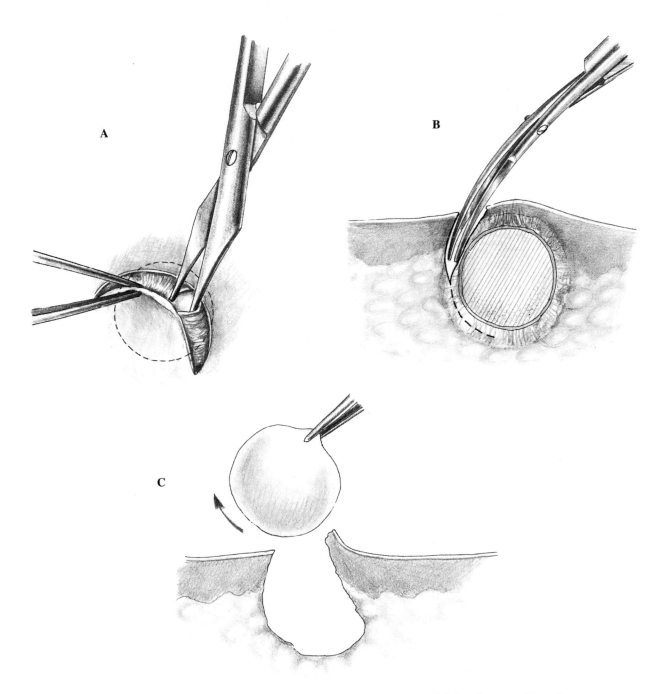

Fig. 26-6. Removal of slightly moveable cyst. **A,** Incision curved, slightly off center. Dissection through fibrous tissue to cyst wall. **B,** Dissection around cyst. **C,** Removal of cyst in toto.

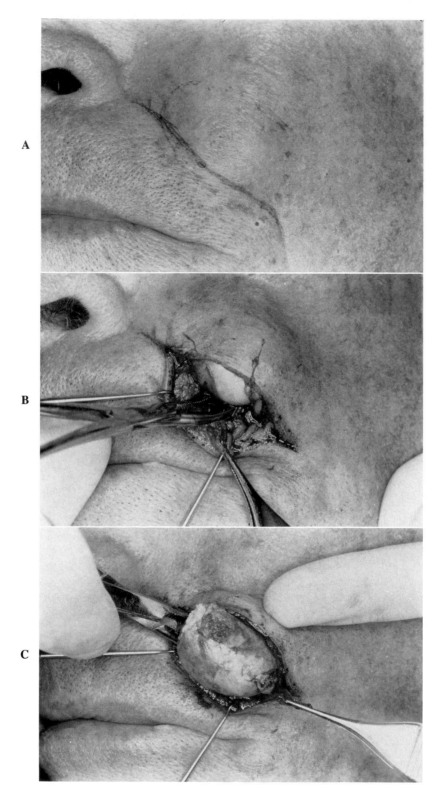

Fig. 26-7. A, Epidermal cyst on cheek. Note planned incision line on one side of cyst, which will blend into melolabial crease. Dotted line represents palpable extent of cyst. **B,** Dissection of cyst by small curved hemostat. Note use of skin hooks to hold tissue to side. **C,** Further extraction of cyst. Note small rupture superiorly.

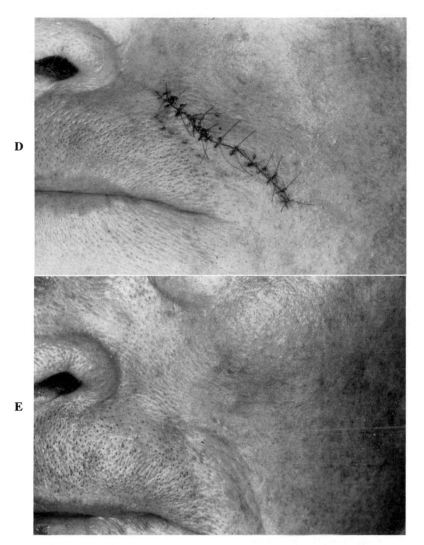

Fig. 26-7, cont'd. D, Wound sutured. **E,** Healed result at 6 months.

Occasionally it is possible to remove a cyst so that the incision line is hidden some distance from the actual cyst. This was described by Peinert and Courtiss, who called it "excision from a distance"[35] (Fig. 26-8). When within a hair-bearing area, an incision should be parallel to the direction of the follicles (which are oblique to the skin surface) so as not to transect the hair follicles beneath the surface of the skin. The length of the incision should be approximately equal to the distance between the incision and the lesion to be removed. Excision from a distance requires dissection through the normal tissue that exists between the incision line and the cyst. This requires retractors, a good light source, suction, and at least one assistant. In addition, considerable time may be spent trying to dissect out the cyst, probably more than if a simple incision overlying the cyst is performed. The punctum is not removed by excision from a distance, but this is sometimes unnecessary

anyway. In a report on 21 epidermal cysts removed in this manner, only 1 patient required further surgery for complete removal of the cyst.[35] Other problems encountered may be nerve damage or hematoma formation. The former may be minimized by gentle dissection and the latter by good hemostasis and a pressure bandage. It is impossible to close the dead space in an excision from a distance; however, the slightly sunken area of the tissue (caused by removal of a cyst) seems to fill in, probably because of the tissue forces in the area.

Fig. 26-9 shows removal of an epidermal cyst through the inside of the upper lip. This obviates the need for a cutaneous incision. The upper lip is one place on the face on which one can safely do this without injuring nerves or muscle insertions. After the incision is made in the mucosa, one should be careful to dissect through the underlying muscle in the direction of the fibers. Since in the upper lip

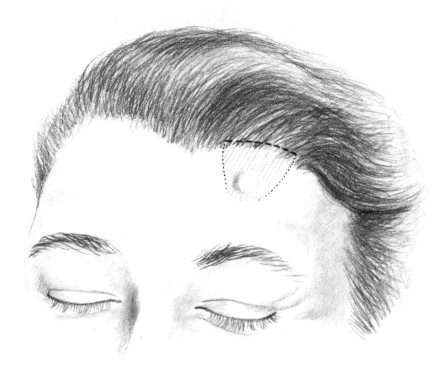

Fig. 26-8. Excision at distance for cyst on forehead. Incision line *(dashed line)* is within hairline. After incision, undermining and tunnelling to cyst is performed thus dissecting it free from *below* skin and removing it through incision above hairline. This prevents noticeable incision line on forehead.

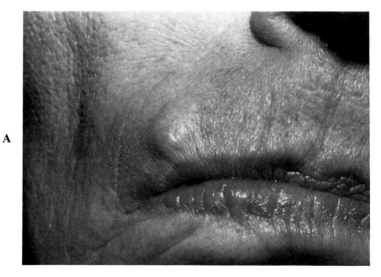

Fig. 26-9. A, Epidermal cyst in upper lip.

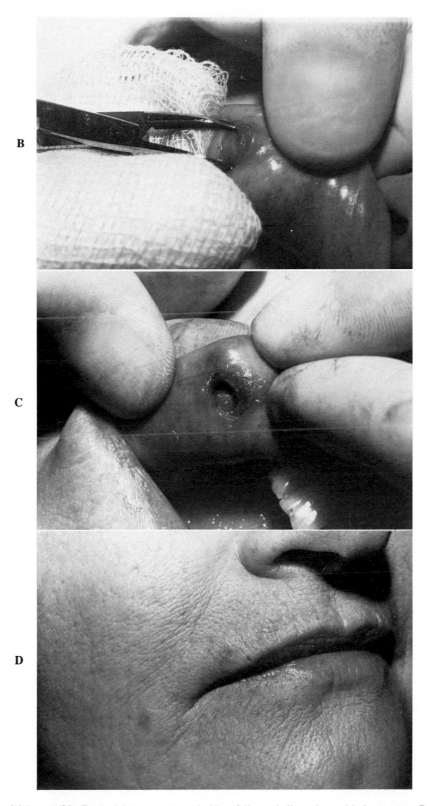

Fig. 26-9, cont'd. B, Incision on mucosal side of lip and dissection with hemostat. Cyst wall appearing between tips of hemostat. **C,** Wound after removal of cyst, subsequently sutured with 4.0 silk. **D,** Healed result in 1 week. Cutaneous incisions were unnecessary. (Operation was performed with Dr. Charles Bartholome.)

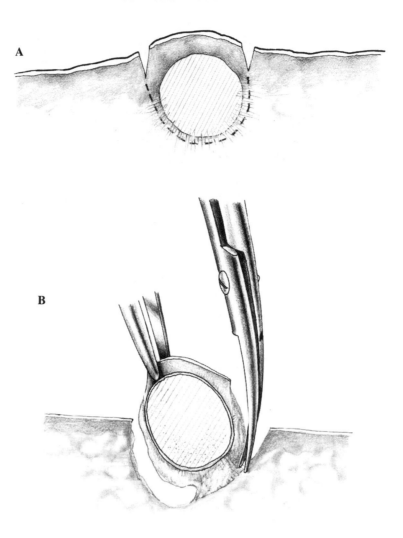

Fig. 26-10. A, Incisions to remove nonmoveable cyst. Note amount of epidermis incised is slightly smaller than fixed area shown by radiating lines. **B,** Cyst and surrounding fibrous tissue are excised with scissors.

these fibers are mostly oriented circumferentially, this is easy to do. I removed two lesions in this manner with excellent cosmetic and functional results. The overlying punctum was not removed but seemed to disappear with time.

Nonmoveable cysts. (Fig. 26-2, *C*) The nonmoveable fixed cyst is removed by excision of the cyst and surrounding fibrous tissue (Fig. 26-10). A fusiform piece of skin overlying the cyst is excised along with the cyst, since separating the cyst from surrounding fibrous tissue is difficult. The wound is then closed in the standard manner with buried dermal-subdermal sutures and percutaneous sutures or with the deep figure-eight suture.

Alternative techniques of epidermal cyst removal. Besides the techniques already mentioned, other methods for removal of epidermal cysts have been described. Perhaps the most discussed is the Danna procedure, as originally described in 1945.[4,5] A diathermy needle is placed through the skin overlying an epidermal cyst, and the tip of the needle

descends until it barely protrudes into the cyst cavity. The current is turned on. The electrodesiccating current is used for small cysts, whereas the electrocoagulating current must be used on larger cysts with thicker walls. A ring of necrosis ensues, which causes a small plug of skin and cyst lining to slough out. The contents of the cyst are left to work their way out over the next few weeks. The cyst wall shrinks by itself gradually over time and becomes level with the skin surface in most cases. At this point, it blends imperceptibly with the skin. Out of 20 cases reported by Danna,[4] leveling off with the skin occurred in 18. In two other cases, a small dimple resembling a blackhead appeared, which could be removed in the future (see Fig. 27-2). This procedure was performed without anesthesia; the cosmetic result was thought to be superior to that with excision.

Various modifications of the Danna procedure have been described. Most popular is to excise an overlying plug of skin and cyst wall with a skin biopsy punch.[21,31,34] The cyst

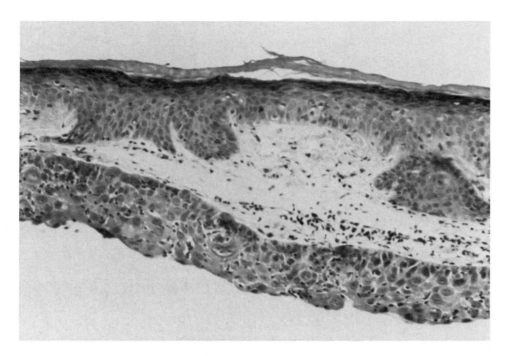

Fig. 26-11. Squamous cell carcinoma in epidermal cyst wall. (Hematoxylin and eosin, × 100.)

contents are then allowed to discharge themselves spontaneously, or they are removed with the cyst wall by means of a small (chalazion) curette. Oliveira et al. described using a skin punch to create a hole in the skin overlying a cyst on the scalp, removing the cyst through the hole, and then replacing the plug of skin back into the hole.[32]

The advantage of Danna's procedure or its modifications is that only a small scar if any results, whereas with an excision, the scar line is sometimes several centimeters long. However, Danna's procedure probably works only if the cyst wall is not firmly attached to the adjacent connective tissue. If this attachment is firm, the cyst wall cannot shrink down, and the cyst refills. It is interesting to note that data on long-term follow-up examinations and recurrence rates are not available either from Danna's or from other published reports of cyst removal methods that are modifications of his procedure.

Another method described for treatment of epidermal cysts is the use of sclerotic or irritant agents. After one expresses the contents of a cyst through a small incision, one places an irritant into the cyst cavity instead of removing the sac. Agents such as phenol,[27] trichloroacetic acid, iodine, silver nitrate sticks, and sodium tetradecyl sulfate (Sotradecol) have been used. Kelley reported success with this method in 30% of cysts when 3% Sotradecol was used; when 5% Sotradecol was used, 77.46% of cysts were eliminated.[16] Thus this method probably does not have an impressively high cure rate.

Mevorah and Bovet excised cysts with overlying skin behind the ear and allowed the resultant wounds to heal by granulation and epidermization.[25] They suggested this method because cysts in this area sometimes go deep and are large, making closure difficult if a significant amount of skin is removed. I have personally not found it necessary to allow wounds from cyst removal to heal by secondary intention if careful dissection is done.

Problems associated with removal of epidermal cysts. Although treatment of epidermal cysts is usually straightforward, problems that merit consideration sometimes arise. Basal or squamous cell carcinomas may arise from epidermal cysts[39] (Fig. 26-11). The reported incidence of such carcinomatous change was about 1.5% in one series,[22] but this figure is probably exaggerated, since it probably included other entities such as proliferating trichilemmal cysts, which are currently thought to be benign tumors.[3,38] A more accurate figure is probably less than 0.1%.

On the pinna, a fluctuant swelling may occur, which resembles an epidermal cyst but in reality is a pseudocyst.[11] The patient is typically a man, and there is no history of antecedent trauma. Its cause is intracartilagenous accumulation of fluid, probably stemming from degeneration of the cartilage. The fluid is yellow, with the consistency of corn oil. On biopsy one sees eosinophilic degeneration of the cartilage with fibrous tissue lining the cartilagenous cavity; thus a pseudocyst is not a true cyst. The treatment is incision and drainage followed by a pressure dressing. Intralesional steroids should not be used because this form of therapy may result in a permanent ear deformity.

Pilar cyst

Pilar cysts are known by a variety of names. Formerly called "sebaceous cysts" and "wens," these lesions are

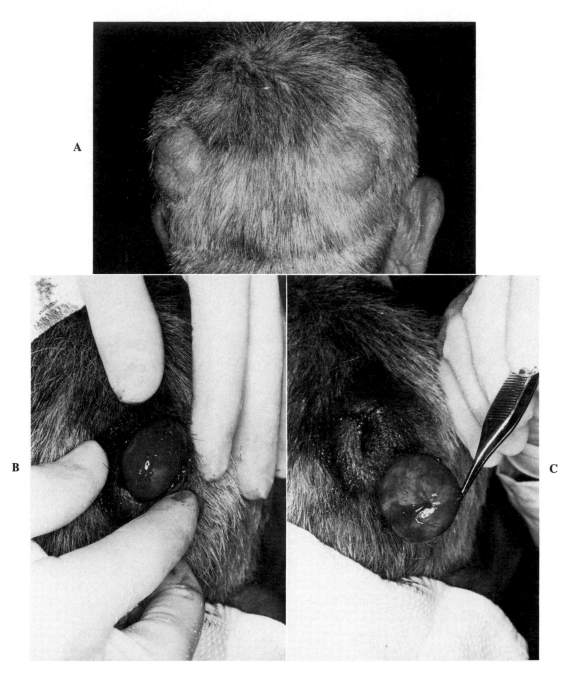

Fig. 26-12. A, Two pilar cysts on scalp. **B,** Dissected cyst just before removal. **C,** Dissected cyst removal in toto. Note crescent incision to one side of skin that had overlain cyst. Also, compare relatively large size of cyst with incision line.

currently referred to as trichilemmal cysts. It is thought that they originate from the middle portion of the hair follicle epithelium. The true sebaceous cyst is a rarity; most of the cysts once called "sebaceous" were actually epidermal cysts.[19]

Clinically pilar cysts are similar to epidermal cysts but less common, comprising only about 15% of all cysts. These cysts are rare on the face, trunk, or extremities; 90% of all pilar cysts occur on the scalp.[24] When they occur on the scalp, they may grow to a very large size (several centimeters) and may induce by underlying pressure an overlying alopecia, which is frequently reversible on cyst removal (Fig. 26-12, *A*).

The contents of the pilar cyst are fairly odorless and not as cheesy in texture as those of the epidermal cyst.

Histopathology. Pilar cysts are lined by an epidermis that

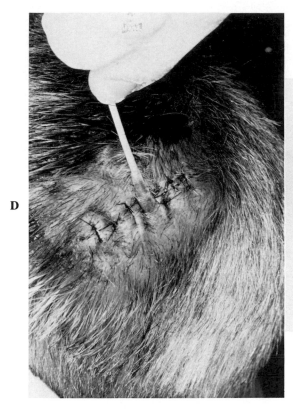

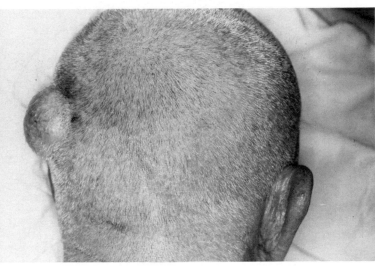

Fig. 26-12, cont'd. D, Incision line closed with some deep figure-eight sutures (see Fig. 11-21). Note cotton-tipped applicator rolled over incision line to express blood. **E,** Healed result 1 month postoperatively. Alopecia (shown in Fig. 26-12, *A*) overlying removed cyst has regressed despite fact that no overlying skin was excised.

encloses amorphous material. This epidermis keratinizes in a manner similar to the trichilemmal keratinization characteristic of the external root sheath of hair. Pale staining cells float off without a granular layer. Occasionally hybrid cysts occur, which have features of both pilar and epidermal cysts.[10,19,24]

A variant of the pilar (trichilemmal) cyst that occurs on the scalp, mostly in women, is the proliferating trichilemmal cyst.[3] Often there is a history of trauma. This entity clinically resembles a pilar cyst but histologically may be misinterpreted as a squamous cell carcinoma. Although the growth itself is benign and self-limiting, epidermal hyperplasia with cellular atypia is present. Thus these lesions have been called proliferating epidermoid cysts, pilar tumors, or even squamous cell carcinomas in sebaceous cysts. As is true with a pilar (trichilemmal) cyst, the keratinization in the proliferating trichilemmal cyst is trichilemmal.

Treatment. The treatment for pilar cysts is similar to that for epidermal cysts. These cysts tend to have thicker, more well-defined walls than epidermal cysts, and they tend not to be firmly attached to the surrounding connective tissue. Therefore usually dissection and extraction of the cyst in toto is easily accomplished; rarely is it necessary to sacrifice overlying normal skin (Fig. 26-12). Extraction through small holes, such as biopsy punches, does not work as well as it does with epidermal cysts.

Dermoid cysts

Dermoid cysts are rare cysts similar to epidermal cysts clinically but having no overlying punctum. Usually the diagnosis is made by the dermatopathologist and not by the physician removing the lesion. These cysts appear at an early age and occur mainly on the face, especially in embryonal fusion planes. Dermoid cysts are thus throught to be caused by sequestration of skin during the closure of embryonic fusion planes. They are generally freely moveable and not attached to the overlying skin.

Histopathology. Dermoid cysts are lined by a nontortuous epidermis; like epidermal cysts, dermoid cysts contain keratin. However, they have in addition fully developed adnexal structures coming off the cyst wall. Usually hair follicles, but also sebaceous glands, eccrine glands, or even apocrine glands may be associated with the cyst wall.

Treatment. Surgical excision is best. This type of cyst can be dissected out with or without overlying epidermis.

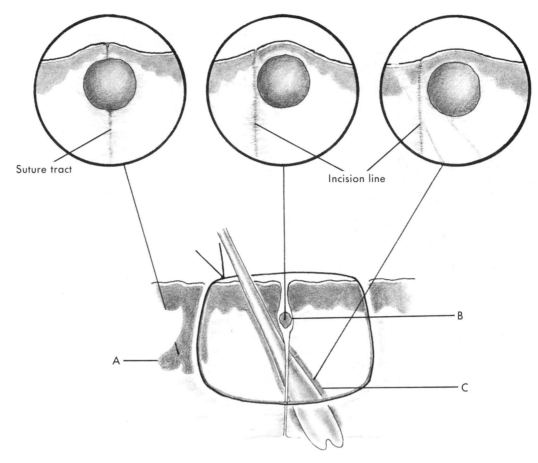

Fig. 26-13. Pathogenesis of milia in incision. *A,* Epidermization of suture tract. *B,* Implantation of epidermal fragment. *C,* Transection of hair follicle with subsequent continued growth of external root sheath cells.

Milia

Milia are cysts that appear as small (1 to 2 mm), usually multiple, whitish, rounded lesions, almost always on the face. Histologically milia appear similar to epidermal cysts.

Cause. Most of the time milia arise spontaneously, with no clear-cut reason for their appearance. Some investigators, however, state that there is a relationship between milia and vellus hair follicles.[9,22] Vellus hairs are fine hairs (thinner than terminal hairs), the follicles of which are small and frequently lack sebaceous glands. Epithelial buds project from the sides of hair follicles at the point where the sebaceous glands normally attach. Epstein and Kligman think that these buds sometimes get separated from follicles and then form milia.[9]

Milia may be associated with trauma, such as dermabrasion (Fig. 13-10); certain blistering diseases, such as porphyria cutanea tarda or epidermolysis bullosa; or wounds allowed to heal by secondary intention. All these situations have in common the fact that the epidermis has been denuded and allowed to heal spontaneously by reepithelialization. The milia appear once the new epidermis has formed.

In these circumstances, biopsies do not show a relationship between milia and the follicular apparatus. Therefore milia are not caused by plugged follicles.[9] Cords of relatively undifferentiated epithelial cells may grow down from the epidermis or from epithelial appendages and possibly cause milia. These strands of cells may result from traumatized, transected (and thus isolated) follicular structures or ducts from sebaceous and eccrine glands. In dermabrasion one should be aware also of the possibility of embedding epidermis at the time of sanding.

Milia may arise in association with wounds closed by sutures, appearing either immediately adjacent to the incision line or at the point of percutaneous puncture by the suture needle (Fig. 26-13). Such milia may be caused by ingrowth of epidermis along suture tracts (Fig. 26-13, *A*) or perhaps by transection of follicles at the time of surgery (Fig. 26-13, *C*), either by the scalpel, the suture, or the suture needle. Another possible reason for milia formation may be inadvertent implantation of epidermis in the wound at the time of surgery before wound closure (Fig. 26-13, *B*).

Treatment. The treatment of milia is simple, and local

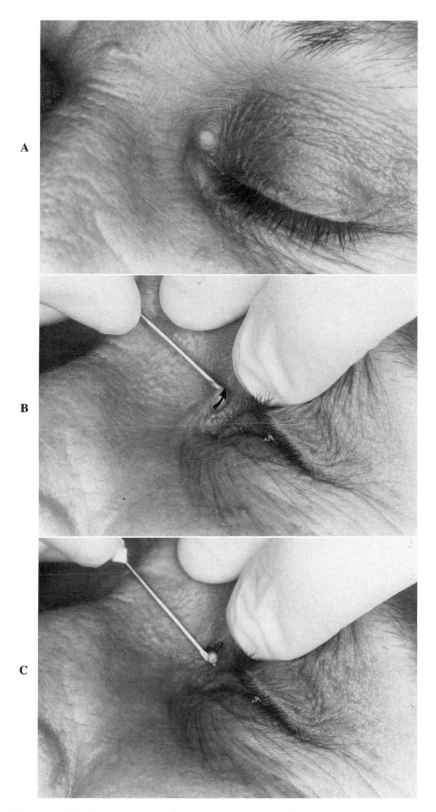

Fig. 26-14. A, Milial cyst at medial side of left upper eyelid. **B,** Creation of small slit in roof with 21-gauge needle. Note direction of movement of needle tip *(arrow)*. **C,** Globoid keratin mass is teased out with needle.

Continued.

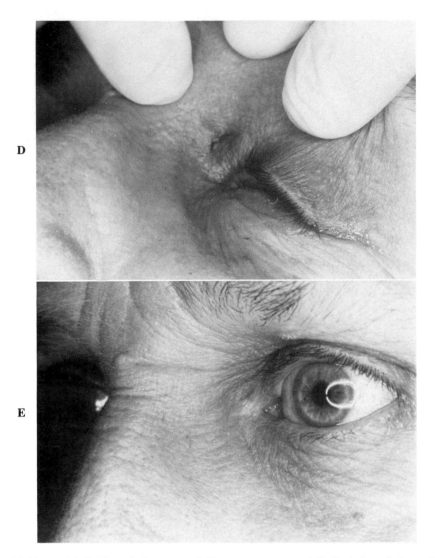

Fig. 26-14, cont'd. D, Wound after removal. No sutures were used. **E,** Healed result 3 months after removal.

anesthesia is not required (Fig. 26-14). The top of the small papule is incised with either a no. 11 scalpel blade or a needle (usually 21-gauge or larger) (Fig. 26-14, *B*). The small globoid whitish mass is then removed (Fig. 26-14, *C*). I have found that its removal is easily accomplished by teasing it out with a needle tip or using a comedo extractor. The resultant small wound (Fig. 26-14, *D*) is allowed to heal by itself. Usually the cosmetic results are excellent (Fig. 26-14, *E*).

Steatocystoma multiplex

Steatocystoma multiplex is a condition in which numerous cystic lesions occur on the anterior trunk and the proximal arms and legs. Usually they first appear in early childhood or adolescence, and the patient develops more with increasing age. These cysts appear as moderately firm, fluctuant nodules that are usually relatively small (5 mm), al-

though the size is variable, ranging from a few millimeters to 2 or 3 cm. They are filled with a yellowish, oily fluid that contains esters and sebum but not free fatty acids.[6] Often there is a familial predisposition with dominant inheritance, although nonfamilial cases may occur.

Cause. Steatocystoma multiplex may be caused by malformation of the pilosebaceous duct junction, which results in dilation of the sebaceous duct and subsequent cyst formation.

Histopathology. One sees a tortuous cystic cavity lined by squamous epithelium without a granular layer. The sebaceous glands are either attached to the cyst cavity or are immediately adjacent. Sometimes vellus hairs are seen within the cyst cavity.

Treatment. Management of the patient with steatocystoma multiplex is usually a dilemma. This is because of the large number (often hundreds) of lesions frequently present,

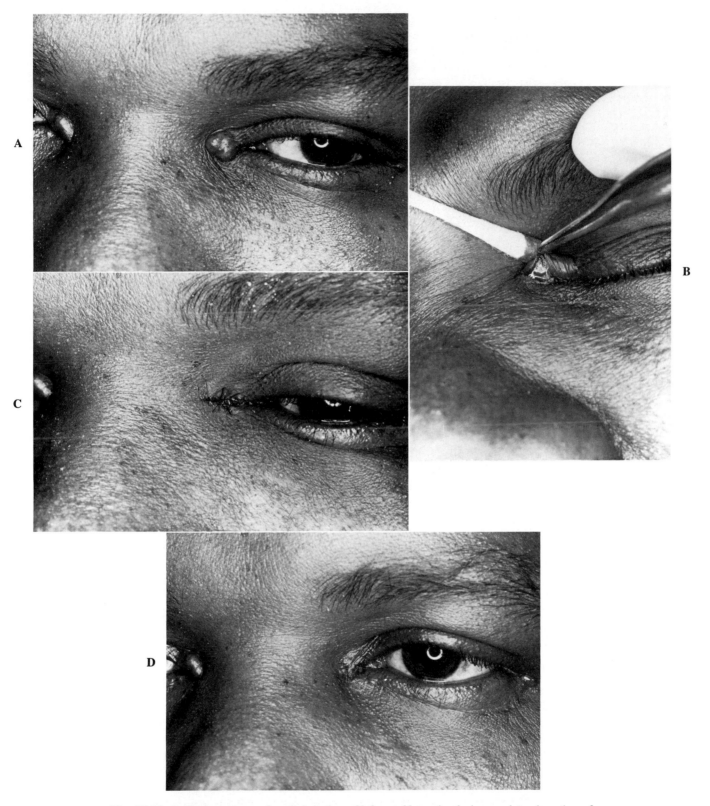

Fig. 26-15. A, Hydrocystoma of medial canthus of left eye. Note other lesions on lateral canthus of left eye and medial canthus of right eye. **B,** Incision made at base of hydrocystoma and intact cyst exposed. Epidermis is being lifted after having been dissected off cyst by blunt scissors. **C,** After cyst is dissected totally free, epidermis is sutured without trimming of excess tissue. **D,** Healed result 3 months after operation.

as well as the fact that more will eventually appear. Treatment is usually medically unnecessary, since these cysts are not painful and rarely get inflamed or infected; however, the patient may desire removal for cosmetic reasons. Since the cysts in steatocystoma multiplex occur mostly on the anterior trunk, where results from excision are notoriously poor, patients should be counseled regarding the benefits versus the poor cosmetic results to be expected from treatment in this area.

Excision offers the patient the best chance for cure of individual lesions. Nevertheless, because of the multitude of lesions present, this is usually impractical. Incision, drainage, and electrocautery can also be effective.[7] Cryosurgery may also be useful.[30]

Hidrocystoma

A hidrocystoma is an uncommon cystic lesion derived from the eccrine duct, the apocrine duct, or the apocrine gland. Usually the patient presents with multiple lesions, more or less symmetrically distributed on the face—most commonly in the periorbital skin. The lesions are round, tense, soft, small (1 to 3 mm) papules in otherwise normal skin.

The cause of hidrocystomas is unknown but is thought to be enlargement (cystic dilation) of the apocrine duct, apocrine gland, or eccrine duct. This condition has a familial tendency, and profuse sweating seems to make it worse.

Histopathology. A cystic cavity lined with secretory cells exists in the dermis. Differentiation between a cyst arising from the apocrine duct and one arising from the eccrine duct can be difficult. If the cyst originates from the apocrine gland, decapitation secretion may be seen.

Treatment. Incision with dissection of this cyst is preferred over excision without dissection. If one is careful, the clear cyst can be separated intact from the overlying epidermis and the surrounding stroma. The overlying epidermis is then sutured into place (Fig. 26-15). Removal in this manner leads to an excellent cosmetic result and little or no likelihood of recurrence. Simple incision and drainage of hidrocystomas result in recurrence.

DIGITAL MYXOID CYST

Myxoid cysts occur as cystic lesions, usually just distal to the distal interphalangeal joints, commonly of the hands and less commonly of the toes (Fig. 26-16). They were initially described by Hyde in 1883.[14] These cystic lesions almost always occur to one side of the midline because the extensor tendon displaces laterally lesions arising in the midline. Most frequently these cysts appear as single lesions, but occasionally several digits are involved. The cyst itself is smooth, shiny, translucent, and of variable size but usually about 0.5 cm. The overlying epidermis appears to be thinned. On puncture and expression of the contents, a clear jellylike substance appears, which is largely hyal-

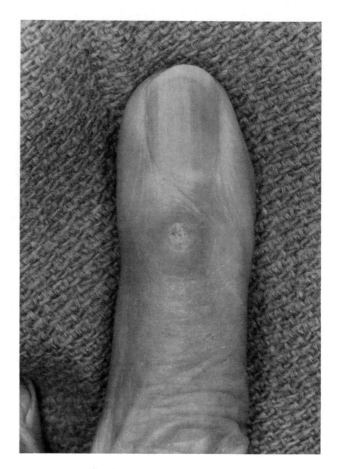

Fig. 26-16. Myxoid cyst of digit.

uronic acid.[15] Myxoid cysts occur more frequently in women than in men, mostly in the late 40s or early 50s; they are usually associated with x-ray findings of osteoarthritis or at least osteophytosis.[18,28] Therefore they may arise from irritation of the synovial lining caused by osteophytes within degenerative interphalangeal joints. Other theories regarding their pathogenesis include mucoid degeneration within the connective tissue and embryonic rests.

Myxoid cysts can be painful and may cause nail deformities such as longitudinal grooving. This grooving can occur as long as 6 months before the appearance of the myxoid cyst and thus may herald the appearance of the cyst itself.[1]

Although some myxoid cysts arise spontaneously without an apparent true connection with the joint space,[36] most probably arise from the synovial lining of adjacent joints. A 1942 study showed that iodopyracet (Diodrast) injected into a myxoid cyst flowed into the joint space, as visualized on an x-ray film.[7] Another study[17] in 1951 demonstrated by careful pathologic dissection that a myxoid cyst was connected with the joint synovium via a small stalk. This has subsequently been confirmed by others.[18,28] Finally a connection was shown between the synovium and digital myxoid cysts by the injection of methylene blue into the joint space.[29] After injection the myxoid cysts also turned blue.

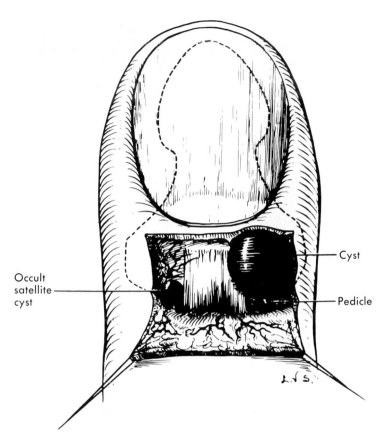

Occult
satellite
cyst

Cyst

Pedicle

ᴌᴠs.

Fig. 26-17. Appearance of digital myxoid cyst after injection of methylene blue into joint space and after skin flap has been raised. Note presence of additional occult satellite cyst and pedicle attachment to joint space. (From Newmeyer, W.L., Kilgore, E.S., Jr., and Graham, W.P., III: Plast. Reconstr. Surg. **53**:313, 1974.)

Histopathology. It is important to appreciate that myxoid cysts are not true cysts in the sense that a well-defined epidermal wall encloses some substance. Instead, mucinous material is seen lying free within the dermis. Therefore this lesion is really a pseudocyst. Cleftlike spaces are initially present, which coalesce to form a larger multiloculated cystic space. This space contains mucin, which is largely hyaluronic acid.

Treatment. The definitive treatment of digital myxoid cysts depends on one's belief about their true etiology. If these cysts, as most authorities currently believe, arise from and are connected with the adjacent joint space, then careful dissection is the treatment of choice, removing both the cyst and its stalk connection to the synovium.

Goldman et al. treated two patients with methylene blue–assisted surgery.[12] After digital nerve block anesthesia is obtained (but before incision), a solution of methylene blue, saline, and hydrogen peroxide is injected inferiorly into the distal interphalangeal joint space. The hydrogen peroxide facilitates movement of the dye into the cyst via its stalk, which connects with the joint space. This technique frequently shows multiple cysts, which have sometimes not been noted clinically (Fig. 26-17). Moreover, the methylene blue helps to identify the stalk.

After injection of the methylene blue a flap is raised on the dorsum of the finger. Two cutaneous incisions are made proximally as extensions of the proximal nail folds to the proximal interphalangeal joint. Hemostasis is achieved by means of a Penrose drain, which encircles the digit proximally and is clamped with a hemostat. It is a good idea to place gauze underneath the Penrose drain to help even out the pressure on underlying arteries. When the flap is turned back, the underlying cysts with their attached stalks can be easily seen, since they are bluish (Fig. 26-17). Sometimes the cysts can be separated from the overlying epidermis if careful dissection is performed. Care should be taken not to injure the extensor tendon or the nail matrix. Osteophytes are almost always present, but their removal is probably unnecessary.[28] The flap is then sutured into place. If the skin overlying the cyst is very thin, it may need to be excised. The resultant surgical defect can usually be easily closed as part of the flap. After surgery the finger is dressed and splinted in the position of function, slightly flexed. Immobilization is continued for 2 to 3 weeks.

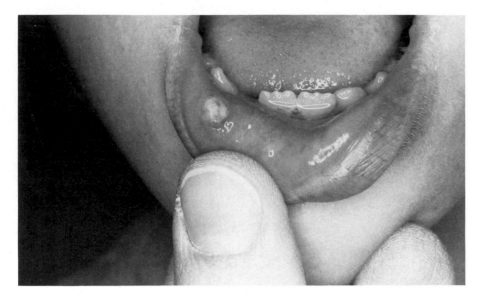

Fig. 26-18. Mucous cyst.

The two patients treated by Goldman et al. with this technique were cured.[12] In contrast, five lesions treated by standard surgical excision recurred. Other authors also report similar successful results (100% cure) without methylene blue injection but with careful dissection of the cyst and its attached stalk.[18,28]

In one report on the use of an en bloc excision of the proximal nail fold for myxoid cysts, the cyst with its overlying skin was removed and the surgical defect allowed to heal by granulation and epidermization.[36] The author reported no recurrences in 5 cases so treated. Other physicians advise skin grafts after such en bloc excisions.

The use of intralesional steroid injections into myxoid cysts is widely practiced. However, when patients are followed-up for long periods of time, such cysts are frequently seen to recur after temporary disappearance.[8] However, because a significant minority of such cysts may completely disappear with such injections, this should be the initial form of therapy to preclude surgery. In the study of Goldman et al. 13 of 31 cysts (42%) were injected without recurrence.[12]

Epstein recommends puncturing the myxoid cyst with a sterile needle and expressing its contents.[8] Repeated needlings were necessary for successful treatment to preclude recurrence. Of 40 cysts treated by this approach, 29 (73%) completely regressed. Of those that failed, most were reduced to small cysts acceptable to patients.

MUCOUS CYST

A clear to bluish cyst that commonly occurs inside the lower lip is the mucous cyst (mucocele) (Fig. 26-18). This cyst varies between 2 and 10 mm in diameter and is solitary. It is soft and causes the patient no discomfort. It may occur at any age. Rarely mucous cysts occur in the buccal mucosa or tongue.

Cause. Mucous cysts are probably caused by sialomucin that has spilled into the submucosa subsequent to rupture of a mucous duct. Rupture of the mucous duct is probably set off by minor trauma. The sialomucin produces inflammation, which is walled off by fibrous tissue, producing a cyst.

Histopathology. A cystic space is surrounded by granulation, fibrosis, or both.

Treatment. Mucous cysts are readily treated by marsupialization. The roof should be removed in toto and the cyst evacuated of its contents, which appear as a clear watery fluid. The lining is then destroyed by electrodesiccation. Excision may also be performed but is often unnecessary.

REFERENCES

1. Anderson, C.R.: Longitudinal grooving of the nails caused by synovial lesions, Arch. Dermatol. Syph. **55:**828, 1947.
2. Bieter, R.N.: Applied pharmacology of local anesthetics, Am. J. Surg. **34:**500, 1936.
3. Brownstein, M.H., and Arluk, D.J.: Proliferating trichilemmal cyst: a simulant of squamous cell carcinoma, Cancer **48:** 1207, 1981.
4. Danna, J.A.: A simple treatment for sebaceous cyst, New Orleans Med. Surg. J. **98:**5, 1945.
5. Danna, J.A.: The treatment of sebaceous cyst by electrosurgical marsupialization, Ann. Sur. **123:**952, 1946.
6. Egbert, B.M., Price, N.M., and Segal, R.J.: Steatocystoma multiplex: report of a florid case and a review, Arch. Dermatol. **115:**334, 1979.
7. Eliassow, A., and Frank, S.B.: Pathogenesis of synovial lesions of the skin, Arch. Dermatol. Syph. **46:**691, 1942.
8. Epstein, E.: A simple technique for managing digital mucous cysts, Arch. Dermatol. **115:**1315, 1979.

9. Epstein, W.L., and Kligman, A.M.: The pathogenesis of milia and benign tumors of the skin, J. Invest. Dermatol. **26:**1, 1956.

10. Epstein, W.L., and Kligman, A.M.: Epithelial cysts in buried human skin, A.M.A. Arch. Dermatol. **76:**437, 1957.

11. Glamb, R., and Kim, R.: Pseudocyst of the auricle, J. Am. Acad. Derm. **11:**58, 1984.

12. Goldman, J.A., et al.: Digital mucinous pseudocysts, Arthritis Rheum. **20:**997, 1977.

13. Greer, K.E.: Epidermal inclusion cyst of the sole, Arch. Dermatol. **109:**251, 1974.

14. Hyde, J.N. In Ormsby, O.S.: Synovial lesions of the skin: clinical report, J. Cutan. Dis. **31:**943, 1913.

15. Johnson, W.C., Graham, J.H., and Helwig, E.B: Cutaneous myxoid cyst: a clinicopathological and histochemical study, J.A.M.A. **191:**15, 1965.

16. Kelley, E.F.: Treatment of sebaceous cysts, N.Y. State J. Med. **50:**679, 1950.

17. King, E.S.J.: Mucous cysts of the fingers, Aust. N.Z. J. Surg. **21:**121, 1951.

18. Kleinert, H.E., et al.: Etiology and treatment of the so-called mucous cyst of the finger, J. Bone Joint Surg. **54A:**1455, 1972.

19. Kligman, A.M.: The myth of the sebaceous cyst, Arch. Dermatol. **89:**253, 1964.

20. Krull, E.A.: The "little" curet [surgical gems], J. Dermatol. Surg. Oncol. **4:**656, 1978.

21. Lieblich, L.M., Geronemus, R.G., and Gibbs, R.C.: Use of a biopsy punch for removal of epithelial cysts, J. Dermatol. Surg. Oncol. **8:**1059, 1982.

22. Love, W.R., and Montgomery, H.: Epithelial cysts, Arch. Dermatol. Syph. **47:**185, 1943.

23. Massanari, R.M.: Abscess culture [letter], J.A.M.A. **250:** 1216, 1983.

24. McGavran, M.H., and Binnington, B.: Keratinous cysts of the skin, Arch. Dermatol. **94:**499, 1966.

25. Mevorah, B., and Bovet, R.: Treatment of retroauricular keratinous cysts, J. Dermatol. Surg. Oncol. **10:**40, 1984.

26. Montagna, W., Chase, H.B., Melaragno, H.P.: The skin of hairless mice. I. The formation of cysts and the distribution of lipids, J. Invest. Dermatol. **19:**83, 1952.

27. Moore, C., and Greer, D.M., Jr.: Sebaceous cyst extraction through mini-incisions, Br. J. Plast. Surg. **28:**307, 1975.

28. Nasca, R.J., and Gould, J.S.: Mucous cysts of the digits, South. Med. J. **76:**1142, 1983.

29. Newmeyer, W.L., Kilgore, E.S., Jr., and Graham, W.P., III: Mucous cysts: the dorsal distal interphalangeal joint ganglion, Plast. Reconstr. Surg. **53:**313, 1974.

30. Notowicz, A.: Treatment of lesions of steatocystoma multiplex and other epidermal cysts by cryosurgery (cryo corner), J. Dermatol. Surg. Oncol. **6:**98, 1980.

31. O'Keeffe, P.J.: Trephining sebaceous cysts, Br. J. Plast. Surg. **25:**411, 1972.

32. Oliveira, A.S., et al.: A simple method of excising tricholemmal cysts from the scalp, J. Dermatol. Surg. Oncol. **5:** 625, 1979.

33. Olsen, C., and Forscher, B.K.: Soluble collagen in acute inflammation, Proc. Soc. Exp. Biol. N.Y. **111:**126, 1962.

34. Patton, H.S.: An alternate method for removing sebaceous cysts, Surg. Gynecol. Obstet. **117:**645, 1963.

35. Peinert, R.A., and Courtiss, E.H.: Excision from a distance: a technique for removal of benign subcutaneous lesions, Plast. Reconstr. Surg. **72:**94, 1983.

36. Salasche, S.J.: Myxoid cysts of the proximal nail fold: a surgical approach, J. Dermatol. Surg. Oncol. **10:**35, 1984.

37. Vivakananthan, C.: Minimal incision for removing sebaceous cysts, Br. J. Plast. Surg. **25:**60, 1972.

38. Wilson Jones, E.: Proliferating epidermoid cysts, Arch. Dermatol. **94:**11, 1966.

39. Yaffe, H.S.: Squamous cell carcinoma arising in an epidermal cyst [letter], Arch. Dermatol. **118:**961, 1982.

27

Lesions of
Epidermal Appendages

ACNE VULGARIS

Acne vulgaris commonly affects the face, chest, and upper back in adolescence and early adulthood. It is characterized by three types of lesions: comedones, pustules, and cysts. The formation of all three types of lesions is caused by blockage of the follicular apparatus. Comedones are the smallest acne lesions. If they are formed with the orifices of the follicles open, they are commonly known as blackheads; if they have closed orifices, they are called uninflamed papules or whiteheads. Whether open or closed, the follicle is occluded with keratin. Such an occluded follicle may develop a small area of weakness in its wall and allow its contents (including fatty acids) to spill over into the surrounding dermis. This results in a heightened inflammatory response and is the genesis of an inflamed papule that eventually may become an acne pustule. Keratin may also be extruded into the surrounding tissue, causing a foreign body reaction. If the ruptured contents become walled off, an acne cyst eventuates. This last lesion may be quiescent and felt as a slightly fluctuant nodule under the skin; or it may become inflamed, in which case it becomes larger, more fluctuant and erythematous.

Surgery for active acne

The surgical management of active acne is based on the premise that mechanical removal of the contents of blocked follicles shortens the lesion duration and prevents additional inflammatory events from occurring. Although comedo removal by pressure extraction is widely accepted as an adjunct to topical or systemic acne treatment both because it is based on common sense and because it has been highly rated by generations of dermatologists, there are few good controlled studies that attest to the efficacy of acne surgery.[9] In one study it was found that pressure extraction of comedones on one half of the forehead in 20 patients prevented

the development of inflamed acne lesions in most patients.[4] In patients with cystic acne, however, pressure extraction of inflamed lesions appeared to make the acne worse. Nevertheless, many patients complain of pruritus, and for this reason as well as for cosmesis acne surgery may be beneficial.

Comedo removal. Comedones are removed by means of pressure with a comedo extractor (pressure extraction). The pressure exerted by this instrument is evenly distributed circumferentially around the lesion on the surface of the skin. This generates pressure forces within the dermis that impinge on the follicle and push the follicular contents out through the follicular opening. If the follicle wall is weak or if there is resistance at the follicular opening, the follicle wall may rupture, spilling its contents into the dermis. This is to be avoided, since it may lead to an inflammatory reaction and cyst formation. For closed comedones (whiteheads), the top of the lesion is first gently nicked either with a no. 11 blade or with a sterile 21-gauge (or larger) syringe needle. Open comedones (blackheads) do not have an epidermal covering, and therefore their contents can be simply extruded by pressure without additional tissue manipulation. Several lesions can be removed at one sitting.

The use of a suction machine to "vacuum out" comedones has been described.[10,11] A glass medicine dropper is used at the end of the suction hose. The tapered glass tip is pressed down over the acne lesion, thus creating both an external positive pressure mechanically and a negative internal pressure by means of suction. As one pushes gently with the medicine dropper, probably less pressure needs to be applied to the skin around a comedo to extract the follicular contents because of the addition of suction. This is less painful for patients and possibly results in less likelihood of development of inflamed acne lesions.

Pustules and cysts. More exuberant pustules and cysts can

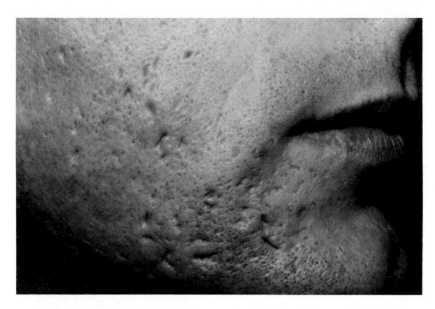

Fig. 27-1. Deep "ice-pick" acne scars.

also be drained, but usually these are not manipulated, because inflammation will probably result or be made worse. If the patient is extremely bothered by these lesions (especially cysts), they can be injected with triamcinolone acetonide (2.5 mg-5 mg/ml), which is preferable to open drainage and hastens resolution.

Dermabrasion. Dermabrasion may be used on patients with active pustular acne, and it has been my observation that this procedure eradicates the lesions. Thus dermabrasion can be considered therapeutic in this situation as a means of draining multiple lesions. However, I do not use this procedure unless there are also shallow scars from previous acne lesions that can benefit from the dermabrasion.

Skin grafting. As an extreme measure for cystic acne on the back, excision with skin grafting has been reported.[13] In my experience this is unnecessary. Medical management properly given with newer retinoids or antibiotics almost always brings recalcitrant acne under control, obviating the need for such extreme measures.

Surgery for acne scars

The scars resulting from acne are of various depths, and the best method of correction is the procedure that gives the maximal improvement with the least subsequent problem. Shallow scars can be dealt with by dermabrasion, dermaplaning (to be discussed in a later volume),[12] or collagen injection. Deep scars, so-called ice-pick scars (Fig. 27-1), are difficult to correct.

Deep pits and scars caused by acne can be sometimes managed by excision and closure. The pits can be excised by means of a skin punch or scalpel blade. However, in patients with very oily skin with patulous pores, excision of deep pits or scars is frequently unsuccessful. The sutures tend to cause suture marks, and the wounds often tend to get infected. Excision of deep pits in such patients seems to work best at the time of a dermabrasion. The pits are excised and sutured closed immediately after the dermabrasion. This leads, in my experience, to imperceptible scars.

Keratin-filled pits, like acne scars, may also be removed by a skin punch (Fig. 27-2). Such pits may be caused by previous acne cysts or large epidermal cysts.

Some authorities recommend using small autotransplants from the postauricular scalp or posterior earlobe. They are placed into recipient sites on the face prepared by using the skin punch to remove deep acne scars. The recipient graft site will be about 0.5 mm larger than the dermal punch size used to produce the surgical defect. Therefore a donor punch 0.5 to 0.75 mm larger than the punch used to create the recipient site provides a skin graft with a tighter fit into the recipient area and should be used. The skin grafts can be held in place by adhesive skin-closure strips. Dermabrasion can be done at a later time following grafting to help the graft blend in more with the surrounding skin. My experience with this technique is that it is only moderately successful. Some grafts do very well and become imperceptible scars; however, other grafts become hypertrophic and may develop cysts if remnants of epithelium are left in the recipient sites. In addition, this technique works less well in those patients with patulous pores who frequently need improvement the most.

ACNE KELOIDALIS NUCHAE

Acne keloidalis nuchae (dermatitis papillaris capillitii, sycosis nuchae) is a chronic folliculitis of the nape of the neck just beneath the hairline with extension into the scalp. This condition usually occurs in blacks, predominantly

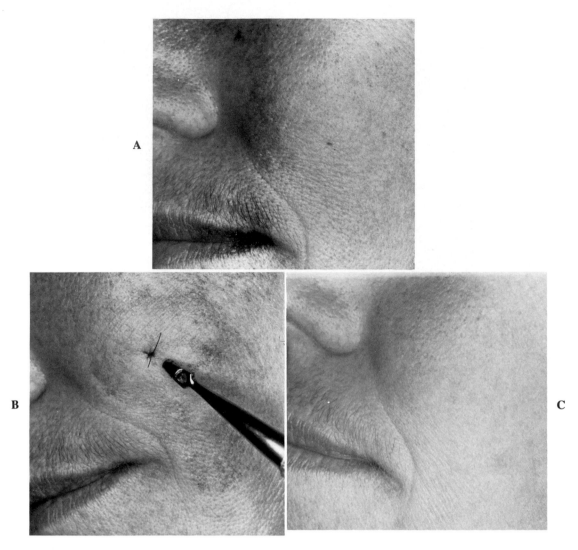

Fig. 27-2. A, Small, depressed, keratin-filled pit on cheek. **B,** Removed with small (2 mm) punch. Defect sutured with one suture, so long axis falls along line of maximal skin tension. **C,** Healed result 6 months later. Surgical scar is difficult to detect.

men. Initially one sees folliculitis, which gives rise to follicular papules, pustules, and abscesses. When the folliculitis is chronic, fibrous tissue forms, and nodular areas appear. Follicular papules perforated by tufts of hair and patchy alopecia may be seen. Any pustules that form tend to recur, and the condition is usually intractable unless treated adequately. Histopathologically, one sees a chronic granulomatous inflammation.

Patients with acne keloidalis nuchae are prone to follicular occlusion processes elsewhere on the body such as acne, sycosis barbae, hidradentitis suppurativa, and folliculitis decalvans. The curliness of the hair may potentiate this problem. Either clipped hairs remain embedded as foreign bodies, or the hairs themselves grow entirely underneath the skin.

Treatment

If few and early, lesions can be treated by antibiotics and the injection of triamcinolone acetonide (10 mg/ml). This aids in the resolution of purulence and small papules. It is wise to get bacterial cultures before prescribing antibiotics. Occasionally, as in hidradentitis suppurativa, anaerobic organisms are an important contributor to the ongoing process. Any easily seen embedded hairs should be removed.

If the process is widespread (Fig. 27-3, *A*), total excision of the affected tissue may be considered. Before the day of excision, any purulent drainage should be brought under control by the use of systemic antibiotics. After local anesthesia has been achieved, the total infected area including fibrous tissue down into subcutaneous fat is removed. (Fig. 27-3, *B*).

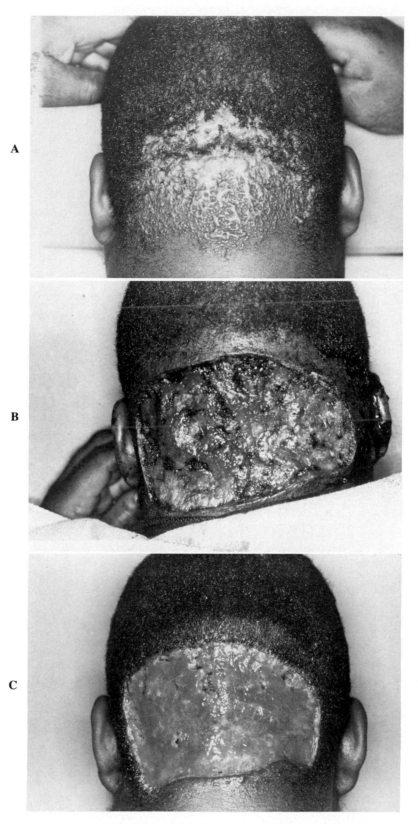

Fig. 27-3. A, Acne keloidalis nuchae. **B,** Excision of involved area into underlying fat. Wound allowed to heal by secondary intention. **C,** Granulation tissue in wound at 3 weeks after surgery.
Continued.

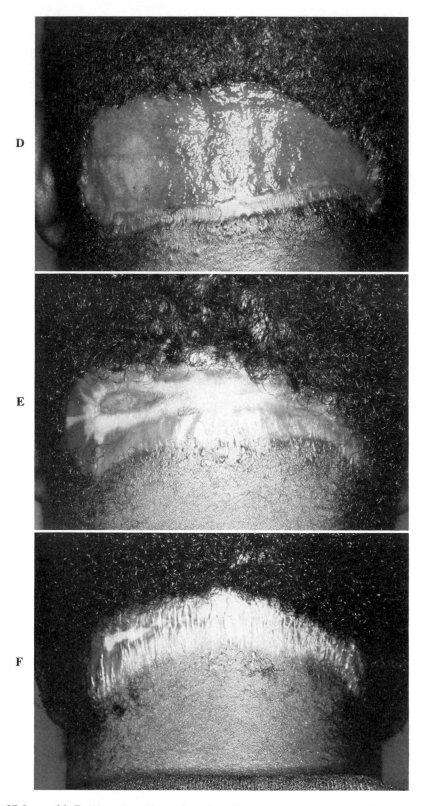

Fig. 27-3, cont'd. D, Wound smaller at 6 weeks following surgery as a result of contraction. Note advancing epidermal edge at lower border of wound. **E,** Almost completely healed wound (except for small area on left) 10 weeks after surgery. Injection of Kenalog-10 given at this time and monthly for 3 months. **F,** Final healed scar at 6 months following surgery. There was no evidence of recurrence of disease process and no keloid formation.

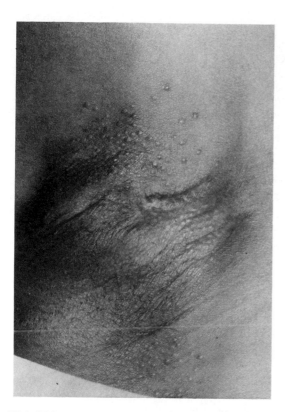

Fig. 27-4. Hidradenitis suppurativa associated with Fox-Fordyce disease (small papules in axilla). Note also the linear bands that are result of fibrosed epithelialized tracts underneath skin surface.

The resultant defect can be allowed to heal by secondary intention (Fig. 27-3, *C* through *E*). Alternatively, it can be grafted or sutured primarily. I prefer to allow the wound to heal by secondary intention, since the cosmetic result is usually good and there are few problems. A skin graft usually gives a sunken appearance, since in this case it overlies a very deep wound. One author[5] advises primarily closing the large wounds by having the patient bend his head back and using bolsters. However, the resultant scar from this technique inevitably spreads and gives about the same appearance as one that results from secondary intention healing. In addition, if one feels compelled to suture a wound, it is possible that not enough tissue will be taken to include all involved areas.

I have personally treated four patients using the technique shown in Fig. 27-3, *A* through *E*. Three of the four patients had no further problem with the area and had good cosmetic results, especially when the hair was grown slightly longer to cover the scar. One patient had two recurrences at the edge of the treated area, but has been in remission for the past 2 years after one major excision and two minor excisions confined to the areas of recurrences. All of the patients are grateful because they had had problems for years in this area.

HIDRADENITIS SUPPURATIVA

Hidradenitis suppurativa (HS) is a chronic inflammatory process that develops on the apocrine gland-bearing areas of the body: the axilla, the areola of the breast, and the anogenital region. Initially a slightly erythematous, tender nodule appears that resembles a furuncle. With time this swelling may resolve, but it often recurs or progresses to a larger abscesslike swelling that may drain by itself. A fistulous opening then commonly occurs. With repeated bouts of swelling and draining, the process extends to adjacent apocrine gland-bearing skin. Eventually many of these abscesslike swellings intercommunicate by way of epidermized tracts. Fibrous bands may then form that are best felt by palpation rather than visualized (Fig. 27-4).

Obese women appear to be affected most frequently, mainly in the axilla. Men are affected most often in the groin. Many patients with HS have other associated follicular occlusion diseases such as acne, folliculitis decalvans, or Fox-Fordyce disease (Fig. 27-4).

The pathogenesis of HS is unclear. Plugging of the apocrine gland orifice followed by dilation of the duct with inflammation probably occurs initially. Infection may then occur. The organisms usually cultured are *Staphylococcus aureus,* β-hemolytic *Streptococcus,* and *Proteus mirabilis.* Also, frequently overlooked are a number of anaerobes.[1] These latter bacteria promote the subcutaneous extension of this disease process.

HS, especially if chronic and in the perineal area, may be associated with development of squamous cell carcinoma.

Histopathology

Abscess formation with acute and chronic inflammation is present. If the abscess is deep, sinus tracts lined by epidermis extend into the subcutaneous tissue. Granulation tissue containing foreign body giant cells may also be present.

Treatment

Although medical management of HS may be possible if the lesions are small and not extensive, surgical removal of diseased tissue is the surest, most successful form of therapy. However, before surgery can be contemplated, the infection and drainage should first be brought under control by use of suitable antibiotics. Abscessed lesions should be cultured for anaerobes and aerobes.[6] Pathology laboratories are reluctant to perform sensitivities on anaerobic organisms if they have been cultured from the perirectal area, since many of these anaerobes are part of the normal flora in that area. However, such sensitivity results may be critical to the selection of antibiotics, so the treating physician should insist on the performance of sensitivity tests. Organisms that are part of the normal flora may become pathogenic in certain circumstances. This apparently is true in HS.

The medical treatment of the infection that occurs with

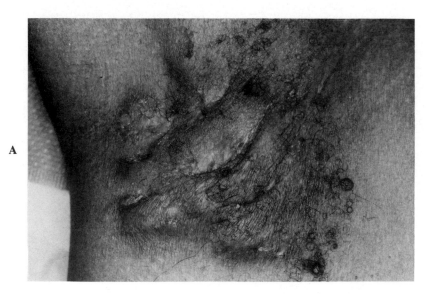

Fig. 27-5. A, Hidradenitis suppurativa of axilla.

HS is directed at both the aerobic *and* anaerobic organisms present. Usually this requires a combination of two antibiotics given simultaneously. For the anaerobes, I usually empirically begin by prescribing metronidazole (Flagyl) while awaiting culture results. In addition, a broad-spectrum antibiotic such as a cephalosporin (Keflex) is used for the gram-positive and gram-negative organisms that are also invariably present. Other suitable antibiotics useful in combination with a cephalosporin for HS are clindamycin (Cleocin) or cefoxitin (Mefoxin).[1] Both the latter drugs have significant activity against anaerobes. Trimethoprim-sulfamethoxazole (Bactrim or Septra) is an alternative antibiotic to a cephalosporin for patients who are allergic to penicillin.

Once infection has been brought under control, surgery can be planned. I favor the exteriorization (marsupialization) procedure.[8] The affected areas are first anesthetized with a suitable local anesthetic. A probe is inserted into the sinus tract opening and used to define the affected areas. The skin overlying the sinus tracts and abscesses is removed with scissors. The mushy contents are curetted with a dermal curette, and the base of the wound is completely coagulated by electrocoagulation. If thick scar tissue exists, it is best to remove this as well. The resultant wound is allowed to heal by means of granulation and epidermization. Skin grafts and flaps can usually be avoided by means of this procedure.

In the axilla significant fibrous tissue may form in response to HS. Simple exteriorization fails to remove this tissue; if it is not removed, recurrences of the basic process can develop. Therefore I recommend full-thickness removal of tissue to fat in this area and allowance of the subsequent wound formed to heal by secondary intention (Fig. 27-5).

In a study[7] of 10 patients with bilateral HS, results after full-thickness excision were compared when one axilla was skin grafted and the other axilla was allowed to heal by secondary intention. Better cosmetic results were obtained with healing by secondary intention. In addition, most patients preferred the healing by secondary intention to skin grafts.

Recent claims have been made regarding the usefulness of systemic retinoids for HS.[2] Isotretinoin (Accutane) has been beneficial for cystic acne. Therefore its use for HS, another follicular occlusive disease, seems reasonable. Clinical studies to date, however, have not shown clear evidence of benefit for extensive disease.[3]

SYRINGOMA

Syringomas appear as small (1 to 2 mm) discrete papules usually on the lower eyelids of women. However, on occasion these lesions are widespread on the cheeks, forehead, and (rarely) on the anterior neck (Fig. 27-6) or trunk. Syringomas are flesh-colored or slightly yellowish and soft.

Histopathology

Microscopically syringomas appear as dilated, cystic, eccrine sweat ducts, some of which have tails resembling commas, giving a "tadpole" appearance to the ducts. Usually these ducts are lined by two layers of cells and contain amorphous debris. The stroma appears fibrous.

Treatment

There is no good treatment for syringomas short of total excision of each lesion, which is usually not feasible. Electrodesiccation of each lesion sometimes suffices. The CO_2 laser is perhaps best suited for destruction of individual lesions, since it offers minimal normal tissue destruction and pinpoint accuracy.

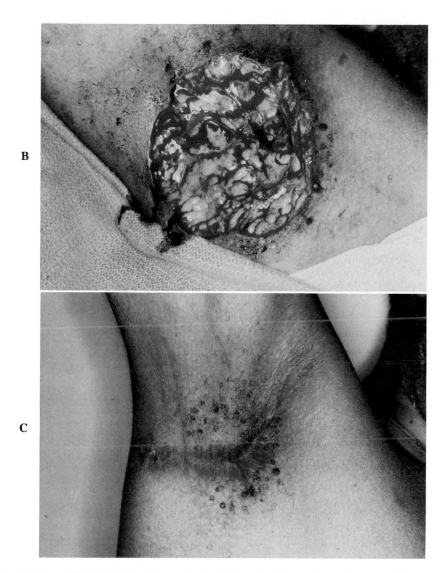

Fig. 27-5, cont'd. B, Extirpation to fat including all fibrous tissue. Extent of tissue removal laterally was determined in part by probing epithelialized tracts. Wound was allowed to heal by secondary intention. **C,** Healed result 6 months later. Patient had full range of motion in arm.

TRICHOEPITHELIOMA

Trichoepitheliomas usually occur as multiple lesions on the central face, especially around the eyelids (Fig. 27-7). The lesions are flesh-colored and usually about 2 to 6 mm in diameter. Multiple trichoepitheliomas can be inherited as an autosomal dominant trait. Solitary trichoepithelioma can also occur, usually on the face, and is nonhereditary.

Histopathology

Tumor aggregates of basophilic cells similar to the cells found in basal cell carcinoma comprise a trichoepithelioma. These cells are usually arranged in a lacelike network.

When branching off a follicular structure, these cell aggregates often have an antlerlike appearance. Horn cysts are usually present. It can be difficult, if not impossible, on occasion to differentiate microscopically a trichoepithelioma from a basal cell carcinoma.

Treatment

Therapy for multiple trichoepitheliomas is limited by the cosmetic results. Removal of the lesions superficially results in their regrowth. However, deeper excisions leave more scarring.

I have found that the loop electrode on the electrosurgical apparatus (set on the cutting current) works well on

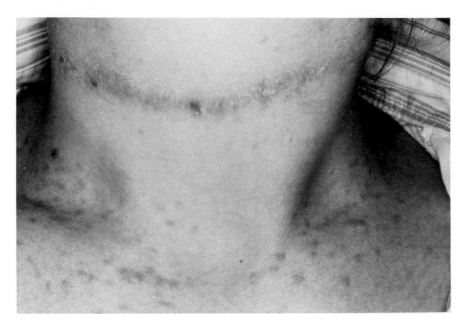

Fig. 27-6. Syringomas of neck and supraclavicular area. Linear scar is result of attempted ("plastic") surgical extirpation performed elsewhere 1½ years previously. This is unacceptable cosmetic result for both patient and physician.

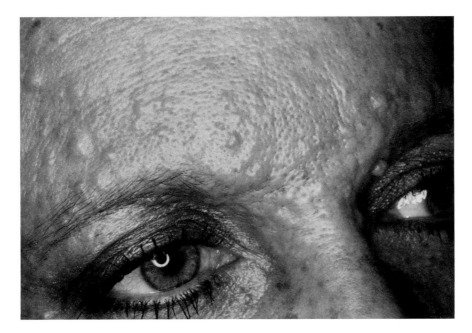

Fig. 27-7. Multiple trichoepitheliomas.

trichoepitheliomas. This minimizes tissue destruction. The lesions are removed as flush as possible with the skin surface. The field of involvement is then dermabraded with a diamond fraise. This procedure results in marked improvement but not total ablation. Patients are usually quite appreciative.

The CO_2 laser may also be useful in removing multiple trichoepitheliomas. This instrument is precise and results in minimal tissue damage. However, whether the short- or long-term results with the laser are better than those with the electrosurgical apparatus with dermabrasion has yet to be established.

REFERENCES

1. Brenner, D.E., and Lookingbill, D.P.: Anaerobic microorganisms in chronic suppurative hidradenitis [letter], Lancet **2**: 921, 1980.
2. Dicken, C.L., Powell, S.T., and Spear, K.L.: Evaluation of isotretinoin treatment of hidradenitis suppurativa, J. Am. Acad. Derm. **11**:500, 1984.
3. Jones, D.H., Cunliffe, W.J., and King, K.: Hidradenitis suppurativa—lack of success with 13-cis-retinoic acid [letter], Br. J. Dermatol. **107**:252, 1982.
4. Lowney, E.D., et al.: Value of comedo extraction in treatment of acne vulgaris, J.A.M.A. **189**:1000, 1964.
5. Malherbe, W.D.F.: Dermatome dermaplaning and sycosis nuchae excision, Clin. Plast. Surg. **4**:289, 1977.
6. Massanari, R.M.: Abscess culture [letter], J.A.M.A. **250**: 1216, 1983.
7. Morgan, W.P., Harding, K.G., and Hughes, L.E.: A comparison of skin grafting and healing by granulation, following axillary excision for hidradenitis suppurativa, Ann. R. Coll. Surg. (Engl.) **65**:235, 1983.
8. Mullins, J.F., McCash, W.B., and Boudreau, R.F.: Treatment of chronic hidradenitis suppurativa: surgical modification, Postgrad. Med. **26**:805, 1959.
9. Olsen, T.G.: Therapy of acne, Med. Clin. North Am. **66**(4): 851, 1982.
10. Pierce, H.E.: Sebo-suction—an effective adjunctive treatment for comedone acne (surgical gems), J. Dermatol. Surg. Oncol. **9**:955, 1983.
11. Potts, L.W., Jr.: Comedone extraction by aspiration: new therapy for acne, Cutis **6**:669, 1970.
12. Spira, M.: Treatment of acne pitting and scarring, Plast. Reconstr. Surg. **60**:38, 1977.
13. Weinrauch, L., et al.: Surgical treatment of severe acne conglobata, J. Dermatol. Surg. Oncol. **7**:492, 1981.

28

Foreign Materials

TATTOOS

Tattoos are frequently presented for removal, usually for cosmetic reasons. They are produced by the introduction of insoluble pigments into the dermis and result in permanent designs or inscriptions. Two types of tattoos are recognized: those produced by professional tattoo artists and those produced by amateurs. The professional tattoo artist uses special equipment that places pigments at a uniform level within the dermis. The amateur, on the other hand, frequently uses a needle to pierce the skin and introduce the pigment; the relatively crude methodology places the pigment at a nonuniform level in the dermis. Because some of the pigment placed by the amateur may be deep, "homemade" tattoos are notoriously more difficult to remove. Also, since these tattoos are often self-inflicted, they are usually placed on highly mobile areas such as the forearms or fingers—areas that are prone to noticeable scar formation.

The pigments that are inserted to produce tattoos include India ink (black), chrome green, cobalt blue, cinnabar (a pigment containing red mercuric sulfide), and cadmium sulfide (yellow). The last is sometimes combined with cinnabar to produce a brighter red and may cause a photosensitivity reaction. Mercury may cause chronic inflammation in tattoos, either by a delayed hypersensitivity type of reaction or by stimulating inflammatory cells by some unknown mechanism.[1] With time, tattoos tend to blur and fade, probably because of pigment migration or phagocytosis by cells.

Histopathology. Diffuse granules of pigment exist in the dermis both within macrophages and extracellularly. An inflammatory reaction is absent.

Occasionally tattoo pigments cause allergic or granulomatous reactions. In photoallergic reactions, such as that to cadmium sulfide, a lymphoid inflammatory infiltrate is present. In granulomatous reactions, as can occur with chrome green, cobalt blue, or mercuric sulfide, an epithelial cell granuloma or a foreign body granuloma is present.

Treatment. Every patient desiring removal of a tattoo should be warned that the cosmetic result may be no better or even worse than the tattoo itself. If tattoos are small, simple excision is satisfactory, although the resultant scars usually spread somewhat with time. When patients have a reaction to the tattoo, only that portion with the offending pigment need be removed (Fig. 28-1). Removal for this reason is a medical, not cosmetic, necessity. Tattoos that cannot be easily excised are best removed by light dermabrasion or by laser treatment.

SILICONE AND PARAFFIN

Both silicone and paraffin were widely used in injections to correct depressions or provide elevations in the skin. Occasionally reactions were seen. See Chapter 18 for a discussion of this topic.

MISCELLANEOUS FOREIGN OBJECTS

Occasionally various foreign objects (for example, glass, wood, or metal) become embedded within or below the dermis, frequently without the patient's knowledge. The overlying skin may then form a nonhealing ulcer or granulation tissue resembling a pyogenic granuloma. Diagnostic x-rays might not confirm the presence of a foreign body unless it is metal or leaded glass. When such lesions occur, especially on the feet, one should suspect the presence of foreign bodies. Feet are more likely to be exposed to the embedding of extraneous substances because people walk around barefoot.

To establish the presence of a foreign body, the wound is probed with a small hemostat. Usually a sinus tract can be found that leads from the wound to the foreign substance. Extraction is then a simple procedure (Fig. 28-2). Complete wound healing will then occur.

REFERENCE

1. Abel, E.A., Silberberg, I., and Queen, D.: Studies of chronic inflammation in a red tattoo by electron microscopy and histochemistry, Acta Dermatol. Venereol. **52**:453, 1972.

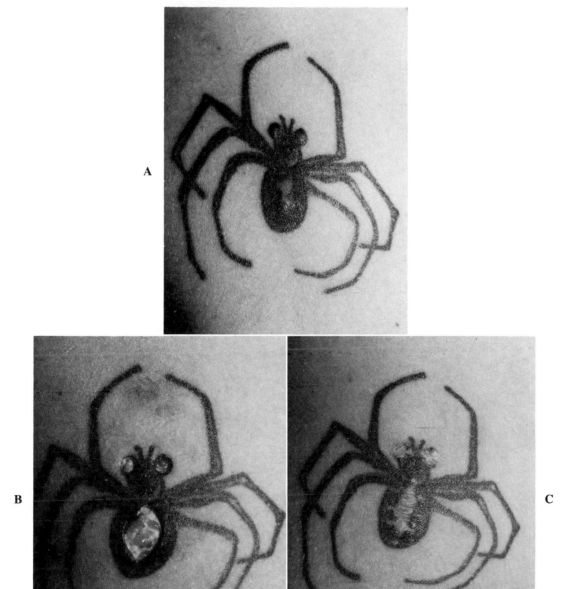

Fig. 28-1. A, Black widow spider tattoo with inflammatory reaction in its red portion (eyes and hourglass). **B,** Excision of inflamed portions of tattoo. **C,** Healed result 3 months later.

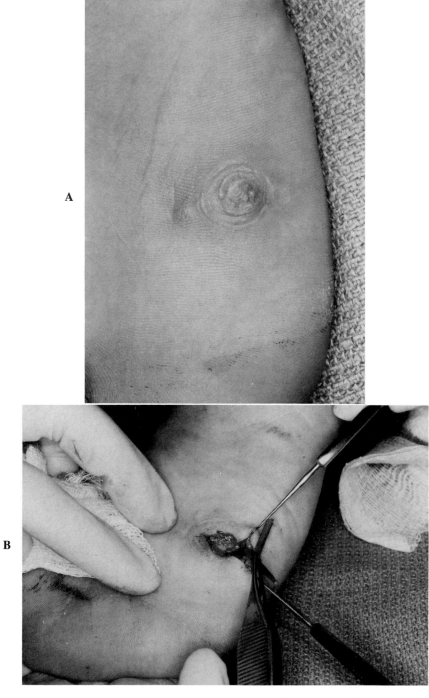

Fig. 28-2. A, Recurrent keratotic area on bottom of foot, underlying which was granulation tissue. **B,** Probing of wound after hyperkeratotic roof was removed, revealing wooden splinter. Patient was unaware of implantation.

PREOPERATIVE EVALUATION FORM FOR CUTANEOUS SURGERY

Patient's name:

Date:

Problem number:

SUBJECTIVE

History of problem:

Review of systems:

Allergies to drugs (anesthetics, antibiotics, pain medications, or topical salves)	No Yes (drug	)
Bleeding problems or anemia (transfusions)	No Yes (type	)
Diabetes	No Yes (treatment	)
Double jointed	No Yes	
Emotional problems	No Yes (treatment	)
Fainting/dizziness	No Yes (cause	)
Glaucoma	No Yes (treatment	)
Heart problems	No Yes (type	)
Hepatitis	No Yes (type	)
High blood pressure	No Yes (treatment	)
Keloid or hypertrophic scar formation	No Yes (site	)
Liver problems	No Yes (type	)
Pacemaker or artificial heart valve	No Yes (type	)

Pigmentary problems	No
	Yes (type)
Pregnancy	No
	Yes (EDC)
Rheumatic fever	No
	Yes (treatment)
Seizures	No
	Yes (treatment)
Wound healing problems	No
	Yes (treatment)

| Other medical conditions: | No | | |
| | Yes | Condition | Treatment |

| Medications (other than above): | No | | |
| | Yes | Medication | Reason |

Past medical problems:

| Prior hospitalization | No | | | |
| | Yes | Reason | Date | Place |

| Prior surgery | No | | | |
| | Yes | Operation | Date | Place |

| Previous radiation (x-ray or grenz ray) treatment | No | |
| | Yes (Anatomic site) |

OBJECTIVE

Physical examination

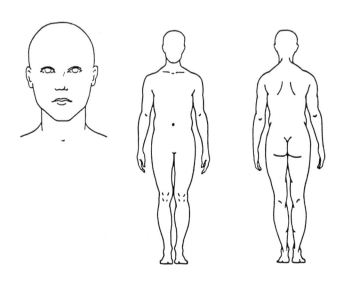

Cutaneous surgical problem (please draw
and label anatomic site)

Cutaneous examination

    Pigmentation

      Facial skin   porous

                                            smooth

      Scars   normal

                                            abnormal

    Palms (for skin cancer patients)

      Keratoses   No

                                            Yes

      Pits   No

                                            Yes

    Signs of radiation (x-ray) damage   No

                                            Yes

    Signs of solar damage   No

                                            Yes

Neurologic examination in area of surgery   normal
    (describe anatomic area examined)   abnormal

Visual acuity (if eyelids included in   OD: OS:
    surgery)

Vital signs   B.P.

                                            H.R.

                                          R.R.

Appearance   well nourished

                                            not well nourished

HEENT   normal

                                            abnormal

Chest   normal

                                            abnormal

Heart

    Rhythm   regular

                                            irregular

    Murmurs   No

                                            Yes (describe:

Abdomen   normal

                                            abnormal

Extremities   normal

                                            abnormal

Laboratory data

    Hematocrit

    Prothrombin time

    Partial thromboplastin time

    Surface hepatitis antigen

    X-ray

    Culture

    Other

ASSESSMENT (include reasons for selecting
   operative procedure)

PLAN

   Diagnostic studies:

   Surgical procedures:

Physician's signature: _____

B

PERMISSION FOR SURGERY AND PHOTOGRAPHY

I, _____, hereby authorize Dr. _____ and/
or designated associates and assistants to perform the following operation(s) on me: _____
_____
_____ .

The nature and purpose of the operations as well as the therapeutic alternatives have been explained to me. Dr. _____ has fully explained to me what will happen during the surgery and has answered all my questions. In addition, I understand that complications such as infection or bleeding can occur and that a scar, although probably minimal, will occur.

I also give Dr. _____ permission to take photographs of my skin lesion and/or any tissue removed before, during, and/or immediately after the operation, and on subsequent office visits. I understand that these photographs may be used for educational purposes and may be published in professional journals or medical books. In such an event I will not be identified by name. Furthermore, I expect no compensation for these photographs and waive all rights to any claims for payment or royalties. I also release Dr. _____ from any liability in connection with the use of such photographs. Further restrictions of photographs include the following:
_____ .

_____   _____
(Witness)   (Patient's signature)

_____   _____
(Witness)   (Date)   (Time)

                                                          _____
                                                          (Signature of person authorized to consent for
                                                          patient. If parents, both must sign.)

                                                          _____

SAMPLE OPERATIVE REPORT

Patient: Doe, John   Status of patient: Outpatient

Patient number: 150-42-31   Place of surgery: Outpatient Surgical Facility, Division of Dermatology

Date of surgery: 9/17/86   Anesthesia started: 8:50 AM

Procedure started: 9:00 AM

Procedure ended: 10:00 AM

Operation: Excision of basal cell carcinoma from forehead and repair of surgical defect with complex closure

Surgeon: Richard G. Bennett, M.D.   Nurse: Elnora Tabila, R.N.

Assisting surgeon(s): Stuart Kaplan, M.D.

Location: Forehead

Preoperative diagnosis: Basal cell carcinoma

Postoperative diagnosis: Basal cell carcinoma

Preoperative medication: Valium 5 mg p.o.

Anesthetic: 8 ml of Xylocaine 1% with epinephrine 1:100,000

Anesthetist: Stuart Kaplan, M.D.

Preparation: The diagnosis, procedure, benefits, risks, advantages, disadvantages, alternative procedures, and consequences of refusal of treatment were discussed with the patient before the administration of any medication. Proper informed consent was obtained. The patient was brought into the operating room and placed in the supine position. The skin surrounding the tumor on the forehead was infiltrated with local anesthetic. The operative field was cleansed with soap, prepped with Betadine solution, and then draped to maintain a sterile operative field.

Procedure: The tumor was debulked with a No. 4 Fox curette to delineate the gross margins. The skin was then incised with a No. 15 blade in a circular manner around the previously delineated margins with a margin of normal skin measuring approximately 5 mm in all directions. The incision was carried in depth to the deep (muscle) fascia. Bleeding vessels were electrocoagulated with biterminal high-frequency electrosurgery. The surgical wound was then closed along the lines of maximal tension with 4-0 Vicryl dermal-subcutaneous sutures. Dog ears were repaired at the lateral margins of the wound. The cutaneous margins were approximated with a running intradermal suture of 5-0 Prolene. The ends of this suture were secured with sterile skin tapes. The epidermal edges were also secured with sterile skin tapes. A sterile pressure dressing was then applied to the wound.

Size and extent of surgical defect: 4 × 2.5 cm with extension in depth to deep (muscle) fascia

Estimated blood loss: Minimal

Complications: None

Condition of patient after surgery: Excellent

Disposition of specimen: The specimen was sent to Dr. Marc Chalet for pathologic examination.

Disposition of patient: Patient was discharged ambulatory to home at 10:15 AM with written postoperative dressing instructions and the physician's home phone number. The patient was instructed to return in 5 days for examination of the wound.

Postoperative medication(s): Plain Tylenol, 2 tablets q4h p.r.n. pain

Stuart Kaplan
_____
(Assistant surgeon)

Richard G. Bennett
_____
(Surgeon)

FROM THE DESK OF

RICHARD G. BENNETT, M.D.
DEPARTMENT OF MEDICINE/DERMATOLOGY
RM. 52-121 CHS/UCLA SCHOOL OF MEDICINE
LOS ANGELES, CA 90024
(213) 825-6911

INSTRUCTIONS FOR POSTOPERATIVE WOUND CARE

1. Cleanse wound with **hydrogen peroxide** using Q-tips.

2. Dry wound with **gauze** and apply **Polysporin Ointment** using Q-tips.

3. Cover with **Telfa and gauze cut to size and apply nonallergic tape** (paper tape).

4. Change dressing _____ times daily

You may get your wound wet. If you wish to shampoo your hair, we recommend a mild shampoo (such as Johnson's Baby Shampoo).

If bleeding occurs, apply 20 minutes of *constant* pressure.

UCLA DIVISION OF DERMATOLOGY
DERMATOLOGIC SURGERY LOG (_____)
FACILITY

KEY:
HOSP — Hospitalized
PC — Procedure Card
RC — Recall Card
OR — Operative Report

CASE NO.	DATE	PATIENT NAME			ID	DIAG-NOSIS	ANATOMIC SITE	PROCEDURE	PRE-OP MEDS	TIME	SIZE (CM)		ANATOMIC EXTENT	OPERATIVE COMPLICATIONS	DISPOSITION (INCLUDING POSTOP MEDS)	SUR-GEON(S)	SURGICAL SPECIMEN		POSTOP COMPLI-CATIONS	PC	RC	OR
			SEX	AGE	PHONE NO.	PREOP BX NO.			ANES-THETIC (TOTAL MGM)	START-ED / FIN-ISHED	PRE-OP / POST-OP		DEPTH		CONDITION	NURSE	HOSP DX	NO.	M A R G I N			

2959 MED/ (185) CG 08619-m-

APPENDIX

F

SURGICAL EMERGENCIES

I. SUGGESTED INVENTORY FOR EMERGENCY
CART
A. Equipment

1. Ambu bag with tracheostomy tube adapter
2. Arm board
3. Cardiac arrest board
4. Cardiac defibrillator-monitor
5. Curved hemostat
6. Endotracheal tube adapter
7. Endotracheal tubes (small, medium, and large)
8. Flashlight
9. IV pole
10. Laryngoscope with light source
11. Needle holder
12. Oropharyngeal airway (adult and child sizes)
13. Oxygen tank with mask and tubing
14. Pickups
15. Scissors
16. Sphygmomanometer
17. Stethoscope
18. Suction apparatus
19. Tourniquet

B. Emergency supplies

1. Blood drawing supplies and tubes
2. Blood gas kits
3. ECG paste
4. Gauze 2 × 2 inches, 4 × 4 inches
5. IV additive labels
6. IV tubing with microdrip set
7. Local anesthetics (1% lidocaine with
   epinephrine 1:100,000)
8. Needles—scalp vein and/or angiocath
9. Needles: 14 ga × 1½ inches
            18 ga × 1½ inches
            20 ga × 1 inch
            25 ga × 1 inch
10. Record sheet for emergency treatment with
    pen and clipboard (should include flow sheet
    for vital signs, time, symptoms, drugs)
11. Skin disinfectants (e.g., alcohol swabs)

780

12. Sterile gloves
13. Sterile towels
14. Suction tubing
15. Sutures: 4-0 Nylon
            4-0 Silk
16. Syringes: 3 cc, 12 cc
17. Tape

C. Medications

1. Aminophylline 250 mg/10 cc; 2 amps
2. Amyl nitrite 2 amps
3. Metaraminol (Aramine) 10 mg/cc in 10 cc vial; 1 vial
4. Aromatic spirits of ammonia; 1 bottle
5. Atropine sulfate 0.4 mg/cc in 2 cc vial; 2 vials
6. Diphenhydramine (Benadryl) 50 mg/cc in 1 cc amps; 2 amps
7. Calcium chloride 10% solution in 10 cc amp; 2 amps
8. Calcium gluconate 100 mg/cc in 10 cc (10% solution) preloaded syringe; 2 syringes
9. Prochlorperazine (Compazine) 5 mg/cc in 10 cc vial; 1 vial
10. Dextrose 50% 50 cc preloaded syringe; 2 syringes
11. Dextrose 5% 500 cc bottles; 2 bottles
12. Dextrose 5% ¼ normal saline; 1 bottle
13. Meperidine (Demerol) 100 mg/ml in 1 cc (10% solution) preloaded syringe; 10 syringes
14. Epinephrine 1:1000 in 1 cc amp; 2 amps
15. Epinephrine 1:10,000 (0.1 mg/cc) in 10 cc syringe preloaded with intracardiac needles; 2 syringes
16. Glucose, instant
17. Isoproterenol (Isuprel) 1:5000 in 1 ml amp; 1 amp
18. Lidocaine 2% solution in 5 cc prepackaged syringes containing 100 mg; 4 syringes
19. Morphine sulfate 10 mg/tube; 2 tubes
20. Naloxone (Narcan) 0.4 mg/cc in 10 cc vials; 1 vial
21. Nitroglycerin tablets, 1 bottle
22. Sodium pentobarbital (Nembutal) 100 mg in 2 cc amp; 4 amps
23. Procainamide (Pronestyl) 100 mg/ml in 10 ml vials; 1 vial
24. Sodium chloride (isotonic) 30 cc vial; 1 vial
25. Sodium bicarbonate 50 mEq/50 cc prepackaged syringe; 4 syringes
26. Solu-Cortef 250 mg vial; 2 vials
27. Chlorpromazine (Thorazine) 25 mg/cc amps; 2 amps
28. Diazepam (Valium) 5 mg/cc in 2 cc amp or 2 cc prepackaged syringe; 2 amps or 2 syringes
29. Water, sterile 30 cc vial; 1 vial

II. EMERGENCY PROBLEMS AND TREATMENT

Problem	Cause	Symptoms	Signs	Treatment
Allergic reaction	Allergy to medication	Pruritus	Urticaria, edema	Apply tourniquet if possible Epinephrine 1:1000 subcutaneous 0.2 to 0.5 cc
Anaphylaxis	Allergy to medication	Vomiting/pruritus	Low blood pressure, pallor, thready pulse, edema, urticaria (hoarseness, wheezing, stridor, difficulty breathing)	Apply tourniquet (if possible). Epinephrine 1:1000 subcutaneous 0.2 to 0.5 cc Benadryl 50 mg IV or IM Steroid IV Consider tracheotomy
Anesthetic toxicity	Rapid injection or absorption	Numbness in tongue and lips	Drowsiness, tremors, seizures, respiratory depression, coma, hypotension, bradycardia	For seizures: Valium 10 mg IV For decreased blood pressure: Metaraminol (Aramine) 0.5 to 1 cc IV over 2 or 3 min For decreased cardiac output: Isoproterenol (Isuprel) 1 to 2 mg (5 to 10 cc) diluted in 250 to 500 mg D5W; infuse at a rate to increase heart rate to 60 beats/min
Cardiac spasm or infarction	Coronary disease	Shortness of breath, chest pain, apprehension	Diaphoresis, clutching chest	Administer nitroglycerin if prescribed, monitor pulse and blood pressure. For infarction, administer Demerol 50 to 75 mg IM, establish IV, give O_2
Cardiopulmonary arrest	Cardiac standstill or fibrillation	—	Loss of consciousness, no pulse or respiration	CPR (see section III of this outline)
Epinephrine toxicity	Rapid injection or absorption	Palpitation, headache	Increased blood pressure, dilated pupils, tachycardia	Thorazine 25 mg/10 cc saline at 2 mg q.15 sec IV to maximum 15 mg; consider Nembutal 100 mg IV
Hypoglycemia (and insulin shock)	Decreased blood sugar	Weakness, trembling	Normal blood pressure, tachycardia, sweating	Carbohydrate; 50 cc of 50% glucose IV
Seizures	Seizure disorder, anesthetic toxicity	—	Loss of consciousness, muscular rigidity	Prevent injury: Valium 10 mg at 5 mg/min IV
Syncope (vasovagal)	Fright	Weakness	Pallor, perspiration, hypotension, unconsciousness, initial tachycardia, bradycardia, loss of consciousness	Elevate legs, cold towel around neck, aromatic ammonia, take pulse and blood pressure, determine cause; consider atropine 0.5 mg IV if severe and prolonged

III. CARDIOPULMONARY RESUSCITATION (CPR)

A. Basic life support
  1. Recognition: "shake and shout," check respirations and carotid pulse
  2. Summon help
     a. Phone numbers: rescue squad
                       emergency room
     b. Nearest oxygen
     c. Nearest defibrillator
  3. Place patient supine on hard surface
  4. Establish airway: tilt head, check for and remove foreign body and/or dentures from mouth
  5. Respirations: four quick breaths, then ventilate (remember to pinch nose closed) 12 to 15 times per minute
  6. External cardiac compression: 60 per minute (depress sternum 1 inch in infants, 1.5 inches in children, 1.5 to 2 inches in adults). If one rescuer, 15 compressions (at a rate of 80 beats per minute) followed by 2 breaths; if two rescuers, 5 compressions (at a rate of 60 beats per minute) followed by 1 breath

B. Advanced life support

  1. Airway: bag-valve mask or endotracheal intubation
  2. Establish an IV line with 5% dextrose in water (D5W)
  3. Cardiac monitor: defibrillation at up to 400 joules
  4. Oxygen 100% at high flow rate
  5. Administration of drugs:

Drug	*Purpose*	*Dosage*
1. Sodium bicarbonate	Reverse acidosis	1 mEq per kg followed by ½ initial dose (0.5 mEq per kg) every 10 min; each 50 cc amp contains 44.6 mEq
2. Lidocaine	Decrease ventricular irritability	1 mg/kg bolus; then 2 to 3 mg/min drip: then repeat bolus every 10 min at ⅔ mg/kg to total dose of 225 mg
3. Epinephrine	Cardiac stimulant, prepare heart for countershock	5 cc to 10 cc of 1 : 10,000 solution; repeat at 5-min intervals
4. Calcium chloride	Cardiac stimulant	3 to 4 cc of a 10% solution
5. Procainamide	Decrease ventricular irritability if lidocaine fails	100 mg/5 min IV to total dose of 1 g
6. Betylium tosylate	Depresses ventricular irritability if lidocaine fails	5 mg/kg IV
7. Isoproterenol	Cardiac stimulant	1 mg vial into 250 cc D5W gives 4 μg/per cc; infuse at 0.4 μg/min and increase to 20 μg/min if necessary
8. Atropine	Reverse bradycardia	0.5 mg IV q5 min until a heart rate of 60 beats/min is achieved or until 2 mg total injected

G

SUGGESTED SURGICAL EQUIPMENT

1. Alcohol dispenser
2. Camera equipment
3. Cannister for gauze
4. Cardiac monitor*
5. Chair, adjustable with wheels
6. Defibrillator
7. Dermabrader
8. Dermabrasion mask
9. Dermatome*
10. Electrosurgical unit (biterminal) with reusable, sterilizable handles
11. Emergency cart
12. Laser (carbon dioxide)*
13. Liquid nitrogen spray apparatus*
14. Liquid nitrogen tank*
15. Mayo stand
16. Mirror, hand
17. Narcotic lock box
18. Nitrous oxide equipment*
19. Otoscope
20. Oxygen tank
21. Power supply, independent
22. Pillows
23. Platform*
24. Shaw scalpel*
25. Soap dispenser with foot control
26. Sphygmomanometer
27. Steam sterilizer
28. Suction machine
29. Surgical light, reflective
30. Surgical power table
31. Trays to soak instruments
32. Ultrasonic cleaner*
33. Wastebucket with wheels, kick
34. Wheelchair*

*Optional

APPENDIX

H

SUGGESTED SURGICAL INSTRUMENTS

1. Anoscope
2. Blade breaker and holder (Castroviejo)*
3. Blade extractor
4. Caliper (Jameson)
5. Chalazion clamp, small
6. Chalazion clamp, medium
7. Chalazion clamp, large
8. Comedo expressor (Schamberg)
9. Curette, dermal (Fox) 3 mm
10. Curette, dermal (Fox) 4 mm
11. Curette, eye (Meyhoefer)
12. Curette, eye (Skeele)*
13. Forceps, 4¾ inches, serrated (Adson)
14. Forceps, 4¾ inches, 1 × 2 inches, toothed (Adson)
15. Forceps, grasping (Allis)
16. Forceps, 3¼ inches serrated (Bishop-Harman)
17. Forceps, 3¼ inches, 1 × 2 inches, toothed (Bishop-Harman)
18. Forceps, jeweler's
19. Forceps, sponge
20. Fraize, diamond
21. Hemostat, 5 inches, curved mosquito (Halsted)
22. Hemostat, 5 inches, straight mosquito (Halsted)
23. Hemostat, 4 inches, curved (Hartmann)
24. Hemostat, 4 inches, straight (Hartmann)
25. Nail splitter with anvil action
26. Nasal speculum
27. Needle holder, smooth-jawed (Castroviejo)
28. Needle holder, smooth-jawed (Webster)
29. Probe and groove director
30. Scalpel handle, No. 3 (Bard-Parker)
31. Scalpel handle, 4 inches, knurled (Beaver)*
32. Scissors, 5½ inches, bandage (Lister)
33. Scissors, delicate (Castroviejo)
34. Scissors, universal bandage
35. Scissors, straight iris 3½ inches, extra delicate
36. Scissors, 5 inches, curved undermining (Metzenbaum)
37. Scissors, suture removal (Shortbent)
38. Scissors, 3½ inches, straight tenotomy (Stevens)
39. Scissors, 3½ inches, curved tenotomy (Stevens)
40. Skin hook, single (Converse)
41. Skin hook, single (Frazier)

*Optional

42. Skin hook, double (Guthrie)
43. Skin punch, cutaneous (Keyes)
44. Skin punch, hair transplant
45. Skin punch, straight (Loo trephine)
46. Towel clamp (Backhaus)
47. Vaginal speculum

I

SUGGESTED SURGICAL SUPPLIES

1. Adhesive bandages (e.g., Coverlet) strips, spots, patches
2. Applicators, 6 inches, wooden with cotton tip (sterile, unsterile)
3. Autoclave steam indicator bags
4. Blades, carbon steel scalpel (No. 15, No. 11)
5. Blades, stainless steel (Beaver, No. 67)
6. Collagen, injectable
7. Cotton balls
8. Dressings, nonadhesive (e.g., Telfa) 4 × 8 inches
9. Drapes, surgical (e.g., Converters Fenestrated Towel by American Converters)
10. Drains, Penrose
11. Elastic wrap bandages (e.g., Ace Wrap) 3 inches, 6 inches
12. Electrode tip, disposable electrosurgical
13. Emesis basin
14. Eyedropper
15. Eye pads
16. Film (e.g., Kodachrome ASA 25 or 64)
17. Gauze, nonadhesive (e.g., Vaseline Gauze) 1 × 3 inches, 3 × 8 inches
18. Gauze packing
19. Gauze sponges (3 × 3 inches, 4 × 4 inches) 12 ply, 16 ply
20. Gauze-type outerwrap, stretchable (e.g., Kling) 2 inches, 4 inches
21. Gelfoam, dental size
22. Gloves (sterile, unsterile)
23. Gowns, surgical
24. Hair covers
25. Instrument milk
26. Instrument soap
27. Masks
28. Medications: Adhesive remover (e.g., Detachol)
    Aluminum chloride 35% in isopropyl alcohol 50%
    Ammonia inhalants
    Acetone
    Alcohol
    Benadryl (50 mg/cc)
    Betadine swab sticks
    Bonney Blue marking dye
    Boric acid ophthalmic solution 5%
    Compazine 5 mg/cc
    Compound tincture of benzoin
    Croton oil
    Diazepam (Valium) 5 mg/cc, 5 mg tablets
    Duranest 1% plain
    Erythromycin 250 mg tablets
    Gentian violet 1% solution

Green soap
Hydrogen peroxide 3% solution
Lidocaine 1% plain, 1% with 1:100,000 epinephrine, 1% with 1:200,000 epinephrine
Meperidine 50 mg/cc
Monsel's solution
Ointment, sterile
Ophthalmic topical anesthetic (e.g., Pontocaine)
Ophthalmic rinse solution (e.g., Dacriose)
Oxygen
Podophylline
Polysporin ointment
Polysporin ophthalmic ointment
Phenergan 50 mg/cc
Phenol
Septisol
Sodium chloride (saline), 30 cc injectable
Tetracycline, 250 mg capsules
Triamcinolone acetonide 10 mg/cc, 40 mg/cc, injectable
Trichloracetic acid 30% and 50%
Tylenol
Tylenol 3
Vistaril 25 mg/cc
Water, sterile 30 cc
Zephiran pads

29. Needles, disposable surgical, No. 16, No. 18, No. 30 gauge (1½ inches, 1 inch)
30. Net surgical covering or stockinette
31. Oxycel, cotton type
32. Pen light
33. Pillow cases
34. Razor blades, Gillette Blue
35. Razors, surgical prep
36. Scrub brushes (Betadine)
37. Scrub suits, shirts, and pants
38. Sheets, sterile and disposable for surgical tray
39. Suction tubing
40. Sutures: 6-0 nylon, black with plastic needle (e.g., P-1)
            6-0 nylon, clear with plastic needle (e.g., P-1)
            5-0 nylon, black with plastic needle (e.g., P-3)
            4-0 nylon, black with plastic needle (e.g., P-3)
            3-0 nylon, black with skin needle (e.g., FS-2)
            5-0 Prolene, blue with plastic needle (e.g., P-3)
            4-0 absorbable suture with skin needle (e.g., FS-2)
            5-0 absorbable suture with plastic needle (e.g., P-3)
            4-0 chromic catgut with skin needle (e.g., FS-2)
            5-0 silk, dermal with skin needle (e.g., FS-2)
            4-0 silk, dermal with skin needle (e.g., FS-2)
41. Staple remover
42. Staples (regular)
43. Suction tubing
44. Sutureless skin closures (e.g., Steri-Strips)
45. Surgical log book
46. Syringes 5 cc, 3 cc, 1 cc with Luer-Lok
47. Table paper
48. Tape, cloth or plastic

49. Tape, paper—micropore (½ inch, 1 inch) brown
50. Tongue depressors
51. Toothbrushes, denture
52. Toothpicks
53. Towels, surgical muslin
54. Trash bags (plastic liners), red for nonsharp surgical waste
55. Vaseline gauze (3 inches, 1 inch)
56. Waste containers for sharp, disposable, surgical materials (e.g., needles and blades)

HAND-TYING KNOTS

Technique I: two-handed tying

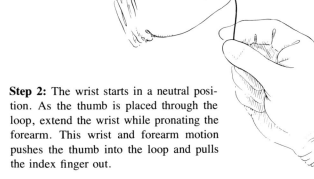

Step 1: Grasp the short end of the suture in the nontying hand. Hold the long end in the middle, ring, and little fingers of the tying hand, about 10 cm (4 in) from the fixed point. The index finger and thumb must be free. Engage the suture with the index finger of the tying hand as shown, and then place the thumb through the loop formed.

Step 2: The wrist starts in a neutral position. As the thumb is placed through the loop, extend the wrist while pronating the forearm. This wrist and forearm motion pushes the thumb into the loop and pulls the index finger out.

From Van Way, C.W., III, and Buerk, C.A.: Pocket manual of basic surgical skills, St. Louis, 1986, The C.V. Mosby Co. Drawings by F. Dennis Giddings.

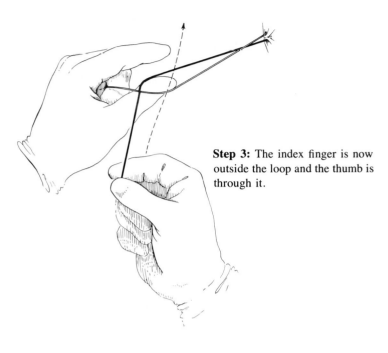

Step 3: The index finger is now outside the loop and the thumb is through it.

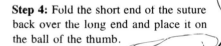

Step 4: Fold the short end of the suture back over the long end and place it on the ball of the thumb.

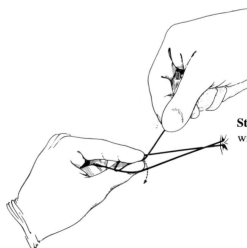

Step 5: Grasp the short end of the suture with the index finger and thumb.

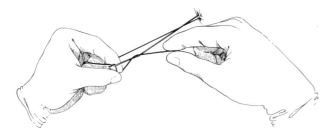

Step 6: Flex the wrist.

Step 7: When the wrist flexes through the midposition, release the short end of the suture with the nontying hand. The short end passes through the loop as the wrist continues to flex. Bring the non-tying hand down to grasp the short end of the suture.

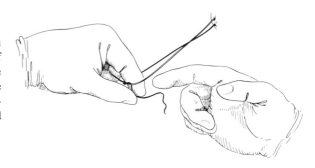

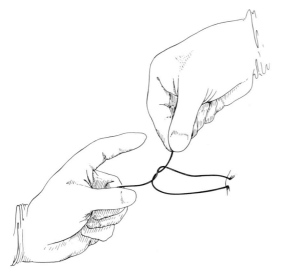

Step 8: The nontying hand then grasps the short end of the suture and begins to tighten the knot.

Step 9: Use the index finger of the tying hand to push the knot down to the fixed point and tighten it. This avoids tension on the fixed point, which may be a relatively fragile vessel, or on some other structure that might be damaged by excessive tension. Tighten the knot flat as shown, even if it is necessary to cross the hands to do so; if the first throw is not placed flat, the completed knot may slip.

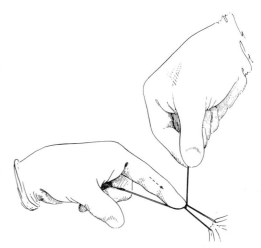

Step 10: Begin the second half of the technique from the final position reached after tightening the first throw and without changing either hand's grasp on the suture. Engage the suture with the thumb of the tying hand.

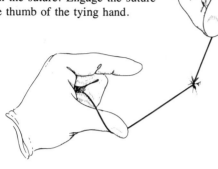

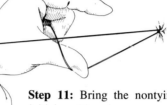

Step 11: Bring the nontying hand from its initial position down across the tying hand in such a way as to bring the short end of the suture across the web between the thumb and index finger of the tying hand. This forms a loop into which the index finger will be placed.

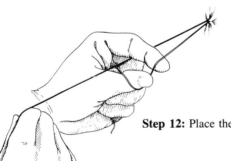

Step 12: Place the index finger into the loop.

Step 13: Flex the wrist. This pushes the index finger further into the loop while withdrawing the thumb. Then move the nontying hand back toward its original position, folding the short end of the suture along the ball of the index finger.

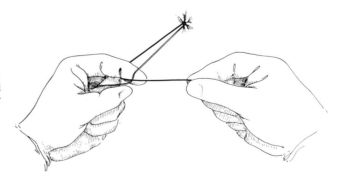

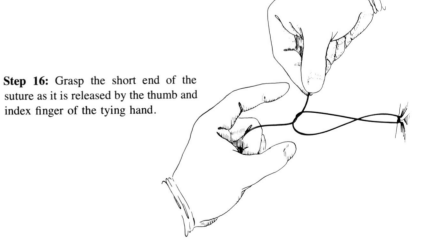

Step 14: Grasp the short end of the suture with the thumb and index finger. Keep the wrist flexed.

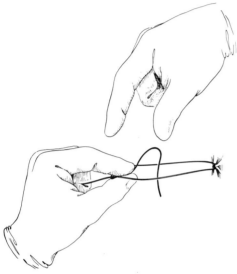

Step 15: Release the short end of the suture and extend the wrist. This brings the short end through the loop. Move the nontying hand up.

Step 16: Grasp the short end of the suture as it is released by the thumb and index finger of the tying hand.

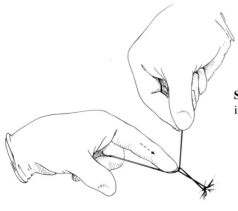

Step 17: Push the knot down with the index finger of the tying hand.

Technique II: one-handed tying

Step 1: In contrast to the two-handed tie, grasp the short end of the suture with the middle finger of the tying hand and the long end with the nontying hand. Pass the index finger of the tying hand under the short end of the suture. The palm of the tying hand faces down. Notice that the suture is crossed at the fixed point.

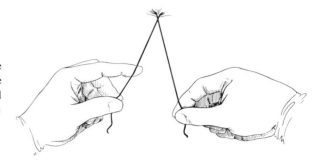

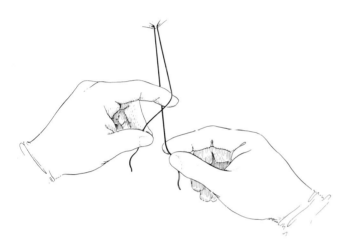

Step 2: With the nontying hand, bring the long end of the suture up to the palmar aspect of the distal interphalangeal joint of the index finger of the tying hand.

Step 3: Without otherwise moving the hands, strongly flex the index finger of the tying hand. In doing this, it is important to keep the thumb and middle finger, which are grasping the short end of the suture, firmly extended.

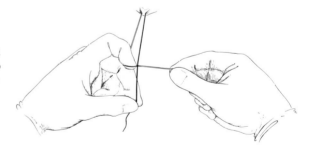

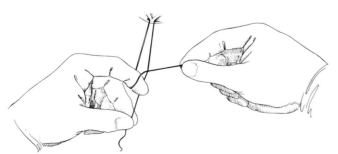

Step 4: Move the index finger up and over the short end of the suture, which should still be held fixed by the thumb and middle finger.

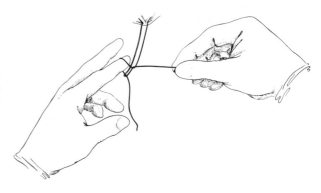

Step 5: With the index finger, pull the short end of the suture through the loop formed by the long end, while the thumb and middle finger release the short end. The middle finger moves up next to the index finger, where it will secure the short end.

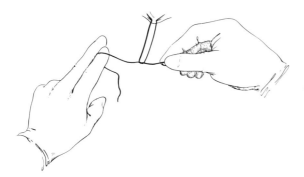

Step 6: Secure the short end of the suture between the middle and index fingers.

Step 7: Bring the thumb over to the middle finger to grasp the short end of the suture and push the knot down with the index finger.

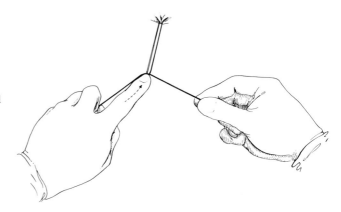

Note: The second half of Technique II is the same as the first half of Technique III (through Step 7).

Technique III: one-handed tying (alternative)

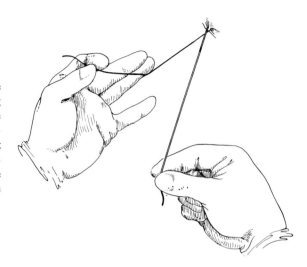

Step 1: Cross the suture at the fixed point. Grasp the short end between the thumb and index finger of the tying hand. Supinate the forearm so that the palm of the tying hand faces up. Position the short end of the suture so that it travels from the thumb and index finger, across the palmar aspect of the fingers, and around the ring finger to the fixed point.

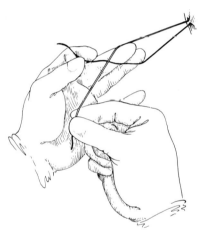

Step 2: Cross the nontying hand in front of the tying hand to position the end of the suture along the radial aspect of the middle finger, crossing the short end of the suture at a point about halfway from the thumb to the ring finger.

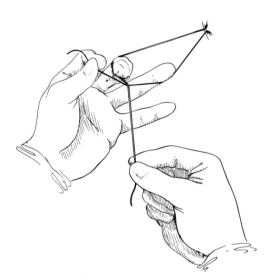

Step 3: Strongly flex the middle finger.

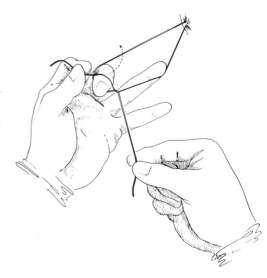

Step 4: Pass the tip of the long finger under the short end of the suture between the crossing of the long end and the point at which it is grasped by the thumb. Extend the finger slightly, so that the back of the middle finger touches the short end of the suture.

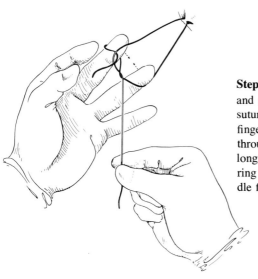

Step 5: Extend the middle finger and release the short end of the suture with the thumb and index finger. This brings the short end through the loop formed by the long end of the suture. Move the ring finger over against the middle finger.

Step 6: Moving the ring finger over against the middle finger secures the short end of the suture.

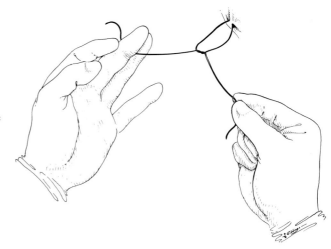

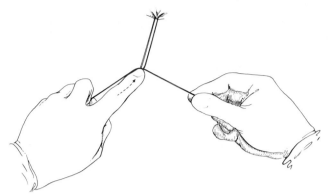

Step 7: Grasp the short end of the suture between the thumb and middle finger of the tying hand and push the knot down with the index finger.

Step 8: Begin the second half of the technique by grasping the short end of the suture between the thumb and index finger of the tying hand. The palm faces up. Bring the long end of the suture close to the ulnar aspect of the ring finger.

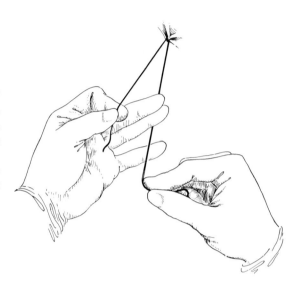

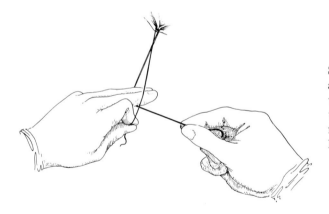

Step 9: Move the nontying hand and pronate the tying hand, wrapping the long end of the suture around the ring and middle fingers at their distal interphalangeal joints.

Step 10: Strongly flex the ring and middle fingers. Keeping the thumb firmly extended, pronate the hand somewhat (not fully). The ring and middle fingers pull the long end of the suture away from the point at which it crosses the short end. Move the nontying hand slightly toward the tying hand to allow the ring and middle fingers to pull the long end of the suture in toward the palm of the tying hand. Notice the position at which the short and long ends of the suture cross. It is well away from the tying hand. This is the most difficult part of the technique.

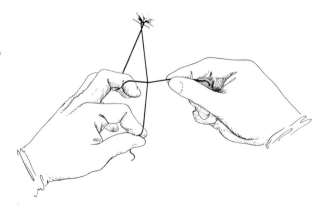

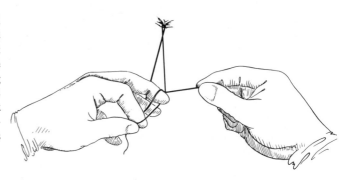

Step 11: Separate the ring and middle fingers slightly and extend them somewhat. Grasp the short end of the suture between the point at which it crosses the long end and the point at which it is held by the thumb and index finger. This maneuver is relatively easy, if the previous step was performed properly.

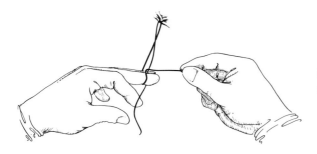

Step 12: While holding the short end of the suture between the ring and middle fingers, release it with the thumb and index fingers.

Step 13: Pull the short end of the suture through the loop in the long end. This is easier to do if the forearm is pronated.

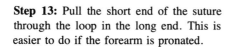

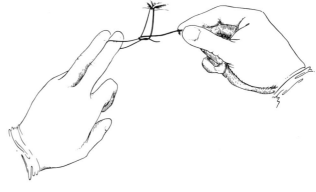

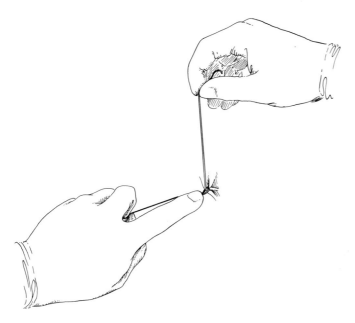

Step 14: Bring the thumb over to grasp the suture with the middle finger while pushing the knot down with the index finger. Notice that the second half of the knot is pushed down flat and forms a square knot with the first half.

INDEX

Dunphy, J.E., 19
Duoderm, 329
Duranest; *see* Etidocaine
Dysplasia, definition of, 670
Dysplastic nevus syndrome, 672, 675-676

E

Ear, 103-105
  cartilage of, 109
  dressings for, 343
  elongated slits in, repair of, 611
  excisional surgery of, 427
  muscles of, 115
  repair of, Tagliacozzi method for, 8-9
  sensory distribution of, 127
Ear piercing, 611-615
Earlobe, split, repair of, 611, 615
Edema
  following surgery, 501
  near surgical wounds, 511
Edwin Smith Papyrus, 18
  wound suturing and, 4
Efudex; *see* 5-Fluorouracil
EGF; *see* Epidermal growth factor
Ehlers-Danlos syndrome type VI, 41
Elase, 166
Elastic fibers, 44
Elasticity, skin, dog-ears and, 473
Electric current, definition of, 555
Electricity
  history of, in medicine, 554-555
  static, 555, 556
  theory of, 555-559
  wound healing and, 85
Electrocautery, 564-565
  for acquired nevocytic nevus, 674
  clinical applications of, 565
  definition of, 553, 564
  equipment for, 564-565
  heat produced by, 564-565, 579
Electrocoagulation, 541, 574-575; *see also* Electrosurgery; High-frequency electrosurgery
  bleeding stopped with, 534
  curettage and, 532
Electrocution, high-frequency electrosurgical units as cause of, 587
Electrodes, patient-indifferent, 565-566
  burns from, 585-586
Electrodesiccation, 541, 574, 575*T*; *see also* Electrosurgery; High-frequency electrosurgery
  for acquired nevocytic nevus, 673
  curettage of warts and, 703
  historical background of, 573
Electrofulguration, 571, 574-575; *see also* Electrosurgery; High-frequency electrosurgery
Electrolysis
  clinical applications of, 562-564
  definition of, 553, 561
  equipment for, 561
  history of, 554
Electromagnetic induction, 555, 557
Electromagnetic radiation and waveforms in high-frequency electrosurgery, 566, 570
Electron drift speed, 555-556
Electrosurgery
  curettage and, 532

Electrosurgery—cont'd
  curettage and—cont'd
    bleeding stopped with, 534
    for malignant lesions, 536, 537, 538, 541-542
  curettage following, 542-543
  definition of, 553
  high-frequency; *see* High-frequency electrosurgery
  for telangiectasias, 602
  wound healing and, 578-579
Electrosurgical devices, electrocution from, 587
Electrosurgical units
  high-frequency, 565-566, 579-580
  pacemaker interference by, 586-587
  patient-monitoring devices' interference by, 587
  ventricular fibrillation and, 587
Electrotomy, 575; *see also* High-frequency electrosurgery
EMLA, 231
Endotherm, 573
Endothermy, 575; *see also* Diathermy; High-frequency electrosurgery
Enterobacteriaceae, 319
Enucleation of corns, 693
Environment, wound healing and, 75
Enzymes, proteolytic, for wound infection, 166
Epidermal cells, migrating
  morphologic changes in, 46-47
  rate of, 48
  substrate attachment of, 47-48
Epidermal cell elongation, biopsy specimens and, 529-530
Epidermal cyst(s)
  clinical appearance of, 734
  etiology of, 734
  freely moveable, 736
    removal of, 737, 739
  histopathology of, 734-735
  infected
    drainage of, 735
    treatment of, 735-736
  inflamed, treatment of, 735
  moderately moveable, 737
    removal of, 739, 743, 746
  nonmoveable, 736-737
    removal of, 746
  removal of, 736-747
    alternative techniques for, 746-748
    carcinomatous change following, 747
  treatment of, 735-747
  in upper lip, removal of, 744, 746
Epidermal growth factor, 51, 59
Epidermal invagination, biopsy specimens and, 529
Epidermis
  layers of, 20
  migration of
    mechanisms of, 48
    under a scab, 48
    in wound healing, 46-49
  proliferation of, 51
  relaxation of, 56
  resurfacing of, 51-52
  surface, lesions of, 692-706
  tensile strength of wounds and, 70
  thickness of, 21
Epidermization, 56
  definition of, 25
  rate of, 317
Epi-Lock, 328